Textbook of

Reproductive Medicine

Second Edition

Textbook of
Reproductive Medicine

Second Edition

Edited by

Bruce R. Carr, MD
Paul C. MacDonald Professor of Obstetrics and Gynecology
Director, Division of Reproductive Endocrinology
Department of Obstetrics and Gynecology
University of Texas Southwestern Medical Center at Dallas
Dallas, Texas

Richard E. Blackwell, PhD, MD
Professor of Obstetrics and Gynecology
Department of Obstetrics and Gynecology
University of Alabama at Birmingham
Birmingham, Alabama

With 42 contributors

APPLETON & LANGE
Stamford, Connecticut

Notice: The authors and the publisher of this volume have taken care to make certain that the doses of drugs and schedules of treatment are correct and compatible with the standards generally accepted at the time of publication. Nevertheless, as new information becomes available, changes in treatment and in the use of drugs become necessary. The reader is advised to carefully consult the instruction and information material included in the package insert of each drug or therapeutic agent before administration. This advice is especially important when using, administering, or recommending new or infrequently used drugs. The authors and publisher disclaim all responsibility for any liability, loss, injury, or damage incurred as a consequence, directly or indirectly, of the use and application of any of the contents of this volume.

Prentice Hall International (UK) Limited, *London*
Prentice Hall of Australia Pty. Limited, *Sydney*
Prentice Hall Canada, Inc., *Toronto*
Prentice Hall Hispanoamericana, S.A., *Mexico*
Prentice Hall of India Private Limited, *New Delhi*
Prentice Hall of Japan, Inc., *Tokyo*
Simon & Schuster Asia Pte. Ltd., *Singapore*
Editora Prentice Hall do Brasil Ltda., *Rio de Janeiro*
Prentice Hall, *Upper Saddle River, New Jersey*

Library of Congress Cataloging-in-Publication Data

Textbook of reproductive medicine / edited by Bruce R. Carr, Richard
    E. Blackwell. — 2nd ed.
        p.   cm.
    Includes bibliographical references and index.
    ISBN 0-8385-8893-X (Case : alk. paper)
    1. Endocrine gynecology.   2. Infertility—Endocrine aspects.
3. Infertility.   I. Carr, Bruce R.   II. Blackwell, Richard E.
    [DNLM: 1. Reproduction—physiology.   2. Genital Diseases, Female.
3. Reproduction Techniques.   WQ 205 T3556 1998]
RG159.T49   1998
618.1—dc21
DNLM/DLC
for Library of Congress   97-37910
                                                              CIP

Acquisitions Editor: Jane Licht
Developmental Editor: Beth P. Broadhurst
Production Editor: Sondra Greenfield

ISBN 0-8385-8893-X
90000
9 780838 588932

PRINTED IN THE UNITED STATES OF AMERICA

CONTENTS

CONTRIBUTORS

Aydin Arici, MD
Associate Professor
Division of Reproductive Endocrinology
Department of Obstetrics and Gynecology
Yale University School of Medicine
New Haven, Connecticut
Chapter 31, "Diagnosis and Management of Tubal Disease"

Ricardo Azziz, MD, MPH
Professor
Division of Reproductive Biology and Endocrinology
Department of Obstetrics and Gynecology
University of Alabama at Birmingham
Birmingham, Alabama
Chapter 18, "Disorders of the Adrenal Cortex"
Chapter 21, "Endocrine Alterations in Female Obesity"

G. William Bates, MD
Clinical Professor
Department of Obstetrics and Gynecology
Vanderbilt University
Nashville, Tennessee
Chapter 5, "Normal and Abnormal Puberty"

Richard E. Blackwell, PhD, MD
Professor of Obstetrics and Gynecology
Department of Obstetrics and Gynecology
University of Alabama at Birmingham
Birmingham, Alabama
Chapter 9, "Neuroendocrinology of Reproduction"
Chapter 10, "Hormonal Regulation of Breast Physiology"
Chapter 15, "Anovulation of CNS Origin: Anatomic Causes"
Chapter 22, "Breast Disease"
Chapter 24, "Chronic Pelvic Pain: Origin, Physiology, Evaluation, and Treatment"
Chapter 26, "Reproductive Medicine and the Managed Care Market"
Chapter 29, "Ovulation Induction"
Chapter 35, "Infertility and Pregnancy Loss: Psychological Aspects of Treatment"
Chapter 36, "Contraception"

Larry R. Boots, PhD
Professor
Director, Obstetrics and Gynecology Research and Diagnosis Laboratory
Division of Reproductive Endocrinology
Department of Obstetrics and Gynecology
University of Alabama at Birmingham
Birmingham, Alabama
Chapter 8, "Laboratory Assessment of Reproductive Hormones"

Karen D. Bradshaw, MD
Associate Professor
Associate Division Director
Division of Reproductive Endocrinology
Department of Obstetrics and Gynecology
University of Texas Southwestern Medical Center
Dallas, Texas
Chapter 27, "Diagnostic Evaluation and Treatment Algorithms for the Infertile Couple"

Serdar E. Bulun, MD
Assistant Professor
Division of Reproductive Endocrinology and Green Center for Reproductive Biology Sciences
Department of Obsteterics and Gynecology
University of Texas Southwestern Medical Center
Dallas, Texas
Chapter 7, "The Molecular Basis of Hormone Action"

William Byrd, PhD
Associate Professor
Division of Reproductive Endocrinology
Department of Obstetrics and Gynecology
University of Texas Southwestern Medical Center
Dallas, Texas
Chapter 1, "Fertilization, Embryogenesis, and Implantation"

Bruce R. Carr, MD
Paul C. MacDonald Professor of Obstetrics and
Gynecology
Director, Division of Reproductive Endocrinology
Department of Obstetrics and Gynecology
University of Texas Southwestern Medical Center at Dallas
Dallas, Texas
Chapter 11, "The Ovary"
Chapter 12, "The Normal Menstrual Cycle:
The Coordinated Events of the Hypothalamic–
Pituitary–Ovarian Axis and the Female
Reproductive Tract"
Chapter 27, "Diagnostic Evaluation and Treatment
Algorithms for the Infertile Couple"
Chapter 36, "Contraception"

R. Jeffrey Chang, MD
Professor
Division of Reproductive Endocrinology
Department of Reproductive Medicine
University of California, San Diego
La Jolla, California
Chapter 15, "Anovulation of CNS Origin: Anatomic
Causes"

Samuel J. Chantilis, MD
Assistant Professor
Director of Invitro Fertilization
Division of Reproductive Endocrinology
Department of Obstetrics and Gynecology
University of Texas Southwestern Medical Center
Dallas, Texas
Chapter 27, "Diagnostic Evaluation and Treatment
Algorithms for the Infertile Couple"

Owen K. Davis, MD
Associate Professor
Division of Reproductive Medicine and Infertility
Department of Obstetrics and Gynecology
Cornell University Medical College
Associate Attending Obstetrician—Gynecologist
The New York Hospital
New York, New York
Chapter 33, "Assisted Reproductive Technology"

Victor Y. Fujimoto, MD
Assistant Professor
Division of Reproductive Endocrinology and Infertility
Department of Obstetrics and Gynecology
University of Washington
Seattle, Washington
Chapter 6, "Normal and Abnormal Sexual
Development"

Barbara Gower, PhD
Assistant Professor
Division of Physiology and Metabolism
Department of Nutritional Sciences
University of Alabama at Birmingham
Birmingham, Alabama
Chapter 21, "Endocrine Alterations in Female
Obesity"

James E. Griffin, MD
Professor
Interim Chief of Endocrinology
Division of Endocrinology and Metabolism
Department of Internal Medicine
University of Texas Southwestern Medical Center
Dallas, Texas
Chapter 13, "The Physiology of the Testis and Male
Reproductive Tract and Disorders of Testicular
Function"

Michael M. Guarnaccia, MD
Instructor/Fellow
Division of Reproductive Endocrinology
Department of Obstetrics and Gynecology
Yale University School of Medicine
New Haven, Connecticut
Chapter 32, "Diagnosis and Management of
Endometriosis"

David S. Guzick, MD, PhD
Professor and Chairman
Department of Obstetrics and Gynecology
University of Rochester
Rochester, New York
Chapter 25, "Clinical Trials for the Reproductive
Endocrinologist: Design, Power Analysis, and
Biostatistics"

Karen R. Hammond, MSN, CRNP
Obstetrics and Gynecology Nurse Practicioner and
Nurse coordinator
Division of Reproductive Biology and
Endocrinology
Department of Obstetrics and Gynecology
University of Alabama at Birmingham
Birmingham, Alabama
Chapter 22, "Breast Disease"
Chapter 29, "Ovulation Induction"

Patricia Honea-Fleming, PhD
Private Practice
Birmingham, Alabama
Chapter 35, "Infertility and Pregnancy Loss:
Psychological Aspects of Treatment"

Eric S. Knockenhauer, MD
University of Alabama at Birmingham
Birmingham, Alabama
Chapter 15, "Anovulation of CNS Origin: Anatomic Causes"

William H. Kutteh, MD, PhD
Associate Professor and Director
Division of Reproductive Endocrinology
Department of Obstetrics and Gynecology
University of Tennessee, Memphis
The Reproductive Medicine and Genetics Center
Memphis, Tennessee
Chapter 34, "Recurrent Pregnancy Loss"

James H. Liu, MD
Professor and Head
Division of Reproductive Endocrinology and Infertility
Department of Obstetrics and Gynecology
University of Cincinnati
Cincinnati, Ohio
Chapter 16, "Anovulation of CNS Origin: Functional and Miscellaneous Causes"

Rogerio A. Lobo, MD
Willard C. Rappleye Professor and Chairman
Division of Reproductive Endocrinology and Infertility
Department of Obstetrics and Gynecology
Columbia University College of Physicians and Surgeons
Director, Sloan Hospital for Women
The Presbyterian Hospital in the City of New York
Department of Obstetrics and Gynecology
Columbia-Presbyterian Medical Center
New York, New York
Chapter 20, "Hirsutism and Virilism"

John D. McConnell, MD
Professor and Chairman
Department of Urology
University of Texas Southwestern Medical Center
Dallas, Texas
Chapter 28, "Diagnosis and Treatment of Male Infertility"

Carole R. Mendelson, PhD
Professor
Departments of Biochemistry and Obstetrics and Gynecology
University of Texas Southwestern Medical Center
Dallas, Texas
Chapter 7, "The Molecular Basis of Hormone Action"

David L. Olive, MD
Professor and Chief
Division of Reproductive Endocrinology
Department of Obstetrics and Gynecology
Professor and Section Chief
Division of Reproductive Endocrinology
Department of Obstetrics and Gynecology
Center for Reproductive Medicine
Yale University School of Medicine
New Haven, Connecticut
Chapter 32, "Diagnosis and Management of Endometriosis"

C. Richard Parker, Jr., PhD
Professor
Division of Reproductive Biology and Endocrinology
Department of Obstetrics and Gynecology
University of Alabama at Birmingham
Birmingham, Alabama
Chapter 2, "The Endocrinology of Pregnancy"

Robert W. Rebar, MD
Professor and Chair
Department of Obstetrics and Gynecology
University of Cincinnati College of Medicine
Chief
Department of Obstetrics and Gynecology
University Hospital
Cincinnati, Ohio
Chapter 14, "Assessment of the Female Patient"

Robert L. Reid, MD, FRCS(C)
Professor and Head
Division of Reproductive Endocrinology and Infertility
Department of Obstetrics and Gynaecology
Queen's University
Head
Division of Reproductive Endocrinology and Infertility
Department of Obstetrics and Gynaecology
Kingston General Hospital
Kingston, Ontario, Canada
Chapter 23, "Psychological Aspects of Menstruation: Premenstrual Syndrome"

Zev Rosenwaks, MD
Professor
Division of Reproductive Medicine and Infertility
Department of Obstetrics and Gynecology
Cornell University Medical College
Director, The Center for Reproductive Medicine and Infertility
Department of Obstetrics and Gynecology
The New York Hospital–Cornell Medical Center
New York, New York
Chapter 33, "Assisted Reproductive Technology"

Isaac Schiff, MD
Joe Vincent Meigs Professor of Gynecology
Harvard Medical School
Chief, Obstetrics and Gynecology
Obstetrics and Gynecology Service
Massachusetts General Hospital
Boston, Massachusetts
Chapter 37, "Physiology of the Climacteric"

Machelle M. Seibel, MD
Associate Clinical Professor of Surgery (Gynecology)
Harvard Medical School
Medical Director
Faulkner Centre for Reproductive Medicine
Boston, Massachusetts
Chapter 19, "Ovarian Dysfunction and Anovulation"

Levent M. Senturk, MD
Postdoctoral Fellow
Division of Reproductive Endocrinology
Department of Obstetrics and Gynecology
Yale University School of Medicine
New Haven, Connecticut
Chapter 31, "Diagnosis and Management of Tubal Disease"

Evan R. Simpson, PhD
Prince Henry's Institute of Medical Research
Monash Medical Centre
Clayton, Victoria
Australia
Chapter 7, "The Molecular Basis of Hormone Action"

Scott M. Slayden, MD
Instructor and Fellow
Division of Reproductive Biology and Endocrinology
Department of Obstetrics and Gynecology
University of Alabama at Birmingham
Birmingham, Alabama
Chapter 10, "Hormonal Regulation of Breast Physiology"
Chapter 15, "Anovulation of CNS Origin: Anatomic Causes"

Michael R. Soules, MD
Professor and Director
Division of Reproductive Endocrinology and Infertility
Department of Obstetrics and Gynecology
University of Washington
Seattle, Washington
Chapter 6, "Normal and Abnormal Sexual Development"

Michael P. Steinkampf, MD
Professor and Director
Division of Reproductive Endocrinology
Department of Obstetrics and Gynecology
University of Alabama at Birmingham
Birmingham, Alabama
Chapter 29, "Ovulation Induction"
Chapter 33, "Assisted Reproductive Technology"
Chapter 36, "Contraception"

Dale Stovall, MD
Associate Professor
Division of Reproductive Endocrinology
Department of Obstetrics and Gynecology
University of Iowa College of Medicine
Iowa City, Iowa
Chapter 25, "Clinical Trials for the Reproductive Endocrinologist: Design, Power Analysis, and Biostatistics"

Earl W. Stradtman, Jr., MD
Clinical Assistant Professor
Divisions of Reproductive Endocrinology and Biology and Medical and Surgical Gynecology
Department of Obstetrics and Gynecology
University of Alabama at Birmingham
Birmingham, Alabama
Chapter 4, "Genetics in Reproduction"
Chapter 17, "Thyroid Dysfunction and Ovulatory Disorders"

Ian H. Thorneycroft, MD
Professor and Chairman
Department of Obstetrics and Gynecology
University of South Alabama
Mobile, Alabama
Chapter 38, "Hormonal Treatment of Menopausal Women: Risks and Benefits"

Brian W. Walsh, MD
Assistant Professor
Department of Obstetrics, Gynecology, and Reproductive Biology
Harvard Medical School
Director, Menopause Center
Department of Obstetrics and Gynecology
Brigham & Women's Hospital
Boston, Massachusetts
Chapter 37, "Physiology of the Climacteric"

Craig A. Winkel, MD
Professor and Chairman
Department of Obstetrics and Gynecology
Georgetown University
Washington, DC
Chapter 30, "Diagnosis and Treatment of Uterine Pathology"

R. Ann Word, MD
Associate Professor
Division of Reproductive Endocrinology
Department of Obstetrics and Gynecology
University of Texas Southwestern Medical Center
Dallas, Texas
Chapter 3, "Parturition"

J. Benjamin Younger, MD
Professor Emeritus
Division of Reproductive Biology and Endocrinology
Department of Obstetrics and Gynecology
University of Alabama School of Medicine
Birmingham, Alabama
Chapter 10, "Hormonal Regulation of Breast Physiology"

PREFACE TO
SECOND EDITION

Reproductive medicine has continued its relentless growth since the preparation of the first edition of this text. We now have available new generations of dopamine agonists for the treatment of pituitary tumors and hyperprolactinemic syndromes, highly purified urinary and recombinant gonadotropins for ovulation induction, significant advances in the use of transvaginal ultrasonography, and an exploding new technology in the field of minimally invasive surgery. Accompanying these advances has been a steady improvement in the pregnancy rate with assisted reproductive technology and the introduction of intracytoplasmic sperm injection for the treatment of male infertility.

In addition to these scientific changes there has been a redirection of the specialty of obstetrics and gynecology and reproductive medicine. Gynecologists now deal with the general area of women's medicine and are assuming a greater role in the diagnosis and treatment of diseases of the breast. These new roles are assumed in an environment of changing health care delivery, managed care. The new health care is delivered through the use of algorithms that are based on evidence-based medicine and cost-effective analysis. The outcomes of these treatments are subjected to rigorous statistical analysis, and each of these areas is dealt with in new chapters added to the text.

It is still the purpose of this book to furnish the practicing obstetrician/gynecologist with a sound scientific basis for diagnosing and managing contemporary reproductive endocrine and infertility problems. The book continues to utilize the strength of numerous clinicians and scientist from many institutions including our own, the University of Texas Southwestern Medical Center at Dallas and the University of Alabama Medical School at Birmingham, to achieve this goal.

PREFACE TO FIRST EDITION

Reproductive medicine has experienced tremendous growth over the last twenty years. The 1970s saw the development and refinement of radioimmunologic techniques that enabled hormones to be detected and quantified in serum and urine. This has enabled investigators to evaluate the primate menstrual cycle, isolate and structure the hypothalamic releasing and inhibiting hormones, and establish the ovarian regulation of ovulatory function. The late 1970s and early 1980s saw the development of sonography, computed axial tomography, and magnetic resonance imaging, which allowed clinicians to evaluate and treat such lesions as prolactinomas and carry out ovulation induction with greater safety and efficacy. The 1980s also saw the development of laser technology, operative laparoscopy, and hysteroscopy, which allowed surgeons to treat gynecologic pathology with far less morbidity. Assisted reproductive technology also flourished during this period, allowing us to manipulate gametes outside the human body and achieve pregnancy in those who would have been viewed as sterile in the past. Finally, in the late 1980s and early 1990s, the use of molecular biology has allowed us to unravel many of the dilemmas of reproductive medicine such as the inheritance pattern of the adrenal hyperplasias and the molecular basis of hypogonadotropism. Concomitant with these developments was the evolution of reproductive endocrinology and infertility into a subspecialty.

All of these developments have resulted in an incredible accumulation of new information about reproductive medicine. Therefore, it is the goal of this textbook to furnish the practicing obstetrician/gynecologist with a sound scientific basis for diagnosing and managing contemporary reproductive endocrine/infertility problems. The book utilizes the strengths of numerous clinicians and scientists from many institutions including our own, the University of Texas Southwestern Medical Center at Dallas and the University of Alabama Medical School at Birmingham, to achieve this goal.

ACKNOWLEDGMENTS

This book is dedicated to our mentors, Dr. Paul C. MacDonald and Dr. Roger Guillemin. The excellent science research and teaching done in laboratories such as theirs forms the foundation for this *Textbook of Reproductive Medicine.* We would also like to thank our respective wives, Phyllis Carr and Kathryn Blackwell for their support and cooperation during the preparation of this book.

Finally, the publication of this book would not have been possible without the help of our associates who contributed to it and the administrative staff who helped prepare it. We wish to express our thanks to Darlene Farmer (Dr. Carr's administrative assistant) and Murrill Lynch (Dr. Blackwell's administrative associate).

Chapter 1

FERTILIZATION, EMBRYOGENESIS, AND IMPLANTATION

William Byrd

Gamete maturation, fertilization, embryo development, and implantation are among the most complex achievements of mammalian development. This chapter is intended as a review of the recent advances in gametogenesis, fertilization, and preimplantation development. Many problems in our understanding of these processes reflect the difficulties of trying to study these events in vitro. With the advent of successful animal and human in vitro fertilization, considerable attention and research has focused on this area with a concomitant increase in our knowledge of the subject.

GAMETE MATURATION AND FERTILIZATION

Maturation of the Oocyte

At birth, the ovaries of women may contain as many as 400,000 haploid oocytes. During the reproductive life span of a woman, only 400 to 500 oocytes will ovulate, while the remaining oocytes undergo atresia.[1–3] Primordial germ cells originate in the gut endoderm and migrate through the dorsal mesentery into the genital ridges and then undergo mitotic proliferation. Following mitosis, oocytes begin meiosis and arrest in prophase I of meiosis during the fourth to seventh month of fetal development (see Chap 11). The majority of oocyte loss will occur prior to birth.[2,3] In the human, oocytes are arrested in diplotene (also referred to as dictyate or diffuse diplotene) for several years in the absence of an appropriate stimulus such as puberty. The primordial follicle consists of an oocyte (approximately 20 μm) with a single layer of flattened cells surrounding it. While the oocyte is in meiotic arrest, there is continued growth of the oocyte and granulosa cell proliferation, resulting in several granulosa cell layers. This layered oocyte forms the secondary follicle. The outermost layers, apposed to the basement membrane that underlies the theca interna, comprise most of the granulosa cells. Finally, formation of a fluid-filled antrum or chamber in the follicle marks the completion of oocyte growth and formation of the Graafian follicle. The granulosa cells immediately surrounding the oocyte that attach it to the follicular wall are the cumulus oophorus. The innermost layers of granulosa cells around the oocyte become columnar and form the corona radiata. The outermost cells will form the cumulus mass. Separating the oocyte from the granulosa cells is a non-cellular porous layer of glycoproteins secreted by the oocyte and the granulosa cells, the zona pellucida, which separates it from the surrounding cumulus cells[4–6] (Fig 1–1). The zona pellucida plays a pivotal role in fertilization and later in establishing a microenvironment for the developing embryo. During its growing phase, the volume of the oocyte will increase approximately 300-fold to become one of the largest cells in the body.[7]

Throughout development, the ovary contains several growing oocytes at different stages of development.[8] There has been considerable interest in the mechanism by which these oocytes are recruited into the pool of oocytes that might be ovulated and how nuclear and cytoplasmic maturation is controlled. Oocytes from antral follicles are competent to resume meiosis after isolation from their follicles, but oocytes from preantral follicles are not.[9] This suggests that different mechanisms to control the resumption of meiosis exist. The completion of nuclear maturation is a two-step process where the oocyte first becomes competent to undergo germinal vesicle breakdown and progress to metaphase I of meiosis. This is followed by a second step, where the oocyte attains the ability to complete meiosis to metaphase II. The first evidence that the granulosa cells had some role

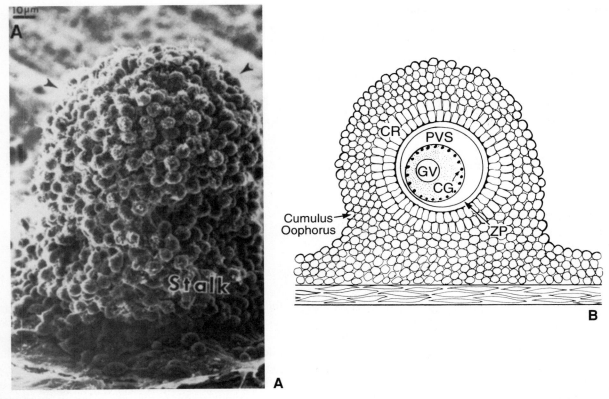

Figure 1–1. A. Scanning electron micrograph of an intact mouse granulosa complex grown for 7 days in vitro. The oocyte is contained within the ball of granulosa cells as indicated by the arrowheads. Photomicrograph courtesy of Dr John Eppig. *(Reproduced, with permission, from Eppig J, et al. Dev Biol. 140:307, 1990.)* **B.** Representation of this cumulus–granulosa–oocyte complex. Abbreviations: CR, corona radiata; CB, cortical granules; ZP, zona pellucida; GV, germinal vesicle; PVS, perivitelline space.

in the development or regulation of oocyte development was the observation of gap junctions.[10–12] Processes from the surrounding cumulus cells pass through the zona pellucida and form gap junctions with the oocyte plasma membrane.[10,11,13–15] Since the cumulus cells have no blood supply, there must be metabolic cooperation between these cumulus cells and oocyte with both metabolic and electrical coupling through the gap junctions.[10,11,16,17]

In response to an endogenous or exogenous luteinizing hormone (LH) surge, the oocyte–cumulus complex undergoes a series of events preparing it for fertilization and nuclear maturation. Maintenance of meiotic arrest is controlled by cAMP generated in the surrounding granulosa cells. Withdrawal of the cytoplasmic processes results in a decrease in cAMP in the oocyte. Deprived of exogenous cAMP, oocyte phosphodiesterase activity lowers cAMP levels, which probably provides the trigger for the resumption of meiosis.[18] Spontaneous maturation of oocytes in vitro can be blocked by the addition of membrane-permeable analogs of cyclic AMP.[7] Similarly, activating adenyl cyclase with agents such as forskolin increases levels of cyclic AMP in the oocyte and prevents maturation in

vitro.[7] While other molecules such as calmodulin are probably involved in this process, their mechanisms of action and relevance in vivo is not yet clear.[7,18]

Once meiosis is resumed, germinal vesicle breakdown occurs. The first metaphase spindle is formed in an eccentric position in the oocyte. The first division results in the formation of daughter cells with a disproportionate amount of cytoplasm and a small polar body. The oocyte enters into the second meiotic division and arrests at the second metaphase, just before ovulation in the human (see Chap 11). In addition to the morphologic changes, there is a decrease in mitotic activity.[19] Resumption of metabolic activity is dependent upon subsequent fertilization. If fertilization does not occur within 6 to 24 hr following ovulation, the oocyte will degenerate.[3]

In response to the LH surge, the cumulus cells surrounding the zona pellucida retract their cellular processes from the oocyte. Disruption of the gap junctions induces cortical maturation with migration of cortical granules from the subcortical cytoplasm to the oocyte cortex.[15,20,21] Concomitant with these meiotic events is the expansion of the cumulus mass and an accumulation of fluid in the antral chamber of the follicle. The cumulus cells are embedded in a matrix of glycosaminoglycans and expansion is primarily due to the secretion of additional matrix by granulosa cells. The density of cells in the cumulus decreases from approximately one million/mm^3 to less than 100,000/mm^3.[22] Dispersion of the outer granulosa cells does not affect the innermost two to three layers of cells around the oocyte that form the corona radiata. The expansion of the cumulus causes a separation of the oocyte–cumulus mass from the follicular wall so the complex is free in the chamber prior to ovulation.

Maturation of Spermatozoa

Traditionally, research on sperm maturation has focused on the testis. Spermatozoa reach the caudal epididymis approximately 72 days after initiation of spermatogenesis (see Chapters 13 and 28). The sperm cell found in the epididymis is highly specialized, consisting of two major components. The head has all the specialized structures required for fertilization, while the flagellum provides energy and motility. The mature spermatozoon consists of a haploid, membrane-bound nucleus capped by a large vesicle of proteolytic enzymes at the anterior portion of the head, the acrosome.[23] This vesicle is closely apposed to the nucleus on its inner boundary and the plasma membrane on its outer boundary. The tail consists of a central axoneme made of a 9 + 9 + 2 complex of microtubules and surrounding dense fibers. The proximal end of the flagellum is surrounded by mitochondria. The acquisition of the ability of the sperm to fertilize an oocyte is dependent upon in vitro or in vivo maturation of sperm following ejaculation or surgical recovery from the epididymis. Mammalian sperm recovered from the testis have not acquired the ability to fertilize eggs in vitro. Testicular sperm are either motionless or weakly motile. It is commonly accepted that a gradual acquisition of motility and fertility, or the ability to bind to the zona pellucida, occurs as sperm pass through the epididymal ducts.[24–28] Epididymal and testicular sperm obtained from males with obstructed ducts has been shown to have some fertilizing ability.[29] However, the fertility potential of sperm from males with normal epididymis has not been studied.

Prior to ejaculation, sperm undergo several changes. The plasma membrane is the most pronounced site of change during epididymal maturation. These include changes in lipid composition,[30–32] lectin binding site distribution,[33–35] diffusion rates of membrane proteins and lipid,[36,37] and intramembranous membrane distribution.[38,39] These changes may enhance the ability of sperm to bind to the zona pellucida, undergo capacitation and the acrosome reaction, and alter calcium permeability and membrane fluidity.[27,40]

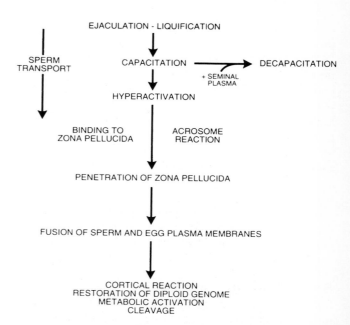

Figure 1–2. Sequence of events in the maturation of spermatozoa and the subsequent fertilization of an oocyte.

Freshly ejaculated sperm require maturation in vitro or in vivo before fertilization can occur[27,41–45] (Fig 1–2). The series of maturational events leading to a sperm capable of fertilizing an oocyte is called capacitation.[43] In the past, studies of human sperm capacitation have been limited by the lack of suitable bioassays for sperm function and the limitations on human in vitro fertilization. Similarly, studies with other mammalian species suffer since much of the comparative literature has focused on epididymal sperm, which has not been exposed to seminal plasma. However, with the advent of human in vitro fertilization programs and resultant technologies more attention has been focused on human sperm capacitation.

Capacitation cannot be viewed as a singular event, but rather as a continuum of events that result in a spermatozoon capable of undergoing an acrosome reaction, the end marker for capacitation.[27,44,45] Upon ejaculation, the human sperm surface is first exposed to seminal plasma. Studies have demonstrated that seminal plasma is more than just a vehicle for spermatozoa. It plays an important role in initiation of motility and modification of the sperm surface.[44,45] Cell surface alterations are a major part of capacitation. Components in seminal plasma can inhibit or block capacitation and fertilization.[46] However, since spermatozoa that are to have a functional role in fertilization must leave the seminal plasma and migrate into cervical mucus, any long-term influence of seminal plasma must be minimal. It is known that long-term exposure to seminal plasma has a deleterious effect on sperm motility and fertility.[46,47] Indeed, long-term exposure (greater than 30 min) to seminal plasma inhibits the ability of sperm to penetrate cervical mucus.[48]

Several other modifications occur during capacitation.[39,49–52] During capacitation, spermatozoa maintain an ionic environment that changes with time. Initially there is a high intracellular potassium and low sodium concentration when compared to the external ion concentrations. During capacitation there is a decrease in intracellular potassium concomitant with an increase in sodium. Permeability to calcium, which is essential to the acrosome reaction, increases during capacitation probably due to loss or alteration of surface molecules. These ionic changes are probably regulated by one or all of the following: (1) a calcium ATPase capable of pumping calcium out of the cell, (2) a sodium–calcium exchanger, or (3) a calcium channel.[27,53–55]

Sperm Transport and Motility

Sperm transport, selection, and survival after deposition in the vagina are an essential prerequisite to fertilization. Several different factors influence how many fertile sperm will reach the ampulla. Unfortunately, the study of this subject has been limited almost entirely to observations in laboratory and domestic animals. Survival in the acidic environment of the vagina requires a rapid transport of sperm from the ejaculate into the cervical mucus. There is a marked reduction in sperm motility if sperm are left in the vagina for longer than 30 min, and almost no motility after 2 hr of exposure to this acidic environment. Migration of sperm out of the seminal fluid can occur within 1 to 3 min following ejaculation.[56] There are both anatomic and physiological mechanisms throughout the reproductive tract that effectively select and limit the number of sperm that pass through the female reproductive tract. Anatomic barriers such as the cervix and cervical mucus act as a screening mechanism. At a microscopic level, cervical mucus appears as a base network of fibrous macromolecules with fluid-filled interstitial spaces. These spaces are small compared to sperm, so the sperm must push their way through the mucus.[57] The number of sperm deposited in the vagina can be reduced from as many as 10^7 sperm in the vagina to less than 10^4 sperm in the uterus and only 10^2 sperm at the site of fertilization.[58,59] Human sperm in an ejaculate are a heterogeneous population with regard to motility, age, and morphology, which can influence survival and selection. Capacitation need not occur at the same rate within a population of sperm.[60,61] With deposition and slow release of sperm from cervical mucus, it would be advantageous to have sperm that complete the capacitation process at different times. Antisperm antibodies either on the sperm or in the reproductive tract fluids can reduce the number of sperm by complement fixation or immobilization. Local infections in either the male or female can affect sperm motility.

Infertility is often the result of either inadequate numbers of motile sperm introduced into the female reproductive tract or a barrier to sperm transport in the female (see Chapter 25). Bypassing the cervix with intrauterine or intrafallopian insemination of sperm can result in pregnancies in couples with different types of infertility, even in cases with less than one million motile cells in the ejaculate.[62–64]

Sperm transport from the cervix to the site of fertilization in the fimbria of the fallopian tubes consists of two components. There can be rapid transport of sperm, even nonmotile sperm, within 5 to 15 min following insemination in rabbits.[58,59] Since sperm migrate through midcycle cervical mucus at a rate of 2 to 3 mm/min,[65] there must be other mechanisms to transport sperm to the ampulla. A possible mechanism to explain passive movement of sperm could be uterine and tubal muscular activity. Following insemination, the cervical mucus and cervical crypts are populated with sperm and constitute a sperm reservoir from which slow release of sperm may occur over prolonged periods.[48,49] Sperm may retain their fertilizing capacity in human cervical mucus for as long as 48 hr and their motility for as long as 120 hr.[66] The rate of sperm passage through the cervix is regulated by sperm motility, muscular activity, the consistency and production of cervical mucus, and time of storage in the cervical crypts. Further passage through the uterus appears to be more dependent upon muscular activity than on sperm motility.[59] Further reduction of sperm numbers occurs during passage through the oviducts.[67] It must be considered that sperm are actively swimming through the fluid secretions of the female reproductive tract as well as the egg investments. The viscosity and composition of these fluids will have an influence on sperm motility.[68] In addition, sperm movement in the oviduct is the result of intrinsic motility, ciliary beat and fluid flow, and muscular activity of the oviduct. The intrinsic motility of the sperm is regulated by flagellar structure, energy sources, and ionic regulation and eventually capacitation. A question that has not yet been answered is the possibility of some sort of chemotaxis or "luring" of the sperm to the egg.[69] It can be shown in vitro that chemotraction of sperm by follicular fluid is possible in a small (2 to 12%) percentage of sperm.[70] This suggests that only capacitated sperm can respond to chemotactic signals and that this responsiveness is only for a limited period of time.

Since visualization of sperm motility in vivo is impractical, analysis of sperm motility patterns has relied on the recovery of a few motile sperm from the site of fertilization or a description of sperm capacitated in vitro. In vivo, as sperm become capacitated they undergo changes in motility in the oviduct called hyperactivation[44] that are believed to be a prerequisite to fertilization. As implied by the term, hyperactivation describes an extremely active movement of the sperm and perhaps provides a

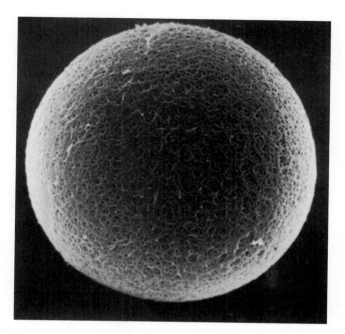

Figure 1–3. Hamster zona pellucida. The surface of the zona pellucida exhibits a fenestrated, multilayered appearance. (× 1500). (*Reproduced, with permission, from Phillips DM, et al. J Exp Zool. 213:1, 1980.*)

thrusting power for penetration of the oocyte. Sperm move rapidly in complex patterns related to flagellar bends and beat.[57,66] Several functions that hyperactivation could be involved in are: (1) the detachment of the sperm from the epithelial walls of the reproductive tract; (2) facilitation of migration; (3) expansion of the area that sperm traverse to enhance the chance of successful fertilization; (4) generation of forces to help penetrate the cumulus mass and zona pellucida.[57]

Sperm and Oocyte Interaction at Fertilization

Penetration of Oocyte Investments. During ovulation, the cumulus mass and oocyte are extruded from the follicle and rapidly transported through the ostium of the oviduct into the ampulla by ciliary action and rhythmic contraction of the fimbriated folds within 2 to 3 min of ovulation.[2,3] The cumulus then reaches the ampullary-isthmic junction, where fertilization occurs. At the time of ovulation there are approximately 20,000 cells present surrounding the oocyte. Transmission electron microscopy of these granulosa cells suggests that they may also possess steroidosynthetic capability.[71] The purpose of this cumulus mass comprised of granulosa cells and hyaluronic acid[72] may be to aid in the transport of the egg to the ampulla.[73] The precise role of the cumulus mass in fertilization is not understood. The presence of cumulus cells is not necessary for fertilization of oocytes in vivo[74] or in vitro[27,44] in several mammals. However, the fertility

of these denuded oocytes in less than intact cumulus masses suggests that these cells play some role in the fertilization process. While sperm have hyaluronidase in the acrosome, evidence suggests that premature release of this enzyme by an acrosome reaction would result in immobilization in the cumulus mass. Several investigators have documented that acrosome-intact sperm can penetrate directly through the cumulus mass to the zona pellucida.[75–79] Evidence to suggest that hyaluronidase was not needed for cumulus penetration was provided by Talbot and co-workers,[77] who demonstrated that both sea urchin and frog spermatozoa, which lack hyaluronidase, can penetrate the cumulus mass of the hamster. Following fertilization, there is a dispersal of the surrounding granulosa cells from the embryo approximately 24 hr after ovulation.[59]

Binding and Penetration of the Zona. The process of sperm penetration of the zona pellucida is a unique, species-specific process dependent upon receptors in the zona that control sperm binding and the acrosome reaction (Fig 1–3). This series of events enables motile sperm to penetrate the noncellular glycoprotein coat and fuse with the underlying oocyte. While the sperm acrosome reaction may occur spontaneously in the reproductive tract or in vitro,[27,61] these reactions may be of little physiological importance. Evidence suggests that the acrosome reaction occurs in all species on or near the zona pellucida.[7,80] Free-swimming sperm that have been recovered from the ampulla are usually acrosome intact.[81] Sperm associated with the cumulus usually have intact acrosomes or are undergoing an acrosome reaction, while sperm bound to the zona have begun or are undergoing an acrosome reaction.[82] There are a variety of glycosaminoglycans, fatty acids, hormones, and neurotransmitters that have been suggested as possible acrosome-inducing components.[82] The physiologic concentration of these acrosomal inducers in vivo is unknown. It is difficult to differentiate between inducers that directly influence capacitation and inducers that directly initiate the acrosome reaction.[83]

Following penetration of the cumulus mass, sperm bind to the zona pellucida in a species-specific manner.[84–87] Most of our knowledge of sperm–egg interaction has been elucidated through studies of other animal species. The initial step in sperm–egg interaction in mammals is a loose attachment between the zona pellucida and the sperm head that precedes a much tighter binding to the zona.[84–87] In the mouse, approximately 2000 sperm can bind to the zona surface in about 10 to 15 min at sperm concentrations of 10^5 to 10^6 sperm/ml.[87] However, this concentration is never seen in vivo. The affinity for spermatozoa is imparted by receptors in the zona pellucida.[5,88] The best-described system for studying sperm–zona interaction has been the mouse.[7] The zona pellucida of the mouse is composed of three sulfated glycoproteins (ZP1, ZP2, ZP3) of 200, 120, and 83 kD, respectively.[7,89–91] Each of these glycoproteins has a specific function. The basic structural unit of the zona pellucida consists of ZP2–ZP3 dimers filaments that are cross-linked by ZP1.[5] Both ZP2 and ZP3 are present in equimolar amounts and make up about 80 percent of the total zona protein. ZP2 apparently acts as a secondary sperm receptor and is modified after fertilization to provide a block to polyspermy. The ZP3 molecule consists of a polypeptide chain to which N-linked oligosaccharides chains, as well as O-linked oligosaccharides, are attached.[92] ZP3 mediates the initial binding of sperm to the zona via the oligosaccharide component. The polypeptide component is required for induction of the acrosome reaction. [5,7,89,90]

The human zona pellucida is comprised of three glycoproteins as in the mouse.[93–95] Chamberlin and Dean[96] used mouse ZP3 sperm receptor genes to isolate its human homolog. ZP3 function is similar to the mouse, and it has been shown that recombinant human ZP3 induces the acrosome reaction.[97] There are certain features of both transcripts that are conserved. The similarity of certain regions suggests that the more highly conserved areas may serve a role in the structural integrity of the zona pellucida. The more heterogeneous areas may be involved in providing species specificity.

While there is little question that ZP3 is the receptor to which sperm bind, there is conflicting evidence for the reciprocal receptor on the sperm. Shur and colleagues[98,99] presented evidence that β-1,4-galactosyltransferase is the molecule on the sperm that mediates adhesion to the N-acetylglucosamine group of the oligosaccharides of ZP3. Several other sperm surface receptors have been proposed. These include a 56-kD protein (SP 56),[100] involvement of a tyrosine-phosphorylated protein (P95),[101] proteinase-like α mannoside,[102] galactosyl receptors,[103] α mannosidase,[104] and lectin-like fucose binding protein.[105]

The acrosome reaction is an exocytotic event that involves multiple fusions between the outer acrosomal membrane with the overlying plasma membrane and fusion to form vesicles. This allows the contents of the acrosomal granule to escape. The inner acrosomal membrane remains and is attached at the equatorial segment. The net effect of the acrosomal reaction is the exposure of the acrosomal contents, which are utilized in the penetration of the zona pellucida. The ionic events that regulate the acrosome reaction are beginning to be understood. Calcium influx is an absolute prerequisite for the acrosome reaction.[27,44,82,106,107] Incubation in a calcium-free medium blocks the acrosome reaction.[108] Incubation with calcium ionophores in other conditions that promote calcium entry will induce reaction. This is presumed to be an increase in intracellular calcium and intercellular pH.

All evidence suggests the acrosome reaction is initiated by the zona as a consequence of induced entry of external calcium.[27] ZP3 may mediate the acrosome reaction by G proteins to increase calcium permeability and stimulate acrosome reaction.[106] Evidence to support the role of G proteins is that the acrosome reaction can be induced by intact zonae or solubilized zonae. Acrosomal induction by zonae is inhibited by pertussis toxin, a specific inhibitor of G proteins.[109–111] Changes in intracellular pH and calcium levels which precede zona pellucida–mediated acrosomal exocytosis are also blocked by pertussis toxin. This suggests that G proteins may be involved in the regulation of these ionic changes.[106] Interestingly, several other molecules can induce the acrosome reaction, such as progesterone.[112] Sperm surface components undergo rearrangement during fertilization. The antigen PT-1 in the guinea pig, located in the posterior flagellar region of epididymal sperm, migrates to the midpiece region during capacitation.[37] Following the acrosome reaction, another surface antigen of guinea pig sperm, PH20, migrates from the posterior head region to the anterior region of the sperm head to the inner acrosomal membrane.[113] Rearrangement of the surface antigens may be involved in mediating zona binding. At the very least, the migration of these molecules to new sites or domains indicates the dynamic membrane changes.

Fusion of the Acrosome-Reacted Sperm with the Oocyte. Penetration of the zona pellucida relies on both mechanical and enzymatic processes. Following the acrosome reaction, acrosin and possibly other enzymes from the acrosomal granule are involved in the penetration of the zona pellucida.[27,44] The sperm that pass the zona are very active. Increased or vigorous motility may facilitate penetration. After the sperm cross the perivitelline space, they become closely opposed to the egg plasma membrane at the region of the equatorial segment. The egg membrane is now characterized by a number of short microvilla (0.3 to 1 μm in length). The point of fusion is probably the segment of the sperm plasma membrane that remains over the restricted equatorial region[24,44,114,115] (Fig 1–4). Following fusion, the sperm membrane remains as part of a mosaic membrane on the egg surface.

Antibody inhibition studies have suggested the possibility of several candidates that could mediate sperm binding and fusion to the oolemma. In the guinea pig, PH30, or fertilin, is one of the proteins that has been implicated in fusion.[116] Proteolytic conversion of PH30 is a prerequisite to the sperm acquiring the ability to fuse with the egg, and inhibitory studies using monoclonal antibodies showed that sperm–egg fusion can be inhibited in vitro.[116] The cloning of cDNAs to encoding fertilin have shown the presence of a domain that would

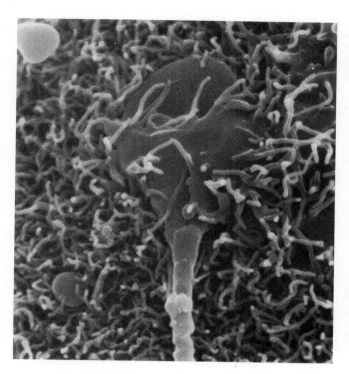

Figure 1–4. Scanning electron micrograph of a human spermatozoon fusing with the surface of a hamster oocyte in vitro. There appear to be oocyte microvilli and membrane over the equatorial surface of the acrosome (× 7000). *(Reproduced, with permission, from Phillips DM. In:* Elements of Mammalian Fertilization. *Boca Raton, Fla., CRC Press, 1991.)*

have a high affinity for integrin receptors on the egg surface.[117] The presence of integrins has been established on the egg oolemma, suggesting that this could be a mechanism for sperm–oocyte binding.[118–120]

The Cortical Reaction, Zona Pellucida Modifications, and the Block to Polyspermy.

Mechanisms exist in all mammalian eggs to block or limit the penetration of supernumerary sperm after the initial sperm has fused with the oocyte. Fusion of sperm and egg membrane triggers three key events: the cortical reaction and the block to polyspermy, nuclear activation and completion of meiosis, and metabolic activation of the oocyte. Following fusion, there is an increase in egg inositol 1,4,5-triphosphate (IP3) that stimulates the release of intracellular calcium and induces the cortical reaction.[20] Ultrastructurally, the cortical reaction can be seen as a fusion of cortical granules (300 to 600 nm in diameter) with the overlying plasma membrane. The exocytotic release of the contents of the cortical granules into the perivitelline space results in a modification of the overlying zona pellucida and a block to further sperm entry through the zona.[20,27,44] The membranes of cortical granules are then incorporated into the plasma

membrane.[44,121] This reaction spreads from the point of sperm fusion around the egg in a wavelike front. The cortical granules release either individually or after coalescence of several small granules.

Modifications to the zona pellucida also result in a loss of sperm binding.[122,123] Since the inhibition of sperm binding by cortical granule exocytosis can be blocked by trypsin inhibitors, a trypsin-like protease has been implicated in this reaction.[85,122] This loss in binding is correlated with alterations in the molecular properties of ZP2 and ZP3.[5,7] Cortical granule exocytosis modifies the zona pellucida so that it is unable to bind sperm and the acrosome-reacted sperm already bound cannot penetrate the zona. One component of the cortical granule contents is a protease that causes cleavage of the ZP2.[21] Following cortical granule exocytosis, there is an increased resistance of the zona pellucida to the enzymatic and chemical digestion, called zona hardening.[124,125]

There is evidence that the egg must be at a certain state of development to undergo a proper cortical reaction and block to polyspermy. Immaturity of the oocytes at the time of penetration and excessive aging of oocytes in culture could result in a partial or incomplete block to polyspermy.

The human oocyte seems to rely heavily upon the zona reaction to block further successful sperm penetration. Reinsemination experiments using human oocytes and embryos demonstrate that plasma membrane receptivity to sperm occurs about 2 hr after insemination.[126] However, polyspermy in the human oocyte can occur if oocytes are inseminated at rather high sperm concentrations in vitro. In mature oocytes, fertilization in vitro can result in a polyspermy rate as high as 5 percent.[127] A summary of the fertilization pathway is depicted in Figure 1–5.

Sperm Decondensation, Pronuclear Formation, and Fusion.

After fusion of the sperm, its contents, including the sperm nucleus, centriole, mitochondria, and tail components, are incorporated into the ooplasm.[16,128] During spermatogenesis, compaction of nuclear DNA material takes place when somatic histones are replaced by sperm-specific histones and protamines, which have a high percentage of basic amino acids. There is also extensive sulfhydryl cross-linking of the nuclear proteins that results in an ever greater rigidity of the sperm head.[27] A rapid breakdown of the nuclear membrane results in exposure of the sperm nucleus to the cytoplasm and allows factors in the oocyte to modulate nuclear decondensation and dispersion. Following dispersion, a pronuclear envelope forms within the next few hours.[128] The nucleus increases in size and approximately eight nucleoli are formed within it.[129] The flagellum is incorporated into the ooplasm and rapidly dispersed. At this

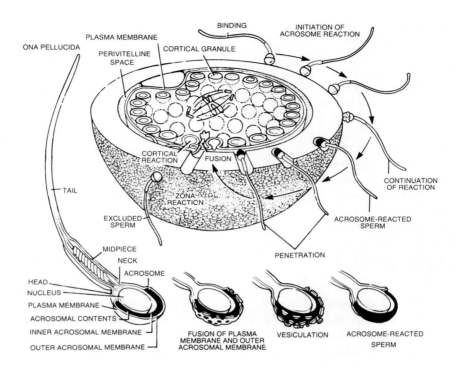

Figure 1–5. Fertilization pathway. After the spermatozoon binds to the zona pellucida, the acrosome reaction takes place (see detail at the bottom). The outer membrane of the acrosome fuses at several points with the plasma membrane surrounding the sperm head. Those fused membranes from vesicles that are eventually sloughed from the head, exposing the proteolytic enzymes of the acrosomal granule. The enzymes digest a pathway through the zona pellucida, enabling the sperm to advance to the egg surface. Eventually, the sperm fuses with the egg membrane, completing the fertilization process. This fusion triggers the cortical and zona reactions. The zona as a result of enzyme modification becomes impermeable to further sperm penetration and polyspermy. *(Reproduced, with permission, from Wassarman PM.* Sci Am. *259:1988.)*

same time, resumption of anaphase and telophase of the second meiotic division of the oocyte with the formation of the second polar body occurs. The second polar body is persistent and can often be found associated with the cleaving embryo. The female pronucleus develops near the site of the second polar body extrusion. Both pronuclei become synthetically active as evidenced by the formation of several nucleoli within them.

Pronuclear fusion in most mammalian species consists of migration of the pronuclei into the interior of the egg,[27,128] and there is close apposition of the nuclear membranes. Chromosomes condense at prophase before nuclear membrane breakdown. Following breakdown of the membranes, maternal and paternal chromosomes mingle on the mitotic spindle. Fertilization can be considered complete with the formation of the first mitotic spindle.

Metabolic Activation. The ovulated oocyte is metabolically inactive before fertilization or parthenogenetic activation. The mammalian oocyte contains an extensive store of material synthesized during oogenesis that will be utilized during development. Following fertilization, there is a limited activation of several metabolic path-

ways concomitant with increased protein and nucleic acid synthesis.[125] During the initial stages of cleavage, there is an absence of RNA synthesis. In the mouse oocyte, there is approximately 200 times more RNA and 1000 times more ribosomal RNA than somatic cells.[7]

The molecular mechanism for activation is as yet unknown. In marine invertebrates and the frog, egg activation is accompanied by an increase in intracellular pH. In the mouse, there is no evidence to suggest that internal pH changes with egg activation.[130] It is known that fertilization results in initiation of a series of calcium transients, probably released from the endoplasmic reticulum, that continue up through pronuclear formation.[131] Whether these signals are part of the mechanism for activation remains to be demonstrated.

PREIMPLANTATION DEVELOPMENT

Fertilization and cleavage take place in the ampulla. The cleaving embryo moves slowly down the fallopian tube over the next 3 days. Embryos are carried by oviductal fluid. Embryo transport would be under the control of the tube and ciliary movement. There is a slow, discontinuous transit through the ampulla to the ampullary-isthmic junction. Approximately 72 hr after ovulation, the embryo is transported through the isthmus and uterotubal junction.[2,3] Additional time is required for the embryo to reach the uterus.[59]

Most mammalian embryos, including the human embryo, can be cultured from the pronuclear stage to the hatching blastocyst in vitro.[2,3,132] While these early developmental events can take place independently of maternal signals or communication, as evidenced by the successful transfer of blastocyst stage embryos to primed host uteri, there still has to be coordination of the developmental stage and endometrial development for successful implantation. Cleavage occurs slowly in mammals compared to other organisms. The time from fertilization to the first cleavage is approximately 18 to 36 hr.[2,133] During later cleavage, blastomeres begin a process of compaction, merging into a single mass of cells. Before compaction, the blastomeres are spherical. During compaction, the cell membranes become flattened against each other. This early event is marked by the formation of gap junctions between the outer blastomeres.[134] The adhesion and compaction of the morula cells and the appearance of tight junctions and adhesion molecules (ovumorulin) regulate the accumulation of blastocoele fluid. Sodium-potassium ATPase becomes distributed in the outer plasma membrane of the mouse trophectoderm. This Na-K ATPase establishes a sodium gradient that causes an osmotic accumulation of fluid in the blastocoele cavity at approximately 120 hr of development. The cells have now become partitioned between the inner cell mass, which will make up the embryo proper. The flattened epithelial trophectoderm cells around the periphery form the trophoblast, which will make up the extraembryonic structures. The polar trophectoderm covers the inner cell mass and the mural trophectoderm surrounds the fluid-filled blastocoele cavity. At this time, there is no expansion of the cavity.

Regulation of Gene Expression

A central question in developmental biology is the developmental potency of the early blastomeres and regulation of gene expression in the pre-implantation embryo. Restriction of the ability of a blastomere to form certain cell structures is called determination. From work by Tarkowski and Wroblewska,[135] the mouse embryo's cell fate to differentiate into trophectoderm or inner cell mass begins to occur at the morula stage (16- to 32-cell stage). There is a full loss of totipotency occurring about the time of blastocyst expansion.

Gene expression is effectively arrested when the oocyte progresses to metaphase II of meiosis. Following fertilization and the restoration of the diploid genome, both copies of maternal and paternal chromosomes will be present, which represents the transition point for new gene products. Initially, maternal RNA stored in the zygote can support protein synthesis up through the 8-cell stage,[136] although most maternal mRNA is depleted by the end of the late 2-cell stage.[137,138] Extensive changes in protein synthesis occur during the late 1-cell and 2-cell stages. The switch from maternal to zygotic control of gene expression varies in different mammals; the mouse switches at the 2-cell stage, humans at 4 cells, and cattle and sheep at 8 to 16 cells.[139]

IMPLANTATION

Implantation, one of the most poorly understood processes in reproductive biology, depends upon the synchronization of the embryo's developmental stage with the maturing uterine endometrium. A successful interaction results in the physical attachment of the embryo, which is essential for further development. Critical to this process is the differentiation of specialized extraembryonic epithelial cells (trophoblastic cells) and the inner cell mass (ICM) while the blastocyst is still unattached. Differentiation of the embryo proper will not begin until after the development of the first placental structures. The invasion of the endometrial wall by a genetically distinct trophoblast requires a delicate balance that allows this invasive process to continue while maintaining the uterine tissues required for support of the development of the implanted embryo.

The current feeling is that in response to ovarian hormones and other factors the uterus matures from a nonreceptive to a receptive stage in regard to implantation. The result of a receptive uterus is the embryo becoming fixed or implanted in the endometrium. The chances of a fertile couple producing viable offspring in any one menstrual cycle is about 20 to 25 percent.[140] Following human in vitro fertilization and embryo transfer, implantation has been shown to be inefficient, with less than 10 percent of all fertilized embryos (on a per embryo basis) resulting in a clinical pregnancy. Since errors in implantation are one of the major contributors to infertility, it is appropriate to understand the contributing factors in implantation. Again, as with fertilization and early development, much of our understanding of implantation is derived from comparative studies with other mammals, in particular the mouse and rat.

Factors That Control Endometrial Changes at the Site of Implantation

The most obvious feature of the menstrual cycle is the periodic endometrial shedding. The epithelial cells lining the remains of the glands in the basal stroma proliferate and resurface the endothelium under the influence of estrogen.

Following the early proliferative phase, the stroma becomes highly vascularized, the arteries spiralize, and the uterine glands develop. Following ovulation, the endometrium enters a secretory phase regulated in the luteal phase by progesterone and estrogen, which primes the uterus for implantation.[140] There is further thickening of the endometrium during the luteal phase with vascularization and accumulation of secretions in the uterine glands. The earliest identifiable sign of implantation is an increase in the endothelial vascularization and stromal differentiation of the predecidual cells.[8] In this reaction, fibroblast-like cells are transformed into decidual cells. Decidual cells are characterized by their epithelioid appearance and the appearance of polyploid nuclei. These cells accumulate glycogen and lipid and develop extensive cell–cell contacts. There is considerable evidence that changes in the endometrium are triggered by prostaglandins. Indomethacin, an inhibitor of prostaglandin biosynthesis, can inhibit development of vascular permeability.[8] Snabes and Harper[141] suggest that the prostaglandins involved in implantation are produced by the endometrium. Harper[141] suggests that the trophoblast as a result of its interaction with the endometrium "traumatizes" it and stimulates prostaglandin synthesis. As a result, the endometrium becomes edematous due to increased vascular permeability. The cells that typically undergo these changes are found adjacent to the embryo and constitute the decidua.

Role of Substances Released by the Endometrium and/or Embryos

Uterine secretion changes in volume and content during the period preceding implantation. Secretions of the endometrium may play a role in the support of unattached blastocysts and recognition of the blastocyst before implantation. The endometrial response to the blastocyst is reminiscent of the changes common to the inflammatory response. These responses include the production of prostaglandins, changes in capillary permeability, and infiltration of leukocytes.

At the same time the endometrium is undergoing modification, there are a number of changes occurring in the trophoblast.[142] Many studies have examined the role of uterine secretions on the blastocyst before implantation.[140] These secretions could be working directly on the blastocysts as informational signals, or they could be acting indirectly by serving as nutrients or modulators. The human embryo blastocyst remains in the uterine luminal secretions for approximately 72 hr.[143] However, this window of implantation can be delayed in other species. Large mammals such as horses and pigs have blastocysts that can remain in the uterus for several days; the armadillo can delay implantation up to 16 weeks; and the sable can delay implantation for up to 7 months. Some species show prolonged implantation times due to lactation. The delayed implantation can be induced by the removal of the litter or the injection of estrogen.[144]

There may be a role for growth factors and other substances produced by either the embryo or endometrium. Mouse embryos can grow to blastocysts in the reproductive tract of steroid-depleted mice. However, there is a considerable loss of viability and a reduction in cell number in these mice cultured in utero.[145] There is evidence that, in addition to the paracrine factors released by the reproductive tract, growth factors and other compounds of embryonic origin may act as autocrine regulators of development. Evidence to support autocrine regulation is supported by evidence that embryos can develop to blastocysts in vitro without complex media and additives.[132] Evidence to suggest that paracrine regulation is also involved is that the development and mitotic activity of these embryos occurs at much slower rate.[146] Autocrine regulation can be shown to have an influence in embryonic growth by crowding experiments. Development of single embryos in culture can be improved by culturing multiple embryos in the same volume.[147,148] Addition of epidermal growth factor or transforming growth factor to single embryos improves development.[148] This would suggest that culture of human embryos in vitro could be improved by co-culture[149] with cells that may produce paracrine growth factors or by culture in a smaller volume of medium or co-culturing with other human oocytes.

Synchrony

For successful embryo implantation, there must be a synchrony between the embryo and endometrium. As discussed earlier, human embryos arrive in the endometrial cavity on day 18 or 19 of an idealized menstrual cycle, assuming the LH surge occurred on day 14. By transfer of 4- to 16-cell embryos into defined endometrial environments, the window of implantation can be determined. In a review of donated oocytes by Rosenwaks,[150] the optimal window for replacement in several studies was 16 to 19 days. If oocytes were transferred from 20 to 24 days, no pregnancies were observed.

Hatching, Apposition, Attachment, and Invasion

Mammalian embryos hatch from their zonae pellucidae before attachment by either hatching or zona lysis. The human blastocyst is free in the uterus approximately 72 hr before it hatches and attaches to the endometrium. While the single-chambered human uterus is capable of supporting several conceptuses, it usually has only one implantation site in the upper, posterior wall of the uterus near the midsagittal plate.[151] Cells in the endometrium are induced to build up stores of nutrients

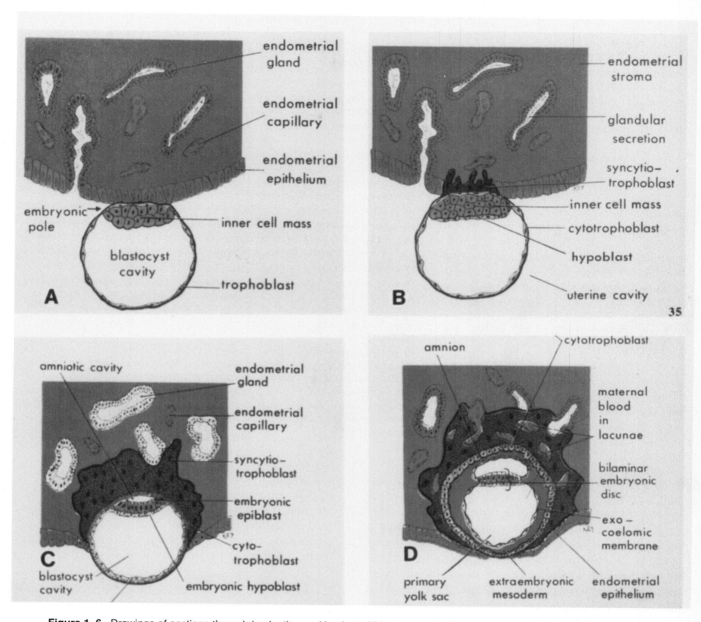

Figure 1–6. Drawings of sections through implanting and implanted blastocysts. **A.** Blastocyst attached to the endometrial epithelium at the embryonic pole of the blastocysts. **B.** The syncytiotrophoblast has penetrated the epithelium and started to invade the endometrial stroma. **C.** The blastocyst has partially implanted in the endometrium at about 8 days of development. Note the slit-like amniotic cavity. **D.** Blastocyst completely implanted in the endometrium at about 9 days of development. Note the spaces or lacunae appearing in the syncytiotrophoblast. These soon begin to communicate with the endometrial vessels. *(Reproduced, with permission, from Moore KL. The Developing Human, 4th ed. Philadelphia, Pa., W. B. Saunders, 1988.)*

that are later released into the extracellular spaces. Attachment of the trophoblast occurs about 6 to 7 days after fertilization,[152] with the embryonic pole of the blastocyst aligned with the endometrium (Fig 1–6). Attachment signifies the invasive stage and initiates stromal cell transformation to decidual cells. There have been several factors identified that are produced during the period of implantation that may be necessary for at-

tachment, implantation, or growth. These include colony stimulating factor (CSF-1), growth factors, leukemia inhibiting factor (LIF), the interleukin family, cytokines, corticotropin releasing factor (CRF), platelet aggregation factor (PAF), and prostaglandins. The number of factors makes the elucidation of their function somewhat difficult; a list of these factors and some of their activities appears in Table 1–1. This process involves cellular pro-

TABLE 1–1. FACTORS INVOLVED IN IMPLANTATION

Factor	Possible Action(s)
Leukemia inhibitory factor (LIF)	Glycoprotein found in embryos and endometrium. May be involved in blastocyst growth and implantation[153,154]
Interleukin (IL)-1 system	IL-1 alpha and beta secreted by the embryos at the time of implantation, and may mediate or modulate prostaglandin synthesis[154]
Colony-stimulating factor (CSF-1)	Stimulates growth and differentiation of stem cells. May regulate trophoblast proliferation and differentiation. Secreted by the glandular epithelium of endometrium[155]
Epidermal growth factor (EGF)	Receptors for EGF have been found on the trophoblast. Probably involved in trophoblast outgrowth and implantation[156,157]
Corticotropin releasing factor (CRF)	Regulates inflammatory response. High concentrations have been found at the site of implantation and it has been implicated in an increase in capillary permeability[158]
Estrogen	Plays a role in stimulating implantation when injected into lactating female mice[153]
Platelet aggregation factor (PAF)	Released from embryos, PAF stimulates release of prostaglandins, which in turn may act on stromal cells to produce more PAF and prostaglandins. PAF has also been shown to increase the implantation potential of mice and human embryos[159]
Prostaglandins (PGE_2)	Involved in implantation response[158]
Transforming growth factors	Polypeptides that may be involved in embryonic development, particularly the proliferation and proteolytic activity of trophoblastic cells. TGF may enhance extracellular matrix production and even modulate maternal/embryonic immune response[153,157]
Urokinase type-plasminogen activator (u-PA)	Thought to play a role in extracellular proteolysis such as invasive growth of trophoblast[153]
Integrins	Invading interstitial cells require a matrix to adhere to and migrate. The integrins are transmembrane glycoproteins composed of alpha and beta subunits which bind to both laminin and fibronectin. These integrins are found both on the trophoblast as well as the decidua[160–162]
Extracellular matrix proteins	Collagen, laminin, and fibronectin have been shown to promote in vitro attachment and outgrowth of mouse blastocysts. Found on both the trophoblast and the decidua cells[163–166]

liferation and differentiation including increases in vascular permeability. Microvilli on the endometrial surface will interdigitate with those of the embryo, forming junctions. Following this attachment phase, the embryo can no longer be flushed from the surface of the endometrium. In humans, the trophoblast overlying the embryonic disc differentiates into the syncytiotrophoblast, which proliferates and penetrates between the epithelial cells. Eventually, the syncytiotrophoblast penetrates deeply into the uterine wall to contact maternal blood vessels. Interactions between embryonic and maternal blood vessels results in the formation of the vascular supply of the placenta.

CONCLUSION

Development of an individual begins with the fertilization of an oocyte and restoration of the diploid state. Fertilization stimulates the completion of meiosis and egg activation, which is followed by syngamy and the first cleavage. There must be a clear understanding of the interrelationships during this process to further our knowledge. While hindered with experimental in vitro and animal models, our understanding of human fertilization and preimplantation development is rapidly progressing. The knowledge gained from these and future studies have far-reaching consequences. We can also expect some debate and discussion on the newer advances in the field for both medical and social issues.

REFERENCES

1. Baker T. Oogenesis and ovulation. In: Austin C, Short R, eds. *Reproduction in Mammals.* Cambridge, U.K., Cambridge University Press, 1982; 1:17–45
2. Edwards RG. Early human development: From the oocyte to implantation. In: Phillip EE, Barnes J, Newton M, Heineman W, eds. *Scientific Foundations of Obstetrics and Gynecology.* Chicago, Ill., Medical Books Ltd., 1977: 175-253
3. Edwards RG. *Conception in the Human Female.* New York, N.Y., Academic Press, 1980
4. Dunbar BS. Morphological, biochemical and immunochemical characterization of the mammalian zona pellucida. In: Hartmann JF, ed. *Mechanism and Control of Animal Fertilization.* New York, N.Y., Academic Press, 1983: 139-157

5. Bleil JD. Sperm receptors of mammalian eggs. In: Wassarman PM, ed. *Elements of Mammalian Fertilization.* Boca Raton, Fla., CRC Press, 1991:134–151

6. Barros C, Crosby JA, Moreno RD: Early steps of sperm–egg interactions during mammalian fertilization. *Cell Biol Int.* 20:33, 1996

7. Wassarman PM. The mammalian ovum. In: Knobil E, Neil JD, et al, eds. *The Physiology of Reproduction.* New York, N.Y., Raven Press, 1988; 1:69–102

8. Hodgen GD, Itskovitz J. Recognition and maintenance of pregnancy. In: Knobil E, Neill JD, et al., eds. *The Physiology of Reproduction.* New York, N. Y., Raven Press, 1988; 1:1995–2021

9. Eppig JJ: Coordination of nuclear and cytoplasmic oocyte maturation in eutherian mammals. *Reprod Fertil Dev.* 8:485, 1996

10. Anderson E. Comparative aspects of the ultrastructure of the female gamete. *Int Rev Cytol.* 4(suppl.):1, 1974

11. Anderson E, Albertini DF. Gap junctions between the oocyte and companion follicle cells in the mammalian ovary. *J Cell Biol.* 71:680, 1976

12. Gilula NB, Epstein ML, Beers WH. Cell to cell communication and ovulation. A study of the cumulus–oocyte complex. *J Cell Biol.* 78:58, 1977

13. Baca M. Zamboni L. The fine structure of human follicular oocytes. *J Ultrastruct Res.* 19:354, 1967

14. Zamboni L. *Fine Morphology of Mammalian Fertilization.* New York, N.Y., Harper and Row, 1971

15. Szollosi D, Gerard M. Cytoplasmic changes in the mammalian oocytes during the preovulatory period. In: Beier HM, Linder HR, eds. *Fertilization of the Human Egg In Vitro.* Berlin, FRG, Springer-Verlag, 1983: 35–56

16. Meck FB, Albright JT, Botticelli CR. The fine structure of granulosa cell nexus in rat ovarian follicles. *Anat Rec.* 175:107, 1973

17. Amsterdam A, Josephs R, Liberman ME, Linder HR. Organization of intramembranous particles in freeze-cleaved gap junctions of rat graafian follicles. *J Cell Sci.* 21:93, 1976

18. Schultz, RM. Meiotic maturation of mammalian oocytes. In: Wassarman PM, ed. *Elements of Mammalian Fertilization.* Boca Raton, Fla., CRC Press, 1991: 78–105

19. Heller DT, Schultz RM. Ribonucleoside metabolism by mouse oocytes: metabolic cooperativity between the fully grown oocyte and cumulus cells. *J Exp Zool.* 214:355, 1980

20. Ducibella T. Mammalian egg cortical granules and the cortical reaction. In: Wassarman PM, ed. *Elements of Mammalian Fertilization.* Boca Raton, Fla., CRC Press, 1991: 206–231

21. Ducibella T, Kurasawa S, Rangarajan S, et al. Precocious loss of cortical granules during mouse oocyte meiotic maturation and correlation with an egg-induced modification of the zona pellucida. *Dev. Biol.* 137:46, 1990

22. Testart J, Thebault A, Frydman R, Papiernik E. Oocyte and cumulus oophorus changes inside the human follicle cultured with gonadotropins. In: Hafez ESE, Semm K, eds. *In Vitro Fertilization and Embryo Transfer.* 1982: 181–198

23. Fawcett DW, Bedford JM (eds). *The Spermatozoon. Maturation, Motility, Surface Properties and Comparative Aspects.* Baltimore, Md., Urban & Schwarzenberg, 1979

24. Eddy EM. The spermatozoon. In: Knobil E, Neill JD, Ewing LL, et al, eds. *The Physiology of Reproduction.* New York, N.Y., Raven Press, 1988; 1:27–68.

25. Eddy EM, O'Brien DA, Welch JE. Mammalian sperm development in vivo and in vitro. In: Wassarman PM, ed. *Elements of Mammalian Fertilization.* Boca Raton, Fla., CRC Press, 1991: 1–28

26. Florman HM, Babcock DF. Progress toward understanding the molecular basis of capacitation. In: Wassarman PM, ed. *Elements of Mammalian Fertilization.* Boca Raton, Fla., CRC Press, 1991: 105–132

27. Yanagimachi R. Mammalian fertilization. In: Knobil E, Neill JD, et al, eds. *The Physiology of Reproduction.* New York, N.Y., Raven Press, 1988; 1:135–186

28. Hoskins DD, Vijayaraghavan S. A new theory on the acquisition of sperm motility during epididymal transit. In: Gagnon C, ed. *Controls of Sperm Motility: Biological and Clinical Aspects.* Boca Raton, Fla., CRC Press, 1991: 53–62

29. Silber SJ. Apparent fertility of human spermatozoa from the caput epididymis. *J Androl.* 10:263, 1989

30. Davis BK. Timing of fertilization in mammals: Sperm cholesterol/phospholipid ratio as a determinant of the capacitation interval. *Proc Natl Acad Sci USA.* 78:7560, 1981

31. Langlais J, Zollinger M, Plante L, et al. Localization of cholesterol sulfate in human spermatozoa in support of a hypothesis for the mechanism of capacitation. *Proc Natl Acad Sci USA.* 78:7266, 1981

32. Go KJ, Wolf DP. Albumin-mediated changes in sperm sterol content during capacitation. *Biol Reprod.* 32:145, 1985

33. Koehler KJ. Lectins as probes of spermatozoa surface. *Arch Androl.* 6:197, 1981

34. Ahuja KK. Carbohydrate determinants involved in mammalian fertilization. *Am J Anat.* 174:207, 1985

35. Deplech S, Hamamah S, Pisselet CL, Courot M. Differential localization of glycoconjugates having affinity for concanavalin A on the surface of the sperm head in the testis, the epididymis and the ejaculate of the ram. *J Exp Zool.* 245:59, 1988

36. O'Rand MG. Changes in sperm surface properties correlated with capacitation. In: Fawcett DW, Bedford JM, eds. *The Spermatozoon.* 1979: 195–204

37. Myles DG, Primakoff P, Koppel DE. A localized surface protein of guinea pig sperm exhibits free diffusion in its domain. *J Cell Biol.* 98:1905, 1984

38. Koehler JK, Gaddum-Rosse P. Media induced alterations of the membrane associated particles of the guinea pig sperm tail. *J Ultrastruct Res.* 51:106, 1975

39. Friend DS. Freeze-fracture alterations in guinea pig sperm membranes preceding gamete fusion. In: Gilula NB, ed. *Membrane–Membrane Interactions.* New York, N.Y., Raven Press, 1980: 153–165

40. Orgebin-Crist M-C, Fournier-Delpech S. Sperm–egg interaction. Evidence for maturational changes during epididymal transit. *J Androl.* 3:429, 1982

41. Austin CR. Observations on the penetration of sperm into the mammalian egg. *Aust J Sci Res (B)*. 4:581, 1951

42. Chang MC. Fertilizing capacity of spermatozoa deposited into the fallopian tubes. *Nature*. 168:697, 1951

43. Austin CR. The capacitation of mammalian sperm. *Nature*. 170:326, 1952

44. Yanagimachi R. Mechanisms of fertilization in mammals. In: Mastroianni L, Biggers JD, eds. *Fertilization and Embryonic Development In Vitro*. New York, N.Y., Plenum Press, 1981: 81–182

45. Bedford JM. Sperm capacitation and fertilization in mammals. *Biol Reprod*. 2(suppl.) 2:128, 1970

46. Kanwar KC, Yanagimachi R, Lopata A. Effects of human seminal plasma on the fertilizing capacity of human spermatozoa. *Fertil Steril*. 31:321, 1979

47. Wolf DP, Sokoloski JE. Characterization of the sperm penetration bioassay. *J Androl*. 3:445, 1982

48. Mortimer D. From the semen to the oocyte: The long route in vivo and the in vitro short cut. In: Tesart J, Frydman R, eds. *Human In Vitro Fertilization*. New York, N.Y., Elsevier Science Publishers, 1985: 93–107

49. Stein DM, Fraser LR. Cyclic nucleotide metabolism in mouse epididymal spermatozoa during capacitation in vitro. *Gamete Res*. 10:283, 1984

50. Friend DS, Orci L, Perrelet A, Yanagimachi R. Membrane particle changes attending the acrosome reaction in guinea pig spermatozoa. *J Cell Biol*. 74:561, 1977

51. Kinsey WH, Koehler JK. Cell surface charges associated with in vitro capacitation of hamster sperm. *J Ultrastruct Res*. 64:1, 1978

52. Bearer EL, Friend DS. Modifications of anionic-lipid domains preceding membrane fusion in guinea pig sperm. *J Cell Biol*. 92:604, 1982

53. Fraser LR, Ahuja KK. Metabolic and surface events in fertilization. *Gamete Res*. 20:491, 1988

54. Uesugi S, Yamazoe S. Presence of sodium-potassium stimulated ATPase in boar epididymal spermatozoa. *Nature*. 209:403, 1966

55. Quinn PJ, White IG. Distribution of adenosine triphosphatase activity in ram and bull spermatozoa. *J Reprod Fertil*. 15:447, 1968

56. Bronson RA, Cooper GW, Rosenfeld DC. Factors affecting the population of the female reproductive tract by spermatozoa: their diagnosis and treatment. *Semin Reprod Endo*. 4:371, 1986

57. Katz DF, Drobnis EZ, Overstreet JW. Factors regulating mammalian sperm migration through the female reproductive tract and oocyte vestments. *Gamete Res*. 22:443, 1989

58. Settledge DSF, Motoshima M, Tredway DR. Sperm transport from the external cervical os to the fallopian tubes in women: A time and quantitative study. *Fertil Steril*. 24:655, 1973

59. Harper MJK. Gamete and zygote transport. In: Knobil E, Neill JD, et al, eds. *The Physiology of Reproduction*. New York, N.Y., Raven Press, 1988; 1:103–134

60. Yanagimachi R. Zona-free hamster eggs: Their use in assessing fertilizing capacity and examining chromosomes of human spermatozoa. *Gamete Res*. 10:178, 1984

61. Byrd W, Tsu J, Wolf DP. Kinetics of spontaneous and induced acrosomal loss in human sperm incubated under capacitating and noncapacitating conditions. *Gamete Res*. 22:109, 1989

62. Byrd W, Ackerman GE, Carr BR, et al. Treatment of refractory infertility by transcervical intrauterine insemination of washed spermatozoa. *Fertil Steril*. 48:921, 1987

63. Kerin J, Byrd W. Supracervical placement of spermatozoa: utility of intrauterine and tubal insemination. In: Soules MR, ed. *Controversies in Reproductive Endocrinology and Infertility*. New York, N.Y., Elsevier, 1989: 183–204

64. Moghissi KS. Sperm migration through the human cervix. In: Elstein M, Moghissi KS, Borth R, eds. *Cervical Mucus in Human Reproduction*. Copenhagen, Denmark, Scriptor, 1972: 128–152

65. Gould JE, Overstreet JW, Hanson FW. Assessment of human sperm function after recovery from the female reproductive tract. *Biol Reprod*. 31:188, 1984

66. Drobnis EZ, Katz DF. Videomicroscopy of mammalian fertilization. In: Wassarman PM, ed. *Elements of Mammalian Fertilization*. Boca Raton, Fla., CRC Press, 1991: 270–300

67. Mortimer D, Templeton AA. Sperm transport in the human female reproductive tract in relation to semen analysis characteristics and time of ovulation. *J Reprod Fertil*. 64:401, 1982

68. Katz DF, Drobnis EZ, Overstreet JW. Factors regulating mammalian sperm migration through the female reproductive tract and oocyte vestments. *Gamete Res*. 22:443, 1989

69. Snell WJ, White JM. The molecules of mammalian fertilization. *Cell*. 85:629, 1996

70. Cohen-Dayen A, Tur-Kaspa I, Dor J, et al. Sperm capacitation in humans is transient and correlates with chemotactic responsiveness to follicular factors. *Proc Natl Acad Sci USA*. 92:11039, 1995

71. Motta PM, Nottola SA, Pereda J, et al. Ultrastructure of human cumulus oophorus: A transmission electron microscopic study on oviductal oocytes and fertilized eggs. *Hum Reprod*. 10:2361, 1995

72. Piko L. Gamete structure and sperm entry in mammals. In: Metz CB, Monroy A, eds. *Fertilization*. New York, N.Y., Academic Press, 1969; 2:325–403

73. Blandau RJ. Gamete transport-comparative aspects. In: Hafez ESE, Blandau RJ, eds. *The Mammalian Oviduct*. Chicago, Ill., University of Chicago Press, 1969: 129–162

74. Moore HDM, Bedford JM. An in vivo analysis of factors influencing the fertilization of hamster eggs. *Biol Reprod*. 19:879, 1978

75. Storey BT, Lee MA, Muller C, et al. Binding of mouse spermatozoa to the zonae pellucidae of mouse eggs in cumulus: Evidence that the acrosome remains substantially intact. *Biol Reprod*. 31:1119, 1984

76. Talbot P. Sperm penetration through oocyte investments in mammals. *Am J Anat*. 174:331, 1985

77. Talbot P, DiCarlantonio G, Zao P, et al. Motile cells lacking hyaluronidase can penetrate the hamster oocyte cumulus complex. *Dev Biol*. 108:387, 1985

78. Cherr GN, Lambert H, Meizel S, Katz DF. In vitro studies of the golden hamster sperm acrosome reaction: Completion on the zona pellucida and induction by homologous solubilized zonae pellucidae. *Dev Biol.* 114:119, 1986

79. Cummins JM, Yanagimachi R. Development of ability to penetrate the cumulus oophorous by hamster spermatozoa capacitated in vitro, in relation to the timing of the acrosome reaction. *Gamete Res.* 15:187, 1986

80. Meizel S. Molecules that initiate or help stimulate the acrosome reaction by their interaction with the mammalian sperm surface. *Am J Anat.* 174:285, 1985

81. Cummins JM, Yanagimachi R. Sperm–egg ratios and the site of the acrosome reaction during in vivo fertilization in the hamster. *Gamete Res.* 5:239, 1982

82. Kopf GS, Gerton GL. The mammalian sperm acrosome and the acrosome reaction. In: Wassarman PM, ed. *Elements of Mammalian Fertilization.* Boca Raton, Fla., CRC Press, 1991: 153–203

83. Cornett LE, Meizel S. Stimulation of in vitro activation and the acrosome reaction of hamster spermatozoa by catecholamines. *Proc Natl Acad Sci USA.* 75:4954, 1978

84. Hartmann JF, Gwatkin RBL, Hutchison CF. Early contact interactions between mammalian gametes in vitro: Evidence that the vitellus influences adherence between sperm and zona pellucida. *Prod Natl Acad Sci USA.* 69:2767, 1972

85. Gwatkin RBL, Williams DT. Receptor activity of the solubilized hamster and mouse zona pellucida before and after the zona reaction. *J Reprod Fertil.* 49:55, 1976

86. Hartmann JF. Mammalian fertilization: Gamete surface interactions in vitro. In: Hartmann JR, ed. *Mechanism and Control of Animal Fertilization.* New York, N.Y., Academic Press, 1983: 325–364

87. Florman HM, Saling PM, Storey B. Fertilization of mouse eggs in vitro. Time resolution of the reactions preceding penetration of the zona pellucida. *J Androl.* 3:373, 1982

88. O'Rand MG. Sperm–egg recognition and barriers to interspecies fertilization. *Gamete Res.* 19:315, 1988

89. Wassarman PM. Profile of a mammalian sperm receptor. *Development.* 108:1, 1990

90. Wassarman PM. The biology and chemistry of fertilization. *Science.* 235:553, 1987

91. Barros C, Crosby JA, Moreno RD. Early steps of sperm–egg interactions during mammalian fertilization. *Cell Biol Int.* 20:33, 1996

92. Salzmann GS, Greve JM, Roller RJ, Wassarman PM. Biosynthesis of the sperm receptor during oogenesis in the mouse. *EMBO J.* 2:1451, 1983

93. Sacco AG, Yurewicz EC, Subramanian MG, DeMayo JF. Zona pellucida composition: Species cross reactivity and contraceptive potential of antiserum to a purified pig zona antigen (PPZA). *Biol Reprod.* 25:997, 1981

94. Bleil J, Wassarman P. Structure and function of the zona pellucida: Identification and characterizations of the proteins of the mouse oocyte's zona pellucida. *Dev Biol.* 76:185, 1980

95. Shabanowitz RB, O'Rand MG. Characterization of the human zona pellucida from fertilized and unfertilized eggs. *J Reprod Fertil.* 82:151, 1988

96. Chamberlin ME, Dean J. Genomic organization of a sex specific gene: The primary sperm receptor of the mouse zona pellucida. *Dev Biol.* 1989

97. Van Duin M, Polma JE, DeBreet IT, et al. Recombinant human zona pellucida protein ZP3 by Chinese hamster ovary cells induces the human sperm acrosome reaction and promotes sperm-egg fusion. *Biol Reprod.* 51:607, 1994

98. Shur BD, Hall NG. A role for mouse sperm surface galactosyltransferase in sperm binding to the egg zona pellucida. *J Cell Biol.* 95:574, 1982

99. Lopez LC, Bayna EM, Litoff D, et al. Receptor function of mouse sperm surface galactosyltransferase during fertilization. *J Cell Biol.* 101:1501, 1985

100. Bookbinder LH, Cheng A, Bleil JD. Tissue- and species-specific expression of sp56, a mouse sperm fertilization protein. *Science.* 269:86, 1995

101. Leyton L, Sailing P. 95 kD sperm proteins bind ZP3 and serve as tyrosine kinase substrates in response to zona binding. *Cell.* 57:1123, 1989

102. Benau DA, Storey BT. Zona-binding site sensitive to trypsin inhibitors. *Biol Reprod.* 32:282, 1987

103. Abdullah M, Kierszenbaum AC. Identification of rat testis galactosyl receptors using antibodies to liver asialoglycoprotein receptor: Purification and localization on surfaces of spermatogenic cells and sperm. *J Cell Biol.* 108:367, 1989

104. Tulsiani DR, Skudlarek MD, Orgebin-Crist M-C. Novel α-D-mannosidase of rat sperm plasma membranes: Characterization of potential role in sperm–egg interactions. *J Cell Biol.* 109:1257, 1989

105. O'Rand MG, Widgren EE, Fisher SJ. Characterization of the rabbit sperm membrane autoantigen, RSA, as a lectinlike zona binding protein. *Dev Biol.* 129:231, 1988

106. Kopf GS. Regulation of sperm function by guanine nucleotide-binding regulatory proteins. In: Hazeltine F, ed. *Meiotic Inhibition: Molecular Control of Meiosis.* New York, N.Y., Alan R. Liss, 1988: 357–386

107. Fraser LR. Cellular biology of capacitation and the acrosome reaction. *Hum Reprod.* 10:22, 1995

108. Green DPL. The activation of proteolysis in the acrosome reaction of guinea pig spermatozoa. *J Cell Sci.* 32:153, 1978

109. Florman HM, Tombes RM, First NL, Babcock DF. An adhesion associated against from the zona pellucida activates G protein promoted elevation in calcium and pH that mediates mammalian sperm acrosomal exocytosis. *Dev Biol.* 135:133, 1989

110. Endo Y, Lee MA, Kopf GS. Evidence for the role of a guanine nucleotide binding regulatory protein in the zona pellucida induced mouse sperm acrosome reaction. *Dev Biol.* 119:210, 1987

111. Endo Y, Lee MA, Kopf GS. Characterization of an islet-activating protein-sensitive site in mouse sperm that is involved in the zona pellucida-induced acrosome reaction. *Dev Biol.* 129:12, 1988

112. Blackmore PF, Beebe SJ, Danforth FR, Alexander NJ. Progesterone and 17 α-hydroxyprogesterone. Novel stimulation of calcium influx in human sperm. *J Biol Chem.* 265:1376, 1990

113. Cowan AE, Primakoff P, Myles DG. Sperm exocytosis increases the amount of PH-20 antigen on the surface of guinea pig sperm. *J Cell Biol.* 103:1289, 1986

114. Bedford JM, Moore HDM, Franklin LE. Significance of the equatorial segment of the acrosome of the spermatozoon in eutherian mammals. *Exp Cell Res.* 119:119, 1979

115. Shalgi R, Phillips DM. Mechanics of sperm entry in cycling hamsters. *J Ultrastruct Res.* 71:154, 1980

116. Primakoff P, Hyatt H, Tredick-Kline J. Identification and purification of a sperm surface protein with a potential role in sperm–egg membrane fusion. *J Cell Biol.* 104:141, 1987

117. Blobel CP, Wolfsberg TG, Turck CW, et al. A potential fusion peptide and an integrin ligand domain in a protein active in sperm–egg fusion. *Nature.* 356:248, 1992

118. Almeida EAC, Huovila APJ, Sutherland AE, et al. Mouse egg integrin α6β1 functions as a sperm receptor. *Cell.* 81:1095, 1995

119. Bronson RA, Gailit J, Bronson S, Oula L. Echistatin, a disintegrin, inhibits sperm–oolemmal adhesion but not oocyte penetration. *Fertil Steril.* 64:414, 1995

120. Evans JP, Schultz RM, Kopf GS. Mouse sperm–egg plasma membrane interactions: Analysis of roles of egg integrins and the mouse sperm homologue of PH-30 (fertilin) β. *J Cell Sci.* 108: 3267, 1995

121. Schuel H. Secretory functions of egg cortical granules in fertilization and development: A critical review. *Gamete Res.* 1:299, 1978

122. Wolf DP, Hamada M. Induction of zonal and egg plasma membrane blocks to sperm penetration in mouse eggs with cortical granule exudate. *Biol Reprod.* 17:350, 1977

123. Gwatkin RBL. *Fertilization Mechanisms in Man and Mammals.* New York, N.Y., Plenum Press, 1977

124. Wolf DP. The mammalian egg's block to polyspermy. In: Mastroianni L, Biggers JD, eds. *Fertilization and Early Embryonic Development In Vitro.* New York, N.Y., Plenum Press, 1981: 183–197

125. Wolf DP. The ovum before and after fertilization. In: Zaneveld LJD, Chatterton RT, eds. *Biochemistry of Mammalian Development.* New York, N.Y., John Wiley & Sons, 1982: 231–259

126. Sengoku K, Tamate K, Horikawa M, et al. Plasma membrane block to polyspermy in human oocytes and preimplantation embryos. *J Reprod Fertil.* 105:85, 1995

127. Wolf DP, Byrd W, Dandekar P, Quigley MM. Sperm concentration and the fertilization of human eggs in vitro. *Biol Reprod.* 31:837, 1984

128. Longo FJ. Fertilization. A comparative ultrastructural review. *Biol Reprod.* 9:149, 1973

129. Soupart P, Strong PA. Ultrastructural observation on human oocytes fertilized in vitro. *Fertil Steril.* 25:11, 1974

130. Phillips KP, Baltz JM. Intracellular pH change does not accompany egg activation in the mouse. *Mol Reprod Dev.* 45:52, 1996

131. Kline D. Activation of the mouse egg. *Theriogenology.* 45:81, 1996

132. Byrd W, Wolf DP. Oogenesis, fertilization and early development. In: Wolf DP, Quigley MM, eds. *Human In Vitro Fertilization and Embryo Transfer.* New York, N.Y., Plenum Press, 1984: 213–273

133. Steptoe PC, Edwards RG, Purdy JM. Human blastocysts grown in culture. *Nature.* 229:132, 1971

134. Pederson RA. Early mammalian embryogenesis. In: Knobil E, Neill JD, et al, eds. *The Physiology of Reproduction.* New York, N.Y., Raven Press, 1988; 1:187–230

135. Tarkowski AK, Wroblewska J. Development of blastomeres of mouse eggs isolated at the 4- and 8-cell stage. *J Embryol Exp Morphol.* 18:155, 1967

136. Piko L, Clegg KB. Quantitative changes in total RNA, total poly(a) and ribosomes in early mouse embryos. *Develop Biol.* 89:362, 1982

137. Latham KE, Garrels JI, Chang C, et al. Quantitative analysis of protein synthesis in mouse embryos. I. Extensive reprogramming at the one-and two-cell stages. *Development.* 112:921, 1991

138. Nothias J, Majumder S, Kaneko KJ, DePamphilis ML. Regulation of gene expression at the beginning of mammalian development. *J Biol Chem.* 270:22077, 1995

139. Schultz GA, Heyner S. Gene expression in preimplantation mammalian embryos. *Mut Res.* 296:17, 1992

140. Webb PD, Glasser SR. Implantation. In: Wolf DP, Quigley MM, eds. *Human In Vitro Fertilization and Embryo Transfer.* New York, N.Y., Plenum Press, 1984: 341–363

141. Snabes MC, Harper MJK. Site of action of indomethacin on implantation in the rabbit. *J Reprod Fert.* 71:559, 1984

142. Lindenberg S, Hyttel P, Sjogren A, Greve T. A comparative study of attachment of human, bovine and mouse blastocysts to uterine epithelial monolayers. *Human Reprod.* 4:446, 1989

143. Croxatto HB, Diaz S, Fuentealba B, et al. The time interval between ovulation and egg recovery from the uterus in normal women. *Fertil Steril.* 23:447, 1972

144. McLaren A. A study of blastocysts during delay and subsequent implantation in lactating mice. *J Endocrinol.* 42:453, 1968

145. Roblero LS, Garavagno AC. Effect of oestradiol-17β and progesterone on oviductal transport and early development of mouse embryos. *J Reprod Fertil.* 57:91, 1979

146. Bowman P, McLaren A. Cleavage rate of mouse embryos in vivo and vitro. *J Embryol Exp Morphol.* 24:203, 1970

147. Angle MJ, Byrd W, Johnston JM. Factors effecting embryo production of platelet aggregation factor in culture. Presented at the 44th Annual Meeting of The American Fertility Society, 1988, p. 158

148. Paria BC, Dey SK. Preimplantation embryo development in vitro: Cooperative interactions among embryos and role of growth factors. *Proc Natl Acad Sci USA.* 87: 4576, 1990

149. Wiemer KE, Cohen J, Wilker SR, et al. Coculture of human zygotes on fetal bovine uterine fibroblasts: Embryonic morphology and implantation. *Fertil Steril.* 52:503, 1989

150. Rosenwaks Z. Donor eggs: Their application in modern reproductive technologies. *Fertil Steril.* 47:895, 1987

151. Gardner RL. Location and orientation of implantation. In: Edwards RG, ed. *Establishing a Successful Human Pregnancy.* New York, N.Y., Raven Press, 1990: 225–238

152. Hertwig AT, Rock J. Two human ova of the pre-villous stage having a development age of about seven and nine days respectively. *Contributions to Embryology.* 31:65, 1945

153. Bulleti C, Polli V, Licastro F, Parmeggiani R. Endometrial and embryonic factors involved in successful implantation. *Ann NY Acad Sci.* 734:221, 1994

154. Polan ML, Simón C, Frances A, et al. Role of embryonic factors in human implantation. *Hum Reprod.* 10:22, 1995

155. Pollard JW, Hunt JS, Wiktor JW, Stanley ER. A pregnancy defect in the osteopetrotic (op/op) mouse demonstrates the requirement for CSF-1 in female fertility. *Devel Biol.* 148:273, 1991

156. Cross JC, Werb Z, Fisher SJ. Implantation and the placenta: key pieces of the development puzzle. *Science.* 266:1508, 1994

157. Paria BC, Dey SK. Preimplantation embryo development in vitro: cooperative interactions among embryos and role of growth factors. *Proc Natl Acad Sci USA.* 87:4756, 1990

158. Psychoyos A, Nikas G, Gravanis A. The role of prostaglandins in blastocyst implantation. *Hum Reprod.* 10:30, 1995

159. Ryan JP, O'Neill C, Ammit AJ, Roberts CG. Metabolic and developmental responses of preimplantation embryos to platelet activating factor (PAF). *Reprod Fertil Dev.* 4:387, 1992

160. Burrows TD, King A, Smith SK, Loke YW. Human trophoblast adhesion to matrix proteins: Inhibition and signal transduction. *Mol Hum Reprod.* 10:2489, 1995

161. Shiokawa S, Yoshimura Y, Nagamatsu S, et al. Function of β_1 integrins on human decidual cells during implantation. *Biol Reprod.* 54:745, 1996

162. Shiokawa S, Yoshimura Y, Nagamatsu S, et al. Expression of β_1 integrins in human endometrial stromal and decidual cells. *J Clin Endocrinol Metab.* 481:1533, 1986

163. Armant DR, Kaplan HA, Lennarz WJ. Cell interactions with laminin and its proteolytic fragments during outgrowth of mouse primary trophoblast cells. *Develop Biol.* 116:519, 1986

164. Turpeenniemi-Hujanen T, Ronnberg L, Kauppila A, Puistola U. Laminin in the human embryo implantation: Analogy to the invasion by malignant cells. *Fertil Steril.* 58:105, 1992

165. Romagnano L, Babiarz B. Mechanisms of murine trophoblast interaction with laminin. *Biol Reprod.* 49:374, 1993

166. Burrows TD, King A, Smith SK, Loke YW. Human trophoblast adhesion to matrix proteins: Inhibition and signal transduction. *Mol Hum Reprod.* 10:2489, 1995

Chapter 2

THE ENDOCRINOLOGY OF PREGNANCY

C. Richard Parker, Jr.

The consequences of pregnancy on the maternal endocrine milieu are substantial. Most of the changes have been clearly linked to either maintenance of the uterine environment in a state that is favorable for continuance of the pregnancy or modification of maternal homeostasis to ensure proper nutritional support for the developing fetus and preparation for lactation after delivery. Most, if not all, of the endocrine changes in the pregnant woman are directly attributable to hormonal signals emanating from the fetoplacental unit. Unquestionably, estrogens and progesterone are among the most important hormones for implantation and pregnancy maintenance in humans and other species, and many endocrine changes during pregnancy are a consequence of the altered production of estrogen and progesterone.

ESTROGEN/PROGESTIN PRODUCTION IN PREGNANCY

Whereas pregnancy maintenance in later pregnancy (≈8 wk to term) is independent of the ovary[1] and is achieved via estrogen and progesterone production in the fetoplacental unit, early pregnancy is dependent upon hormonal interactions between the trophoblast and ovary for maintenance of estrogen and progesterone production. Thus, pregnancies with deficient or absent ovarian function should be supplemented with exogenous progesterone (and possibly estrogen) therapy for up to the first 10 to 12 wk of gestation; 1 to 2 mg estradiol and 50 to 100 mg progesterone/day have proved successful in pregnancies achieved through assisted reproduction techniques with donor eggs.[2,3]

In contrast to the expected decline in maternal serum levels of estrogens, progesterone, and 17OH-progesterone that usually occurs 10 to 12 days after ovulation in the infertile ovarian cycle (Fig 2–1), with fertilization and implantation, production of these steroids is maintained and increased somewhat for the first 6 to 8 wk of pregnancy (Fig 2–2) by the corpus luteum under the influence of human chorionic gonadotropin (hCG) produced in trophoblast (detailed elsewhere). The demise of the steroidogenic capacity of the corpus luteum of pregnancy occurs at about 8 to 10 wk of gestation and is heralded by a reduction in maternal serum levels of hCG and of 17OH-progesterone but no decline in serum levels of progesterone. For the duration of pregnancy, maternal serum levels of progesterone and estrogens are maintained by de novo placental progesterone formation, possibly under the influence of hCG, and by placental aromatization of estrogen precursors provided by maternal and fetal adrenal cortices.[4,5] The pattern of maternal serum progesterone and estrogens (estrone, estradiol-17β, and estriol) throughout the latter two thirds of normal pregnancy are shown in Figure 2–3.

Whereas the placenta is capable of producing progesterone somewhat autonomously, the placenta is an incomplete endocrine tissue with respect to estrogen production,[6] primarily as a consequence of lacking 17-hydroxylase/17,20-desmolase activities that are essential for conversion of pregnenolone or progesterone (C-21 steroids) into androgens (C-19 steroids). Consequently, placental estrogen production is ultimately dependent upon the rate of adrenal steroidogenesis of both mother and fetus. The interactions among maternal, fetal, and placental compartments in estrogen and progesterone formation are illustrated in Figure 2–4.

Progesterone

Trophoblastic tissue usually has very low capacity for de novo cholesterol biosynthesis.[7] Thus, as indicated earlier, progesterone normally is produced in placenta (as it is in corpus luteum) from cholesterol contained in low-density lipoprotein (LDL).[8–11] In steroidogenic tissues of humans and several other species, circulating LDL is assimilated via the classical LDL receptor pathway, which then

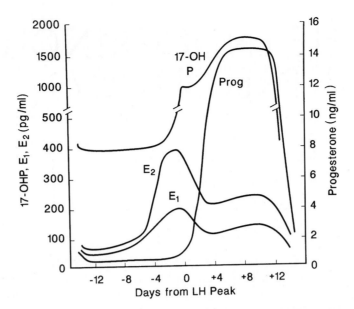

Figure 2–1. Serum levels of estrone (E₁), estradiol (E₂), 17-hydroxyprogesterone (17-OHP), and progesterone (P) in women during the ovulatory cycle. Data are presented in relation to the timing of the LH surge. (*Adapted from Carr BR, Parker CR Jr, Madden JD, et al.* J Clin Endocrinol Metab. *49:346, 1979, and unpublished studies of the author.*)

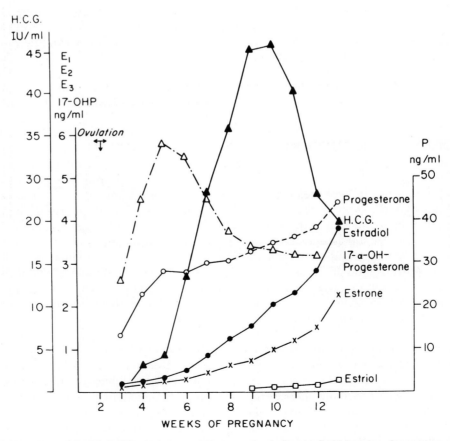

Figure 2–2. Serum levels of estrogens, progestins, and hCG in women during the first trimester of pregnancy. (*Reproduced, with permission, from Tulchinsky D, Hobel CJ.* Am J Obstet Gynecol. *17:884, 1973.*)

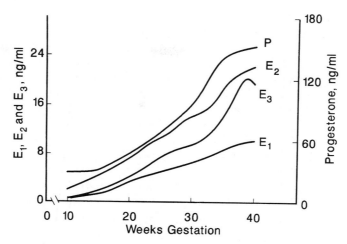

Figure 2–3. Serum levels of estrone (E$_1$), estradiol (E$_2$), estriol (E$_3$), and progesterone (P) in women during the second and third trimester of normal pregnancy. (*Adapted from Parker CR Jr, Illingworth DR, Bissonnette J, Carr BR. N Engl J Med. 314:557, 1986, and unpublished studies of the author.*)

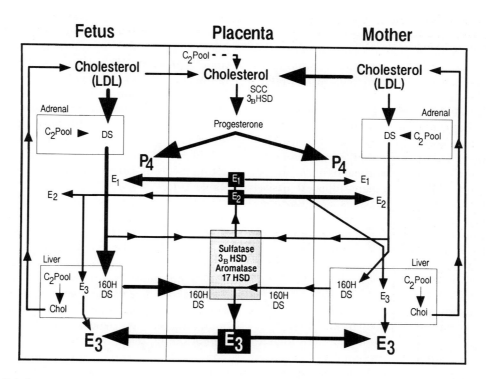

Figure 2–4. Relative contributions of the fetal, placental, and maternal compartments to estrogen and progesterone production in human pregnancy.

provides the cholesterol in such lipoprotein particles for use by the cells for substrate in steroid formation and probably other purposes as well.[12,13] Usually, maternal LDL is present in high quantities,[14] and thus abundant substrate is available to the placenta, which also has an abundance of LDL receptors.[15] However, in circumstances of absent or negligible maternal serum LDL, placental progesterone formation may be compromised. For example, in a

case of hypobetalipoproteinemia the abnormally low, yet still substantial, quantities of progesterone produced[16] likely were achieved by a compensatory increase in de novo cholesterol synthesis in placenta or utilization of fetal LDL and/or maternal high-density lipoprotein (HDL). Neither fetal well-being nor the status of estrogen production in pregnancy appears to be important to orderly formation of progesterone in trophoblast. Thus, progesterone production is not attenuated by fetal anencephaly,[17] which gives rise to impaired fetal estrogen precursor production,[18,19] or, at least acutely, by fetal demise.[20] Indeed, progesterone production is striking in molar pregnancies and choriocarcinoma.[21]

In addition to serving to prepare the uterus for implantation, progesterone also appears to serve other functions once pregnancy is established. Progesterone appears to be important in maintaining uterine quiescence during pregnancy by actions on uterine smooth muscle.[22] Progesterone also can be inhibitory to uterine prostaglandin production,[23] which would otherwise promote uterine contractions and cervical ripening. Progesterone also may play a role in maintaining pregnancy by virtue of inhibiting T lymphocyte cell-mediated processes that occur in graft rejection.[24] Thus, the high local concentration of progesterone probably contributes to the immunologically privileged status of the pregnant uterus. Also, progesterone plays an important role in remodeling the cellular architecture and secretory activity of the lining of the cervix to create a barrier to penetration of pathogens into the uterus. Although it has been proposed that progesterone may serve as an important substrate for production of glucocorticoids in the fetal adrenal, such a role seems unlikely since the fetal adrenal has an exceptionally high rate of LDL cholesterol uptake, a high rate of de novo cholesterol biosynthesis, and the ability to produce prodigious quantities of cortisol in cell culture in the absence of added progesterone.[13] Moreover, despite the finding that adrenal tissue of anencephalic fetuses contains, on a weight-adjusted basis, normal levels of steroidogenic enzymes and enzyme mRNA[25] and essentially normal rates of placental progesterone formation in such circumstances, umbilical cord serum levels of glucocorticoids and mineralocorticoids in anencephalics are subnormal.[17,26,27]

Estrogens

The high rate of estrogen production in human pregnancy is unparalleled in the mammalian kingdom. Urinary estriol excretion at term is about 1000-fold higher than in nonpregnant women.[28] In nonpregnant premenopausal women, serum levels of estrone and estradiol range from 0.05 to 0.4 ng/ml, whereas estriol is virtually undetectable (<0.01 ng/ml). During pregnancy, however, serum levels of estrone and estradiol rise from 0.5 to 1 ng/ml in the first few weeks of pregnancy, when they are derived from the corpus luteum, to 10 to 30 ng/ml at term,[29–31] being produced primarily in the placenta from maternal and fetal adrenal precursor, dehydroepiandrosterone sulfate (DS). Although maternal and fetal adrenals contribute about equally to maternal serum estrone and estradiol, the fetal adrenal, by means of 16-hydroxylation of DS in fetal liver, is the source of

about 90 percent of estriol produced in pregnancy.[6] The critical role of the adrenals, particularly the fetal adrenal, in estrogen production in pregnancy is supported by many lines of evidence. Intrauterine fetal demise leads to a rapid decline in maternal estrogen levels, particularly of estriol.[32] Fetal anencephaly with attendant fetal adrenal maldevelopment is associated with strikingly reduced maternal serum estriol.[17,33] Also, fetal and maternal adrenal suppression after glucocorticoid administration to the mother leads to rapid reduction of maternal serum estrogen levels.[34] Lastly, absence of maternal LDL (which might be expected to impair maternal adrenal steroidogenic capacity) but heterozygosity for hypobetalipoproteinemia in the fetus was recently shown to be associated with a marked reduction in estradiol but a less striking reduction in estriol levels in maternal serum.[16]

In addition to the discordant contribution of maternal and fetal precursors to placental estrogen formation, the three major estrogens appear to be released into maternal and fetal blood differentially. Whereas estradiol is released in greater proportion into maternal blood, estrone is preferentially released into the umbilical vessels in humans.[35–37] The reason for this divergence is unclear but may relate to differential redox potentials in maternal and fetal compartments or to a steroid carrier system in placenta. As is the case with progesterone,[17] fetal serum levels of unconjugated estriol far exceed those in maternal blood.[35,38] The differences in fetal and maternal serum levels of estrogens and progesterone are shown in Table 2–1.

As can be seen, whereas E_2 is the predominant unconjugated estrogen in maternal serum, E_3 predominates in the fetus. The E_1/E_2 ratio in maternal serum is approximately 0.5, and that in umbilical cord serum is about 2.0. Although the serum concentration of E_1 and E_2 might vary significantly from individual to individual, the ratios noted above for fetal and maternal sera are reasonably consistent in normal pregnancies, both at term and in midgestation. Also, whereas the E_3/E_2 ratio in maternal serum during the third trimester is ≤1, that in umbilical cord serum is >10. Another estrogen, estetrol, which is the 15α-hydroxylated derivative of E_3, also is present in ma-

TABLE 2–1. CONCENTRATIONS OF UNCONJUGATED ESTROGENS AND PROGESTERONE IN MATERNAL VENOUS AND UMBILICAL CORD SERA AT TERM

	E_1	E_2	E_3	P
Maternal	10–13	18–24	15–20	100–140
Fetal	10–15	5–7	90–115	500–1000

Hormone values are in ng/ml and are representative of the range of mean values obtained in various published and unpublished studies of the author. Abbreviations: E_1, estrone; E_2, estradiol; E_3, estriol; P, progesterone.

ternal plasma; this unique estrogen appears to derive solely from fetal precursors.[39]

Since maternal estrogens, especially E_3 and estetrol, are largely derived from fetal precursors, it was once thought that monitoring of maternal serum or urinary estrogens might provide a means of assessing fetal well-being. Although such an approach was based upon sound theoretical grounds and low or declining estrogen levels often correctly identified fetuses whose status was deteriorating,[32,39–41] such a prognostic device has been found largely to be impractical, even in medical centers equipped to provide rapid turnaround of test results. This is due to the finding that maternal serum levels of estriol vary substantially over the course of a day[42] and maternal serum estrogen levels can be artificially increased, despite fetal jeopardy, in women having renal disease.[43,44]

Apart from a deteriorating intrauterine environment, there are several other circumstances in which there are low levels of estrogens in maternal serum and urine. Any developmental defect in which fetal adrenal function is compromised, ie, anencephaly or congenital absence of adrenal, will be associated with markedly low levels of maternal estrogens, particularly E_3.[17,33] Also, adrenal suppression due to glucocorticoid treatment leads to low maternal estrogen levels.[34] Antibiotics that affect gastrointestinal flora, and thus impair hydrolysis of biliary estrogen conjugates, can lead to reduced urinary estrogen levels without necessarily altering estrogen levels in maternal serum.[45] Estrogen levels are severely reduced in cases of placental sulfatase deficiency.[46,47] In this X-linked syndrome, which primarily affects males and has a frequency of 1/2000 to 6000 pregnancies, there is inability of the placenta to hydrolyze the sulfate moiety from DS or 16OH-DS, which is required prior to conversion to estrogens. Many pregnancies affected by this disorder proceed beyond term and are resistant to labor induction and require cesarean section.[47] A past history of postterm pregnancies, cesarean sections, and ichthyosis in relatives should be sufficient to lead the physician to perform antenatal testing. Low levels of maternal serum or urinary estrogens, increased DS and low estrogen levels in amniotic fluid, and failure of maternal estrogen levels to rise appropriately after a bolus IV injection of DS are predictive of the disorder.[47] Although there is merit to studies that use estrogen measurements in investigating the biochemistry and physiology of normal and abnormal pregnancy, estrogen measurements purely for assessment of fetal well-being seem to be a poor substitute for other modern monitoring techniques.

In addition to the causes mentioned of hypoestrogenism in pregnancy, another cause of estrogen deficiency in pregnancy has recently been described—placental aromatase deficiency due to mutations in the fetal aromatase gene (reviewed in reference 48). Unlike the situations in which estrogen production is reduced due to diminished fetal adrenal DS production or to inability to cleave the sulfate moiety of DS or 16-OH-DS, fetal aromatase deficiency is likely associated with high rates of adrenal androgen production and placental sulfatase activity as occurs normally. In such circumstances, the failure of the placenta to convert the substantial supply of maternally and fetally derived adrenal androgens into estrogens instead gives rise to accentuated conversion of such precursors into more potent androgens. Consequently, this rare disorder has been found to be associated with maternal virilization during the latter half of pregnancy and masculinization of affected female fetuses in utero. Sexual differentiation in utero of an affected male was apparently normal.

Whereas human pregnancy is uniquely characterized by the massive levels of estrogen produced, the exact roles of estrogen in pregnancy are unclear. Based upon the observations that pregnancies with marked estrogen deficiency, as in those complicated by fetal anencephaly or placental sulfatase deficiency, often proceed substantially beyond term,[47,49] it seems likely that estrogens are important in the timely onset of parturition. A definitive role in this process for estrogen, however, is not established in humans. The stimulatory effects of estrogen on phospholipid synthesis and turnover, prostaglandin production, and enhanced formation of lysosomes in the uterine endometrium, as well as estrogen modulation of adrenergic mechanisms in uterine myometrium, may be means whereby estrogen might act in the timing of labor onset.[50] Estrogens also stimulate uterine blood flow,[51] which is clearly important in maintaining a favorable intrauterine environment. Estrogens also are important in preparing the breast for lactation[52] and impact other hormonal systems, such as the renin–angiotensin system,[53] and stimulate production of hormone-binding globulins in liver such as CBG[54] and TBG.[55] There also is evidence that estrogen plays a role in fetal development and organ maturation, such as, along with other substances, increasing the capacity for fetal lung surfactant production (discussed by Parker et al[38]).

PLACENTAL PROTEIN/PEPTIDE HORMONES

Human Chorionic Gonadotropin

The chorionic gonadotropin, hCG, is a glycoprotein having a molecular mass of approximately 38,000 Da. It is structurally related to the pituitary hormones luteinizing hormone (LH), follicle-stimulating hormone (FSH), and thyrotropin-stimulating hormone (TSH), being composed of two noncovalently linked subunits, alpha (α) and beta (β), that are encoded by two separate mRNAs.[56–58] The α-subunit of hCG, which is encoded by one gene from chromosome 6[57] or 18,[58] contains 92 amino acids, has a mass of 16,000 Da, and is virtually identical to that of LH, FSH, and TSH. The β-subunit of hCG, which confers biologic specificity to the molecule by virtue of containing the bulk of the determinants required for binding to cell surface receptors,[59] has a molecular weight of 23,000 Da and shares considerable sequence homology with β-LH, which is somewhat smaller. A family of eight genes on chromosome 19 code for the β-subunits of hCG and LH: one for LH and seven for hCG, of which only two or three are actively expressed.[57,60,61] The unique sequence of the extended C-terminal portion of β-hCG confers immunologic specificity to hCG, allowing it to be quantified in radioimmunoassays (RIAs) distinct from LH when antisera against the hCG β-subunit are utilized. Because of the extensive glycosylation of hCG,[62] this hormone has a long half-life in the circulation[63,64] and is thus preferable to LH when administered to stimulate the gonads in vivo.

Although it was initially proposed to derive from the cytotrophoblast, intact hCG is now recognized to be produced primarily by the syncytiotrophoblastic cells.[65,66] hCG is produced by all types of trophoblastic tissues, including that from hydatidiform mole, chorioadenoma destruens (invasive mole), and choriocarcinoma, even that not associated with recent pregnancy.[67] In addition, hCG can be produced by fetal tissues[68] and is also believed to be a secretory product of the adult human pituitary[69]; the role of extratrophoblastic hCG is unclear. Although excess free β-hCG appears to be produced in the first few weeks of gestation,[70,71] thereafter the α-subunit is produced in excess of the β-subunit, and the α-to-β synthetic ratio appears to increase with advancing gestation.[70] Thus, most hCG in the circulation during the majority of pregnancy is either intact hCG or free α-hCG, with little, if any, β-hCG present in serum. Only intact hCG has biologic activity; the α- or β-subunits cannot stimulate steroid production in target tissues.[72]

The most widely recognized roles of hCG are (1) stimulating the corpus luteum to produce progesterone, estrogens, and relaxin; and (2) maintaining corpus luteum life span beyond the normal 10 to 14 days.[73–75] A role for hCG in placental steroidogenesis is controversial. In addition to stimulating enzymes involved in steroidogenesis, hCG also increases LDL uptake in corpus luteum.[76] hCG appears to be responsible for early masculinization of male fetuses by virtue of stimulating testosterone secretion by the fetal testis[77,78]; a role of hCG in ovarian development is not established. Subsequent fetal gonadal stimulation probably is achieved by fetal pituitary LH and FSH, the plasma concentrations of which are not maximal until 20 to 25 wk and then decline thereafter.[79] The studies of several investigators are suggestive that hCG also is immunosuppressive and that the high local concentrations of hCG (perhaps in concert

with progesterone) in placenta may be important in preventing the rejection of the fetal allograft by the maternal host.[80–82] The direct immunosuppressive actions of hCG have, however, been the subject of continuing debate since highly purified hCG has been found by some investigators to be without activity in this regard.[83,84] In addition, hCG appears to possess thyrotropic activity, although such effects are minor compared to those of equivalent amounts of TSH.[85,86]

Placental production of hCG appears to be autonomous of extraplacental influences. Production of hCG in vitro has been found to be augmented by cyclic AMP,[87] epidermal growth factor,[88] and the LH-releasing factor gonadotropin-releasing hormone (GnRH).[89,90] It also has been found that GnRH antagonists inhibit placental hCG and progesterone production in vitro.[91] Indeed, it is feasible that GnRH, produced in cytotrophoblast,[92,93] is the trophic stimulus to hCG production in neighboring syncytiotrophoblast. Maximal placental concentrations of GnRH occur at the time of maximal hCG production and then decline after 20 weeks of gestation.[94] It is also possible that the increasing production of placental progesterone and/or estrogens act via a negative feedback mechanism to reduce placental hCG production at the end of the first trimester.[95,96] Such an arrangement is analogous to GnRH regulation of pituitary LH production.

Detectable amounts of hCG are produced as early as 6 days after ovulation,[71,97] and with implantation there is a dramatic progressive rise in maternal serum hCG levels (Fig 2–5). During the first 4 to 5 wk of pregnancy, serum hCG levels double each 1.3 to 2.0 days,[97–99] achieving maximal levels of 10,000 to 100,000 mIU/ml (First International Reference Preparation) at 8 to 10 wk of pregnancy, which then decline to 10,000 to 20,000 mIU/ml by 20 wk and remain reasonably stable throughout the remainder of pregnancy.[100] The serum concentration of hCG at the time of the first expected menses after ovulation ranges from 50 to 250 mIU/ml.[97]

The clinical utility of hCG measurement is based upon the finding that deviation from normal levels early in pregnancy can be diagnostic of several disorders. In cases of suspected ectopic pregnancy, hCG analysis can establish the presence or absence of pregnancy and, if values are abnormally low and fail to rise appropriately, can be diagnostic of ectopic pregnancy in a vast majority of cases.[101–104] Confirmation of intrauterine pregnancy is now possible at serum hCG titers of about 2000 mIU/ml by use of vaginal ultrasound. hCG measurements can be of utility in predicting the outcome of patients with threatened abortion. In one study, it was found that most women with threatened abortion did ultimately abort if serum hCG levels were less than 10,000 mIU/ml (2nd International Standard); among patients who did not abort, all had hCG levels

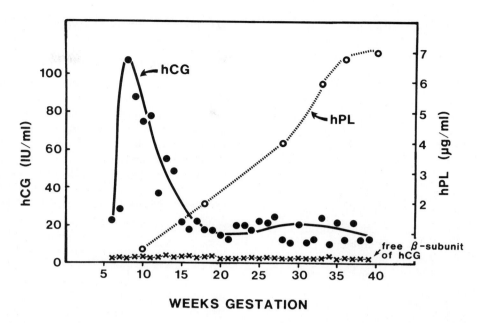

Figure 2–5. Serum levels of hCG and hPL in women during pregnancy. (*Reproduced, with permission, from Pritchard JA, MacDonald PC, Gant NF. Williams Obstetrics, 17th ed. New York, Appleton-Century-Crofts, 1985, p 121.*)

greater than 10,000 mIU/ml at the time the threatened abortion was first considered.[105] Others also have found that women having first-trimester abortions generally had hCG levels that declined to low levels and/or failed to rise at an appropriate rate.[71,106,107] In addition to serving as a diagnostic aid in gestational trophoblastic disease (values often exceed 200,000 mIU/ml[108–110]), serum hCG levels are extremely useful in monitoring response to therapy. In general, serum hCG should be undetectable (<5 mIUfirst IRP/ml) within 13 to 15 weeks after evacuation of molar pregnancy.[108–110] Many patients who will ultimately be found to have persistent trophoblastic disease or choriocarcinoma, however, might be identified much earlier based upon the failure of their hCG levels to decline in an orderly fashion.[110] It has even been proposed that women who develop persistent disease might often be identified at the time of evacuation by virtue of having excessive levels of the free β-subunit in relation to total hCG levels in serum.[111] Although the theoretical basis for such an association is unclear, several investigators have recently found that women pregnant with fetuses having trisomy 21 tend to have increased serum hCG levels in early pregnancy.[112,113] The utility of hCG measurements, alone or in conjunction with α-fetoprotein and estriol, in the diagnosis of chromosomal abnormalities is, however, not firmly established.[113]

Recently, a fragment of the β-subunit of hCG that consists of residues 6–40 disulfide linked to residues 55–92 and two N-linked sugar chains lacking sialic acid has been found in urine.[114] High levels of this β-core fragment have been detected in urine of pregnant women and women having trophoblastic disease and certain other cancers.[114–116] Since little if any β-core fragment is detectable in serum, it has been assumed that the peptide in urine primarily represents a degradation product of intact hCG or of β-subunit that is formed in kidney and possibly other tissues.[117] A recent study in which it has been proposed that serum β-core fragment is masked by associated macromolecules, thus preventing its detection in RIAs,[118] again raises questions about the origin and pathophysiological significance of this interesting substance.

Human Chorionic Somatomammotropin

Human chorionic somatomammotropin (hCS), initially termed human placental lactogen (hPL), was isolated in the early 1960s from human placenta and found to have lactogenic activities in experimental animals.[119–121] This single-chain polypeptide contains 191 amino acids and two disulfide bonds and has a molecular weight of approximately 22,000 Da; the amino acid sequence of hCS shares up to 96 percent homology with human growth hormone (hGH) and about 67 percent homology with human prolactin.[122,123] The growth hormone/hCS gene family on chromosome 17 consists of five genes, two coding for hGH and three for hCS.[124] Two of the hCS genes appear to be expressed at equivalent rates in term placenta and produce identical final products[125]; the other hCS gene is a pseudogene.

hCS appears to be produced exclusively by syncytiotrophoblast cells, suggesting it is a product of fully differentiated trophoblast.[66,126] Since the concentration of hCS mRNA in syncytial cells remains relatively constant throughout gestation,[127] the increasing placental content of hCS and the progressive rise in maternal serum hCS levels during gestation appear to be due to increasing numbers of such cells as the trophoblast grows during gestation.[128,129] Thus, serum hCS levels correlate well with placental mass and, due to its short half-life[130] in contrast to that of hCG, hCS would seem to be a potentially useful marker of placental function. hCS is measurable in maternal serum early in pregnancy (though not as early as hCG), and serum levels rise continually thereafter in contrast to those of hCG (Fig 2–5). At term, hCS is the most abundant protein secretory product of the placenta; maternal serum levels range from 5 to 15 μg/ml,[128,129] and about 20 percent of the translatable mRNA in term placenta is that of hCS.[131]

The regulation of synthesis and secretion during pregnancy and the physiological role of hCS are, for the most part, unclear. Most studies have failed to demonstrate a role of other hormones, neuropeptides, and neurotransmitters as stimulators or inhibitors of hCS production. Placental hCS production, aside from being related to placental mass and viability, may be regulated to a degree by nutritional factors. Thus, maternal starvation leads to increased maternal levels of hCS.[132,133] Transient hypo- and hyperglycemia has been shown in some,[134,135] but not all, studies to increase and decrease hCS levels, respectively, in women. Whether the effects noted above are attributable to glucose or insulin titers is unclear. Regulation of hCS production by nutritional factors seems, however, to fit in with its postulated role in regulating maternal metabolism, particularly of lipid and carbohydrates.[136] hCS has been shown to be lipolytic in humans[137] and other species, to augment insulin release in response to carbohydrate load in humans,[136,138] and to augment glucose utilization in adipose tissue.[139] Such actions could serve to ensure adequate energy stores for the mother and glucose for the fetus in states of nutritional deprivation and accentuate establishment of energy stores in the fed state. Whereas hCS has structural homology to GH and prolactin, the growth-promoting and lactogenic activity of this protein appears to be very limited in humans. Since normal pregnancies and well-developed infants have occurred in circumstances of very low-to-absent hPL production due to gene defects,[140–142] it seems possible that hCS might serve as an evolutionary redundancy for pituitary GH and prolactin rather than a critical element for pregnancy maintenance. It is not known, however, whether the above pregnancies would have had good outcomes in the face of nutritional deprivation.

Soon after its initial identification and establishment of hCS as a placental secretory product, numerous studies were conducted in the 1960s and 1970s to determine whether maternal serum hCS (hPL) levels might provide insights into fetoplacental health. The findings of many such studies[143–147] are summarized in Table 2–2.

A consideration of the findings described leads one to the view that maternal serum hCS levels are primarily related to placental size and/or the integrity of the utero/placental vasculature. Consequently, impending fetal demise will not necessarily be heralded by low levels of hCS. On the other hand, low or declining hCS levels often are associated with "placental insufficiency" or disruption in delivery of the peptide to the maternal bloodstream. Such phenomena are now readily recognized by other means of monitoring, suggesting hCS measurement currently is of marginal utility in the management of obstetric complications. There is, however, much to be learned about the physiological role of this substance in fetal development and pregnancy homeostasis.

TABLE 2–2. RELATION OF MATERNAL hCS LEVELS TO PREGNANCY CONDITIONS

Pregnancy Condition	Maternal Serum hCS (hPL) Levels
Diabetes mellitus	Normal to high, even with IUFD
Rh disease	Normal to high, even with IUFD
Dysmaturity	Often reduced
Multiple gestation	High
Pregnancy-induced hypertension	Often low, severity related
Fetal distress	Often low if due to causes other than nuccal cords
Late first/second trimester abortion	Low in most cases after bleeding
Growth retardation	Low
Molar pregnancy	Normal to high

IUFD (intrauterine Fetal Demise)

Human Chorionic Thyrotropin

In the late 1960s, a proteinaceous substance that shared several characteristics with pituitary TSH was isolated from human placenta.[148,149] Despite initial enthusiasm about the potential significance of human chorionic thyrotropin (hCT), subsequent studies have failed to confirm its existence and/or secretion by the placenta.[150,151] Thus, it has been suggested that the mild hyperthyroid state in early pregnancy and in some cases of hydatidiform mole and choriocarcinoma is likely attributable to the weak thyroid-stimulating activity of hCG.[85,86,151]

Pro-opiomelanocortin-Related Peptides

The presence of pro-opiomelanocortin-related peptides (POMC)-derived peptides in human placenta, including corticotropin (ACTH), β-lipotropin, and β-endorphin, was first suggested in the 1970s.[152–154] Subsequently, the pla-

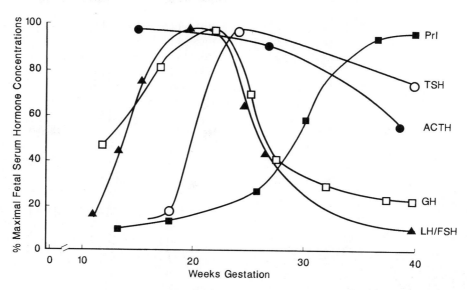

Figure 2–8. Ontogeny of pituitary hormones in human fetal serum.[79, 257–259]

of POMC peptides in fetal blood. High levels of ACTH have been found at midgestation, and thereafter plasma ACTH levels appear to decline[260]; confirmation of this paradoxical pattern is presently lacking. Developmental patterns in fetal blood of β-endorphin; β-lipotropin; or α-MSH, which appears to exist as a deacetylated form in fetal pituitary,[261] are not established.

Gonads

Steroid production in the human fetal testis, morphologically identifiable by 6 to 7 wk gestation, is initiated before 10 wk gestation, is maximal at 15 to 16 wk, and then declines dramatically to low levels by 20 to 25 wk.[257,262] Since fetal plasma gonadotropin levels are low at the time of increasing steroidogenic activity of the testis,[79,257] it seems likely that hCG, which is present in high quantities in fetal blood at this time,[263] is responsible for the differentiation and early steroid secretion by the fetal testis. The early fetal testis contains abundant hCG receptors, and hCG clearly augments steroid secretion in vitro.[264,265] The period of maximal testosterone production in vivo is accompanied by maximal levels of testicular hCG receptors,[264,265] LDL binding, and de novo cholesterol biosynthesis[266] in vitro. On the other hand, it is likely that continued gonadal activity, at least through 15 to 20 wk, is dependent upon the transient surge of fetal pituitary gonadotropin secretion that occurs at this time.[79,257,263] The importance of fetal pituitary gonadotropins in fetal testicular function is exemplified by the defects in sexual maturation that frequently occur in anencephalic fetuses: decreased numbers of Leydig cells, hypoplastic external genitalia, and undescended testes.[267]

Production of testosterone and the Müllerian-inhibiting factor (MIF) by the testis of the early male fetus accomplishes male sexual differentiation: stimulation of embryonic Wolffian duct system (testosterone) and external genitalia (5α-dihydrotestosterone) and regression of the Müllerian ducts.

The fetal ovary, morphologically distinct by 7 to 8 wk gestation, appears to have the capacity for steroid production during the first and second trimesters.[268–270] On the other hand, hormone production by the fetal ovary does not appear to play a role in female sexual maturation: Wolffian ducts regress spontaneously in the absence of testosterone, and development of the Müllerian duct system and the female external genitalia can occur even in the agonadal fetus.[271]

Thyroid

Since the placenta is essentially impermeable to thyroid hormones and TSH,[258] the fetal thyroid system develops and functions autonomously of the maternal compartment. By 10 to 12 wk gestation, the fetal thyroid is histologically distinct, concentrates radioiodine, and can synthesize iodothyronines; the fetal pituitary contains TSH and the fetal hypothalamus contains TRH.[249,250,258] Nevertheless, pituitary secretion of TSH and thyroid hormone production is limited until about 18 to 20 wk gestation (Fig 2–9). Thereafter, probably in response to increased release of hypothalamic TRH (and possibly pancreatic TRH[272]) and/or increased pituitary sensitivity, a marked increase in TSH secretion occurs through about 28 to 30 wk.[258,273] Thyroid production of T_4 is increased, beginning at about 20 wk, progressively through term, despite the slight decline in TSH levels from 30 to 40 wk. T_3 formation, however, is limited until the last few weeks of gestation; the bulk of hepatic metabolism of T_4 proceeds through reverse T_3, resulting in high levels of reverse T_3 in fetal serum during

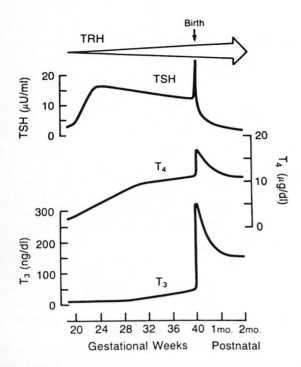

Figure 2–9. Ontogeny of TSH, thyroxine (T$_4$) and tri-iodothyronine (T$_3$) in fetal and neonatal serum. The increasing impact of TRH on the pituitary–thyroid axis also is depicted. (*Reproduced, with permission, from Fisher DA. Clin Perinatol. 10:615, 1983.*)

the second and early third trimester.[273,274] The decline in reverse T$_3$ and the increase in T$_3$ levels in fetal blood that occurs during the last 10 wk of gestation likely are the result of glucocorticoid actions on thyroid-metabolizing enzyme systems in fetal liver.[275] A striking surge in TSH, T$_4$, and T$_3$ levels in serum occurs shortly after birth (Fig 2–9).

Adrenal Cortex

Because of its involvement in estrogen production in human pregnancy and its importance in the onset of par-

turition, at least in the sheep,[276] the adrenal has been the most widely studied endocrine tissue of the fetus. The human fetal adrenal is disproportionately large and contains a unique zone, the fetal zone, which comprises about 80 percent of the cortical mass at term. The fetal zone then regresses soon after birth.[277] The changes in adrenal volume throughout fetal life and into young adulthood are graphically depicted in Figure 2–10. Although there are no data to demonstrate common mechanisms, there are interesting parallels between the growth and pattern of androgen production by the fetal adrenal and the adrenal during puberty.[278]

The inner fetal zone is composed of eosinophilic cells having a relatively large cytoplasmic/nuclear ratio. The outer zone cells, thought to give rise to the three zones of cells of the postnatal adrenal, compose the neocortex and have a smaller cytoplasmic/nuclear ratio. With culture, however, the morphologic differences between the two fetal adrenal cell types disappear.[279] In addition to the histologic differences in the two cortical zones of the fetal adrenal, the zones differ with respect to several functional characteristics (Table 2–3).

Based upon the results of numerous studies utilizing organotypic or cell culture of fetal zone tissue, it is clear that the fetal zone produces the full complement of steroids produced by the adult adrenal. Yet, as a result of the low levels of 3β-HSD/delta^{4,5}-isomerase,[280] which may be due in part to estrogen inhibition of this pathway,[281] and the presence of high levels of dehydroepiandrosterone sulfotransferase,[282] the fetal zone primarily produces delta^5-sulfated steroids such as DS and pregnenolone sulfate and relatively little gluco- or mineralocorticoids Indeed, it appears that even in the neocortex, there is little 3β-HSD/delta^{4,5}-isomerase until the later stages of gestation.[280] The neocortex, on the other hand, primarily produces C$_{21}$ delta^4 steroids such as cortisol and little of the delta^5-sulfated steroids.[283] Interestingly, when exposed to ACTH in culture fetal zone production of DS, usually high already, is

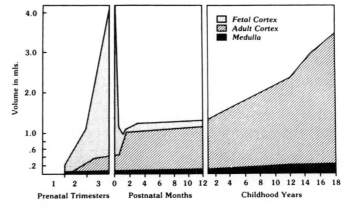

Figure 2-10. Size of the adrenal gland and its component parts during fetal life, infancy, and childhood. (*Reproduced, with permission, from Carr BR, Simpson ER. Endocrine Rev. 2:306, 1981.*)

TABLE 2–3. FUNCTIONAL ASPECTS OF FETAL AND NEOCORTICAL ZONES OF THE HUMAN FETAL ADRENAL

	Fetal Zone	Neocortex
Major steroid	DS	F
Adenyl cyclase	1X	2X
Protein kinase	2X	1X
LDL binding	2X	1X
Cholesterol synthesis	2X	1X
3β-HSD	1X	3X
P450$_{17\alpha}$	3X	1X

enhanced only slightly, whereas production of cortisol is increased three- to fivefold compared to initial rates of secretion. On the other hand, ACTH treatment of neocortex cells substantially increases DS production, as well as cortisol synthesis (Fig 2–11).

It seems clear that the fetal adrenal is dependent upon ACTH in vivo. The adrenal of anencephalic infants, who have deficient production of ACTH,[255,256] is very small[284] and produces low amounts of steroids.[18,19,26] Fetal ACTH and adrenal steroidogenesis are suppressed by maternal glucocorticosteroid therapy,[34] whereas fetal production of 17OH-progesterone is increased markedly in circumstances of congenital adrenal hyperplasia due to 21-hydroxylase deficiency.[285] Yet, ACTH treatment of fetal adrenal tissue in vitro leads to a pattern of steroid production that differs from that produced at the initiation of culture (Fig 2–11), as well as from that seen in umbilical cord blood (high DS, low cortisol). Thus, it is conceivable that factors in addition to ACTH are important regulators of the fetal adrenal in vivo.

Several hormones, including hCG, GH, hPL, and prolactin, as well as ACTH-related peptides derived from POMC, have been studied for their potential role as modulators of fetal adrenal growth and/or steroidogenesis. To date, there is little convincing evidence that non-POMC hormones influence the human fetal adrenal.[13] The possibility that N-terminal fragments of POMC and large-molecular-weight forms of POMC fragments that contain the ACTH sequence, which had been shown to be active in studies of adrenal tissue from experimental animals[286] and, therefore, might regulate fetal adrenal function, has yet to be addressed fully. Peptides, other than ACTH$_{1-39}$, that stimulate DS and cortisol production by human fetal adrenal tissue have been detected in fetal pituitary extracts; one appeared to be similar to ACTH$_{1-38}$, whereas the other appeared to be unrelated to ACTH or MSH.[287] An 18 amino acid sequence (POMC 79-96) that is part of the joining peptide of POMC was reported to stimulate adrenal androgen production[288]; in subsequent studies, it has been found to be without activity in cultures of fetal[289] or adult[290] human adrenal tissues.

Apart from responding to ACTH and possibly to other POMC-derived peptides, the fetal adrenal, like other steroidogenic tissues, may be regulated by cytokines and growth factors.[291–294] Both fibroblast growth factor and epidermal growth factor have been shown to stimulate proliferation of fetal adrenal cells,[291] as has conditioned medium from human placental cultures,[292] which likely contains a host of growth factors.[170] On the other hand, ACTH is generally considered antimitotic to the fetal adrenal.[295] Interestingly, however, ACTH has been found to interfere with the inhibitory effects of transforming growth factor-β on proliferation of cultured fetal adrenal cells.[296]

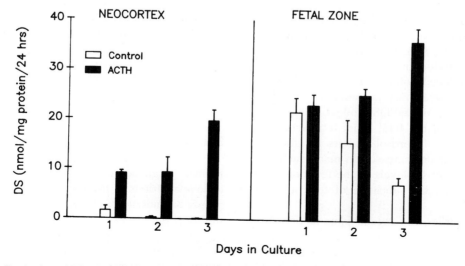

Figure 2–11. Production of DS and cortisol by fetal zone and neocortical zone tissue of the human fetal adrenal gland during culture in the presence and absence of ACTH. (*Reproduced, with permission, from Doody KM, Carr BR, Rainey WE, et al.* Endocrinology. *126:2487, 1990.*)

Although the fetal adrenal expresses a high rate of de novo cholesterol biosynthesis in vitro and can support steroidogenesis in the absence of exogenous precursors, it also possesses extensive capacity for uptake and metabolism of LDL, which are increased by ACTH.[297,298] Moreover, adrenal steroidogenesis in vitro is preferentially enhanced in the presence of LDL compared to that seen with HDL or very low-density lipoprotein (VLDL).[299] Indirect in vivo evidence for a role of LDL cholesterol in fetal adrenal steroidogenesis, which is substantial, is derived from several observations[19,300–304] of an inverse correlation between concentrations of adrenal steroids and LDL cholesterol (but not HDL or VLDL cholesterol) in fetal blood (Fig 2–12). Thus, it appears likely that, in vivo, the fetal adrenal obtains cholesterol for use in steroidogenesis via the LDL receptor pathway, and the rate of adrenal LDL uptake for steroid production, in turn, regulates fetal plasma LDL concentrations.

In addition to the extensive in vitro studies of the human fetal adrenal, there have been many in vivo analyses of fetal adrenal activity during normal and abnormal pregnancy. In uncomplicated pregnancies, umbilical cord plasma levels of DS and cortisol are reasonably stable during the late second and early third trimester. During the last 6 to 10 wk of gestation, however, there are striking increases in the concentrations of DS and cortisol in fetal blood.[305,306] Fetal plasma cortisol is derived both from fetal as well as maternal adrenals,[307] which makes it difficult to correlate fetal adrenal activity with fetal plasma cortisol levels in various physiologic or pathophysiologic circumstances. On the other hand, fetal plasma DS, which arises from fetal adrenal production, appears to be indicative of fetal responses to pregnancy conditions. For example, umbilical cord plasma levels of DS have been found to be reduced in pregnancies with specific medical complications such as hypertension, Rh disease, and syphilis,[302,303,308] as well as in pregnancies in which fetal growth is retarded.[309] In such circumstances, characterized by reduced fetal DS levels, often there is subnormal estrogen production[32,39–41,45,310] and morphologic evidence for reduced volume of the fetal zone of the fetal adrenal.[310] Whereas several pregnancy complications give rise to reduced fetal DS production and possible maldevelopment of the fetal zone, fetal serum or newborn urinary levels of cortisol and its metabolites seem to be normal or even increased in many such circumstances.[302,303,311] Cortisol levels in the fetus or newborn, however, may not be indicative of fetal adrenal activity.

As mentioned earlier, the mechanisms responsible for the growth and pattern of steroidogenesis by the human fetal adrenal are not established. Although short-term correlations between fetal pituitary ACTH production and fetal adrenal activity are evident, eg, after

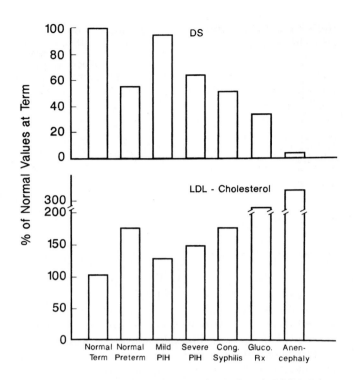

Figure 2–12. Inverse relation between fetal adrenal activity and LDL cholesterol. Umbilical cord levels of DS and LDL cholesterol are plotted in relation to values in normal newborns at term. Physiologic and pharmacologic reductions in fetal adrenal DS production result in corresponding increases in fetal plasma levels of LDL cholesterol. (*Data from refs. 19, 300–304, and unpublished observations of the author.*)

maternal glucocorticoid treatment, there is little established concerning fetal pituitary ACTH production in relation to pregnancy complications. Somewhat paradoxically, fetal plasma immunoreactive ACTH levels appear to decline over the latter half of gestation,[260] whereas fetal adrenal growth and steroid production, particularly that of the fetal zone, is markedly enhanced. Consequently, there is much yet to learn about the control of growth and function of the fetal adrenal in normal and complicated pregnancy.

SUMMARY

Human pregnancy is characterized by numerous physiologic adaptations in the maternal compartment. Many of these adaptations are in response to the altered hormonal milieu of pregnancy. There are changes in the rate of formation and/or clearance of most, if not all, hormones that are usually secreted in the nonpregnant state. The discovery of redundant production in the placenta of hormones that are identical or structurally similar to those found in the pituitary and hypothalamus has opened up new avenues of research. Whereas great strides have been made in defining the endocrine changes that occur during pregnancy, our understanding of the causes for such changes is less well developed. Great insights into the normal regulation of the maternal, placental, and fetal endocrine units have been made in the past based on the results of studies of pregnancies that are complicated by maternal, placental, and fetal abnormalities. Continued study of pregnancy anomalies likely will be the source of new discoveries about the endocrinology of pregnancy.

REFERENCES

1. Csapo AI, Pulkkinen MO, Wiest WG. Effects of luteectomy and progesterone replacement therapy in early pregnant patients. *Am J Obstet Gynecol.* 115:759, 1973
2. Schmidt CL, de Ziedler D, Gagliardi CL, et al. Transfer of cryopreserved-thawed embryos: The natural cycle versus controlled preparation of the endometrium with gonadotropin-releasing hormone agonist and exogenous estradiol and progesterone (GEEP). *Fertil Steril.* 52:609, 1989
3. Sauer MV, Paulson RJ, Lobo RA. A preliminary report on oocyte donation extending reproductive potential to women over 40. *N Engl J Med.* 323:1157, 1990
4. Siiteri PK, MacDonald PC. The utilization of circulating dehydroisoandrosterone sulfate for estrogen synthesis during human pregnancy. *Steroids.* 2:713, 1963
5. Siiteri PK, MacDonald PC. Placental estrogen biosynthesis during human pregnancy. *J Clin Endocrinol Metab.* 26:751, 1966
6. Simpson ER, MacDonald PC. Endocrine physiology of the placenta. *Annu Rev Physiol.* 43:163, 1981
7. Zelewski L, Villee CA. The biosynthesis of squalene, lanosterol, and cholesterol by minced human placenta. *Biochemistry.* 5:1805, 1966
8. Hellig H, Gattereau D, Lefebvre Y, Bolté E. Steroid production from plasma cholesterol. I. Conversion of plasma cholesterol to placental progesterone in humans. *J Clin Endocrinol Metab.* 30:624, 1970
9. Winkel CA, Snyder JM, MacDonald PC, Simpson ER. Regulation of cholesterol and progesterone synthesis in human placental cells in culture by serum lipoproteins. *Endocrinology.* 106:1054, 1980
10. Carr BR, Sadler RK, Rochelle DB, et al. Plasma lipoprotein regulation of progesterone biosynthesis by human corpus luteum tissue in organ culture. *J Clin Endocrinol Metab.* 52:875, 1981
11. Soto E, Silavin SL, Tureck RW, Strauss JF III. Stimulation of progesterone synthesis in luteinized human granulosa cells by human chorionic gonadotropin and 8-bromoadenosine 3',5'-monophosphate: The effect of low density lipoprotein. *J Clin Endocrinol Metab.* 58:831, 1984
12. Brown MS, Kovanen PT, Goldstein JL. Receptor-mediated uptake of lipoprotein-cholesterol and its utilization for steroid synthesis in the adrenal cortex. *Recent Prog Horm Res.* 35:215, 1979
13. Carr BR, Simpson ER. Lipoprotein utilization and cholesterol synthesis by the human fetal adrenal gland. *Endocrine Rev.* 2:306, 1981
14. Desoye G, Schweditsch MO, Pfeiffer P, et al. Correlation of hormones with lipid and lipoprotein levels during normal pregnancy and postpartum. *J Clin Endocrinol Metab.* 64:702, 1987
15. Malassine A, Besse C, Roche A, et al. Ultrastructural visualization of the internalization of low density lipoprotein by human placental cells. *Histochemistry.* 87:457, 1987
16. Parker CR Jr, Illingworth DR, Bissonnette J, Carr BR. Endocrine changes during pregnancy in a patient with homozygous familial hypobetalipoproteinemia. *N Engl J Med.* 314:557, 1986
17. Parker CR Jr, Carr BR, Casey ML, Gant NF, MacDonald PC. Extra-adrenal deoxycorticosterone production in hypoestrogenic pregnancies: Serum concentrations of progesterone and deoxycorticosterone in anencephalic fetuses and in women pregnant with an anencephalic fetus. *Am J Obstet Gynecol.* 147:415, 1983
18. Easterling WE Jr, Simmer HH, Dignam WJ, et al. Neutral C_{19}-steroids and steroid sulfates in human pregnancy. II. Dehydroepiandrosterone sulfate, 16-hydroxydehydroepiandrosterone, and 16-hydroxydehydroepiandrosterone sulfate in maternal and fetal blood of pregnancies with anencephalic and normal fetuses. *Steroids.* 8:157, 1966
19. Parker CR Jr, Carr BR, Winkel CA, et al. Hypercholesterolemia due to elevated low density lipoprotein-cholesterol in newborns with anencephaly and adrenal atrophy. *J Clin Endocrinol Metab.* 57:37, 1983
20. MacDonald PC, Cutrer S, MacDonald C, et al. Regulation of extra-adrenal steroid 21-hydroxylase activity. Increased conversion of plasma progesterone to deoxycorticosterone during estrogen treatment of women pregnant with a dead fetus. *J Clin Invest.* 69:469, 1982
21. Teoh ES, Das NP, Dawood MY, Ratsum SS. Serum progesterone and serum chorionic gonadotropin in hydatidiform mole and choriocarcinoma. *Acta Endocrinol.* 70:791, 1972
22. Roberts JM, Lewis VL, Riemer RK. Hormonal control of uterine adrenergic response. In: Bottari J, Thomas P, Vokser A, Vokser R, eds. *Uterine Contractility.* New York, N.Y., Masson Publishing Co., 1984: 161–173
23. Cane EM, Villee CA. The synthesis of prostaglandin F by human endometrium in organ culture. *Prostaglandins.* 9:281, 1975
24. Siiteri PK, Fobres F, Clemens LE, et al. Progesterone and maintenance of pregnancy: Is progesterone nature's immunosuppressant? *Ann NY Acad Sci.* 286:384, 1977
25. Simpson ER, Carr BR, John ME, et al. Cholesterol metabolism in the adrenals of normal and anencephalic fetuses. In: Albrecht E, Pepe GJ, eds. *Perinatal Endocrinology.* Ithaca, N.Y., Perinatology Press, 1985: 161–173
26. Montserrat De MF, Osathanondh R, Tulchinsky D. Plasma cortisol and cortisone in pregnancies with normal and anencephalic fetuses. *J Clin Endocrinol Metab.* 43:80, 1976
27. Parker CR Jr, Carr BR, Winkel CA, et al. Umbilical cord plasma concentrations of deoxycorticosterone sulfate in anencephalic fetuses. *Am J Obstet Gynecol.* 150:754, 1984

28. Brown JB. Urinary excretion of oestrogen during pregnancy, lactation and the re-establishment of menstruation. *Lancet.* 1:704, 1956

29. Loriaux H, Ruder J, Knab DR, Lipsett MB. Estrone sulfate, estrone, estradiol and estriol plasma levels in human pregnancy. *J Clin Endocrinol Metab.* 35:887, 1972

30. Tulchinsky D, Hobel CJ, Yeager E, Marshall JR. Plasma estrone, estradiol, estriol, progesterone, and 17-hydroxyprogesterone in human pregnancy. I. Normal pregnancy. *Am J Obstet Gynecol.* 112:1095, 1972

31. Tulchinsky D, Hobel CJ. Plasma human chorionic gonadotropin, estrone, estradiol, estriol, progesterone, and 17-hydroxyprogesterone in human pregnancy. III. Early normal pregnancy. *Am J Obstet Gynecol.* 117:884, 1973

32. Beischer NA, Brown JB. Current status of estrogen assays in obstetrics and gynecology. II. Estrogen assays in late pregnancy. *Obstet Gynecol Surv.* 27:303, 1972

33. Tulchinsky D, Osathanondh R, Belisle S, Ryan KJ. Plasma estrone, estradiol, estriol and their precursors in pregnancies with anencephalic fetuses. *J Clin Endocrinol Metab.* 45:1100, 1977

34. Simmer HH, Tulchinsky D, Gold EM, et al. On the regulation of estrogen production by cortisol and ACTH in human pregnancy at term. *Am J Obstet Gynecol.* 119:283, 1974

35. Tulchinsky D. Placental secretion of unconjugated estrone, estradiol and estriol into the maternal and the fetal circulation. *J Clin Endocrinol Metab.* 36:1079, 1973

36. Gurpide E, Marks C, de Ziegler, D, et al. Asymmetric release of estrone and estradiol derived from labeled precursors in perfused human placentas. *Am J Obstet Gynecol.* 144:551, 1982

37. Patten FT, Anderson ABM, Turnbull AC. Human fetal and maternal plasma oestrogens and the onset of labor. *J Obstet Gynecol Br Commonw.* 80:952, 1973

38. Parker CR Jr, Hankins GD, Guzick DS, et al. Ontogeny of unconjugated estriol in fetal blood and the relation of estriol levels at birth to the development of respiratory distress syndrome. *Pediatr Res.* 21:386, 1987

39. Tulchinsky D, Frigoletto FD Jr, Ryan KJ, Fishman J. Plasma estetrol as an index of fetal well-being. *J Clin Endocrinol Metab.* 40:560, 1975

40. Goebelsmann U, Freeman RK, Mestmann JH, et al. Estriol in pregnancy. II. Daily urinary estriol assays in the management of the pregnant diabetic woman. *Am J Obstet Gynecol.* 115:795, 1973

41. Long PA, Abell DA, Beischer NA. Fetal growth and placental function assessed by urinary estriol excretion before the onset of pre-eclampsia. *Am J Obstet Gynecol.* 135:344, 1979

42. Patrick J, Challis J, Campbell K, et al. Circadian rhythms in maternal plasma cortisol and estriol concentrations at 30 to 31, 34 to 35, and 38 to 39 weeks of gestational age. *Am J Obstet Gynecol.* 136:325, 1980

43. Rothchild SB, Tulchinsky D, Fencl M deM, et al. Estriol determinations in diabetic pregnancies complicated by nephropathy. *Am J Obstet Gynecol.* 134:772, 1979

44. Carrington ER, Oesterling MJ, Adams FM. Renal clearance of estriol in complicated pregnancies. *Am J Obstet Gynecol.* 106:1131, 1970

45. Levitz M, Young BK. Estrogens in pregnancy. *Vitam Horm.* 35:109, 1977

46. France JT, Liggins GC. Placental sulfatase deficiency. *J Clin Endocrinol Metab.* 29:138, 1969

47. Bradshaw KD, Carr BR. Placental sulfatase deficiency: maternal and fetal expression of steroid sulfatase deficiency and X-linked ichthyosis. *Obstet Gynecol Surv.* 41:401, 1986

48. Bulun SE. Aromatase deficiency in women and men: Would you have predicted the phenotypes? *J Clin Endocrinol Metab.* 81:867, 1996

49. Malpas P. Postmaturity and malformations of the foetus. *J Obstet Gynecol Br Emp.* 40:1046, 1933

50. Casey ML, Winkel CA, Porter JC, MacDonald PC. Endocrine regulation of the initiation and maintenance of parturition. *Clin Perinatol.* 10:709, 1983

51. Resnik R, Killam AP, Battaglia FC, et al. The stimulation of uterine blood flow by various estrogens. *Endocrinology.* 94:1192, 1974

52. Martin RH, Oakey RE. The role of antenatal oestrogen in postpartum human lactogenesis: evidence from oestrogen-deficient pregnancies. *Clin Endocrinol.* 17:403, 1982

53. Carr BR, Gant NF. The endocrinology of pregnancy-induced hypertension. *Clin Perinatol.* 10:737, 1983

54. Doe RP, Fernandez R, Seal US. Measurement of corticosteroid binding globulin in man. *J Clin Endocrinol Metab.* 14:1029, 1964

55. Dowling JT, Freinkel N, Ingbar SH. The effect of estrogens upon the peripheral metabolism of thyroxine. *J Clin Invest.* 39:1119, 1960

56. Bahl OP, Carlsen RB, Bellisario R, Swaminatnar L. Human chorionic gonadotropin: amino acid sequence of the α and β subunits. *Biochem Biophys Res Comm.* 48:416, 1972

57. Naylor SL, Chin WW, Goodman HM, et al. Chromosome assignment of genes encoding the α and β subunits of glycoprotein hormones in man and mouse. *Somatic Cell Mol Genet.* 9:757, 1983

58. Hardin JW, Riser ME, Trent JM, Kohler PO. The chorionic gonadotropin α-subunit gene is on human chromosome 18 in JEG cells. *Proc Natl Acad Sci USA.* 80:6282, 1983

59. Strickland TW, Puett D. Contribution of subunits to the function of luteinizing hormone/human chorionic gonadotropin recombinants. *Endocrinology.* 109:1933, 1981

60. Talmadge K, Boorstein WR, Fiddes JC. The human genome contains seven genes for the β-subunit of chorionic gonadotropin but only one gene for the β-subunit of luteinizing hormone. *DNA.* 2:281, 1983

61. Talmadge K, Boorstein WR, Vamvakopoulos NC, et al. Only three of the seven human chorionic gonadotropin beta subunit genes can be expressed in the placenta. *Nucleic Acids Res.* 12:8415, 1984

62. Endo Y, Yamashita K, Tachibana Y, Tojo S, Kobata A. Structures of the asparagine-linked sugar chains of human chorionic gonadotropin. *J Biochem.* 85:669, 1979

63. Yen SSC, Llerena O, Little B, Pearson OH. Disappearance rates of endogenous luteinizing hormone and chorionic gonadotropin in man. *J Clin Endocrinol Metab.* 28:1763, 1968

64. Midgley AR Jr, Jaffe RB. Regulation of human gonadotropins. II. Disappearance of hCG following delivery. *J Clin Endocrinol Metab.* 28:1712, 1968

65. Dreskin RB, Spicer SS, Greene WB. Ultrastructural localization of chorionic gonadotropin in human term placenta. *J Histochem Cytochem.* 18:862,1970

66. Hoshina M, Boothby M, Hussa R, et al. Linkage of human chorionic gonadotropin and placental lactogen biosynthesis to trophoblast differentiation and tumorigenesis. *Placenta.* 6:163, 1985

67. Morrow CP. Postmolar trophoblastic disease: Diagnosis, management, and prognosis. *Clin Obstet Gynecol.* 27: 211, 1984

68. McGregor WG, Kuhn RW, Jaffe RB. Biologically active chorionic gonadotropin: Synthesis by the human fetus. *Science.* 220:306, 1983

69. Odell WD, Griffin J. Pulsatile secretion of human chorionic gonadotropin in normal adults. *N Engl J Med.* 317: 1688, 1987

70. Cole LA, Kroll TG, Ruddon RW, Hussa RO. Differential occurrence of free beta and free alpha subunits of human chorionic gonadotropin (hCG) in pregnancy sera. *J Clin Endocrinol Metab.* 58:1200, 1984

71. Hay DL. Discordant and variable production of human chorionic gonadotropin and its free α- and β-subunits in early pregnancy. *J Clin Endocrinol Metab.* 61:1195, 1985

72. Catt KJ, Dufau ML, Tsuruhara T. Absence of intrinsic biological activity in LH and hCG subunits. *J Clin Endocrinol Metab.* 36:73, 1973

73. Garner PR, Armstrong DT. The effect of human chorionic gonadotropin and estradiol-17β on the maintenance of the human corpus luteum of early pregnancy. *Am J Obstet Gynecol.* 128:469, 1977

74. Bryant-Greenwood GD. Relaxin as a new hormone. *Endocrine Rev.* 3:62, 1982

75. Hanson FW, Powell JE, Stevens VC. Effects of HCG and human pituitary LH on steroid secretion and functional life of the human corpus luteum. *J Clin Endocrinol Metab.* 32:211, 1971

76. Golos TG, Soto EA, Tureck RW, Strauss JF. Human chorionic gonadotropin and 8-bromo-adenosine 3',5'-monophosphate stimulate [^{125}I] low density lipoprotein uptake and metabolism by luteinized human granulosa cells in culture. *J Clin Endocrinol Metab.* 61:633, 1985

77. Reyes FI, Winter JSD, Faiman C. Studies on human sexual development. I. Fetal gonadal and adrenal sex steroids. *J Clin Endocrinol Metab.* 37:74, 1973

78. Huhtaniemi IT, Korenbrot CC, Jaffe RB. HCG binding and stimulation of testosterone biosynthesis in the human fetal testis. *J Clin Endocrinol Metab.* 44:963, 1977

79. Kaplan SL, Grumbach MM, Aubert ML. The ontogenesis of pituitary hormones and hypothalamic factors in the human fetus. Maturation of central nervous system regulation of anterior pituitary function. *Recent Prog Horm Res.* 32:161, 1976

80. Billingham RE. Transplantation immunity and the maternal–fetal relation. *N Engl J Med.* 270:667, 1964

81. Pearse WH, Kaiman H. Human chorionic gonadotropin and skin homograft survival. *Am J Obstet Gynecol.* 98:572, 1967

82. Contractor SF, Davies H. Effect of human chorionic somatomammotrophin and human chorionic gonadotropin on phytohaemagglutinin-induced lymphocyte transformation. *Nature.* 243:284, 1973

83. Gundert D, Merz WE, Hilgenfeldt U, Brossmer R. Inability of highly purified preparations of human chorionic gonadotropin to inhibit the phytohemagglutinin-induced stimulation of lymphocytes. *FEBS Lett.* 53: 309, 1975

84. Pattillo RA, Shalaby MR, Hussa RO, et al. Effect of crude and purified hCG on lymphocyte blastogenesis. *Obstet Gynecol.* 47:557, 1976

85. Kenimer JG, Hershman JM, Higgins HP. The thyrotropin in hydatidiform moles is human chorionic gonadotropin. *J Clin Endocrinol Metab.* 40:482, 1975

86. Taliadouros GS, Canfield RE, Nisula BC. Thyroid-stimulating activity of chorionic gonadotropin and luteinizing hormone. *J Clin Endocrinol Metab.* 47:855, 1978

87. Hussa RO, Story MT, Pattillo RA. Cyclic adenosine monophosphate stimulates secretion of human chorionic gonadotropin and estrogens by human trophoblast *in vitro.* *J Clin Endocrinol Metab.* 38:338, 1974

88. Benveniste R, Speeg KV, Carpenter G, et al. Epidermal growth factor stimulates secretion of human chorionic gonadotropin by cultured human choriocarcinoma cells. *J Clin Endocrinol Metab.* 46:169, 1978

89. Khodr G, Siler-Khodr TM. The effect of luteinizing hormone-releasing factor on human chorionic gonadotropin secretion. *Fertil Steril.* 30:301, 1978

90. Siler-Khodr TM, Khodr GS. Dose response analysis of GnRH stimulation of hCG release from human term placenta. *Biol Reprod.* 25:353, 1981

91. Siler-Khodr TM, Khodr GS, Vickery BH, Nestor JJ. Inhibition of hCG, αhCG and progesterone release from human placental tissue *in vitro* by a GnRH antagonist. *Life Sci.* 32:2741, 1983

92. Gibbons JM, Mitnick M, Chieffo V. *In vitro* biosynthesis of TSH- and LH-releasing factors by the human placenta. *Am J Obstet Gynecol.* 121:127, 1975

93. Khodr GS, Siler-Khodr TM. Placental luteinizing hormone-releasing factor and its synthesis. *Science.* 207:315, 1980

94. Siler-Khodr TM, Khodr GS. Content of luteinizing hormone releasing factor in the human placenta. *Am J Obstet Gynecol.* 130:216, 1978

95. Wilson EA, Jawad MJ, Dickson LR. Suppression of human chorionic gonadotropin by progestational steroids. *Am J Obstet Gynecol.* 138:708, 1980

96. Iwashita M, Watanabe M, Adachi T, et al. Effect of gonadal steroids on gonadotropin-releasing hormones stimulated human chorionic gonadotropin release by trophoblast cells. *Placenta.* 10:103, 1989

97. Lenton EA, Neal LM, Sulaiman R. Plasma concentrations of human chorionic gonadotropin from the time of implantation until the second week of pregnancy. *Fertil Steril.* 37:773, 1982

98. Marshall JR, Hammond CB, Ross GT, et al. Plasma and urinary chorionic gonadotropin during early human pregnancy. *Obstet Gynecol.* 32:760, 1968

99. Pittaway DE, Reisch RL, Wentz AC. Doubling times of human chorionic gonadotropin increase in early viable intrauterine pregnancies. *Am J Obstet Gynecol.* 152:299, 1985

100. Braunstein GD, Rasor J, Adler D, et al. Serum human chorionic gonadotropin levels throughout normal pregnancy. *Am J Obstet Gynecol.* 126:678, 1976

101. Kosasa TS, Taymor ML, Goldstein DP, Levesque LA. Use of a radioimmunoassay specific for human chorionic gonadotropin in the diagnosis of early ectopic pregnancy. *Obstet Gynecol.* 42:868, 1973

102. Kadar N, Caldwell BV, Romero R. A method of screening for ectopic pregnancy and its indications. *Obstet Gynecol.* 58:162, 1981

103. Romero R, Kadar N, Copel JA, et al. The value of serial human chorionic gonadotropin testing as a diagnostic tool in ectopic pregnancy. *Am J Obstet Gynecol.* 155:392, 1986

104. Barnea ER, Oelsner G, Benveniste R, et al. Progesterone, estradiol, and α-human chorionic gonadotropin secretion in patients with ectopic pregnancy. *J Clin Endocrinol Metab.* 62:529, 1986

105. Nygren KG, Johansson EDB, Wide L. Evaluation of the prognosis of threatened abortion from the peripheral plasma levels of progesterone, estradiol and human chorionic gonadotropin. *Am J Obstet Gynecol.* 116:916, 1973

106. Jouppila P, Huhtaniemi I, Tapanainen J. Early pregnancy failure. Study by ultrasonic and hormonal methods. *Obstet Gynecol.* 55:42, 1980

107. Jovanovic L, Dawood MY, Landesman R, Saxena BB. Hormonal profile as a prognostic index of early threatened abortion. *Am J Obstet Gynecol.* 130:274, 1978

108. Goldstein DP, Pastorfide GB, Osathanondh R, Kosasa TS. A rapid solid-phase radioimmunoassay specific for human chorionic gonadotropin in gestational trophoblastic disease. *Obstet Gynecol.* 45:527, 1975

109. Ho Yuen B, Cannon W. Molar pregnancy in British Columbia. Estimated incidence and postevacuation regression patterns of the beta subunit of human chorionic gonadotropin. *Am J Obstet Gynecol.* 139:316, 1981

110. Schlaerth JB, Morrow CP, Kletzky OA, et al. Prognostic characteristics of the serum radioimmunoassay beta subunit human chorionic gonadotropin titer regression curve following molar pregnancy. *Obstet Gynecol.* 58:478, 1981

111. Khazaeli MB, Hedavat MM, Hatch KD, et al. Radioimmunoassay of free β-subunit of human chorionic gonadotropin as a prognostic test for persistent trophoblastic disease in molar pregnancy. *Am J Obstet Gynecol.* 155:320, 1986

112. Bogart MH, Pandian MR, Jones OW. Abnormal maternal serum chorionic gonadotropin levels in pregnancies with fetal chromosome abnormalities. *Prenat Diagn.* 7:623, 1987

113. Heyl PS, Miller W, Canick JA. Maternal serum screening for aneuploid pregnancy by alpha-fetoprotein, hCG, and unconjugated estriol. *Obstet Gynecol.* 76:1025, 1990

114. Birken S, Armstrong EG, Kolks MA, et al. Structure of the human chorionic gonadotropin β-subunit fragment from pregnancy urine. *Endocrinology.* 123:572, 1988

115. Cole LA, Wang YX, Elliott M, et al. Urinary hCG free β-subunit and β-core fragment: a new marker of gynecological cancers. *Cancer Res.* 48:1356, 1988

116. Akar AH, Wehmann RE, Blithe DL, et al. A radioimmunoassay for the core fragment of the human chorionic gonadotropin β-subunit. *J Clin Endocrinol Metab.* 66:538, 1988

117. Wehmann RE, Blithe DL, Akar AH, Nisula BC. Disparity between β-core levels in pregnancy urine and serum: Implications for the origin of urinary β-core. *J Clin Endocrinol Metab.* 70:371, 1990

118. Kardana A, Cole LA. Serum HCG β-core fragment is masked by associated macromolecules. *J Clin Endocrinol Metab.* 71:1393, 1990

119. Ito Y, Higashi K. Studies on the prolactin-like substance in human placenta II. *Endocrinol Jpn.* 8:279, 1961

120. Josimovich JB, MacLaren JA. Presence in the human placenta and term serum of a highly lactogenic substance immunologically related to pituitary growth hormone. *Endocrinology.* 71:209, 1962

121. Cohen H, Grumbach MM, Kaplan SL. Preparation of human chorionic "growth hormone-prolactin." *Proc Soc Exp Biol Med.* 117:438, 1964

122. Bewley TA, Dixon JS, Li CH. Sequence comparison of human pituitary growth hormone, human chorionic somatomammotropin, and ovine pituitary growth and lactogenic hormones. *Int J Pept Protein Res.* 4:281, 1972

123. Cooke NE, Coit D, Shine J, et al. Human prolactin cDNA structural analysis and evolutionary comparisons. *J Biol Chem.* 256:4007, 1981

124. Owerbach D, Rutter WJ, Martial JA, et al. Genes for growth hormone chorionic somatomammotropin and growth hormone-like gene on chromosome 17 in humans. *Science.* 209:289, 1980

125. Barrera-Saldana HA, Seeburg PH, Saunders GF. Two structurally different genes produce the same secreted human placental lactogen hormone. *J Biol Chem.* 258:3787, 1983

126. McWilliams D, Boime I. Cytological localization of placental lactogen messenger ribonucleic acid in syncytiotrophoblast layers of human placenta. *Endocrinology.* 107:761, 1980

127. Hoshina M, Boothby M, Boime I. Cytological localization of chorionic gonadotropin α and placental lactogen mRNAs during development of the human placenta. *J Cell Biol.* 93:190, 1982

128. Spellacy WN, Carlson KL, Birk SA. Dynamics of human placental lactogen. *Am J Obstet Gynecol.* 96:1164, 1966

129. Friesen HG, Suwa S, Pare P. Synthesis and secretion of placental lactogen and other proteins by the placenta. *Recent Prog Horm Res.* 25:161, 1969

130. Kaplan SL, Gurpide E, Sciarra JJ, Grumbach MM. Metabolic clearance rate and production rate of chorionic growth hormone-prolactin in late pregnancy. *J Clin Endocrinol Metab.* 28:1450, 1968

131. McWilliams D, Callahan RC, Boime I. Human placental lactogen mRNA and its structural genes during pregnancy: Quantitation with a complementary DNA. *Proc Natl Acad Sci USA.* 74:1024, 1977

132. Tyson JE, Austin KL, Farinholt JW. Prolonged nutritional deprivation in pregnancy: Changes in human chorionic somatomammotropin and growth hormone secretion. *Am J Obstet Gynecol.* 109:1080, 1971

133. Kim YJ, Felig P. Plasma chorionic somatomammotropin levels during starvation in mid-pregnancy. *J Clin Endocrinol Metab.* 32:864, 1971

134. Spellacy WN, Buhi WC, Schram JD, et al. Control of human chorionic somatomammotropin levels during pregnancy. *Obstet Gynecol.* 37:567, 1971

135. Gaspard U, Sandront H, Luyckx A. Glucose–insulin interaction and the modulation of human placental lactogen (HPL) secretion during pregnancy. *J Obstet Gynecol Br Commonw.* 81:201, 1974

136. Grumbach MM, Kaplan SL, Sciarra JJ, Burr IM. Chorionic growth hormone-prolactin (CGP): Secretion, disposition, biological activity in man, and postulated function as the "growth hormone" of the second half of pregnancy. *Ann NY Acad Sci.* 148:501, 1968

137. Grumbach MM, Kaplan SL, Abrams CL, et al. Plasma free fatty acid response to the administration of chorionic "growth hormone-prolactin." *J Clin Endocrinol Metab.* 26:478, 1966

138. Beck P, Daughaday WH. Human placental lactogen: Studies of its acute metabolic effects and disposition in normal man. *J Clin Invest.* 46:103, 1967

139. Felber JP, Zaragoza N, Benuzzi-Badoni M, Genazzani AR. The double effect of human chorionic somatomammotropin (HCS) and pregnancy on lipogenesis and on lipolysis in the isolated rat epididymal fat pad and fat pad cells. *Horm Metab Res.* 4:293, 1972

140. Nielsen PV, Pedersen H, Kampmann EM. Absence of human placental lactogen in an otherwise uneventful pregnancy. *Am J Obstet Gynecol.* 135:322, 1979

141. Sideri M, de Virgiliis G, Guidobono F, et al. Immunologically undetectable human placental lactogen in a normal pregnancy. Case report. *Br J Obstet Gynecol.* 90:771, 1983

142. Parks JS, Nielsen PV, Sexton LA, Jorgensen EH. An effect of gene dosage on production of human chorionic somatomammotropin. *J Clin Endocrinol Metab.* 60:994, 1985

143. Saxena BN, Emerson K Jr, Selenkow HA. Serum placental lactogen (HPL) levels as an index of placental function. *N Engl J Med.* 281:225, 1969

144. Sanger W, Desjardins P, Friesen HG. Human placental lactogen. An index of placental function. *Obstet Gynecol.* 36:222, 1970

145. Spellacy WN, Teoh ES, Buhi WC, et al. Value of human chorionic somatomammotropin in managing high-risk pregnancies. *Am J Obstet Gynecol.* 109:588, 1971

146. Lindberg BS, Nilsson BA. Human placental lactogen (HPL) levels in abnormal pregnancies. *J Obstet Gynecol Br Commonw.* 80:1046, 1973

147. England P, Fergusson JC, Lorrimer D, et al. Human placental lactogen: The watchdog of fetal distress. *Lancet.* (Jan. 5):5, 1974

148. Hershman JM, Starnes WR. Extraction and characterization of a thyrotropic material from the human placenta. *J Clin Invest.* 48:923, 1969

149. Hennen G, Pierce JG, Freychet P. Human chorionic thyrotropin: Further characterization and study of its secretion during pregnancy. *J Clin Endocrinol Metab.* 29:581, 1969

150. Harada A, Hershman JM. Extraction of human chorionic thyrotropin (hCT) from term placentas: Failure to recover thyrotropic activity. *J Clin Endocrinol Metab.* 47:681, 1978

151. Harada A, Hershman JM, Reed AW, et al. Comparison of thyroid stimulators and thyroid hormone concentrations in the sera of pregnant women. *J Clin Endocrinol Metab.* 48:793, 1979

152. Rees LH, Burke CW, Chard T, et al. Possible placental origin of ACTH in normal human pregnancy. *Nature.* 254:620, 1975

153. Genazzani AR, Fraioli F, Hurlimann J, et al. Immunoreactive ACTH and cortisol plasma levels during pregnancy. Detection and partial purification of corticotropin-like placental hormone. The human chorionic corticotropin (hCC). *Clin Endocrinol.* 4:1, 1975

154. Nakai Y, Nakao K, Oli S, Imura H. Presence of immunoreactive β-lipotropin and β-endorphin in human placenta. *Life Sci.* 23:2013, 1978

155. Odagiri ED, Sherrell BJ, Mount CD, et al. Human placental immunoreactive corticotropin, lipotropin and β-endorphin: Evidence for a common precursor. *Proc Natl Acad Sci USA.* 76:2027, 1979

156. Liotta A, Osathanondh R, Ryan KJ, Krieger DT. Presence of corticotropin in human placenta: Demonstration of in vitro synthesis. *Endocrinology.* 101:1551, 1977

157. Liotta A, Krieger DT. In vitro biosynthesis and comparative posttranslational processing of immunoreactive precursor corticotropin/β-endorphin by human placental and pituitary cells. *Endocrinology.* 106:1504, 1980

158. Petraglia F, Sawchenko P, Rivier J, Vale W. Evidence for local stimulation of ACTH secretion by corticotropin-releasing factor in human placenta. *Nature.* 328:717, 1987

159. Margioris AN, Grino M, Protos P, et al. Corticotropin-releasing hormone and oxytocin stimulate the release of placental proopiomelanocortin peptides. *J Clin Endocrinol Metab.* 66:922, 1988

160. Shibasaki T, Odagin E, Shizume K, Lind N. Corticotropin-releasing factor like activity in human placental extract. *J Clin Endocrinol Metab.* 55:384, 1982

161. Grino M, Chrousos GP, Margioris AN. The corticotropin releasing hormone gene is expressed in human placenta. *Biochem Biophys Res Comm.* 148:1208, 1987

162. Robinson BG, Emanuel RL, Frim DM, Majzoub JA. Glucocorticoid stimulates expression of corticotropin-releasing hormone gene in human placenta. *Proc Natl Acad Sci USA.* 85:5244, 1988

163. Jones SA, Brooks AN, Challis JRG. Steroids modulate corticotropin-releasing hormone production in human fetal membranes and placenta. *J Clin Endocrinol Metab.* 68:825, 1989

164. Liu KS, Wang CY, Mills N, et al. Insulin-related genes expressed in human placenta from normal and diabetic pregnancies. *Proc Natl Acad Sci USA.* 82:3868, 1985

165. Shen SJ, Wang CY, Nelson KK, et al. Expression of insulin-like growth factor II in human placentas from normal and diabetic pregnancies. *Proc Natl Acad Sci USA.* 83:9179, 1986

166. Wang CY, Daimon M, Shen SJ, et al. Insulin-like growth factor I mRNA in the developing human placenta and in term placenta of diabetics. *Mol Endocrinol.* 2:217, 1988

167. Rutanen EM, Bohn H, Seppala M. Radioimmunoassay of placental protein 12: Levels in amniotic fluid, cord blood and serum of healthy adults, pregnant women and patients with trophoblastic disease. *Am J Obstet Gynecol.* 144:460, 1982

168. Koistinen R, Kalkkinen N, Huhtala M-L, et al. Placental protein 12 is a decidual protein that binds somatomedin and has an identical N-terminal amino acid sequence with somatomedin-binding protein from human amniotic fluid. *Endocrinology.* 118:1375, 1986

169. Fields PA, Larkin LH. Purification and immunohistochemical localization of relaxin in the human term placenta. *J Clin Endocrinol Metab.* 52:79, 1981

170. Petraglia F, Calza L, Garuti GC, et al. New aspects of placental endocrinology. *J Endocrinol Invest.* 13:353, 1990

171. Shambaugh G, Kubek M, Wilber JF. Thyrotropin-releasing hormone activity in the human placenta. *J Clin Endocrinol Metab.* 48:483, 1979

172. Nakazawa K, Makino T, Iizuka R, et al. Immuno-histochemical study on oxytocin-like substance in the human placenta. *Endocrinol Jpn.* 31:763, 1984

173. Watkins WB, Yen SSC. Somatostatin in cytotrophoblast of the immature human placenta, localization by immunoperoxidase cytochemistry. *J Clin Endocrinol Metab.* 50:969, 1980

174. Lemaire S, Valette A, Chouinard L, et al. Purification and identification of multiple forms of dynorphin in human placenta. *Neuropeptides.* 3:181, 1983

175. Rama SBV, Barnwell SL, Tayeb OS, et al. Occurrence of methionine enkephalin in human placental villus. *Biochem Pharmacol.* 29:475, 1980

176. Petraglia F, Calza L, Giardino L, et al. Identification of immunoreactive neuropeptide-Y in human placenta: Localization, secretion, and binding sites. *Endocrinology.* 124:2016, 1989

177. Baird A, Wehremberg B, Bohlen P, Ling N. Immunoreactive and biologically active growth hormone-releasing factor in the rat placenta. *Endocrinology.* 117:1598, 1985

178. Maslar IA, Riddick DH. Prolactin production by human endometrium during the normal menstrual cycle. *Am J Obstet Gynecol.* 135:751, 1979

179. Golander A, Hurley T, Barrett J, Handwerger S. Synthesis of prolactin by human decidua in vitro. *J Endocrinol.* 82:263, 1979

180. Riddick DH, Luciano AA, Kusmik WF, Maslar IA. De novo synthesis of prolactin by human decidua. *Life Sci.* 23:1913, 1978

181. Takahashi H, Nabeshima Y, Nabeshima Y, et al. Molecular cloning and nucleotide sequence of DNA complementary to human decidual prolactin nRNA. *J Biochem.* 95:1491, 1984

182. Riddick DH, Luciano AA, Kusmik WF, Maslar IA. Evidence for a nonpituitary source of amniotic fluid prolactin. *Fertil Steril.* 31:35, 1979

183. Bigazzi M, Ronga R, Lancranjan I, et al. A pregnancy in an acromegalic woman during bromocriptine treatment: Effects on growth hormone and prolactin in the maternal, fetal, and amniotic compartments. *J Clin Endocrinol Metab.* 48:9, 1979

184. Rosenberg SM, Maslar IA, Riddick DH. Decidual production of prolactin in late gestation: Further evidence for a decidual source of amniotic fluid prolactin. *Am J Obstet Gynecol.* 138:681, 1980

185. Kletzky OA, Rossman F, Bertolli SI, et al. Dynamics of human chorionic gonadotropin, prolactin, and growth hormone in serum and amniotic fluid throughout normal human pregnancy. *Am J Obstet Gynecol.* 151:878, 1985

186. Lee DW, Markoff E. Synthesis and release of glycosylated prolactin by human decidua in vitro. *J Clin Endocrinol Metab.* 62:990, 1986

187. Luciano AA, Varner MW. Decidual, amniotic fluid, maternal and fetal prolactin in normal and abnormal pregnancies. *Obstet Gynecol.* 63:384, 1984

188. Fukamatsu Y, Tomita K, Fukuta T. Further evidence of prolactin production from human decidua and its transport across fetal membrane. *Gynecol Obstet Invest.* 17:309, 1984

189. Golander A, Barrett J, Hurley T, et al. Failure of bromocriptine, dopamine, and thyrotropin-releasing hormone to affect prolactin secretion by human decidual tissue in vitro. *J Clin Endocrinol Metab.* 49:787, 1979

190. Daly DC, Maslar IA, Riddick DH. Prolactin production during in vitro decidualization of proliferative endometrium. *Am J Obstet Gynecol.* 145:672, 1983

191. Daly DC, Maslar IA, Riddick DH. Term decidua response to estradiol and progesterone. *Am J Obstet Gynecol.* 145:679, 1983

192. Ogren L, Talamantes F. Prolactins of pregnancy and their cellular source. *Int Rev Cytol.* 112:1,1988

193. Johnson JWC, Tyson JE, Mitzner W, et al. Amniotic fluid prolactin and fetal lung maturation. *Am J Obstet Gynecol.* 153:372, 1985

194. Hatjis CG, Wu CH, Gabbe SG. Amniotic fluid prolactin levels and lecithin/sphingomyelin ratios during the third trimester of human gestation. *Am J Obstet Gynecol.* 139:435, 1981

195. Saller DN, Canick JA. Maternal serum screening for fetal Down syndrome: Clinical aspects. *Clin Obstet Gynecol.* 39:783, 1996

196. Saller DN, Canick JA. Maternal serum screening for fetal Down syndrome: The detection of other pathologies. *Clin Obstet Gynecol.* 39:793, 1996

197. Gemzell CA. Blood levels of 17-hydroxycorticosteroids in normal pregnancy. *J Clin Endocrinol Metab.* 13:898, 1953

198. Nolten WE, Lindheimer MD, Oparil S, Ehrlich EN. Desoxycorticosterone in normal pregnancy. I. Sequential studies of the secretory patterns of desoxycorticosterone, aldosterone, and cortisol. *Am J Obstet Gynecol.* 132:414, 1978

199. Carr BR, Parker CR Jr, Madden JD, et al. Maternal plasma adrenocorticotropin and cortisol relationships throughout human pregnancy. *Am J Obstet Gynecol.* 139:416, 1981

200. Burke CW, Roulet F. Increased exposure of tissues to cortisol in late pregnancy. *Br Med J.* 1:657, 1970

201. Carr BR, Parker CR Jr, Madden JD, et al. Plasma levels of adrenocorticotropin and cortisol in women receiving oral contraceptive steroid treatment. *J Clin Endocrinol Metab.* 49:346, 1979

202. Weir RJ, Paintin DB, Brown JJ, et al. A serial study in pregnancy of the plasma concentrations of renin, corticosteroids, electrolytes, and proteins and of haematocrit and plasma volume. *J Obstet Gynecol Br Commonw.* 78:590, 1971

203. Gant NF, Daley GL, Chand S, et al. A study of angiotensin II pressor response throughout primigravid pregnancy. *J Clin Invest.* 52:2682, 1973

204. Parker CR Jr, Everett RB, Quirk JG, et al. Hormone production in pregnancy in the primigravida. II. Plasma concentrations of deoxycorticosterone throughout pregnancy in normal women and in women who developed pregnancy-induced hypertension. *Am J Obstet Gynecol.* 138:626, 1980

205. Winkel CA, Milewich L, Parker CR Jr, et al. Conversion of plasma progesterone by deoxycorticosterone in men, nonpregnant and pregnant women and adrenalectomized subjects. Evidence for steroid 21-hydroxylase in non-adrenal tissues. *J Clin Invest.* 66:803, 1980

206. Winkel CA, Simpson ER, Milewich L, MacDonald PC. Deoxycorticosterone (DOC) biosynthesis in human kidney. Potential for the formation of a potent mineralocorticosteroid in its site of action. *Proc Natl Acad Sci USA.* 77:7069, 1980

207. Milewich L, Gomez-Sanchez C, Madden JD, et al. Dehydroisoandrosterone sulfate in peripheral blood of premenopausal, pregnant and postmenopausal women and men. *J Ster Biochem.* 9:1159, 1978

208. Grimes EM, Fayez JA, Miller GL. Cushing's syndrome and pregnancy. *Obstet Gynecol.* 42:550, 1973

209. van der Spuy ZM, Jacobs HS. Management of endocrine disorders in pregnancy. II. Pituitary, ovarian and adrenal disease. *Postgrad Med J.* 60:312, 1984

210. Brent F. Addison's disease and pregnancy. *Am J Surg.* 79:645, 1950

211. Kreines K, Devaux WD. Neonatal adrenal insufficiency associated with maternal Cushing's syndrome. *Pediatrics.* 47:516, 1971

212. Burrow GN. Hyperthyroidism during pregnancy. *N Engl J Med.* 298:150, 1978

213. Fisher DA, Lehman H, Lackey C. Placental transport of thyroxine. *J Clin Endocrinol Metab.* 24:393, 1964

214. Zakarija M, McKenzie JM. Pregnancy associated changes in the thyroid stimulating antibody of Graves' disease and the relationship to neonatal hyperthyroidism. *J Clin Endocrinol Metab.* 57:1036, 1983

215. Cheron RG, Kaplan MM, Larsen PR, et al. Neonatal thyroid function after propylthiouracil therapy for maternal Graves' disease. *N Engl J Med.* 304:525, 1981

216. Pekonen F, Teramo K, Ikonen E, et al. Women on thyroid hormone therapy: Pregnancy course, fetal outcome, and amniotic fluid thyroid hormone level. *Obstet Gynecol.* 63:635, 1984

217. Van der Spuy ZM, Jacobs HS. Management of endocrine disorders in pregnancy. I. Thyroid and parathyroid disease. *Postgrad Med J.* 60:245, 1984

218. Shauberger CW, Pitkin RM. Maternal–perinatal calcium relationships. *Obstet Gynecol.* 53:74, 1979

219. Pitkin RM, Reynolds WA, Williams GA, Hargis GK. Calcium metabolism in pregnancy: A longitudinal study. *Am J Obstet Gynecol.* 133:781, 1979

220. Drake TS, Kaplan RA, Lewis TA. The physiologic hyperparathyroidism of pregnancy: Is it primary or secondary? *Obstet Gynecol.* 53:746, 1979

221. Pitkin RM. Endocrine regulation of calcium homeostasis during pregnancy. *Clin Perinatol.* 10:575, 1983

222. Kumar R, Cohen WR, Silva P, Epstein FH. Elevated 1,25-dihydroxyvitamin D plasma levels in normal human pregnancy and lactation. *J Clin Invest.* 63:342, 1979

223. Lowe DK, Orwoll ES, McClung MR, et al. Hyperparathyroidism and pregnancy. *Am J Surg.* 145:611, 1983

224. Juan D. Hypocalcemia. Differential diagnosis and mechanisms. *Arch Intern Med.* 139:1166, 1979

225. Landing BH, Kamoshita S. Congenital hyperparathyroidism secondary to maternal hypoparathyroidism. *J Pediatr.* 77:842, 1970

226. Ludwig GD. Hyperparathyroidism in relation to pregnancy. *N Engl J Med.* 267:637, 1962

227. Johnstone RE II, Kreindler T, Johnstone RE. Hyperparathyroidism during pregnancy. *Obstet Gynecol.* 40:580, 1972

228. Costrini NV, Kalkhoff RK. Relative effects of pregnancy, estradiol and progesterone on plasma insulin and pancreatic islet insulin secretion. *J Clin Invest.* 50:992, 1971

229. Kalkhoff RK. Metabolic effects of progesterone. *Am J Obstet Gynecol.* 142:735, 1982

230. Cousins L, Rigg L, Hollingsworth D, et al. The 24-hour excursion and diurnal rhythm of glucose insulin and C-peptide in normal pregnancy. *Am J Obstet Gynecol.* 136:483, 1980

231. Phelps RL, Metzger BE, Freinkel N. Carbohydrate metabolism in pregnancy: XVII. Diurnal profiles of plasma glucose, insulin, free fatty acids, triglycerides, cholesterol and individual amino acids in late normal pregnancy. *Am J Obstet Gynecol.* 140:730, 1981

232. Hollingsworth DR. Alterations of maternal metabolism in normal and diabetic pregnancies: Differences in insulin-dependent, non-insulin-dependent, and gestational diabetes. *Am J Obstet Gynecol.* 146:417, 1983

233. Delaney JJ, Ptacek J. Three decades of experience with diabetic pregnancies. *Am J Obstet Gynecol.* 106:550, 1970

234. Soler NG, Soler SM, Malins JM. Neonatal morbidity among infants of diabetic mothers. *Diabetes Care.* 1:340, 1978

235. Reyes FI, Winter JS, Faiman C. Pituitary gonadotropin function during human pregnancy. Serum FSH and LH levels before and after LHRH administration. *J Clin Endocrinol Metab.* 42:590, 1976

236. Genazzani AR, Facchinetti F, Parrini D. β-Lipotropin and β-endorphin plasma levels during pregnancy. *Clin Endocrinol.* 14:409, 1981

237. Goland RS, Wardlaw SL, Stark RI, Frantz AG. Human plasma β-endorphin during pregnancy, labor and delivery. *J Clin Endocrinol Metab.* 52:74, 1981

238. Campbell EA, Linton EA, Wolfe CDA, et al. Plasma corticotropin-releasing hormone concentrations during pregnancy and parturition. *J Clin Endocrinol Metab.* 64:1054, 1987

239. Goland RS, Wardlaw SL, Blum M, et al. Biologically active corticotropin-releasing hormone in maternal and

fetal plasma during pregnancy. *Am J Obstet Gynecol.* 159:884, 1988

240. Goluboff LG, Ezrin C. Effect of pregnancy on the somatotroph and the prolactin cell of the human adenohypophysis. *J Clin Endocrinol Metab.* 29:1533, 1969

241. Spellacy WN, Buhi WC, Birk SA. Human growth hormone and placental lactogen levels in midpregnancy and late postpartum. *Obstet Gynecol.* 36:238, 1970

242. Tyson JE, Hwang P, Guyda H, Friesen HG. Studies of prolactin secretion in human pregnancy. *Am J Obstet Gynecol.* 113:14, 1972

243. Rigg LA, Lein A, Yen SSC. The pattern of increase in circulating prolactin levels during human gestation. *Am J Obstet Gynecol.* 129:454, 1977

244. Franks S. Regulation of prolactin secretion by oestrogens: Physiological and pathological significance. *Clin Sci.* 65:457, 1983

245. Liu J, Rebar RW, Yen SSC. Neuroendocrine control of the postpartum period. *Clin Perinatol.* 10:723, 1983

246. Thliveris JA, Currie RW. Observations on the hypothalamohypophyseal portal vasculature in the developing human fetus. *Am J Anat.* 157:441, 1980

247. Hyyppa M. Hypothalamic monoamines in human fetuses. *Neuroendocrinology.* 9:257, 1972

248. Nobin A, Bjorklund A. Topography of the monoamine neuron systems in the human brain as revealed in fetuses. *Acta Physiol Scand.* 388(Suppl.):1, 1973

249. Winters AJ, Eskay RL, Porter JC. Concentration and distribution of TRH and LRH in the human fetal brain. *J Clin Endocrinol Metab.* 39:960, 1974

250. Baker BL, Jaffe RB. The genesis of cell types in the adenohypophysis of the human fetus as observed with immunocytochemistry. *Am J Anat.* 143:137, 1975

251. Fisher DA. Maternal–fetal neurohypophyseal system. *Clin Perinatol.* 10:695, 1983

252. Bugnon C, Fellman D, Gouget A, et al. Corticoliberin neurons: Cytophysiology, phylogeny and ontogeny. *J Steroid Biochem.* 20:183, 1984

253. Ackland J, Ratter S, Bourne G, Rees LH. Proopiomelanocortin peptides in the human fetal pituitary. *Regul Peptides.* 6:51, 1983

254. Siler-Khodr TM, Morgenstern LL, Greenwood FC. Hormone synthesis and release from human fetal adenohypophyses in vitro. *J Clin Endocrinol Metab.* 39:891, 1974

255. Hayek A, Driscoll SG, Warshaw JB. Endocrine studies in anencephaly. *J Clin Invest.* 52:1636, 1973

256. Allen JP, Greer MA, McGilvra R, et al. Endocrine function in an anencephalic infant. *J Clin Endocrinol Metab.* 38:94, 1974

257. Reyes FI, Boroditsky RS, Winter JSO, Faiman C. Studies on human sexual development. II. Fetal and maternal serum gonadotropin and sex steroid concentrations. *J Clin Endocrinol Metab.* 38:612, 1974

258. Fisher DA, Dussault JH, Sack J, Chopra IJ. Ontogenesis of hypothalamic–pituitary–thyroid function and metabolism in man, sheep and rat. *Recent Prog Horm Res.* 33:59, 1977

259. Winters AJ, Colston C, MacDonald PC, Porter JC. Fetal plasma prolactin levels. *J Clin Endocrinol Metab.* 41:626, 1975

260. Winters AJ, Oliver C, Colston C, et al. Plasma ACTH levels in the human fetus and neonate as related to age and parturition. *J Clin Endocrinol Metab.* 39:269, 1974

261. Tilders FJH, Parker CR Jr, Barnea A, Porter JC. The major immunoreactive α-melanocyte-stimulating hormone (α-MSH)-like substance found in human fetal pituitary tissue is not α-MSH but may be a desacetyl-α-MSH (adrenocorticotropin 1-13 NH_2). *J Clin Endocrinol Metab.* 52:319, 1981

262. Tapanainen J, Kellokumpu-Lehtinen P, Pelliniemi L, Huhtaniemi I. Age-related changes in endogenous steroids of human fetal testis during early and midpregnancy. *J Clin Endocrinol Metab.* 52:98, 1981

263. Kaplan SL, Grumbach MM. Pituitary and placental gonadotropins and sex steroids in the human and subhuman primate fetus. *Clin Endocrinol Metab.* 7:487, 1978

264. Huhtaniemi IT, Korenbrot CC, Jaffe RB. hCG binding and stimulation of testosterone biosynthesis in the human fetal testis. *J Clin Endocrinol Metab.* 44:963, 1977

265. Molsberry RL, Carr BR, Mendelson CR, Simpson ER. Human chorionic gonadotropin binding to human fetal testes as a function of gestational age. *J Clin Endocrinol Metab.* 55:791, 1982

266. Carr BR, Parker CR Jr, Ohashi M, et al. Regulation of human fetal testicular secretion of testosterone: Low-density lipoprotein-cholesterol and cholesterol synthesized de novo as steroid precursor. *Am J Obstet Gynecol.* 146:241, 1983

267. Bearn JG. Anencephaly and the development of the male genital tract. *Acta Paediatr Acad Sci Hung.* 9:159, 1968

268. Bloch E. Metabolism of 4-^{14}C-progesterone by human fetal testis and ovaries. *Endocrinology.* 74:833, 1964

269. Jungmann RA, Schweppe JS. Biosynthesis of sterols and steroids from acetate-^{14}C by human fetal ovaries. *J Clin Endocrinol Metab.* 28:1599, 1968

270. Payne AH, Jaffe RB. Androgen formation from pregnenolone sulfate by the human fetal ovary. *J Clin Endocrinol Metab.* 39:300, 1974

271. Jost A. Problems of fetal endocrinology. The gonadal and hypophyseal hormones. *Rec Prog Horm Res.* 8:379, 1953

272. Koivusalo F. Evidence of thyrotropin releasing hormone activity in autopsy pancreata from newborns. *J Clin Endocrinol Metab.* 53:734, 1981

273. Klein AH, Oddie TH, Parslow M, et al. Developmental changes in pituitary thyroid function in the human fetus and newborn. *Early Hum Dev.* 6:321, 1982

274. Isaac RM, Hayek A, Standefer JC, Eaton RP. Reverse tri-iodothyronine to tri-iodothyronine ratio and gestational age. *J Pediatr.* 94:477, 1979

275. Osathanondh R, Chopra IJ, Tulchinsky D. Effects of dexamethasone on fetal and maternal thyroxine, triiodothyronine, reverse triiodothyronine and thyrotropin levels. *J Clin Endocrinol Metab.* 47:1236, 1978

276. Challis JRG, Brooks AN. Maturation and activation of hypothalamic–pituitary–adrenal function in fetal sheep. *Endocrine Rev.* 10:182, 1989

277. Johannison E. The foetal adrenal cortex in the human. *Acta Endocrinol.* 58(Suppl. 130):7, 1968

278. Adams JB. Control of secretion and the function of C_{19}delta^5-steroids of the human adrenal gland. *Mol Cell Endocrinol.* 41:1, 1985

279. Fujieda K, Faiman C, Reyes FI, et al. The control of steroidogenesis by human fetal adrenal cells in tissue culture. II. Comparison of morphology and steroid production in cells of the fetal and definitive zones. *J Clin Endocrinol Metab.* 53:401, 1981

280. Parker CR Jr, Faye-Petersen O, Stankovic AK, et al. Immunohistochemical evaluation of the cellular localization and ontogeny of 3β-hydroxysteroid dehydrogenase/delta 5-4 isomerase in the human fetal adrenal gland. *Endocrine Res.* 21:69, 1995

281. Fujieda K, Faiman C, Reyes FI, Winter JSD. The control of steroidogenesis by human fetal adrenal cells in tissue culture. The effects of exposure to placental steroids. *J Clin Endocrinol Metab.* 54:89, 1982

282. Parker CR Jr, Stankovic AK, Falany CN, et al. Immunocytochemical analyses of dehydroepiandrosterone sulfotransferase in cultured human fetal adrenal cells. *J Clin Endocrinol Metab.* 80:1027, 1995

283. Pepe GJ, Albrecht ED. Regulation of the primate fetal adrenal cortex. *Endocrine Rev.* 11:151,1990

284. Benirschke K. Adrenals in anencephaly and hydroencephaly. *Obstet Gynecol.* 8:412, 1956

285. Pang S, Levine LS, Decerquist LL, et al. Amniotic fluid concentrations of delta^{4}delta^5 steroids in fetuses with congenital adrenal hyperplasia due to 21-hydroxylase deficiency and in anencephalic fetuses. *J Clin Endocrinol Metab.* 51:223, 1980

286. Roebuck MM, Jones CT, Holland D, Silman R. In vitro effects of high molecular weight forms of ACTH on the fetal sheep adrenal. *Nature.* 284:616, 1980

287. Brubaker PL, Baird AL, Bennett HPJ, et al. Corticotropic peptides in the human fetal pituitary. *Endocrinology.* 111:1150, 1982

288. Parker L, Lifrak E, Shively J, et al. Human adrenal gland cortical androgen-stimulating hormone (CASH) is identical with a portion of the joining peptide of pituitary pro-opiomelanocortin (POMC). Proceedings of the 71st Annual Meeting of the Endocrine Society, 1989, abstract 299

289. Mellon SH, Shively JE, Miller WL. Human proopiomelanocortin-(79-96), a proposed androgen stimulatory hormone, does not affect steroidogenesis in cultured human fetal adrenal cells. *J Clin Endocrinol Metab.* 72:19, 1991

290. Penhoat A, Sanchez P, Jaillard C, et al. Human proopiomelanocortin-(79-96), a proposed cortical androgen stimulating hormone, does not affect steroidogenesis in cultured human adult adrenal cells. *J Clin Endocrinol Metab.* 72:23, 1991

291. Krickard K, Ill CR, Jaffe RB. Control of proliferation of human fetal adrenal cells in vitro. *J Clin Endocrinol Metab.* 53:790, 1981

292. Riopel L, Branchaud CL, Goodyer CG, et al. Effect of placental factors on growth and function of the human fetal adrenal in vitro. *Biol Reprod.* 41:779, 1989

293. Jaattela M, Carpen D, Stenman U-H, Saksela E. Regulation of ACTH-induced steroidogenesis in human fetal adrenals by TNF-α. *Mol Cell Endocrinol.* 68:R31, 1990

294. Stankovic AK, Parker CR Jr. Effects of transforming growth factor-β on human fetal adrenal steroid production. *Mol Cell Endocrinol.* 99:145, 1994

295. Simonian MH, Gill GN. Regulation of the fetal human adrenal cortex: Effects of adrenocorticotropin on growth and function of monolayer cultures of fetal and definitive zone cells. *Endocrinology.* 108:1769, 1981

296. Stankovic AK, Grizzle WE, Stockard CR, Parker CR Jr. Interactions between transforming growth factor β and adrenocorticotropin in growth regulation of human fetal zone cells: Possible involvement of adenylate cyclase. *Am J Physiol.* 266:E495, 1994

297. Mason JI, Rainey WE. Steroidogenesis in the human fetal adrenal: A role for cholesterol synthesized de novo. *J Clin Endocrinol Metab.* 64:140, 1987

298. Carr BR, Ohashi M, Simpson ER. Low density lipoprotein binding and de novo synthesis of cholesterol in the neocortex and fetal zones of the human fetal adrenal. *Endocrinology.* 110:1994, 1982

299. Carr BR, Parker CR Jr, Milewich L, et al. The role of low density, high density, and very low density lipoproteins in steroidogenesis by the human fetal adrenal gland. *Endocrinology.* 106:1854, 1980

300. Parker CR Jr, Simpson ER, Bilheimer DW, et al. Inverse relation between low-density lipoprotein-cholesterol and dehydroisoandrosterone sulfate in human fetal plasma. *Science.* 208:512, 1980

301. Parker CR Jr, Carr BR, Simpson ER, MacDonald PC. Decline in the concentration of low-density lipoprotein-cholesterol in human fetal plasma near term. *Metabolism.* 32:919, 1983

302. Parker CR Jr, Hankins GDV, Carr BR, et al. The effect of hypertension in pregnant women on fetal adrenal function and fetal plasma lipoprotein-cholesterol metabolism. *Am J Obstet Gynecol.* 150:263, 1984

303. Parker CR Jr, Wendel GD. The effects of syphilis on endocrine function of the fetoplacental unit. *Am J Obstet Gynecol.* 159:1327, 1988

304. Parker CR Jr, Atkinson MW, Owen J, Andrews AA. Dynamics of the fetal adrenal, cholesterol, and apolipoprotein B responses to antenatal betamethasone therapy. *Am J Obstet Gynecol.* 174:562, 1996

305. Parker CR Jr, Leveno KJ, Carr BR, et al. Umbilical cord plasma levels of dehydroepiandrosterone sulfate during human gestation. *J Clin Endocrinol Metab.* 54:1216, 1982

306. Murphy BEP. Human fetal serum cortisol levels related to gestational age: Evidence of a midgestational fall and steep late gestational rise, independent of sex or mode of delivery. *Am J Obstet Gynecol.* 144:276, 1982

307. Beitins IZ, Bayard F, Ances IG, et al. The metabolic clearance rate, blood production, interconversion, and transplacental passage of cortisol and cortisone in pregnancy near term. *Pediatric Res.* 7:509, 1973

308. Cleary RE, Depp R, Pion R. Relation of C_{19} steroid sulfates in cord plasma to maternal urinary estriol. *Am J Obstet Gynecol.* 106:534, 1970

309. Parker CR Jr, Buchina ES, Barefoot TK. Abnormal adrenal steroidogenesis in growth-retarded newborn infants. *Pediatrics.* 50:515, 1994

310. Bech K. Morphology of the fetal adrenal cortex, and maternal urinary oestriol excretion in pregnancy. *Acta Obstet Gynecol Scand.* 50:215, 1971

311. Reynolds JW, Mirkin BL. Urinary steroid levels in newborn infants with intra-uterine growth retardation. *J Clin Endocrinol Metab.* 36:576, 1973

Chapter 3

PARTURITION

R. Ann Word

The mechanism of the onset of human labor is unknown. The endocrinologic events that precede parturition in animals are complex and vary markedly from species to species. In most other species, certain lesions of the hypothalamus prevent labor, and specific hormonal changes induce labor. No hormonal event is known to initiate human parturition. Whereas measurements of hormones, neurotransmitters, peptides, and other biochemical compounds in human plasma, placenta, or fetal membranes may pose reasonable hypotheses, testing these hypotheses requires experimentation. Experimentation, however, in human pregnancy is difficult. The relevance of results obtained from experiments conducted in other animal species to human parturition will always be questionable. Nevertheless, these studies may be extremely valuable in the development of strategies to prevent preterm birth. In this chapter, we will highlight the key endocrinologic events believed to accompany the parturitional process in all species, and discuss current issues related to human parturition.

PARTURITION IN SHEEP

The physiologic sequence of events leading to the initiation of parturition in sheep has been well defined.[1,2] Late in sheep gestation, at a critical time in fetal maturation, there is an increase in the secretion of cortisol by the fetal adrenal cortex. The increase in cortisol secretion is primarily due to an increase in the number of corticotropin (ACTH) receptors in the fetal adrenal since the levels of immunoreactive ACTH in fetal blood do not increase at this time. Fetal-produced cortisol acts upon trophoblasts to induce the synthesis of the microsomal monoxygenase enzyme, 17α-hydroxylase. This enzyme directs steroid biosynthesis in the sheep placenta toward an increase in estrogen formation and a decline in progesterone secretion (Fig 3–1). The withdrawal of progesterone, together with increasing levels of estrogen, effect increased prostaglandin formation, the formation of gap junctions between myometrial cells, cervical ripening, and the commencement of parturition in sheep.

Fetal-induced progesterone withdrawal in sheep occurs by way of several complex pathways. In sheep placenta, as in other steroidogenic organs, cholesterol is converted to pregnenolone in a reaction catalyzed by the mitochondrial enzyme, cholesterol side-chain cleavage. The predominant pathway for progesterone withdrawal is by way of the diversion of pregnenolone away from progesterone biosynthesis toward estrogen biosynthesis. Before the time of the increase in placental steroid 17α-hydroxylase activity, pregnenolone is converted to progesterone, which is secreted from the trophoblasts. After the fetal cortisol-induced stimulation of placental 17α-hydroxylase, pregnenolone is converted to 17α-hydroxypregnenolone and dehydroepiandrosterone. In this manner, pregnenolone is diverted from progesterone biosynthesis toward estrogen biosynthesis. Dehydroepiandrosterone, then, is converted to androstenedione (by the action of steroid 3β-hydroxysteroid dehydrogenase) and then to estrogen by cytochrome P_{450}-aromatase in placenta. Progesterone formed from pregnenolone is also converted to 17α-hydroxyprogesterone, thus contributing to progesterone withdrawal. These alterations in steroidogenesis result in marked attenuation of progesterone secretion.

The supply of C_{19}-steroid precursors (dehydroepiandrosterone and androstenedione) formed de novo in placenta is rate limiting for estrogen formation in the sheep placenta (Fig 3–2). Androstenedione arises primarily from dehydroepiandrosterone and not from 17α-hydroxyprogesterone because 17α-hydroxypregnenolone is the preferred substrate for 17,20-desmolase compared with 17α-hydroxyprogesterone. Thus, an increase in fetal cortisol-induced synthesis of a single protein (17α-hydroxylase/17,20 desmolase) results in an adequate supply of immediate precursors of estrogen in sheep placenta and progesterone withdrawal.[3]

Differences in Sheep and Human Parturition

It seems that, in sheep, the mature fetus provides the initial signal to commence parturition. It is reasonable to suggest that the conceptus (fetus, placenta, or fetal membranes)

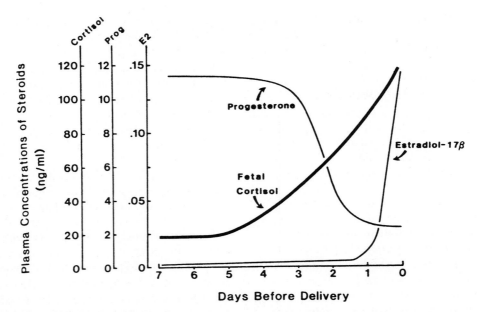

Figure 3–1. Endocrinology of sheep parturition. An increase in fetal cortisol production precedes the decline in progesterone biosynthesis and concomitant increase in estrogen biosynthesis. (*Reproduced, with permission, from Cunningham FG, MacDonald PC, Gant NF, eds.* Williams Obstetrics, *18th ed. Norwalk, Conn., Appleton & Lange, 1989: 191.*)

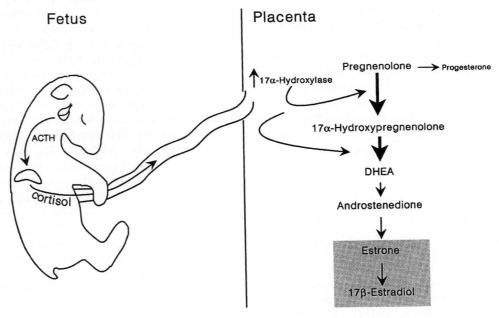

Figure 3–2. Regulation of hormonal secretion by 17α-hydroxylase in sheep placenta. Increases in fetal ACTH stimulate the fetal adrenal to secrete cortisol. Cortisol acts on trophoblast to increase synthesis of placental 17α-hydroxylase. 17α-Hydroxylase diverts pregnenolone from progesterone synthesis toward estrogen biosynthesis. Progesterone is further metabolized by 17α-hydroxylase to 17α-hydroxyprogesterone (not shown).

triggers the onset of labor when maturity is adequate for extrauterine life. Direct evidence gained from several animal species including sheep and the intermediate lengths of gestation of pregnancies in animals crossed from breeds of different gestational lengths is suggestive that the concep-

tus must influence the length of gestation.[4,5] There are, however, crucial differences between the endocrinology of human and sheep parturition: (1) In the human, there is not a significant increase in cortisol formation by the fetal adrenal before the onset of labor; (2) the infusion of ACTH or cortisol into the fetus does not result in labor in the human as it does in the sheep; (3) dexamethasone treatment in human pregnancy causes a pronounced decrease in estrogen formation but no change in the levels of progesterone; (4) there is no decrease in the rate of secretion or the blood levels of progesterone before the onset of labor in the human; (5) placental progesterone production in sheep pregnancy is small compared with that in the human; (6) steroid 17α-hydroxylase is not expressed in the human placenta; and (7) intrauterine prostaglandin formation during sheep parturition[6] is at least 20 times that produced in uterine tissues during human labor.[7]

As stated, there is no reduction in progesterone levels in maternal or fetal blood before the onset of spontaneous parturition during normal human pregnancy. Currently, there is no substantial evidence for alterations in progesterone metabolism, sequestration of progesterone, or for alterations in a progesterone-binding protein or receptor numbers to account for some hidden form of progesterone withdrawal as the signal for human parturition. Indeed, a woman with homozygous familial abetalipoproteinemia conceived and maintained a successful pregnancy with the spontaneous onset of labor and delivery despite very low levels of progesterone.[8] Actually, progesterone withdrawal alone may not be sufficient to initiate parturition. For example, mice with an induced null mutation in 5α-reductase I suffer reproductive problems including delayed parturition.[9] In 67 percent of mice, parturition was delayed despite normal progesterone withdrawal and timely induction of uterine oxytocin receptors.[9] The defect could be rescued by systemic delivery of antiprogestins and 5α-reduced androgens. In mice, 5α-reductase I is expressed in the endometrial glandular epithelium and in the endocervical glands. The expression pattern of 5α-reductase I in human reproductive tissues is not known; but if similar to that of mice, mutations in nature may be observed only in women with delayed cervical ripening or postterm pregnancy.

Recently, it has been proposed that TGF-β (or some other protein) may act as an endogenous antiprogestin to oppose the genomic actions of progesterone.[10] Evidence for increases in TGF-β or increased activation of latent TGF-β in human reproductive tissues prior to the onset of labor is lacking.

Although progesterone levels do not decline prior to spontaneous parturition in women, artificially induced progesterone withdrawal does effect abortion or labor in human pregnancy. For example, removal of the corpus luteum in early human pregnancy results in abortion; in other abnormal conditions such as ectopic pregnancy and fetal demise, a decrease in progesterone formation may precede the onset of uterine contractions and evacuation of uterine contents. Pharmacologically induced inhibition of progesterone action or progesterone formation in human pregnancy also causes abortion early in pregnancy and results in an increased sensitivity to oxytocin and $PGF_{2\alpha}$ in late gestation. The administration of progesterone to women in preterm labor, however, does not arrest preterm labor.

PROPOSED SEQUENCE OF EVENTS IN HUMAN PARTURITION

Clearly, the mechanisms of progesterone maintenance of human pregnancy and the sequence of events that herald the onset of spontaneous labor in women remain largely undefined. A number of hypotheses have been proposed (Table 3–1). None have been proven, and

TABLE 3–1. THEORIES REGARDING THE INITIATION OF PARTURITION IN WOMEN

	Source	Agent	Evidence
Maternal	Hypothalamus/pituitary	Oxytocin	Maternal hypophysectomy results in no or very low plasma oxytocin; onset of labor is normal
	Myometrium, paracrine	Increased oxytocin receptors	Oxytocin knockout mice deliver at term
	Decidua, autocrine/paracrine	Increased oxytocin and oxytocin receptors result in increased PG synthesis	Oxytocin knockout mice deliver at term
Fetus	Hypothalamus/pituitary	Fetal cortisol	Onset of labor is normal in fetal anencephaly, although variability of gestation is increased; mean gestational length is normal in fetal adrenal hypoplasia
	Endocrine	Oxytocin	Fetal-derived oxytocin may activate receptors in decidua and myometrium
	Fetal kidneys	PAF or other stimulator of PG synthesis	Onset of labor is term in fetal renal agenesis
	Fetal lungs	PAF or surfactant to stimulate PG synthesis	Onset of labor is normal in tracheal atresia
Amnion	Paracrine	PGs	Labor occurs at term with amnion bands
	Endocrine/paracrine	Progesterone metabolism	None

several experiments of nature fail to support a major role of some of these suggested mechanisms. The next section discusses the proposed mechanisms.

Fetal-Derived Signals

It has been proposed that a signal derived from the fetal hypothalamic–pituitary–adrenal axis signals the onset of labor as it does in other species (Table 3–1 and Fig 3–2). In pregnancies complicated by fetal anencephaly without polyhydramnios, the mean gestational length is 40 weeks; but the variance is greater than in normal fetuses, suggesting that the pituitary has a modulating effect on the duration of pregnancy.[11] In the human, there is no significant increase in cortisol formation by the fetal adrenal before the onset of labor, and the infusion of ACTH or cortisol into the fetus does not result in labor in the human as it does in the sheep. There is no fetal cortisol in pregnancies complicated by fetal adrenal hypoplasia; yet labor and delivery occur at term. In addition, it has been proposed that a signal from the fetal kidney or lung (eg, platelet activating factor, or PAF) signals prostaglandin synthesis in amnion cells and thereby effects parturition).[12] In pregnancies complicated by renal agenesis or tracheal atresia, however, there is no PAF and no surfactant stimulating PG synthesis in amnion; yet the onset of labor occurs at term.

Prostaglandins

Although many elements involved in parturition are unknown, it is believed that prostaglandins are somehow involved in the normal onset and progression of labor. Prostaglandins are synthesized in every tissue of the body, including the uterus and conceptus. In general, prostaglandins act within or near the tissue in which they are synthesized. They are metabolized close to their site of synthesis and usually enter the systemic circulation as inactive products. Even if they enter the circulation un-

metabolized, one circulation through the lungs ensures almost complete inactivation. Prostaglandins can be considered local agents whose production, actions, and degradation are confined within the uterus. The strongest evidence in support of a causative influence of prostaglandins on the onset of labor is provided by the observation that pharmacologic treatment with prostaglandins results in the induction of labor at all stages of gestation. Direct evidence relating to endogenous prostaglandins is far more difficult to assess.

There is a five- to tenfold increase in the concentration of free arachidonic acid in amniotic fluid during labor, and the concentration of this prostaglandin precursor continues to increase as a function of the progress of labor.[13,14] The rate of release of arachidonic acid is believed to be the rate-limiting step in prostaglandin formation in many tissues; thus, the regulation of arachidonic acid release in uterine and extrauterine tissue is important in our understanding of the timing and origin of increased prostaglandin formation during human parturition. Early in labor, the free arachidonic acid that enters amniotic fluid arises, at least in part, by release from glycerophospholipids in the fetal membranes by way of the action of phospholipases in these tissues.[15] Amnion assimilates arachidonic acid from amniotic fluid[16]; in fact, in the later stages of labor the content of arachidonic acid in the amnion is equal to or greater than that of membranes before labor. The net increase in arachidonic acid in the amnion *during labor* most likely accumulates from arachidonic acid that has been released from activated macrophage-like decidua, the probable source of amniotic fluid arachidonic acid.[17]

During labor, there is a striking increase in the concentration of both PGE_2 and $PGF_{2\alpha}$ in amniotic fluid (Fig 3–3). There is also an increase in the concentration of a metabolite of $PGF_{2\alpha}$, 13,14-dihydro-15-keto-$PGF_{2\alpha}$ (PGFM), in amniotic fluid and in maternal blood and

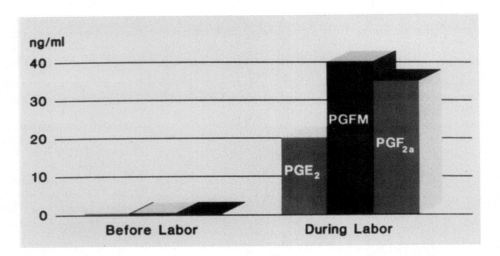

Figure 3–3. Amniotic fluid concentrations of PGE_2, $PGF_{2\alpha}$, and PGFM during late pregnancy.

urine during labor (for review, see Casey and MacDonald[7] and Mitchell[18]). It is doubtful that significant amounts of nonmetabolized PGE_2 pass through the membranes to reach the myometrium. Moreover, PGE_2 does not effect contraction of human myometrium in vitro.[19] The prostaglandin that gains access to the myometrium during parturition is mainly $PGF_{2\alpha}$, and it is believed that this prostaglandin is predominantly derived from the uterine decidua.[20] A further argument against amnion as a prime factor in the initiation of labor is the fact that labor occurs normally in pregnancies in which the amnion is detached from the chorion-forming constricting bands.

Whereas all investigators agree that PGE_2 and $PGF_{2\alpha}$ can act pharmacologically as uterine contractants when administered to pregnant women at any stage of gestation, it has not been established that prostaglandins serve as the physiologic uterotonins of parturition or that prostaglandins are obligatorily involved in parturition. In women, it is difficult to prove that changes in amniotic fluid prostaglandin concentrations actually precede the onset of labor or that changes in the activities of prostaglandin synthetic enzymes cause, rather than result from, the onset of labor. The possibility exists that prostaglandins are produced in increased amounts as a consequence of labor and are not required for the commencement of labor. The immediate challenge is to further define the role of prostaglandins in human parturition and the signal mechanisms by which prostaglandins are synthesized and metabolized.

Oxytocin

Oxytocin has been postulated to facilitate mammalian reproduction at several levels. In addition to milk ejection in response to suckling and uterine contractions during labor, oxytocin is believed to play important roles elsewhere in both males and females. Oxytocin is synthesized in the hypothalamic paraventricular and supraoptic nuclei during late embryogenesis[21] and is released into the circulation via the posterior pituitary. Oxytocin is also synthesized in the corpus luteum, uterus,[22,23] placenta,[24] amnion,[25] and testis.[26,27] Whereas posterior pituitary-derived oxytocin appears to regulate milk ejection, production of oxytocin in the uterus and/or placenta may initiate and maintain parturition.[22–24,28] Oxytocin and oxytocin receptor mRNA levels in the rodent uterus increase dramatically during gestation, and at parturition, oxytocin receptors are present in the myometrium and decidua of rats and humans, the number of which increases dramatically shortly before the onset of labor.[27–31] This receptor is notable for its exquisite responsiveness to gonadal and adrenal steroids[32] and for its downregulation by exogenous oxytocin administration.[33] The sensitivity of the myometrium to oxytocin, therefore, changes more dramatically in preparation for labor than do the circulating levels of the hormone. Oxytocin also stimulates the

production of PGE_2 and $PGF_{2\alpha}$ from human and rat decidua.[30,34]

A physiologic role for oxytocin during the initiation of human parturition, however, is not accepted universally. Studies of women and sheep have demonstrated that levels of oxytocin in maternal plasma increase only with the second stage of labor.[35,36] The infusion of oxytocin is relatively ineffective in inducing labor in human pregnancies, except in those relatively late in gestation when cervical ripening has occurred. Thus, oxytocin may act to maximize the myometrial forces involved in the expulsive phase of labor, and it may effect uterine contractions after delivery, thereby acting to decrease blood loss.

Mice carrying a deletion of the oxytocin-coding region are both viable and fertile.[37] Females lacking oxytocin have no obvious deficits in fertility or reproduction, including gestation and parturition. Although oxytocin-deficient females demonstrate normal maternal behavior, all offspring die shortly after birth because of the dam's inability to nurse. Postpartum injections of oxytocin to the oxytocin-deficient mothers restore milk ejection and rescue the offspring.[37] Thus, despite the multiple reproductive activities that have been attributed to oxytocin, oxytocin plays an essential role only in milk ejection in the mouse. It is likely that oxytocin plays a similar role in human reproduction and is not responsible for the initiation or maintenance of labor.

Endothelin

Endothelins are a family of sarafotoxin-like peptides that are potent vasoconstrictors. A host of smooth muscle tissues (stomach,[38] duodenum,[38] colon,[38] and trachea[39]) contract in response to treatment with endothelin-1. Similarly, human uterine tissues obtained from nonpregnant and pregnant women respond to endothelin-1 with forceful contractions (Fig 3–4); and endothelin-1 acts to cause an increase in intracellular calcium and myosin light-chain phosphorylation in human myometrial smooth muscle cells in culture.[40] mRNA levels for preproendothelin are present in relatively large amounts in human amnions of normal pregnancies and in amnion cells in monolayer culture.[41] The half-life of endothelin-1 in blood, however, is approximately 1 to 2 min, and endothelin increases the production of vasodilatory agents, including atrial natriuretic peptide, prostacyclin, and endothelium-derived relaxing factor, all of which may serve to counter the actions of endothelin-1.[38] Whereas immunoreactive endothelin is present in human amniotic fluid (in a concentration 10 to 100 times that in plasma), it seems unlikely that amnion serves as the primary source of a uterotonin that would cause the myometrial contractions of labor, but that possibility cannot be excluded.[42] The physiologic or pathophysiologic role for this family of fascinating peptides in human reproduction is yet to be established.

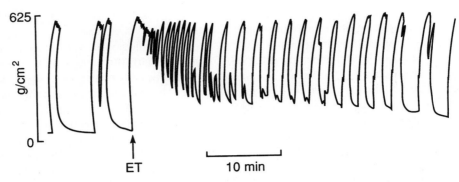

Figure 3–4. Effect of endothelin (10^{-8} M) on contraction of human myometrial uterine smooth muscle. Uterine smooth muscle strips from the longitudinal layer of uteri were obtained from premenopausal women at the time of hysterectomy. The amplitude of contraction is correlated directly with force; a scale of force normalized to tissue cross-sectional area is provided. (*Reproduced, with permission, from Garfield RE, et al, eds, 1990: 45.*[69])

COMMON THEMES IN PARTURITION AMONG ALL SPECIES

In all species, pregnancy is characterized by a relatively firm, rigid cervix and the striking absence of coordinated uterine contractions. At term, the cervix softens, and uterine contractions become synchronous. Cervical ripening and coordination of uterine contractions are processes common to parturition in all species. Cervical ripening is a process whereby the cervix transforms from a rigid organ occluding the uterine cavity to a stretchable and retractable part of the birth canal. The regulation of cervical ripening is not well understood and has received relatively little attention in the literature (discussed later). Coordinated uterine contractions require the muscle fibers to be interconnected electrically, facilitating the spread of excitation throughout the myometrium. This is achieved by the formation of gap junctions between muscle fibers, transforming the myometrium into a cohesive electrical and metabolic unit.[43] Myometrial gap junctions are present in all species studied during term and preterm labor and will be discussed further.

MYOMETRIUM

Physiology of Uterine Contractions

Uterine smooth muscle belongs to a broad class of smooth muscles termed phasic smooth muscle. Phasic smooth muscle is characterized by generation of action potentials, spontaneous contractile activity that is independent of extrinsic innervation, and the presence of gap junctions that serve to electrically couple adjoining myocytes. The degree of shortening in smooth muscle is of greater magnitude than that of skeletal muscle; yet, the rate of force development is slower. The forces in the smooth muscle cells can be multidirectional rather than

always aligned with the axis of the muscle fibers as in skeletal muscle.[44] This facilitates expulsive forces irrespective of fetal lie and presentation.

Muscle contraction occurs as a result of the cyclic interaction of myosin with actin filaments. Myosin, composed of two heavy-chain subunits (200 kD) and two pairs of light-chain (20 and 17 kD), is arranged in its hexameric form into thick filaments. Each heavy chain consists of an α-helical carboxy-terminal region and an amino-terminal globular head region that contains an actin-binding site, an ATP hydrolysis site, and one each of the two types of light chains (Fig 3–5). The tail regions of the heavy chains intertwine to form the backbone of the bipolar thick filaments from which the two head regions protrude and interact with filamentous actin to form a cross bridge. Muscle myosin is an actin-activated MgATPase.[45] Activation of smooth muscle myosin MgATPase activity requires phosphorylation of the 20-kD

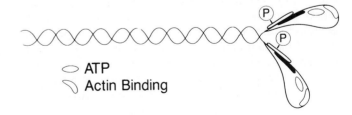

⬭ ATP
⤸ Actin Binding

Figure 3–5. Schematic drawing of the myosin phosphorylation system. Myosin is composed of two heavy-chain subunits arranged in rod-shaped α-helical coils that end in globular head projections. Two types of light-chain subunits are bound to the neck region of each myosin head. Phosphorylation of one type of light-chain subunit (the regulatory light chain) is indicated by the circled P. Myosin phosphorylation is catalyzed by Ca^{2+}/calmodulin-dependent myosin light-chain kinase and dephosphorylation by myosin light-chain phosphatase. (*Reproduced, with permission, from Garfield RE, et al, eds, 1990: 45.*[69])

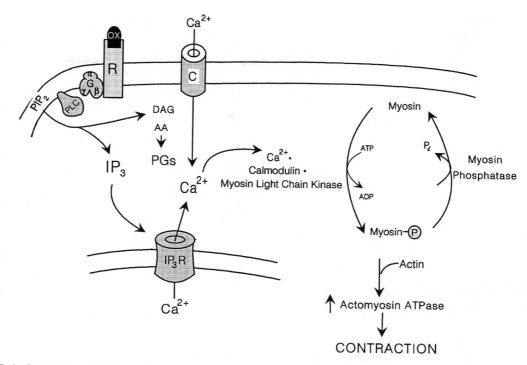

Figure 3–6. Scheme for initiation of smooth muscle contraction via myosin light chain phosphorylation. Increases in intracellular $[Ca^{2+}]$ occur by ligand/receptor-activated phosphatidylinositol hydrolysis, IP_3 formation, and release of Ca^{2+} from IP_3-sensitive stores and/or by influx of extracellular Ca^{2+} via plasma membrane Ca^{2+} channels (C). Oxytocin receptor with its heterotrimeric G protein complex is illustrated. This increase in cytoplasmic $[Ca^{2+}]$ is the primary event that initiates the activation of smooth muscle contractile elements by Ca^{2+}/calmodulin/myosin light chain kinase-dependent phosphorylation of myosin light chain (myosin-(P)). Phosphorylated myosin undergoes ATP-dependent cyclic interactions with actin to produce contraction. Phosphorylation is reversed by myosin phosphatase. Additional regulation may occur by regulatory proteins associated with the IP_3 receptor (IP_3R), G-proteins (G) associated with ligand receptors, or phospholipase C (PLC), and regulation of myosin light-chain kinase or phosphatase activities.

regulatory light chain of myosin (Fig 3–6). The regulation of contraction by myosin light chain phosphorylation is applicable to all smooth muscle types and of central importance in the biochemical regulation of relaxation and contraction in myometrium. Cytoplasmic Ca^{2+} is believed to be the primary determinant for regulation of myosin light chain phosphorylation. The increase in cytoplasmic free Ca^{2+} via influx of extracellular Ca^{2+} or through mobilization of intracellular Ca^{2+} stores can be induced by two distinct mechanisms of excitation–contraction coupling: (1) electromechanical coupling, mediated through depolarization of the surface membrane by action potentials or high K^+ solutions; and (2) pharmacomechanical coupling, a mechanism by which agents mediate an increase in the intracellular Ca^{2+} concentration independent of cell surface membrane potentials. Electromechanical coupling (depolarization of the plasma membrane by action potentials) is the major signaling pathway involved in the spontaneous contractions of uterine smooth muscle. Pharmacomechanical coupling (by way of oxytocin, for example) involves Ca^{2+} influx via receptor-operated Ca^{2+} channels

and receptor-mediated inositol trisphosphate formation with release of Ca^{2+} from intracellular stores in the sarcoplasmic reticulum (Fig 3–6).

Contractile stimulation results in an increase in the cytoplasmic Ca^{2+} concentration. Ca^{2+} binds to calmodulin, forming a Ca^{2+}/calmodulin complex[34] that activates myosin light-chain kinase. Myosin light-chain kinase catalyzes the phosphorylation of the 20-kD regulatory light chain subunit of myosin, resulting in activation of actomyosin MgATPase, initiation of cross-bridge cycling and mechanical output (force generation and muscle shortening).[46–48] Sequestration or extrusion of Ca^{2+} from the cell results in inactivation of myosin light-chain kinase, dephosphorylation of myosin by myosin light-chain phosphatase, inactivation of myosin MgATPase, and relaxation of the muscle (Fig 3–6). In relaxed conditions, the free cytoplasmic Ca^{2+} concentration is low (110 to 150 nmol). Thus, very little Ca^{2+} is bound to calmodulin, and myosin light chain kinase is minimally activated, resulting in low amounts of phosphorylated myosin light-chain. Increases in cytoplasmic Ca^{2+} result in activation of myosin light-chain kinase and myosin light-chain phosphorylation.

Is Nitric Oxide Involved in Human Parturition?

Although many investigations regarding parturition in the past have focused on contractile substances that lead to the onset of labor in women, none have been identified as physiologic mediators of parturition. Recently, it has been proposed that parturition represents withdrawal or retreat from uterine quiescence and pregnancy maintenance, rather than increased contractile stimulation.[49] It has been proposed that nitric oxide (NO) may be an endogenous uterine relaxant that contributes to uterine quiescence during pregnancy prior to term, and that relief of NO action may lead to retreat from uterine quiescence with the onset of spontaneous uterine contractions of labor.[50,51]

In the vasculature, endothelial NO or atrial peptides signal smooth muscle relaxation by intracellular increases in guanosine 3',5'-monophosphate (cyclic GMP or cGMP) (Fig 3–7). The downstream target for cGMP is believed to be the cGMP-dependent protein kinase (PKG), which mediates the vasorelaxant effects of cGMP (Fig 3–7).[52–54] Whereas increases in cGMP correlate with relaxation in a time- and concentration-dependent manner in vascular smooth muscle,[55] the role of cGMP as a uterine relaxant is not as well established. For example, there is no correlation between increases in cGMP and relaxation in myometrial smooth muscle,[56,57] and increases in cGMP that effect almost complete relaxation of tonic smooth muscles have relatively little effect in uterine smooth muscle.[56,58] It is feasible, however, that NO, produced from nerve plexi, decidua,[50,51] or other resident cells of the myometrium (eg, macrophages[59]) could diffuse to myometrial smooth muscle cells, activate soluble guanylate cyclase, and increase cellular levels of cGMP. Thus, NO-induced cGMP elevation may effect uterine relaxation in a manner analogous to NO action in the vasculature. Yallampalli et al[60] found that L-arginine, the substrate for NO, caused a rapid and substantial relaxation of spontaneous contractions in myometrium from pregnant rats but not from nonpregnant animals. The effects were reversed by L-nitro-arginine methyl ester (L-NAME), an inhibitor of NO-synthase. Further investigations, however, indicated that this relaxation response may be nonspecific because treatment with other basic amino acids (D-arginine, lysine, and ornithine, 3 mmol) also resulted in similar patterns of relaxation.[61] Moreover, treatment of myometrial tissues with L-arginine (3 mmol, pH neutralized to 7.6) or ornithine hydrochloride (pH 7.0) did not result in relaxation. Using a buffered physiologic solution that effectively buffers the change in pH induced by L-arginine, relaxation responses to L-arginine are not observed.[61] Neither L-arginine nor inhibitors of NO synthase alter contractility of human myometrial smooth muscle strips.[62]

Others have found that myometrium during pregnancy is insensitive to relaxation by cGMP compared with either nonpregnant myometrium or vascular tissue.[63–65] The lack of sensitivity to relaxation has been correlated with decreased expression of PKG in myometrial tissues.[65] In vivo, NO synthase inhibitors do not affect uterine contractility, and neither NO synthase inhibitors nor NO donors alter the timing of parturition.[66–68] Taken together, these data provide evidence that the NO-cGMP-signaling pathway is probably not involved in the physiologic maintenance of uterine quiescence during pregnancy. NO, however, dramatically affects uterine blood flow and is an important modulator of vascular reactivity during pregnancy.

Gap Junctions

The optimum functioning of the myometrium during labor is due to its ability to develop well-coordinated synchronous contractions, which requires highly developed cell-to-cell coupling (for review, see Garfield et al[69,70]). Structures called gap junctions, consisting of two symmetrical portions of plasma membrane from two opposing cells, are thought to be largely responsible for this coupling. Gap junctions are formed when intramembranous proteins from the opposing cell membranes align themselves, thereby creating pores from the cytoplasm of one cell to the cytoplasm of the other. These pores provide sites for low-resistance electrical or ionic coupling between cells, as well as a pathway for transport of metabolites directly between cells. Evidence suggests that gap junctions can exist in an open or closed state,

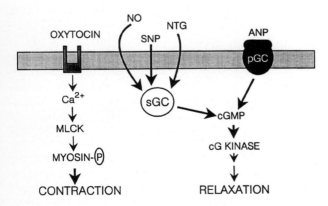

Figure 3–7. Nitric oxide-induced smooth muscle relaxation. The scheme for contraction is illustrated on the left with oxytocin binding to its receptor initiating activation of myosin light chain kinase (MLCK), myosin phosphorylation, and contraction. Nitric oxide (NO), sodium nitroprusside (SNP), or nitroglycerin (NTG) activates soluble guanylate cyclase (sGC) to increase cellular levels of cGMP. Increases in cGMP may also arise by way of particulate guanylate cyclases of atrial natriuretic peptide (ANP) receptors. Increases in cGMP activate cGMP-dependent protein kinase, which leads to decreases in intracellular Ca^{2+} and relaxation.

thus providing for a rapid control of coupling. The mechanism controlling this is not known, although coupling can be affected by changes in both CA^{2+} and pH. In rats, guinea pigs, sheep, and humans, the number of gap junctions is low or absent throughout pregnancy but at term increases dramatically; thus, at delivery of the fetus their frequency of occurrence and size reach a maximum. A decline begins 24 hr later.[69] In rabbits and rats, estrogens promote and progesterone inhibits formation of gap junctions. To what extent these steroids regulate gap junction formation in humans is unknown.

CERVICAL RIPENING

Whereas the uterine fundus is composed predominantly of smooth muscle cells, the predominant element in the cervix is collagen, fibrils of which are bound into dense bundles that confer tissue rigidity. The collagen is embedded in a ground substance of large-molecular-weight proteoglycan complexes that consist of a core protein to which are attached glycosaminoglycan branches.[70] These are long chains of highly negatively charged repeating disaccharides containing one hexosamine (glucosamine or galactosamine) and one uronic acid (glucuronic or iduronic). The cervix contains a variety of glycosaminoglycan branches, such as heparin, heparin sulfate, chondroitin, and dermatan sulfate, the latter being the most abundant in women. Cervical ripening is a qualitative change in the glycosaminoglycan content of the ground substance, namely, a replacement of those with a strong binding affinity to collagen (iduronic sulfates) with those of lower affinity and more hydrophilic properties (ie, hyaluronic acid) so that the water content of the tissue increases.[71,72] In addition, there is also a reduced collagen concentration and an increase in cervical collagenase activity during cervical ripening.[72,73] Thus, the tissue changes of cervical ripening are complex and are more accurately described as a remodeling of cervical architecture than simple collagenolysis.

Cervical tissues are also subject to endocrine control, much of which is similar to the control of myometrial contractility. Cervical collagenase activity is inhibited by progesterone and increased by estradiol. The origin of collagenase is suspected to be from both cervical fibroblasts and immune cells that infiltrate the cervix with the onset of parturition (Fig 3–8).[74] These inflammatory cells synthesize and secrete interleukin-1, which has numerous biologic effects on various target cells. IL-1 accelerates the production of collagenase and simultaneously decreases the biosynthesis of tissue inhibitor metalloproteinase. It also promotes production of other matrix metalloproteinases such as stromelysin.[74,75] IL-1 induces rapid induction of IL-8, which further stimulates

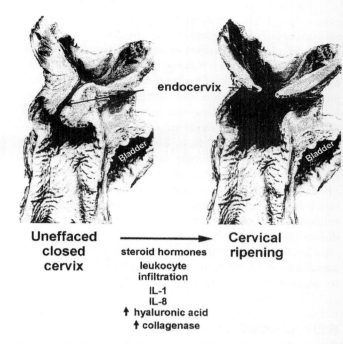

Figure 3–8. Cervical ripening. Prior to parturition, the cervix transforms from an uneffaced, rigid organ to a thin, retractable tissue by interactions with steroid hormones and immune modulators. This results in remodeling of the cervical architecture, effacement, and ultimately cervical dilation. (Modified drawing from the Hunterian Anatomical Museum, University of Glasgow.)

prostaglandin production and massive infiltration of neutrophils.[75,76] Although antiprogestins result in a highly responsive myometrium that responds readily to exogenous stimuli in human pregnancy, antiprogestins per se have little stimulatory effect on uterine contractions.[77,78] Nevertheless, antiprogestins, even at low doses, cause marked cervical ripening in all species tested, including humans.[79,80] In summary, the biochemical cascade of events involved in cervical ripening is not completely understood. Results indicate that complex interactions between cervical fibroblasts, neutrophils, and other immune cells, together with estrogen, progesterone, and inflammatory mediators, are important in remodeling of the cervical architecture for well-timed effacement and dilation during parturition.

SUMMARY

The endocrinologic and biomolecular events that signal the onset of labor are complex and vary from species to species. It is remarkable that human pregnancy is maintained for some 38 postovulatory wk without uterine contractions. Although in some species the fetus is responsible for timing its birth by initiating endocrine events that bring about the spontaneous onset of labor, there is not convincing evidence for this in human pregnancy. Human parturition is not preceded by dramatic changes in the concentration of progesterone or estrogens in the maternal circulation or of cortisol in the fetal circulation. The uterine quiescence of human pregnancy may depend upon tonic inhibition of prostaglandin synthesis in uterine tissues, but it has not been demonstrated that prostaglandins are obligatorily involved in the parturitional process. Nitric oxide may be important in maintaining uterine blood flow during pregnancy but is probably not the physiologic mediator of uterine quiescence. More work is required to understand the mechanisms by which human pregnancy is maintained and the processes by which pregnancy maintenance is withdrawn to bring about timely initiation of labor and delivery. A definition of the biochemistry of labor is important not only in the prevention of prematurity but also in the management of those pregnancies complicated by maternal or fetal jeopardy.

REFERENCES

1. Liggins G. Fetal influences on myometrial contractility. *Clin Obstet Gynecol.* 16:148, 1973

2. Liggins GC, Fairclough RJ, Grieves SA, et al. The mechanism of initiation of parturition in the ewe. *Recent Prog Horm Res.* 29:111, 1973

3. France JT, Magness RR, Murry BA, et al. The regulation of ovine placental steroid 17α-hydroxylase and aromatase by glucocorticoid. *Mol Endocrinol.* 2:193, 1988

4. Liggins GC, Fairclough RJ, Grieves SA, et al. Parturition in the sheep. In: Knight J, O'Connor M, eds. *The Fetus and Birth.* Ciba Foundation Symposium 47. Amsterdam, Elsevier, 1977: 5

5. Challis JRG, Olson DM. Parturition. In: Knobil E, Neill J, eds. *The Physiology of Reproduction.* New York, Raven Press, 1988: 2177

6. Flower RJ. The role of prostaglandins in parturition, with special reference to the rat. In: Knight J, O'Conner M, eds. *The Fetus and Birth.* Ciba Foundation Symposium 47. Amsterdam, Elsevier, 1977: 297

7. Casey ML, MacDonald P. Decidual activation: The role of prostaglandins in labor. In: McNellis D, Challis JRG, MacDonald PC, et al, eds. *Cellular and Integrative Mechanisms in the Onset of Labor.* An NICHD workshop. Ithaca, NY, Perinatology Press, 1988: 141

8. Parker CR Jr, Illingworth DR, Bissonette J, Carr BR. Endocrinology of pregnancy in abetalipoproteinemia: Studies in a patient with homozygous familial hypobetalipoproteinemia. *N Eng J Med.* 314:557, 1986

9. Mahendroo MS, Cala KM, Russell DW. 5α-Reduced androgens play a key role in murine parturition. *Mol Endocrinol.* 10:380, 1996

10. Casey ML, MacDonald PC. Transforming growth factor β acts as a gene-specific antiprogestin. 40th annual meeting. *Proc Soc Gynecol Invest.* 69, 1993

11. Honnebier WM, Swaab DF. The influence of anencephaly upon intrauterine growth of the fetus and placenta and upon gestation length. *J Obstet Gynaecol Brit Comm.* 80: 577, 1973

12. Muguruma K, Hisashi N, Kawano Y, Johnston J. Platelet-activating factor in reproduction. *Infert Reprod Med Clin North Am.* 8:1, 1997

13. Keirse MJNC, Hicks BR, Mitchell MD, Turnbull, A. Increase in the prostaglandin precursor, arachidonic acid in amniotic fluid during spontaneous labour. *Br J Obstet Gynaecol.* 84:743, 1977

14. MacDonald PC, Schultz FM, Duenhoelter JH, et al. Initiation of human parturition. I. Mechanism of action of arachidonic acid. *Obstet Gynecol.* 44:29, 1974

15. Okita JR, MacDonald PC, Johnston JM. Mobilization of arachidonic acid from specific glycerophospholipids of human fetal membranes during early labor. *J Biol Chem.* 247:14029, 1982

16. Okita JR, MacDonald PC, Johnston JM. Initiation of human parturition. XIV. Increase in the diacylglycerol content of amnion during parturition. *Am J Obstet Gynecol.* 147:477, 1983

17. Casey ML, MacDonald PC. Biomolecular mechanisms in human parturition: Activation of uterine decidua. In: d'Arcangues C, Fraser LS, Newton JR, Odlind V, eds. *Contraception and Mechanisms of Endometrial Bleeding.* Cambridge University Press, 1990: 305

18. Mitchell MD. Sources of eicosanoids within the uterus during pregnancy. In: McNellis D, Challis JRG, MacDonald PC, et al, eds. *Cellular and Integrative Mechanisms in the Onset of Labor.* An NICHD workshop. Ithaca, NY, Perinatology Press, 1988: 165

19. Word RA, Kamm KE, Casey ML. Contractile effects of prostaglandins, oxytocin, and endothelin-1 in human myometrium in vitro: Refractoriness of myometrial tissue of pregnant women to prostaglandins E_2 and F_2. *J Clin Endocrinol Metab.* 75:1027, 1992.

20. Casey ML, MacDonald PC. Biomolecular processes in the initiation of parturition: Decidual activation. *Clin Obstet Gynecol.* 31:533, 1988

21. Fuchs AR, Fuchs F, Husslein P, et al. Oxytocin receptors and human parturition: A dual role for oxytocin in the initiation of labor. *Science.* 214:1396, 1982

22. Laurent FM, Hindelang C, Klein JM, et al. Expression of the oxytocin and vasopressin genes in the rat hypothalamus during development: an in situ hybridization study. *Dev Brain Res.* 46:145, 1989

23. Lefebvre DL, Giaid A, Bennet H, et al. Oxytocin gene expression in rat uterus. *Science.* 256:1553, 1992

24. Lefebvre DL, Farookhi R, Larcher A, et al. Uterine oxytocin gene expression. I. Induction during pseudopregnancy and the estrous cycle. *Endocrinology.* 134:2556, 1994

25. Lefebvre DL, Giaid A, Zingg HH. Expression of the oxytocin gene in rat placenta. *Endocrinology.* 130:1185, 1992

26. Chibbar R, Miller FD, Mitchell BF. Synthesis of oxytocin in amnion, chorion, and decidua may influence the timing of human parturition. *J Clin Invest.* 91:185, 1993

27. Foo NC, Carter DA, Murphy D, Ivell R. Vasopressin and oxytocin gene expression in rat testis. *Endocrinology.* 128:2118, 1991

28. Ang HL, Ungefroren H, DeBree F, et al. Testicular oxytocin gene expression in seminiferous tubules of cattle and transgenic mice. *Endocrinology.* 128:2110, 1991

29. Larcher A, Necullcea J, Breton C, et al. Oxytocin receptor gene expression in the rat uterus during pregnancy and the estrous cycle and in response to gonadal steroid treatment. *Endocrinology.* 136:5350, 1995

30. Challis JRG, Lye SJ. Parturition. In: Knobil E, Neill JD, eds. *The Physiology of Reproduction,* 2nd ed. New York, Raven Press, 1994: 985–1031

31. Robinson G, Evans JJ. Oxytocin has a role in gonadotropin regulation in rats. *J Endocrinol.* 125:425, 1990

32. Chibbar R, Miller FD, Mitchell BF. Synthesis of oxytocin in amnion, chorion, and decidua may influence the timing of human parturition. *J Clin Invest.* 91:185, 1993

33. Barberis C, Tribollet E. Vasopressin and oxytocin receptors in the central nervous system. *Crit Rev Neurobiol.* 10:119, 1996

34. Insel TR, Young L, Witt DM, Crews D. Gonadal steroids have paradoxical effects on brain oxytocin receptors. *J Neuroendocrinol.* 5:619, 1993

35. Witt DM, Insel TR. A selective oxytocin antagonist attenuates progesterone facilitation of female sexual behavior. *Endocrinology.* 138:3269, 1991

36. Glatz TH, Weitzman RE, Eliot RJ, et al. Ovine maternal and fetal plasma oxytocin concentrations before and during parturition. *Endocrinology.* 108:1328, 1981

37. Leake RD, Weitzman RE, Glatz TH, Fisher DA. Plasma oxytocin concentration in man, nonpregnant women and pregnant women before and during spontaneous labor. *J Clin Endocrinol Metab.* 53:730, 1981

38. Nishimori K, Young LJ, Guo Q, et al. Oxytocin is required for nursing but is not essential for parturition or reproductive behavior. *Proc Natl Acad Sci.* 93:11699, 1996

39. De Nucci G, Thomas R, D'Orleans-Juste P, et al. Pressor effects of circulating endothelin are limited by its removal in the pulmonary circulation and by the release of prostacyclin and endothelium derived relaxing factor. *Proc Natl Acad Sci.* 85:9797, 1988

40. Uchida Y, Ninomiya H, Saotome M, et al. Endothelin, a novel vasoconstrictor peptide, as potent bronchoconstrictor. *Eur J Pharmacol.* 154:227, 1988

41. Word RA, Kamm KE, Stull JT, Casey ML. Endothelin increases cytoplasmic calcium and myosin phosphorylation in human myometrium. *Am J Obstet Gynecol.* 162:1103, 1991

42. Sunnergren K, Word RA, Sambrook JF, et al. Expression and regulation of endothelin precursor mRNA in avascular human amnion. *Mol Cell Endocrinol.* 68:R7, 1990

43. Casey ML, Word RA, MacDonald PC. Endothelin-1 gene expression and regulation of endothelin mRNA and protein biosynthesis in avascular human amnion: Potential source of amniotic fluid endothelin. *J Biol Chem.* 266:5762, 1991

44. Garfield RE, Blennerhassett MG, Miller SM. Control of myometrial contractility: Role and regulation of gap junctions. *Oxf Rev Reprod Biol.* 10:436, 1988

45. Hartshorne DJ, Gorecka A. Biochemistry of the contractile proteins of smooth muscle. In: Bohr DF, Somlyo AP, Sparks HV Jr, eds. *Handbook of Physiology. The Cardiovascular System,* vol. 2. *Vascular Smooth Muscle.* Bethesda, Md., Am Physiol Soc, 1980: 93

46. Word RA, Kamm KE. Regulation of smooth muscle contraction by myosin phosphorylation. In: Carston ME, ed. *Smooth Muscle Contraction.* Rensselaer, N.Y. Sterling Drug, 1996

47. Kamm KE, Stull JT. Activation of smooth muscle contraction: Relation between myosin phosphorylation and stiffness. *Science.* 232:280, 1986

48. Word RA. Myosin phosphorylation and the control of myometrial contraction/relaxation. In: Sanborn B, Monga M, eds. *Current Concepts in the Regulation of Uterine Contractile Activity. Seminars in Perinatology.* Philadelphia, W. B. Saunders, 1995: 3

49. Word RA, Kamm KE, Casey ML, Stull JT. Contractile elements and myosin light chain phosphorylation in myometrial tissues from nonpregnant and pregnant women. *J Clin Invest.* 92:29, 1993

50. Natuzzi ES, Ursell PC, Harrison M, et al. Nitric oxide synthase activity in the pregnant uterus decreases at parturition. *Biochem Biophys Res Comm.* 194:1, 1993

51. Sladek SM, Regenstein AC, Lykins D, Roberts JM. Nitric oxide synthase activity in pregnant rabbit uterus decreases on the last day of pregnancy. *Am J Obstet Gynecol.* 169:1285, 1993

52. Francis SH, Noblett BD, Todd BW, et al. Relaxation of vascular and tracheal smooth muscle by cyclic nucleotide analogs that preferentially activate purified cGMP-dependent protein kinase. *Mol Pharmacol.* 34:505, 1988

53. Cornwell TL, Lincoln TM. Regulation of intracellular Ca^{2+} levels in cultured vascular smooth muscle cells. Reduction of Ca^{2+} by atriopeptin and 8-bromo-cyclic GMP is mediated by cyclic GMP-dependent protein kinase. *J Biol Chem.* 264:1146, 1989

54. Lincoln TM, Cornwell TL. Intracellular cyclic GMP receptor proteins. *FASEB J.* 7:328, 1993

55. Kukovetz WR, Holzmann S, Wurm A, Poch G. Evidence for cyclic GMP-mediated relaxant effects of nitrocompounds in coronary smooth muscle. *Naunyn-Schm Arch Pharmacol.* 310: 129, 1979

56. Diamond J. β-adrenoceptors, cAMP and cGMP in control of uterine motility. In: Carsten ME, Miller JD, eds. *Uterine Function: Molecular and Cellular Aspects.* New York, Plenum Press, 1990: 255

57. Diamond J. Lack of correlation between cyclic GMP elevation and relaxation of nonvascular smooth muscle by nitroglycerin, nitroprusside, hydroxylamine and sodium azide. *J Pharmacol Exp Ther.* 225:422, 1983

58. Word RA, Casey ML, Kamm KE, Stull JT. Effects of cGMP on $[Ca^{2+}]$, myosin light chain phosphorylation, and contraction in human myometrium. *Am J Physiol.* 260:C861, 1991

59. Stewart IJ, Mitchell BS. Macrophages and other endocytic cells in the mouse uterus during the second half of pregnancy and into the postpartum period. *J Anat.* 181:119, 1992

60. Yallampalli C, Izumi H, Byam-Smith M, Garfield RE. An L-arginine–nitric oxide–cyclic guanosine monophosphate system exists in the uterus and inhibits contractility during pregnancy. *Am J Obstet Gynecol.* 170:175, 1994

61. Kato S, Word RA. Effect of basic amino acids and alkaline pH on uterine contractility in vitro. *J Soc Gynecol Invest.* 2:179, 1995

62. Jones GD, Poston L. The role of endogenous nitric oxide synthesis in contractility of term or preterm human myometrium. *Br J Obstet Gynecol.* 104:241, 1997

63. Potvin W, Varma DR. Refractoriness of the gravid rat uterus to tocolytic and biochemical effects of atrial natriuretic peptide. *Br J Pharmacol.* 100:341, 1990

64. Potvin W, Varma DR. Down-regulation of myometrial atrial natriuretic factor receptors by progesterone and pregnancy and up-regulation by oestrogen in rats. *J Endocrinol.* 131:259, 1991

65. Word RA, Cornwell TL. Regulation of cyclic GMP-induced relaxation and cGMP-dependent protein kinase in myometrium during pregnancy. *Am J Physiol.* In press, 1997

66. Ahokas RA, Mercer BM, Sibai BM. Enhanced endothelium-derived relaxing factor activity in pregnant, spontaneously hypertensive rats. *Am J Obstet Gynecol.* 165:801, 1991

67. Diket AL, Peirce MR, Munshi UK, et al. Nitric oxide inhibition causes intrauterine growth retardation and hind-limb disruptions in rats. *Am J Obstet Gynecol.* 171: 1243, 1994

68. Molnar M, Hertelendy F. *N*-nitro-L-arginine, an inhibitor of nitric oxide synthesis, increases blood pressure in rats and reverses the pregnancy-induced refractoriness to vasopressor agents. *Am J Obstet Gynecol.* 166:1560, 1992

69. Garfield RE, Tabb T, Thilander G. Intercellular coupling and modulation of uterine contractility. In: Garfield RE, ed. *Uterine Contractility.* Norwell, Mass., Serono Symposia, 1990: 21

70. Obrink B. A study of the interactions between monomeric tropocollagen and glycosaminoglycan. *Eur J Biochem.* 33:387, 1973

71. Kleissl HP, van der Rest M, Naftolin F, et al. Collagen changes in the human cervix at parturition. *Am J Obstet Gynecol.* 130:748, 1978

72. Granstrom L, Ekman G, Ulmsten U, Malmstrom A. Changes in the connective tissue of corpus and cervix uteri during ripening and labour in term pregnancy. *Br J Obstet Gynecol.* 96:1198, 1989

73. Junqueira LCU, Zugaib M, Montes GS, et al. Morphologic and histochemical evidence for the occurrence of collagenolysis and for the role of neutrophilic polymorphonuclear leukocytes during cervical dilatation. *Am J Obstet Gynecol.* 138:273, 1980

74. Kelly RW, Leask R, Calder AA. Choriodecidual production of interleukin-8 and mechanism of parturition. *Lancet.* 339:776, 1992

75. Osmers RGW, Blaser J, Kuhn W, Tschesche H. Interleukin-8 synthesis and the onset of labor. *Obstet Gynecol.* 86:223, 1995

76. El Maradny E, Kanayama N, Halim A, et al. The effect of interleukin-1 in rabbit cervical ripening. *Eur J Obstet Gynecol Reprod Biol.* 60:75, 1995

77. Bydeman M, Swahn ML. Progesterone receptor blockage. Effect on uterine contractility and early pregnancy. *Contraception.* 32:45, 1985

78. Elger W, Fähnrich M, Beier S, et al. Endometrial and myometrial effects of progesterone-antagonists in pregnant guinea pigs. *Am J Obstet Gynecol.* 157:1065, 1987

79. Chwalisz K, Elger W. Induction of labour with antigestagens in the rat and guinea pig. *J Steroid Biochem.* 25 (suppl.):1315, 1986

80. Frydman R, Fernandez H, Pons JC, Ulmann A. Mifepriston (zRU 486) and therapeutic late pregnancy termination: A double-blind study of two different doses. *Hum Reprod.* 3:803, 1988

Chapter 4

GENETICS IN REPRODUCTION

Earl W. Stradtman, Jr.

For you created my inmost being; you knit me together in my mother's womb. I praise you because I am fearfully and wonderfully made; your works are wonderful, I know that full well.[1]

The role of genetics is becoming increasingly important in clinical medicine and in science. Techniques of molecular biology can detect point gene mutations, can amplify a gene sequence from a single copy to nanogram quantities in less than a day, and enable scientists to sequence the human genome. The impact of genetics in reproductive medicine is far-reaching. Knowledge of molecular mechanisms of hormonal production and regulation is exploding. The obstetrician–gynecologist, as caretaker of the mother and the unborn child, is expected to identify inheritable risk factors that could result in an adverse pregnancy outcome. Patients with disorders of sexual development may have gonads of uncertain malignant potential. As normal and mutant genes are sequenced and cloned, diagnosis of genetic disorders should become increasingly accurate. This chapter reviews the principles of molecular genetics, cytogenetics, patterns of inheritance, and selected clinical disorders, and summarizes some of the recent advances in molecular genetics that should enhance the management and counseling of our patients.

MOLECULAR STRUCTURE OF DNA

Native deoxyribonucleic acid (DNA) exists as a double helix of two nucleotide chains, a nucleotide being a five-carbon sugar–phosphate unit covalently linked to an inwardly directed nitrogenous base.[2,3] The bases are the purines adenine (A) and guanine (G) and the pyrimidines cytosine (C) and thymine (T), and each base has a unique complement with which it will pair in parallel planes by hydrogen bonding, or hybridization, as a base pair (bp). The primary DNA structure, based on the hybridization between complementary nucleotide strands, provides a template for the exact replication of new DNA strands or the transcription into ribonucleic acid (RNA) and translation into protein, aids complementary strands in finding each other, and helps maintain the double helical, or secondary, DNA structure. The secondary structure guards against damage and promotes repair. The tertiary structure involves the coiling of 146 bp of DNA around basic regulatory proteins called histones, and the DNA-protein unit is called a nucleosome. The role of histones is under active investigation, but this intricate coiling process seems to allow compression of long DNA strands into compact units.

Directionality is also important in DNA structure: the deoxyribose units are covalently linked by phosphate groups bound to the 5' hydroxyl group of one unit to the 3' hydroxyl of the next, and since A pairs only with T, and C only with G, a linear arrangement such as ACCTG can pair only with its complement TGGAC in the opposite direction. The notation of the sequence written another way is as follows:

$$5'\text{-ACCTG-}3'$$
$$3'\text{-TGGAC-}5'$$

If even one base has no complement in the sister strand, complete hybridization will not occur. This precision in the matching of base pairs forms the basis of many of the diagnostic techniques of modern molecular biology.

HUMAN CHROMOSOMES

Chromosomes are the highest order of DNA coiling. Normal human somatic cells have 46 chromosomes, 44 autosomes, and 2 sex chromosomes. The chromosomes occur in homologous pairs, to which the germ cell from each parent contributes one chromosome. Each human gamete, therefore, contains 23 or a haploid (n) number of

TABLE 4–1. SYMBOLS FOR CHROMOSOME NOMENCLATURE (PARTIAL LIST)

A–G	The chromosome groups
1–22	The autosome numbers
X, Y	The sex chromosomes
/	Diagonal line indicates mosaicism, eg, 46/47 designates a mosaic with 46-chromosome and 47-chromosome cell lines
del	Deletion
der	Derivative of chromosome
i	Isochromosome
ins	Insertion
inv	Inversion
mar	Marker of chromosome
p	Short arm of chromosome
q	Long arm of chromosome
r	Ring chromosome
s	Satellite
t	Translocation
rcp	Reciprocal translocation
rob	Robertsonian translocation
ter	Terminal (may also be written as pter or qter)
->	From -> to
+ or –	Placed before the chromosome number, these symbols indicate addition (+) or loss (–) of a whole chromosome; eg, +21 indicates an extra chromosome 21, as in Down syndrome. Placed after the chromosome number, these symbols indicate increase or decrease in the length of a chromosome part; eg, 5p– indicates a loss of part of the short arm of chromosome 5, as in cri du chat syndrome

(Reproduced, with permission, from Thompson JS, Thompson MW. Genetics in Medicine, 4th ed. Philadelphia, W. B. Saunders Co., 1986: 10.)

chromosomes. The embryo contains a diploid number (2n) of chromosomes, or 23 homologous pairs, having received one homologue from each parent. Chromosomes exist for most of the cell cycle in a diffuse state, invisible during normal light microscopy, and are unwound and available for transcription and translation. During metaphase of mitosis, the chromosomes become coiled and dense enough to view under the light microscope when stained. Table 4–1 gives symbols for chromosome nomenclature.

MITOSIS

Mitosis is cell division in which one cell gives rise to two cells genetically identical to the parent cell. This process of cell multiplication transforms a single-cell human embryo, for example, into an adult human being. No more of the genetic information needed for protein synthesis and to regulate cell processes is present in an adult than in the embryo.

The cell cycle is composed of the following phases: G_0, the resting phase; G_1, the first gap phase; S, the phase of DNA synthesis; G_2, the second gap phase; and M, or mitosis.[4] Mitosis comprises five phases (Fig 4–1): interphase, prophase, metaphase, anaphase, and telophase.

Interphase is a resting phase between cell divisions in which metabolic processes and DNA replication occur, specifically in the S phase of the cell cycle, resulting in 4n chromosomes. The cell enters prophase when the chromosomes begin to condense and are just visible by staining. The appearance of chromatids, pairs of thin parallel strands joined at the centromere, characterizes prophase. In addition, the nuclear membrane dissipates, the centriole replicates, and each one moves toward opposite poles of the cell. In metaphase the chromosomes are their most dense and align themselves at the equatorial plate of the cell. The spindle forms and consists of microtubules that connect the centrioles to the kinetochores of the centromeres to prepare for chromosomal migration to opposite poles. In anaphase the centromeres divide, the sister chromatids separate, and the spindle contracts (possibly by actin–myosin interactions), pulling the now daughter chromosomes to opposite poles of the cell. Once the daughter chromosomes arrive at the poles, telophase begins. Cytokinesis, or division of the cell membrane, ensues with an invagination at the equatorial plate which culminates in cleavage of the membrane into two daughter cells with 2n chromosomes. A disturbance of chromosomal separation could cause an unbalanced number of chromosomes to occur in the daughter cells, which enter interphase and the remainder of the cell cycle.

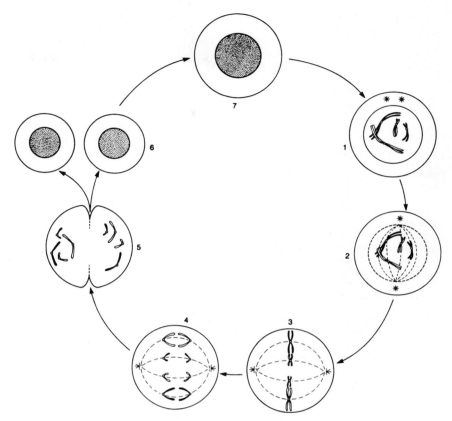

Figure 4–1. Stages of mitosis. Diagrams show two representative pairs of chromosomes. (1 = prophase; 2 = prometaphase; 3 = metaphase; 4 = anaphase; 5 = telophase; 6, 7 = interphase.) *(Reproduced, with permission, from Thompson MW, McInnes RR, Willard HF. Thompson and Thompson:* Genetics in Medicine, *5th ed. Philadelphia, W. B. Saunders Co., 1991: 22.)*

MEIOSIS

Meiosis is reduction cell division, which occurs only in gametogenesis (see Chapter 1). A primary spermatocyte, for example, with a diploid (2n) chromosomal complement replicates its DNA (4n) and ultimately becomes 4 haploid (n) sperm. Fertilization with a haploid oocyte results in a diploid zygote. In contrast to mitosis, in which two daughter cells are genetically identical to the parent cell, meiosis results in four daughter cells that have half the genetic complement of the parent (see Chapter 11).

Meiosis consists of two phases. Meiosis I involves a reduction division (Fig 4–2); in meiosis II no DNA duplication occurs but joined chromatids separate at the centromere, ending in haploid constituents (Fig 4–3).

Meiosis I

Prophase of Meiosis I. Duplication of DNA has occurred by this stage of meiosis I, resulting in a 4n complement.

Leptotene (4n). Leptotene (Greek *leptos*, slender, thin + *tainia*, band, tape) is the first stage of the prophase of meiosis I and is characterized by thin filamentous chromosomes arranged at random as they begin to condense. The outlines of meiotic chromosomes have alternating thick and thin regions called chromomeres, which form specific patterns for each chromosome.

Zygotene (4n). Zygotene (Greek *zygon*, joining + *tainia*) involves the joining (synapsis) of homologous chromosomes, which is absent in mitosis. The homologues align themselves in parallel according to corresponding points on each chromosome. An exception to crossing over between homologous chromosomes is that which occurs between the short arms of X and Y. The distal portion of the Y short arm (Yp) is largely homologous with Xp, thus undergoing crossing over during meiosis at about 20 to 30 times the normal rate between homologous X chromosomes. Apparent autosomal inheritance of genes in this region has coined the term "pseudoautosomal region" of Y.

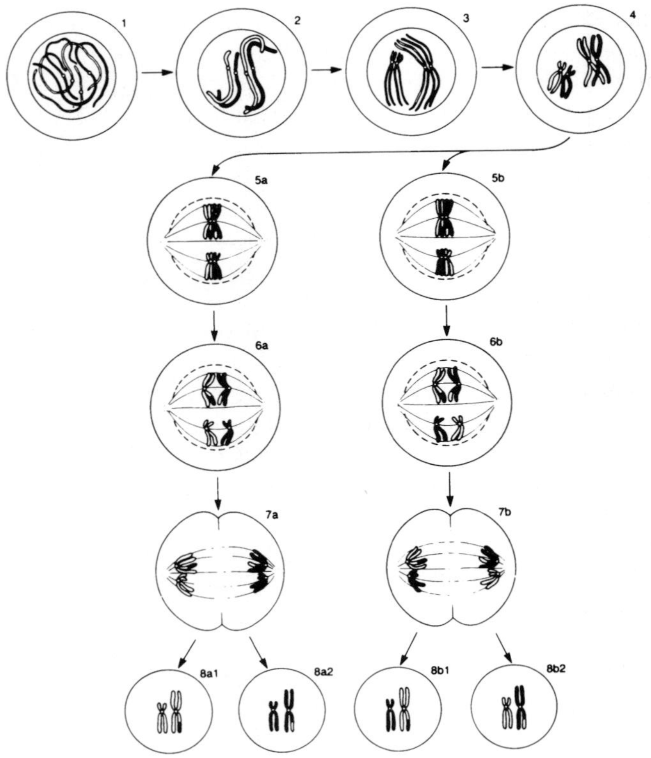

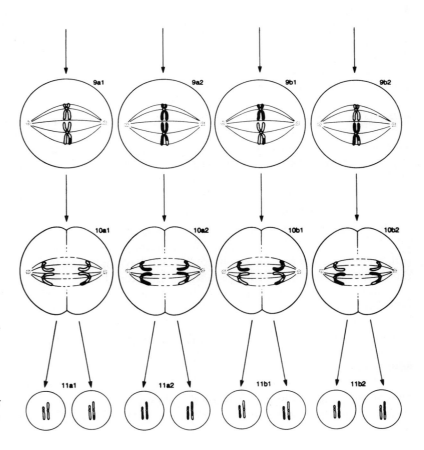

Figure 4–2. Stages of meiosis I. Diagrams show two representative pairs of chromosomes. Crossing over is shown in 4, 5a, and 5b; a and b illustrate alternate arrangements of chromosomal pairs following a single crossing-over event in the plates below. (1–4 = stages of prophase I: 1 = leptotene; 2 = zygotene; 3 = pachytene; 4 = diplotene and diakinesis. 5A and 5B = metaphase I; 6A and 6B = anaphase I; 7A and 7B = telophase I; 8A1, 8A2, 8B1, and 8B2 = possible chromosomal arrangements at completion of meiosis I.) *(Reproduced, with permission, from Thompson MW, McInnes RR, Willard HF. Thompson and Thompson:* Genetics in Medicine, *5th ed. Philadelphia, W. B. Saunders Co., 1991: 24.)*

Figure 4–3. Stages of meiosis II. Sequences a and b indicate possible arrangements of chromosomal arms following a single crossing-over event. (9 = metaphase II; 10 = anaphase II; 11 = eight possible gamete combinations at completion of meiosis II. *(Reproduced, with permission, from Thompson, MW, McInnes, RR, Willard, HF. Thompson and Thompson:* Genetics in Medicine, *5th ed. Philadelphia, W. B. Saunders Co., 1991: 25.)*

Pachytene (4n). During pachytene (Greek *pachys*, thick + *tainia*) the chromosomes thicken, coil tightly, and stain intensely, and the chrommomeres are more evident. What had appeared to be bivalents, or paired homologous chromosomes, are tetrads, which represent two chromatids per homologous chromosome. This stage is important because crossing over occurs and allows exchange of homologous parts of 2 of the 4 chromatids.

Diplotene (4n). In diplotene (Greek *diplous*, double + *tainia*) the chromosomes shorten and thicken, and each homologue begins to separate from its mate, but each chromosome (2 chromatids each) has an intact centromere. As the chromosomes separate, the parts of the arms which have crossed over, the chiasmata (*chiasma*, cross), overlap and hold the chromatid arms in close association to allow crossing over to be completed. At the conclusion of diplotene, chromosomes separate distinctly, and the chiasmata start to terminalize, or draw to the ends of the chromosomes.

Diakinesis (4n). Diakinesis (Greek *dia*, through + *kinesis*, movement) marks the last stage of prophase of meiosis I. The chromosomes coil and stain more densely, and terminalization is complete.

Metaphase I (4n). As in mitosis, the nuclear membrane disappears, and the chromosomes become aligned along the equatorial plate of the cell. In mitosis, duplicated chromatids (4n) are aligned at the equatorial plate without homologous pairing, but in meiosis, duplicated paired homologous chromosomes (4n) are aligned together.

Anaphase I (4n). Anaphase I begins with the separation of homologous chromosomes, or bivalents, toward opposite poles. Although homologous pairing occurs, the original parental chromosomes are sorted independently, so that a new cell has an equal chance of receiving the paternal or maternal chromosome. The separation of homologous chromosomes, which explains gene segregation, and the random arrangement of parental chromosomes, which explains independent assortment, demonstrate Mendelian laws of inheritance in meiosis I. The remainder of anaphase I is analogous to mitosis.

Telophase I (4n -> 2n). The mechanism of telophase I is similar to mitosis. This stage marks the completion of meiosis I in which each of two new cells has a haploid number of chromosomes. It should be noted that the term "haploid" refers to the number of chromosomes, not the number of copies of DNA. Strictly speaking, each chromosome contains 2 chromatids, but only one of the two homologous chromosomes remains in each cell.

Meiosis II

No interphase or DNA replication precedes meiosis II. The process parallels mitosis in that the centromeres divide and the chromatids migrate to opposite poles of the cell (Fig 4–3). Except for regions of crossing over in meiosis I, the chromatids in the daughter cells are identical. Thus, in meiosis, one replication of DNA ultimately results in 4 haploid daughter cells.

A significant feature of meiosis is the phenomenon of crossing over (Fig 4–2, sections 4, 5a, 5b). Since portions of chromosomal arms are translocated to the homologue, genetic variation can be increased. With independent assortment of parental chromosomes, 2^{23} or about 8 million combinations are possible in the gamete of one individual.[4]

GENETICS OF GAMETOGENESIS

Besides the differences in gamete production between spermatogenesis and oogenesis, aspects of meiosis differ in age of onset and tempo between males and females. Primordial germ cells migrate from the endoderm of the yolk sac to the genital ridges, associate with somatic cells, and form undifferentiated gonads. At the initial writing of this chapter in 1993, the location of testicular determining factor (TDF), a major determinant of testicular differentiation, was inferred to be on Yp. Recent evidence has confirmed that within TDF lies the sex-determining region of Y (*SRY*), the gene for determination of maleness, although other genes are necessary for complete testicular development (discussed later). In the absence of TDF and in the presence of putative ovarian determining genes, ovaries develop (see Chap 6).

Spermatogenesis begins at puberty and lasts potentially throughout the lifetime of an adult male in the Sertoli cell–seminiferous tubule complex. The genetic and cellular changes proceed from the periphery of the seminiferous tubule toward the lumen over about 64 to 75 days. Spermatogonia line the basement membrane of the tubule and are mitotically active stem cells; some are self-replenishing and others become primary spermatocytes, which enter meiosis. The end products of meiosis I are two secondary spermatocytes, which contain 23 chromosomes each. These cells promptly enter meiosis II, which is complete upon the formation of four spermatids. Spermiogenesis, the maturation of spermatids to spermatozoa, continues in a luminal direction, releasing flagellated sperm into the lumen. The older the father, the more cell divisions of the spermatogonia have occurred, and the greater is the likelihood that alterations in DNA may have occurred. Autosomal dominant disorders have been reported more frequently in offspring of men over 55 yr old (see section on paternal age below), after controlling for maternal age and birth order. An error of chromosome segregation in meiosis I causes four chromosomally unbalanced sperm, and in meiosis II two unbalanced and two normally balanced sperm result. Mitochondrial DNA is present in the sperm tailpiece and is not transferred to the zygote. In summary, gametogenesis in the male begins at puberty and may continue throughout adult life.

In contrast, meiosis in the female begins in fetal life, arrests in the second trimester, and resumes after puberty. Primordial germ cells in the cortex of the fetal ovary proliferate into oogonia, the germ cells around which follicles develop. Primary oocytes enter prophase of meiosis I asynchronously between 8 and 13 wk of gestation[5] and become arrested in the dictyotene (Greek *diktyon*, net + *taina*) stage[4] by about 28 wk. Follicular atresia in a chromosomally competent female begins at about 24 wk and oogonial atresia at about 28 wk of gestation, and no oogonia are usually present at birth. The number of primary oocytes is maximal at 6 to 7 million at about 20 wk of gestation, and follicular atresia reduces the number to about 1 to 2 million at term and about 300,000 at puberty. After puberty has occurred, follicle-stimulating hormone (FSH) recruits a cohort of follicles for each ovulatory cycle. After the midcycle luteinizing hormone (LH) surge but before oocyte release, meiosis I resumes by an incompletely understood mechanism, releasing the first polar body which transforms the primary oocyte into a secondary oocyte. The purported meiosis inhibitor may originate from the granulosa cells, since oocytes free from granulosa can complete meiosis. Meiosis II proceeds promptly but is suspended until fertilization occurs, whereupon the second polar body is extruded, resulting in a haploid ovum. Several important contrasts between the genetics of spermatogenesis and oogenesis should be emphasized. Oogenesis is maximal in midfetal life, limiting the number of gametes a woman will have in her lifetime. Unlike the four similar-sized sperm produced, the ovum receives most of the cytoplasm, compared to the polar bodies. Errors in chromosomal segregation in meiosis I or II in women cause abnormal ova. Moreover, the lengthy arrest of meiosis I for about 12 to 50 yr may predispose to errors in meiosis. The only source of mitochondrial DNA for the zygote is cytoplasm of the ovum, and mutations in the maternal template are likely to be transferred to the offspring.

CYTOGENETICS

The karyotype is a photomicrograph of the total number of chromosomes per cell of an individual, and karyotyping is the analysis of the abnormalities of chromosome number, structure, or rearrangement that can be evaluated by light microscopy. The centromere, a constriction of the chromosome, separates the chromosome into short (p) and long (q) arms. Each chromosome has a characteristic length and a location of the centromere which has given rise to systems for identification. Chromosomes in which the centromere is located in the middle are called metacentric; closer to one end than the other, submetacentric; and very close to one end, acrocentric.[6] The chromosomal portions of material in the short arms of acrocentric chromosomes are called satellites and staining may be helpful in cytogenetic diagnosis. Before chromosomal staining or banding techniques allowed individual identification of each chromosome, they were organized into groups of similar length and centromeric location, the Denver classification (groups A to G). Figure 4–4 shows a normal human male karyotype with both the chromosomal nomenclature according to the Denver Conference of 1960 and the current standard numerical classification based on the Paris Conference in 1971.[4]

Cytogenetic analysis requires that nucleated somatic cells multiply in culture. Peripheral blood leukocytes (PBL) are the most readily available source, but fetal cells in amniotic fluid, skin fibroblasts, or tissue sample are also adequate. Cell cultures of PBL are more short lived and may be less sensitive than other tissues in the detection of mosaicisms, such as detecting a Y cell line on mixed gonadal dysgenesis. A sample of PBL is heparinized, the buffy coat separated, placed in cell culture medium, and treated with a mitogen to stimulate proliferation, such as phytohemagglutinin.[4] After about 72 hr, dilute colchicine, which binds to tubulin, inactivates the spindle, and prevents the centromeres from dividing, is added to arrest the mitoses in metaphase. Chromosomes are the most densely coiled and folded in metaphase and are optimal for analysis by light microscopy. Addition of a hypo-osmotic solution causes swelling and rupture of the cells, and the chromosomes usually separate enough to analyze.

Staining of chromomeres gives the appearance of bands along the arms which are characteristic for each chromosome. Heterochromatin is noncoding chromatin that stains differently from normal euchromatin. Q banding uses quinacrine mustard or a similar agent to produce bright and dim fluorescent bands (Q bands). The heterochromatic region of Yq characteristically fluoresces brightly and documents at least that Y fragment. G banding is performed by treating the chromosomes with trypsin to denature the chromosomal protein and by staining with Giemsa. The patterns of dark and light bands (G bands) determine the chromosomal "signature." The dark G bands correspond to the bright Q bands. R banding results from heat pretreatment of the

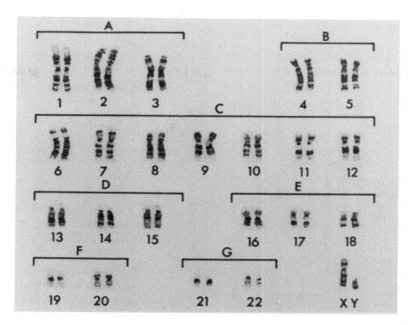

Figure 4–4.   Normal human male karyotype (46,XY) using Giemsa banding (G banding). Homologous somatic chromosomes 1–22 and the sex chromosomes are labeled individually according to the current Paris Conference nomenclature, and are grouped according to Denver Conference nomenclature previously used. *(Reproduced, with permission, from Thompson JS, Thompson MW. Genetics in Medicine, 4th ed. Philadelphia, W. B. Saunders Co., 1986: 12.)*

chromosomes followed by Giemsa staining, giving reverse bands from G banding. C banding stains the centromere and other heterochromatin. NOR (nucleolar organizing regions) staining selectively stains the 18S and 28S ribosomal genes in the satellites of the acrocentric chromosomes.

Since prophase and prometaphase chromosomes are not coiled as densely as those in metaphase, the stained bands will be farther apart. Since the greater distance between bands allows greater resolution of each band, more bands can be analyzed. So-called high-resolution banding (800 to 1400 bands) permits greater precision in determining the breakpoint of a rearrangement or abnormal chromosomal morphology than by metaphase (about 200) analysis. The cell cycle is blocked in the S phase and the block removed in late prophase or prometaphase.

Alterations in chromosome morphology are described by standard terminology. Table 4–1 lists the abbreviations and descriptions of the most common terms of cytogenetic nomenclature. These terms apply to the actual chromosomal mapping sites. For example, 45,X/ 46,XY denotes mixed gonadal dysgenesis, a mosaicism containing the two cell lines 45,X and 46,XY. The term 46,XY, del 15q11-q12 refers to a deletion on the long arm of chromosome 15, including positions q11 and q12, which occurs in Prader–Willi syndrome.

SEX CHROMOSOMES

X Chromosome

X Chromatin.   In 1949[4] Barr and Bertram found that a chromatin mass was present more often in the nerve cells of female cats than in males. Barr and associates later noted this X chromatin, or Barr, body in most somatic mammalian cells, including human cells. Since all but one X chromosome is inactive during interphase in somatic cells, X chromatin represents the condensed, inactivated X chromosome(s). Therefore, the number of X chromatin masses should be one less than the total number of X chromosomes in the karyotype, regardless of the number of Y chromosomes. For example, in 45,X and 46,XY, there are no X chromatin masses; in 46,XX, there is one; in 47,XXX, there are two; and so forth. However, in female germ cells both X chromosomes remain active, but the single X in male germ cells is inactivated.

X chromatin is most conveniently evaluated by a buccal smear, a fixed stained smear of cells from the epithelium of the inside of the cheek. The percentage of cells exhibiting X chromatin is recorded. Although the buccal smear may be useful, it is now performed infrequently by laboratories, and its precision depends in part on the quality control of the laboratory. In general, more complete information about the chromosomal constitution of an individual can be obtained by karyotype analysis than by the buccal smear.

X Chromosome Inactivation (Lyon Hypothesis).

Why does a woman who is homozygous for a gene express no more gene product than an individual with only one X (eg, 46,XY and 45,X)? Why is a woman who is homozygous for an X-linked disorder no more severely affected than a hemizygous individual? These two enigmatic questions about X chromosomal inheritance have been explained by the hypothesis of X chromosome inactivation.

Mary Lyon has recently reviewed[7] the hypothesis she originally stated[8] in 1962, which is based on the following observations in human somatic cells:[3]

1. X inactivation appears to occur early in embryonic life. A normal human female contains a mosaicism of cells with only one active X chromosome per cell. Inactive X chromosomes are dense and replicate late, thus forming the X chromatin mass at interphase. The timing of inactivation in human embryonic life is uncertain but inactivation has been detected in the implanted blastocyst by days 9 to 12 of embryonic life.
2. X inactivation is essentially complete and appears to proceed from an inactivation center throughout the length of X. Studies of X-autosome translocations in mice have shown that not only does the translocated portion of X not containing the inactivation center remain activated, but the autosomal fragment translocated to X will be inactivated. However, in humans at least 2 genes on distal Xp are not inactivated: Xg[a] blood group antigen and steroid sulfatase, and some genes on Xq26 that maintain ovarian function, are spared. The nature of the spreading signal is unknown, but 5-methylation of cysteine DNA residues may occur. Therefore, X inactivation is an active process requiring a signal and does not result from just a loss of activity.
3. Random X inactivation generally occurs: that is, either X[m] or X[p] may be inactivated. However, exceptions to this principle are as follows: a structurally abnormal X (as with a deletion) will usually be inactivated, but in an X-autosome translocation the structurally normal chromosome is inactivated; nonrandom inactivation may also depend upon the embryological age and type of tissue.
4. X inactivation is permanent and clonally propagated. Inactivation may affect either X[m] or X[p] in different cell lines in the same individual, but once inactivation occurs, the cell line retains the inactivated chromosome.
5. Based on X-autosome translocations in mice, X reactivation with aging has been reported.[7] The significance of this phenomenon in humans has yet to be determined.

Clinical results of X inactivation are dosage compensation, variable expression in heterozygous females, and mosaicism. X inactivation explains why a 46,XX female produces the same amount of gene product from X as a 46,XY male, but it alone does not account for abnormal phenotypes in 45,X or 47,XXY individuals. Two possible explanations are that the initiation of the abnormalities occurs prior to X inactivation and that the original X inactivation was nonrandom in cell lines with an abnormal number of chromosomes. Although random X inactivation might be thought to produce equivalent proportions of cells expressing and not expressing an abnormal X-linked gene, carrier females can exhibit phenotypes ranging from incomplete to complete expression. A symptomatic carrier is called a manifesting heterozygote, who is said to have unfavorable Lyonization. Differential X inactivation results in mosaicism with respect to the active X. Cell culture of fibroblasts may demonstrate each population of cells with its own gene expression. Some genes are not inactivated, such as the Xg blood group and steroid sulfatase. Interestingly, these genes have been mapped to distal Xp, which may not be inactivated and may indicate the mechanism of meiotic pairing with Y.

Y Chromosome

Since a normal Y chromosome seems to be necessary for testicular development and male fertility, genes encoding for testicular determining factor(s) (TDF) and spermatogenesis would be expected to be found on Y. Indeed, the "Holy Grail" of current research on Y has been the discovery and mapping of these genes.

The Y chromosome comprises about 60 million base pairs (bp), or about 1 percent of the human genome.[9] Y is cytogenetically divided into three portions: the short arm (Yp), the centromere, and the long arm (Yq) (Fig 4–5A). The specificity of cytogenetic and molecular markers depends upon the uniqueness of the portion of Y to which they bind, and the sensitivities depend upon the amount of DNA necessary for detection. Since Y fragments may have partial deletions, testing with a panel of markers to various regions of Y may increase the predictive value of a negative result.

Yp. Yp contains several important regions, and none of Yp fluoresces with quinacrine staining. The distal end of Yp comprises about 2.5 million bp and is largely homologous with Xp. These homologous regions undergo crossing over during meiosis, at about 20 to 30 times the normal rate between homologous X chromosomes. Apparent "autosomal inheritance" of genes in this region has brought about the term "pseudoautosomal region" of Y. Using various Y DNA probes, a molecular map has been proposed for the regions presumably including TDF (*SRY*) and other important functional regions of Yp (Fig 4–5B).

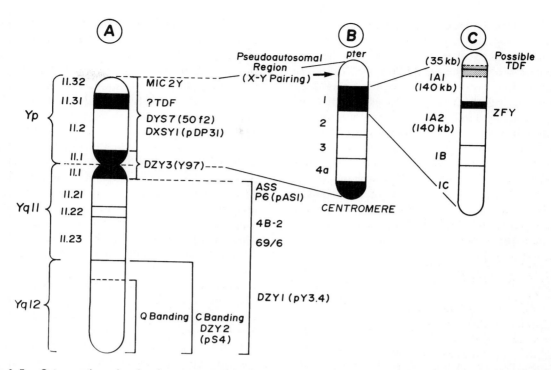

Figure 4–5. Cytogenetic and molecular anatomy of the human Y chromosome. **A.** Cytogenetic and partial molecular map of the Y chromosome. The euchromatic short arm, Yp, contains the pseudoautosomal and probably the testicular-determining regions. The shaded area represents the heterochromatic centromere, which contains Y-specific alphoid sequences that fluoresce with quinacrine staining. Yq11 is the nonfluorescing euchromatic proximal long arm. Most of Yq12, the heterochromatic distal long arm, fluoresces with quinacrine, and the whole segment is identified with C-banding. *(Adapted, with permission, from McDonough PG, Tho SPT, Trill JJ, et al. Use of two different deoxyribonucleic acid probes to detect Y chromosome deoxyribonucleic acid in subjects with normal and altered Y chromosomes.* Am J Obstet Gynecol. *154:744, 1986; and Tho SPT, McDonough PG. Use of Y DNA probes to identify children at risk for dysgenetic gonadal tumors.* Clin Obstet Gynecol. *30:674, 1987.)* **B, C.** Detailed representative molecular map of the short arm of the Y chromosome (Yp), emphasizing the pseudoautosomal pairing region and the putative testicular- or sex-determining region of Y (*SRY*). The pseudoautosomal pairing region on distal Yp undergoes crossing over with its homologous region on Xp at meiosis. ZFY (zinc-finger Y), spanning segments 1A1 and 1A2, was a previous candidate for *SRY. SRY* is currently thought to reside within a 35-kb segment of distal 1A1. Please see text for details. *(Adapted, with permission, from McLaren A. The making of male mice.* Nature. *351:96, 1991.)*

The TDF gene or genes probably either direct or modulate the development of Sertoli cells and have been postulated to reside on Yp. Mapping of the putative TDF gene has been accelerated by study of at least two abnormalities in nature: 46,XX sex-reversed (SXR) males and 46,XY females (eg, Swyer's syndrome).[10] Page et al[11] performed chromosomal mapping of the deletions or breakpoints, which indicate missing or translocated TDF. Their results suggested that TDF, formerly hypothesized within the region of zinc-finger Y (ZFY, Fig 4–5C), is located proximal to the pseudoautosomal region and distal to ZFY within 1A2 (Fig 4–5C). The ZFY gene encodes a protein with multiple finger-like domains, is homologous with a similar gene on X (ZFX), and had been initially thought to contain TDF. More recently, Koopman and colleagues[12] isolated the human gene *SRY*, which is now considered TDF and has been mapped to a 35-kb segment in region 1A1

(Fig 4–5C) just proximal to the pseudoautosomal boundary region of Y (PABY). Incorporation of the mouse homologue *SRY* into the genome of chromosomally female mice induced both testicular and phenotypic male development.

Y-specific probes have hybridized with DNA from 60 to 80 percent of 46,XX males. Failure of hybridization in the remaining males may occur in the presence of a very small portion of Y to which no probes are available, 46,XX/46,XY (or altered Y) chimeras in which the 46,XX cell line was preferentially selected for testing, or true hermaphroditism with 46,XX karyotypes, which have generally shown no hybridization with the available Y DNA probes. In situ hybridization has shown translocation to Xp in some patients, suggesting a paternal error in meiosis I or Y-autosome translocations. As Y DNA in this region continues to be sequenced, the structure of TDF will likely be completed.

Y probes defining regions proximal to region 1 have identified single-copy DNA which is either Y-specific or which also hybridizes to other chromosomes. In the most proximal region, probes have been hybridized to repeating segments of DNA, suggesting that the further distal on Yp, Y-specific single-copy DNA is present. Most but not all 46,XY females have a cytogenetically normal Y, but some patients have small deletions or alterations in Y. Some patients in both groups have not hybridized with Y-specific probes, but the failure to detect a deletion or alteration may result from the insufficient power of the probes to resolve micro- or point mutations or from a mutation of an autosomal gene which permits testicular development without *SRY*. The complexity of testicular development was demonstrated in a recent interesting report, in which a patient with ambiguous genitalia, ovotestes, and a 46,XY karyotype underwent testing of peripheral blood leukocytes for the presence of PABY, ZFY, and *SRY* and gonadal tissue for *SRY*.[13] All three parts of *SRY* were present in leukocytic DNA. The sequenced *SRY* products from the patient and the father were identical with the published sequence. In the PCR product of the patient's gonadal DNA, the wild-type and two postzygotic point mutations were present, which always occurred together. One mutation was silent and the other encoded for an amino acid substitution from leucine to histidine in part of the gonadal tissue, which was presumed to confer a loss of the testicular-determining function of the gonad. Other studies have indicated that other genes are involved in testis expression, including *SRY*-related high-mobility group (HMG) box gene (*Sox9*), mutations of which have been associated with autosomal sex reversal and campomelic dysplasia, a disorder with severe skeletal malformations resulting in death by about 2 years of age.[14] The protein encoded by *SRY* has a DNA-binding sequence, the HMG box, which suggests that it is a transcriptional factor that changes the expression of other genes by binding to their DNA and causing a conformational change.[15] Most sex-reversing mutations of *SRY* reduce its binding to DNA or the bending it causes, and the mutations seem to prevent that change from occurring. The genes steroidogenic factor 1 (*SF-1*) and Wilms' tumor 1 (*WT1*) are necessary for early gonadal development and for the formation of the adrenals and kidneys, respectively. A proposed explanation has been that *SRY* and other genes operate in sequence or in a cascade, each one regulating another "downstream." In summary, successful testicular development is complex and depends upon not only *SRY*, which appears to be the necessary and sufficient gene on Y, but also upon other genes, implied by the presence of a normal *SRY* in most females with 46,XY pure gonadal dysgenesis and its absence in a small number of phenotypic 46,XY and 46,XX males.[16]

Y Centromere. The centromere fluoresces with quinacrine staining. The centromeric region DYZ3 represents tandemly arranged repeating units of 170 bp, called alphoid sequences (Fig 4–5A). Alphoid sequences probably occur in most chromosomes but are chromosome specific. The probe Y97 defines a Y-specific 5.5-kb fragment product of an *Eco*RI digest present in about 100 copies on the Y centromere.

Yq. Quinacrine staining cytogenetically separates Yq into two segments: the nonfluorescent euchromatic (band Yq11) and fluorescent heterochromatic (band Yq12) regions (Fig 4–5A). As noted in Table 4–2, three probes to single-copy sequences in the euchromatic region have been cloned: pAS1 (or ASSP6), 4B-2, and 69/6. About 60 to 70 percent of Y DNA consists of repeating segments, or heterochromatin, which vary in length according to the individual. These DNA sequences seem unrelated to TDF, because normal phenotypic males may have deletions of Yq12. DZY1 and DZY2 are Y-specific and have been used for clinical diagnosis.

TABLE 4–2. REPRESENTATIVE DNA PROBES TO REGIONS OF Y

Y Region	DNA Probe	Restriction Enzyme	Cytogenetic Map
Yp	MIC 2Y		Yp 11.32
	Putative TDF gene (*SRY*)	*Hind*III, *Eco*R1, *Bam*HI, *Sal*I	Yp 11.31 - 11.2 (or just proximal to pseudoautosomal region)
	Y-280[10]	*Hind*III	Yp
	Y-286[10]	*Hind*III, *Eco*R1	Yp (and Yq)
	p50 f2 (or DYS7)		Yp 11.2
	pDP 31 (or DXYS 1)	*Taq*1	Yp 11.2
Y centromere	Y 97 (or DYZ 3)	*Eco*R1	Yp 11.1, Yq 11.1
Yq11 (euchromatic)	pAS1 (or ASS P6)	*Eco*R1	Yq 11.21
	4B-2	*Eco*R1, *Hind*III	Yq 11.22
	69/6	*Eco*R1	Yq 11.23
Yq12 (heterochromatic)	pY 3.4 (or DYZ 1)	*Hae*III	Yq12
	pS4 (or DYZ 2)	*Hae*III, *Mbo*I	Yq12

D = DNA; X = X chromosome; Y = Y chromosome; S = single copy; Z = repetitive copy DNA; 1,2,3,... = published order of cloned sequence.

TABLE 4–3. PATTERNS OF GENETIC INHERITANCE

Inheritance Pattern	Type of Disorder	Risk of Affected Offspring	Risk of Carrier Offspring	Examples	Comments
Mendelian (single-gene) disorders	Autosomal recessive (AR)	1:4 in obligate carrier parents	1:2 in obligate carrier parents	Sickle-cell disease Cystic fibrosis Tay–Sachs disease 21-OHase deficiency	Homozygotes for abnormal allele are symptomatic Heterozygotes are usually asymptomatic carriers Risk increased with consanguinity
	Autosomal dominant (AD)	1:2 with affected parent	Not applicable	Neurofibromatosis Huntington's chorea Achondroplasia Marfan syndrome	Heterozygotes and homozygotes express trait Penetrance—expression of abnormal gene in an offspring (qualitative) Expressivity—degree to which an offspring will manifest the abnormal trait (quantitative) Spontaneous mutation rate may be significant and vary by disorder
	X-linked recessive (XLR)	1:2 for child at risk (46,XY; 45,X, homozygote) given carrier mother	1:2 for carrier daughter given carrier mother	Hemophilia A Duchenne muscular dystrophy Red-green colorblindness	Females with intact 2nd X usually are asymptomatic Symptomatic: 46,XY; 45,X; homozygous female Spontaneous mutation rate may be significant Transmission may appear to skip generation
	X-linked dominant (XLD)	1:2 for child given affected parent	Not applicable	Ornithine transcarbamylase deficiency Incontinentia pigmenti Fragile X syndrome	Single gene on X will be expressed
Chromosomal abnormality	Translocation, inversion, insertion, deletion, shift, ring, isochromosome, mosaicism, chimera	Depends on anomaly (see text)	Variable	45,X/46,XY gonadal dysgenesis	See text
Multifactorial		Depends on anomaly (see text)	Variable	Neural tube defect (NTD)	See text

H-Y antigen, previously thought to be TDF, is probably located on Yq and may be related to spermatogenesis in man. In mouse, H-Y protein is related to spermatogenesis, not testis formation. Another important Y-specific testicular product is Müllerian inhibiting factor (MIF), or anti-Müllerian hormone (AMH), a peptide hormone produced by Sertoli cells, which completes Müllerian regression by about wk 10 of fetal life. The MIF gene has been mapped to Yp19.

INHERITANCE PATTERNS

Inherited disorders are generally classified into one of three categories: single-gene (Mendelian) disorders, chromosomal abnormalities, or multifactorial or polygenic inheritance. The types of disorders in each category are summarized in Table 4–3. When a suspected abnormality is encountered in the patient's personal or family history, it is helpful to obtain a detailed pedigree. Published experience suggests that discussing each family member, living or dead, and any offspring is more likely to identify an abnormality than by asking general questions, such as "Has anyone in your family had any birth defects?" For more details about constructing a pedigree and about inheritance patterns, the reader may consult other sources.[3,17]

Single-Gene Disorders

Mendelian disorders are caused by a single mutant gene and are classified by chromosomal location and expression.

Autosomal disorders result from mutations on chromosomes 1 through 22, and sex- (or X-) linked disorders from mutations on X. In a dominant disorder, expression of a trait requires that only one of the two homologous genes be mutant (heterozygosity), but a recessive disorder requires two mutant genes for expression (homozygosity). Traits, but not genes, are dominant or recessive, because carrier states are often detectable in heterozygotes, as with sickle hemoglobin. Mutational mechanisms include deletion, insertion, or substitution. These changes can affect translation into protein in one of several ways. If the change in DNA encodes for a different amino acid (missense mutation), the amino acid sequence of the protein product will be altered, which may affect its properties. If the base change results in a stop codon (nonsense mutation), a truncated abnormal protein is produced. Deletion of one base pair may cause a shift in the reading frame (frame shift mutation) and usually produce an abnormal protein as well.

Chromosomal Anomalies

Chromosomal anomalies are gross, genomic alterations in chromosomal number or structure and are usually detectable by cytogenetic techniques. Euploidy refers to the presence of the normal diploid number of chromosomes. Polyploidy is the presence of multiples of the haploid number of chromosomes other than diploidy (2n), such as triploidy (3n = 69) or tetraploidy (4n = 92). Aneuploidy is an abnormal chromosome number other than a multiple of n, such as trisomy (2n + 1) or monosomy (2n − 1). Aneuploidy usually results from nondisjunction, or the failure of chromosomes to separate during cell division. The causes of nondisjunction are unclear, but the risks are increased with advancing maternal age, suggesting that alterations may be increased with prolongation of arrest of prophase of meiosis I. Nondisjunction may occur in meiosis I or II with different consequences. If nondisjunction occurs in meiosis I, two of the four gametes will have two homologous chromosomes and the other two will lack either one. Nondisjunction in meiosis II results in one gamete lacking either chromosome, another with two chromosomes from the same parent, and two with one chromosome each from the other parent. Fertilization of gametes from a meiotic I error will always have trisomic or monosomic offspring, whereas fertilization of gametes from a meiotic II error will result in monosomy in 25 percent, trisomy in 25 percent, and euploidy in 50 percent of conceptuses.

Anaphase lag is nondisjunction that occurs in mitosis that leads to mosaicism, or daughter cell lines with an unbalanced number of chromosomes (45,X/47,XXX). An autosomic trisomic cell line is more likely to persist than a monosomic one; X chromosome monosomy is the most common surviving monosomic cell line.

Structural chromosomal abnormalities may involve one or more chromosomes. Translocations are the most common types of structural chromosomal abnormalities, the most common being reciprocal and Robertsonian translocations. A reciprocal translocation represents an exchange of chromosomal material between chromosomal arms at the respective breakpoints, leaving the total amount of genetic material unchanged. Robertsonian translocations involve the joining of two acrosomic chromosomes (those in which the centromere is located near the end of chromosome) at short arms or at centromere (chromosomes 13, 14, 15, 21, 22). Chromosomal rearrangements may be balanced so that a parent may have complete genomic DNA, a balanced complement of genes. However, during meiosis, gametes of translocation carriers become unbalanced and may lead to chromosomally abnormal liveborn or stillborn offspring, pregnancy losses, normal children, and carrier children. Karyotyping could be done on affected offspring or the pregnancy losses, but since this information is usually unavailable, the parents are usually karyotyped, in hopes of finding a carrier of a balanced chromosomal rearrangement.

Inversions, insertions, deletions, duplications, ring chromosomes, and isochromosomes are the other major chromosomal anomalies. An inversion involves two breaks in a single chromosome; a pericentric inversion involves the centromere, a paracentric inversion does not. An insertion requires at least three breaks in two chromosomes. A deletion is the loss of chromosomal material. Duplications involve attachment of a duplicated chromosomal arm to the end of the parent arm. Ring chromosomes are special cases of deletions in which terminal deletions occur and the remaining ends rejoin. Rings are often unstable through cell division unless they contain a centromere. Isochromosomes occur when an abnormal cleavage of the centromere results in the loss of either the short or the long arm and persistence of the other.

Detection of subtle deletions and other anomalies that often accompany these anomalies may require higher resolution banding than that provided with routine karyotyping, even with special dyes or fluorochromes. High-resolution banding is achieved by arresting chromosomal condensation prior to metaphase, so that the arms will be longer and the staining bands will be farther apart. The requesting physician should communicate the clinical impressions to the laboratory. If a mosaicism is suspected, then at least 50 cells should be counted or other tissue obtained. Some high-volume laboratories may karyotype only a few cells. Some disorders such as Prader–Willi syndrome have deletions that may require high-resolution banding for detection.

Multifactorial Inheritance

Multifactorial inheritance does not follow strict Mendelian laws and is thought to involve multiple genes with or without influence from environmental factors. Recurrence risks usually depend upon the relationship between the fetus at risk and the affected family member, and perhaps the sex and number of previously affected family members.

Example: Neural Tube Defect. The background risk in the United States, in general, for neural tube defect (NTD) is 1 to 2 per 1000 live births. In the Southeast United States, the risk is 3 to 4 per 1000, and in the United Kingdom about 8 per 1000. With a positive family history on the maternal side, the risk is 10 per 1000; and on the paternal side, 5 per 1000. With a previously affected child, the risk is 20 per 1000; with two previously affected children, it climbs to 60 per 1000. Typical recurrence risks for multifactorial disorders with a previously affected child range from about 2 to 6 percent but depend upon the specific disorder.

NTD can be associated with specific syndromes, such as with Mendelian inheritance patterns (Meckel–Gruber syndrome) or with chromosomal anomalies (certain trisomies—about 1 percent recurrence risk with full trisomy). In the case in which an otherwise multifactorial disorder occurs as part of a syndrome, the recurrence risk is usually governed by that of the syndrome. When there is no identifiable syndrome, the risk follows that of the multifactorial disorder.

PRENATAL GENETIC DIAGNOSTIC TESTING

Since the 1960s, the increasing expectations of parents for a "perfect" child, the ability to evaluate the fetus with increasing accuracy, and the legalization of abortion have fostered the development of techniques with more diagnostic accuracy about the fetus than before 1960. Having the information, however, has not altered the ethical and moral decisions that the knowledge makes possible. Indeed, the obstetrician-gynecologist has come under increasing medicolegal pressure to identify patients at risk for fetal abnormalities and provide or recommend further genetic counseling. The risk of a fetal anomaly may be increased because of a chronic maternal disease (eg, diabetes mellitus), a history of exposure to a risk factor (retinoic acid), an affected family member (neural tube defect), or demographic or ethnic status (Ashkenazi Jewish ancestry).

Preconception or antenatal counseling may be indicated for a variety of reasons, which may be initiated by the patient's concern or elicited by the physician's thorough family and medical history. Many physicians have begun to use detailed questionnaires at the initial office visit, both for obstetric and gynecologic patients. Construction of a pedigree involves all close relatives, living or dead, and helps avoid missing inheritable disorders or pregnancy losses. Compared to risk assessment from history or mathematical principles alone, laboratory techniques such as cytogenetics, enzyme analysis, high-resolution ultrasound, and molecular analysis may provide increased diagnostic accuracy about the fetus. Molecular analyses have even made possible prenatal diagnosis in future pregnancies from stored tissue samples (eg, blood or skin fibroblasts) from affected family members in the event of their death. The usual invasive procedures by which tissue samples are obtained for testing of existing pregnancies are amniocentesis and chorionic villus sampling.

Amniocentesis

Diagnostic amniocentesis involves the removal of amniotic fluid for prenatal diagnosis and should be a familiar procedure to obstetrician–gynecologists. In the first half of pregnancy, amniotic fluid reflects the composition of maternal plasma.[18] As pregnancy progresses, phospholipids and desquamated cells (amniocytes) from the fetal epidermal, respiratory, and gastrointestinal epithelia accumulate. The ionic composition changes throughout pregnancy, and the mean volume at 12 wk is about 50 ml. Any interruption in the epidermal or vascular integrity, such as with a neural tube defect, may allow exudation of fetal serum into the fluid. The factors regulating amniotic fluid volume are probably multiple, but a significant source seems to be the amnion and transudation across the fetal skin. After about 4 mo of gestation, fetal urine output and swallowing appear to affect the flux. Because changes in the fetus may affect amniotic fluid volume or composition, sampling of the fluid may provide diagnostic information.

The main components of amniotic fluid are the amniocytes and the fluid itself. The karyotype of nucleated amniocytes grown in cell culture generally reflects the fetal karyotype. Because the success of cell culture depends upon how well the amniocytes proliferate, poorly growing cell lines, such as mosaicisms, may be underrepresented. Rarely do maternal cells proliferate preferentially to amniocytes resulting in an inappropriate 46,XX karyotype. Amniocytes can also be tested for enzymatic activity in cases of suspected congenital enzyme deficiencies. Prenatal diagnosis is also aided by analysis of amniotic fluid constituents, such as alpha-fetoprotein (AFP) and acetylcholinesterase (AChE). Specific components, such as 17-hydroxyprogesterone in the diagnosis of 21-hydroxylase deficiency, can be measured as needed.

Recommendations for timing of amniocentesis seek to balance fetal safety against the maternal risk of abortion, which increases with gestational age. Amniocentesis can technically be done any time in gestation that an adequate fluid sample can be obtained and leave enough fluid for fetal survival. Amniocentesis traditionally has been performed between about 14 and 17 wk of gestation so that the cytogenetic analysis can be completed before 20 wk of pregnancy for a relatively safe abortion. In order to diagnose fetal abnormalities at an earlier gestational age for a less risky abortion, early amniocentesis has been performed between 7 and 15 wk of gestation,[19,20] with results comparable to standard amniocentesis. Because studies have defined "early amniocentesis" by different ranges of gestational ages, interpretation of the data should take these differences into account. In a recent review of studies of early amniocentesis,[21] the recommended technique involved ultrasound-guided aspiration of about 1 cc of amniotic fluid per week of gestational age. Successful amniocenteses were accomplished with one needle insertion in 89 to 96 percent of pregnancies, and repeat procedures were needed in only 0.6 to 3.5 percent. Bleeding after amniocentesis occurred in 0.6 to 5 percent of procedures, but one third had bleeding prior to amniocentesis. Delayed complications were noted in about 2.8 percent of patients. Premature rupture of membranes occurred in about 1.1 percent of patients, and the risk increased with a coexisting viral syndrome or vomiting. Procedure-related pregnancy loss rates ranged from 0.4 to 2.3 percent. Perinatal complications and congenital anomalies were not increased over those of the general population. The authors suggested possible confounding risk factors in early pregnancy diagnostic procedures: selection bias requiring early prenatal care may contribute to pregnancy loss; advanced maternal age, longer observation times, and specific indications for early diagnostic testing may appear to increase loss rates; and abnormal symptoms prior to amniocentesis may adversely influence pregnancy outcomes. As with routine amniocentesis, early amniocentesis had a low rate of maternal contamination and pseudomosaicism, and allowed for testing of amniotic fluid AFP and AChE, unlike CVS. Culture failure rates ranged from 0.32 to 1.6 percent. Despite lower numbers of amniocytes with decreasing gestational age, modified culture techniques have allowed a mean culture time of 8.8 days. Detection of chromosomal abnormalities was reported from 1.1 to 3.3 percent, with culture artifacts usually less than 1 percent.

Good data regarding amniotic fluid levels of AFP and AChE are available as early as 13 wk, and data from earlier than 13 wk should be forthcoming. Amniotic fluid AFP below 0.6 multiples of the median (MOM) was associated with aneuploidy (trisomy 21) in 8.7 percent of the samples tested at 10 to 15 wk of gestation (n = 476).[22] The interpretation of AChE detected in samples from 11 to 14 wk is currently unclear. An inconclusive band on electrophoresis for AChE was found in 10.6 percent of samples, higher than the 2.5 percent rate later in gestation, and was associated with 20 percent of fetal anomalies, compared with 56 percent. Burton and colleagues[23] reported 5 unexplained false-positive assays for AChE in 93 samples from 11 to 14 wk (5.4 percent) with normal AFP, suggesting that detection of AChE before 15 wk with normal AFP does not likely indicate an open neural tube defect.

Rebello and colleagues[20] compared karyotypes of 114 consecutive amniotic fluid samples taken from 12 to 14 wk of gestation with 114 samples taken from pregnancies 15 wk or later. A difference of about 1 percent was found between the early and standard amniocentesis groups, regarding times to harvest (12.2 versus 10.6 days, respectively) and times to report (21.8 versus 20.8, respectively). No difference was found between pregnancy loss rate, procedure failure, pseudomosaicism, maternal cell contamination, or cytogenetic anomalies.

Improved amniocyte culture techniques have made karyotyping possible with as little as 10 ml of fluid. As more amniocenteses are performed, normative data for alpha-fetoprotein levels in maternal serum and amniotic fluid can be established. Indications for amniocentesis are similar to those for chorionic villus sampling, but analysis of the amniotic fluid itself can be performed only by amniocentesis. The procedure-related pregnancy loss rate of amniocentesis should be no greater than 1 in 200 (0.5 percent).

Chorionic Villus Sampling

Chorionic villus sampling (CVS) was developed out of a felt need to diagnose fetal abnormalities in the first trimester and provide abortion at a less risky gestational age than that available with amniocentesis. CVS can be used for the same chromosomal, enzymatic, or genetic indications as amniocentesis but not when analysis of amniotic fluid is required, such as AFP. Chorionic villi are part of the trophoblast, which derives from the same progenitor cells as the fetus, and theoretically the genetic findings should be as representative of the fetus as amniocentesis is. The villi are sampled from the chorion frondosum, which can be accessed transcervically before the chorion laeve fuses with the basalis at 11 to 12 wk. Villi can be obtained transcervically, transabdominally, and transvaginally. Transcervical sampling was reported first,[24] but transabdominal and transvaginal sampling appear to complement the former technique in some cases of fundal placentas or anteflexed uteri and retroflexed uteri.

Some of the concerns about CVS have included obtaining an adequate number of cells, success of cell growth in culture, how well the karyotype of the villi correlates with that of the fetus, maternal safety, and risk of fetal loss. Failure of amniocytes and villus cells (mesenchymal core cells) to grow in culture is rare. In fact, CVS cultures usually grow more rapidly (5 to 8 days) than amniocytes. Rapid "in situ" karyotype preparations can be performed with cytotrophoblast cells, but the metaphases have been reported as poorer than those from cell cultures. Maternal contamination is also rare but should be minimized by dissecting villi from decidua under a dissecting microscope.

Abnormal karyotypes of villi do not always correlate with the fetal karyotype. A seven-center collaborative study in the United States[25] obtained cytogenetic diagnoses on 6008 of 6033 (99.6 percent) successful CVS samples. Of the 1671 cases evaluated by direct and culture methods, 9 (0.54 percent) had discrepancies. Seven of the 9 had abnormal direct preparations that were normal by trophoblast cell culture, as well as in 5 of 7 cultures of amniotic fluid or fetal tissue. Two of the 9 normal direct studies had an abnormal karyotype (tetraploidy and nonmosaic trisomy 18) in cell culture. Mosaicism was found in 0 of 852 control patients but in 50 of the 6008 cases (23 direct, 23 cell culture, 4 both) (0.83 percent for CVS, compared to 0.25 percent usually reported[26] with amniocentesis). In 7 of 30 (23.3 percent) that underwent culture of amniotic fluid or fetal blood, the mosaicism was confirmed. None of 10 (0 percent) direct preparations were verified, but 7 of 18 cultures were (38.9 percent). Pseudomosaicism was defined as the presence of an aneuploidy in only one cell of a direct study or culture or in multiple cells of a single culture. Pseudomosaicism was found in 107 of 6008 samples (1.8 percent, versus 1.3 percent with amniocentesis) and was not thought to be clinically significant. Overall, the direct method seems to have higher false-positive and false-negative rates than cell culture. Maternal cell contamination occurred in only 2 of 3884 (0.05 percent) direct karyotypes and in 35 of 3777 (0.93 percent) cell cultures. Follow-up amniocentesis may be required to resolve a discrepancy from CVS in 1 percent or less of patients.

At least three recent prospective trials have compared CVS and amniocentesis. In a prospective controlled NICHD study[27] comparing amniocenteses (n = 651) with transcervical CVS (n = 2235), amniocentesis resulted in cytogenetic diagnoses in 99.4 percent of cases and CVS in 97.8 percent (P <0.05). (Randomization was not offered for ethical considerations.) CVS was unsuccessful in 49 patients (n = 40 with sample <1 mg villi, and n = 9 with laboratory failure). Amniocentesis was performed in 0.8 percent (n = 17) of women who had had an ambiguous diagnosis from CVS. Aneuploidy was diagnosed in 1.8 percent of pregnancies evaluated with CVS, compared to 1.4 percent by amniocentesis. Two diagnoses of aneuploidy were falsely positive in normal infants.

No diagnostic errors occurred regarding major aneuploidies (21, 13, and 18), sex chromosome aneuploidies, chromosomal structure, or fetal sex, but the phenotypes were ascertained by newborn examinations alone. The excess procedure-related loss rate of CVS over amniocentesis was 0.8 (80 percent confidence interval = 0.6 to 2.2 percent), not statistically significant. The loss rate of chromosomally normal fetuses after one CVS attempt was 2.9 percent and increased proportionally to 10.8 percent with three or four passes.

In the Canadian Collaborative CVS–Amniocentesis Trial Group,[28] 2787 women were randomized to either transcervical CVS (n = 1391) or amniocentesis (n = 1396). Maternal cell contamination of the cell culture did not result in a diagnostic error in either study. The procedure-adjusted loss rate for CVS was 7.6 percent compared with 7.0 percent for amniocentesis, not statistically significant. Other fetal or neonatal outcomes, such as preterm delivery, growth retardation, and gestational age-related mean birthweights, were similar between the groups. Unlike the NICHD study, aneuploidy was present in 4.5 percent of CVS karyotypes and 2.4 percent of amniocenteses (P <0.01). The procedure-related fetal loss rate from transcervical CVS ranges between 3 and 4 percent. The same rate with abdominal CVS has ranged between 2 and 3 percent, but fewer centers have been performing the procedure.

In the Medical Research Council European trial of CVS,[29] 3248 women seeking prenatal diagnosis were recruited prospectively and randomized between CVS (n = 1609) and amniocentesis (n = 1592), as long as the diagnosis could be made by either method (3201 singleton pregnancies with known follow-up were ultimately analyzed). CVS was performed transcervically in 72 percent and transabdominally in 28 percent of women. The mean gestational age for performing CVS was 71 days (35 to 59), compared with 112 (105 to 122) for amniocentesis. Patients undergoing CVS had more than one insertion (31 versus 6 percent) than with amniocentesis, required second procedures more often (100 versus 35), and diagnosed mosaicisms more frequently (9 versus 2.9 percent). No statistical comparisons between these groups were reported. Nonmosaic karyotypic anomalies were found in 3.5 percent of CVS and in 2.7 percent of amniotic fluid samples. Nonmosaic trisomy 18 was diagnosed more frequently by CVS (n = 10) than by amniocentesis (n = 3), suggesting placental aneuploidy unrelated to the fetus, but 4 fetal karyotypes confirmed the diagnosis. Mosaic abnormalities were found in 1.6 percent (n = 18) and 1.2 percent (n = 12) of CVS and amniotic fluid samples. Since chromosomal rearrangements were diagnosed more often in CVS samples than expected for advanced maternal age, confirmation by amniotic fluid or fetal blood sampling and karyotyping of the parents was recommended.

Only 3 cases of maternal cell contamination in CVS samples and 2 in amniotic fluid were suspected, for a rate of about 0.5 percent. Regarding pregnancy outcome, first-trimester CVS reduced the chance of a normal live-born child by 4.6 percent (95 percent CI 1.6 to 7.5, P <0.01) compared to amniocentesis. This difference was attributed to more spontaneous fetal deaths before 20 wk, elective abortions for chromosomal anomalies, and delivery between 20 and 28 wk gestation, than amniocentesis. The analyses were unable demonstrate that the fetal loss rate was different depending on the route of sampling, and failed to show an increase in fetal limb abnormalities after sampling between 56 and 66 days.

In summary, CVS has been associated with a low rate of fetal loss, comparable to or possibly slightly greater than amniocentesis. Inadequate tissue sampling requiring repeat sampling seems more likely. CVS may detect a placental aneuploidy, which may not reflect the fetal karyotype, and require a second diagnostic procedure. The optimal route of sampling has not been determined, but skill is required in all methods because placental sites will have a variety of presentations. Tissue samples from CVS can be used for cytogenetic, enzymatic, or molecular analysis. Testing of the amniotic fluid, for example for AFP, contraindicates CVS. With the increasing availability of amniocentesis between 10 and 14 weeks, the utility of CVS may become more limited than it is now.

CLINICAL APPLICATIONS OF MOLECULAR BIOLOGY TECHNIQUES

Review of Molecular Biology

The advent of techniques in molecular biology has allowed investigators to increase the precision by which diagnoses of certain genetic disorders can be made, above that which can be deduced from classical principles, empiric associations, or cytogenetic analyses.[2] Understanding the following terms can help illustrate the major principles of molecular biology.

Gene Structure. Chromosomes comprise linear arrangements of genes, the structural and functional units of inheritance, interspersed with other nucleotide sequences. Genes are DNA sequences that are transcribed into RNA and translated into proteins. Normally, each member of a gene pair (allele) derives from its respective parent chromosome; genes segregate to separate chromosomes, never the same one. Genes also undergo independent assortment during meiosis, that is, homologous genes on the maternal and paternal chromosomes in an individual recombine randomly.[4] About two thirds of human DNA is single copy, but less than 5 percent encodes for the estimated 10,000 to 100,000 genes. The re-

maining DNA is composed of repetitive sequences of uncertain significance, but characteristic segment lengths have been helpful in gene mapping and clinical diagnosis.

The human genes consist of exons and introns, sequences that result in coding or no coding, respectively, for amino acids (Fig 4–6). A gene with four exons would have three introns. The nucleotide sequence determines the direction of transcription, which occurs from the 5' (left or upstream) to the 3' (right or downstream) deoxyribose units.

The region 5' to the initiation of transcription (initiation codon) is called the 5' untranslated region and contains the promoter, a nucleotide sequence located about 300 to 400 bp 5' to the initiation codon. The region 3' to the end of transcription (stop codon) is designated the 3' untranslated region. The promoter fixes the start of transcription and may control the amount of RNA available and tissue specificity of transcription. The promoter may contain consensus sequences, such as TATA (or "TATA box"), about 25 to 30 bp 5' to the initiation codon, and seems to designate the initiation, or "cap," site. A modified nucleotide (7-methyl guanosine) is added to cap the 5' end of the RNA. Occasionally, the sequence CCAAT ("cat box") is located 75 to 80 bp 5' to the initiation codon and appears to regulate gene expression. Enhancers of transcription usually lie in the 5' untranslated region, but may be found within the gene itself or distant from the gene in either direction.

Other consensus sequences determine the positions of the introns. Introns usually begin with GT (splice donor sites) and end with AT sequences (splice acceptor sites). Splicing is the removal of introns and rejoining of exons. The consensus sequence AATAA in the 3' untranslated region is the signal for polyadenylation of RNA. The addition of multiple adenosine units (poly A tail) to the 3' end of RNA is necessary to permit it to leave the nucleus. Regulators of gene expression may exist on the same (*cis*-acting elements) chromosome or a different (*trans*-acting factors) one.

In principle, every nucleated somatic cell contains identical DNA (excluding random mutations), but certain genes are expressed only in specific tissues. The various regions of DNA exposed to RNA polymerase (the enzyme that transcribes DNA to messenger RNA) may be tissue specific and related to its tertiary structure. Alternately, tissue-specific elements in the 5' untranslated region may help regulate gene expression.

Transcription. RNA is similar to DNA except that it is single-stranded, ribose replaces deoxyribose, and uracil (U) is substituted for thymine. RNA occurs in three forms: messenger RNA (mRNA), transfer RNA (tRNA), and ribosomal RNA (rRNA). Transcription requires separation of double-stranded DNA (dsDNA) into single strands (ssDNA). The nuclear enzyme RNA polymerase II (pol II) unwinds a small portion of dsDNA and transcribes ssDNA into mRNA in the 5' to 3' direction (Fig 4–7).

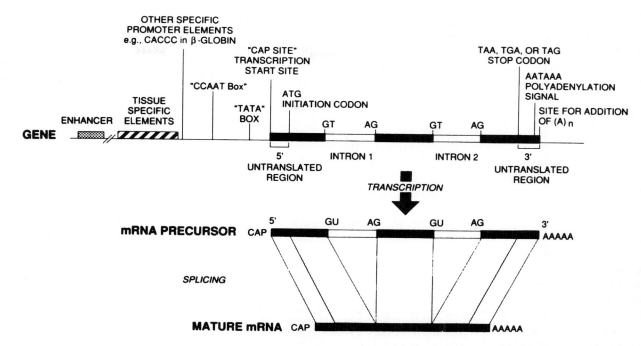

Figure 4–6. Structure of a model gene with its regulatory elements and transcription products. This gene has three exons and two introns, which begin with GT and end with AG. Note that **GT** in DNA is transcribed to G**U** in RNA. The introns are spliced out of the precursor mRNA resulting in the mature message product. Promoter elements and enhancers may be tissue specific. *(Reproduced, with permission, from Gelehrter TD, Collins FS.* Principles of Medical Genetics. *Baltimore, Williams and Wilkins, 1990: 91.)*

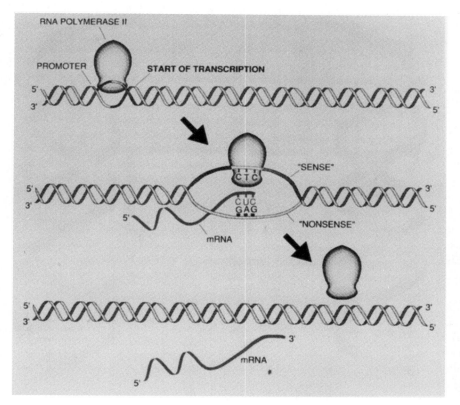

Figure 4–7. Transcription of DNA into RNA. RNA polymerase II recognizes the specific promoter sequence at the 5' end of a gene and transcribes DNA into mRNA in the same 5' to 3' direction as the DNA is read. The resulting "sense" strand of RNA has a sequence parallel to the 5' to 3' strand, whereas the complementary 3' to 5' "nonsense" strand serves as the template. *(Reproduced, with permission, from Gelehrter TD, Collins FS.* Principles of Medical Genetics. *Baltimore, Williams and Wilkins, 1990: 14.)*

TABLE 4-4.   THE GENETIC CODE TRIPLET tRNA CODONS CORRESPONDING TO AMINO ACIDS

Position 1 (5′ end)	Position 2				Position 3 (3′ end)
	U	C	A	G	
U	Phe	Ser	Tyr	Cys	U
	Phe	Ser	Tyr	Cys	C
	Leu	Ser	STOP	STOP	A
	Leu	Ser	STOP	Trp	G
C	Leu	Pro	His	Arg	U
	Leu	Pro	His	Arg	C
	Leu	Pro	Gln	Arg	A
	Leu	Pro	Gln	Arg	G
A	Ile	Thr	Asn	Ser	U
	Ile	Thr	Asn	Ser	C
	Ile	Thr	Lys	Arg	A
	Met	Thr	Lys	Arg	G
G	Val	Ala	Asp	Gly	U
	Val	Ala	Asp	Gly	C
	Val	Ala	Glu	Gly	A
	Val	Ala	Glu	Gly	G

Ala = alanine; Arg = arginine; Asn = asparagine; Asp = aspartic acid; Cys = cysteine, Gln = glutamine; Glu = glutamic acid; Gly = glycine; His = histidine; Ile = isoleucine; Leu = leucine; Lys = lysine; Met = methionine; Phe = phenylalanine; Pro = proline; Ser = serine; Thr = threonine; Trp = tryptophan; Val = valine.
(Reproduced, with permission, from Gelehrter, TD, Collins, FS. Principles of Medical Genetics. *Baltimore, Williams and Wilkins, 1990: 15.)*

Because of the complementarity of DNA, the strand that ultimately encodes for the protein is designated the "sense" strand and the complementary strand, the "antisense" strand. The pol II enzyme uses the antisense template so that the mRNA will reflect the order of the sense strand. As transcription occurs, pol II adds nucleotides to the growing chain and ultimately releases the completed mRNA. The dsDNA reforms and resumes the double helix. Complementary DNA (cDNA) is made from an RNA template by reverse transcriptase and is antisense. Upon completion of transcription, the introns are spliced out at the donor and acceptor consensus sites noted earlier. The AATAAA sequence initiates polyadenylation, resulting in mRNA without introns containing the poly-A tail.

Translation. The translation of mRNA into protein is based on the triplet genetic code, in which amino acids are encoded by an ordered sequence of three nucleotides (codon) (Table 4–4). With 4 nucleotides arranged in three possible sequences, 4^3 or 64 possible combinations exist. The association of more than one codon with each of the 20 amino acids is called a degenerate code.

Specific consensus sequences mark the sites of initiation and termination of translation. The gene codon ATG (AUG for RNA) signals the start of translation, and any of three codons (TAA, TAG, or TGA) signals the end. Proper recognition of these, or any, codons requires that they be read "in frame." A reading frame is one of the three possible ways of interpreting or translating codons, and an open reading frame refers to a series of codons without a stop codon. For example, the sequence -UUU-CCC- could be read -UUU-CCC-, -UUU-CCC-, or -UUU-CCC- depending on the initiation site. An open reading frame is required until the protein is translated. If a stop codon occurs prematurely, then a truncated defective protein would likely result. If a base substitution occurs that alters the amino acid sequence, the protein could be altered significantly. An example of a base substitution resulting in a marked alteration in protein product is in hemoglobin S. Substitution of thymine for adenine changes the encoded amino acid from glutamic acid to valine at the sixth amino acid, causing a conformational change and sickling of the β-chain of hemoglobin.

Translation of mRNA to protein actually occurs in the cytoplasm on the ribosomes (Fig 4–8). Presumably, the poly-A tail facilitates movement from the nucleus to the cytoplasm. After identification of the initiation codon (AUG) by rRNA, translation proceeds in the 5' to 3' direction, corresponding to the amino terminus and the carboxy terminus of the protein, respectively. The tRNA links a specific codon (called an anticodon) complementary to that on mRNA to each amino acid, according to the genetic code. When an anticodon on tRNA hybridizes to its complement, the linked amino acid is enzymatically added to the growing peptide chain. The ribosome proceeds along the mRNA until a stop codon is reached, and the completed protein is released. To the extent that certain proteins, such as insulin, are synthesized in precursor forms, they are modified to produce the biologically active form.

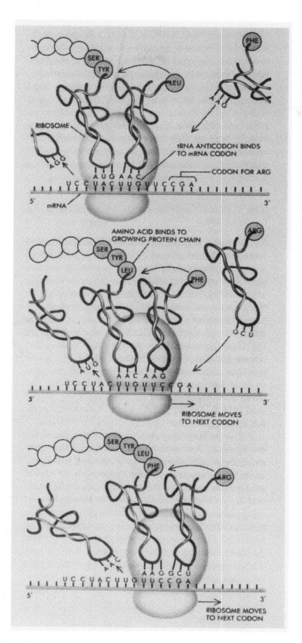

Figure 4–8. Translation of RNA into protein. As the ribosome moves along the growing polypeptide chain, the triplet codon on mRNA undergoes base pairing with the anticodons of transfer RNA linked to amino acids. The amino acid is added to the protein and the transfer RNA is released from mRNA. *(Reproduced, with permission, from Watson JD, Tooze J, Kurtz D. Elucidation of the genetic code. In: Recombinant DNA: A Short Course. New York, Scientific American Books, 1983: 37.)*

Recombinant DNA Technology

Restriction Enzymes. Much of recombinant DNA technology derives from the complementarity of its base pairs. As noted, complementarity refers to the unique pairing of different nucleotide bases with one and only one

counterpart. The discovery of restriction enzymes catapulted progress in molecular biology. Restriction enzymes are bacterial enzymes that cleave specific nucleotide sequences, based on a unique nucleotide order and number of bases. The sequences are palindromic, meaning that the order of bases (5' to 3') is the same along the sense strand as on the antisense strand in the same direction. The likelihood of occurrence of a given sequence is indirectly proportional to its length, so enzymes that cut longer sequences cut farther apart and produce longer fragments. In any individual the cut sites are specific and produce fragments of reproducible length. The term "restriction" indicates that the cutting is restricted to foreign DNA.

For example, the enzyme *Eco*RI (from *E coli* RY13) cuts the sequence

$$5'\text{-}G^*AATTC\text{-}3'$$
$$3'\text{-}CTTAA^*G\text{-}5'$$

at the *, giving

$$5'\text{-}G \quad AATTC\text{-}3'$$
$$3'\text{-}CTTAA \quad G\text{-}5'$$

*Eco*RI will only cut the 6-nucleotide sequence ("6-cutter") between the guanine and adenine. If a mutation alters the cut site (eg, **C** for A, giving GCATTC), the restriction enzyme will not recognize the altered site and pass on to the next site, producing a longer fragment compared with that cut at the unaltered site. The unpaired bases resulting from the cleavage form "sticky" ends, which promote binding with other sequences for cloning.

Molecular Probes

Probes are DNA sequences complementary to the sense strand of a gene or to RNA and can be derived by several methods. Probes are usually labeled (with radioactivity or an enzyme) to identify the sequence in question. If a mutant gene is sought and if the normal gene has been cloned, then the probe can be constructed from a portion of the gene sequence common to both genes. If the gene has not been cloned, then producing a probe can be involved. If a gene is likely to be expressed in a tissue, then obtaining cDNA clones may be possible. Using the genetic code to deduce possible cDNA sequences from a limited amino acid sequence of the protein product, short (14 to 30 bp) ssDNA sequences, or oligonucleotides, can be synthesized. Because the genetic code is degenerate, many combinations may need to be produced and used to screen for hybridization. The reader is referred to additional sources for more specific information about cloning and probe production.[3]

Blotting Techniques

In general, blotting techniques allow detection and characterization of molecular fragments. Three types of blots have been developed to analyze their respective species:

Southern blots for DNA, Northern blots for RNA, and Western blots for protein. Detection requires a known complement to the substance of interest, such as a cDNA probe for DNA or RNA or a monoclonal antibody raised against its epitope. The probe must be labeled, usually radioactively, so that its binding can be identified. Characterization requires electrophoretic separation of the fragments of various sizes so that a probe can hybridize or an antibody can bind to its complement, which can be visualized as a single band migrating a reproducible distance on a gel. The intensity of the band is an approximate indication of concentration of the unknown species compared to a standard. Electrophoresis is a method of separating molecular fragments through a "sieve" or matrix (gel) based on molecular size or weight. Movement of the frag-

ments occurs upon exposure to an electrical field placed across the gel. The net charge on the fragments determines, in part, the direction of migration. The rapidity of the movement is determined by the molecular weight. The blot itself consists of DNA, RNA, or protein fragments bound to a solid phase, such as a nitrocellulose membrane.

Southern Blots. Southern blotting uses probes, or ssDNA sequences from genes of interest, to detect its complement within genomic DNA, the number of copies of the sequence, and the possibility of mutations. Because the blot can be hybridized many times and over a period of years, DNA can be stored for diagnostic testing in the future.

The Southern blot is performed as outlined in Figure 4–9. Double-stranded genomic DNA is extracted from

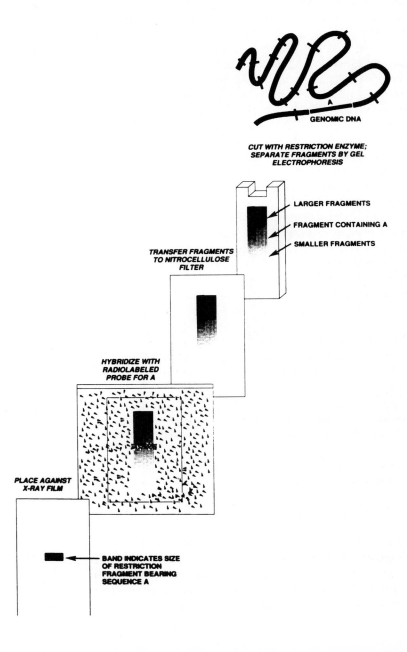

Figure 4–9. Southern blotting. This technique allows detection of a specific genomic fragment (denoted as gene *A*) in a mixture of about 1 million fragments. *(Reproduced, with permission, from Gelehrter TD, Collins FS. Principles of Medical Genetics. Baltimore, Williams and Wilkins, 1990: 77.)*

nucleated cells, such as leukocytes. The DNA is cut with a restriction enzyme into many fragments, which are separated by electrophoresis on an agarose gel. Electrophoresis separates molecular fragments through a "sieve" or matrix (gel) based on molecular size or weight. Movement of the fragments occurs when fragments are exposed to an electrical field placed across the gel, and the net charge on the fragments determines, in part, toward which pole they will move. The rapidity of the movement is inversely proportional to the molecular size. Control sequences of known length are added to the gel as a standard. Ethidium bromide is added to visualize the DNA by ultraviolet light by insinuating itself, or intercalating, between bp. The gel appears as a smear, because it cannot resolve the many DNA fragments from cut genomic DNA. DNA must be single stranded to hybridize with a probe, so the gel is denatured with alkali. The DNA in the gel is transferred by capillary action to a nitrocellulose membrane, the Southern blot, to which it is permanently bound by baking. A labeled DNA probe—usually labeled with radioactive ^{32}P—is denatured and hybridized to the membrane. After washing the blot to remove nonspecifically hybridized probe, the blot is placed next to x-ray film for an extended period of time and developed, a process called autoradiography. A band results wherever the probe has hybridized, indicating the presence of the DNA sequence or gene. If the restriction enzyme leaves the gene intact, one band should result, but if it cuts within the gene, two or more bands usually occur. Mutations that can be detected are single-point mutations if they occur within the restriction site and any rearrangement at least 50 to 100 bp, which would result in a change in band size. The greater the intensity of the band, compared with single-copy control sequences, the greater the number of copies of the gene are present. Homozygosity or heterozygosity may be determined as well.

Northern and Western Blots. Northern blotting is similar to Southern blotting, except that cDNA probes hybridize with RNA fragments. Preservation of RNA is challenging because of RNases, cellular enzymes that can rapidly degrade RNA. Tissue must be snap frozen to minimize degradation. Northern blotting is used to determine gene transcriptional activity. Western blotting is a sensitive technique that ultimately determines mRNA translation into protein. Protein fragments are separated by electrophoresis and hybridized with labeled antibodies. The remainder of the process is in principle similar to Southern blotting.

Restriction-Fragment Length Polymorphisms

Polymorphisms are benign normal mutations of DNA segment length, which are transmitted in a Mendelian manner. When a polymorphic gene is linked closely with a restriction site, the restriction endonuclease produces

a fragment of different length than the wild-type gene, but the fragment length must be great enough for the gel to resolve the difference in fragment length or size. However, if the polymorphism affects the restriction site, the enzyme will not recognize it, pass on to the next site, and produce a longer fragment than if the site was recognized (Fig 4–10).

By definition, alteration of the restriction site does not adversely affect the individual, only fragment size in vitro. In order for a band to be visualized, a probe must hybridize to a portion of the fragment. The bands that result from the action of restriction endonucleases are called restriction fragments, and polymorphisms that result in a gain or loss of a restriction site will usually be the most informative in diagnosis. Therefore, restriction fragment-linked polymorphisms (RFLPs) are mutations that alter restriction sites, but not the biologic activity of genes, and lead to fragments of different length than those associated with the normal gene.

Linkage disequilibrium is a factor in how informative an RFLP can be. During meiotic crossing over, the farther apart two genes reside on a given chromosome, the more likely they are to cross over. The closer the genes are, the more likely they are to remain linked during crossing over. Linkage disequilibrium refers to the likelihood that two closely linked genes will remain

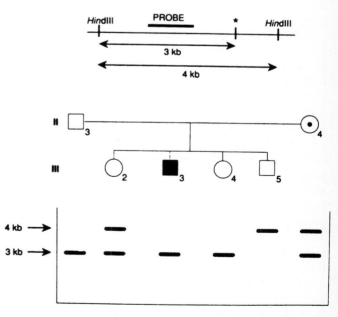

Figure 4–10. Diagram of an RFLP in an intron of the factor VIII gene as it relates to a family with a carrier mother and affected son. In the upper figure the asterisk indicates a polymorphic site, a benign mutation on one of the alleles of the gene, causing a difference in cut sites by the restriction enzyme *Hind*III, resulting in different fragment lengths. The results from the Southern blot indicate that individual III-2 is not a carrier for hemoglobin A. *(Reproduced, with permission, from Gelehrter TD, Collins FS.* Principles of Medical Genetics. *Baltimore, Williams and Wilkins, 1990: 81.)*

linked. In order for RFLPs to be informative, a particular fragment length must uniquely segregate with the mutant gene, or disease state, and another fragment with the normal gene or absence of disease. In addition, an informative RFLP requires heterozygosity in the family: at least one affected, one heterozygous, and one unaffected member. Since the gene itself cannot be tested, family studies must be used. It is important to emphasize that the RFLP does not cause the disorder, but is just linked to a fragment that segregates with the disorder. The sequence of the gene in question need not be known, nor need it be linked to the restriction site. The closer the mutation is to the restriction site, the more likely the fragment will segregate with the disorder and will be informative.

In Situ Hybridization

In situ hybridization involves the detection and localization of nucleic acid or protein in intact tissue. The technique is most commonly used with metaphase chromosomes for gene mapping[3] and with tissues to detect mRNA transcript. The benefits of this procedure are its relative ease of execution, the requirement of relatively small quantities of sample, the production of a visual signal, and its ability to localize a gene to a band with high-resolution banding. Its disadvantages include the requirement of a known gene sequence, relative insensitivity compared with Southern or Northern blotting, and its semiquantitative signal.

When used for gene mapping, molecular probes for cloned gene sequences are labeled usually with radioactive isotopes such as tritium, or with a fluorescent marker by hybridizing fluorescent streptavidin to a biotinylated cDNA probe. The latter technique, fluorescent in situ hybridization (FISH), has become a powerful tool used in reproductive genetics, analysis of tumor DNA, and mapping the human genome.[30] After metaphase chromosomes are fixed on a slide and denatured, the labeled probe is allowed to hybridize. The image is recorded with autoradiography or by fluorescence microscopy, and the intense focus of signal is the location of the gene sequence on the chromosome. Initially, FISH was used only with metaphase chromosomes whose bands range in size from 1 to 5 megabases (Mb), thus limiting the resolution to detecting DNA sequences at least 1 Mb apart. More recently, the resolution has been increased by using FISH with interphase nuclei, free chromatin, DNA fibers, and mechanically stretched chromosomes,[31] which has permitted detection of sequences separated by as little as a few kilobases. By using dyes with different colors, more than one DNA sequence can be localized simultaneously and, if contained on the same chromosome, their relative positions can be determined. With its sensitivity and resolution, FISH has been used to detect microdeletions and microduplications.

An interesting adaptation of FISH called chromosome orientation and direction fluorescence in situ hybridization (COD-FISH) has been used to detect pericentric inversions.[32] A single-stranded probe is hybridized to one and only one chromatid of a metaphase chromosome aligning with the 5'-to-3' direction. Since an inversion contains reversed DNA sequences, the probe would be detected as a change in direction of the signal within the inversion, compared to a reference probe outside the inversion on the chromosome.

The uses of FISH in reproductive genetics have been numerous. FISH can been used to screen for multiple aneuploidies or polyploidies, such as in prenatal diagnosis in uncultured chorionic villus cells and amniotic fluid cells.[33] Over 10,000 cases have been evaluated with FISH resulting in 90 percent of attempted analyses giving informative results with high detection rate and low false-positive and false-negative rates. Some unresolved problems include occasional technical failures, mixture of maternal blood, and up to 20 percent uninformative scoring results. Presently, FISH should probably be viewed as an adjunct to classic cytogenetics and might best be used as a screening test. Chromosomal rearrangements have been detected, such as in a recent report of a patient with clinical Down syndrome with an apparently normal karyotype.[34] FISH detected an unbalanced translocation t(15;21)(q26;q22.1) of paternal origin, the balanced form of which was found in the father, brother, sister, and her fetus. Finally, FISH holds promise for forensic use in sexual molestation and assault cases. A prospective blinded controlled study used FISH to detect sperm and non-sperm male cells in cervicovaginal smears from 40 women after reported postcoital intervals.[35] FISH, using X and Y chromosome-specific probes, identified sperm and/or non-sperm male cells in all specimens from women who reported having had intercourse for up to 3 weeks after intercourse, even when the partner had had a vasectomy. In comparison, cytology identified sperm in 41 percent of women who had reported having had intercourse and none beyond 2 weeks.

Since detection of a gene in genomic DNA tells nothing about the gene function on a particular tissue, in situ hybridization can also be used to assess mRNA transcription in cells. Formalin-fixed tissues can be tested, but with most molecular biology techniques, snap-frozen tissues avoid molecular alterations by fixatives and RNA degradation by RNases. Since a cDNA probe hybridizes with sense DNA and mRNA, essentially all of the cytoplasmic signal represents transcript and at most two copies of the gene give a minimal nuclear signal. Documentation of mRNA and translation into protein, using monoclonal antibodies, help confirm gene activity in cells.

Polymerase Chain Reaction

Polymerase chain reaction (PCR) allows rapid, exponential amplification of a DNA sequence (gene) from as little as a single copy of the sequence. Southern blotting requires about 5 to 7 µg of DNA and about a week to perform, but PCR can amplify ng amounts of DNA within a day.

Gene amplification by PCR requires that the gene sequence or the borders of the gene (primers) be available. Primers are 20- to 30-bp strands of ssDNA, which are complementary to the 3' ends of each strand of the dsDNA to be amplified. PCR involves three steps: denaturing the DNA into single strands by heating, hybridization of the primers by cooling, and synthesis of the complementary strand by reheating (Fig 4–11). The necessary primers, substrates, probe, and restriction enzyme are placed into a chamber (thermal cycler) programmed to change temperatures quickly. Upon heating to 94 °C, DNA denatures into single strands. Abrupt cooling to 37 to 55 °C allows the primers preferentially to hybridize with the complementary ends of the DNA sequence in question before the entire DNA molecule rehybridizes. At 72 °C, a DNA polymerase (such as *Taq* I [*Thermus aquaticus*] polymerase) adds the triphosphate nucleotides to the ends of the primers and completes the synthesis of the new complementary DNA strands. Since *Taq* I is stable at 72 °C, the cycles can be repeated without replenishment of the enzyme. With each PCR cycle one strand of dsDNA gives rise to two strands of dsDNA, such that the final number of dsDNA strands will be 2^n, n being the number of cycles. In less than a day, 30 PCR cycles can produce over 1 million copies of the gene, which can be identified without using a probe on a Southern blot. Sequences a few kb in length up to 10 kb have been successfully amplified. Factors complicating PCR amplification include incomplete strand formation and contamination with DNA from within the laboratory environment.

Applications. PCR has a variety of uses in clinical genetic diagnosis. It can amplify a suspected gene from as little as a single copy of genomic DNA, thus requiring a minimal specimen. PCR can be used to identify RFLPs for clinical genetic diagnosis. In diseases with point or other small mutations that Southern blot analysis cannot resolve, oligonucleotide probes synthesized for the normal and mutated genes are called allele-specific oligonucleotide probes. These probes can be hybridized to PCR products in dot blots. In an autosomal recessive disorder, the affected person would hybridize only the mutated probe, a heterozygous person both probes, and a homozygous unaffected person the normal probe. In diseases such as cystic fibrosis the most common mutations can be sought. In disorders involving mutations in different sites of a gene amplification of several segments can be accomplished with multiplex PCR.

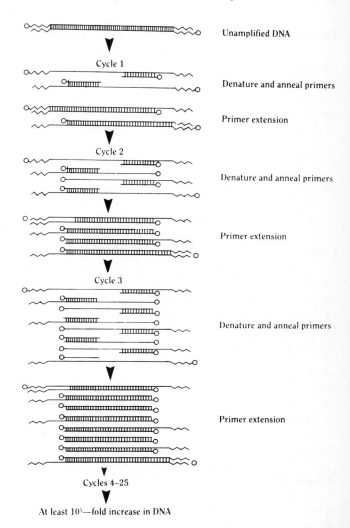

Figure 4–11. Diagram of the polymerase chain reaction (PCR). Oligonucleotide primers are represented by small rectangles on the inner aspect of the single strands of DNA, and complementary base pairing is illustrated by crosshatching. *(Reproduced, with permission, from GeneAmp Polymerase Chain Reaction Diagram, Perkin-Elmer Corporation, Norwalk, Ct., Spring 1990, p 4.)*

Although Southern blot analysis has been used in the diagnosis of infectious diseases, PCR has recently been successfully applied. Human immunodeficiency virus (HIV), Lyme disease, and human papillomavirus (HPV) are among several diseases that can be diagnosed with PCR.

Other uses for PCR in molecular biology include gene mapping, cloning, DNA sequencing, and amplifying DNA or RNA from a single cell. PCR has also been used in denaturing gradient gel electrophoresis, which can detect single-bp mutations that alter the DNA melting point. Clinical PCR can amplify a sequence from genomic DNA from an embryonic blastomere for diagnosis of a molecular defect (eg, sickle-cell disease) or for fetal sexing using Y-specific probes.

Summary. The ability to diagnose carrier states and exclude affected fetuses has improved from classical Mendelian principles to a relatively high degree of certainty, largely because genes are being mapped and sequenced and probes developed. Table 4–5 lists representative diseases for which molecular techniques have improved the diagnostic accuracy over that of standard techniques. When probes for actual genes (or critical regions) are not available, then family linkage studies need to be performed and usually require DNA from an affected family member. Forethought should be given to obtaining blood or tissue from such individuals in the event that prenatal testing is desired at a later time.

Hypervariable Minisatellite Regions or Variable Number Tandem Repeats

Although most RFLPs result from a gain or loss of a restriction site, the number of noncoding repeating DNA sequences usually varies according to the individual. Hypervariable minisatellite regions, or variable number tandem repeats (VNTRs), are sequences of several hundred copies of DNA that do not encode for protein. If a restriction site is near tandem repeats, it may give rise to fragments of a characteristic size for an individual. This technique already has forensic applications for DNA "fingerprinting"[36] in combination with PCR.

Selected Clinical Genetic Disorders

Androgen Insensitivity Syndrome. The gene for the human androgen receptor (hAR) has been mapped to the X chromosome (Xq11-12),[37,38] and abnormalities in androgen receptor action comprise the various clinical presentations of the androgen insensitivity syndrome (AIS) (see Chap 13). Genetic males present with a spectrum of phenotypes from normal external female genitalia (complete AIS, Fig 4–12) to incomplete masculinization or normal but infertile males (incomplete AIS, Fig 4–13). In the classic paper by Morris,[39] genetic males had female external genitalia, female breast development, an absent proximal vagina and other Müllerian structures, and abdominal or inguinal testes. They may have absent or minimal axillary or pubic hair, and the breast tissue, which is often prominent, usually has glandular abnormalities. Serum testosterone (T) and other androgen levels are normal or elevated, and T and dihydrotestosterone (DHT) may bind normally or abnormally to androgen receptors. Serum luteinizing hormone (LH) values are normal or elevated because of androgen insensitivity, and follicle stimulating hormone (FSH) levels are normal or elevated. Common presenting symptoms include an inguinal mass or amenorrhea. Patients with complete AIS are raised as females. Because the risk of malignant gonadal neoplasia appears to be small and since puberty is negotiated more smoothly with the endogenous gonadal steroids, gonadectomy is delayed until puberty is completed. If the diagnosis is made prior to completion of puberty, close observation is nevertheless prudent.

Patients with incomplete AIS may present with female, ambiguous, or male genitalia in infancy. Since androgen production and aromatization to estrogens are not impaired, patients with incomplete AIS may have findings similar to complete AIS or phallic enlargement at birth and varying degrees of feminization or virilization at puberty. Syndromes of partial androgen insensitivity with azoospermia include Lubs, Gilbert–Dreyfus, Reifenstein, and Rosewater syndromes, listed in order of increasing androgen expression.[40] In summary, impaired androgen action at or beyond its receptor is the mechanism of action in AIS (Fig 4–14). Removal of cryptorchid gonads is usually indicated when the diagnosis is made to avoid heterosexual development.

The hAR gene, like other steroid receptor genes, contains N-terminal, DNA-binding, and steroid-binding domains, and the receptors have a high degree of sequence homology. Chang and associates[41] and Lubahn et al[42,43] cloned hAR cDNAs that were translated into a 76-kD protein. Tilley and colleagues[44] isolated the cDNA for the entire hAR gene, which should produce a protein of 917 amino acids weighing 98.9 kd. The N-terminal domain probably serves a regulatory function and is encoded by exon 1 (1586 bp), the DNA-binding domain by exons 2 and 3 (152 and 117 bp, respectively), and the steroid-binding domain by 5 exons ranging from 131 to 288 bp. Three cDNA probes have been used to study the hAR gene. The hAR-1 (718 bp) hybridizes with the DNA-binding and part of the steroid-binding domain, hAR-2 (490 bp) with the remainder of the steroid-binding domain, and hAR-3 (575 bp) with part of the N-terminal domain.

AIS appears to include a heterogeneous group of genetic and clinical disorders (Table 4–6). Quantitative or qualitative differences in the androgen receptor number, binding, or postreceptor action seem to account for the phenotypes.[45,46] Brown and associates[47] studied hAR binding in cultured skin fibroblasts of patients with complete AIS and found that some patients' cells demonstrated absence of binding of androgen to hAR (hAR–) or normal binding (hAR+). PCR was used to amplify separate exons of the hAR gene, and point mutations were found in 3 patients. After the cDNA of each patient was translated into mutant protein, the protein products from 2 hAR– patients exhibited no androgen binding, but the protein from the hAR+ patient bound androgen. To date, much research has been done regarding the androgen insensitivity syndrome and the human androgen receptor. In general, complete or gross deletions of the androgen recep-

TABLE 4–5. REPRESENTATIVE GENETIC DISORDERS IN WHICH MOLECULAR TECHNIQUES CAN FACILITATE DIAGNOSIS OF CARRIER STATE OR AN AFFECTED INDIVIDUAL

Cystic Fibrosis[70–72]

Heterogeneous AR disorder, most common severe AR genetic disease in Caucasians

Carrier rate as high as 1/20 to 1/22 Caucasians, incidence about 1/1500 to 1/2500 Caucasians, 1/17,000 blacks; gene frequency about 1/50

CF gene is located on chromosome 7 (7q31.3-q32), about 250,000 bp and 24 exons

CF gene was determined and sequenced before actual defective protein was known (reverse genetics)

Most common mutation (about 70 percent) involves a 3-bp deletion resulting in deletion of a phenylalanine amino acid at position 508 (DF_{508}) on the cystic fibrosis transmembrane regulator protein (CFTR). The remaining 30 percent of mutations are varied, presumably accounting for the heterogeneous nature of the disease. This transmembrane protein is thought to have about 1480 amino acids with MW 168,138 D and participates in ATP binding and perhaps regulation of chloride channels.

Historically, antenatal detection of CF in families with a previously affected child was based on elevated amniotic fluid microvillar intestinal enzymes (presumably associated with meconium ileus) in the second trimester (γ-glutamyl-transpeptidase, aminopeptidase M, and alkaline phosphatase). The timing of the testing is critical, from 17 to 18 weeks gestation

Currently, probes exist to regions involving the 3-bp deletion and using the polymerase chain reaction to amplify small copy numbers of DNA, prenatal diagnosis can be made when this common deletion exists. A negative test could reduce the chances of having an affected child from 25 percent, empirically, to 1 to 2 percent or less. With the mutations known and available probes, carrier screening could potentially be undertaken, though it would be impractical now. In vitro gene therapy studies have shown promising results

21-Hydroxylase Deficiency—Congenital Adrenal Hyperplasia[51,73–75]

Incidence varies: (classic forms) average about 1/10,000 (1/400 to 1/700, Yu'pik Eskimos; 1/5000, Switzerland; 1/67,000, Maryland); carrier frequency as high as 1/12, 1/36

Nonclassic forms: 0.3 percent Caucasians, 3 percent Ashkenazi Jews

AR inheritance

Heterogeneous disorder probably resulting from different mutations: salt-wasting, virilizing, late-onset (nonclassical), and cryptic

Severity may result from type of mutation: Mutation involving termination of protein formation would produce a nonfunctioning enzyme (eg, classical), whereas a small deletion or substitution may produce an enzyme with reduced function (eg, nonclassical)

CA21H-A (pseudogene) and CA21H-B (active gene) located adjacent to C4-A and C4-B, respectively, on chromosome 6p (within the histocompatibility complex); thus HLA linkages were noted historically

Probes are available for the cytochrome $P-450_{C-21OH}$ enzyme for use in prenatal testing,[76] which would allow fetal adrenal suppression to optimize development of female external genitalia (investigational)

Sickle-Cell Anemia[76]

Incidence 1/400 U.S. blacks, AR inheritance

Point mutation (GAG to GTG) in β-globin gene (11p12) resulting in amino acid substitution of valine for glutamic acid, which predisposes the hemoglobin chain to the conformational change, sickling

Blacks and patients of Mediterranean origin should be considered for testing for hemoglobinopathies. When carrier parents are noted, prenatal testing can be offered

Appropriate probes and primers are now available so that PCR can be used to amplify the region in question to determine the presence of the base substitution. In fact, polar bodies and blastomere cells have been removed from embryos and prenatal diagnosis made by PCR

Other hemoglobinopathies can be diagnosed as well

Hemophilia A[76]

Incidence 1/8500 male births. Inheritance XLR

Problem with prenatal diagnosis is that assays of F VIII can change with pregnancy, so that carrier states by this method have to be performed prior to pregnancy

Defect is in Factor VIII production (F VIII = VIII C (determined by X) + VIII R (determined by autosome); gene maps to proximal Xq28

Most mutations seem to be point mutations in the C and G nucleotides

Probes available (extragenic probes DX13 and St14 hybridize to distal Xq28, as well as intragenic probes), which can be used for prenatal diagnosis

Duchenne Muscular Dystrophy[24,25]

Incidence 1/3300 male births. Inheritance XLR. Carrier rate 1/100,000 women

Very large gene for protein of interest, dystrophin, mapped to Xp21.2 (2.3 Mbp)

Effect of mutation determines severity: deletion causing termination of dystrophin (frameshift) results in severe disease (DMD); deletion causing shortened, partially functional segment of dystrophin (inframe) results in mild disease (Becker's muscular dystrophy)

Historically, carrier, prenatal, and neonatal detection involved assays of CPK or LDH (isoenzyme 5) levels in nonpregnant maternal serum, amniotic fluid, or infant serum, but false-positives and false-negatives can occur

In presumed carrier females, a diagnostic approach involves immunochemistry for dystrophin in muscle and, if abnormal, PCR, Southern blotting, and linkage studies

Similar techniques can be applied to amniocytes or chorionic villi

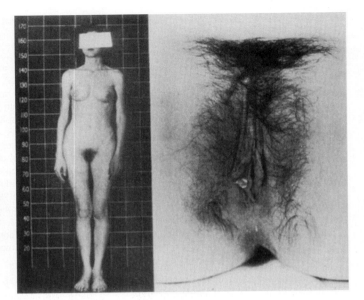

Figure 4–12.   A patient with complete androgen insensitivity syndrome, receptor (+). Note the prominent breast development, female body habitus, decreased pubic hair, and blind vaginal pouch. *(Reproduced, with permission, from Brown TR. Male pseudohermaphroditism: Defects in androgen-dependent target tissues. Semin Reprod Endocrinol. 5:251, 1987.)*

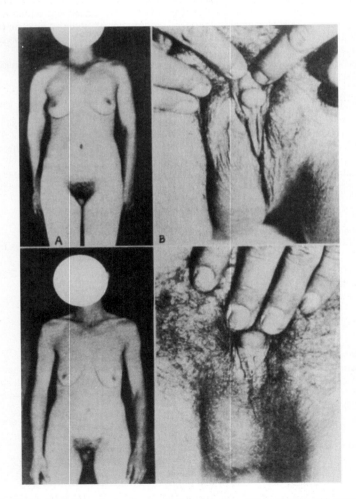

Figure 4–13.   Two siblings with incomplete androgen insensitivity syndrome. *(Reproduced, with permission, from Brown TR. Male pseudohermaphroditism: Defects in androgen-dependent target tissues. Semin Reprod Endocrinol. 5:251, 1987.)*

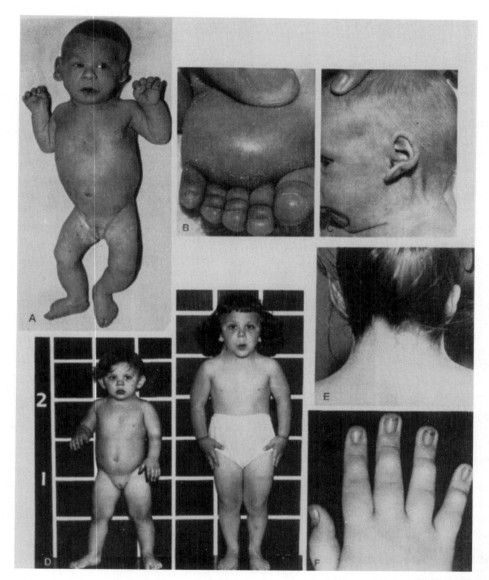

Figure 4–15.   Phenotypic abnormalities in 45,X gonadal dysgenesis (Turner syndrome). **A–C.** One-month-old girl. Note lymphedema, prominent ears, and loose skin folds in posterior neck with low nuchal hair line. **D.** Same patient at ages 2 and 4, with height ages of 17 mo and 3 yr, respectively. **E.** Low nuchal hairline and residual lateral neck web. **F.** Narrow, hyperconvex, deep-set fingernails; residual puffiness. *(Reproduced, with permission, from Jones KL.* Smith's Recognizable Patterns of Human Malformation, *4th ed. Philadelphia, W. B. Saunders Co., 1988: 77.)*

should be plotted on a growth curve specifically for patients with Turner syndrome. Growth hormone therapy has become standard in many countries and when growth decreases below the 5th percentile, usually between ages 2 and 5, patients should be evaluated for treatment. Consideration should be given to referring the patient and her family to a pediatric endocrinologist or other physician with expertise in growth evaluation and treatment in Turner syndrome when growth failure occurs. The initial growth hormone dose has been 0.05 mg/kg body weight per day. At age 9 to 12 adding an anabolic steroid, such as oxandrolone at 0.0625 mg/kg body weight per day, has been recommended. Excessive doses can cause virilization. Treatment is usually continued until bone age exceeds 15 yr or growth velocity decreases to less than 2 cm/yr. Final adult heights of greater than 153 cm, a gain in predicted height of more than 10 cm or about 60 inches, have been achieved. Estradiol affords no growth velocity enhancement and has been shown to reduce final adult height by a mean of 4 to 5 cm if begun before age 12 yr rather than delaying to age 14. The recommended time for initiation of estrogen therapy is

TABLE 4–7. SOMATIC AND OTHER ANOMALIES IN 45,X AND MOSAICISMS WITH AND WITHOUT A VARIANT X

Anomaly	Comments
Short stature	Intrauterine growth retardation Low birthweight Normal linear growth rate, 3rd percentile Usually less than 63 inches (160 cm)
Lymphatic obstruction	Pterygium colli (webbed neck, possibly a result of fetal cystic hygroma) Lymphedema usually of lower extremities—may be helped by support hose or diuretics
Cardiovascular–renal anomalies	Coarctation of the aorta Ventricular septal defect Labile hypertension in some adults Horseshoe kidney Unilateral renal agenesis
Craniofacial abnormalities	High arched palate Brachycephaly (disproportionate shortness of head) Abnormal dentition Otitis media common—may progress to mastoiditis and cholesteatoma Conductive and sensorineural hearing loss Strabismus, amblyopia, and ptosis common
Skeletal abnormalities	Short 4th metacarpal Cubitus valgus (deviation of forearm laterally or toward radius) Shield chest (widely spaced nipples) Recommend orthopedic evaluation
Dermatological abnormalities	Multiple pigmented nevi Nail hypoplasia Low nuchal hairline Predisposition to keloid formation
Gonadal failure	Sexual infantilism May have secondary sexual characteristics or menses for limited number of years Rare pregnancies can occur
Endocrinopathies	Glucose intolerance[77,78] Autoimmune thyroiditis [46,X, i(Xq) or 45,X/46,X, i(Xq)] and some 45,X patients

TABLE 4–8. CLINICAL OBSERVATIONS ABOUT PRESUMED 45,X INDIVIDUALS

1. Bilateral streak gonad formation occurs
2. Short stature (less than 63 inches) is the rule, regardless of the size of the X chromosome deletion
3. In 11 to 12 percent of patients limited ovarian estrogen production occurs but is benign
4. High levels of pulsatile gonadotropins may result in swings of estrogen production, leading to dysfunctional uterine bleeding or ovarian cyst formation
5. Patients with isochromosome Xq anomalies [46,X, i (Xq) or 45,X/46,X, i (Xq)] are prone to autoimmune thyroiditis and thyroid carcinoma. Ten to 30 percent of patients with Turner syndrome develop primary hypothyroidism associated with antithyroid antibodies
6. Patients rarely conceive but aneuploidy may occur in up to 50 percent of pregnancies
7. Any masculinization suggests a Y cell line and potential malignant tumor formation
8. Suggested follow-up for 45,X patients in whom a Y cell line cannot be excluded is annual measurement of β-hCG, α-fetoprotein, and anteroposterior films of the pelvis to rule out calcification from a gonadoblastoma
9. Exclusion of cardiovascular renal anomalies should be done (eg, renal ultrasound, excretory urogram, palpation of carotid and lower extremity pulses)
10. Preservation of the uterus should be considered because pregnancies can occur with donor oocytes or embryos
11. Patients should be followed to rule out hypertension, especially if hormonal therapy includes oral contraceptives
12. In the absence of Y chromosome or fragments and masculinization, gonadectomy need not be performed. Y DNA without cytogenetically evident Y chromosomal material may not require gonadectomy until gene for gonadoblastoma is determined

(Based, with permission, upon McDonough PG. Disorders of gonadal differentiation and sex chromosome anomalies. Semin Reprod Endocrinol. 5:221, 1987.)

TABLE 4–9. SOMATIC AND GONADAL PHENOTYPES OF 45,X/46,XY INDIVIDUALS WITH OR WITHOUT VARIANT Y[57,79]

Somatic Phenotype	Gonadal Phenotype
Stigmata of Turner syndrome with sexual infantilism	Bilateral intra-abdominal streak gonads
Newborn with or without stigmata of Turner syndrome with clitoromegaly and masculinization at puberty	Unilateral streak gonad and contralateral intra-abdominal testis
Newborn with sexual ambiguity	Unilateral streak gonad with inguinal, labial, or scrotal gonad
Male with short stature with or without stigmata of Turner syndrome with testicular failure	Bilateral hypoplastic or normal scrotal testes

(Based, with permission, upon McDonough PG. Disorders of gonadal differentiation and sex chromosome anomalies. Semin Reprod Endocrinol. 5:221, 1987.)

about age 14 to 15 yr, after counseling with the patient and her family. Because spontaneous puberty can occur, obtaining serum FSH and/or LH levels should be considered prior to starting therapy.[65] Natural estrogens are preferred, and the dose should be started low, as 0.3 mg of conjugated estrogens or esterified estrogens or 0.5 mg of micronized estradiol daily, to simulate physiologic puberty without prematurely closing the epiphyses. The dose can be gradually increased to 1.25 mg conjugated or esterified estrogens or 2 mg micronized estradiol daily, since this gradual increase seems to result in a smoother course and more natural breast contour than starting with maintenance doses. Once estrogen breakthrough bleeding occurs or about 2 yr of estrogen replacement has been given, a progestin such as medroxyprogesterone acetate (MPA) 5 to 10 mg daily for about 14 days/mo should be added to cycle the endometrium.

In addition to hormone replacement therapy, optimal bone density is achieved with adequate calcium supplementation (suggested doses of 1000 to 1500 mg daily) and regular weight-bearing exercise. Infants with the Turner phenotype have an increased risk of congenital hip dislocation, which may be associated with degenerative hip arthritis in older women. About 10 percent of girls develop scoliosis, most commonly in adolescence, so that an initial orthopedic evaluation should be considered. Growth hormone therapy results in adequate bone density through mid-adolescence. The bone mineral density of the lumbar spine and hips correlates with the duration of hormone replacement therapy, and perhaps should be measured at the initial evaluation and then repeated in 3 yr. If no change in bone density has occurred, then follow-up measurements may be made less often. If bone density has decreased, then osteoporosis management should be undertaken.

Turner syndrome patients who are surgical candidates have special considerations. Narrow endotracheal tubes are often needed. Their risk of keloid formation is increased, compared to unaffected patients, so that elective surgery, even ear piercing, should be carefully considered before proceeding.

Combination oral contraceptives, because they contain synthetic estrogens and have had associated cardiovas-cular side effects, should be used and monitored cautiously for maintenance therapy only as long as no hypertension or cardiovascular–renal anomalies or their sequelae contraindicate their use. Annual assessments of blood pressure, serum lipids, highly sensitive serum TSH level, and perhaps blood glucose and liver function tests should be done. Abnormal uterine bleeding should be evaluated by pelvic ultrasonography and/or endometrial biopsy; but the need for routine endometrial biopsies in patients who have received years of oral contraceptives or MPA 10 mg for 14 days/mo is unclear. Women with Turner syndrome have a higher mortality than unaffected women, with a mean age at death of 69 yr. About 50 percent of affected patients died of cardiovascular disease and 20 percent of cancer.

Mixed Gonadal Dysgenesis (Y Chromosome Mosaicism With or Without a Variant Y). Patients with mixed gonadal dysgenesis have a mosaicism containing an X chromosome monosomy and a diploid cell line with a normal or an altered Y chromosome: 45,X/46,XY or 45,X/46,X variant Y. These patients present with a spectrum of somatic and gonadal phenotypes listed in Table 4–9.

The prevalence of mosaicism and variant Y chromosomes in this disorder suggests that early mitotic errors in a 46,XY individual may alter the Y chromosome, and anaphase lag may give rise to daughter cell lines containing missing or abnormal Y chromosomes.[9] The proportion of 45,X patients having a cytogenetically undetectable normal or variant Y-bearing cell line is currently a subject of investigation.

The goals of clinical management are to establish a sex of rearing, to provide acceptable external genitalia as early in life as possible, to identify somatic anomalies, to remove gonads with the potential of malignant tumor formation, to institute hormonal therapy when appropriate, and to identify other family members at risk.[66] A male gender assignment is usually made only if the phallus is sufficiently developed to allow urination while standing and coitus. A female sex of rearing is usually chosen when these criteria are not met. Gender assignment is urgent and preferably should be performed before the infant leaves the hospital. In general, reconstructive surgery is safe and can be performed within the first few weeks of life,[67] even before the neonate is discharged.[68] A delayed change in the gender assignment may cause uncertainty in the family about the validity of the original sex of rearing. Psychological counseling of the patient and family are essential to establishing a gender identity and a supportive family. Somatic anomalies as in the Turner phenotype should be sought, and hormonal replacement therapy should be instituted in a manner similar to that in patients with 45,X gonadal dysgenesis. In children with dysgenetic gonads associated with a cell line containing a Y chromosome, pericentromeric fragments, or a Y marker, who are at risk for malignant transformation or in whom the gonad is discordant with the sex of rearing, gonadectomy is the treatment of choice. Patients with virilization or gonadoblastoma should be evaluated for low-frequency Y-chromosome mosaicism. Gonads may be absent, dysgenetic, hypoplastic, or relatively normal and should be located. Gonads palpable in the inguinal canals or labioscrotal pouches of children with an intended female sex of rearing are usually easily palpated and removed. Intra-abdominal gonads may be small streaks, but they may extend for quite a distance and require careful dissection. Until the role of gonadectomy by operative laparoscopy has been established, laparotomy should be considered standard surgical therapy. Although McDonough and associates[69] found normal paternal karyotypes in study subjects (n = 20) having mixed gonadal dysgenesis with cytogenetically normal or abnormal Y chromosomes, questions of the inheritance of an abnormal Y have not been completely answered.

The DNA of some phenotypic 45,X males has hybridized with Y-specific probes, indicating the presence of Y as otherwise undetectable separate or translocated fragments. McDonough and associates[69] tested the sensitivity and specificity of Y probes 4B-2 and DYZ2 in detecting Y DNA in patients with mixed gonadal dysgenesis (Fig 4–5A). Twenty patients (n = 19 with 45,X/46,XY) with normal (n = 8) and altered Y (n = 12) DNA were studied. Digestion of DNA from normal 46,XY males with *Hae*III results in two male-specific fragments, 3.4 and 2.1 kb in length, which are not present in a digestion of normal 46,XX DNA. In mixtures of 46,XX and 46,XY DNA, these two bands could be detected in as low a fraction as 0.30 (600 ng) of male DNA. A similar digest probed with DYZ2 showed a 2.1-kb band in both sexes, but digestion with *Mbo*I gave tenfold greater hybridization 2.3-kb band, which was detectable to as little as 2.5 ng of male DNA (1:400 ratio of male:45,X DNA). Hybridization with Y-specific probes offers greater sensitivity than digestion alone, which requires less time than probing. DYZ2 hybridized with DNA from patients (n = 8) with a cytogenetically intact Y, even at a level of mosaicism of 10 percent of 46,XY; it hybridized at a reduced intensity with altered heterochromatin (C-banding but no Q-banding); and it failed to hybridize in the absence of

Q- and C-banding. Hybridization of 4B-2 paralleled that of DYZ2 except that the former did hybridize with 3 of the patients and the latter did not. These results indicate that the regions defined by C- and Q-banding on Yq do not overlap, and that C-banding extends more proximally than Q-banding. Although patients without C- or Q-banding were cytogenetically indistinguishable, the Y probes seemed to detect deletions beyond the resolution of cytogenetics.

XY Gonadal Dysgenesis (Swyer's Syndrome). Patients with 46,XY gonadal dysgenesis, or Swyer's syndrome, have streak gonads, normal stature, and a sexually infantile phenotype with Müllerian structures present.[47] The inheritance is usually sporadic but can be autosomal dominant or X-linked recessive. Unlike 45,X patients, stigmata of Turner syndrome are rare. As many as 20 to 30 percent of patients are at risk for malignant gonadal tumor formation and should undergo gonadectomy soon after the diagnosis is made. Despite the presence of Y, these patients presumably lack testicular-determining genes or the genes are not expressed after early embryonic life. The presence of Müllerian structures indicates that MIF was not produced after about 6 wk of fetal life. Patients are raised as females and hormonal replacement therapy is instituted as in 45,X patients. Continued study of 46,XY females and 45,X or 46,XX males may ultimately disclose the locations of TDF and factors related to malignant gonadal tumor transformation.

In summary, the role of Y-specific DNA probes in detecting occult Y segments is still investigational. Molecular techniques such as PCR, chromosome walking, pulsed field gel electrophoresis, in situ hybridization, and gene sequencing should enable investigators eventually to identify all genes for testicular determination, spermatogenesis, and for malignant gonadal tumor formation.

CONCLUSIONS

As the level of molecular resolution and the refinement of micromanipulation techniques advance, the ability of scientists to study the anatomy of the human genome, to understand its regulation of cellular processes, and to treat genetic disorders prior to implantation will improve and change the face of clinical medicine. Compared to the resolution afforded by cytogenetics only 30 to 40 yr ago, we now can potentially detect alterations in single nucleic acids using techniques of molecular biology. The ability to diagnose carrier states and exclude affected fetuses has improved from classical Mendelian principles to a relatively high degree of certainty, largely because genes are being mapped and sequenced and probes developed. When probes for genes (or critical regions) are not available, then family linkage studies are needed and usually require DNA from an affected family member. Forethought should be given to obtaining blood or tissue from such individuals in the event that prenatal testing is desired at a later time.

The goal of the Human Genome Project is to sequence human DNA in its entirety. Assuming that goal is ultimately achieved, the processes of regulation of transcription, translation, and secretion; the regulation of developmental genes; the timing of gene transcription and inactivation; and the signal for the first mitosis will still need to be understood. Knowing all the potential flaws in genetic, embryonic, and fetal development, it is miraculous that reproduction is successful as often as it is and that we exist.

Acknowledgments

The author acknowledges the following physicians and friends for their contributions to this chapter: Dr. Larry Layman for his guidance in preparing the sections on molecular biology; Dr. Richard E. Blackwell for the opportunity to write this chapter; and Dr. Paul G. McDonough, my fellowship director and mentor, who cultivated and has sustained my interest in the genetics of reproduction.

REFERENCES

1. Psalm 139:13–14. In: Barker K, ed. *The NIV Study Bible, New International Version.* Grand Rapids, Mich., Zondervan Bible Publishers, 1985: 932
2. Layman LC. Basic concepts of molecular biology as applied to pediatric and adolescent gynecology. *Obstet Gynecol Clin North Am.* 19:1, 1992
3. Gelehrter TD, Collins FS. *Principles of Medical Genetics.* Baltimore, Williams and Wilkins, 1990: 9–23
4. Thompson JS, Thompson MW. *Genetics in Medicine,* 4th ed. Philadelphia, W. B. Saunders Co., 1986: 6–26
5. Adashi EY. The ovarian life cycle. In: *Reproductive Endocrinology,* 3rd ed. Philadelphia, W. B. Saunders Co., 1991: 181–237
6. Garver KL, Marchese SG. *Genetic Counseling for Clinicians.* Chicago, Year Book Medical Publishers, 1986: 13–18
7. Lyon MF. The William Allan Memorial Award address: X-chromosome inactivation and the location and expression of X-linked genes. *Am J Hum Genet.* 42:8, 1988
8. Lyon MF. Sex chromosome and gene action in the mammalian X chromosome. *Am J Hum Genet.* 14:135, 1962
9. Tho SPT, McDonough PG. Use of Y DNA probes to identify children at risk for dysgenetic gonadal tumors. *Clin Obstet Gynecol.* 30:671, 1987
10. Muller U. Mapping of testis-determining locus on Yp by the molecular genetic analysis of XX males and XY females. *Development.* 101(Suppl.):51, 1987
11. Page DC, Mosher R, Simpson EM, et al. The sex-determining region of the human Y chromosome encodes a finger protein. *Cell.* 51:1091, 1987
12. Koopman P, Gubbay J, Vivian N, et al. Male development of chromosomally female mice transgenic for *SRY. Nature.* 351:117, 1991
13. Braun A, Kammerer S, Cleve H, et al. True hermaphroditism in a 46,XY individual, caused by a postzygotic somatic point mutation in the male gonadal sex-determining locus (SRY): Molecular genetics and histological findings in a sporadic case. *Am J Hum Genet.* 52:578, 1993
14. Ramkissoon Y, Goodfellow P. Early steps in mammalian sex determination. *Curr Opin Genet Devel.* 6:316, 1996
15. Marx J, Williams N. Special news report: Sex determination. Tracing how the sexes develop. *Science.* 269:1822, 1995
16. McElreavey K, Barbaux S, Ion A, et al. The genetic basis of murine and human sex determination: A review. *Heredity.* 75:599, 1995
17. Thompson MW, McInnes RR, Willard HF. Thompson and Thompson: *Genetics in Medicine,* 5th ed. Philadelphia, W. B. Saunders Co., 1991
18. Pritchard JA, MacDonald PC, Gant NF. *Williams Obstetrics,* 17th ed. Norwalk, Conn., Appleton-Century-Crofts, 1985: 169–170
19. Wathen NC, Cass PL, Kitau MJ, Chard T. Human chorionic gonadotropin and alpha-fetoprotein levels in matched samples of amniotic fluid, extraembryonic coelomic fluid, and maternal serum in the first trimester of pregnancy. *Prenat Diagn.* 11:145, 1991
20. Rebello MT, Gray CT, Rooney DE, et al. Cytogenetic studies of amniotic fluid taken before the 15th week of pregnancy for earlier diagnosis: A report of 114 consecutive cases. *Prenat Diagn.* 11:35, 1991
21. Penso CA, Frigoletto FD. Early amniocentesis. *Semin Perinatol.* 14:465, 1990
22. Drugan A, Snyer FN, Greb A, et al. Amniotic fluid alpha-fetoprotein and acetylcholinesterase in early genetic amniocentesis. *Obstet Gynecol.* 72:35, 1988
23. Burton OK, Nelson LH, Pettenati MJ. False-positive acetylcholinesterase with early amniocentesis. *Obstet Gynecol.* 74:607, 1989
24. Elias S, Simpson JL. Sampling the chorionic villi. *Contemp Obstet Gynecol.* 11, 1991
25. Ledbetter DH, Martin AO, Verlinsky Y, et al. Cytogenetic results of chorionic villus sampling: High success rate and diagnostic accuracy in the United States collaborative study. *Am J Obstet Gynecol.* 162:495, 1990
26. Hsu LYF, Perlis TE. United States survey on chromosome mosaicism and pseudomosaicism in prenatal diagnosis. *Prenat Diagn.* 4:97, 1984
27. Rhoads GG, Jackson LG, Schlesselman SE, et al. The safety and efficacy of chorionic villus sampling for early prenatal diagnosis of cytogenetic abnormalities. *N Engl J Med.* 320:609, 1989
28. Canadian Collaborative CVS–Amniocentesis Clinical Trial Group. Multicentre randomised clinical trial of chorionic villus sampling and amniocentesis. *Lancet.* 1:1, 1989
29. MRC Working Party on the Evaluation of Chorionic Villus Sampling. Medical Research Council European Trial of Chorionic Villus Sampling. *Lancet.* 337:1491, 1991

30. Sawicki MP, Samara G, Hurwitz M. Human Genome Project. *Am J Surg.* 165:258, 1993

31. Palotie A, Heiskanen M, Laan M, et al. High-resolution fluorescence in situ hybridization: A new approach in genome mapping. *Ann Med.* 28:101, 1996

32. Bailey SM, Meyne J, Cornforth MN, et al. A new method for detecting pericentric inversions using COD-FISH. *Cytogenet Cell Genet.* 75:248, 1996

33. Philip J, Bryndorf T, Christensen B. Prenatal aneuploidy detection in interphase cells by fluorescence in situ hybridization. *Prenat Diagn.* 14:1203, 1994

34. Nadal M, Moreno S, Pritchard M, et al. Down syndrome: Characterisation of a case with partial trisomy of chromosome 21 owing to a paternal balanced translocation (15;21)(q26;q22.1) by FISH. *J Med Genet.* 34:50, 1997

35. Roa PN, Collins KA, Geisinger KR, et al. Identification of male epithelial cells in routine postcoital cervicovaginal smears using fluorescence in situ hybridization. *Am J Clin Pathol.* 104:32, 1995

36. Jeffreys AJ, Wilson V, Thein SL. Hypervariable "mini-satellite" regions in human DNA. *Nature.* 314:67, 1985

37. Brown CJ, Goss SJ, Lubahn DB, et al. Androgen receptor locus on the X chromosome: Regional localization to Xq11-12 and description of a DNA polymorphism. *Am J Hum Genet.* 44:264, 1989

38. McKusick V. Testicular feminization syndrome (313700). *Online Mendelian Inheritance in Man (OMIM).* Online database accessible through Howard Hughes Foundation, Welch Library, Johns Hopkins Hospital, Baltimore, Md. Last edited October 14, 1991

39. Morris JM. The syndrome of testicular feminization in male pseudohermaphrodites. *Am J Obstet Gynecol.* 65:1192, 1953

40. Jaffe RB. Disorders of sexual development. In: Yen SSC, Jaffe RB, eds. *Reproductive Endocrinology. Physiology, Pathophysiology, and Clinical Management,* 3rd ed. Philadelphia, W. B. Saunders Co., 1991: 480–510

41. Chang C, Kokontis J, Kiao S. Molecular cloning of human and rat complementary DNA encoding androgen receptors. *Science.* 240:324, 1988

42. Lubahn DB, Joseph DR, Sar M, et al. The human androgen receptor: Complementary deoxyribonucleic acid cloning, sequence analysis, and gene expression in prostate. *Mol Endocrinol.* 2:1265, 1988

43. Lubahn DB, Joseph DR, Sullivan PM, et al. Cloning of the human androgen receptor complementary DNA and localization to the X chromosome. *Science.* 240:327, 1988

44. Tilley WD, Marcelli M, Wilson JD, McPhaul MJ. Characterization and expression of a cDNA encoding the human androgen receptor. *Proc Nat Acad Sci USA.* 86:327, 1989

45. DiLauro SD, Behzadian A, Tho SPT, McDonough PG. Probing genomic deoxyribonucleic acid for gene rearrangement in 14 patients with androgen insensitivity syndrome. *Fertil Steril.* 55:481, 1991

46. Pereira RR, Brinkmann AO, Ring D, Hodgins MB. Partial androgen insensitivity as a cause of genital maldevelopment. *Helv Paediatr Acta.* 39:255, 1984

47. Brown TR, Lubahn DB, Wilson EM, et al. Functional characterization of naturally occurring mutant androgen receptors from subjects with complete androgen insensitivity. *Mol Endocrinol.* 4:1759, 1990

48. Brinkmann A, Jenster G, Ris-Stalpers C, et al. Molecular basis of androgen insensitivity. *Steroids.* 61:172, 1996

49. Bruggenwirth S, Nedel S, Werde EA, et al. Molecular basis of androgen insensitivity. *J Steroid Biochem Mol Biol.* 58:569, 1996.

50. Balducci R, Ghirri P, Brown TR, et al. A clinician looks at androgen resistance. *Steroids.* 61:205, 1996

51. McDonough PG. Disorders of gonadal differentiation and sex chromosome anomalies. *Semin Reprod Endocrinol.* 5:221, 1987

52. Butler WJ, McDonough PG. The spectrum of gonadal dysgenesis. *Contemp Obstet Gynecol.* 29:57, 1984

53. Turner HH. A syndrome of infantilism, congenital webbed neck and cubitus valgus. *Endocrinology.* 23:566, 1938

54. Ford CE, Jones KW, Polani PE. A sex chromosome anomaly in a case of gonadal dysgenesis (Turner's syndrome). *Lancet.* 1:711, 1959

55. Jones KL. *Smith's Recognizable Patterns of Human Malformation,* 4th ed. Philadelphia, W. B. Saunders Co., 1988: 77–79

56. Singh RP, Carr DH. The anatomy and histology of XO human embryos and fetuses. *Anat Rec.* 155:369, 1966

57. Migeon BR, Kennedy JF. Evidence for the inactivation of an X chromosome early in the development of the human female. *Am J Hum Genet.* 27:233, 1975

58. Gartler SM, Liskay RM, Gant N. Two functional X chromosomes in human fetal oocytes. *Exp Cell Res.* 82:464, 1973

59. Cuniff C, Jones KL, Benirschke K. Ovarian dysgenesis in individuals with chromosomal abnormalities. *Hum Genet.* 86:552, 1991

60. Hook EB, Warburton D. The distribution of chromosomal genotypes associated with Turner's syndrome: Livebirth prevalence rates and evidence for diminished fetal mortality and severity in genotypes associated with structural X abnormalities or mosaicism. *Hum Genet.* 64:24, 1983

61. Sanger R, Tippett P, Gavin J, et al. Xg groups and sex chromosome abnormalities in people of northern European ancestry. An addendum. *J Med Genet.* 14:210, 1977

62. Hassold T, Kumlin E, Takeesu N, Leppert M. Determination of parental origin of sex chromosome monosomy using restriction fragment length polymorphisms. *Am J Hum Genet.* 37:965, 1985

63. Page DC, de la Chapelle A. The paternal origin of X chromosomes in XX males determined using restriction fragment length polymorphisms. *Am J Hum Genet.* 36:656, 1984

64. Saenger P. Turner's syndrome. *N Engl J Med.* 335:1749, 1996

65. Rosenfeld RG, Tesch LG, Rodriguez-Rigau LJ, et al. Recommendations for diagnosis, treatment, and management of individuals with Turner syndrome. *Endocrinologist.* 4:351, 1994

66. Stradtman EW. Female gender reconstruction surgery for ambiguous genitalia in children and adolescents. *Curr Opin Obstet Gynecol.* 3:805, 1991

67. Sharp RJ, Holder TM, Howard CP, Grunt JA. Neonatal genital reconstruction. *J Pediatr Surg.* 22:168, 1987

68. Donahoe PK, Hendren WH. Perineal reconstruction in ambiguous genitalia infants raised as females. *Ann Surg.* 200:363, 1984

69. McDonough PG, Tho SPT, Trill JJ, et al. Use of two different deoxyribonucleic acid probes to detect Y chromosome deoxyribonucleic acid in subjects with normal and altered Y chromosomes. *Am J Obstet Gynecol.* 154:737, 1986

70. McKusick V, et al. *Online Mendelian Inheritance in Man (OMIM).* Online database accessible through Howard Hughes Foundation, Welch Library, Johns Hopkins Hospital, Baltimore, Md. Last edited October 14, 1991

71. Kerem E, Corey M, Kerem B, et al. The relation between genotype and phenotype in cystic fibrosis—Analysis of the most common mutation (delta-F_{508}). *N Engl J Med.* 323:1517, 1990

72. Lemna WK, Feldman GL, Kerem B, et al. Mutation analysis for heterozygote detection and the prenatal diagnosis of cystic fibrosis. *N Engl J Med.* 322:291, 1990

73. Drucker S, New M. Nonclassical adrenal hyperplasia due to 21-hydroxylase deficiency. *Pediatr Clin North Am.* 34:1067, 1987

74. White PC, New MI, Dupont B. Congenital adrenal hyperplasia. Parts I and II. *N Engl J Med.* 316:1519, 1987

75. Meyers CM, Elias S. Genetic screening for Mendelian disorders. *Contemp Obstet Gynecol.* 35:56, 1990

76. Reindollar RH, Lewis JB, White PC, et al. Prenatal diagnosis of 21-hydroxylase deficiency by the complementary deoxyribonucleic acid probe for cytochrome $P-450_{C-21OH}$. *Am J Obstet Gynecol.* 158:545, 1988

77. Costin G, Kogut MD. Carbohydrate intolerance in gonadal dysgenesis: Evidence for insulin resistance and hyperglucagonemia. *Horm Res.* 25:260, 1985

78. Rasio E, Antaki A, Van-Campenhout J. Diabetes mellitus in gonadal dysgenesis: Studies of insulin and growth hormone secretion. *Eur J Clin Invest.* 6:59, 1976

79. McDonough PG, Tho PT. The spectrum of 45,X/46,XY gonadal dysgenesis and its implications: A study of 19 patients. *Pediatr Adolesc Gynecol.* 1:1, 1983

Chapter 5

NORMAL AND ABNORMAL PUBERTY

G. William Bates

Puberty is the physical, emotional, and sexual transition from childhood to adulthood. Although the initiation of puberty is almost imperceptible and the transition from sexual immaturity to sexual maturity occurs gradually, puberty is punctuated by well-defined events and milestones.[1] The hypothalamic–pituitary–gonadal axis functions during fetal life and during the first few weeks following birth. The reproductive endocrine system then becomes quiescent. Puberty is the reawakening of the reproductive endocrine system, which leads to full secondary sexual maturation with capacity for reproduction. The mechanism(s) for holding reproductive function in abeyance during childhood is unknown. Moreover, the neuroendocrine events that trigger puberty are unidentified.

Recordings of the age of onset of secondary sexual maturation suggest that the age of onset of menarche in girls and voice changes in boys has been decreasing over the past century.[2,3] The decreasing age of secondary sexual maturation has been attributed to improved nutrition associated with the industrialization of Western culture. However, the age of onset of menarche seems to have stabilized during the past decade.[4]

In this chapter, the physical changes in girls and boys at puberty will be presented first, followed by the hormonal events of puberty. The chapter will conclude with discussions of evaluation of the adolescent, delayed puberty, and precocious puberty.

PHYSICAL CHANGES IN GIRLS

Physical changes in girls at the expected time of puberty occur in an orderly, predictable sequence. The events, age, and hormone(s) responsible for the sequence of secondary sexual maturation in girls are presented in Table 5–1. The developmental events of puberty in girls and boys were first described and codified by Marshall and Tanner.[5,6]

Breast Development

Breast development is usually the first physical manifestation of secondary sexual maturation in girls. With the beginning of estradiol secretion by the ovarian follicles, the breast bud rises on the chest wall. First, the nipples and areolae enlarge and elevate. Then, the breast mounds begin to form on the chest wall. Breast budding may occur as early as 8 yr and may be delayed for up to 13 yr. In most girls, breast budding will begin by 10 yr.

With increasing estradiol secretion, the breasts begin to take on an adult configuration. Ovulation, with consequent progesterone secretion, leads to full breast development with rounding of the lateral quadrants of the breasts. Breast development is usually completed by 14 yr. These events are presented in Figure 5–1.

Sexual Hair Growth

Pubic hair growth begins in most girls within 6 mo of the appearance of the breast bud. Sexual hair growth results from exposure of the hair follicles on the mons pubis and labia majora to androgens—particularly testosterone. Synergism exists between androgens and estrogens to stimulate sexual hair growth. In girls with Turner syndrome, where the ovaries are unable to secrete estradiol, there is adequate adrenal androgen secretion to stimulate sexual hair growth. However, pubic hair does not fully appear until exogenous estrogens are administered.[7]

Pubic hair appears first on the inner aspects of the labia majora and then progresses to fill the pubic triangle. Coincident with pubic hair growth, there is continued breast development.

TABLE 5–1. SEQUENCE OF SEXUAL MATURATION IN GIRLS

Event	Age (yr)	Hormone(s)
Breast budding	10–11	Estradiol
Sexual hair growth	10.5–11.5	Androgens
Growth spurt	11–12	Growth hormone
Menarche	11.5–13	Estradiol
Adult breast	12.5–15	Progesterone
Adult sexual hair	13.5–16	Androgens

Axillary hair in girls usually appears within 1 yr of the appearance of pubic hair. In American girls, this manifestation begins by 13 yr. Full axillary hair growth is not completed until age 14 to 15 yr in most girls.

Breast development is the first physical manifestation of puberty in most girls. However, in approximately 15 percent of girls pubic hair will be the first manifestation of puberty.[8] If the interval between the appearance of pubic hair and breast development is longer than 6 mo, the physician should suspect an androgen excess disorder. This will be discussed in more detail.

Along with appearance of sexual hair, the apocrine glands of the mons pubis and axillae enlarge and begin secreting volatile organic acids that produce an "adult body odor." In conditions of androgen excess and precocious puberty, the adult body odor may be the first sign of precocious puberty noted by parents of a young girl or boy.

Growth Spurt

Girls and boys grow at a similar rate of approximately 6 cm/yr during childhood. Predictable changes occur in the fusion of epiphyseal plates between the shafts of long bones and in the ossification centers.[9,10] Thus, bone age can be assigned from the changes in epiphyseal fusion and ossification. These bone changes correlate better with secondary sexual development than does chronological age. To obtain a bone age, an x-ray of the left hand and wrist is compared with Bayley–Pinneau tables or the Gruelich and Pyle[11] atlas of skeletal maturation. These tables are useful in assessing delayed sexual maturation and precocious sexual maturation. An example of a hand film showing open epiphyseal plates is presented in Figure 5–2.

Soon after breast development begins in girls and testicular enlargement begins in boys, the rate of growth accelerates to a maximal rate of 9 cm/yr in girls and 10 cm/yr in boys. Growth is both stimulated and arrested by sex-steroid hormones.[12] Estrogens stimulate long bone growth in girls in concert with the action of growth hormone. However, with maximal estrogen secretion, epiphyseal closure occurs and further long bone growth is arrested. Since boys begin testosterone secretion about 2 yr after girls begin estradiol secretion, boys are taller as adults compared with girls because of the longer time for basal childhood growth.

In girls with precocious puberty, there is premature secretion of estradiol with resultant stimulation of long

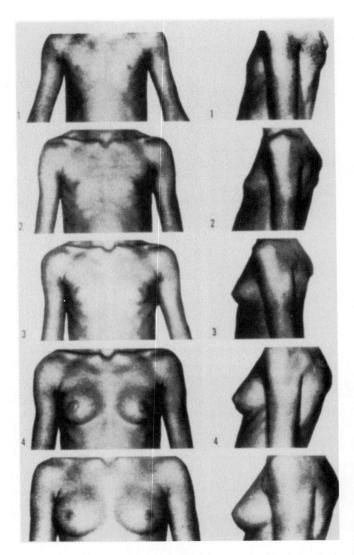

Figure 5–1. Sequence of breast development in girls during the process of puberty. The Tanner stage of breast development is indicated by the number. *(Reprinted, with permission, from Marshall WA, Tanner JM.* Arch Dis Child. *44:291, 1969.)*

bone growth and epiphyseal closure. The adult height is truncated because there is inadequate time for full basal childhood growth.

In delayed puberty, some girls may be taller than peers but this is usually not the case. In boys with delayed puberty, the pubertal process is accelerated and expected adult height is achieved.

Breast development usually correlates with a bone age of 11 yr regardless of chronological age; menarche usually correlates with a bone age of 13 yr regardless of chronological age. A bone age of 13 yr in boys correlates with testicular enlargement and the appearance of pubic hair. These facts can be reassuring to parents whose children have delayed puberty.[13]

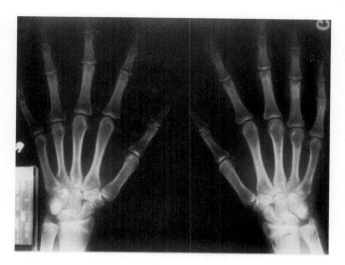

Figure 5–2.   Hand x-ray of a 15-yr-old girl with isolated gonadotropin deficiency. She is 65 in tall. The epiphyses have not closed, and an adult height of 66 in is forecast.

Other Somatic Changes

As girls begin the pubertal process, there are other changes in the body habitus. The body is composed of more fat and less lean body mass as a percentage of total body mass. When full secondary sexual maturation has been attained and ovulation established, most girls will have 25 to 27 percent of their body mass as fat.[14] This fat accumulates on the hips, around the anterior thighs, and around the midriff. Girls develop broader hips relative to shoulders while boys develop wide shoulders relative to hips. These somatic differences are driven by the differential effects of estradiol and testosterone. Boys have greater physical strength than girls after full sexual maturation has been achieved.

Menarche

The first menstrual period can be recalled by most adult women. Although menarche can come as a surprise, for most girls the first menstrual period is an expected event. Menarche marks impending ovulation. Most girls will begin ovulating within 6 to 9 mo of menarche and regular ovulatory cycles are established within 1 to 2 yr of menarche.[15] The mean age for menarche for girls in the United States is 12.8 yr. Menarche can occur as early as 10 yr and as late as 16 yr.

PHYSICAL CHANGES IN BOYS

Testicular and Penile Enlargement

The first evidence of secondary sexual development in boys is enlargement of the testicles.[6] This event begins at a mean age of 11 yr. The prepubertal testicles measure less than 2.5 cm in length and usually less than 15 cc in volume. With the beginning of gonadotropin secretion from the anterior pituitary gland, the Leydig cells of the testicles begin to enlarge and secrete testosterone. Testosterone has a direct effect on the seminiferous tubules of the testicles, thus giving rise to increased testicular size. Within 4 yr of beginning testicular enlargement, the testicles have reached adult size.

Elongation and enlargement of the penis begins within 1 yr of testicular enlargement. Full development of the external genitalia is completed by age 15 yr.

Sexual Hair Growth

The appearance of pubic hair marks the first visible manifestation of male secondary sexual maturation. Pubic hair appears about 6 mo after the beginning of testicular enlargement. The first pubic hair appears at the root of the penis and spreads out across the mons pubis and on the surface of the scrotum. Axillary hair growth begins about 18 mo after pubic hair growth begins.

Facial hair appears at about 15 yr. The first facial hair begins on the lateral corners of the upper lip and spreads medially. Next comes sideburn hair, followed by hair on the chin. Full facial hair development is usually not completed until about age 20 yr. This is the final event in completion of male secondary sexual development.

Spermarche

Motile spermatozoa can be found in urine by age 13.5 to 14 yr. The first conscious ejaculation occurs by 14.5 yr and usually presents as a nocturnal emission.[16,17] With the first ejaculation, full reproductive capacity has been attained.

Other Changes

With testosterone secretion by the testicles, the voice begins to deepen as the larynx enlarges. The musculoskeletal system takes on an adult masculine configuration. In about 40 percent of boys, there will be gynecomastia, a source of embarrassment for a developing boy. However, the physician can provide reassurance that the enlarging breasts will begin involution as sexual maturation progresses.[18] With beginning testosterone secretion, some testosterone is converted by aromatization to estradiol. Estradiol causes initial breast enlargement.

By age 14 yr, regular ovulatory cycles have been established in most girls; by age 15 yr, regular, frequent erections with ejaculation of semen have been established in most boys. Thus, full sexual maturity with the capacity for reproduction has been achieved.

EMOTIONAL CHANGES OF ADOLESCENCE

Moodiness and associated behavioral changes are common at puberty. Certain behaviors, such as depressive affect, are relatively rare before adolescence yet occur with

96 Textbook of Reproductive Medicine

relative frequency at puberty. In girls age 10 to 15 yr, there is a fourfold increased incidence in depression that resolves in most girls beyond age 15 yr. Warren and Brooks-Gunn demonstrated correlation of changes in behavioral patterns as there were changes in hormone secretory patterns.[19] Some investigators suggest drug use in adolescence may be an inadvertent form of self-medication for depression.[20]

HORMONAL CHANGES AT PUBERTY

The mechanism(s) for restraining puberty and the endocrine events that initiate the onset of secondary sexual maturation are unknown, but theories have been proposed.[21] A proposed mechanism is presented in Figure 5–3. Puberty is held in abeyance until age 10 yr in girls and 11 yr in boys. The hypothalamic–pituitary–gonadal axis functions during fetal life and during the first few weeks after birth. Then, the hypothalamic–pituitary–gonadal axis becomes relatively quiescent, although neural inhibition is rarely absolute during childhood. There are detectable levels of gonadotropins and estrogens during childhood, and evidence of ovarian follicular development is found frequently throughout childhood.

At approximately 6 yr, adrenarche begins. The adrenal glands begin secreting increasing quantities of de-

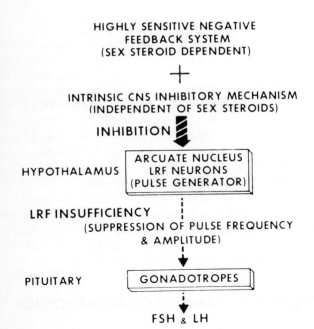

Figure 5–3. Proposed mechanism for the restraint of puberty. *(Reprinted, with permission, from Reiter EO, Grumbach MM. Annu Rev Physiol. 44:595,1982.)*

hydroepiandrosterone (DHEA) and dehydroepiandrosterone sulfate (DS). The role of these adrenal hormones in subsequent secondary sexual development is unknown. However, in some girls these adrenal androgens will stimulate the growth of sexual hair prior to the onset of breast development.

By age 8 to 9 yr, the anterior pituitary gland begins secreting gonadotropin hormones—follicle-stimulating hormone (FSH) and luteinizing hormone (LH). The secretion of gonadotropin is under control of the pulsatile secretion of gonadotropin-releasing hormone (GnRH) from the medial basal hypothalamus.

Three lines of evidence suggest that pulsatile secretion of GnRH is required for initiation of puberty.[22] First, pulsatile changes occur in FSH and LH secretion in peripubertal boys and girls during sleep. Second, the intravenous administration of GnRH in a pulsatile fashion initiates puberty in women with olfactory hypoplasia associated with delayed puberty. Third, chronic administration of long-acting GnRH to children with central precocious puberty will arrest pubertal development and hold further secondary sexual development in abeyance until long-acting GnRH is withdrawn.

Early studies of LH secretion showed that humans as well as animals release LH into the circulation in a series of pulses.[23–25] Studies in animals have shown that each LH pulse is the result of a pulse of GnRH from the hypothalamus. On the basis of these data, we make the assumption that LH pulses reflect hypothalamic GnRH secretion in humans. GnRH pulse frequency is lower in prepubertal children than in children in early puberty.[26]

Two critical elements, sleep and adequate body fat, are essential for the initiation of secondary sexual development. Boyar et al[27] and Katz et al[28] described the gonadotropin secretory pattern in prepubertal, intrapubertal, and sexually mature adolescents. These investigators found that the release of gonadotropins, especially the release of LH, is sleep entrained and occurs during Stage IV sleep stages (Fig 5–4). Once secondary sexual maturation is completed, there is no further relationship between sleep and gonadotropin release. From the neuroendocrine perspective, the resurgence of the reproductive system at puberty is initiated by the sleep-entrained secretion of gonadotropins that are stimulated by the release of GnRH.

Apter et al[29] compared GnRH activity in prepubertal girls and sexually mature adolescent girls and found greater GnRH in the prepubertal years. Thus, there is GnRH activity prior to measurable changes in sex-steroid hormones.

Adolescents require long hours of sleep. Their demand for sleep increases during the intrapubertal years and lessens after full sexual maturation is achieved. The

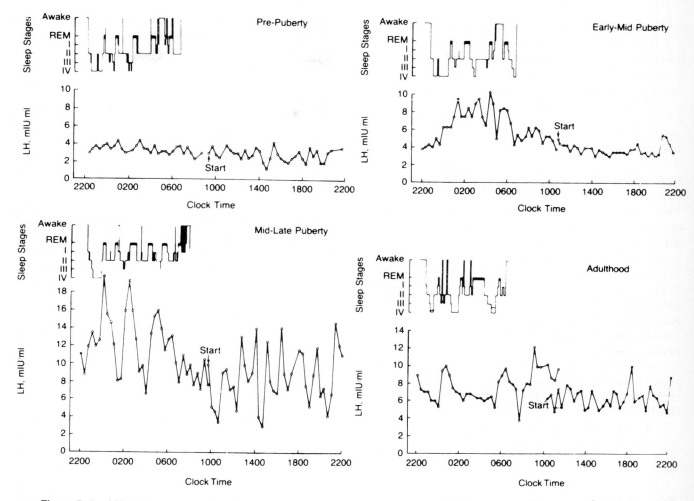

Figure 5–4. LH secretory pattern over 24 hr during the stages of puberty. Note the relationship between LH secretion and sleep during midpuberty. *(Reprinted, with permission, from Katz J, Boyar RM, Finklestein JW, et al. Psychosom Med. 40:549, 1978.)*

relationship between sleep and gonadotropin secretion is presented in Figure 5–3.

Frisch and Revelle[30] proposed a theory that girls must attain a critical body weight before puberty begins. According to this theory, breast budding, growth spurt, and menarche occur with increasing body fat and change in the lean:fat ratio. In prepubertal girls, the lean:fat ratio is 5:1. With the onset of puberty, the lean:fat ratio decreases to 3:1 and is maintained at that level as ovulatory cycles are established. Menarche occurs when the percentage of body mass as body fat reaches 21 percent; ovulatory cycles are established and maintained when body mass is 24 percent body fat.[31]

In clinical practice, the observation is made frequently that plump girls begin breast development early and that slender girls have delayed breast development. Moreover, plump—but not morbidly obese girls—may have early menarche; slender girls may have delayed

menarche. Several clinical conditions seen in adolescent girls who present with amenorrhea can be related to alterations in body weight that interfere with the physiological secretion of GnRH and gonadotropins.

How does body fat alter the neuroendocrine mechanism(s) that triggers hypothalamic–pituitary function? There is accumulating evidence that body fat plays a direct and indirect role in sex-steroid hormone production and metabolism. When Fishman et al[32] infused radiolabeled estradiol into three groups of women (obese women, women of normal body weight, and women with anorexia nervosa), they found differences in the metabolism of estradiol between the three groups. Obese women excreted estriol as the major metabolite of estradiol, while women with anorexia nervosa excreted 2-hydroxyestradiol (a catechol estrogen) as the major metabolite of estradiol. Thus, in women with a low percentage of body fat, the pathway for estradiol metabolism is directed toward the production of catechol estrogens. Adashi et al[33] found that the administration of catechol estrogens to hypogonadal women results in a decrease in the amplitude and pulse frequency of pituitary gonadotropin secretion.

De Ridder et al[34] reported that body fat distribution, rather than body fat mass, influenced the onset of puberty. Girls with fat predominantly localized on the hips had the highest levels of sex steroids and gonadotropins. This finding was interpreted to indicate that this fat distribution was the result of ovarian activity. On the other hand, girls with predominantly abdominal fat were more obese and showed increased plasma levels of estradiol and a lower androgen:estrogen ratio, which was interpreted as resulting from increased estrogen production by extraglandular aromatization of androgens in obese girls.

In a later longitudinal study of 68 school girls, de Ridder et al[35] found that control of the onset of puberty and maturation of the hypothalamic–pituitary–gonadal axis are partially independent. Body fat distribution, rather than body fat mass, was more important to the onset of puberty in girls

Undernutrition delays the onset of sexual maturation in boys similar to the delaying effects of undernutrition on menarche.[36,37] In the male, the weight gain required to initiate puberty is less than in girls. At full sexual maturation, the male will have approximately 15 to 17 percent of body mass as fat, whereas the female will have approximately 24 to 26 percent of body mass as body fat.

Role of the Pineal Gland in Puberty

Since the first description of a boy with precocious puberty associated with a neoplasm invading the pineal gland, it has been postulated that the pineal gland secretes a substance that delays secondary sexual maturation until adolescence.[38] In rodents, melatonin appears to inhibit LH and FSH secretion and play a role in reproductive function. Human data are conflicting and no conclusions can be drawn.[39]

DELAYED SEXUAL MATURATION AND AMENORRHEA

The adolescent girl with delayed secondary sexual development or menstrual abnormalities is usually brought to the physician by her mother.[40] By the time an abnormality of puberty or a menstrual disorder is recognized by an adolescent girl and her parents, the girl has a concept of secondary sexual development, menstruation, and reproductive function. These concepts are well established, even if secondary sexual development has not begun. It is important that the physician who first evaluates a young woman with abnormal secondary sexual development or menstrual dysfunction communicate with the adolescent woman. Too often, the parent(s) becomes the focus of the discussion and the adolescent simply becomes the subject of the discussion.

History of Secondary Sexual Development

The young woman should provide as much of the history as possible. If communication is conducted through the parent(s), the patient becomes a third party to the conversation. She is reduced to only yes or no answers with interspersed grunts. This situation can be avoided by allowing the patient to recite the history.

The physician obtaining the history should be comfortable inquiring about breast development, sexual hair growth, development of libidinal desire, and menstruation. If the physician is uncomfortable asking these questions of adolescents (in private with the adolescent or in the presence of the adolescent and parents), the adolescent girl will feel ill at ease. Open communication at the time of the initial visit will allow for further open communication later with the adolescent girl, the physician, and her parents.

The physician begins obtaining the history by inquiring about the stages of secondary sexual development.[41] By following the expected stages of secondary sexual development, the history is logical for the physician to formulate a cause for delayed maturation or amenorrhea and makes the line of reasoning logical for the patient as she knows what is happening to her peers and the sequence of these events. Inquire about breast development first, followed by the onset of sexual hair growth, the growth spurt, menstruation, established cycles, and the effects of cycles on the breasts, skin, mood, and affect.

If no secondary sexual development has occurred by age 13 to 14 yr, this fact suggests that the hypothalamic–pituitary axis has failed to secrete GnRH and/or gonadotropins or that the ovaries have failed to respond to the hypothalamic–pituitary signal.

If secondary sexual development has occurred partially, ie, breast development has begun but not been completed and sexual hair growth has begun but not been completed, the pubertal process was initiated but interrupted prior to completion of sexual maturation.

If menstruation has occurred but cyclic menses have not developed, this suggests that hypothalamic–pituitary–ovarian function was interrupted before ovulation was fully established.

If full sexual maturation has occurred, ie, there is full breast development with full sexual hair growth, and if there is history of menstrual molimina (cyclic breast fullness, cyclic mood changes, cyclic acne, and pelvic abdominal bloating), it is likely that full secondary sexual maturation and function have occurred but there is obstruction of the genital outflow tract or absence of the uterus.[42]

Libidinal desire stems from cyclic sex-steroid hormone secretion and is usually established with ovulation.[43] The presence or absence of libidinal desire is helpful in developing a differential diagnosis of delayed puberty or amenorrhea.

Illicit drug use—especially use of marijuana—can alter hypothalamic–pituitary function to produce cessation of ovarian function.[44] Other illicit drugs have less effect on secondary sexual development and the menstrual cycle.

Alterations in body weight, both rapid weight gain and rapid weight loss, interfere with estrogen metabolism to produce alterations in secondary sexual maturation and amenorrhea. Body weight alterations can result both from low caloric intake and exercise.

Physical Examination

A thorough physical examination must be performed with special reference to the development of secondary sexual characteristics, the integument, the senses, and vital signs. No effort should be made to avoid performing a pelvic examination; if this is the first pelvic examination for a young woman, it must be performed with reassurance and sensitivity.

The general body habitus should be evaluated first. Obesity and slimness are associated with delayed sexual development and amenorrhea. Excessively tall adolescent girls may have a 46,XY karyotype; excessively short girls may have a 45,X karyotype (Turner syndrome) or a 46,XX/45,X mosaic karyotype. Abnormalities in the shape of the skull, scoliosis, limb defects, and spacing of the nipples can be found in association with delayed sexual development and amenorrhea.

When the vital signs are obtained, be aware that hypertension in an adolescent with delayed sexual maturation is associated with the enzyme defect 17-hydroxylase deficiency. Hormonal studies are required to establish this diagnosis, but the finding of hypertension makes this a likely cause of sexual infantilism and amenorrhea.

Abnormalities of specific cranial nerves are associated with conditions of delayed sexual development and amenorrhea. The history of poorly developed senses of taste and smell and the physical finding of anosmia or hyposmia is a clue to the condition of Kallmann syndrome (DeMorsier syndrome in females). This will be described in more detail. A history of high-frequency hearing loss is associated with partial deletion of the long arm of one X chromosome. In this condition, there is premature ovarian failure that may present as complete lack of secondary sexual development and amenorrhea, partial secondary sexual development with amenorrhea, or the establishment of complete secondary sexual maturation with ovulation followed by secondary amenorrhea due to premature ovarian failure.

A history of visual disturbances can be associated with pituitary adenomas or other benign tumors that impinge on the optic chiasm. In patients with prolactin-secreting adenomas, amenorrhea (or arrested sexual function in males) may be secondary; in patients with hamartomas or craniopharyngiomas, arrested sexual maturation may be primary. In patients with visual field disturbances, the presenting symptom may be difficulty driving an automobile. Severe visual field defects may be detected by gross evaluation of visual fields; subtle visual field defects must be evaluated by special visual field testing.

Changes in the integument may give clues to the etiology of delayed secondary sexual development or amenorrhea. Young women with acne and hirsutism likely have an underlying androgen excess disorder. Women with absence of sexual hair or sparse sexual hair and presence of breast development may have a 46,XY karyotype with a deficiency of androgen receptors. Hypopigmented skin can be associated with pituitary failure; vitiligo (patchy areas of depigmented skin) may be associated with immunologic ovarian failure. Hyperpigmented skin can be associated with cortisol excess when the adrenal glands are hyperstimulated by excess adrenocorticotropic hormone. Sallow skin color can be found in young men and women with chronic diseases while skin with a yellow cast may be found in association with anorexia nervosa. Acanthosis nigricans is found in areas of skin folds (on the posterior neck, between the breasts, in the intertriginous areas of the thighs, and on the elbows and knees). The finding of acanthosis nigricans is associated with androgen excess and insulin-resistant diabetes mellitus.

The thyroid gland must be palpated as a routine in evaluation of young women with amenorrhea. Both hypo- and hyperthyroidism can present in association with amenorrhea. It is difficult to differentiate the two conditions on the basis of the consistency of the thyroid gland alone. However, in hyperthyroidism the gland may be pulsatile and elicit bruits to auscultation. In thyroiditis, the thyroid gland may be tender to palpation. Thyroiditis can be associated with immunologic premature gonadal failure.

Breast examination is essential to understanding the causes of abnormal sexual development in girls and boys and amenorrhea in girls. Breast development is dependent upon estrogen production in early female puberty and progesterone production in later female puberty. Estrogens stimulate the ductal elements of the breasts, while progesterone stimulates the acinar elements of the breasts. Estrogens alone produce tubular-appearing breasts; progesterone produces rounding of the breasts. A deficiency in estrogen exposure causes breast underdevelopment. Truncated or delayed breast development is often found in adolescent girls with premature ovarian failure; failure of breast development is often found in women with hypothalamic–pituitary dysfunction. The physical characteristics of the nipples and areolae provide clues to the hormonal environment to which they have been exposed. The nipples and areolae are rich in estrogen receptors; conditions of estrogen excess lead to protuberance of the nipples and areolae, while conditions of estrogen deficiency lead to small, pale nipples and areolae. This is especially seen in anorexia nervosa. In adolescent males, gynecomastia occurs in about 40 percent to a limited extent. Breast enlargement in an adolescent male can lead to ridicule and embarrassment. In all but a few adolescent males, this is a transitory occurrence and can be managed by providing reassurance. However, in a few, where gynecomastia persists, endocrine evaluation and surgical management may be required.

Few abnormalities of the heart and lungs coexist with conditions of delayed sexual maturation and amenorrhea. Adolescent women with Turner syndrome may have coarctation of the aorta with its characteristic auscultatory changes. However, this diagnosis is obvious from other physical findings.

On abdominal examination, pay particular attention to the inguinal canals. Inguinal hernia in an adolescent female may be a clue to the diagnosis of androgen insensitivity syndrome.

Examination of the external and internal genitalia is essential to evaluate delayed sexual maturation and amenorrhea. Is pubic hair present? Absence of pubic hair with breast development is found in androgen insensitivity syndrome. Presence of pubic hair in the absence of breast development can be a clue to precocious adrenarche or adrenal hyperplasia. If pubic hair is excessive and the clitoris is enlarged, there is usually an androgen excess condition. In the androgen insensitivity syndrome, the external genitalia appear female. Yet, on careful inspection the labia majora and labia minora are hypoplastic. In conditions of estrogen deficiency, the vaginal mucosa is pale, thin, dry, and lacks rugation. The cervical mucus is absent in conditions of estrogen deficiency; the cervical mucus is abundant in conditions of estrogen excess.

In genital tract anomalies, the hymen may appear imperforate. When the imperforate hymen is the cause of amenorrhea, the hymen will be bulging. When the vagina (and usually the uterus) is absent, the hymen will be flat. This is an important point for clinical differentiation.

In the adolescent male, attention should be paid to body habitus, beard growth, penile and testicular enlargement, and prostatic enlargement. In excessively tall males with delayed or truncated sexual development, the clinician should consider the possibility of Klinefelter syndrome (47,XXY). If sexual development is delayed, the possibility of hypothalamic–pituitary failure or testicular failure must be evaluated.

Laboratory Evaluation of Delayed Puberty and Amenorrhea

The physician should quickly establish the role of the hypothalamus, pituitary gland, and gonads in conditions of delayed puberty and amenorrhea. The best method to isolate the roles of these glands is to measure FSH and LH. If the problem is hypothalamic–pituitary dysfunction, FSH and LH will be in the low range; if the problem is gonadal failure, FSH and LH will be elevated as in menopausal women. Adolescent women with ovarian failure who have never been exposed to estrogens will not have hot flushes, and adolescent women with hypothalamic–pituitary dysfunction will not have hot flushes. Therefore, this is not a useful clinical clue in differentiating between these causes of amenorrhea.

Some physicians recommend a progestin challenge test as the first step in the diagnostic evaluation of amenorrhea. The response to the progestin challenge test is dependent upon previous estrogen exposure of the endometrium. If the endometrium has been stimulated previously by estrogens, the administration of progestin will produce withdrawal bleeding from the endometrium. However, if the endometrium has not been previously exposed to estrogens prior to the progestin administration there will be no withdrawal bleeding. The progestin challenge test provides information only about previous endometrial estrogen exposure. The knowledgeable clinician can predict the response to the progestin challenge test by evaluating the cervical mucus. If the mucus is abundant, thin, clear, and watery, there will be a positive response to progestin withdrawal. On the other hand, if the cervical mucus is scant, the progestin challenge test will be negative.

Prolactin measurement should be a routine part of the laboratory evaluation of delayed puberty and amenorrhea. Hyperprolactinemia, in the absence of galactorrhea, can exist as a cause of delayed puberty or amenorrhea. In conditions of hyperprolactinemia, FSH and LH are suppressed from providing an adequate signal to stimulate gonadal function.

Primary hypothyroidism is a rare cause of delayed puberty and adolescent amenorrhea. In this condition, there may be hyperprolactinemia. However, thyroid function studies (thyroid-stimulating hormone [TSH], T_3, T_4) should not be obtained as a routine part of the evaluation.

If there is clinical evidence of androgen excess (hirsutism, excessive acne; anatomic alterations of the genitalia), then androstenedione, testosterone, and dehydroepiandrosterone sulfate should be obtained as part of the initial laboratory evaluation.

Imaging, chromosomal, and stimulation studies should be reserved until the initial studies have been obtained and interpreted. The rush to be "complete" at the time of initial evaluation may cause the physician to order expensive, irrelevant tests.

If an adolescent male or female has hypogonadotropic hypogonadism (low FSH and LH) or hyperprolactinemia, it is appropriate to follow up with a lateral skull film to evaluate the sella turcica and suprasellar area of the skull. Lesions such as craniopharyngioma, hamartoma, and prolactin-secreting pituitary adenomas may produce abnormal calcification of the sella turcica on lateral skull film. The follow-up study should be a magnetic resonance imaging study of the hypothalamic–pituitary area of the brain.

Chromosomal studies should be obtained in adolescent males and females who exhibit evidence of premature gonadal failure or those who have an intersex problem. Particular attention should be paid to the X chromosomes in girls. Deletion of a fragment of the long arm of one X chromosome can result in premature ovarian failure with resultant truncated secondary sexual development or amenorrhea. The presence of a Y chromosome in a person raised as a female denotes an intersex problem. An extra X chromosome in a male (47,XXY) is evidence of the Klinefelter syndrome associated with hypogonadism.[45]

It is difficult for the clinician to distinguish hypothalamic dysfunction from pituitary dysfunction when amenorrhea or gonadal failure in a male exists. The differential diagnosis can be further elucidated by intravenous bolus injection of GnRH (100 µg) and measuring FSH and LH at 10-min intervals for 60 min. In conditions of hypothalamic dysfunction, there will be a rise in FSH and LH; in conditions of pituitary dysfunction, FSH and LH will remain at the basal level. This test is rarely indicated in the evaluation of amenorrhea.

CAUSES OF DELAYED PUBERTY AND AMENORRHEA

Hypothalamic–Pituitary Dysfunction

Hypothalamic–pituitary dysfunction occurs with increasing frequency as a cause of primary and secondary amenorrhea.[46] The gonadotropin signals from the pituitary gland are inadequate to produce follicular maturation with subsequent sex-steroid hormone secretion. The causes of hypothalamic pituitary dysfunction are presented in Table 5–2.

Kallmann syndrome is a condition of hypoplasia of the olfactory tracts with coexisting dysfunction of the arcuate nucleus of the hypothalamus.[47] The hypothalamus cannot secrete GnRH. Because of the olfactory tract hypoplasia, the affected individual cannot smell and has absent or poorly developed sense of taste. In this condition, there is little or no secondary sexual development. The disorder occurs more commonly in boys than in girls. In girls, the condition is called DeMorsier syndrome.[48] The diagnosis can be made in the ambulatory setting by challenging the patient to recognize common odors such as coffee, rubbing alcohol, or ether.

TABLE 5–2.   CAUSES OF HYPOTHALAMIC–PITUITARY DYSFUNCTION

Functional Causes
  Low body weight
  Exercise-induced amenorrhea
  Marijuana-induced amenorrhea
  Stress

Pituitary Failure (Primary and Secondary)
  Isolated GnRH deficiency
  Sheehan syndrome
  Kallmann (DeMorsier) syndrome

Neoplastic Disorders
  Craniopharyngioma
  Pituitary prolactinoma

Sheehan syndrome is rare in adolescent women. This condition occurs when the pituitary gland sustains infarction and loses the ability to secrete pituitary tropic hormones.[49] In addition to gonadal dysfunction, thyroid and adrenal dysfunction usually coexist as well. Pituitary infarction is most likely to occur in association with obstetrical hemorrhage leading to shock.

Craniopharyngioma is a benign neoplasm located between the hypothalamus and pituitary gland that interferes with portal blood flow between the hypothalamus and pituitary gland.[50] This diagnosis is suspected by the finding of calcification in the area described on lateral skull film. Follow-up evaluation is made by magnetic resonance imaging. Secondary sexual development can be initiated and completed by administration of exogenous sex-steroid hormones or pulsatile GnRH. Ovulation and spermatogenesis can be induced by administration of human menopausal gonadotropin (hMG) or pulsatile GnRH when reproductive function is desired. Since the tumor must be removed surgically, the physician must proceed with caution in advising surgery. Unless the patient is suffering from chronic, debilitating headache, surgical removal may not be necessary.

Isolated gonadotropin deficiency is a rare condition similar to Kallmann syndrome in which the hypothalamus does not secrete GnRH. It may be a variant of Kallmann syndrome. The diagnosis is made by priming the pituitary gland with exogenous estrogens and injecting later a bolus of GnRH. A person with this disorder will not secrete FSH and LH from the pituitary gland. Isolated gonadotropin deficiency presents as sexual infantilism. There is usually no breast development and only sparse pubic hair in girls and poor genital development with sparse pubic hair in boys.

Low body weight, exercise-induced amenorrhea, and stress-induced amenorrhea can be grouped because the pathophysiology is similar.[51–54] In each of these conditions, there is interference with pulsatile release of GnRH—both amplitude and pulse frequency are altered—such that gonadotropin release from the pituitary gland does not adequately stimulate follicular development. There are varying degrees of ovarian dysfunction in these disorders, ranging from short luteal phase of an ovulatory reproductive cycle to amenorrhea. The mechanism(s) for these alterations are poorly understood. When low body weight, exercise-induced amenorrhea, or stress-induced amenorrhea is suspected, the adolescent woman should be counseled to change behavior or alter coping skills to restore cyclic reproductive function.

Problems with low body weight are seen with increasing frequency in clinical practice. Young women should be encouraged to attain and maintain their ideal body weight. This problem is seen rarely in adolescent males.

Marijuana use is widespread in modern society. Marijuana finds its way into high schools and middle schools so it cannot be assumed that adolescent males with truncated secondary sexual development and adolescent women with amenorrhea, delayed sexual development, or incomplete sexual development do not use the drug. Marijuana blocks release of GnRH. Thus, gonadotropin stimulation of the testicles and ovaries is truncated or absent. The effects of marijuana on reproductive function are self-limiting. When the drug is discontinued, cyclic reproductive function is restored in women and normal sexual function is restored in men.

Hyperprolactinemia rarely is associated with delayed sexual maturation and primary amenorrhea but must be considered in any adolescent woman with secondary amenorrhea and adolescent man with impotence.[55] Galactorrhea may or may not be a clinical finding in women. The diagnosis is established by the finding of prolactin excess in plasma. If the plasma prolactin exceeds 100 ng/ml, imaging studies of the sella turcica are warranted.

Treatment of hypothalamic–pituitary dysfunction must be directed to the underlying cause. Those with Kallmann syndrome, craniopharyngioma, Sheehan syndrome, and isolated gonadotropin deficiency require exogenous hormone replacement to establish secondary sexual maturation (if it has failed to occur) and will require replacement with pulsatile GnRH or hMG to induce spermatogenesis or ovulation when reproduction is desired.

Women with low body weight, exercise-induced amenorrhea, and stress-induced amenorrhea will have spontaneous resumption of hypothalamic–pituitary function when they change behavior and lifestyle. The problem is self-limiting. However, it is often difficult to convince adolescent women and their parents that lifestyle and behavior can produce hypothalamic–pituitary dysfunction and can be the cause of truncated puberty and amenorrhea. Women with these conditions are at risk for the development of osteoporosis. Women with exercise-induced amenorrhea—especially ballerinas, competitive runners, and gymnasts—are at increased risk for fractures of the vertebral column and calcaneus.[56,57] Consideration must be given to exogenous estrogen replacement for protection from osteoporosis. Yet, the underlying causes cannot be allowed to go ignored.

Marijuana-induced amenorrhea and testicular dysfunction are self-limiting and are reversed promptly after drug use is discontinued. It is the skillful physician who can elicit the history of marijuana use and counsel the adolescent to stop the practice of drug use.

Ovarian Failure

Ovarian failure in adolescents is most commonly the result of chromosomal deletions, especially deletions of the X chromosome or fragments of the long arm of the X chromosome. Less common causes of ovarian failure in adolescents result from the toxic effects of alkylating chemotherapy on the ovarian follicular membranes when administered for the treatment of childhood and adolescent neoplasms and the rare gonadotropin-resistant ovary syndrome (Savage syndrome). These conditions will be discussed in this section.

Turner syndrome (45,X gonadal dysgenesis) is the most frequent cause of premature ovarian failure.[58,59] The defect results from the absence of one of the two X chromosomes. The short arm of the X chromosome (designated p) carries somatic information necessary for full adult height and development of the skeletal and cardiovascular systems. The long arm of the X chromosome (designated q) carries information necessary for maintenance of ovarian follicles in an arrested state for future maturation and ovulation.

In Turner syndrome, the absence of an X chromosome causes both skeletal and cardiovascular abnormalities and premature atresia of ovarian follicles. At birth, girls with Turner syndrome have characteristic physical findings of lymphedema, shield chest, and cubitus valgus (increased carrying angle of the arms). Most have ovarian failure at birth. The oocytes that normally migrate to the ovarian stroma by midgestation do not fully migrate in female fetuses with Turner syndrome. However, those oocytes that do migrate undergo atresia prior to birth due to the absence of the long arm of the X chromosome. Gonadotropins are in the menopausal range at birth.[60]

The physical characteristics that distinguish Turner syndrome are recognized prior to puberty. Therefore, the failure to undergo secondary sexual maturation can be anticipated and exogenous hormone replacement administration initiated to coincide with the expected time of secondary sexual maturation to prevent embarrassing delay in breast development and sexual hair growth. Since short stature is a feature of Turner syndrome, estrogen administration must be begun at a low dosage to prevent premature epiphyseal closure. By giving estradiol-17β at a dosage of 0.5 mg/day for 6 to 9 mo and then increasing the dosage to 1 mg/day until breast development accelerates, maximal height can be achieved.

There is no rationale for estrogen as growth-promoting therapy. In patients in whom estrogen therapy was initiated on or before 12 yr of age, the degree of improvement in final height was significantly less (approximately 4 to 5 cm) than in those in whom therapy was started after 14 yr of age.[61]

Other X chromosomal disorders include the mosaic Turner syndrome (45,X/46,XX karyotype), in which some of the cell lines have a normal chromosomal complement. In the mosaic Turner syndrome, there may be partial or even full secondary sexual maturation before ovarian failure occurs. There are some case reports of pregnancy in women with mosaic Turner syndrome. In the mosaic Turner syndrome, women are usually short of stature but not as short as women with Turner syndrome.

A variant of Turner syndrome is Sweyer syndrome (46,XY karyotype). These individuals have female external and internal genitalia. The testicles are dysgenetic. During embryogenesis, the dysgenetic testicles fail to secrete Müllerian duct-inhibiting factor and testosterone. At birth, the sexual assignment is female. At the expected time of puberty, there is no secondary sexual development, which leads to the diagnosis. When the diagnosis is established, the dysgenetic testicles should be removed because of the incidence (>25 percent) of developing gonadoblastoma. Management is otherwise the same as in other adolescent women with ovarian failure.

Long-arm deletion of the X chromosome (46XXq–) is a variant of gonadal failure in which the extent of deletion of the long arm of the X chromosome determines the time of onset and extent of ovarian failure.[62] If all of the long arm is deleted, there will be ovarian failure at the time of birth as in Turner syndrome. On the other hand, if there is fragmentary deletion of the long arm, then secondary sexual maturation may be complete. Pregnancies occur commonly in women with small fragmentary deletions of the long arm of the X chromosome.

Alkylating chemotherapy administered for childhood leukemia, lymphoma, and other childhood and adolescent neoplasms has toxic effects on the follicular membrane of the ovarian follicles and on the germinal epithelium of the testicles.[63] Many young women and men have gonadal failure following several courses of alkylating chemotherapy.

Gonadotropin-resistant ovary syndrome is rare in adolescent women but is seen with increasing frequency in adult women.[64] In this poorly understood disorder, the ovarian follicles are present within the ovarian stroma but do not bind FSH. Thus, FSH and LH are elevated in the menopausal range despite the presence of ovarian follicles. There is no known associated chromosomal abnormality with the gonadotropin-resistant ovary syndrome. The diagnosis is made by histologic confirmation of ovarian follicles within the ovarian stroma. However, ovarian biopsy is not recommended to make the diagnosis as it can produce periovarian adhesions and compromise later reproduction. In the gonadotropin-resistant ovary syndrome, there have been a number of case reports of pregnancy in women who were receiving exogenous estrogen and progestin therapy.

The diagnosis of ovarian failure can be suspected when an adolescent woman complains of hot flushes. However, many do not have this complaint until they have first received exogenous estrogen replacement and experienced estrogen withdrawal. A combination of hypergonadotropic hypogonadism and exogenous estrogen exposure seems to be prerequisite for hot flushes.

Ovarian failure is treated by estrogen and progestin replacement. If left untreated, adolescent women with ovarian failure will develop early, profound osteoporosis. The same applies in males with testicular failure. This can be prevented by timely administration of exogenous estrogen for women and testosterone for men. Moreover, estrogen is necessary to stimulate breast development, facilitate sexual hair growth, and initiate menses. After secondary sexual maturation has reached that which is compatible with an adolescent woman ready to establish cyclic ovulatory cycles, progesterone should be added to the estrogen replacement regimen.

Ovarian failure formerly carried a hopeless prognosis for pregnancy. With the advances in assisted reproductive technology, oocyte donation and embryo transfer open new vistas for adolescent women with ovarian failure and adult women with premature ovarian failure.[65] This technology can be applied even in women with Sweyer syndrome.

Anatomic Defects

The internal genital tract forms from the fusion and canalization of the Müllerian ducts during the first 8 to 12 wk of fetal life. Failure of formation, fusion, and canalization of the Müllerian ducts or failure of canalization of the urogenital sinus will result in primary amenorrhea. Anatomic defects of the genital tract have no effect on ovarian function. In adolescent women with genital tract abnormalities, there will be no interference with secondary sexual maturation. In some adolescent women, ovulatory cycles may be established before the diagnosis of genital tract atresia or obstruction is made.

The most common anatomic defects of the genital tract are imperforate hymen and Müllerian agenesis (Rokitansky–Kuster–Hauser syndrome) and complete androgen-resistant syndrome (testicular feminization).[66] The adolescent woman with imperforate hymen presents with a history of cyclic pelvic pain and a bluish bulge at the perineum. These symptoms begin once cyclic menses are established. The diagnosis is simple to make on the basis of history and physical examination.

Müllerian agenesis is most often painless since the uterus and vagina are congenitally absent. On rare occasions (10 percent of cases), the uterus will be present and the vagina absent. In this situation, there is cyclic abdominal pain and an abdominal mass. In total Müllerian agenesis, there is full secondary sexual maturation with cyclic ovulation.

Treatment of the imperforate hymen requires only a simple hymenotomy. Treatment of vaginal agenesis is controversial. Some advocate pressure dilatation of the genital tract to create a vagina (Frank procedure and Ingram procedure), while others advocate the creation of a neovagina by transplanting a split-thickness skin graft from the hip to the vaginal space. The vaginal space is opened at the time the skin graft is taken, and the graft is placed around a vaginal prosthesis. After several months, the neovagina takes on the secretory characteristics of natural vaginal epithelium.[42]

In the rare situation where the uterus and cervix are present, a neovagina can be surgically created and connected to the uterus. This procedure has resulted in pregnancy and birth of a healthy child.[67,68]

Intrauterine adhesions (Asherman syndrome) is usually an acquired condition that results following curettage of the endometrial cavity[69] and has been associated with tuberculous endometritis. This condition can produce amenorrhea but will not interfere with secondary sexual development or ovulation.

Other Conditions

Polycystic ovarian disease and late-onset adrenal hyperplasia do not fit conveniently into other classifications of delayed puberty and amenorrhea. These disorders do not present often as primary amenorrhea but may present as secondary amenorrhea.[70] (See Chapter 19.)

Late-onset adrenal hyperplasia[71] is another condition not uncommon to adolescent women that presents with irregular cycles, acne, hirsutism, or secondary amenorrhea. In the common form of this disorder, there is deficiency of the enzyme 21-hydroxylase. (See Chapter 18.)

PRECOCIOUS PUBERTY

If a girl develops secondary sexual characteristics before age 8 yr or a boy develops secondary sexual characteristics before age 9 yr, the child is considered to have sexual precocity.[72] Precocious sexual development can result from hypothalamic–pituitary stimulation of the gonads, in which case secondary sexual development will follow the expected normal sequence of puberty. On the other hand, precocious sexual development can result from inappropriate hormone secretion, in which case pubertal development will deviate from the expected norm. Modern classification of precocious sexual development divides the conditions into: (1) central precocious puberty; (2) peripheral precocious puberty; and (3) contrasexual precocious puberty.

Classifications

Central Precocious Puberty. **Idiopathic precocious puberty** is the most frequent type of premature secondary sexual maturation in girls and occurs only rarely in boys.[73] In idiopathic precocious puberty, the appearance of developmental milestones occurs in the expected way with the time of appearance following the expected time line. An example of a 6-yr-old girl with central precocious puberty is presented in Figure 5–5. Moreover, in idiopathic precocious puberty there is no evidence of central nervous system lesions, which could stimulate GnRH release or block inhibition of GnRH secretion until the expected time.

Girls with idiopathic precocious puberty first will have breast development, followed by sexual hair growth, followed by menarche, and concluded by ovulation. The growth spurt will occur at the appropriate time in the sequence of sexual development. Precocious puberty in girls does not compromise reproductive function and does not portend premature menopause. Although these girls will be taller than their peers at the time secondary sexual development begins, they will be short as adults because of the premature sexual development.

Boys with idiopathic precocious puberty will have testicular enlargement, followed by penile enlargement and the appearance of pubic hair, and followed by ejaculation of seminal fluid. Like girls, boys with idiopathic precocious puberty will be short as adults.

Hormonal studies in children with idiopathic precocious puberty will be consistent with values found in adolescents with normal pubertal development. Pituitary gonadotropin secretory patterns will mimic those found in normal pubertal children and are sleep entrained.

Central nervous system tumors and inflammatory disorders can initiate hypothalamic–pituitary function to stimulate gonadal sex-steroid secretion. Lesions associated with precocious puberty are craniopharyngiomas, hamartomas, gliomas, and ependymomas.[74] Hamartomas are unique. They may secrete ectopic GnRH.[75]

Precocious puberty has been reported in association with encephalitis, meningitis, sarcoidosis of the

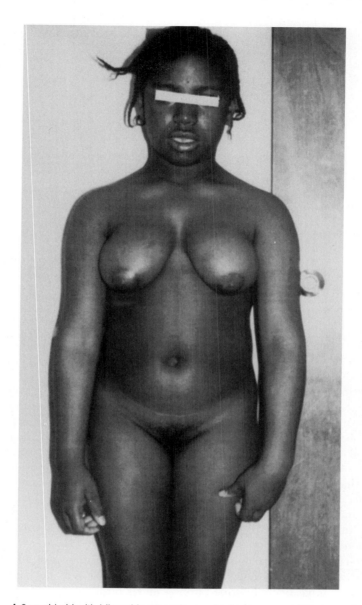

Figure 5–5.   A 6-yr-old girl with idiopathic precocious puberty. Her menarche occurred at age 7 yr.

hypothalamic–pituitary axis, and tuberculosis of the hypothalamus.[76] Inflammatory diseases tend to be self-limiting. When the inflammation subsides, hypothalamic secretion of GnRH usually abates and secondary sexual development is arrested until the appropriate time.

Central nervous system tumors that are localized in the area of the hypothalamus are difficult to treat by neurosurgical methods. The lesions are often inaccessible and attempts at surgical removal can produce lasting side effects. Unless there are indications other than precocious puberty, these lesions are best left alone and the precocious puberty managed by medical means.

Peripheral Precocious Puberty. Any source of human chorionic gonadotropin (hCG) remote from the hypothalamic–pituitary axis or any source of sex-steroid hormones not stimulated by gonadotropin will produce precocious puberty. Because the stimulation of secondary sexual development is not of central nervous system origin, it is classified as peripheral precocious puberty. Ectopic hCG from germ cell or hepatic tumors will stimulate the gonads to secrete sex-steroid hormones. However, since hCG secretion does not occur in a pulsatile fashion, the progression of puberty will not occur in the expected sequence or in the expected time frame. Moreover, autonomous secretion of sex-steroid hormones

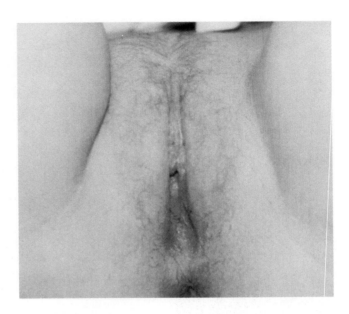

Figure 5–6.   Precocious sexual hair growth in a 7-yr-old girl with adrenal hyperplasia—21-hydroxylase type. The diagnosis was made by finding an elevated DS and 17-hydroxyprogesterone. ACTH stimulation test confirmed the diagnosis.

by the gonads or adrenal glands will stimulate development of secondary sex characteristics.[77]

McCune–Albright syndrome causes precocious puberty in both males and females.[78] The etiology of this disorder is due to a mutation of the $G_s\alpha$ increasing adenylate cyclase activation (see Chapter 7). In addition to precocious secondary sexual development, there is polyostotic fibrous dysplasia of bone with characteristic sclerosis of the basal skull and café au lait spots with irregular borders on the skin surfaces.

Gonadotropin-independent precocity is a syndrome marked by precocious pubertal development in the absence of pubertal levels of gonadotropins. This unique form of sexual maturation has been described in both girls with McCune–Albright syndrome and boys in whom there is a male family history of precocious puberty. This condition is unaltered by administration of long-acting GnRH.[79]

The sex-steroid hormone secretion is autonomous rather than under the control of hypothalamic–pituitary gonadotropin secretion. In girls, there will be follicular cysts of the ovaries and in boys there will be testicular enlargement. Other endocrinopathies have been reported in association with McCune–Albright syndrome. These include gigantism, hyperthyroidism, and Cushing syndrome.

Adrenal hyperplasia (21-hydroxylase deficiency and 11-β hydroxylase deficiency) causes precocious puberty in the male characterized by penile enlargement, enlargement of the muscular limb–shoulder girdle, and the appearance of pubic and axillary hair.[80] Because the adrenal glands are the source of androgens and are not under the control of hypothalamic–pituitary gonadotropin secretion, the testicles will be small (prepubertal) in size. This is a characteristic feature and can lead the clinician to suspect the diagnosis. In girls, adrenal hyperplasia presents with precocious pubic hair (Fig 5–6), axillary hair, and associated acne. Breast development, if present, will be truncated. Both boys and girls with this condition will be taller than their peers but will have short adult height because of premature epiphyseal closure if therapy is not instituted promptly.

The diagnosis of adrenal hyperplasia is established by the findings of elevated DS, 17-hydroxyprogesterone, and a positive corticotropin (ACTH) stimulation test.[81] Rarely, the adrenal hyperplasia is due to 11-β hydroxylase deficiency. In this situation, there will be less virilization than that found in 21-hydroxylase deficiency.

Autonomous ovarian cysts can be a cause of precocious sexual development in girls.[78] During childhood, ovarian follicles are stimulated by pituitary gonadotropins but do not secrete sufficient estradiol to stimulate breast growth or vaginal maturation. Some follicular cysts in children secrete sufficient estradiol to stimulate estrogen-dependent tissues. Once hypothalamic–pituitary gonadotropin secretory function and ectopic hCG secretion have been excluded as causal, the diagnosis of autonomous ovarian cyst formation can be considered. In this condition, vaginal ultrasound examination will reveal small (8 to 10 mm) follicular cysts in the ovaries.

Exogenous sex-steroid hormones can stimulate dependent tissues and produce precocious secondary

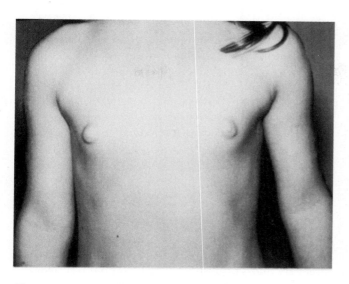

Figure 5–7. Precocious thelarche in a 5-yr-old girl. All hormonal studies were normal. Her pubertal development began at age 10 yr.

sexual development. Girls may be exposed to estrogens by mistaking oral contraceptive tablets for candy or through cosmetics that contain estrogens. Moreover, there have been reported cases of precocious sexual development as the result of estrogen ingestion through the food chain. Estrogens have been fed to cattle and poultry for the purpose of forcing weight gain and fat marbling. These estrogens may be sequestered in the tissue of animals and fowl and stimulate estrogen-dependent tissues in children.[82]

Boys who are exposed to exogenous estrogens will develop gynecomastia. This condition is self-limiting and will remiss when testosterone production begins and the source of estrogens is removed. Exogenous androgens are not as available as exogenous estrogens. It is less

likely for a child to be exposed to exogenous testosterone and become virilized.

Limited pubertal development occurs more commonly in girls than in boys. Pubertal development can be limited to precocious thelarche, precocious adrenarche, and, rarely, precocious menarche.

Precocious thelarche usually begins by age 3 yr with the appearance of the breast bud.[83] Progression of breast development is slow, and full breast development as seen in pubertal girls is not achieved (Fig 5–7). Moreover, there is no sexual hair growth associated with premature thelarche. This finding differentiates the condition from central precocious puberty.

Precocious adrenarche usually begins by age 5 yr with the signs of pubic hair growth and an adult body odor.[84] There may be limited, mild acne on the face. There is no associated breast development (Fig 5–8). In precocious adrenarche, DS may be elevated but other androgens and adrenal hormone metabolites are within normal limits. An ACTH stimulation test will be normal. These hormonal findings serve to differentiate precocious adrenarche from adrenal hyperplasia.

Precocious menarche with menstrual bleeding in the absence of other signs of puberty has been reported in a few girls. The etiology and pathogenesis are unknown. The condition is self-limiting and does not interfere with normal pubertal progression.

Contrasexual Precocious Puberty. If a male is stimulated by estrogens or a female is stimulated by androgens, contrasexual development will occur. In males, estrogen production can occur in androgen insensitivity syndrome, leading to gynecomastia, and there is one reported case of excess aromatase activity in a male leading to feminization.

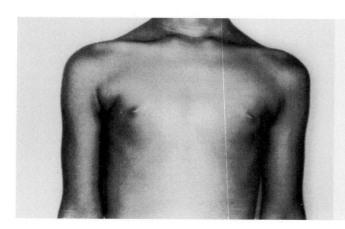
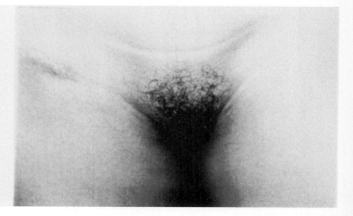

Figure 5–8. Precocious adrenarche in a 6-yr-old girl. Note the Tanner stage 3 sexual hair growth and the absence of breast development. Her DS was at the upper limits of normal for her age.

In girls, virilization during early childhood should be considered abnormal and a source of androgens should be sought. Most commonly, virilization of a girl is the result of adrenal hyperplasia.

Evaluation

The evaluation of a child with precocious sexual development should begin with a medical history and physical examination. The physician should focus on the age of onset of sexual maturation, the sequence of appearance of secondary sexual characteristics, and the rate of growth. Exogenous sources of hormones should be considered in the evaluation, and the possibility of central nervous system tumors or inflammation should be excluded.

The initial evaluation should include a bone film of the left hand and wrist to establish bone age and forecast future growth potential and measurement of gonadotropins, androgens, and estradiol. A lateral skull film will reveal suprasellar calcification if present. This finding could be a clue to the presence of central nervous system tumors or inflammatory disorders. A magnetic resonance imaging study of the hypothalamic–pituitary region is not warranted on initial evaluation and should be selected only when there is suspicion of a central nervous system lesion.

In idiopathic precocious puberty, the gonadotropin secretory pattern will be identical to that found in normal intrapubertal adolescents, and the gonadal response to gonadotropin secretion will be similar. Moreover, the response to GnRH injection will be the same as that found in normal adolescents.

In peripheral precocious puberty, the hypothalamic–pituitary gonadotropin secretory pattern will be similar to that found in prepubertal children. However, sex-steroid hormones will be elevated as the result of ectopic stimulation of the gonads or adrenal glands or autonomous adrenal or gonadal hormone secretion.

Treatment

Once a cause for precocious puberty has been established, treatment options are then considered.[85,86] If the precocious puberty is idiopathic, the physician may elect to treat or not treat depending upon the age of the child and the emotional adjustment of the child and parents to the precocious sexual development. Consideration *must* be given to bone age and predicted adult height.

Idiopathic precocious puberty is best managed by administration of long-acting GnRH agonists.[87] These agents downregulate the GnRH pulses, which prevents pulsatile release of gonadotropins. GnRH agonists will arrest secondary sexual development and hold it in abeyance until withdrawn.

GnRH agonists will also arrest central precocious puberty where the pituitary gonadotropin secretion is dependent upon hypothalamic GnRH secretion. In conditions of ectopic GnRH, GnRH agonists will have no effect and other treatment methods must be sought.

In the case of a central nervous system tumor causing precocious sexual development, surgical management of the lesion is advised *only* if there are other neurosurgical indications such as intractable headache, visual field disturbances, or recurrent nausea and vomiting.

Peripheral precocious puberty is managed best by attacking the source of sex-steroid hormones. In some cases, the source of hormones can be blocked by administration of enzyme inhibitors such as testolactone, which blocks aromatization of androgens to estrogens,[88] or ketoconazole,[89] which blocks C-17,20 lyase, thus preventing the synthesis of androgens from progesterone. Medroxyprogesterone acetate has been the classical treatment for all forms of precocious puberty until the discovery and synthesis of long-acting GnRH agonists. Medroxyprogesterone acetate still has a place in the treatment of precocious puberty, although it is limited today.[90] Medroxyprogesterone acetate downregulates estrogen receptors. Therefore, it has the action to blunt the effects of estrogens and slow the rate of secondary sexual development.

In conditions of tumors that secrete ectopic hCG or steroid hormones, surgical removal is the treatment of choice. In conditions of adrenal hyperplasia, administration of glucocorticoid hormones will prevent the production of excess androgens.

SUMMARY

Puberty is the reawakening of the hypothalamic–pituitary–gonadal axis some 9 to 10 yr following birth. The events of secondary sexual maturation and the attainment of reproductive capacity occur in a logical, predictable sequence. Puberty can be delayed due to late reawakening of the hypothalamic–pituitary–gonadal axis or abnormalities of the endocrine systems. Puberty can be advanced by the premature function of the hypothalamic–pituitary–gonadal axis, resulting in precocious puberty. Evaluation of delayed or precocious puberty should be conducted in a logical, systematic way. Problems of adolescent boys and girls should be handled in a sensitive manner.

REFERENCES

1. Finkelstein JW. The endocrinology of adolescence. *Ped Clin N Am.* 27:53, 1980
2. Tanner JM. Trend toward earlier menarche in London, Oslo, Copenhagen, the Netherlands, and Hungary. *Nature.* 243:95, 1973

3. Zacharias L, Wurtman RJ. Age at menarche. *N Engl J Med.* 280:868, 1969

4. Wyshak G, Frisch RE. Evidence for a secular trend in age of menarche. *N Engl J Med.* 306:1033, 1982

5. Marshall WA, Tanner JM. Variations in the pattern of pubertal changes in girls. *Arch Dis Child.* 44:291, 1969

6. Marshall WA, Tanner JM. Variations in the pattern of pubertal changes in boys. *Arch Dis Child.* 45:13, 1970

7. Sklar CS, Kaplan SL, Grumbach MM. Evidence for dissociation between adrenarche and gonadarche: Studies in patients with idiopathic precocious puberty, gonadal dysgenesis, isolated gonadotropin deficiency, and constitutionally delayed growth and adolescence. *J Clin Endocrinol Metab.* 51:548, 1980

8. Wheeler MD. Physical changes of puberty. *Endocrinol Metab Clin N Am.* 20:1, 1991

9. Zacharias L, Rand WM, Wurtman RJ. A prospective study of sexual development and growth in American girls: The statistics of menarche. *Obstet Gynecol Surv.* 31:325, 1976

10. Martha PM Jr, Reiter EO. Pubertal growth and growth hormone secretion. *Endocrinol Metab Clin N Am.* 20:165, 1991

11. Greulich WW, Pyle SI. *Radiographic Atlas of Skeletal Development of the Hand and Wrist*, 2nd ed. Stanford, Calif., Stanford University Press, 1959

12. Fried RI, Smith EE. Postmenarchal growth patterns. *J Pediatr.* 61:562, 1962

13. Rosenfield RL. The diagnosis and management of delayed puberty. *J Clin Endocrinol Metab.* 70:559, 1990

14. Frisch RE. Fatness, menarche, and female fertility. *Perspect Biol Med.* 28:611, 1985

15. Talbert LM, Hammond MG, Groff T, Udry JR. Relationship of age and pubertal development to ovulation in adolescent girls. *Obstet Gynecol.* 66:542, 1985

16. Hirsch M, Shemesh J, Modan M, Lunenfeld B. Emission of spermatozoa: Age of onset. *Int J Androl.* 2:289, 1979

17. Carlier JG, Steeno OP. Oigarche: The age at first ejaculation. *Andrologia.* 17:104, 1985

18. Large DM, Anderson DC. Twenty-four hour profiles of circulating androgens and oestrogens in male puberty with and without gynaecomastia. *Clin Endocrinol.* 11:505,1979

19. Warren MP, Brooks-Gunn J. Mood and behavior at adolescence: Evidence for hormonal factors. *J Clin Endocrinol Metab.* 69:77, 1989

20. Deykin EY, Levy JC, Wells V. Adolescent depression, alcohol, and drug abuse. *Am J Public Health.* 77:178, 1987

21. Reiter EO, Grumbach MM. Neuroendocrine control mechanisms and the onset of puberty. *Annu Rev Physiol.* 44:595, 1982

22. Ross GT. Disorders of the ovary and female reproductive tract. In: Wilson JD, Foster DW, eds. *Williams Textbook of Endocrinology*, 7th ed. Philadelphia, Pa., W. B. Saunders, 1985: 206

23. Knobil E, Plant TM, Wildt L, et al. Control of the rhesus monkey menstrual cycle: Permissive role of the hypothalamic gonadotropin-releasing hormone. *Science.* 207:1371, 1980

24. Oerter KE, Uriatre MN4, Rose SR, et al. Gonadotropin secretory dynamics during puberty in normal girls and boys. *J Clin Endocrinol Metab.* 71:1251, 1990

25. Marshall JC, Kelch RP. Gonadotropin-releasing hormone: Role of pulsatile secretion in the regulation of reproduction. *N Engl J Med.* 315:1459, 1986

26. Wu FCW, Butler GE, Kelnar CJH, Sellar RE. Patterns of pulsatile luteinizing hormone secretion before and during the onset of puberty in boys: A study using an immunoradiometric assay. *J Clin Endocrinol Metab.* 70:629, 1990

27. Boyar RM, Finkelstein JW, David R, et al. Twenty-four hour patterns of plasma luteinizing hormone and follicle stimulating hormone in sexual precocity. *N Engl J Med.* 289:282, 1973

28. Katz J, Boyar RM, Finkelstein JW, et al. Weight and circadian luteinizing hormone secretory pattern in anorexia nervosa. *Psychosom Med.* 40:549, 1987

29. Apter D, Bützow TL, Laughlin GA, Yen SSC. Gonadotropin-releasing hormone pulse generator activity in girls: Pulsatile and diurnal patterns of circulating gonadotropins. *J Clin Endocrinol Metab.* 76:940, 1993

30. Frisch RE, Revelle R. Height and weight at menarche and a hypothesis of critical weights and adolescent events. *Science.* 169:397, 1970

31. Frisch RE. Body weight and reproduction. *Science.* 246:432, 1989

32. Fishman J, Boyar RM, Hellman L. Influence of body weight gain on estradiol metabolism in young women. *J Clin Endocrinol Metab.* 41:988, 1975

33. Adashi EY, Rakoff J, Divers W, et al. The effect of acutely administered 2-hydroxyesterone on the release of gonadotropin and prolactin before and after estrogen priming in hypogonadal women. *Life Sci.* 25:2051, 1979

34. DeRidder CM, Bruning PF, Zonderland ML, et al. Body fat mass, body fat distribution, and plasma hormones in early puberty in females. *J Clin Endocrinol Metab.* 70:888, 1990

35. DeRidder CM, Thijssen JHH, Bruning PF, et al. Body fat mass, body fat distribution, and pubertal development: A longitudinal study of physical and hormonal sexual maturation in girls. *J Clin Endocrinol Metab.* 75:442, 1992

36. Tanner JW. *Growth at Adolescence*, 2nd ed. Oxford, U.K., Blackwell, 1962

37. Ghafoorunissa H. Undernutrition and fertility of male rats. *J Reprod Fert.* 59:317, 1980

38. Heubner JO. *Dtsch Med Wochenschr.* 24:214, 1899

39. Reiter RJ. Pineal melatonin: Cell biology of its synthesis and of its physiological interactions. *Endocrine Rev.* 12:151, 1991

40. Neinstein LS. Menstrual problems in adolescents. *Med Clin N Am.* 17:1181, 1990

41. Bates GW. Disorders of puberty. *Contemp Ob/Gyn.* 19:165, 1982

42. Wiser WL, Bates GW. Management of vaginal agenesis: A report of 92 cases. *Surg Gynecol Obstet.* 159:108, 1984

43. Bates GW. Estrogen and sexual function. *Medical Aspects of Human Sexuality.* June:11, 1990

44. Asch RH, Smith CG, Siler-Kohdr TM, Pauerstein CJ. Effects of Δ^9-tetrahydrocannabinol during the follicular phase of the rhesus monkey (*Macaca mulatta*). *J Clin Endocrinol Metab.* 52:50, 1981

45. Schwartz ID, Root AW. The Klinefelter syndrome of testicular dysgenesis. *Endocrinol Metab Clin N Am.* 20:153, 1991

46. Vigersky JRA, Andersen AE, Thompson RH, et al. Hypothalamic dysfunction in secondary amenorrhea associated with simple weight loss. *N Eng J Med.* 297:1141, 1977

47. Kallmann FJ, Schoenfeld WA, Barrera SE. The genetic aspects of primary eunuchoidism. *Am J Ment Defic.* 48:203, 1944

48. DeMorsier G, Gauthier G. La dysplasie olfacto genitale. *Patho Biol.* 11:1267, 1963

49. Sheehan HL. Simmond's disease due to post-partum necrosis of the anterior pituitary. *Q J Med.* 32:277, 1940

50. Banna M, Hoare RD, Stanley P, Till K. Craniopharyngioma in children. *J Pediatr.* 83:781, 1980

51. Bates GW. The hypothalamus. In: Aiman EJ, ed. *Infertility: Diagnosis and Management.* New York, N.Y., Springer-Verlag, 1984: 31

52. Warren MP. The effect of exercise on pubertal progression and reproductive function in girls. *J Clin Endocrinol Metab.* 51:1150, 1980

53. Stager JM, Wigglesworth JK, Hatler LK. Interpreting the relationship between age of menarche and prepubertal training. *Med Sci Sports Exer.* 22:54, 1990

54. Axelrod J, Reisine TD. Stress hormones: Their interaction and regulation. *Science.* 224:452, 1984

55. Quigley ME, Judd SJ, Gilliland GB, Yen SSC. Functional studies of dopamine control of prolactin secretion in normal women and women with hyperprolactinemic pituitary microadenoma. *J Clin Endocrinol Metab.* 50:994, 1980

56. Warren MP, Brooks-Gunn J, Hamilton LH, et al. Scoliosis and fractures in young ballet dancers. Relation to delayed menarche and secondary amenorrhea. *N Engl J Med.* 314:1348, 1986

57. Drinkwater BL, Nilson K, Ott S, Chesnutt CH. Bone mineral density after resumption of menses in amenorrheic athletes. *JAMA.* 256:380, 1986

58. Turner HH. A syndrome of infantilism, congenital webbed neck, and cubitus valgus. *Endocrinology.* 23:566, 1938

59. Reindollar RH, Byrd JR, McDonough PG. Delayed sexual development: A study of 252 patients. *Am J Obstet Gynecol.* 140:371, 1981

60. Lippe B. Turner syndrome. *Endocrinol Metab Clin N Am.* 20:121, 1990

61. Saenger P. Turner's syndrome. *N Engl J Med.* 335:1749, 1996

62. Krauss CM, Turksoy RN, Atkins L, et al. Familial premature ovarian failure due to an interstitial deletion of the long arm of the X chromosome. *N Engl J Med.* 317:125, 1987

63. Siris ES, Leventhal BG, Vaitukiatis JL. Effects of childhood leukemia and chemotherapy on puberty and reproductive function in girls. *N Engl J Med.* 294:1143, 1976

64. Aiman J, Smentek C. Premature ovarian failure. *Obstet Gynecol.* 66:9, 1985

65. Sauer MV, Paulson RJ, Lobo RA. A preliminary report on oocyte donation extending reproductive potential to women over 40. *N Engl J Med.* 323:1157, 1990

66. Griffin JE, Edwards C, Madden JD, et al. Congenital absence of the vagina. The Mayer–Rokitansky–Kuster–Hauser syndrome. *Ann Intern Med.* 85:224, 1976

67. Bates GW, Wiser WL. A technique for uterine conservation in adolescent women with vaginal agenesis and a functional uterus. *Obstet Gynecol.* 66:290, 1985

68. Hampton HL, Meeks GR, Bates GW, Wiser WL. Pregnancy after successful vaginoplasty and cervical stenting for partial atresia of the cervix. *Obstet Gynecol.* 76(suppl.):900, 1990

69. Asherman JG. Amenorrhea traumatica (atretica). *J Obstet Gynaecol Br Emp.* 55:23, 1948

70. Bates GU. Hirsutism and androgen excess in childhood and adolescence. *Ped Clin N Am.* 28:513, 1983

71. White PC, New MI, Dupont B. Congenital adrenal hyperplasia. *N Engl J Med.* 316:1519, 1987

72. Wheeler MD, Styne DM. Diagnosis and management of precocious puberty. *Ped Clin N Am.* 37:1255, 1990

73. Root AW, Shulman DI. Isosexual precocity: Current concepts and recent advances. *Fertil Steril.* 45:749, 1986

74. Styne DM, Grumbach MM. Puberty in the male and female. Its physiology and disorders. In: Yen SSC, Jaffe RW, eds. *Reproductive Endocrinology. Physiology, Pathophysiology, and Clinical Management.* 2nd ed. Philadelphia, Pa., W. B. Saunders, 1986: 313

75. Judge DM, Kulin HE, Page R, et al. Hypothalamic hamartoma: A source of luteinizing-hormone-releasing factor in precocious puberty. *N Engl J Med.* 296:7, 1977

76. Asherson RA, Jackson WPA, Lewis B. Abnormalities of development associated with hypothalamic calcification after tuberculosis meningitis. *Br Med J.* 2:839, 1965

77. Chasalow FI, Granoff AB, Tse TF. Adrenal steroid secretion in girls with pseudoprecocious puberty due to autonomous ovarian cysts. *J Clin Endocrinol Metab.* 63:828, 1986

78. Lee PA, Van Dop C, Migeon CJ. McCune–Albright syndrome. Long-term follow-up. *JAMA.* 256:2980, 1986

79. Boepple PA, Frisch LS, Wierman ME, et al. The natural history of autonomous gonadal function, adrenarche, and central puberty in gonadotropin-independent puberty. *J Clin Endocrinol Metab.* 75:1550, 1992

80. Cutler GB, Laue L. Congenital adrenal hyperplasia due to 21-hydroxylase deficiency. *N Engl J Med.* 323:1806, 1990

81. Siegel SF, Finegold DN, Lanes R, Lee PA. ACTH stimulation tests and plasma dehydroepiandrosterone sulfate levels in women with hirsutism. *N Engl J Med.* 323:849, 1990

82. Bongiovanni AM. An epidemic of premature thelarche in Puerto Rico. *J Pediatr.* 103:245, 1983

83. Beck W. Hormonal pattern of plasma LH, FSH, and prolactin in girls with premature thelarche and advanced bone age: A synonym for precocious puberty. *Horm Metab Res.* 12:101, 1980

84. Oberfield SE, Mayes DM, Levine LS. Adrenal steroidogenic function in a black and Hispanic population with precocious pubarche. *J Clin Endocrinol Metab.* 70:76, 1990

85. Klech RP. Management of precocious puberty. *N Engl J Med.* 312:1057, 1985

86. Kaplan SL, Grumbach MM. Pathophysiology and treatment of sexual precocity. *J Clin Endocrinol Metab.* 71:785, 1990

87. Conn PM, Crowley WF. Gonadotropin-releasing hormone and its analogues. *N Engl J Med.* 324:93, 1991

88. Feuillan PP, Foster CM, Pescovitz OH, et al. Treatment of precocious puberty in the McCune–Albright syndrome with the aromatase inhibitor testolactone. *N Engl J Med.* 315:1115, 1986

89. Holland FJ, Fishman L, Bailey JD, Fazekas ATA. Ketoconazole in the management of precocious puberty not responsive to LHRH-analogue therapy. *N Engl J Med.* 312:1023, 1985

90. Grumbach MM, Kaplan SL. Recent advances in the diagnosis and management of sexual precocity. *Acta Paediatr Jpn.* 30(suppl.):155, 1988

Chapter 6

NORMAL AND ABNORMAL SEXUAL DEVELOPMENT

Victor Y. Fujimoto and Michael R. Soules

Human sexual development is more than the secondary sexual development that occurs at puberty. Adults refer to puberty as the time of the "hormone surge," when girls develop breasts and boys experience muscle hypertrophy. Actually, sexual development begins much earlier—at conception, when the chromosomal sex is determined (males 46,XY, females 46,XX). Sex determination, however, depends not only upon the chromosomal determinants but also upon appropriate gonadal development, hormone production, and end-organ responsiveness. The anatomic differences between the sexes are determined by the amounts and types of steroid hormones secreted by the gonads and the ability of the embryo and fetus to respond appropriately to these hormones. A person's sexual identity as a male or female usually corresponds to the maleness or femaleness of the other aspects of their sexual development; that is, a person who considers himself a male is usually 46,XY and has a penis and testes that primarily secrete testosterone (T). Sexual identity is a product of the other three elements but also includes one's upbringing and environment. Therefore, sexual development should be viewed as occurring over time and comprising four interdependent aspects: genetic, hormonal, anatomic, and sexual identity (Table 6–1).

An understanding of sexual development is pertinent to this book, which focuses on clinical aspects of reproductive medicine. This chapter discusses normal sexual development first and then abnormal sexual development. Each of these major sections is subdivided somewhat arbitrarily into three areas: secondary sexual development, external genitalia, and internal genitalia. Sexual identity is not covered in this chapter.

NORMAL SEXUAL DEVELOPMENT

Genetics

Sex determination in humans is a complicated process that is only partly understood. In general, individuals with a Y chromosome will develop testes regardless of the number of X chromosomes present, and individuals lacking a Y chromosome will develop ovaries.

The gonadal primordium will develop via the default pathway into an ovary unless three gonad-specific cell lineages are changed directly or indirectly by a regulatory Y-chromosome specific regulatory gene that encodes region Y (SRY), a DNA-binding protein whose mechanisms of action remain unknown: (1) the primordial germ cells that originate in the hindgut entoderm and migrate into the gonadal primordium.[1] The germ cells form prospermatogonia in the fetal testis and meiotic oocytes in the fetal ovary. (2) The "supporting cells" that form Sertoli cells in the fetal testis that secrete Müllerian-inhibiting substance (MIS)[2] and H-Y antigen. In the ovary, these supporting cells become granulosa cells. (3) The steroid cell line that forms the testosterone-secreting Leydig cells in the fetal testis and the theca cells of the ovary.

Although it has been known since 1966 that the short arm of the Y chromosome was male determining,[3] the testis-determining factor (TDF) known as SRY itself

TABLE 6–1. LEVELS OF SEXUAL DEVELOPMENT

1. Genetic	46,XX or 46,XY	
2. Anatomic	Gonads: ovary or testis; internal genitalia; external genitalia	
3. Hormonal	Ovary: estradiol; testis: testosterone	
4. Identity	Self-perception as male or female	

has been elusive. For nearly 10 yr, H-Y antigen, the male-specific histocompatibility antigen, was believed to be TDF; however, the hypothesis was abandoned when mice with normal testes were found to be negative for H-Y antigen[4] and the gene for H-Y antigen in humans was mapped to the long arm of the Y chromosome, some distance from SRY on the short arm.[5] Following the development of molecular genetic techniques, the Y chromosome was divided into seven regions, with intervals 1 to 3 arbitrarily assigned to the short arm (Fig 6–1).[6] As far as the structure of the human Y chromosome, the distal tip of the short arm contains sequences homologous with the X chromosome distal short arm. This region of the Y chromosome has been termed the "pseudoautosomal region" because during male meiosis the distal short arm of the X and Y chromosome pair and undergo recombination. In 1987, Page et al[7] identified a gene, now termed ZFY for the zinc finger protein it encodes, on the short arm of the Y chromosome that was thought to be TDF; however, identification of XX males who did not contain this sequence of the Y chromosome[8] excluded ZFY as TDF.

Recent studies have narrowed the sex-determining region of the Y chromosome (termed SRY) to a 35-kilobase sequence within part of region 1 designated as 1A1.[9,10] Recently, the identity of SRY as TDF was clearly demonstrated when XX mice in which SRY gene sequences had been microinjected formed testes.[11] Even though the SRY gene is TDF, it is clear that normal male sexual development is not dependent upon a single gene but rather the interaction of numerous genes, their protein products, and hormones. For instance, it has been proposed that a Y-lined gene (GBY, which has not been cloned) has a function in spermatogenesis and may predispose dysgenic gonads to gonadoblastoma. It now appears that, at least in the mouse, ZFY has a role in germ cell development and H-Y antigen in spermatogenesis.

In the absence of these specific Y chromosome sequences, the indifferent embryonic gonad develops into an ovary. However, if two normal X chromosomes are not present, the ovarian follicles generally degenerate by the time of birth. Therefore, it appears that the X chromosome contains genes responsible for ovarian "maintenance" but not for differentiation. Through correlations of the phenotypic manifestations of specific X chromosome deletions detected by cytogenetic studies, it has been possible to define those regions of the X chromosome critical to ovarian maintenance and other areas that are more variable. The pericentromeric region of the X chromosome, from within band p11 on the short arm to approximately band q21 on the long arm, appears to be essential to ovarian function (Fig 6–2). As a general rule, women with deletions of the X chromosome involving any portion from Xp11 to Xq21 have primary amenorrhea and streak gonads. By contrast, females with deletions of the X chromosome more distal to these regions on either arm of the X chromosome may have either secondary amenorrhea or normal fertility.[12]

Using molecular genetic techniques, numerous genes have been mapped precisely on the X chromosome. Although the DNA sequence of numerous X chromosome genes is known, no specific gene crucial to ovarian maintenance has been postulated, let alone sequenced. The combined use of molecular genetic techniques and cytogenetic studies allowed investigators to define more precisely a large inherited Xq deletion causing premature ovarian failure in a family and propose that band q26 to q27 may contain genes important for ovarian maintenance.[13] This approach may prove to be a model for future studies to detect regions on the X chromosome critical to ovarian function.

X chromosome inactivation, the process by which only a single X chromosome remains active in any diploid somatic cell, results in dosage compensation for X-lined genes in XX females and XY males. The X inactivation center has been mapped to Xq13. Although a model exists to explain some aspects of X inactivation, the process of X inactivation is still not well understood.[14] However, X inactivation and gene dosage compensation appear to play no role in sex determination in humans.

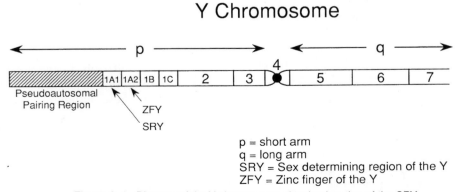

Y Chromosome

p = short arm
q = long arm
SRY = Sex determining region of the Y
ZFY = Zinc finger of the Y

Figure 6–1. Diagram of the Y chromosome showing location of the SRY.

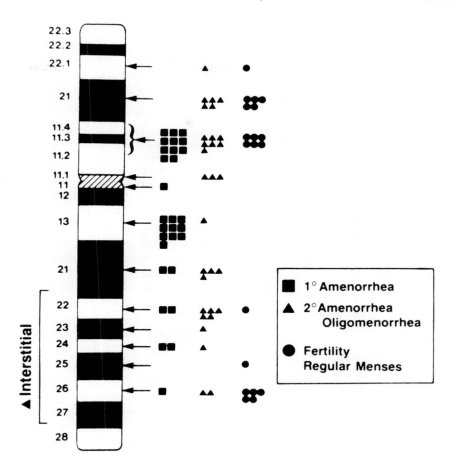

Figure 6–2. Diagram of the X chromosome showing regions that are more and less critical for ovarian function. *(Reprinted, with permission, from Simpson JL, 1990.[12])*

Secondary Sexual Characteristics

A normally functioning ovary or testis is the key element to the development of normal secondary sexual characteristics. Breast and pubic hair development are the primary components of female secondary sexual characteristics. The principal components of male secondary sexual characteristics are the development (growth) of the testes, penis, and pubic hair. These sexual characteristics in young women and men develop as a result of hormonal secretion at puberty, as discussed in Chapter 5.

External Genitalia

Endocrinology. The male and female external genitalia are formed during embryogenesis. At birth, a baby has small, but complete, male or female genitalia. Reproductive hormones secreted at puberty lead to growth of the genitalia but do not alter the anatomy present at infancy.

Androgens are the only class of steroid hormones relevant to the embryogenesis of the external genitalia. In the absence of androgens, female external genitalia

develop. There are no hormones or other products secreted by the ovary that are necessary for the development of female genitalia. The relative deficiency of receptors for luteinizing hormone (LH) and human chorionic gonadotropin (hCG) in the fetal ovary probably accounts for its lack of hormone secretion.[15] Normal female genitalia develop when (1) there are ovaries, (2) there are no functioning gonads, (3) there is androgen insensitivity, or (4) there is inadequate androgen production from testicular tissue.

Absence of the gonads is a situation in which female genitalia can be seen. Absence of the ovary always results in the development of female external genitalia. However, anorchia (absence of the testes) can be associated with either normal female or male external genitalia.

The latter is termed the vanishing testis syndrome. Anorchic males with normal male external genitalia at birth had functioning testes early in gestation that secreted sufficient levels of androgens and MIS to permit normal male genital development but had resorption of the testes later in gestation, resulting in congenital absence of the testes. In other cases of the vanished testis syndrome, the testes are resorbed prior to the secretion of androgen and MIS, resulting in the appearance of normal female external genitalia. Altogether, there is a simplicity to the development of external genitalia: Female anatomy results unless there are adequate levels of androgens that are "recognized" by appropriate tissue receptors.

The androgens responsible for virilization of the external genitalia are T and dihydrotestosterone (DHT). In androgen-responsive cells, some T is converted by the enzyme 5α-reductase to DHT. Both T and DHT have a biologic effect by binding to the androgen receptor, which then becomes active. DHT is twice as potent as T. The inherited condition 5α-reductase deficiency has provided a model in which the relative roles of T and DHT in male sexual development can be distinguished (Table 6–2).[16] From the phenotype of 5α-reductase deficiency, it can be determined that (1) both T and DHT contribute to phallic growth; (2) a urethral opening on the distal phallus, complete scrotal fusion, and testicular descent are partially dependent upon DHT; and (3) body hair (beard) and prostate growth are almost entirely dependent upon DHT.

T levels are detectable in the fetal testis after 6 wk gestation and are maximum at 12 wk of fetal age (8th and 14th wk of pregnancy, respectively). Circulating fetal serum T levels are detectable by 6 wk and peak at 14 to 16 wk (16 to 18 wk gestational age). From 16 to 24 wk, male fetal serum T levels fall. During the last trimester of pregnancy, T levels are indistinguishable in male and female fetuses.[17] Therefore, the testes actively secrete T from about 8 to 24 wk of gestation (Fig 6–3). The stimulatory basis for T secretion by the testes appears to be a combination of hCG and LH. The primary stimulus for testicular T secretion prior to 20 wk gestation is hCG. LH is the primary stimulus after 20 wk.

Testosterone increases in the mother (maternal compartment) during normal pregnancy. Normal range for serum T for a nonpregnant adult female is 40 to 80 ng/dl. In pregnancy, the range is 100 to 300 ng/dl.[18] This increase is largely due to an increase in sex hormone-binding glob-

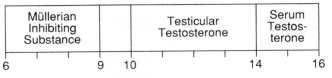

Figure 6–3. The testes secrete both Müllerian-inhibiting substance and testosterone. Müllerian-inhibiting substance is secreted early in fetal life and precedes testosterone secretion. Testosterone secretion by the Leydig cells within the testis leads to an increase in local tissue concentrations prior to achieving measurable levels in the serum.

ulin (SHBG)-bound T, which is not biologically active. Very little, if any, maternal T crosses the placenta because the trophoblastic tissue of the placenta has a high level of aromatizing capacity by which the majority of maternal androgens are converted to estrogens.

Embryology/Anatomy. At about the 8th wk of development, the external genitalia of male and female embryos are indistinguishable. In response to secretion of T and conversion to DHT, the phallic urethra and scrotum form and the midline genital tubercle develops into a penis. Masculinization of the external genitalia takes about 5 wk. By the middle of the second trimester of pregnancy, a male fetus can be easily distinguished by the appearance of external genitalia. The penis continues to grow until birth at a steady rate of 1.4 mm every 2 wk. Therefore, a premature male infant will have an anatomically correct but smaller phallus than a full-term male. The average penile length in term males is 3.5 cm.[19] Without T or other androgens, the undifferentiated genitalia develop as female (Fig 6–4). The distinction between a clitoris and penis are size and the presence or absence of an associated urethra.

Internal Genitalia

While "external genitalia" is a commonly used term, "internal genitalia" is not. In this chapter, the gonads (ovaries and testes) are not considered part of the internal genitalia for several reasons: (1) their embryologic derivation is separate; (2) they both migrate (and, in the case of the testes, leave the pelvis late in fetal life); and (3) the presence and nature of the internal genitalia depend upon their function. The components of female internal genitalia are the vagina, cervix, uterus, and fallopian tubes. The male internal genitalia are the vas deferens, seminal vesicles, and prostate.

Endocrinology. As occurs with the external genitalia, there is a passive (female) and an active (male) pathway for development of the internal genitalia. When ovaries (or no gonads) are present, the paramesonephric ducts,

TABLE 6–2. RELATIVE CONTRIBUTIONS OF T AND DHT IN MASCULINIZATION

	T	DHT
Penile growth	+	+
Sexual hair		+
Phallic urethra		+
Scrotal fusion		+
Testicular descent	+	+
Wolffian maturation	+	
Prostate		+
Male muscle pattern	+	

+ = Dominant effect.

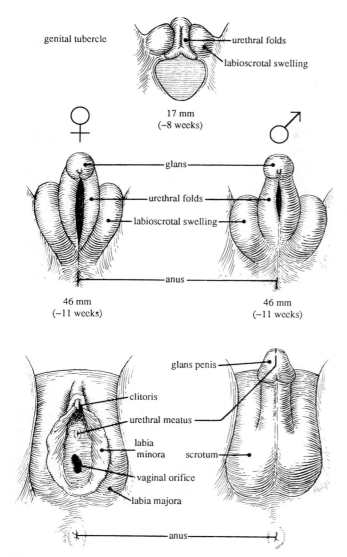

genital tubercle

urethral folds

labioscrotal swelling

17 mm
(~8 weeks)

♀   ♂

glans

urethral folds

labioscrotal swelling

anus

46 mm
(~11 weeks)

46 mm
(~11 weeks)

glans penis

clitoris

urethral meatus

labia
minora

scrotum

vaginal orifice

labia majora

anus

Figure 6–4. Early in fetal development, the external genitalia are in a unisex state and are bipotential. If sufficient circulating levels of testosterone are present in the late first trimester of gestation, then these bipotential genitalia develop into structures associated with a normal male. Without testosterone, the external genitalia develop in the classic female pattern.

better known as the Müllerian ducts, develop into female internal genitalia. When testes are present, the Müllerian ducts regress and the development of the Wolffian ducts is promoted.

During fetal development, T is secreted by the Leydig cells of the testes as discussed earlier. It is important to remember that T concentrations develop in the fetal testis 2 to 4 wk before circulating T can be detected. While it is circulating T that virilizes the external genitalia, it is only the local concentration of T in the vicinity of a testis that is capable of inducing Wolffian duct development.[20] It is presumed that higher local con-

centrations of T occur in the vicinity of the testis than are achieved in the systemic circulation. Clinically, this fact is relevant since females with virilized external genitalia (eg, congenital adrenal hyperplasia) do not have virilization of their internal genitalia; true hermaphrodites, who by definition have both ovarian and testicular tissue, develop Wolffian structures only ipsilateral to the testis. Since the Wolffian (mesonephric) structures do not have the 5α-reductase enzyme and cannot convert T to DHT,[21] it is T alone that promotes the development of the vas deferens and seminal vesicles.

The other critical hormone in the development of the internal genitalia has several synonyms: MIS, anti-Müllerian hormone (AMH), and Müllerian-inhibiting factor (MIF). MIS is a glycoprotein (72 kD) with disulfide bridges that is produced by the Sertoli cells of the fetal testis.[22] The gene has recently been sequenced and mapped to the short arm of chromosome 19. MIS diffuses from the testis, active, in a paracrine fashion to effect Müllerian regression. The atresia of Müllerian structures occurs by breakdown of the basal membrane of the Müllerian ducts followed by condensation of the mesenchyme. MIS is active as early as 6 wk of development, preceding the secretion and effects of T (Fig 6–3). Therefore, the Müllerian ducts are suppressed before the Wolffian ducts are stimulated. Genetic males with the vanishing testes syndrome may or may not have a uterus or male internal genitalia depending upon whether the testes vanished before or after MIS and/or T secretion. The testes continue to secrete MIS throughout fetal development and even into childhood. Its role(s) in other stages of sexual development is unknown.

Embryology/Anatomy. There is a close anatomic and developmental association between the renal system and the internal genitalia. Recall that renal development goes through three phases—pronephric, mesonephric, and metanephric. When renal development progresses to the metanephric stage, the mesonephric system of paired ducts is available for development as internal genitalia. At this stage, the mesonephric ducts are more often called the Wolffian ducts; the pair of paramesonephric ducts are usually called the Müllerian ducts (Fig 6–5). The cranial aspects of the Müllerian ducts develop from coelomic epithelium and the caudal aspects from the Wolffian ducts.

At 6 to 8 wk of development, the internal genitalia of an embryo is indifferent and the embryo is "unisex." In the absence of hormonal influence, the Müllerian ducts develop and the internal genitalia become those of a normal female. The Müllerian system will develop unless MIS is secreted by a testis in the vicinity of a paramesonephric duct. Each Müllerian duct is under the influence of MIS from the ipsilateral testis. If only one

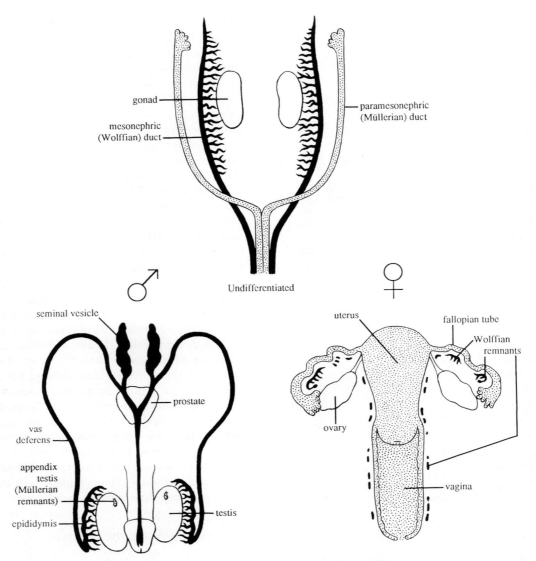

Figure 6–5. In the presence of relatively high local concentrations of testosterone, the mesonephric (Wolffian) ducts develop into the structures comprising the male internal genitalia. Without testosterone, the paramesonephric (Müllerian) ducts develop into the female internal genitalia. *(Redrawn from Netter FH. Reproductive System, vol. 2. In: Oppenheimer E, ed.* The Ciba Collection of Medical Illustrations. *Summit, N.J., CIBA Pharmaceutical Products, 1954: 2.)*

testis is present, a Müllerian duct will develop on the contralateral side.[20] Wolffian ducts partially degenerate if not rescued by T diffusing out from the ipsilateral testis[20] Therefore, a true hermaphrodite with a unilateral testis and a contralateral ovary will have (1) a unicornuate uterus and fallopian tube with Wolffian remnants (hydatid cysts) on the ovarian side; and (2) epididymis, vas deferens, and seminal vesicle on the testicular side. By 12 wk of in utero development, a normal female has fused Müllerian ducts and a normal male has no Müllerian ducts.

Anatomic orientation is reviewed here to clarify the discussion of normal and abnormal Müllerian development. By convention, proximal refers to the segment of

the Müllerian system closest to the introitus (eg, the distal vagina is the segment closest to the cervix; the proximal oviduct is the isthmic portion of the tube). Caudad conveys essentially the same information as proximal, in that it refers to the segment of Müllerian or Wolffian tissue closest to the perineum; cephalad or cranial refers to the opposite pole.

The Müllerian system proceeds through four basic maturation steps: elongation, fusion, canalization, and septal resorption. Fusion proceeds from caudad to cranial. When a fusion defect occurs in vaginal–uterine development, the ducts remain apart from that point cephalad. Normally, there are two solid columns of tissue lying side by side. Canalization of these tissue cords results in a pair of cavities. When the septum between these cavities is absorbed, there is a single vaginal and uterine cavity. The time course of these steps is illustrated in Figure 6–6.

There are several theories of vaginal development. The classic theory is that the proximal one third of the vagina develops from the urogenital sinus and the distal two thirds develop from the Müllerian system. A more plausible theory of vaginal development is that Müllerian tissue extends to the introitus in early development with urogenital sinus squamous epithelium subsequently migrating over the Müllerian tissue remnants up to the level of the cervix. Another argument for the entire vagina to have developed from Müllerian tissue is the fact that vaginal agenesis typically accompanies cervical or uterine agenesis. However, the dimple (1 to 4 cm) of proximal vagina that occasionally forms when there is cervical or uterine agenesis is consistent with a proximal urogenital sinus contribution to vaginal development.

Renal anomalies are commonly associated with Müllerian anomalies because the renal and reproductive systems arise from ducts that are anatomically contiguous. Some Müllerian anomalies are "subtraction anomalies" in that only a portion of Müllerian tissue is absent (eg, uterine agenesis, unicornuate uterus). Renal anomalies occur more frequently in association with these subtraction Müllerian anomalies. The prevalence of renal anomalies has been reported to be as high as 50 percent in women with Müllerian agenesis. In some families, Müllerian and renal anomalies are inherited as an autosomal dominant condition.[23] Although the ovaries are intimately associated with the fallopian tubes and uterus, which are of Müllerian origin, their embryologic origins are separate; therefore, Müllerian anomalies are rarely if ever associated with ovarian anomalies. The ovaries remain in their adnexal position and function normally regardless of deficiencies in the tissues of Müllerian origin.

Testicular migration and descent is a complex process in which the testes are initially close to the male internal genitalia but eventually become part of the external genitalia. During fetal development, the testes remain anchored in the region of the internal inguinal ring while the kidneys migrate cephalad. During the 7th gestational mo, the gubernaculum, which extends from the testis to the base of the scrotum, undergoes a marked

TABLE 6–3. PREVALENCE OF CRYPTORCHIDISM

Age	% Undescended Testis
Premature infant	33
Term infant	4
One mo	1.8
One yr	0.7
Adult	0.5

swelling.[24] The swelling actually consists of a Wharton's jelly-like substance responding to an increase in hyaluronic acid content. The diameter of the gubernaculum actually equals or exceeds that of the testes. The gubernaculum is coated by a thin layer of muscle that eventually becomes the cremasteric. It is speculated that this acute increase in size dilates the inguinal canal to allow for testicular descent. It is primarily DHT that stimulates these changes in the gubernaculum. The actual descent of the testes occurs in a relatively rapid manner and by the 8th gestational mo, the testes are in the scrotum. The gubernaculum regresses, and by birth a short scrotal ligament is the only identifiable remnant.[24]

Physical factors such as increased intra-abdominal pressure also play a role in testicular descent. Therefore, testicular descent can be altered by several different processes, such as defects in androgen synthesis, androgen insensitivity, and anatomic obstruction by an enlarged bladder (eg, prune belly syndrome). Sometimes, normal testicular descent is simply delayed. Table 6–3 lists the prevalence of cryptorchidism (failure of the testes to descend normally into the scrotum).[25] It is common in premature infants since descent occurs relatively late in gestation. It is not until a boy is 1 yr old that he should be considered to have true cryptorchidism. The persistence of intra-abdominal testes increases the risk of malignant degeneration (20 to 40 percent relative risk). Cryptorchidism may also contribute to permanent suppression of spermatogenesis and infertility.

ABNORMAL SEXUAL DEVELOPMENT

This discussion is divided into three sections on abnormal sexual development in relation to (1) secondary sexual characteristics, (2) external genitalia (most often referred to as ambiguous genitalia), and (3) internal genitalia (most often referred to as Müllerian anomalies).

Secondary Sexual Characteristics

Secondary sexual development refers to the growth and development of sexual hair, breast tissue, penis, testes, and scrotum at puberty in both sexes. The primary clinical issues pertaining to secondary sexual development are abnormalities in the timing of their appearance—

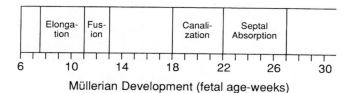

Figure 6–6. Time course for the steps that comprise Müllerian development.

precocious or delayed puberty. These topics are covered in the preceding chapter. The only topic that needs to be addressed here is abnormal development of secondary sexual characteristics in a girl or boy who has otherwise experienced normal pubertal development.

Abnormal Female Secondary Sexual Development.
Interestingly, there are no recognized clinical abnormalities of pubic and axillary hair development in girls who otherwise experience a normal puberty. There can be a lack of sexual hair in young women with the androgen insensitivity syndrome and excess sexual hair (hirsutism) in conditions such as polycystic ovary syndrome. However, both of these clinical entities are not associated with a normal female puberty in which there are normally functioning ovaries.

There are several abnormalities in breast development in girls with normal ovarian function.[26,27] The breasts are apparent during the 5th wk of fetal development as "milk streaks" that run from the axilla to the groin. Normally, only that portion of embryonic breast tissue that rests on the chest wall develops any further. But accessory mammary tissue along the trunk from axilla to groin is present in 2 to 6 percent of adult women. This accessory tissue is usually an ectopic nipple that is small and nonfunctional. More clinically relevant are abnormalities that develop in the pair of primary breasts. A rare congenital abnormality is amastia, complete absence of breast tissue. This is usually unilateral and associated with absence of the pectoral muscle in 90 percent of cases. When there is syndactyly of the fingers of the ipsilateral hand in association with amastia, the term Poland syndrome is used.

More common among breast anomalies are hyperplasia, hypoplasia, and asymmetry (Figs 6–7 to 6–9). All combinations occur: The breasts can be too large (hyperplasia) or too small (hypoplasia), and this can be unilat-

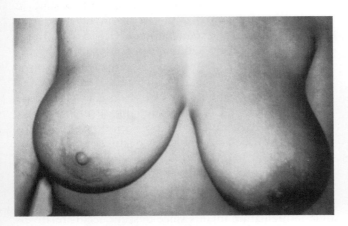

Figure 6–7. Breast hyperplasia.

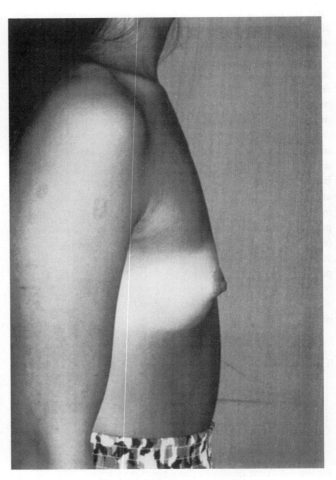

Figure 6–8. Breast hypoplasia.

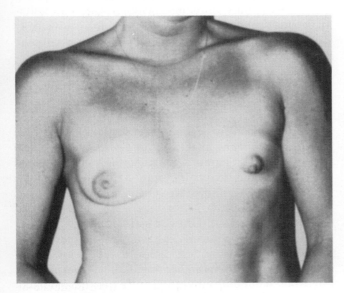

Figure 6–9. Asymmetrical breast development.

eral (asymmetry) or bilateral. For instance, a woman can have bilateral breast hyperplasia, another can have a normal-sized breast with a hypoplastic breast, and a third patient could have breasts that are both within the range of normal size yet differ in size. Although women expect their breasts to be equal in size, a small amount of asymmetry is the norm. When asymmetry is obvious and of cosmetic concern, surgical adjustment is an option.[27] When the problem is one of size, there are operations for augmentation and reduction of breast tissue. The goal of aesthetic breast surgery is the creation of attractive, symmetrical breasts that coincide with the patient's desires for breast size and are in proportion with her body size and other features. Most plastic surgeons recommend operating on both breasts if they are asymmetric to balance the postoperative effect. For example, with hypoplasia and asymmetry the operation would be a bilateral augmentation procedure using breast prostheses of different sizes.

Large breasts (hyperplasia) can cause symptoms beyond cosmetic considerations. Poor posture, neck and shoulder pain, dermatologic conditions, mastalgia, and even brachial plexus nerve compression can occur secondary to breast hyperplasia. At puberty, young women can develop an entity known as giant virginal hypertrophy, which presents as massive breast enlargement.

Hyperplasia can occur after pregnancy if the breasts fail to involute. Some menopausal women can have excessive fat disposition and develop larger, pendulous breasts. Reduction mammoplasty is the recommended procedure for all hyperplastic conditions.

Breast augmentation is primarily performed for cosmetic indications. This statement does not discount cosmetic indications, because body image is important. Breast implants are available in different sizes: They are plastic envelopes that are *re*filled *with silicone or can be injected* with saline. The operation can be successfully performed by placing implants under the breast tissue (submammary) or pectoralis muscle (submuscular). The submuscular implant technique has more postoperative pain but less capsular (scar contraction) formation. Both techniques are acceptable, and plastic surgeons often individualize implant placement and incision location (areolar, inframammary, or axillary).

Abnormal Male Secondary Sexual Development.
There is considerable variation, largely genetic, in the onset and duration of puberty and the degree of secondary sexual development among normal boys. This variation results in a normal range of secondary sexual characteristics in boys during and after puberty. Although marked abnormalities of sexual development in boys are usually a result of androgen deficiency, abnormal male sexual characteristics can also be associated with otherwise normal pubertal development.

Gynecomastia, benign glandular enlargement of the male breast, is a common occurrence at the time of puberty. Between the ages of 10 and 16 yr, approximately 40 to 65 percent of boys develop transient, so-called pubertal, gynecomastia, which spontaneously and gradually regresses within 3 yr in nearly all instances. Because pubertal gynecomastia is common, it is considered normal. The amount of breast tissue is usually less than 4 cm in diameter (Tanner stage II) and asymptomatic (see Chap 5). Uncommonly, pubertal gynecomastia may be excessive and persist into adulthood (persistent pubertal macromastia) and can be familial as well. Persistent pubertal macromastia is usually greater than 6 cm in diameter (Tanner stages II to IV). Gynecomastia must be distinguished from other benign and malignant tumors of the chest wall (lipoma, male breast carcinoma) and may also occur as a result of underlying pathology, such as androgen deficiency. Although the precise pathophysiology is unclear, pubertal gynecomastia occurs in a hormonal milieu of increased estrogen/androgen ratio.[28] In pubertal gynecomastia, this increase is thought to be transient. In persistent pubertal macromastia, the increased estrogen/androgen ratio may be due to an increase in extraglandular aromatization of androgens to estrogens in some cases.[29]

Because spontaneous regression occurs, no therapy other than reassurance is recommended for boys with pubertal gynecomastia. Medical therapy with an estrogen antagonist (eg, tamoxifen) or an aromatase inhibitor (eg, testolactone) can be used to hasten the regression of breast tissue in boys who experience extreme psychosocial distress or symptomatology. Treatment of pubertal macromastia present for more than 4 yr is reduction mammoplasty.

Hypospadias is a condition in which the urethral meatus terminates on the ventral aspect of the penis, proximal to its usual site at the tip of the glans. Rarely, the meatus is located on the dorsum of the penis (epispadias). These conditions result from incomplete fusion of the penile urethral folds and are often associated with absence of the ventral (or, rarely, the dorsal) foreskin, which causes a curvature of the penis known as chordee. Hypospadias occurs in approximately 0.8 percent of males and is often associated with abnormalities in androgen secretion or action, other urogenital tract abnormalities, and malformation syndromes.[30] Most cases of isolated hypospadias are thought to be familial. Hypospadias is considered in more detail later in this chapter under ambiguous genitalia.

Micropenis describes a normally formed penis with a stretched length less than two standard deviations below the mean for age.[19] Micropenis must be differentiated from a normal penis that is concealed in excessive suprapubic fat. The majority of cases of micropenis are associated with fetal/prepubertal androgen deficiency or resistance, and, therefore, patients have evidence of abnormal sexual development. However, some cases of micropenis are idiopathic and associated with normal pubertal development. Micropenis is also considered later in this chapter under ambiguous genitalia.

Macro-orchidism (testicular volume >2 SD or larger than 35 to 40 ml) occurs in 80 percent of postpubertal males and 40 percent of prepubertal males with fragile X syndrome. The fragile X syndrome is an X-linked recessive disorder with moderate to severe mental retardation in affected males. While macro-orchidism is a useful finding that alerts the clinician to the possibility of the fragile X syndrome, it is not specific to this disorder and can be seen in mentally retarded males without fragile X. The increased testicular size is secondary to increased connective tissue and ground substance. Spermatogenesis and fertility are normal in men with the fragile X syndrome.[31]

Cryptorchidism (undescended testes) should be distinguished from *retractile testes*, which are usually located in the scrotum but easily withdraw to a location in the inguinal canal with minimal stimulation; *ectopic testes*, which are located outside the normal path of testicular descent; and *anorchia*, in which the testes are absent.[32] Cryptorchidism is present in 3 to 4 percent of full-term newborn males and is bilateral in 25 percent. Spontaneous testicular descent occurs in all but 0.7 percent of cases by 1 yr of age, after which it is unusual.[25] Cryptorchidism may be associated with fetal and prepubertal androgen deficiency or resistance and numerous malformation syndromes.

However, it can also occur as an isolated finding in the presence of otherwise normal sexual differentiation. Complications of cryptorchidism include impaired spermatogenesis with reduced fertility and increased risk of malignancy. Both hCG and gonadotropin-releasing hormone (GnRH) therapy have been used to induce testicular descent in patients with cryptorchidism. If hormone therapy fails, orchipexy is indicated in an attempt to preserve testicular function and allow easier examination of the testes for malignant degeneration. Despite orchipexy, reduced fertility and the potential for malignant degeneration remain.

Ambiguous Genitalia

Clinical Presentation. One of the universal experiences of human life that spans recorded time and all civilization is the assignment of sex to a child at birth. The external genitalia are examined and a pronouncement is made—"it's a girl" or "it's a boy." In modern Western civilization, it is usually the health care provider performing the delivery who examines the genitalia and makes this pronouncement. This section is devoted to the situation where the external genitalia are neither normal male nor normal female. The clinical picture usually looks like Figure 6–10: The phallus is too large for a female clitoris, yet too small for a male penis; the urethral opening is not

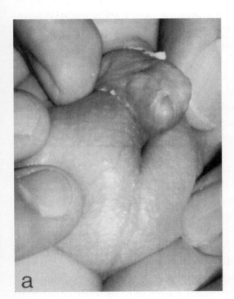 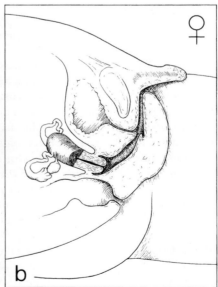 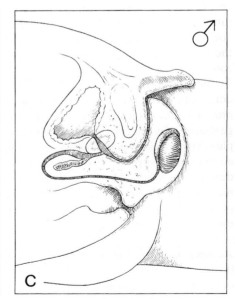

Figure 6–10. A. Photograph of the genitalia of a newborn infant with ambiguous genitalia. The phallus is too large for a normal clitoris and too small for a normal penis. The opening at the base of the phallus through which the infant urinates may be a true urethra or a pseudourethra at the apex of fused labia. The rugated skin below the phallus may be an incompletely fused scrotum or fused labia. **B.** Cross-sectional drawing of the anatomy if the child is female. The fused labia form a pseudourethral opening and cover both the true urethral meatus and the vaginal introitus. **C.** Cross-sectional drawing of the anatomy if the child is male. The opening at the base of the phallus is a urethra and the child has hypospadias. The testis could have descended into the partially fused scrotum, but may be found in the abdominal cavity or the inguinal canal. *(Reprinted, with permission, from Bostwick J III, 1990.)*

at the tip of the phallus but at the base; the perineum either has fused labia or an incompletely developed scrotum. This is the clinical presentation in most ambiguous genitalia cases.

The following phenotypes are considered ambiguous: (1) subphallic urethra with no palpable gonads, (2) subphallic urethra with one palpable gonad, and (3) abnormal phallus with no palpable gonads. It is appropriate at this point to defer assigning the sex of an infant with any one of these findings until further studies can be performed. When one is not certain whether the newborn is a boy or a girl, it should be so stated; to do otherwise is nothing more then guessing. There is considerable turmoil if gender is assigned and later proven incorrect. While it may be difficult for a physician to express uncertainty, it is clearly the best approach until a definite assignment can be made.

Premature infants can have ambiguous genitalia, but caution must be exercised not to over-diagnose underdeveloped genitalia as ambiguous. While ambiguous external genitalia are usually recognized at birth, an older child or even an adult can present with ambiguous genitalia. These are usually tragic cases in which the ambiguity during infancy was either ignored or a male sex assignment was made after a cursory evaluation. The physician and parents were hopeful that the underdeveloped male genitalia would "normalize" over time. In these cases with older patients, the person may have been given a sex assignment, reared as a boy or girl (but ambivalently), and developed only a fragmented sexual identity. Fortunately, late presentations of ambiguous genitalia are rare and most of the time health care providers recognize the need for evaluation shortly after birth that results in correct diagnosis and treatment.

Once it has been decided to defer temporarily gender assignment, a plan needs to be made to identify the proper sex of rearing. First, it must be determined if the genital ambiguity is an isolated problem or part of a complex malformation syndrome. If the baby has multiple anomalies, the primary goal becomes diagnosis of the underlying problem. Many malformation syndromes that include genital ambiguity are life threatening and merit prompt diagnosis. Such disorders may be chromosomal, monogenic, or sporadic in etiology. For example, chromosomal abnormalities such as trisomy 12, triploidy, and 13q-syndrome usually involve severe malformations of the central nervous system, as well as other organ systems. Cryptophthalmos, camptomelic dysplasia, and Smith–Lemli–Opitz syndrome are three autosomal recessive disorders frequently lethal in the neonatal period in which undermasculinization of the male fetuses can cause genital ambiguity. Persistence of the cloaca and exstrophy of the cloaca have associated anomalies of the kidneys and gastrointestinal tract that may require immediate life support and surgical intervention. In any of these instances, assessment by a medial geneticist or dysmorphologist may help in syndrome identification, which delineates the natural history and clarifies the management options for the family.

If no other anomalies are present, the other life-threatening disorder to consider is the salt-wasting form of congenital adrenal hyperplasia (CAH), which occurs when there is a partial enzyme deficiency in the cortisol and aldosterone pathways. Hyponatremia and hyperkalemia can develop within days of birth. When salt wasting is a factor, the clinical presentation is vomiting, poor feeding, hypotension, and lethargy. Electrolytes must be monitored until a definitive diagnosis is made.

In the majority of ambiguous genitalia cases, a clear diagnosis can be made within 3 to 7 days. Considering the relative rarity of ambiguous genitalia, the number of organ systems potentially involved, and the large number of disorders in the differential diagnosis, a team approach is recommended. Members of a gender assessment team should include (1) a psychologist/counselor experienced in intersex disorders, (2) a general pediatrician as the primary physician, (3) a pediatric urologist, (4) a pediatric endocrinologist, (5) a clinical geneticist, and (6) a reproductive endocrinologist. Each specialist brings a different and equally important expertise to the problems of diagnosis and treatment. If an operation is required, the urologist will usually be the surgeon if the child is to be reared as a male, and the gynecologist (reproductive endocrinologist) will be the surgeon if the child is to be raised a female. The team should continue to review each case periodically.

Evaluation. In this section, the presumptive patient is a newborn with ambiguous genitalia. The evaluation should begin with a complete pregnancy history, family history, and physical examination. The history should focus on (1) family members with similar problems, (2) pregnancy history with emphasis on maternal medications, (3) any signs of virilization in the mother, (4) growth and development in utero, and (5) labor and delivery. The physical examination should include evaluation for other congenital malformations and a description of the external genitalia:

1. Phallic size should be measured by stretching the phallus and measuring along the dorsum from symphysis pubis to glans.
2. The location of the urethral meatus should be noted—phallic or on the perineum.
3. The degree of fusion and rugation of the labial/scrotal folds should be recorded.
4. It should be noted if there are gonads in the labial/scrotal area or in the inguinal canal. Newborn testes are 1 to 2 cm in size and can be difficult to palpate, especially in the inguinal canal. They are

also retractable and can move between examinations. A palpable gonad invariably has testicular tissue and is a good indicator of the presence of a Y chromosome.

5. Rectal examination should be performed to determine if there is a small, firm midline pelvic structure, which would indicate a uterus.

6. It is difficult to determine if a vagina is present by physical examination, since it will be hidden behind the fused labia.

The following laboratory tests are usually necessary: (1) serum electrolytes; (2) 17-OH-progesterone (17-OH-P) to evaluate for 21-hydroxylase deficiency; (3) peripheral blood karyotype with G and Q banding; (4) serum hormone levels of T, estradiol androstenedione, and DHEAS; and (5) biopsy of genital skin for androgen binding studies. There are several caveats in relation to these laboratory studies: (1) A karyotype can be ordered "stat" with the results available within less than 1 wk; (2) a buccal smear is useless and should never be performed; (3) for several weeks after birth, both ovaries and testes are active in terms of hormone secretion before becoming quiescent; (4) androstenedione and DHEAS are adrenal androgen hormones that may be elevated if there is an adrenal enzyme deficiency other than 21-hydroxylase; and (5) many endocrine laboratories do not have reference ranges for newborns. Therefore, it is sometimes necessary to send these samples to a regional laboratory.

The following imaging techniques are helpful. Pelvic ultrasound should be performed on all patients to determine if a uterus or other Müllerian structures are present. The uterus is hypertrophied in the neonate, making ultrasound evaluation effective in detecting its presence or absence (Fig 6–11). Renal anatomy, especially the collecting systems and ureters, can be defined with an excretory urogram. A "genital sinogram" can be helpful. This sinogram can radiologically define the lower genitourinary anatomy of a patient with ambiguous genitalia. What appears to be the urethral meatus through which the infant urinates may be the urethra or only the opening at the top of the fused labia. A small feeding tube can be placed into this opening and water-soluble radiopaque media injected. The bladder will be visualized if the opening is the urethra. If the opening was a pseudourethra at the apex of the labial fusion (Fig 6–12), the space behind the labial fusion and vagina will be visualized.

Results of these tests will yield clear and proper diagnosis in most cases. However, the cause of ambiguous genitalia in a particular patient may be elusive even after all testing is complete. In these cases, a diagnostic laparotomy may be necessary to evaluate the gonads and Müllerian or Wolffian structures. In these cases, the na-

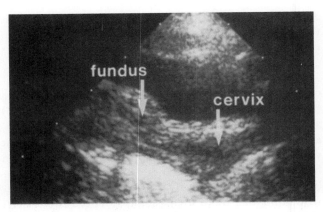

Figure 6–11. Pelvic ultrasound that presents a longitudinal view of the uterus and cervix in a newborn female. The uterus is relatively large, as is found in a reproductive female.

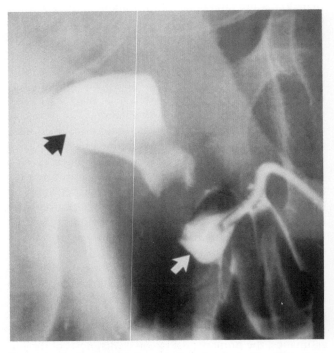

Figure 6–12. Genital sinogram in a female infant with ambiguous genitalia (fused labia). A pediatric feeding tube has been placed through the opening at the apex of the fused labia. Water-soluble media was injected and the space behind the fused labia (white arrow) was visualized. The media diffused through the introitus and visualized the upper vagina as well (black arrow).

ture of the intra-abdominal gonads (ovary or testis?) are often not recognizable, and biopsy with pathology consultation on a frozen section may be necessary. The laparotomy (in conjunction with the other tests) usually leads to a definitive diagnosis; in that case, operative therapy, if necessary, can then be completed prior to abdominal closure.

Etiology. Table 6–4 lists the known diseases and conditions that can cause or are associated with ambiguous genitalia. The table uses traditional terminology: female and male pseudohermaphroditism and true hermaphroditism. This terminology is confusing but unfortunately has persisted in the medical literature. A female pseudohermaphrodite is a 46,XX individual with masculinized external genitalia; a male pseudohermaphrodite is a 46,XY individual with undermasculinization of the external genitalia. Although female pseudohermaphrodites often have ovaries and male pseudohermaphrodites have testes, this relationship is not always present. A true hermaphrodite has both ovarian and testicular tissue present.[33] The karyotype is often, but not always, 46,XX.

To provide some indication of relative frequency of the disorders causing genital ambiguity, Table 6–4 includes a prevalence figure for the cases that have been managed by the gender assessment team at our institution from 1982 to 1990. The prevalence for each diagnosis in Table 6–4 is expressed as a percentage of the total cases managed (n = 64). This team did not necessarily see all patients with ambiguous genitalia in the region, as it only consulted on those cases that were referred. While it is believed that most (if not all) cases of a particular etiology were referred (eg, cloacal exstrophy), other less severe cases may well not have been referred (eg, CAH, maternal androgen exposure).

Certain diagnoses that have been inappropriately considered as a cause of ambiguous genitalia in the past are discussed here to explain their exclusion: (1) uteri hernia inguinal—normal 46,XY males with MIS deficiency who are born with normal male external genitalia; (2) complete androgen insensitivity—46,XY individuals with normal testes, normal female external genitalia, and normal female sexual identity; (3) Müllerian agenesis (Rokitansky syndrome)—46,XX females with normal ovaries and normal female external genitalia; (4) gonadal dysgenesis—individuals with an X chromosome abnormality, streak gonads, and normal female external genitalia.

Pertinent Issues to Sex of Rearing Recommendations.
The recommendation for the sex of rearing of a child with ambiguous genitalia is more complex than simply "making the proper diagnosis." Superficially, it would appear that the sex of rearing should naturally follow from the chromosomal sex or the gonadal type and/or the dominant sex hormone being secreted. But other relevant issues must also be considered. Depending upon the age of the patient, a sexual identity as a male or female may have already been partially or completely established at the time of diagnosis. Even when the child is too young to have acquired a sexual identity, the parents may have become committed to a particular sex of

rearing. The presence of a sexual identity is always considered but weighs heavily when the diagnosis could lead to recommendation of the opposite sex of rearing. Most operative and hormonal treatments can be effective at any age. Hence, age is not a problem in terms of anatomic outcome but is a crucial and often decisive factor in terms of established sexual identity.

Other important issues to be considered in making a sex of rearing recommendation are (1) potential sexual function, (2) potential fertility, (3) anatomic constraints, and (4) available psychosocial support system. The gender assessment team should consider which assignment would be most compatible with normal sexual intercourse as an adult. Another crucial issue that does not apply until adulthood is the potential for an ovary or testis to produce oocytes or spermatozoa. New reproductive technologies (eg, in vitro fertilization) bring a new dimension to the fertility issue. Based upon experience with prior cases with the same diagnosis, the team can usually accurately predict future sexual function and fertility.

The anatomy of the external genitalia is never exactly the same in each patient with ambiguous genitalia. The ability to enhance the anatomy toward maleness or reduce the anatomy toward femaleness should be individually considered for each patient by the surgeons on the team. Obviously, both experience and operative skill are important. In general, it is technically easier to reduce the anatomy toward femaleness than it is to reconstruct tissues toward maleness. Finally, it is important to consider the future support system available to a given patient, such as (1) the presence, knowledge, and capabilities of the parents and family; (2) financial and geographic access to future medical care; and (3) probability of compliance with periodic follow-up. An appropriate decision concerning the sex of rearing should be made only when all of these issues have been thoroughly considered.

Treatment

Operative

TIMING OF PROCEDURES. Several surgical procedures can be performed for problems of abnormal sexual development. Three operations will be considered here: exploratory laparotomy, clitoral reduction (feminizing genitoplasty), and reconstruction of the male phallus. Laparotomy is sometimes necessary to complete the diagnostic process, and is therefore performed in the neonatal period. Reconstruction of the phallus for females is referred to as clitoral reduction. In males, it is referred to as a hypospadias repair. The clitoral reduction should be performed early (age 3 to 6 mo) to reduce

TABLE 6–4. ETIOLOGY OF AMBIGUOUS GENITALIA: CLASSIFICATION OF DISEASES AND CONDITIONS

Disease or Condition	Description	Inheritance	Key(s) to Diagnosis	Optimal Sex of Rearing	Prevalence (%)
Female Pseudohermaphroditism (genotype 46,XX)					
Congenital adrenal hyperplasia (CAH)	Partial 21- and 11-hydroxylase enzyme deficiencies leading to chronic elevations of adrenal androgens; salt wasting can occur in 21-hydroxylase deficiency; in 11-hydroxylase deficiency, hypertension occurs	Autosomal recessive	Elevated serum level of 17-OH-progesterone (21-OHase) or 11 deoxycorticosterone Cmpd-S (11-OHase)	Female	15.3
Adrenogenital syndromes	Partial steroid enzyme deficiencies that lead to abnormal levels of precursor steroid hormones; these enzymes are 3β-ol-dehydrogenase, 17-hydroxylase, and 17-20 desmolase: the adrenal and ovary are both affected	Autosomal recessive	Elevated serum levels of the hormones that precede the enzyme deficiency (eg, progesterone in 17-hydroxylase deficiency)	Female	1.6
Maternal androgen exposure	Fetus was exposed in utero to elevated androgens from maternal ingestion (eg, danazol, nortestosterone, progestins) or maternal virilizing tumor (eg, arrhenoblastoma or luteoma) aromatase deficiency.	Sporadic	Maternal pregnancy history regarding drug ingestion and/or virilization	Female	1.6
Idiopathic clitoromegaly	Ambiguity is limited to clitoral enlargement	Sporadic	Complete evaluation including pregnancy history finds no endocrine abnormalities	Female	4.6
Familial clitoromegaly	Ambiguity is limited to clitoral enlargement	History of other affected family members	Complete evaluation including pregnancy history finds no endocrine abnormalities	Female	0
Associated with urogenital sinus abnormalities (cloacal exstrophy)	Ambiguous genitalia in association with a more severe genital developmental defect	Sporadic	Persistence of the cloaca is associated with imperforate anus and abnormalities of bladder outlet; exstrophy of the cloaca is associated with imperforate anus, bladder exstrophy, omphalocele, and scoliosis; ovaries are present and functioning normally	Female	6.1
Male Pseudohermaphroditism (genotype 46,XY)					
Incomplete androgen insensitivity syndromes (Lubs, Gilbert–Dreyfus, Reifenstein, and Rosewater syndromes)	Presentation varies from nearly normal male genitalia to mildly virilized female genitalia	X-linked recessive	These patients have a normal or elevated serum T; androgen receptor binding and/or function in genital skin is abnormal	Male or female	6.1
5-α-Reductase deficiency (pseudovaginal perineal hypospadias)	There is an enzymatic deficiency in 5-α-reductase whereby T is not intracellularly converted to DHT	Autosomal recessive	Positive family history; increased serum T/DHT ratio; decreased ratio of 5α/5β C21 and C19 steroids in urine; abnormal conversion of T to DHT in genital skin	Male	0
Testosterone biosynthetic defects	There is a defect involving an enzyme in the steroid synthetic pathway between cholesterol and the C-19 androgens	Autosomal recessive	Family history, low testosterone level, and elevated precursor steroid(s); underdeveloped testes	Male or female	3.0

TABLE 6–4. (CONT'D)

Leydig cell resistance	Testes are incapable of producing T; there is a presumption that Leydig cells lack LH receptors	Sporadic	Low T; elevated LH, FSH; underdeveloped but otherwise normal testes	Male	1.6
Testicular regression (vanishing testes syndrome; anorchia)	Testes can regress or "vanish" during fetal development; it can occur: early before MIS or T secretion with normal female genitalia; after MIS but before T secretion with absent Müllerian structures but normal female genitalia; after MIS and some T secretion with ambiguous genitalia	Sporadic	Low serum T level; elevated LH, FSH; no gonads (not even a streak); laparotomy is necessary to make this diagnosis	Male if late regression; female if early regression	1.6
Hypospadias	Urethral opening is not at the tip of the glans penis; the opening can be located anywhere on the penile shaft or at the base of the penis	Sporadic (majority) or part of a syndrome with multiple congenital anomalies (eg, Drash, Cornelia de Lange syndromes)	Testes are usually present in the inguinal canal or scrotum but can have cryptorchidism; the phallus has normal male dimensions; the serum T level is normal	Male	24.6
Micropenis	Only ambiguity of the genitalia is the penile length <2.8 cm (term); urethral opening in normal location	Sporadic	Testes are usually present in the inguinal canal or scrotum but can have cryptorchidism; when seen with bilateral cryptorchidism, hypogonadism is likely; these latter patients should be evaluated for panhypopituitarism; usually have normal serum T level and serum LH, FSH; normal androgen receptor concentration and function	Male (usually)	12.3
Associated with urogenital sinus abnormalities (cloacal exstrophy)	Ambiguous genitalia problem in association with a more severe genital development defect	Sporadic	Persistence of the cloaca is associated with imperforate anus and abnormalities of bladder outlet; exstrophy of the cloaca is associated with imperforate anus, bladder exstrophy, omphalocele, and scoliosis; testes are present and functioning normally	Male (usually)	6.1
Other: Karyotype Variable					
True hermaphrodite	Presentation may vary from ambiguous genitalia to almost normal male to normal female genitalia; some Müllerian structures are usually present	Sporadic	To make the diagnosis, there must be ovarian tissue with primordial follicles and testicular tissue with tubules; the gonads are usually intra-abdominal and a laparotomy is required for a definitive diagnosis; most common karyotype is 46,XX; can be 46,XY or 46,XX/46,XY	Male or female	4.6
Mixed gonadal dysgenesis	Presentation is classic ambiguous genitalia; there is an intra-abdominal unilateral streak gonad and a contralateral testis	Sporadic	Testis is often small and may be normally descended, in the inguinal canal, or in the abdomen; the serum T level can vary from normal female to normal male range; a laparotomy is necessary to make the diagnosis; the karyotype is usually 45,X/45,XY but can be 46,XY	Male or female	10.7

parental anxiety of having a baby whose phenotype does not appear to match her gender assignment. Excision of labial fusion is often performed at the same time. When gender assignment is male, hypospadias surgery is best performed between 6 and 18 mo of age. Orchipexy for undescended testes should be done before 2 yr of age to maximize future testicular function.

EXPLORATORY LAPAROTOMY. In most cases of true hermaphroditism and mixed gonadal dysgenesis, cystoscopy and exploratory laparotomy are performed in the neonatal period to complete the diagnostic process. The nature of the internal genital ducts can be determined, gonadal biopsy can be obtained, and a sample of genital skin can be sent for androgen receptor studies. When streak gonads are encountered, they should be removed. When a true hermaphrodite is to be reared as a male, the ovarian and Müllerian duct tissue is removed at the time of this diagnostic laparotomy. If female gender assignment has been made for a true hermaphrodite, the testicular and Wolffian tissue is excised.

FEMINIZING GENITOPLASTY. The most common operative procedure for ambiguous genitalia in patients who receive a female gender assignment is the feminizing genitoplasty. This procedure has three parts: clitoral reduction, formation of labia, and vaginoplasty. Clitoral reduction has evolved from clitoral amputation[34] to various plication[35,36] and concealment[37] procedures to the current recommended procedure. Although several variations exist, the goals of current clitoral reduction operations are the same: (1) preserve the vascular and nerve supply to the glans clitoris; (2) recess the glans to the inferior aspect of the pubis; and (3) disrupt engorgement (erection) of the corporal bodies by resection and ligation. These goals are achieved by the procedures described by Allen et al[38] and Snyder et al.[39] To afford good exposure of the perineum, the patient is placed in the dorsolithotomy position, which affords good exposure of the perineum. The skin of the phallus is incised and the corporal bodies are exposed. A segment of the corpora cavernosa is resected with preservation of the dorsal neurovascular bundle (it supplies sensation and blood to the glans clitoris). The glans is then recessed to the inferior aspect of the symphysis pubis, and the shaft skin is used to form labia minora.

Attention should then be directed to the labial fusion and the vagina. Depending upon the level at which the vagina enters the urogenital sinus, vaginoplasty can be performed at the same time as clitoral reduction or deferred until the patient is older. This can be determined by careful cystoscopy and a preoperative genital sinogram. With a relatively low vagina (orifice is from the urethra and in a more standard position), a simple excision of the fused labia or use of the Y-V technique incorporating an inverted u-shaped flap can be performed at the time of the initial operation. If the vagina enters the urogenital sinus at the level of the external urinary sphincter, vaginal exteriorization is delayed until about 12 mo of age. For high vaginas, an additional anterior perineal flap can be used to construct the anterior wall of the vagina.[40] The Passerini technique uses the inverted phallic shaft skin to reach the vagina once it has been separated from the urogenital sinus.[41] Postoperatively, a vaginal pack is left for 24 to 36 hr along with a Foley catheter. Labial edema can be significant initially and take several days to resolve.

RECONSTRUCTION OF THE MALE PHALLUS. When male gender assignment has been made, the principles of hypospadias repair are employed. Reconstruction of the urethra with straightening of the corpora can be performed in one[42] or two[43] stages. When the hypospadias is of such severity that a diagnosis of ambiguous genitalia is made, a two-staged operation is recommended. Often, the penis is small and preoperative treatment with T will increase growth, facilitating surgery. Over 150 procedures for the cure of hypospadias have been reported, but only one will be described here. The Belt–Fuqua operation entails a two-stage approach.[43] In the first stage, the chordee is resected to correct the ventral curvature of the corpora. Occasionally, transfer of a corporal wedge of tissue from the dorsal aspect to the ventral aspect is necessary. Success is demonstrated by intraoperatively creating an artificial erection (using a tourniquet at the base of the corpora and injecting saline). Once a satisfactorily straight penile shaft is achieved, the dorsal-hood prepuce is transferred to the ventrum by making a buttonhole. Scrotoplasty (to correct a bifid scrotum) can be performed at this time. The second stage is performed about 6 mo later: Parallel incisions are made on the ventral aspect of the penile shaft that produce a strip of skin that can be tubularized. Enough length should be realized to achieve glanular placement of the meatus. Redundant shaft skin is approximated to cover the neourethra, which results in a circumcised penis. A urethral stent is left in place for 10 to 14 days. Possible surgical complications include fistula formation, urethral stricture, and meatal stenosis. Wound infection can cause complete dehiscence of the repair.

Surgical techniques of genital reconstruction continue to improve. Proper application of these procedures with meticulous technique (optimal magnification, fine suture, and delicate tissue handling) can lead to a successful outcome in most cases.

Hormonal. Hormonal therapy is often necessary in the treatment of many ambiguous genitalia cases. The appropriate hormone therapy is either estrogen or T, dependent upon the sex of rearing. This need for male or female reproductive hormones is present because the child never had a functional gonad in terms of hormone secretion (eg, testicular regression syndrome, Leydig cell resistance, incomplete androgen insensitivity) or the gonads were removed as part of the operative therapy (eg, mixed gonadal dysgenesis, testosterone biosynthetic syndrome, micropenis).

Note that the testes should be removed when they are nonfunctional and/or the sex of rearing is to be female. Likewise, intra-abdominal gonads should be removed whenever there is a Y chromosome in the genotype to prevent malignant transformation (eg, seminoma).[44] The only exception to gonadal extirpation with a Y chromosome would be a functional intra-abdominal ovary in a true hermaphrodite that is to be raised female.

FEMALE HORMONE THERAPY. When the sex of rearing is female and there is no functional ovary, then a plan for estrogen treatment needs to be formulated. The first consideration is the timing of puberty. The target organs at puberty are the epiphyses and the breasts. Since estrogen secretion usually begins between 8 and 10 yr of age in normal puberty, low-dose estrogen therapy should be initiated about age 10. A bone age should be obtained at the initiation of estrogen therapy and annually thereafter as an index of estrogen effect. Height and breast development (Tanner stages) should be noted as well. A daily oral dose of 0.3 mg conjugated equine estrogen (CEE) or its equivalent is recommended. This dose is low enough to be used without a progestin since it generally will not stimulate the endometrium sufficiently to cause menstrual flow. The low daily dose can be continued for 1 to 2 yr. For those patients with a uterus, a progestin can be given to determine the amount of endometrial stimulation and prepare for an increase in estrogen dose. The progestin dose is 5 mg of medroxyprogesterone acetate (MPA) or its equivalent administered daily for 14 days in conjunction with estrogen. At approximately age 12, the estrogen is increased to 0.625 mg CEE daily with the 5 mg MPA administered simultaneously for 14 days each month. This estrogen/progestin dose should be continued for about 1 yr. Some monthly withdrawal flow usually occurs when the CEE dose is increased to 0.625 mg.

The following year, at approximately age 13, the estrogen dose should be increased to 1.25 mg CEE daily to maximize breast development. This dose should be continued for 2 yr, at which time breast development and epiphyseal fusion should be complete. This higher estrogen dose should also be accompanied by 14 days of 5 mg MPA/day each mo. At approximately age 15, the young woman can be placed on a permanent replacement regimen of 0.625 mg CEE daily plus 14 days of 5 mg MPA each mo. When mature adult status is reached, an alternative replacement regimen is standard-dose contraceptives, which can be continued indefinitely.

MALE HORMONE THERAPY. Replacement T therapy is effectively and safely accomplished using long-acting T esters, such as T enanthate or cypionate. Oral androgen preparations carry a risk of liver toxicity in addition to being less potent and less effective. In the future, transdermal T administration may provide a useful alternative to injections in both children and adults. Because overly aggressive androgen treatment in prepubertal children may result in excessive erections and premature closure of the epiphyses, resulting in compromised final adult height, initial doses should be low and bone age should be carefully monitored during therapy.

During infancy and early childhood, T enanthate or cypionate 15 to 25 mg IM every 2 to 3 wk is used to stimulate penile growth in patients with micropenis. The response of the penis is usually quite striking; at times, significant penile growth occurs after a single injection of T. In general, a total of three injections is sufficient. Courses of treatment can be repeated yearly if necessary to keep penile size in the range of normal for age. For induction and maintenance of virilization in older boys, the dose of T enanthate or cypionate is increased gradually to 50 to 100 mg IM every 2 to 3 wk. In adolescents, the testosterone dose is increased over a period of 3 to 4 yr to the adult replacement dosage of 200 mg IM every 10 to 14 days.

Müllerian Anomalies

General Considerations. The presence of a uterus and fallopian tubes indicates that MIS activity did not occur during the critical stages of Müllerian duct development. Therefore, Müllerian anomalies occur in 46,XX women and in 46,XY phenotypic women with androgen insensitivity. In the case of androgen insensitivity syndrome, the regression of the Müllerian ducts may be directly linked to the active secretion of MIS from the embryonic testis. Developmental anomalies of these ducts could be called "ambiguous internal genitalia." Since Müllerian anomalies are internal and more difficult to detect, they usually do not present until after puberty, if at all. For example, a woman with a septate uterus may have normal pregnancies and never have a clinical indication to perform a hysterosalpingogram (HSG); on the other hand, a girl with cervical agenesis and outflow obstruction to the menstrual flow will present within months after her menarche. It is uncertain how many normal women have underdiagnosed uterine anomalies (see Chap 30).

Clinical Issues. The clinical issues pertinent to Müllerian anomalies are listed in Table 6–5.

1. Obstetric problems are the most frequent. Most uterine anomalies (eg, septate uterus, unicornuate uterus, bicornuate uterus, uterus didelphys) are compatible

TABLE 6–5. MÜLLERIAN ANOMALIES: POTENTIAL CLINICAL PROBLEMS

Obstetric
  Recurrent spontaneous abortions
  Incompetent cervix
  Premature labor
  Transverse lie
  Malpresentation
  Prolonged labor—dystocia
  Entrapped placenta
  Postpartum hemorrhage
Amenorrhea
Endometriosis
Dyspareunia/dysmenorrhea
Infertility
Ectopic pregnancy

with normal fertility. There is an increased prevalence of almost every known obstetric complication in patients with uterine anomalies. Often, these are not diagnosed until the time of delivery, when the complication prompts additional investigation that identifies the Müllerian anomaly.

2. The principal clinical feature of Müllerian anomalies is primary amenorrhea. Müllerian anomalies rank second only to gonadal dysgenesis as a cause of primary amenorrhea.

3. Dyspareunia occurs with some Müllerian anomalies. In vaginal dyspareunia in association with a vaginal septum, patients with Müllerian anomalies are predisposed to endometriosis, presumably secondary to retrograde menstruation. Deep dyspareunia also occurs in association with endometriosis.

4. Infertility occurs when there is insufficient Müllerian tissue for conception (eg, Müllerian agenesis) or endometriosis.

5. Ectopic pregnancies are more common in diethylstilbestrol (DES)-induced uterine anomalies.

The diagnosis of Müllerian anomalies can be difficult. For asymptomatic patients, the diagnosis is made as an incidental finding at physical examination or during an unrelated operative procedure. Müllerian anomaly should be suspected if there is a history of certain obstetric problems such as malpresentation or retained placenta. Pelvic pain and a pelvic mass in patients with primary amenorrhea are the only clinical signs that are virtually pathognomonic of Müllerian anomalies; therefore, heightened clinical awareness is usually necessary to diagnose Müllerian anomalies. Many patients with Müllerian anomalies present with the chief complaints of recurrent miscarriage and/or infertility.

Physical examination is the method of diagnosis of vaginal anomalies. The combination of an imaging technique plus endoscopy is usually necessary to make the correct diagnosis of uterine anomaly. The most cost-effective imaging technique is an HSG, in which radiopaque media is injected transcervically into the uterine cavity. This technique outlines the internal uterine anatomy. Laparoscopy is often necessary to delineate the external uterine anatomy. While a combination of transabdominal and transvaginal sonography can usually distinguish the correct uterine anatomy, it is not as accurate as HSG in combination with laparoscopy. In complex cases, laparotomy may be the only way to make the diagnosis.

Associated developmental anomalies of the renal and skeletal systems are common in Müllerian anomalies in 46,XX women. Approximately one third of patients have abnormal kidney formation. Therefore, all women with Müllerian anomalies should have an excretory urography (IVP), renal ultrasound, and/or renal scan to assess their renal anatomy. The excretory urogram is the current method of choice. Skeletal abnormalities can be identified in 10 percent of cases and include wedge vertebrae, fusions, rudimentary vertebral bodies, and scoliosis.

Classification. The classification of Müllerian anomalies (Table 6–6) is based upon the involved segments (uterus, cervix, and/or vagina). There can be defects confined to one level, such as a uterine anomaly with normal vagina, cervix, and fallopian tubes. There can be anomalies that are all inclusive, such as Müllerian agenesis, where the vagina, cervix, and uterus are absent. There can be a combination of vaginal anomalies in association with cervical anomalies.

Müllerian Agenesis. Müllerian agenesis is congenital absence of the vagina, cervix, and uterus (Fig 6–13). Müllerian agenesis in a 46,XX woman with ovaries is known as Mayer–Rokitansky–Kuster–Hauser syndrome.[45] In Rokitansky syndrome, the defective Müllerian embryogenesis occurs early in the development of the upper reproductive tract at the elongation stage. The reported incidence of Müllerian agenesis is 1 in 4000 to 5000 female births. Although the family history of women with Rokitansky syndrome is usually negative for similar anomalies, autosomal dominance inheritance has been reported and may be more common than appreciated. Failure to ascertain other individuals in the family with the gene for Müllerian dysplasia may be secondary to (1) reduced penetrance (some individuals may carry the gene but not express it); (2) variable expressivity (the presence of mild and severe anomalies in the same family); or (3) infertility in those with the most severe anomalies. Characteristically, rudimentary bicornuate cords are seen at the time of laparoscopy or laparotomy in Müllerian agenesis. Congenital absence of the vagina, cervix, and uterus in a 46,XY phenotypic female with testes is known as the androgen insensitivity syndrome or testicular feminization.[16] This is an X-linked recessive disorder in which the

TABLE 6-6. CLASSIFICATION OF MÜLLERIAN ANOMALIES

Anomaly	Description	Pathogenesis	Likelihood of Associated Renal Anomaly	Primary Clinical Problems
Complete Müllerian agenesis (Rokitansky syndrome)	Partial or complete absence of vagina; absent cervix and uterus	Failure of elongation of Müllerian ducts	High	Primary amenorrhea; infertility; sexual dysfunction
Vaginal agenesis: complete or partial	Complete refers to the absence of the entire vagina; partial agenesis can be proximal, in which there is an upper vagina into which the patient menstruates and there is outflow obstruction, or distal, where there are several centimeters of proximal vagina ending in a blind pouch	Either failure of Müllerian ducts to elongate to level of urogenital sinus (complete) or a segmental deletion defect (partial)	High	Primary amenorrhea; dysmenorrhea; endometriosis; infertility; sexual dysfunction
Vaginal septum: longitudinal or transverse	Longitudinal septum usually runs the entire length of the vagina, resulting in two vaginal orifices and two cavities; there are usually two cervices; a transverse vaginal septum is usually found 4 to 8 cm from the introitus and completely blocks the vagina except for small fenestrations	Longitudinal: a septal resorption defect; transverse: a segmental canalization, septal resorption defect	Low	Dyspareunia and sexual dysfunction
Cervical agenesis	Absence of the cervix and cervical canal usually in association with vaginal agenesis; the uterus is usually present	Segmental deletion defect	Medium	Pelvic pain; primary amenorrhea; infertility; sexual dysfunction; endometriosis
Uterine—septate	External contour of the uterus appears normal but internally the myometrium protrudes from the fundus into the cavity for a variable length	Cranial septal resorption defect	Low	Obstetric complications; recurrent spontaneous abortion
Uterine—unicornuate	Uterus that formed from a single Müllerian duct; consists of a single horn and one fallopian tube	Partial (unilateral) elongation defect	High	Obstetric complications
Uterine—bicornuate: symmetrical or asymmetrical	Uterus that formed from two Müllerian ducts that did not fuse above the cervix; the two horns can be of the same or disparate size; may or may not communicate with each other	Cranial fusion defect	Medium	Obstetric complications; recurrent spontaneous abortion; ectopic pregnancy
Uterine—didelphys	Uterus with two horns and two cervices usually in association with a longitudinal vaginal septum	Partial fusion and complete septal resorption defect	Medium	Obstetric complications
Uterine—iatrogenic	Exposure to estrogen (DES) during the first trimester of pregnancy can lead to vaginal, cervical, and uterine anomalies	Estrogen is a teratogen to fetal Müllerian ducts	Low	Spontaneous abortion; premature labor

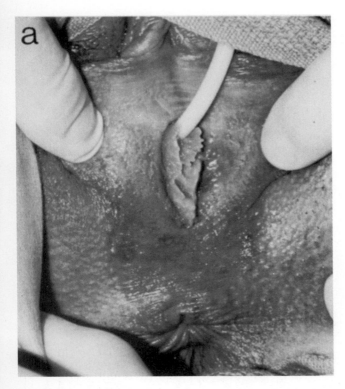
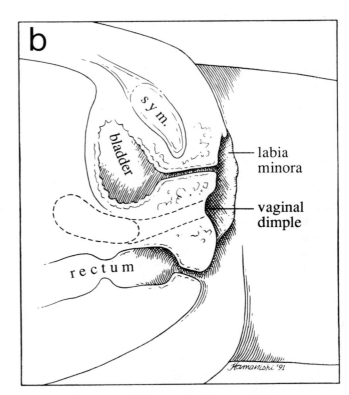

Figure 6–13. Perineum in a young woman with Müllerian agenesis. (**A,** photograph; **B,** drawing.) The bladder and rectal anatomy are normal. The space between the bladder and rectum that is usually occupied by Müllerian structures is made up of loose areolar tissue that extends up to the level of the peritoneal reflection.

Müllerian structures are absent secondary to normal MIS secretion by normal testes.

The absence of Müllerian tissue is complete in both disorders, although some patients have several centimeters of proximal vagina that ends in a blind pouch. They usually present after age 16 for primary amenorrhea. Patients with Rokitansky syndrome and androgen insensitivity undergo normal thelarche. In androgen insensitivity syndrome, normal thelarche occurs due to peripheral aromization of high circulating androgen levels. Pubarche is normal in women with Rokitansky syndrome but not in those with androgen insensitivity due to the absence of a functional androgen receptor. In both disorders, hormone secretion is normal.

The treatment of congenital absence of the vagina is the creation of a functional vagina. Women with Rokitansky syndrome cannot bear children but can provide oocytes for an in vitro fertilization procedure with the embryos transferred to the womb of a gestational surrogate mother. Women with androgen insensitivity also require gonadectomy after completion of puberty and before the age of 20.[44] The only option for childrearing in these women is adoption.

Vaginal Anomalies. Vaginal anomalies are complete or partial absence of the vagina. Distal (complete) vaginal agene-

sis is caused by Rokitansky syndrome or androgen insensitivity. In these cases, a vagina is created either by dilatation or a vaginoplasty. The bicycle seat dilatation method of Ingram is a new version of an older method (the Frank method) that results in a functional vagina in most women.[46] The most common and successful operative vaginoplasty is the McIndoe method, which consists of the insertion of a mold covered by a split-thickness skin graft into a surgically created space between the bladder and rectum.[47] After either of these therapies, a functional vagina with normal length, caliber, and sensation can be expected.

Partial proximal vaginal agenesis is a rare vaginal anomaly in which the proximal vagina is absent and the distal vagina is present. In these cases, menstruation into a blind pouch causes pelvic pain shortly after menarche. Although this diagnosis may be suspected after a pelvic sonogram, it must be confirmed surgically. Operative drainage is necessary and can be combined with a proximal vaginoplasty.

When a longitudinal or transverse vaginal septum is present, the rest of the Müllerian tract is usually present as well. The longitudinal vaginal septum can run down the middle of the vagina from the cervix to the introitus and divide the vagina into two equal cavities or deviate to one side and lead to two asymmetrical vaginal cavities. A longitudinal septum is usually associated with the presence of two cervices and a uterus didelphys, providing an example of a septal resorption defect that occurs caudad and is present throughout the more cranial aspects of the Müllerian system. The longitudinal septum is usually uninterrupted but may be fenestrated. The only indication for operative removal is chronic dyspareunia or the presence of a large window that could lead to obstetrical complications.

A transverse vaginal septum is usually a several millimeters thick, fenestrated membrane that separates the proximal vagina from the distal vagina. A transverse septum is usually sporadic (secondary to a segmental canalization defect) and rarely associated with renal anomalies. Menstrual flow is usually normal. The diagnosis can be confirmed by injecting radiopaque media through the fenestration to visualize the upper vagina and uterus. A longitudinal septum may remain asymptomatic with the diagnosis only incidentally, whereas a transverse vaginal septum usually becomes symptomatic with attempted intercourse. With a transverse septum the distal vagina is often dilated secondary to partial outflow obstruction. A transverse vaginal septum should be adequate to avoid "napkin ring" constriction of the vagina.

Cervical Anomalies. The cervix is part of the uterus. Absence of the cervix when the rest of the uterus is present is know as cervical agenesis. This Müllerian anomaly is rare, occurs sporadically, and is a segmental deletion defect resulting from failure of contact between the Müllerian system and the urogenital sinus. Examination of the external genitalia suggests Müllerian agenesis; however, the presence of a normal-sized uterus distinguishes these patients from those with Müllerian agenesis. These girls present with cyclic pelvic pain shortly after menarche. Retrograde menstruation caused by uterine outflow obstruction *can* result in pelvic endometriosis. These girls can be distinguished from Müllerian agenesis by the presence of both primary amenorrhea and pelvic pain. The uterus is a midline mass palpable on rectal examination and is visible on sonogram as well. The diagnosis of cervical agenesis can be suspected based upon history, physical examination, and radiologic imaging procedures like ultrasound and/or MRI, but a laparotomy is usually necessary to confirm the diagnosis.

The conservative approach to this problem is placement of a drain such as a T-tube into the uterine cavity with the stem brought out the perineum.[48] A cervical canal can thus be created surgically and the drain left in place for weeks to months in an attempt to form a permanent canal by epithelialization over this tract. Overall, the results have been equivocal. A canal forms in approximately 50 percent of cases but obstruction can occur. The current recommendation is hysterectomy with preservation of ovarian function. Treatment for the associated vaginal agenesis is also necessary. Another option that has not yet been reported is long-term sup-

pression of the endometrium using injections of depomedroxyprogesterone acetate or GnRH analog therapy. This therapy would prevent endometriosis and ensuing complications until the patient was ready to conceive. At that time, conception could be attempted using gamete intrafallopian tube transfer techniques. The first pregnancy was reported in a patient with cervical agenesis by Thijssen et al.[49]

Uterine Anomalies. Among other clinical issues, most women with uterine anomalies have an increased incidence of obstetric complications. These complications vary anywhere from spontaneous abortion to pyelonephritis to retained placenta. At one time, an astute observer (Dr. Semmens) classified these obstetric complications into two groups based upon their relative prevalence in relation to specific uterine anomalies.[50] In other words, certain pregnancy complications seemed to occur more frequently with certain uterine anomalies. These groupings, based upon obstetric complications, are clinically helpful (see Chap 30).

Wolffian Abnormalities

While less common than Müllerian anomalies, Wolffian anomalies also occur.

Wolffian Aplasia. The absence of Wolffian duct derivatives may or may not be associated with abnormalities of mesonephric (renal) development. Most commonly, the urinary tract is normal in individuals who lack epididymides, vas deferens, and/or seminal vesicles. Individuals with bilateral defects are infertile.

Failure of Epididymal and Testicular Fusion. Failure of epididymal and testicular fusion is a developmental disorder that results from failure of fusion of the testicular rete cords and mesonephric cords to form the different ducts. If this condition occurs bilaterally, infertility results.

Wolffian Duct Dysgenesis. Occlusion of the lumina of the Wolffian-derived male structures occurs in cystic fibrosis and results in infertility.

In Utero DES Exposure in Males. In utero DES exposure in male fetuses has been associated with an increased incidence of epididymal cysts and possibly infertility.

CONCLUSION

Abnormalities of sexual development are relatively rare. No physician (regardless of specialty) sees these cases on a regular basis. Although the abnormalities are serious and can have major ramifications for an individual's self-perception (sexual identity, fertility), they rarely present as a medical emergency. Most of the time, the clinician has a chance to approach these disorders thoughtfully and in a clear and organized fashion.

REFERENCES

1. Jirasek JE. Principles of reproductive embryology. In: Simpson JL, ed. *Disorders of Sexual Differentiation.* New York, N.Y., Academic Press, 1976: 52–56

2. Cate RL, Mattaliano RJ, Hession C, et al. Isolation of the bovine and human genes for mullerian inhibiting substance and expression of the human gene in animal cells. *Cell.* 45:685, 1986

3. Jacobs PA, Ross A. Structural abnormalities of the Y chromosome in man. *Nature.* 210:352, 1966

4. McLaren A, Simpson E, Tomonari K, et al. Male sexual differentiation in mice lacking H-Y antigen. *Nature.* 312:552, 1984

5. Simpson E, Chandler P, Goulmy E, et al. Separation of the genetic loci for the H-Y antigen and for testis determination on human Y chromosome. *Nature.* 326:876, 1987

6. Vernaud G, Page DC, Simmler MC, et al. A deletion map of the human Y chromosome based on DNA hybridization. *Am J Human Genet.* 38:109, 1986

7. Page DC, Moster R, Simpson EM, et al. The sex-determining region of the human Y chromosome encodes a finger protein. *Cell.* 51:1091, 1987.

8. Palmer MS, Sinclair AH, Berta P, et al. Genetic evidence that ZFY is not the testis-determining factor. *Nature.* 342:937, 1989

9. Sinclair AH, Berta P, Palmer MS, et al. A gene from the human sex-determining region encodes a protein with homology to a conserved DNA-binding motif. *Nature.* 346:240, 1990

10. McLaren A. What makes a man a man? *Nature.* 346:216, 1990

11. Koopman P, Gubbay J, Vivian N, et al. Male development of chromosomally female mice transgenic for SRY. *Nature.* 351:117, 1992.

12. Simpson JL. Localizing ovarian determinants through phenotypic-karyotypic deductions. Progression and pitfalls. In: Rosenfeld RG, Grumbach MM, eds. *Turner Syndrome.* New York, N.Y., Marcel Dekker, 1990: 65–77

13. Krauss CM, Turksoy RN, Atkins L, et al. Familial premature ovarian failure due to an interstitial deletion of the long arm of X chromosome. *N Engl J Med.* 317:125, 1987

14. Lyon MF. The quest for the X-inactivation centre. *Trends Genet.* 7:69, 1991

15. Wilson EA, Jawad MJ. The effect of trophic agents on ovarian steroidogenesis in organ culture. *Fertil Steril.* 32:73, 1979

16. Quigley CA, De Bellis A, Marschke KB, et al. Androgen receptor defects: historical, clinical, and molecular perspectives. *Endocrin Rev.* 16:271, 1995

17. Reyes FI, Winter JSD, Faiman C. Endocrinology of the fetal testis. In: Burger H, de Kretser D, eds. *The Testis,* 2nd ed. New York, N.Y., Raven Press, 1989: 119–142

18. Rivarola MA, Forest MG, Migeon CJ. Testosterone, androstenedione and dehydroepiandrosterone in plasma during pregnancy and at delivery: Concentration and protein binding. *J Clin Endocrinol.* 28:34, 1968

19. Feldman KW, Smith DW. Fetal phallic growth and penile standards for newborn male infants. *J Pediatr.* 86:395, 1975

20. Jost A. Embryonic sexual differentiation (morphology, physiology, abnormalities). In: Jones HW Jr, Scott WW, eds. *Hermaphroditism, Genital Anomalies and Related Endocrine Disorders.* Baltimore, Md., Williams and Wilkins, 1971: 16–64.

21. Grumbach MM, Conte FA. Disorders of sexual differentiation. In: Wilson JD, Foster DW, eds. *Textbook of Endocrinology,* 7th ed. Philadelphia, Pa., W. B. Saunders, 1981: 330–401.

22. Josso N, Picard JY. Anti-Müllerian hormone. *J Physiol Rev.* 66:1038, 1986

23. Biedel CW, Pagon RA, Zapata JO. Müllerian anomalies and renal agenesis: Autosomal dominant urogenital adysplasia. *J Pediatr.* 104:861, 1984

24. Marshall FF, Elder JS. Mechanisms of testicular descent. In: Marshall FF, Elder JS, eds. *Cryptorchidism and Related Anomalies.* New York, N.Y., Praeger Publishers, 1982

25. Rajfer J. Congenital anomalies of the testis. In: Walsh PH, Gittes RF, Perlmutter AD, et al, eds. *Campbell's Urology,* 5th ed. Philadelphia, Pa., W. B. Saunders, 1986: 1947–1968

26. Osborne MP. Breast development and anatomy. In: Harris JR, Hellman S, Henderson IC, Kinne DW, eds. *Breast Diseases.* Philadelphia, Pa., Lippincott, 1987: 1–14

27. Bostwick J III, ed. *Aesthetic and Reconstructive Breast Surgery.* St. Louis, Mo., Mosby Publishers, 1983

28. LaFranchi SH, Parlow AF, Lippe BM, et al. Pubertal gynecomastia and transient elevation of serum estradiol level. *Am J Dis Child.* 129:927, 1975

29. Berkovitz AM, Amiel SA, Millis RD, et al. Familial gynecomastia with increased extraglandular aromatization of plasma carbon 19-steroids. *J Clin Invest.* 75:1763, 1985

30. Sweet RA, Schrott HG, Kurland R, et al. Study of the incidence of hypospadias in Rochester, Minnesota, 1940–1970, and a case control comparison of possible etiologic factors. *Mayo Clin Proc.* 49:52, 1974

31. Hagerman RJ. Fragile X syndrome. *Curr Probl Pediatr.* 17:623, 1987

32. Rezvani I. Cryptorchidism: A pediatrician's view. *Pediatr Clin North Am.* 34:735, 1987

33. Berkovitz GD. Abnormalities of gonadal determination and differentiation. *Semin Perinatol.* 16:289, 1992

34. Gross RE, Randolph J, Crigler JF Jr. Clitorectomy for sexual abnormalities: Indications and techniques. *Surgery.* 59: 300, 1966

35. Glassberg KI, Laungani G. Reduction clitoroplasty. *J Urol.* 17:604, 1981

36. Randolph JG, Hung W. Reduction clitoroplasty in females with hypertrophied clitoris. *J Pediatr Surg.* 5:224, 1970

37. Ansell JS, Rajfer J. A new and simplified method for concealing the hypertrophied clitoris. *J Pediatr Surg.* 16:681, 1981

38. Allen LE, Hardy BE, Churchill BM. The surgical management of the enlarged clitoris. *J Urol.* 128:351, 1982

39. Snyder HM III, Retik AB, Bauer SB, Colodny AH. Feminizing genitoplasty: A synthesis. *J Urol.* 129:1024, 1983

40. Hendren WH, Donahoe PK. Correction of congenital abnormalities of the vagina and perineum. *J Pediatr Surg.* 15:751, 1980

41. Passerini-Glazel G. A new one-stage procedure for clitorovaginoplasty in severely masculinized female pseudohermaphrodites. *J Urol.* 142:565, 1989

42. Duckette JW. Transverse preputial island flap technique for repair of severe hypospadias. *Urol Clin North Am.* 7:423, 1980

43. Fuqua F. Renaissance of a urethroplasty: The belt technique of hypospadias repair. *J Urol.* 106:782, 1971

44. Ulrich U, Keckstein J, Buck G. Removal of gonads in Y-chromosome-bearing gonadal dysgenesis and in androgen insensitivity syndrome by laparoscopic surgery. *Surg Endosc.* 10:422, 1996

45. Fedele L, Dorta M, Brioschi D, et al. Magnetic resonance imaging in Mayer–Rokitansky–Kuster–Hauser syndrome. *Obstet Gynecol.* 76:593, 1990

46. Ingram JM. The bicycle seat stool in the treatment of vaginal agenesis and stenosis: A preliminary report. *Am J Obstet Gynecol.* 140:867, 1981

47. McIndoe A. Treatment of congenital absence and obliterative conditions of vagina. *Br J Plast Surg.* 2:254, 1950

48. Farber M, Marchant DJ. Reconstructive surgery for congenital atresia of uterine cervix. *Fertil Steril.* 27:1277, 1976

49. Thijssen R, Hollander J, Willeimsen W, et al. Successful pregnancy after ZIFT in a patient with congenital cervical atresia. *Obstet Gynecol.* 76:902, 1990

50. Semmens JP. Congenital anomalies of the female genital tract. *Obstet Gynecol.* 19:328, 1962

Chapter 7

THE MOLECULAR BASIS OF HORMONE ACTION

Serdar E. Bulun, Evan R. Simpson, and Carole R. Mendelson

This chapter includes basic information regarding cellular signaling pathways and a synopsis of clinical syndromes associated with gene defects in hormone receptors. It is not the intent to provide a complete database of the known signaling pathways; rather, the chapter familiarizes the reproductive endocrinologist with the molecular mechanisms responsible for the hormone action related to reproductive function.

It is now over 90 yr since Bayliss and Starling originally introduced the term "hormone" to apply to a chemical substance that, after being produced in one part of the body, enters the circulation and is carried to distant organs and tissues to modify their structure and function. The word "hormone" is derived from the Greek, meaning "to excite." However, we now know that not all such chemical messengers have stimulatory effects; a number, in fact, are inhibitory. From the turn of the century until some 30 yr ago, the pursuit of endocrinology was confined to determining the chemical nature and properties of the various compounds that could justifiably be termed hormones and estimating their levels in the blood and other body fluids. During that period, almost nothing was known about their mechanisms of action. It was only with the development of techniques to radiolabel molecules to very high specific activities that it became apparent that the first step in the series of events that lead to a cellular response was the binding of an excitatory substance to a receptor. This event, which was found to occur with high specificity and affinity, served therefore as the initial point of contact between the regulatory ligand and the responsive cell. Indeed, the presence of cellular receptors specific for a particular ligand determines the capacity of a cell to respond to that particular hormone.

Since that time, enormous progress has been made in the characterization of a large number of receptors and also of the second messenger systems to which they are coupled, due in large part to the widespread deployment of the tools of recombinant DNA technology. In general, it can be considered that hormone receptors fall into two categories: those present on the cell surface, which in general interact with hormones that are water soluble such as peptide and protein hormones, as well as prostaglandins, catecholamines, and other neurotransmitters. On the other hand, lipophilic hormones such as steroids, as well as thyroid hormones, retinoic acid, and 1,25 dihydroxyvitamin D_3, interact with receptors primarily localized within the nucleus. To interact with nuclear receptors, therefore, these compounds presumably have to diffuse freely through the lipophilic plasma membrane, cytoplasm, and nuclear membrane to interact with their receptors.

It now has become apparent that many of these substances do not fall into the strict definition of the term "endocrine" in that they are not necessarily produced at a site distal to the target cell. On the contrary, many regulatory substances are produced and secreted by cells proximal to the target cell (eg, neurotransmitters). The term "paracrine" has been coined to define such factors. It also is recognized that some regulatory substances interact with receptors on the surface of the same cells that produce them. Such factors are known as "autocrine" agents. And, finally, it now appears that there are intracellular receptors that interact with ligands present within the same cell and never leave that cell. The term "intracrine" has been introduced to define this type of ligand–receptor interaction.

RECEPTOR PROPERTIES

The function of a receptor is to recognize one particular ligand among all other molecules in the environment of the cell at a given time and, after binding, transmit a signal that ultimately results in a biologic response. Hormones are normally present in the circulation in extremely low concentrations, from 10^{-11} to 10^{-9} mol/L. The receptor must therefore have an *affinity* for the hormone that is of a magnitude appropriate to the circulating levels. The receptor must also bind the hormone with high *specificity* so that it has a greater affinity for one biologically active molecule than for another.

The affinity of a hormone for its receptor results from *noncovalent* binding, primarily in the form of hydrophobic interactions that provide the driving force for the binding reaction, as well as from electrostatic interactions. The latter, which occur between oppositely charged groups on peptide hormones and their receptors, are important for hormone–receptor specificity. The affinity of a hormone–receptor interaction is defined in terms of the *equilibrium dissociation constant (K_d)*. In a system in which there is a single class of binding sites with no interactions among receptors, the K_d is defined as the concentration of hormone required for binding to 50 percent of the receptor sites at equilibrium. The affinity can also be expressed in terms of the *equilibrium association constant (K_a)*, the reciprocal of the K_d.

The binding of hormone to receptor is a *saturable* process; in other words, there is a finite number of receptors for a given hormone on a target cell. In addition, the binding of hormone to receptor must either precede or accompany the biologic response, and the magnitude of the biologic response must be associated, in some manner, with receptor occupancy. Analogs that bind to receptors and elicit the same biologic response as the naturally occurring hormone are termed "agonists." Molecules that bind to receptors but fail to elicit the normal biologic response are termed "competitive antagonists" because they occupy the receptors and prevent the binding of the biologically active molecules. Molecules that bind to receptors, but are less biologically active than the native hormone, are termed "partial agonists." The term "partial antagonist" also applies because partial agonists bind to receptors and prevent the binding of the fully biologically active native hormone.

Relationship of Binding to Biologic Response

The biologic response of a target cell to a hormone is determined by a number of factors, including the concentration of hormone, density of receptors on the cell surface, and affinity of the receptor for the hormone. Normally, the concentration of a particular hormone in the circulation is much lower than the K_d of the hormone–receptor interaction. Therefore, the receptors on a target cell are almost never saturated and an increase in the concentration of circulating hormone results in a proportional increase in the number of occupied receptors.

In a number of examples of peptide hormone binding to cell surface receptors, the response of the target

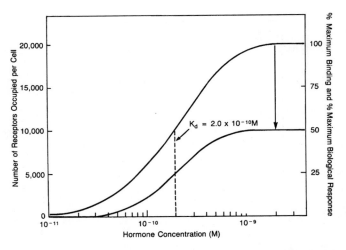

Figure 7–1. Hormone binding and biologic response curves when no spare receptors are present. In this example, the hormone binding and biologic response curves are superimposed over the entire range of hormone concentrations. A 50 percent decrease in receptor number with no change in the K_d of the hormone–receptor interaction will result in an equivalent reduction in the maximum biologic response. *(Reproduced, with permission, from Mendelson CR. Mechanism of hormone action. In: Griffin JE, Ojeda SR, eds. Textbook of Endocrine Physiology. Oxford, UK, Oxford University Press, 1996: 29–65.)*

cell to the hormone is directly proportional to the number of receptor sites occupied, that is, the binding and biologic response curves are superimposable over the entire range of hormone concentrations and a maximum biologic response is achieved when 100 percent of the receptor sites are occupied (Fig 7–1). If the number of cell surface receptors is reduced without a change in the K_d, both the binding and biologic response curves are reduced and remain superimposable.

In the majority of examples, however, the maximum biologic response of a target cell is achieved at concentrations of hormone lower than those required to fully occupy all receptors on that cell. For example, in isolated adipocytes, maximum stimulation of glucose oxidation is achieved at concentrations of insulin such that only 2 to 3 percent of the insulin receptors are occupied. In Leydig cells, maximum stimulation of testosterone synthesis occurs at concentrations of gonadotropin such that only 1 percent of the receptors are occupied. In these systems, >97 percent of the receptors are referred to as *spare receptors*. The term does not imply that these receptors are not being utilized, but rather that a maximum biologic response is achieved when any one of the receptors on a target cell is occupied, on average <3 percent of the time. The proportion of receptors for a particular hormone on a target cell that may be "spared" can vary from one cellular response to another, resulting in a different dose–response curve for each biologic response of a cell to a given hormone.

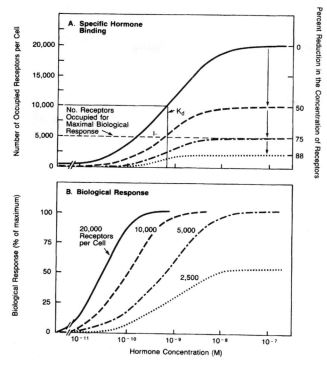

Figure 7–2. Hormone binding (A) and biologic response (B) curves when spare receptors are present. In this example, when the target cell contains its full complement of 20,000 receptors, a maximum biologic response is achieved at concentrations of hormone required to occupy only 25 percent of the cellular receptors. When the number of cellular receptors is reduced to 10,000 or 5000 without a change in the K_d, a maximum biologic response can still be achieved, albeit at progressively increased concentrations of hormone. When the number or cellular receptors is decreased by 88 percent, the maximum biologic response is reduced by 50 percent. *(Reproduced, with permission, from Mendelson CR. Mechanism of hormone action. In: Griffin JE, Ojeda SR, eds. Textbook of Endocrine Physiology. Oxford, UK, Oxford University Press, 1996: 29–65.)*

Let us consider the hormone-binding (Fig 7–2A) and biologic response (Fig 7–2B) curves for a hypothetical target cell that contains spare receptors for a particular biologic response. This hypothetical cell normally contains 20,000 receptors for the hormone. In this example, 75 percent of these receptors are considered spare receptors, because a maximum biologic response is achieved at concentrations of hormone required to occupy only 5000 receptor sites per cell. The question to be addressed is, what happens when the number of cellular receptors is reduced by 50 and 75 percent without a change in receptor affinity? In fact, the maximum biologic response remains unchanged; however, half-maximum response is achieved at progressively increased concentrations of hormone. When the number of cellular receptors is reduced below 75 percent to, say, 12 percent of the original, then the maximum biologic response is reduced proportionately.

From this example, one can see that the greater the proportion of spare receptors involved in a particular biologic response the more sensitive is the target cell to the hormone, that is, the lower the concentration of hormone required to achieve half-maximum biologic response. In addition to increasing the sensitivity of the target cell for the hormone, spare receptors also serve to prolong the biologic response of a cell to short bursts of circulating hormones. The hormone–receptor complexes in excess of those required for the maximum biologic response will maintain the response for longer periods as the concentration of hormone in the circulation declines.

PLASMA MEMBRANE RECEPTORS COMPOSED OF SEVEN TRANSMEMBRANE DOMAINS

As indicated, receptors for a large number of regulatory substances are located in the plasma membrane. These include protein and peptide hormones, prostaglandins, catecholamines, and other neurotransmitters. Such receptors are integral membrane proteins that traverse the plasma membrane. The number of transmembrane regions differs from one receptor to the next, ranging from one to many. As indicated earlier, the function of a receptor is to interact with its regulatory ligand. In the case of plasma membrane receptors, this interaction results in the transduction, followed by the amplification, of a signal. This sign generally takes the form of a second messenger molecule, such as cyclic adenosine monophosphate (cAMP) or inositol triphosphate, or calcium ions.

The amino acid sequences of a large number of cell surface receptors have now been deduced by sequencing the cDNA inserts complementary to mRNA encoding these receptors. From these sequences, structural inferences have been made by computer analysis of hydrophobic versus hydrophilic regions and of homologies of amino acid residues. On the basis of these sequence homologies, receptors have been divided into a number of superfamilies. The first of these is a large family of receptors that includes the β- and α-adrenergic receptors, muscarinic cholinergic receptors, and receptors for prostaglandins, gonadotropins, thyrotropin (TSH), corticotropin (ACTH), gonadotropin-releasing hormone (GnRH), angiotensin II, serotonin, and substance P, as well as the receptor mediating the response of the retinal rod cells to light, namely, rhodopsin. These receptors are characterized by having seven transmembrane domains; signal transduction is mediated by a second group of receptor interacting proteins known as guanine nucleotide-binding or G proteins (discussed later). The end result is the synthesis of an intracellular second messenger molecule, such as cAMP or diacylglycerol, which then mediates the activation of kinase, namely, protein kinase A or protein kinase C, respectively. Inositol triphosphate may also be formed, which is responsible for increasing intracellular free calcium ion concentrations ($[Ca^{++}]_i$). A possible consequence of increased $(Ca^{++})_i$ is the liberation of arachidonate from the sn-2 position of glycerophospholipids, with the consequent formation of prostaglandins and other eicosanoids.

A second large group of cell surface receptors is characterized as having a single transmembrane domain and a cytoplasmic tail that contains a protein tyrosine kinase domain. Several families of receptors fall into this category, including the insulin-like growth factor I (IGF-I) family, receptors for the platelet-derived growth factor (PDGF) and colony-stimulating factors, as well as receptors for epidermal growth factor (EGF), HER-2/*neu,* and fibroblast growth factor (FGF). In the case of these receptors, it is apparent that recognition of the excitatory ligand, transduction of the signal, and generation of the second messenger response are all properties of the same receptor protein, which therefore can be classified as a multifunctional molecule having several functional domains, each performing a separate role.

A third group of cell surface receptors lacks any intrinsic kinase activity, but recruits a cytoplasmic tyrosine kinase, such as members of the Src or Jak families, which then mediate the response. Receptors for the class I cytokines belong to this group, as do the receptors for growth hormone (GH) and prolactin. Yet another family of cell-surface receptors possesses not tyrosine, but intrinsic serine/threonine kinase activity, while other receptors, such as those for TNF-α and Interleukin-1β, have no endogenous kinase activity, nor do they recruit an interacting kinase molecule. In all the molecules so far discussed, interaction with the excitatory ligand results in the transduction of some signal leading to the generation of the second messenger molecule. However, it should be borne in mind that not all cell surface receptors have this signal transduction function. In a number of instances, interaction with the ligand serves as a signal for its endocytosis and consequent removal from the circulation. Such is the case for receptors for low-density lipoprotein (LDL), transferrin, α₂-macroglobulin, and chylomicron remnants. In such instances, the receptor–ligand complex translocates to coated pits that then undergo a process of adsorptive endocytosis. This commonly leads to fusion of the endocytotic vesicle with lysosomes and the subsequent degradation either of the ligand itself or the ligand plus the receptor. In examples in which the receptor is not degraded, it may be recycled to the cell surface and undergo this endocytotic recycling process several times (eg, the LDL receptor). Such endocytosis may be a property of some receptors that also have transducing functions. For example, the receptors for EGF and insulin also are internalized along with their ligands,

leading to destruction of ligand–receptor complexes in the lysosome. This process can result in downregulation of such receptors and decreased sensitivity of the target cell to the ligand.

Receptors for Glycoproteins

This subgroup of the seven transmembrane domain family of receptors interacts with large hydrophilic molecules as ligands, namely, the glycoprotein hormones, human chorionic gonadotropin (hCG), luteinizing hormone (LH), follicle-stimulating hormone (FSH), and TSH. The extracellular N-terminal region of these receptors is extremely long and maintains the conformation of the ligand-binding site by forming disulfide bridges. The LH receptor, which mediates the actions of LH and hCG, is a transmembrane polypeptide. The C-terminal half of the protein contains seven hydrophobic regions, each of sufficient length to span the plasma membrane, and therefore traverses the plasma membrane seven times (Fig 7–3). The cytoplasmic loop between the fifth and sixth transmembrane domains is especially large and is involved in interaction with G proteins. The binding of LH or hCG to LH receptors promotes interaction of the receptors with the stimulatory guanine nucleotide-binding protein of adenylate cyclase (G_s). Interaction of the LH receptor with G_s promotes the activation of adenylate cyclase, which gives rise to formation of cAMP (described later). There also is evidence for activation of phospholipase C by LH receptor.

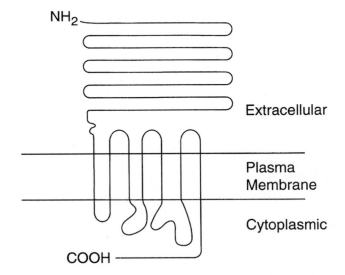

Figure 7–3. Schematic representation of the structure and plasma membrane orientation of the LH/hCG receptor. The receptor comprises two halves of similar size: the extracellular amino terminal half and the membrane-embedded carboxyl terminal half. The carboxyl terminal half contains seven transmembrane domains, three extracellular loops, and three cytoplasmic loops and a carboxyl terminus. This receptor belongs to the superfamily of G protein-coupled receptors.

The receptor for the decapeptide, GnRH, also has been cloned and characterized. This receptor, in common with those previously discussed, has seven hydrophobic regions believed to be transmembrane domains. The extracellular domain of the GnRH receptor, however, is much smaller than those of the glycoprotein receptors. The mechanism of signal transduction by this receptor is similar to that of the LH receptor, namely, interaction with the appropriate G proteins, in this case giving rise to an increase in the levels of cytosolic free calcium ion. Calcium appears to be the intracellular mediator of GnRH action on LH release, which involves calmodulin.

Signal Transduction Mechanisms Utilized by the Seven Transmembrane Domain Receptor Superfamily

The so-called second messenger hypothesis of hormone action was proposed in the early 1960s, when it was discovered that the activation of glycogen phosphorylase by epinephrine and glucagon in liver slices was mediated by the formation of a heat-stable compound, identified as cAMP. Cyclic AMP is formed from Mg^{++} adenosine triphosphate (ATP) by a membrane-associated enzyme, adenylate cyclase. According to this concept, the hormone, or first messenger, carries information from its site of production to the target cell, where it binds to specific receptors on the cell surface. This results in the activation of a membrane-bound enzyme or effector (eg, adenylate cyclase), which generates a soluble intracellular second messenger (eg, cAMP), which then transmits the information to the cellular machinery, resulting in a biologic response. In recent years, a number of other effector/second messenger systems have been discovered that mediate the actions of a variety of hormones on cellular metabolism and function.

Hormone-Sensitive   Adenylate   Cyclase. The hormone-sensitive adenylate cyclase system has at least three components: the receptor (R), a form of guanine nucleotide-binding regulatory protein (G_s or G_i), and the catalytic component (C), namely adenylate cyclase itself, which enzymatically converts $Mg^{++} \cdot ATP$ to cAMP (Fig 7–4). The guanine nucleotide-binding regulatory protein, G_s, mediates the actions of hormones that stimulate adenylate cyclase activity, whereas G_i mediates the action of those hormones that inhibit adenylate cyclase. A number of different types of hormone receptors on a single cell can interact with the same pool of regulatory and catalytic components, and these combined interactions result in either a net stimulation or inhibition of adenylate cyclase activity. As discussed above, G_s and G_i are heterotrimers composed of a unique α-subunit (α_s or α_i) and identical β- and γ-subunits. Numerous different α-subunit proteins have now been characterized, as well as several β- and γ-subunits.

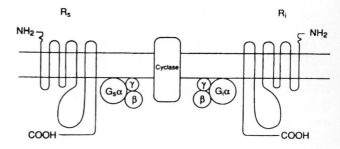

Figure 7–4. Plasma membrane components of hormone-sensitive adenylate cyclase. Hormone-sensitive adenylate cyclase is composed of the following integral proteins of the plasma membrane: receptors for either stimulatory (R_s) or inhibitory (R_i) hormones, the guanine nucleotide-binding regulatory proteins G_s or G_i, and the catalytic component (cyclase). G_s is composed of a unique α-subunit, $M_r \cong 45,000$ and β and γ subunits, $M_r \cong 35,000$ and $10,000$, respectively. G_i has a unique α-subunit, $M_r = 41,000$, and β- and γ-subunits that appear to be similar to those of G_s.

Receptor-Mediated   Stimulation   of   Adenylate Cyclase. The proposed mechanism for the hormonal activation of adenylate cyclase is presented in Figure 7–5.[1] As discussed, G_s has three subunits, α_s, β, and γ. In the inactive state, the guanine nucleotide bound to the α-subunit of G_s is guanosine diphosphate (GDP). The binding hormone (H) to receptor (R) is believed to promote the formation of the ternary complex, $H \cdot R \cdot G$, which facilitates the dissociation of GDP and the binding of GTP to the G_sα-subunit. The binding of GTP to G_sα

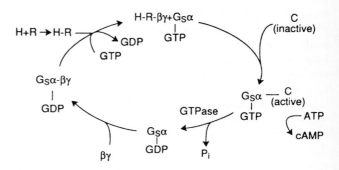

Figure 7–5.   Proposed mechanism for the hormonal activation of adenylate cyclase. G_s is composed of three subunits, α_s, β, and γ (depicted here as G_sα and βγ). In the absence of the binding of a stimulatory hormone to its receptor, the guanine nucleotide GDP is bound to G_sα and adenylate cyclase is in the inactive state. The binding of hormone to receptor facilitates the dissociation of GDP and association of GTP with the α-subunit of G_s. This in turn results in the dissociation of G_sα from the βγ subunits and its association with the catalytic component (C), resulting in adenylate cyclase activation. The activated G_sα contains a GTPase, which hydrolyzes the bound GTP to GDP, resulting in a return of adenylate cyclase to an inactive state. Cholera toxin, which inhibits the GTPase activity, causes a persistent activation of adenylate cyclase.

results in the dissociation of α_s from the $\beta\gamma$-subunits. The $G_s\alpha\bullet$GTP then associates with the catalytic subunit (C) of the adenylate cyclase to form the active holoenzyme ($G_s\alpha\bullet$GTP$\bullet$C). The activated catalytic subunit then converts MG$^{++}\bullet$ATP to cAMP. The activated $G_s\alpha$ contains a GTPase activity, which catalyzes the hydrolysis of GTP to GDP and terminates the cycle of adenylate cyclase activation. Substitution of a nonhydrolyzable analog of GTP (eg, GTPγS), or inhibition of the GTPase activity can result in permanent activation of G proteins. For example, cholera toxin, produced by the bacterial organism *Vibrio cholera*, binds to gangliosides (complex glycolipids) on the cell surface and penetrates the cell membrane. Once within the cell membrane, the toxin catalyzes the adenosine diphosphate (ADP) ribosylation of $G_s\alpha$, which results in inhibition of the GTPase activity (Fig 7–5), causing a persistent activation of adenylate cyclase. In intestinal mucosal cells, the binding of cholera toxin and subsequent activation of adenylate cyclase results in the stimulation of ion (primarily Cl$^-$) and water secretion across the intestinal brush border, causing massive diarrhea. A mutation in the $G_s\alpha$ gene may also give rise to the inhibition of its GTPase activity and ligand-independent stimulation of multiple endocrine glands including gonads. Such is the case in McCune–Albright syndrome, in which a postzygotic mutation becomes manifest as autonomous activation of $G_s\alpha$ in the ovaries, testes, parathyroids, adrenals, and melanocytes of the skin (see Chap 5).

Receptor-Mediated Inhibition of Adenylate Cyclase.

A number of hormones inhibit adenylate cyclase activity. These include catecholamines that bind to α_2-adrenergic receptors, muscarinic–cholinergic agonists, and opioids. These hormones bind to cell surface receptors that interact with the inhibitory guanine nucleotide-binding regulatory protein, G_i. Like $G_s\alpha$, $G_i\alpha$ contains a guanine nucleotide-binding site. The binding of these hormones to their receptors promotes the exchange of GTP for GDP on $G_i\alpha$. This results in the dissociation of α_i from $\beta\gamma$. The inhibition of adenylate cyclase activity appears to be mediated primarily by the interaction of the free $\beta\gamma$-subunits of G_i with the α-subunit of G_s, reducing the concentration of free $G_s\alpha$. Islet-activating protein, one of the toxins of *Bordetella pertussis*, prevents the dissociation of G_i, which results in adenylate cyclase activation, because less free $\beta\gamma$ is available to interact with $G_s\alpha$. Thus, cholera toxin activates adenylate cyclase by promoting the dissociation of G_s, whereas islet-activating protein activates adenylate cyclase by inhibiting the dissociation of G_i. However, there are several examples, including one form of adenylate cyclase, in which the $\beta\gamma$ dimer can also interact directly with an effector molecule to mediate signal transduction.

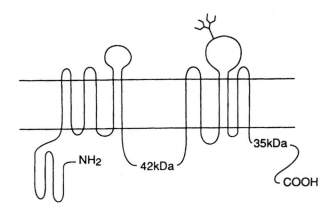

Figure 7–6. Structure of adenylate cyclase deduced from sequencing of the cDNA. The cyclase can be considered to be composed of two halves; each of which has six transmembrane domains, separated by a long cytoplasmic loop. Both the N- and C-termini are intracellular. The extracellular domain is glycosylated.

Structure of Adenylate Cyclase.

The structure of adenylate cyclase has been deduced on the basis of the sequence of cDNA clones (Fig 7–6).[2] The cyclase is a large transmembrane glycoprotein composed of two similar regions, each of which has six transmembrane domains, separated by a long (~42 kDa) cytoplasmic loop. Both the N- and C-termini are intracellular, and the N-terminal portions of each region are quite homologous to each other, as well as to sequences present in guanylate cyclases. Interestingly, the cyclase bears some topologic homology to the multiple drug resistance (MDR) gene product, as well as the cystic fibrosis gene product, both of which are channel proteins.

Cyclic AMP Regulation of Cellular Function.

The major mechanism by which cAMP regulates cellular function is through its binding to cAMP-dependent protein kinase (protein kinase A). The cAMP-dependent protein kinase holoenzyme is composed of a regulatory subunit (R) dimer and two catalytic subunits (C). The R subunit is a cAMP-binding protein, while the C subunit, when free of R, expresses protein kinase activity. Each molecule of R dimer binds four molecules of cAMP. The binding of cAMP to R causes dissociation of the inactive holoenzyme to yield two active catalytic subunits (Fig 7–7). The active free catalytic subunits can now catalyze the phosphorylation of cellular proteins. Protein kinase A catalyzes the transfer of a phosphate from ATP to the hydroxyl groups of serine and, to a lesser extent, threonine residues on cellular proteins. The phosphorylation of enzymes may result in increases or decreases in activity. For example, phosphorylation of hormone-sensitive lipase, cholesteryl esterase, or glycogen phosphorylase results in enzyme activation. On the other hand, phosphorylation of glycogen synthase causes a decrease in enzyme activity.[3]

$$R_2C_2 + 4cAMP \rightarrow R_2 \cdot 4cAMP + 2C$$
$$\text{(inactive)} \qquad\qquad \text{(active)}$$

Figure 7–7.   Mechanism of protein kinase A activation. (R_2 regulatory subunit; C, catalytic subunit.)

The specific responses of various cell types to an increase in cAMP and the activation of protein kinase A is determined by the cellular phenotype and, therefore, by the enzymes and substrates available for regulation. Thus, a major response of a liver cell to an increase in cAMP is the formation of glucose through glycogenolysis and gluconeogenesis. In a fat cell, on the other hand, the primary response to an increase in cAMP is lipolysis of the triglycerides stored in the lipid droplets, giving rise to free fatty acids and glycerol.

In addition to regulating the catalytic activity of enzymes, cAMP also regulates the transcription of specific genes in eukaryotic cells. An effect of cAMP at the level of gene transcription has been found for a number of eukaryotic genes, including steroidogenic P450 genes such as aromatase, 17α-hydroxylase, 21-hydroxylase, and cholesterol side-chain cleavage enzyme. The mechanism by which this occurs in many genes has been uncovered with the discovery of the cAMP-response element binding protein (CREB), which mediates the action of cAMP to regulate specific genes (Fig 7–8). CREB is a member of a large family of DNA-binding proteins, the activating transcription factors (ATF proteins), which bind to a common palindromic DNA sequence TGACGTCA. These proteins serve a role as transcription factors and belong to the group of *trans*-acting regulatory proteins that possess an amino acid motif known as a leucine zipper—a sequence of some five leucines, each separated by seven other amino acids. This zipper-like motif effects dimerization of the protein. CREB interacts with the TGACGTCA sequence, referred to as the cAMP response element (CRE), a *cis*-acting enhancer element in a number of cAMP-stimulated genes, such as vasoactive intestinal peptide (VIP), somatostatin, and PEPCK. CREB also binds to DNA sequences that are similar to the CRE as is found in the aromatase

P450 gene, resulting in an activation of transcription. CREB is activated by phosphorylation via cAMP-dependent protein kinase A at a specific serine residue.

Other Second Messenger Systems: Phospholipid Turnover and Inositol Triphosphate. A significant number of regulatory molecules which bind to seven transmembrane domain receptors exert their actions on cellular metabolism and function by mechanisms that do not involve adenylate cyclase activation or inhibition. Table 7–1 lists hormones that act through cAMP, as well as those that do not. Hormones that act through cAMP-mediated mechanisms include ACTH, glucagon, and the pituitary glycoprotein hormones, LH, FSH, and TSH. The glycoprotein hormone of human placental origin, hCG, which is highly homologous to LH and binds to LH receptors, also increases cAMP formation.

Other hormones, such as α_1-adrenergic agonists, angiotensin II, and some hypothalamic-releasing hormones, act through mechanisms independent of cAMP. Certain hormones may act through a cAMP-mediated mechanism in one tissue and by a cAMP-independent mechanism in another. For example, vasopressin binds to a specific subset of receptors (V_2) on cells of the kidney collecting tubules and loop of Henle to promote sodium and water reabsorption. These actions of vasopressin are mediated by increased cAMP formation and cAMP-dependent protein kinase activation. On the other hand, in the liver vasopressin acts through another subset of receptors (V_1) to enhance glycogenolysis, and this effect is mediated by a cAMP-independent pathway. The catecholamines, epinephrine and norepinephrine, bind to several subsets of receptors present in different relative amounts in various tissues. Binding of catecholamines to β-adrenergic receptors activates adenylate

TABLE 7–1. SIGNAL TRANSDUCTION MECHANISMS EMPLOYED BY HORMONES USING RECEPTORS WITH SEVEN TRANSMEMBRANE DOMAINS

Ligands That Increase cAMP Levels	Ligands That Decrease cAMP Levels	Ligands That Do Not Act Through cAMP-Mediated Mechanisms
Epinephrine and norepinephrine (β-receptors)	α_2-Adrenergic agonists	α_1-Adrenergic agonists
Glycoprotein hormones (LH, hCG, FSH, TSH)	Acetylcholine (muscarinic receptors)	Angiotensin II
Glucagon; ACTH; vasopressin (V_2 receptors)	Opioid peptides	Vasopressin (V_1 receptors)
Dopamine (D1 receptors); corticotropin-releasing hormone; vasoactive intestinal peptide	Dopamine (D_2 receptors); somatostatin	GnRH, TRH
	Substance P	

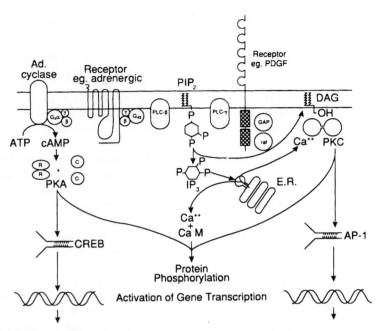

Figure 7–8. Summary of second messenger systems in mammalian cells. In addition to the adenylate cyclase system, metabolism of phosphoinositides plays a key role. The polyphosphoinositides phosphatidylinositol 4-phosphate (PIP) and phosphatidylinositol 4,5-biphosphate (PIP_2) are formed within the plasma membrane from phosphatidylinositol (PI) and ATP in reactions catalyzed by kinases. The binding of hormone to receptor results in the activation of a specific phospholipase C (PLC) within the plasma membrane, which catalyzes the hydrolysis of PIP_2 to form the putative second messengers, inositol triphosphate (IP_3) and diacylglycerol (DAG). The hormone-receptor activation of PLC-β is believed to be mediated by a guanine nucleotide binding regulatory protein, whereas PLC-γ may be activated by receptor tyrosine kinases (eg, the PDGF receptor). The water soluble IP_3 diffuses into the cytoplasm and stimulates the release of calcium from storage sites, primarily within the endoplasmic reticulum. The increased free cytosolic calcium exerts some of its effects on cellular metabolism by binding to calmodulin (CaM). The calcium–calmodulin complex binds to various enzyme or effector proteins, causing changes in their activities. One such protein is phosphorylase kinase, activated by an increase in cytoplasmic calcium ion. The IP_3 is subsequently hydrolyzed by specific phosphates to form the inactive IP_2, IP, and inositol. The DAG remains within the plasma membrane, where it facilitates the activation of protein kinase C (PKC) by calcium ion and phospholipid. The DAG and inositol are utilized for the resynthesis of phosphatidylinositol.

cyclase and increases cAMP formation. Interaction of catecholamines with α_2-adrenergic receptors, on the other hand, inhibits adenylate cyclase, while binding to α_1-adrenergic receptors increases inositol phospholipid turnover with a resulting increase in the levels of free cytosolic calcium ion and an activation of protein kinase C.

In addition to catecholamines acting through α_1-adrenergic receptors, a number of other regulatory ligands cause increased phospholipid turnover, protein kinase C activation, and increased cytosolic free calcium.[4] Hormone receptor interactions that result in the formation of these second messengers include the binding of vasopressin to V_1 receptors and angiotensin II to receptors on liver cells. The proposed mechanism of action of such hormones is presented in Figure 7–8. The binding of hormone to receptor results in the rapid activation of a plasma membrane associated phospholipase. Although enzymes with phospholipase C activity have received the most attention in this regard, phospholipases A and D may also have regulatory functions in certain second messenger systems, particularly those in which metabolites of arachidonic acid are involved. The

phospholipase C in question catalyzes the hydrolysis of a specific inositol phospholipid within the plasma membrane, namely, phosphatidylinositol 4,5-biphosphate (PIP_2), to form the second messengers diacylglycerol (DAG) and inositol 1,4,5-triphosphate (IP_3). The hormonal activation of the specific phospholipase C is mediated by the interaction of the receptor with a specific G protein (G_q).[5] At least three different phospholipase C (PLC) proteins have been characterized, namely, PLC-β, -γ, and -δ. The particular isoform involved in interaction with this family of receptors is PLC-β.[6] The hydrolysis of PIP_2 to form IP_3 is specifically associated with an increase in the levels of free cytosolic calcium ion and the subsequent physiologic response. Furthermore, incubation of permeabilized cells with IP_3 results in a profound increase in the release of calcium ion from intracellular stores, primarily the endoplasmic reticulum. A receptor for IP_3 present on the endoplasmic reticulum has been cloned and characterized. In addition to mediating IP_3-stimulated Ca^{++} influx to the cytosol from the endoplasmic reticulum, this receptor also may act in conjunction with dihydropyridine-gated calcium channels to facilitate Ca^{++}

influx from outside the cell. Once formed, IP_3 is rapidly hydrolyzed to IP_2, IP, and inositol by the actions of specific phosphomonoesterases. The action of the esterase that hydrolyzes IP to inositol is inhibited by lithium ion.

Calcium as a Second Messenger.
The levels of free calcium ion in the cytoplasm are normally quite low ($\approx 10^{-7}$ mol/L) compared to the levels of calcium ion in the extracellular fluid ($\approx 10^{-3}$ mol/L). Within the cell, calcium is stored in relatively high concentrations in the mitochondria and endoplasmic reticulum (sarcoplasmic reticulum of muscle cells). An increase in the levels of free cytosolic calcium ion can have a variety of effects on the cell, including changes in cell motility, contraction of muscle cells, increased release of secretory proteins, and activation of a number of regulatory enzymes. Calcium ion exerts most of these effects in cells by binding to specific calcium binding proteins, such as *calmodulin*. The binding of calcium results in the activation of calmodulin, enabling it to bind to various enzymes or effector molecules, causing a change in their activities. Two enzymes activated by the calcium–calmodulin complex are phosphorylase kinase and myosin light-chain kinase (MLCK), in smooth muscle. Phosphorylase kinase has four subunits, α, β, γ, and δ. The δ-subunit is calmodulin and the γ-subunit is the catalytic component of the enzyme. The α- and β-subunits are phosphorylated by cAMP-dependent protein kinase. Phosphorylase kinase is an example of an enzyme activated by an increase either in intracellular calcium ion (eg, in response to angiotensin II) or cAMP (in response to glucagon). This provides an example of a system in which the actions of cAMP and calcium occur in the same direction. There are also examples in which the actions of calcium and cAMP are opposed. In smooth muscle, MLCK is activated by Ca^{++}-calmodulin, following the increase in cytosolic Ca^{++} triggered by muscarinic cholinergic activation. This results in phosphorylation of myosin light chains and activation of the contraction mechanism. On the other hand, increased cAMP levels resulting from β-adrenergic activation cause phosphorylation of MLCK via protein kinase A. This causes a decrease in the affinity of MLCK for Ca^{++}-calmodulin and decreased kinase activity, with the result that relaxation ensues.

Role of Protein Kinase C.
The other product of the hydrolysis of inositol phospholipids, diacylglycerol, also serves as a second messenger by acting within the cell membrane to activate protein kinase C.[7] Protein kinase C is a phospholipid- and calcium-dependent enzyme that catalyzes the phosphorylation of serine and threonine residues on a number of cellular proteins. Diacylglycerol dramatically increases the affinity of the enzyme for calcium ion and therefore promotes an increase in enzyme activity at resting levels of intracellu-

lar calcium. The diacylglycerol-mediated hormonal activation of protein kinase C can be mimicked by incubating cells with tumor-promoting phorbol esters, which interact with the enzyme at the same site as diacylglycerol. Because phorbol esters are not rapidly degraded, these agents cause long-term activation of protein kinase C.

In addition to phosphorylating serine and threonine residues on enzyme proteins, protein kinase C, like protein kinase A, is capable of mediating the regulation of expression of specific genes. Just as the action of protein kinase A to regulate gene expression is mediated by a transcription factor, namely, CREB, so the action of protein kinase C is mediated by a transcription factor known as AP-1. This is a heterodimer of two related proteins containing leucine-zipper motifs, namely c-Fos and c-Jun, both of which are recognized proto-oncogenes. AP-1 binds to a regulatory element on responsive genes that differs from the CRE by a single nucleotide, namely, TGAC/GTCA. It is now known that a family of protein kinase C isoforms exist, and the roles for the various family members are currently being investigated.

RECEPTORS WITH TYROSINE KINASE ACTIVITY

As mentioned previously, a second large group of cell surface receptors is characterized by having a single transmembrane domain and a cytoplasmic tail that contains a protein tyrosine kinase domain, that is, the ability to phosphorylate tyrosyl residues in specific proteins. Families of receptors that fall into this category include (1) the EGF, HER-2/*neu*, v-*erb*-B family; (2) the insulin IGF-I receptor family; (3) the family that includes receptors for PDGF, c-Fms/CSF-1, and the product of the c-Kit proto-oncogene; and (4) the family of receptors for FGF and int-2. The four families are indicated diagrammatically in Figure 7–9.

Epidermal Growth Factor Receptor Family
The EGF receptor is comprised of a single polypeptide chain of 1186 amino acids. The protein can be divided into three domains: an N-terminal domain of 621 amino acids that contains the EGF binding site; a membrane-spanning domain of 26 hydrophobic amino acids; and a C-terminal cytoplasmic domain of 542 amino acids that shares sequence homology with other tyrosine-specific protein kinases. The tyrosine kinase activity of the receptor is stimulated upon binding of EGF and is believed to mediate most of its actions.[8] The N-terminal region contains many cysteine residues, which are clustered into two regions that may form an EGF-binding cleft. The EGF receptor is found to be overproduced in a number of tumor cell lines, suggesting that overexpression of the

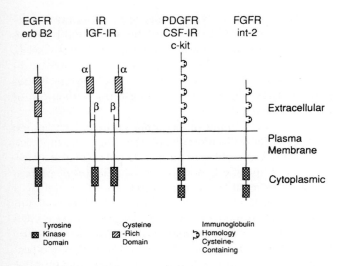

Figure 7–9. Schematic diagram of the four major categories of tyrosine kinase-related receptors that have thus far been defined. These are described in greater detail in the text.

EGF receptor gene may contribute to the phenotype of cellular transformation. It also is of interest that the cytoplasmic portion of the EGF receptor, which encodes the tyrosine kinase, has a very high degree of sequence homology with one of the transforming proteins of the avian erythroblastosis virus, the v-*erb*-B oncogene product.[9] It has been suggested that the v-*erb*-B gene product induces cellular transformation because of the constitutive expression of the tyrosine kinase domain in the absence of expression of the regulatory EGF-binding domain. Another member of this family is HER-2/*neu*, a transmembrane protein homologous to the EGF receptor and the *neu* oncogene. Amplification of HER-2/*neu* (also known as *erb*-B2) occurs in many adenocarcinomas and is overexpressed in nearly 30 percent of human breast cancer patients. A ligand for this receptor has not yet been identified, although ligands for other family members, namely HER-3 and HER-4, are known (eg, heregulin). It is now known that HER-2 can heterodimerize with other members of this family such as HER-3 and HER-4.

Insulin Receptor Family

The polypeptide hormone, insulin, exerts a variety of metabolic and growth-promoting effects on its target cells that are initiated by its interaction with specific plasma membrane receptors. The insulin receptor is a high-molecular-weight glycoprotein that exhibits insulin-dependent tyrosine-specific protein kinase activity. The receptor exists in the plasma membrane as a tetramer consisting of two disulfide-linked heterodimers $(\alpha\beta)_2$.[10] The α- and β-subunits of the insulin receptor are synthesized as part of a single 180-kDa precursor polypeptide chain, which is subsequently proteolytically cleaved

and inserted into the plasma membrane. The α-subunit can be chemically cross-linked to [^{125}I]-labeled insulin and contains the hormone-binding site of the receptor. The β-subunits exhibit insulin-dependent tyrosine kinase activity and contain the membrane-spanning domain. The α-subunit of the receptor does not contain a hydrophobic membrane-spanning sequence and is localized exclusively on the outer face of the plasma membrane. Like the N-terminal extracellular domain of the EGF receptor, the α-chain is rich in cysteine residues.

The receptor for Insulin growth factor-1 is quite similar in primary structure and organization to the insulin receptor. The only regions of significant divergence are in the extracellular cysteine-rich region, believed responsible for ligand binding, and in the C-terminus downstream of the tyrosine kinase. The highest homology is in the tyrosine kinase domain, although the IGF-I receptor has a nine amino acid insertion in the kinase domain as compared to the insulin receptor.

The status of the receptor for IGF-II is somewhat more confusing. The receptor initially characterized as the IGF-II receptor was originally isolated as one of the mannose-6-phosphate receptors. This molecule has a single transmembrane-spanning region and a large extracellular domain, some 2200 amino acids with 15 repeating segments, each containing multiple cysteines. There is a relatively short (164 amino acids) cytoplasmic domain lacking homology to any known protein, including tyrosine kinases. There is evidence to suggest that the role of this receptor is to clear these molecules from the extracellular space rather than serve a second messenger role. It is likely that the biologic actions of IGF-II are mediated by its binding to the IGF-I receptor, since the affinity of IGF-II for IGF-I receptor is only about twofold less than that for IGF-I, whereas the affinity for insulin is 100-fold less.[11]

Platelet-derived Growth Factor, Colony Stimulating Factor-I, c-Kit Receptor Family

The proteins belonging to this family are all receptors that once again contain a single transmembrane-spanning domain and tyrosine kinase domains in their cytosolic tail. The extracellular portions of these receptors have 5 immunoglobulin-like domains with a pattern of cysteines distinct from those of the EGF receptor and insulin receptor families. In addition, their tyrosine kinase domains contain 70 to 100 amino acid insertions compared to the tyrosine kinase domains of the EGF receptor and insulin receptor families, and are consequently divided into two segments. The ligands, PDGF and CSF-I, are both disulfide-linked dimeric molecules. PDGF specifically stimulates the proliferation of mesenchymal cells by acting early in the transition from the quiescent state to G_1. It is released from platelets when they adhere to injured vessels. However, it is also probably produced by endothelial cells and macrophages. The macrophage growth factor, CSF-I, stimulates hemopoietic precursor cells to form colonies containing mononuclear phagocytes. It selectively binds to hemopoietic precursor cells and promotes their differentiation.

Fibroblast Growth Factor Receptor Family

The last receptor family in this group of transmembrane receptors is that which binds FGF, including acidic and basic FGFs, and the int-2 gene product. FGFs appear to be important in angiogenesis and wound-healing, as well as the maintenance of neuronal cell viability. The receptor is a 91-kDa protein with a single transmembrane region. The extracellular portion has three immunoglobulin-like domains found in the PDGF receptor family. The FGF receptor differs from other tyrosine kinase receptors in that the distance between the transmembrane region and the start of the tyrosine kinase domain is longer, some 87 amino acids instead of the 50 amino acids in other receptors of this type. Similar to the PDGF receptor family, the tyrosine kinase domain of the FGF receptor is split by an insert of some 14 amino acids.

Signal Transduction by the Tyrosine Kinase Family of Cell Surface Receptors

A considerable body of evidence exists to support the view that most, if not all, of the actions of this group of receptors are a consequence of the tyrosine kinase activity stimulated upon binding of the ligand. Many of these ligands have growth-promoting activities on their target cells; frequently, overexpression of the receptors can result in the development of a transformed phenotype. Mutations of these receptors, which result in constitutive activation of the tyrosine kinase, also can frequently lead to transformation. An important question that arises then is the nature of the protein substrates for the tyrosine kinase activities of these receptors.

It is now appreciated that these receptors interact to form homo- or heterodimers. In the cases of insulin and IGF-I receptors, these exist as tetramers of two disulfide-linked heterodimers. In this way, transphosphorylation of specific tyrosines on the cognate receptor is mediated by the tyrosine kinase of its partner. These phosphorylated tyrosines, together with the adjacent amino acid sequences, comprise recognition sequences for adaptor proteins which mediate the signal transduction cascade. One such adaptor protein is GRB-2. In common with other adaptor proteins, GRB-2 has a region known as a Src-homology-2 (SH2) domain which recognizes a phosphotyrosine sequence on the receptor and binds to this region. GRB-2 then recruits another protein, SOS, by means of another Src-homology region (SH3) which recognizes a proline-rich region in SOS. SOS, which also is known

as guanine nucleotide releasing factor, activates GTP-binding to Ras by releasing GDP, and this initiates a phosphorylation cascade involving kinases of the MAPKKK, MAPKK, MAPK families.[12] In this case, MAPKKK is Raf, but other possible cascades also have been recognized. Ultimately, the MAPK components activate transcription factors such as members of the Ets family and AP-1, which results in expression of selected genes. In the case of the insulin receptor, and probably also the IGF-I receptor, another adaptor protein, IRS (insulin receptor substrate), intervenes to bind via SH2 domains to phosphotyrosine sequences on the ligand-activated receptor.

Another protein which has SH2 homology domains is PLC-8$_\gamma$, which also recognizes phosphotyrosine motifs on transmembrane receptors and thus is activated to hydrolyze PIP_2 with release of IP_3. Yet another enzyme that appears to be activated by these receptors is phosphatidylinositol-3-kinase, which in addition to its catalytic subunit has a regulatory subunit containing SH2 domains. However, the role of this enzyme in the production of active inositol phosphates from phosphatidylinositol breakdown is not clear at this time, although a role in vesicle transport and secretion is indicated.

In conclusion, it is now evident that the tyrosine kinase family of cell surface receptors can activate in overlapping as well as parallel fashions various second messenger systems that are activated by cell surface receptors that interact with G proteins. Clearly, some of these interactions are additive or synergistic, whereas others are opposing. However, the net result is the integrated control of cellular homeostasis, function, and growth.

THE GUANYLYL CYCLASE RECEPTOR FAMILY

Shortly after the discovery of cAMP, another cyclic nucleotide, namely cyclic guanosine monophosphate (cGMP), was also discovered. Considerable excitement was generated for several years over the possibility that these two cyclic nucleotides might work in opposite fashions to regulate cell metabolism, the so-called Yin–Yang hypothesis. With the failure of efforts to confirm consistent cellular responses to cGMP, however, interest in this molecule as a potential second messenger waned. However, investigations into the role of cGMP have intensified with the recent characterization of several proteins containing guanylate cyclase activity and the clear involvement of this cyclic nucleotide in a number of cell regulatory mechanisms.

Soluble Guanylate Cyclases

The first guanylate cyclase to be characterized was found to be soluble and present in the cytoplasm. This protein is now recognized to be activated by exogenous nitrovasodilators such as nitroglycerine and azide. It was the realization that this soluble guanylate cyclase mediated the rapid vasodilatory effects of nitroglycerine on cardiac vasculature that was in large part responsible for the renewed interest in this enzyme. It now is realized that these nitrovasodilators, as well as a number of endogenous activators of the enzyme—such as acetylcholine, histidine, and endothelin—give rise to a common second messenger signal, namely, the formation of the molecule nitric oxide (NO). NO activates soluble guanylate cyclase, which is a heterodimer of subunits of 82 and 70 kDa, each of which has a heme group that binds the NO, as well as a catalytic site. This activation, in turn, leads to increased levels of cGMP. It now is known that endogenous nitric oxide is formed from the side chain of the amino acid, arginine, via the activity of the enzyme nitric oxide synthase, which requires calcium and ATP. Several forms of this enzyme exist, which are activated by the endogenous stimulators of this pathway such as acetylcholine, histidine, and endothelin.

Membrane-Bound Guanylate Cyclases

In addition to the soluble guanylate cyclase, there are a number of transmembrane receptors that contain guanylate cyclase activity. These receptors bind such ligands as atrial natriuretic peptide (ANP) and related proteins such as brain natriuretic peptide (BNP) through their extracellular domains and mediate induction of guanylate cyclase activity. ANP and BNP induce natriuresis, diuresis, and vasodilation partially or entirely through the increased production of the second messenger, cGMP.[13] The ANP and BNP receptors are proteins of about 130 kd that have at least four distinct domains: ligand binding, transmembrane, kinase-like, and guanylate cyclase catalytic domains. The kinase-like domain appears necessary for ANP stimulation of guanylate cyclase activity. The guanylate cyclase catalytic domain has sequence similarity to domains found in both the α- and β-subunits of the soluble guanylate cyclase and to the intracellular N-terminal region of adenylate cyclase. In addition to these transmembrane guanylate cyclases, there is another type of guanylate cyclase protein present in retinal rod cells, which is responsible for synthesis of the cGMP involved in transduction of the rhodopsin-mediated light-induced signal. This guanylate cyclase is attached to structural elements within the cell.

One question that arises, then, is how does cGMP work in these systems? In the case of the retinal rod cells, there is a cGMP-gated ion channel that allows sodium and calcium ions to enter the cell in the presence of cGMP. Activation of cGMP phosphodiesterase by GTP-bound transduction in response to the light signal results in closure of the channel, thus preventing the uptake of sodium and calcium ions. This results in hyperpolarization of the plasma membrane, which is transmitted to the synaptic terminal at the other end of the cell and conveyed to neurons of the retina. In other cell types, cGMP actions may include activation of a cGMP-dependent phosphodiesterase, which in turn lowers cAMP levels, and activation of cGMP-dependent protein kinases. Thus, cGMP may indeed oppose some effects of cAMP at various times.

OTHER RECEPTOR SIGNAL TRANSDUCTION PATHWAYS

Jak/STAT Pathway

As indicated earlier, a number of receptors lack obvious kinase homology regions in their cytoplasmic domains. In the case of the class I cytokines—interleukin 6 (IL-6), IL-11, leukemia inhibitory factor (LIF), and oncostatin M—the receptor complex contains homo- or heterodimers of a transmembrane component, gp130, which binds a member of the soluble tyrosine kinase family, the Jak kinases.[14] Upon dimerization, the Jak protein is phosphorylated by its partner and, in turn, catalyzes the phosphorylation of the transcription factor STAT3, which has been recruited to a phosphotyrosine recognition site on gp130 via an SH2 domain. These SH2 domains now recognize the newly phosphorylated tyrosine of another STAT3 protein, resulting in formation of a STAT3 homodimer. The STAT3 homodimer translocates to the nucleus where it binds to a DNA sequence element on responsive genes known as a GAS element, resulting in activation of transcription. Similar mechanisms operate to mediate signal transduction from GH and prolactin, except that different members of the Jak and STAT families are employed.

TGFβ, Activin, Inhibin, Müllerian Inhibitory Substance (MIS)

Receptors for this family of ligands have a unique signal transducing mechanism which only now is being elucidated. The cytoplasmic domains of these receptors contain a serine/threonine kinase. Binding of ligand results in heterodimerization of R1 and R2 receptor isoforms and transphosphorylation. Although many of the downstream events are still unclear, the signal appears to be transduced by a series of proteins known as SMADs, which upon activation translocate to the nucleus where they may activate transcription.

TNF-α, Fas

These factors, together with IL-1β, are capable of initiating apoptosis in a variety of cell types.[15] However, TNF-α also has powerful antilipotropic activity and is capable of reversing the adipocyte differentiation process. Unlike Fas and IL-1β, TNF-α also can activate the transcription factor NFκB. These trimeric ligands bind to receptors which also are trimeric. Fas receptor seems to transduce uniquely the apoptotic pathway. These receptors have no intrinsic kinase activities; however, each contains a sequence known as a death domain, which permits recruitment of the death domain-containing proteins, TRADD in the case of the TNF-α receptor and FADD in the case of the Fas receptor. TRADD initiates a series of events leading to activation of NFκB. This involves phosphorylation of the NFκB inhibitory partner, IκB, leading to its dissociation and activation of NFκB. The kinase that phosphorylates IκB is still unknown. FADD initiates a cascade of events leading to apoptosis and cell death, which involves activation of ICE-related proteases. TRADD also initiates a similar sequence of events, but does so by first interacting with FADD. Many of the actions of TNF-α at the cellular level can be mimicked by ceramide, indicating that sphingomyelinase activity is involved; however, the role of sphingomyelinase is still unclear. Work to elucidate the steps involved in each of these pathways is proceeding at a rapid pace.

ALTERATIONS IN RECEPTOR NUMBER AND FUNCTION

As discussed above, changes in concentration of cellular receptors for a specific hormone can markedly alter the sensitivity of the target cell to that hormone; a decrease in the concentration of receptors can decrease sensitivity to the hormone, whereas an increase in receptor concentration can increase the sensitivity of the target cell for the hormone. It is apparent that the concentration of cellular receptors for a specific hormone can vary considerably with the physiologic state. Most commonly, an increase in the level of a specific hormone will cause a decrease in the available number of its cellular receptors. This decrease in available receptors can be due either to a sequestration of receptors away from the cell surface or an actual disappearance or loss of receptors from the cell. This hormonally induced negative regulation of receptors is termed *homologous downregulation* or *desensitization*.[16] Studies of the downregulation of receptors for insulin and EGF by the homologous hormones indicate that downregulation is caused, at least in part, by a clustering of hormone–receptor complexes in coated pits on the cell surface, internalization within coated vesicles, and degradation by lysosomal enzymes. Coated pits and coated vesicles are so named because they contain a protein, clathrin, that forms a "coat" on their cytoplasmic surfaces. There is little doubt that receptor internaliza-

tion provides an important homeostatic mechanism that serves to protect the organism from the potential toxic effects of hormone excess.

Desensitization is defined as a decrease in the responsiveness of a cell to a constant level of hormone or factor upon prolonged exposure. Homologous desensitization can also result from a hormone-induced alteration in the receptor, which uncouples it from some component of the signal transduction pathway. Another form of desensitization, *heterologous desensitization*, occurs when incubation with one agonist reduces the responsiveness of a cell to a number of other agonists that act through different receptors. This phenomenon is most commonly observed with receptors that act through the adenylate cyclase system. Heterologous desensitization reflects a broad pattern of refractoriness that has a slower onset than homologous desensitization.

NUCLEAR RECEPTORS

Members of the nuclear receptor superfamily are ligand-dependent transcription factors that regulate the expression of target genes via binding to specific *cis*-acting elements. The superfamily consists of receptors for steroid hormones (estrogens, progestins, androgens, and corticosteroids), sterol derivatives (1,25 dihydroxyvitamin D_3), and nonsteroids (retinoids and thyroid hormone). It also includes a growing number of structurally related proteins for which ligands have yet to be identified, referred to as "orphan receptors."

Classical steroid hormone receptors compose an important but small component of the nuclear receptor superfamily. Steroids travel in the circulation predominantly bound to several classes of serum proteins. Estrogens and androgens are transported in the circulation bound to testosterone-binding globulin (TeBG), which binds estradiol-17β and testosterone with relatively high affinity ($K_d \approx 10^{-9}$ mol/L). These steroids also are weakly bound to serum albumin. Glucocorticoids and progesterone are bound in the circulation to corticosteroid binding globulin (CBG), also referred to as transcortin (Fig 7–10). Presumably, steroids can freely diffuse across the plasma membranes of all cells but are sequestered only within cells that contain specific intracellular receptors. The steroid binds to its receptor with an affinity ($K_d \approx 10^{-10}$ mol/L) that is at least 10-fold greater than the affinity with which it binds to the serum globulins. Steroid hormone receptors, in the absence of their ligands, are complexed with heat shock proteins and are not able to bind DNA (Fig 7–11). In this unoccupied state, receptors for estrogen, progesterone, androgens, and mineralocortoids are present in the nucleus, whereas the glucocorticoid receptor is found in the cytoplasm. Binding of hormone transforms the receptor

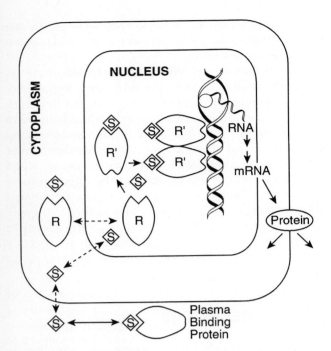

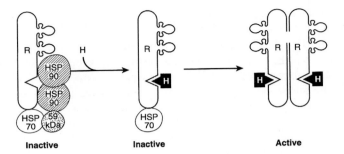

Figure 7–11. Proposed mechanism for hormone-induced activation of the glucocorticoid receptor. The inactive "free" glucocorticoid receptor (R) exists in the cytoplasm as a monomer in association with a protein complex comprised of two molecules of heat shock protein (hsp) 90, one molecule of hsp70, and number of other proteins. After hormone (H) binding, the receptor dissociates from the hsp complex and forms a homodimer with another molecule of glucocorticoid receptor. This process is required for transformation of the receptor to a DNA-binding, transcription modulating state. *(Reproduced, with permission, from Mendelson CR. Mechanism of hormone action. In: Griffin JE, Ojeda SR, eds.* Textbook of Endocrine Physiology. *Oxford, UK, Oxford University Press, 1996: 29–65.)*

Figure 7–10. Schematic representation of a steroid hormone responsive cell. Steroid hormones (S) in the circulation are predominantly bound to specific proteins. Only a small proportion of the circulating steroid is free; it is the unbound steroid that has the capacity to enter cells by free diffusion. Within target cells, the steroids bind with high affinity to specific receptors that are primarily localized within the nucleus. After binding steroid, the receptor (R) undergoes a process of "transformation," which results in an increase in the affinity of the receptor for specific sequences of DNA proximate to steroid-regulated genes. The binding of the receptor as a dimer to these genomic regions can result in increases or decreases in the rates of gene expression. The steroid–receptor complex is believed to increase the rate of transcription of specific genes by causing the formation of a stable preinitiation complex and facilitating the binding of RNA polymerase II to the promoter regions of such genes. This results in the synthesis of RNA molecules that are processed within the nucleus to mRNAs that enter cytoplasm and are translated into specific proteins. *(Reproduced, with permission, from Mendelson CR. Mechanism of hormone action. In: Griffin JE, Ojeda SR, eds.* Textbook of Endocrine Physiology. *Oxford, UK, Oxford University Press, 1996: 29–65.)*

into antive form by mediating the dissociation of heat shock proteins and allowing the dimerization of receptor proteins. The activated receptor is now able to bind the hormone-responsive element in genomic DNA as a homodimer and stimulate, or in some cases repress, the expression of target genes (Fig 7–10).

The second group within the superfamily are the non-steroidal, ligand-activated receptors, which consist of the receptors for thyroid hormone, retinoic acid (RAR), and 1,25 dihydroxyvitamin D_3. These receptors are located in the nucleus in their free or bound state, and are bound to their hormone response elements as homo- or heterodimers with another member of the family, the retinoid-X-receptor (RXR) in the absence or presence of ligand: In the absence of ligand, these receptors act as silencers of the genes with which they interact. Ligand binding, however, dramatically alters the activity of these receptors from transcriptional silencers to transcriptional enhancers.

Orphan receptors constitute the largest component of the nuclear receptor superfamily. These receptors can bind as monomers or as heterodimers to defined DNA motifs and may be constitutively active. Two of the orphan receptors are of particular importance for reproduction: steroidogenic factor-1 (SF-1, also known as Ad4 binding protein) and DAX-1 [DSS (dosage-sensitive sex)-AHC (adrenal hypoplasia congenita)] critical region in the X chromosome, gene-1). SF-1 was originally described by two separate groups for its role in the regulation of the 11-hydroxylase[17] and 21-hydroxylase genes.[18] Knockout of the SF-1 gene in mice results in the failure of gonadal and adrenal development, as well as impaired ventromedial hypothalamic nucleus development and gonadotropin secretion. DAX-1 is another orphan receptor. Mutagenesis of the DAX-1 gene has been reported to be responsible for X-linked AHC and hypogonadotropic hypogonadism.[19] SF-1, immediately followed by DAX-1, is expressed in mouse embryos at very early developmental stages in the hypothalamus, pituitary, adrenals, and gonads suggesting vital roles for both factors in the development of these tissues. DAX-1 also is one of the candidate determining factors of gonadal sex.

Receptor Structure and Molecular Forms
The primary structures of the nuclear receptors have been determined by the use of recombinant DNA tech-

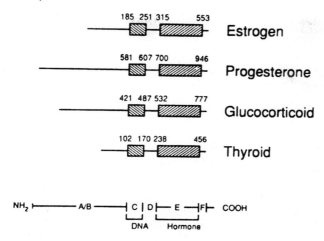

Figure 7–12. Schematic representation of the domain structures of steroid and thyroid hormone receptors. The amino acid sequences of the human estrogen receptor, chicken progesterone receptor, human glucocorticoid receptor, and human thyroid hormone receptor have been found to contain two highly conserved regions (C and E), represented by the striped boxes. The numbers refer to the positions of the amino acid residues from the amino terminus of each protein. Region C, a cysteine-rich region that is the putative DNA binding domain, is highly conserved among the different receptors. Region E, the putative hormone binding domain, has reduced, albeit significant hormology among the various receptors. Region A/B, which is the least conserved in amino acid sequence and length, is important in transcriptional activation.

nology.[20] Amino acid sequence analysis indicates that these receptors share common structural motifs, thus suggesting that they are evolutionarily linked. All these receptor proteins have the same general structure, as well as a high degree of homology in their hormone and DNA binding regions (Fig 7–12). In each case, the ligand binding domain (E) is localized at the carboxy terminus of the molecule. Within the central portion of the protein lies the DNA-binding domain (C), which contains two repeated units enriched in the amino acids Cys, Lys, and Arg. It has been proposed that each of these units is folded into a finger-like structure with a zinc ion at its center. These DNA binding "fingers" have the capacity to insert into a half-turn of DNA. The hydrophilic region (D), which varies in length and sequence among the different receptors, may serve as a hinge between the hormone and DNA binding domains. The carboxy terminal regions of the members of the steroid/thyroid receptor gene family all have a high degree of sequence homology with the v-*erb*-A protein of the oncogenic avian erythroblastosis virus. This is the viral counterpart of c-*erb*-A, which encodes the thyroid hormone receptor.[21]

Of potential importance is the finding that most nuclear receptors are phosphoproteins that can be phosphorylated upon hormone binding. These receptors are substrates for protein kinases, such as protein kinase A. Although the significance of this still is poorly under-

stood, it is known in the case of the progesterone receptor, that inhibition of protein kinase A can block progesterone action. It is likely, therefore, that phosphorylation plays an important, but as yet poorly understood, role in modulating the action of at least one member of this receptor family, the progesterone receptor.[22]

Regulation of Gene Expression by Steroid Hormones

As mentioned earlier, the steroid receptors directly link extracellular signals to transcriptional responses and comprise, in fact, a family of ligand-modulated transcription factors that regulate homeostasis, reproduction, development, and differentiation. Understanding of their mode of action, therefore, requires knowledge of the *cis*-acting elements of the regulated genes, that is, the linear sequence of bases that constitutes a regulatory element on the gene with which these ligand-modulated transcription factors interact. These receptors can be divided into several groups depending upon the sequences of the response elements with which they interact. The first group comprises the glucocorticoid, mineralocorticoid, progesterone, and androgen receptors, which all bind as homodimers to the same double-stranded idealized inverted repeat of a six-nucleotide sequence (half-site) with a three nucleotide spacer, namely, AGAACAnnnTGTTCT. The second group, which comprises receptors for thyroid hormones, retinoids, and 1,25-dihydroxyvitamin D_3, usually bind as heterodimers with RXR to a double-stranded direct hexameric repeat of the sequence AGGTCA separated by a spacer of 1 to 5 nucleotides ($AGGTCAn_{1-5}AGGTCA$). Binding specificity is determined by the number of nucleotides in the spacer. On the other hand, the estrogen receptor binds to an inverted repeat of a half-site identical to that recognized by the thyroid/retinoid/vitamin D_3 receptor subfamily; however, in the case of the estrogen receptor, this is an inverted repeat with a 3-nucleotide spacer, namely AGGTCAnnnTGACCT.[23]

The fact that the glucocorticoid, androgen, mineralocorticoid, and progesterone receptors interact with the same response element implies that specificity of transcription of a target gene, in response to a particular hormone, is governed by whether or not the required hormone receptor is present within that particular cell type. In the case of the thyroid/retinoid/vitamin D_3 receptors, binding specificity is determined in part by the number of nucleotides in the spacer between direct repeats of the half-site.

As discussed, the glucocorticoid receptor binds to its DNA response element as a homodimer to activate transcription of target genes. On the other hand, the glucocorticoid receptor can form a heterodimer with a molecule of c-Jun, which belongs to yet another family of transcription factors, namely, the basic leucine zipper family (bZIP).[24]

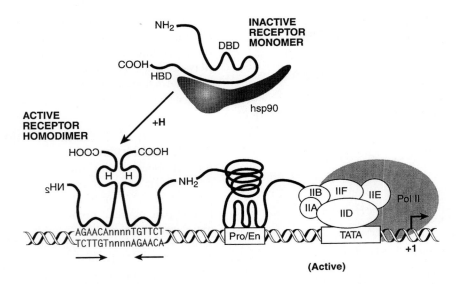

Figure 7–13. Proposed mechanism for regulation of gene transcription by glucocorticoid, progesterone, mineralocorticoid, and androgen receptors. After binding hormone (H), the receptor dissociates from the complex with hsp90 and other proteins, and binds to its hormone response element (HRE) upstream of the target gene as a homodimer. The activated receptor dimer can now interact with other receptor dimers bound to their HREs, with other transcription factors bound to promoter or enhancer elements (Pro/En), and/or directly with the preinitiation complex of proteins which, in turn, facilitates the binding of RNA polymerase II (Pol II) and activation of transcription initiation. It recently has been found that a number of receptors in the steroid receptor superfamily can interact directly with transcriptional initiation factor IIB (TFIIB). Since binding of TFIIB is rate limiting in preinitiation complex assembly, it is suggested that the steroid receptor may facilitate preinitiation complex assembly, through its interaction with TFIIB. *(Reproduced, with permission, from Mendelson CR. Mechanism of hormone action. In: Griffin JE, Ojeda SR, eds.* Textbook of Endocrine Physiology. *Oxford, UK, Oxford University Press, 1996: 29–65.)*

Activated upon phosphorylation by a specific kinase, c-Jun commonly forms a heterodimer with another bZIP protein (c-fos) to form a transcription-activating complex, termed AP-1. The interaction of the glucocorticoid receptor with c-Jun inhibits capacity of AP-1 to activate gene expression. Because activation of the AP-1 transcription factor appears to mediate the collagenolytic response to cytokines such as TNF-α and some of the interleukins, inhibition of AP-1 by heterodimer formation with the glucocorticoid receptor may be important in the action of glucocorticoids to reduce the inflammatory symptoms of rheumatoid arthritis. Finally, co-activator proteins were shown to bind steroid receptors to enhance their transcriptional activity. One such example is steroid receptor co-activator-1 (SRC-1), which increases the transcriptional activity of the estrogen receptor.[25]

Figure 7–13 shows a proposed model of the mechanisms of gene activation by glucocorticoid, mineralocorticoid, androgen, and progesterone receptors. After binding steroid, the receptor is released from the heat shock protein complex and forms a homodimer with another molecule of receptor. The activated receptor binds to its response element in DNA, as well as with other transcription factors and co-activators to form a complex. This complex, in turn, facilitates assembly and/or stabilization of the preinitiation complex (TFIIA, TFIIB, TFIID, TFIIE, TFIIF) bound to the TATA box. This,

in turn, enhances the binding of RNA polymerase II and the initiation of gene transcription.

Tissue-Specific Expression of Hormonally Regulated Genes

The phenotype of a given cell is the result of the complement of genes that are expressed; the expression of a number of these cellular genes will be subject to hormonal regulation. As indicated, because glucocorticoid, mineralocorticoid, progesterone, and androgen receptors share common response elements, the same gene has the potential to respond to the different steroid hormones; the response elicited, therefore, is determined by the receptors present in a given cell. Thus, specificity of response will be determined by receptor phenotype. In addition, a hormone acting through its cellular receptors can regulate the expression of different genes in different tissues. For example, estrogen regulates the expression of the ovalbumin gene in the chick oviduct and the vitellogenin gene in chick liver. Because the estrogen receptors in oviduct and liver tissues are apparently identical, and because the DNA sequences within and surrounding eukaryotic genes should be essentially the same in all cell types of a given organism, there must be other structural features that determine which genes are expressible and available to hormonal regulation. The complement of genes that are expressed in a given cell type is determined at the time of cellular differentiation. It is apparent that such expressible genes exist in so-called "DNase I-sensitive" regions, that is, they reside in regions of the chromatin that are more readily digested in vitro by DNase I than is the bulk of chromosomal DNA. The DNase I-sensitive regions define the structural framework in a given cell for the genes available for expression. Most cellular genes are not expressed and are tightly packaged with histone proteins in higher-order chromosomal structures, rendering them DNase I resistant.

Tissue-specific expression of steroid-responsive genes is also determined by the expression of tissue-restricted transcription factors that interact with response elements in the genomic regions surrounding the gene. These tissue-specific transcription factors may interact with the steroid receptors bound to their response elements, and/or with adaptor proteins (co-activators) that may also bind to the steroid receptors and to the preinitiation complex bound to the TATA box.

ENDOCRINE DISORDERS DUE TO DEFECTS IN SIGNAL TRANSDUCTION

Most of the genetic defects that result in endocrine disorders have been localized to the hormone receptors (Table 7–2). The following are some examples that are relevant to the reproductive endocrinologist. Mutations in the LH receptor gene giving rise to inactivation[26] or autonomous activation of the LH receptor[27] have recently been described. A homozygous inactivating mutation (recessive) in the sixth transmembrane domain of the LH receptor has been found to give rise to Leydig cell hypoplasia with deficient testosterone formation in 46,XY fetuses. This results in male pseudohermaphroditism. Activating heterozygous mutations (dominant) in the sixth transmembrane domain and third cytosolic loop of the LH receptor, on the other hand, become manifest as male-limited precocious puberty (testotoxicosis), which is characterized by increased testosterone synthesis in the absence of testicular stimulation by LH.[27] The female members of these families that carry this mutation are phenotypically normal.

Clinical manifestations of $G_s\alpha$ defects are extremely diverse. Mutations that give rise to autonomous activation of $G_s\alpha$ are manifest as the McCune–Albright syndrome. In this disorder, the mutant $G_s\alpha$ associated with LH, FSH, melanocyte stimulating hormone (MSH), ACTH, TSH, and PTH receptors causes activation of the signaling cascade in an uncontrolled fashion. The mutant $G_s\alpha$ has decreased GTPase activity, leading to constitutive adenylate cyclase activation. This, in turn, gives rise to isosexual precocity in boys and girls, discoloration of the skin, adrenal and thyroid hyperfunction, and cystic bone lesions. On the other hand, certain forms of pseudohypoparathyroidism have been associated with inactivating mutations in the $G_s\alpha$. Most of these patients show hypocalcemia and a characteristic phenotype referred to as Albright's hereditary osteodystrophy, which comprises short stature, skeletal abnormalities, and subcutaneous calcifications. Affected individuals also show resistance to hormones other than PTH. A temperature-sensitive activating mutation in the $G_s\alpha$ in two unrelated boys intriguingly gave rise to a paradoxical combination of testotoxicosis and pseudohypoparathyroidism type Ia, a condition marked by resistance to PTH and TSH.[28] While the $G_s\alpha$ protein with this mutation is quite stable at testicular temperature giving rise to autonomous

TABLE 7–2. ENDOCRINOPATHIES IN HUMANS DUE TO GENE DEFECTS IN SIGNAL TRANSDUCTION

Mutated Gene	Inheritance	Result	Phenotype
LH receptor[26]	Autosomal recessive	Inactivation	Leydig cell hypoplasia (male pseudohermaphroditism)
LH receptor[27]	Autosomal dominant	Activation	Testotoxicosis (familial male-limited precocious puberty)
TSH receptor	Autosomal dominant	Activation	Non-autoimmune autosomal dominant hyperthyroidism
$G_s\alpha$	Postzygotic mutation	Activation	McCune–Albright syndrome (male and female precocious puberty and other endocrine hyperfunction)
$G_s\alpha$[28]	Postzygotic mutation	Temperature-sensitive activation/inactivation	Testotoxicosis and PTH-resistant (pseudo)hypoparathyroidism
$G_s\alpha$	Postzygotic mutation	Inactivation	Pseudohypoparathyroidism
Estrogen receptor[29]	Autosomal recessive	Inactivation	Estrogen resistance (tall stature, continued linear growth and osteoporosis in adult men)
Androgen receptor	X-linked recessive	Inactivation	Androgen resistance (male pseudohermaphroditism)
Glucocorticoid receptor[30]	Autosomal recessive	Inactivation	Glucocorticoid resistance (androgen excess in women)
Vitamin D receptor	Autosomal recessive	Inactivation	Vitamin D resistance (rickets)
Thyroid hormone receptor[31]	Autosomal dominant	Inactivation	Thyroid hormone resistance
Dax-1[19]	X-linked recessive	Inactivation	Adrenal hypoplasia congenita and hypogonadotropic hypogonadism

testosterone secretion, it is rapidly degraded at 37 °C, explaining the PTH and TSH resistance caused by loss of $G_s\alpha$ activity.

Defects in androgen receptors give rise to varying degrees of androgen resistance, which is the most common form of male pseudohermaphroditism. An estrogen receptor defect that is associated with extremely tall stature, continued linear growth during the adult life, and osteoporosis in a 28-year-old man has recently been described.[29] This case report demonstrated the crucial role of estrogen action in men in closure of epiphyses and maintenance of bone mass. Glucocorticoid receptor defects may be manifest in boys as isosexual precocity due to elevated adrenal androgen precursors that are partially converted to testosterone in the periphery. In women, glucocorticoid resistance gives rise to androgen excess by the same mechanism.[30] Anovulation and hirsutism of pubertal onset are common presenting symptoms of glucocorticoid resistance in women. Among the other members of the nuclear receptor superfamily, mutant vitamin D receptors are detected in cases of vitamin D-dependent rickets (type II); and mutations in the thyroid hormone receptor-β are associated with symptoms of hypothyroidism but elevated levels of free T_3 and free T_4.[31]

Various mutations in hormone receptors are also demonstrated in certain neoplasias. Constitutively active forms of mutated estrogen receptors in breast cancer or androgen receptors in prostate cancer are some examples.[32] Somatic mutations in the TSH gene are associated with hyperfunctioning thyroid adenomas.

Finally, no gene defects in the insulin receptor have been demonstrated to date in the most common form of insulin resistance, which is non-insulin-dependent diabetes mellitus associated with obesity. However, in a limited number of women with extremely severe insulin resistance, ovarian hyperthecosis and acanthosis nigricans, mutations in the insulin receptor were found, most of which interfere with its tyrosine kinase activity. In the much more common form of the polycystic ovary syndrome (PCOS) with milder insulin resistance, however, receptor defects could not be demonstrated. In these relatively common conditions that are associated with mild insulin resistance, namely, obesity and PCOS, decreased receptor number on target cells or postreceptor defects (especially failure to activate the receptor tyrosine kinase) are likely mechanisms for insulin resistance.

Following is a list of abbreviations used in this chapter.

ANP	Atrial natriuretic peptide
BNP	Brain natriuretic peptide
CREB	Cyclic AMP response element binding protein
CSF-I	Colony stimulating factor-I
DAX-1	Dosage-sensitive sex adrenal hypoplasia congenital critical region in the X chromosome, gene-1
DAG	Diacylglycerol
EGF	Epidermal growth factor
FADD	Fas-activating death domain
FGF	Fibroblast growth factor
G-protein	GTP-binding protein
GRB-2	Grab-2
HER-2	Human epidermal growth factor receptor-2
ICE	IL-Iβ converting enzyme
IGF-I	Insulin-like growth factor-I
IκB	Inhibitor kappa beta
IL-1β	Interleukin-1β
IP$_3$	Inositol 1,4,5-triphosphate
IRS	Insulin receptor substrate
Jak	Janus kinase
LIF	Leukemia inhibitory factor
MAPKK	Mitogen-activated protein
MLCK	Myosin light chain kinase
NFκB	Nuclear factor kappa beta
NO	Nitric oxide
PDGF	Platelet-derived growth factor
PEPCK	Phosphoenol pyruvate carboxy kinase
PIP$_2$	Phophatidylinositol 4,5-biphosphate
PLCγ	Phospholipase-Cγ
RAR	Retinoic acid receptor
RXR	Retinoid-X receptor
SCR-1	Steroid receptor co-activator-1
SF-1	Steroidogenic factor-1
SH2	Src-homology-2
SMAD	Sma mothers against decapentaplegic
SOS	Son of sevenless (guanine nucleotide exchange factor)
STAT	Signal transducer and activator of transcription
TFIIA	Transcriptional initiation factor-IIA
TNF-α	Tumor necrosis factor-α
TRADD	TNF-α-receptor-activating death domain

CONCLUSIONS AND FUTURE DIRECTIONS

Our understanding of cellular and molecular mechanisms underlying endocrinologic processes grows exponentially. The generated knowledge and technology are applied in every scientific field and eliminate the boundaries between the disciplines. For example, human immunodeficiency virus entry into CD4+ cells was recently shown to require co-factors that were identified as G-protein-coupled seven-transmembrane domain proteins, which belong to a subfamily of chemokine receptors.[33] Furthermore, activation of signal-transduction mechanisms has been found to determine cell survival or death. Thus, it has become apparent that cellular signaling is the key to many vital functions. Although the field of endocrinology increases in complexity with each new scientific development, in reality, this complexity has given rise to increased understanding of the mechanisms of cellular function. The important role of endocrinology has also been recognized by the scientific community, as exemplified by award of the 1994 Nobel Prize in Medicine or Physiology to Drs. Alfred G. Gilman and Martin Rodbell for their work on G-proteins.

The next few years will no doubt witness the characterization of many more receptors; however, of even greater significance will be the new insights gained through understanding the mechanisms whereby transcription of specific genes is switched on and off and the means by which hormone-generated signals regulate these processes. We also will gain new understanding of how the various signal transduction pathways are interrelated, thus leading to comprehension of how different hormones act in coordinate fashion to reinforce each others' actions, or in antagonistic fashion to oppose one another. Lastly, there will be a great increase in our understanding of the molecular basis of endocrine disease by characterization of mutations that alter the properties of receptors and other regulatory proteins. The excitement of endocrinology, awakened at the beginning of this century, will certainly not be extinguished at its close.

REFERENCES

1. Gilman AG. G proteins and dual control of adenylate cyclase. *Cell.* 36:577, 1984
2. Krupinski J, Coussen F, Bakalya HA. Adenylyl cyclase amino-acid sequence: Possible calcium- or transporter-like structure. *Science.* 244:1558, 1989
3. Cohen P. The role of protein phosphorylation in neural and hormonal control of cellular activity. *Nature.* 296:613, 1982
4. Berridge MJ. The molecular basis of communication within the cell. *Sci Am.* 253:142, 1985
5. Smrcka AV, Hepler JR, Brown KO, Sternweis PC. Regulation of polyphosphoinositide-specific phospholipase C activity by purified G_q. *Science.* 251:804, 1991
6. Rhee SG, Ryn SH, Lee SY. Studies of inositol phospholipid-specific phospholipase C. *Science.* 244:546, 1989
7. Kikkawa U, Kishimoto A, Nishizuka Y. The protein kinase C family: Heterogeneity and its implications. *Ann Rev Biochem.* 58:31, 1989
8. Ullrich A, Coussens L, Hayflick JS. Human epidermal growth factor receptor cDNA sequence and aberrant expression of the amplified gene in A431 epidermoid carcinoma cells. *Nature.* 309:418, 1984
9. Downward J, Yarden Y, Mayes E. Close similarity of epidermal growth factor receptor and v-*erb*-B oncogene protein sequences. *Nature.* 307:521, 1984
10. Ebina Y, Ellis L, Jarnagin K. The human insulin receptor cDNA: The structural basis for hormone-activated transmembrane signaling. *Cell.* 40:747, 1985
11. Czech MP. Signal transmission by the insulin-like growth factors. *Cell.* 59:235, 1989
12. Canman CE, Kastan MB. Three paths to stress relief. *Nature.* 384:213, 1996
13. Yamaguchi M, Rutledge LJ, Garbers DL. The primary structure of the rat guanylyl cylcase A/atrial natriuretic peptide receptor gene. *J Biol Chem.* 265:20414, 1990
14. Zhao Y, Nichols JE, Bulun SE, et al. Aromatase P450 gene expression in human adipose tissue: Role of a Jak/STAT pathway in regulation of the adipose-specific promoter. *J Biol Chem.* 270:16449, 1995
15. Nagata S. Apoptosis by death factor. *Cell.* 88:355, 1997
16. Sibley DR, Lefkowitz RJ. Molecular mechanisms of receptor desensitization using the β-adrenergic receptor-coupled adenylate cyclase system as a model. *Nature.* 317:124, 1985
17. Morohashi K, Honda S, Inomata Y, et al. A common *trans*-acting factor, Ad4-binding protein, to the promoters of steroidogenic P-450s. *J Biol Chem.* 267:17913, 1992
18. Parker KL, Schimmer BP. Transcriptional regulation of the adrenal steroidogenic enzymes. *Trends in Endocrinology and Metabolism.* 4:46, 1993
19. Muscatelli F, Strom TM, Walker AP, et al. Mutations in the DAX-1 gene give rise to both X-linked adrenal hypoplasia congenita and hypogonadotropic hypogonadism. *Nature.* 372:672, 1994
20. Green S, Chambon P. A superfamily of potentially oncogenic hormone receptors. *Nature.* 324:615, 1986
21. Weinberger C, Thompson CC, Ong ES. The c-*erb*-A gene encodes a thyroid hormone receptor. *Nature.* 324:641, 1986
22. Denner LA, Schrader WT, O'Malley BW, Weigel NL. Hormonal regulation and identification of chicken progesterone receptor phosphorylation sites. *J Biol Chem.* 265:16548, 1990
23. Forman BM, Samuels HH. Interactions among a subfamily of nuclear hormone receptors: The regulatory zipper model. *Mol Endocrinol.* 4:1293, 1990
24. Yang-Yen HF, Chambard JC, Sun YL. Transcriptional interference between c-Jun and the glucocorticoid receptor: Mutual inhibition of cDNA binding due to direct protein-protein-interaction. *Cell.* 62:1205, 1990
25. McInerney EM, Tsai MJ, O'Malley BW, Katzenellenbogen BS. Analysis of estrogen receptor transcriptional enhancement by a nuclear hormone receptor coactivator. *Proc Natl Acad Sci USA.* 93:10069, 1996
26. Laue LL, Shao-Ming W, Kudo M, et al. Compound heterozygous mutations of the luteinizing hormone receptor gene in leydig cell hypoplasia. *Mol Endocrinol.* 10:987, 1996
27. Kawate N, Kletter GB, Wilson BE, et al. Identification of constitutively activating mutation of the luteinising hormone receptor in a family with male limited gonadotrophin independent precocious puberty (testotoxicosis). *J Med Genet.* 32:553, 1995
28. Iiri T, Herzmark P, Nakamoto JM, et al. Rapid GDP release from Gs alpha in patients with gain and loss of endocrine function. *Nature.* 371:164, 1994

29. Smith EP, Boyd J, Frank GR, et al. Estrogen resistance caused by a mutation in the estrogen-receptor gene in a man. *N Engl J Med*. 331:1056, 1994

30. Stratakis CA, Karl M, Schulte HM, Chrousos GP. Glucocorticosteroid resistance in humans. Elucidation of the molecular mechanisms and implications for pathophysiology. *Ann NY Acad Sci*. 746:362, 1994

31. DeRoux N, Misrahi M, Braunder R, et al. Four families with loss of function mutations of the thyrotropin receptor. *J Clin Endocrinol Metab*. 81:4229, 1996

32. Leslie KK, Tasset DM, Horwitz KB. Functional analysis of a mutant estrogen receptor isolated from T47Dco breast cancer cells. *Am J Obstet Gynecol*. 166:1053, 1992

33. Deng HK, Liu R, Ellmeier W, et al. Identification of a major co-receptor for primary isolates of HIV-1. *Nature*. 381:661, 1996

Chapter 8

LABORATORY ASSESSMENT OF REPRODUCTIVE HORMONES

Larry R. Boots

HISTORICAL BACKGROUND

The early beginnings of reproductive physiology occurred almost simultaneously with the discovery of several hormones and their measurement in relation to various physiologic changes in the reproductive tract.[1,2] From the observation in 1849 that testes from a castrated rooster, when implanted on the intestines, prevented the occurrence of the usual effects of castration, reproductive physiology began to develop. In 1917 and 1922, the estrous cycles of guinea pigs and rodents, respectively, were described. These studies relied on changes in vaginal smears and in 1923 were the basis of the first bioassay in reproductive biology when vaginal cornification was observed to occur in response to the follicular hormone, estrone. Other bioassays were subsequently developed as progesterone and testosterone were isolated and purified in 1929. The discovery and isolation of luteinizing hormone (LH) (1941) and follicle-stimulating hormone (FSH) (1950) were also associated with development of bioassays for their measurement.

All of these procedures for assay of steroids and gonadotropins, after considerable technical skill and effort were expended, still produced highly variable results. Except for bioassays for human chorionic gonadotropin (hCG), few if any of these procedures had any clinical significance.

As more was learned of the chemistry of hormones, clinical assays were developed, but because of low secretion rates 24-hr urine collections were required. These procedures included the Porter–Silber and Zimmerman reactions for 17-ketosteroids, 17-ketogenic steroids, and 17-hydroxycorticosteroids. Each of these groups of excreted steroids were comprised of hormones from multiple sources, causing problems with interpretation of data.

These procedures were also relatively insensitive, required extraction and other manipulations, and were subject to nonspecific interference due to medications and the health status of the patient. Such tests were commonly used in the 1960s and 1970s, but should be totally replaced by more modern procedures.

The greatly improved sensitivity of immunoassays has allowed measurement of most hormones in serum. Consequently, urinary assays have largely disappeared from the laboratory. However, that is not to say that urinary assays gave inaccurate information. In fact, assay of a 24-hr urine sample probably provides the best estimate of the individual's hormone production. While there are many disadvantages to urinary procedures, measurement of new markers such as hCG β-subunit core fragment in pregnancy urine and the development of immunoassay procedures that measure steroid conjugates directly, without extraction, may breathe new life into urinary assay methodology.

THE PRESENT

The majority of hormone assays performed today involve the binding of either naturally occurring binding proteins or antibodies specific for individual hormones to the hormone being measured. Thus, the term "binding assays" (BAs), which include radioimmunoassay (RIA), enzyme immunoassay (EIA) or enzyme-linked immunosorbent assay (ELISA), immunoradiometric assay (IRMA), and competitive protein-binding assay (CPB), was coined. Yalow and Berson[3] and Ekins[4] are generally credited with development of the first BA procedures. Yalow and Berson described an insulin assay that used an antibody as the binder, while Ekins developed an assay for thyroxine using a naturally occurring binding protein, thyroxine-binding globulin. Since 1960, BAs have been developed for all hormones of interest in reproductive biology. They offer the advantages of being highly sensitive, specific, and precise, as well as having a short turnaround time in clinical settings. They are relatively inexpensive in terms of technician time and materials, but require expensive equipment to determine their end points. Of the BAs, radio- and non-radiolabeled assays are both common. There are trade-offs, however, when choosing one type of assay over the other. Most non-radiolabeled procedures are more expensive than radiolabeled assays and, while touted to be easier to perform, in reality require as much technical skill to perform accurately. As disposal of radiolabeled compounds continues to become more difficult and expensive, the non-radiolabeled assays will continue to become more popular. With increasing numbers of reproductive hormone assays becoming available on automated instruments, the use of radiolabeled assays will surely diminish. The most important feature of any assay, however, should be accuracy, and there seems to be little evidence to promote any one of these techniques over another.

FUTURE DEVELOPMENTS

Non-radiolabeled assays will continue to increase in popularity. As automation and advances in detection equipment continue, it will be easier to perform assays away from the laboratory or at least in situations where radiometric analysis is not possible, such as third-world countries or rural areas with poorly equipped laboratories. Terms such as fluoroimmunoassay, bioluminescence, chemiluminescence, liposomal electrochemical immunoassay, bioselective electrodes, and analytical amperometric sensors are common and show promise of the day when a probe may be available that can be placed in the serum sample and almost immediately determine multiple hormone levels. An amperometric technique has been described for hCG[5] that utilizes the catalytic activity of glucose oxidase coupled to a modified immunometric assay. Judging from the large number of applications of this technology outside the field of endocrinology, one can predict increased development of these procedures for hormone measurement.

It has always been a dream of many laboratorians to make the jump from measuring hormone levels in isolated blood samples to real-time evaluation. Several problems exist, including the requirement for exquisite sensitivity of the assay itself, for ultra-sensitive detection instrumentation and routine ability to work with very small volumes of blood. Many of these problems have been solved. In a recent publication, Cantor et al[6] de-

scribed a system utilizing amperometric sensors for near-continuous on-line monitoring of hormone secretion. They were able to detect an amperometric signaling molecule that corresponded closely to immunoactive LH profiles taken at 30-second intervals. This system enables continuous, on-line, real-time evaluation of cell and hormone dynamics.

The subject of serum versus urinary assay will probably be reconsidered. New BAs have been developed that do not require extraction and excessive manipulation of the urine sample. Assays for estrone glucuronide and pregnanediol glucuronide, for instance, are direct assays and in some situations may replace serum estradiol and progesterone assays.[7,8] Reliable results may be obtained from first morning urine collections, which will be more convenient to the patient.

More concern will appear over the relationship of BA data to bioactivity. This has been a recent topic of discussion.[9] With the development of sensitive in vitro bioassays, changes in the biologic potency of hormones over time and varying physiologic conditions have been observed.[10–14] More importantly, changes in the biologic (bioassay) to immunologic (BA) ratio of hormone activity (B/I ratio) have been reported.[15] These observations not only point out a shortcoming of BA studies but also that the endocrine system is even more complex than previously imagined in that glands appear to have the ability to secrete hormones with varying biologic potency. Examples include the increase in the B/I ratio of LH after acute gonadotropic-releasing hormone (GnRH) stimulation and during the physiological LH pulse. The B/I ratio of LH increases during puberty and in women after menopause. Androgens increase the B/I ratio, estrogens decrease it, and polycystic ovarian disease is associated with an increased B/I ratio of LH.

An area of great interest and one that will probably expand is the practical application of home diagnostic products. Glucose levels have been measured by diabetic patients for some time now. Home tests for urinary tract infections and sexually transmitted diseases are also available. More pertinent to reproductive biology are home tests for monitoring time of ovulation and detection of pregnancy.[16,17] These tests need to be used with caution and may not be applicable to all patient settings. Over-the-counter assays have the same requirements as any other laboratory test in terms of proper storage and handling of materials, attention to incubation times while performing the test, and the experience required to interpret the tests' end point. The latter of these problems may be subjective in situations where pregnancy detection is attempted too early or midcycle LH is on the shoulder rather than at its peak. The success of these procedures is dependent upon the patient's ability to obtain a reliable result. If the physician perceives "at-home tests" as being less reliable than laboratory procedures and routinely repeats them, then the patient has wasted time and money.

One last area of interest as the future of laboratory assays unfolds involves the increasingly complex role played by the laboratorian. In the past, the majority of laboratory directors have been responsible for the organization of the laboratory, quality control (QC) of assays, and reporting of the data. Interpretation of all patient data has been reserved solely for the physician. As statistical manipulation of data becomes more common, incorporating corrections for the influence of body weight, age, race, week of gestation, etc, the laboratorian is required to be even more knowledgeable of the relevant physiology and actually makes the interpretation of whether the data are normal or abnormal. The laboratory report may list the actual hormone level, but this in itself is meaningless to the physician. Only with the help of sophisticated computer analysis is the laboratorian able to assess whether a hormone value is normal or abnormal.

PRINCIPLES OF BINDING ASSAYS FOR HORMONE MEASUREMENT

The Basic Principle

All BA procedures are composed of basic reagents including the hormone (H) being measured; the antibody, binding protein, or receptor (B); the radiolabeled hormone (the hormone may be labeled with other nonradioactive substances) or tracer (H^*); and a means of separating bound from free H and H^*. Following the laws of mass action, the binder, B, is mixed with the hormone, H, to form the complex BH (Fig 8–1). A small or tracer quantity of the labeled hormone, H^*, is added and forms the complex BH^*. The quantity of B is always held constant so both H and H^* compete for the limited number of binding sites available on B. As the quantity of unknown hormone, H, increases, less H^* will complex with B. By separating bound (B) from free (F) H^*, a standard curve can be constructed from which the level of unknown hormone in serum or other medium can be estimated (Fig 8–2). The assay is the result of the following reactions:

$$H + B \overset{K_1}{\underset{K_2}{\rightleftharpoons}} HB$$

$$H^* + B \overset{K_3}{\underset{K_4}{\rightleftharpoons}} H^*B$$

The terms K_1 and K_3 are association rate constants while K_2 and K_4 are dissociation rate constants. Because H^* and B are kept constant in the assay, less H^*B complex forms as the total concentration of unknown hormone increases

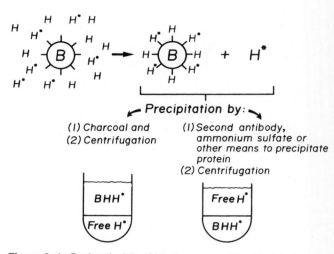

Figure 8–1. Basic principle of binding assays. The binding agent (*B*), which is either an antibody, binding protein, or receptor, complexes with hormone present in the sample being tested or with reference preparation that has been added (*H*) to form *BH* complexes. Simultaneously, or previously, tracer (*H**) is added. The precipitating reagent (antirabbit immunoglobulin [second antibody], charcoal, ammonium sulfate, etc) is then added to separate bound from unbound tracer and one of these is quantitated.

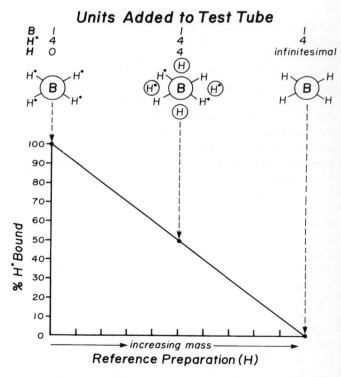

Figure 8–2. As the mass of *H* is increased in the test tubes of the standard curve or as it increases in the sample, the amount of *H** that can bind to the constant and limited number of binding sites on *B* decreases and a standard curve can be constructed.

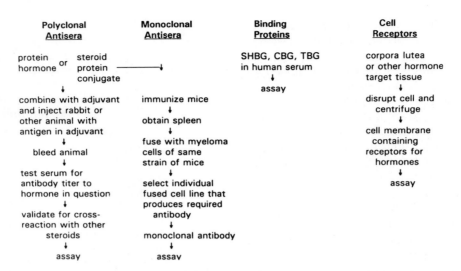

Figure 8–3. Production of the various binding agents for use in assays.

in the serum or urine sample. Extensive discussions of the mathematical analysis of BA systems are available in a number of publications.[18–20]

Binding Reagent

The binding reagent is the central component of the BA. It can be an antibody, a naturally occurring binding protein, or a cell receptor. The most common binding agent is the antibody. The typical immunization procedure[20] produces a polyclonal antiserum (Fig 8–3), ie, one that is likely to be made up of numerous antibodies, each capable of binding with different degrees of success to the hormone being measured or to other hormones. This causes problems of specificity and requires that each antiserum be carefully validated. The advantages of using antibodies as binding agents are many. They usually have high equilibrium constants that allow them to detect very small concentrations of hormone; they may be highly specific and able to distinguish between very similar molecules; and, in addition, they can offer great convenience. Usually, they can be used at high dilutions so that only a few milliliters of undiluted serum will provide binding reagent for many years. Antisera are also stable for many years when stored frozen. The major problems encountered with antisera are the difficulty in producing usable antisera. There is no guarantee that the few rabbits that have been immunized will produce an antibody of sufficient titer, specificity, or affinity to be of any use in an assay. The other problem that may be encountered is that an antibody may recognize an antigenic site on the hormone that is not related to biology activity.

Another method of obtaining antibodies is the production of monoclonal antibodies (MAb).[21] A brief procedure for the production of MAb has been published by Chard.[20] Briefly, a group of mice are immunized as in the production of polyclonal antisera. Antibody-producing cells (spleen cells) from these mice are fused in vitro with myeloma cells from the same strain of mice. The result is a cell line that produces antibody (Fig 8–3). One can then select individual fused cells that produce exactly the antibody desired. These cell lines can then produce antibody indefinitely. Advantages of MAb include production of highly specific antibodies more predictably and consistently than with polyclonal methods. Once a clone has been established, it can produce large quantities of antisera indefinitely. Disadvantages include the expense and sophistication of the facilities needed to produce MAb. It is also true that selection of highly specific antibodies is not always possible. There is no guarantee that the MAb product will be any better than the polyclonal product.

Naturally occurring binding proteins can also be used in BAs (Fig 8–3). The best known of these proteins are cortisol-binding globulin (CBG), sex hormone-binding globulin (SHBG), and thyroxine-binding globulin (TBG). The biggest disadvantage of these proteins in BAs is a poor degree of specificity. In the case of CBG, both corticosteroids and progesterone are bound; with SHBG, estrogens and androgens are bound; and TBG can bind thyroxine and triiodothyronine. Most assays that have utilized naturally occurring, circulating binding proteins have been replaced by immunoassays.

Cell receptors for hormones have been used as binding agents in BAs, but today few if any remain in existence (Fig 8–3). The obvious advantage of cell receptors as binding agents is that a biologically functional site of the hormone should be involved in the assay. This may be of special importance in light of the ongoing dialog over relevance of assay methodology to biologic activity. From a practical standpoint, receptor preparations are difficult to work with. Preparations of receptors are often unstable, a limited number of cell receptors are available, and specificity can still be a problem.

One final consideration of antibody production for use in BAs is the difference in dealing with peptides versus steroids as antigens (Fig 8–4). The development of antibodies for peptide hormone assays occurred first. Peptides are readily immunogenic in an unrelated species, thus the usual procedure of immunizing rabbits or guinea pigs with purified human peptide hormones such as LH, FSH, hCG, and prolactin. Immunoassays for steroid hormones were developed later than those for peptide hormones primarily because steroids are not naturally immunogenic. It was not long, however, before steroids were conjugated to large proteins and specific antisera were produced. Hemisuccinate, chlorocarbonate, or oxime derivatives were prepared and then linked to large, immunogenic proteins such as bovine serum albumin. The steroid protein conjugates are then used in immunization procedures. Antibodies have been produced to almost all steroids of interest. The methods have been reviewed in detail.[22–25]

The assessment of antiserum in the selection process for use in a BA is extremely critical to the development of a good assay. The three criteria generally used are antibody titer, affinity, and specificity. The titer of the antibody is loosely defined as the dilution of the antiserum that provides sufficient binding of labeled antigen and ensures optimal sensitivity in the assay (Fig 8–5). In practical terms, this means that the chosen dilution of antiserum will bind 25 to 50 percent of labeled antigen in the absence of unlabeled antigen.

Once a working titer or dilution has been established, the specificity of the antiserum for the hormone to be measured can be established. This is the most important of all criteria when assessing antisera. The ability of any potential cross-reacting hormone to interfere with binding is determined by the ability of excessive quantities of potentially contaminating hormones to interfere with the antiserum's ability to bind to the labeled hormone being assayed (Fig 8–6). Many antisera cross-react with multiple hormones, and unless they can be neutralized or the sample purified to remove the cross-reacting contaminants the antiserum is not useful in developing an assay.

The affinity of an antibody affects the sensitivity of an assay. Antibody affinity has been discussed[19] in theoretical detail, but for more practical purposes the affinity of the antibody is accepted and the antibody selected dependent upon the sensitivity required. Sensitivity is relevant in some assays but much less so in others.

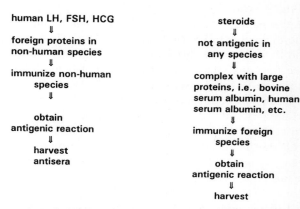

Figure 8–4. Steroids, made antigenic by conjugation with large proteins, can produce antigenic reactions similar to those of the protein hormones, resulting in the production of specific antisera suitable for use in BAs.

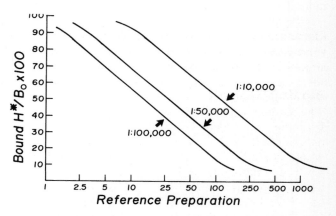

Figure 8–5. Example of how antisera dilution can affect assay sensitivity. Taking 90 percent binding as the minimal limit of detection, at a dilution of 1:10,000 12.5 U of reference preparation can be detected. At dilutions of 1:50,000 and 1:100,000, 3.1 and 1.6 U can be detected, respectively.

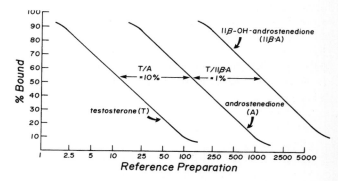

Figure 8–6. To test any antiserum for cross-reaction with other hormones, large quantities are added and tested against the same reference preparation, in this case testosterone. Because there would have to be 1500 U 11β-OH-androstenedione present to act like 15 U testosterone, at 50 percent binding, it cross-reacts only 1.0 percent.

Assay Tracers

As the name "tracer" suggests, these compounds allow one to trace or follow the reactions that occur in the BAs and determine the distribution between the bound and free fractions. Tracers are usually radiolabeled hormone in the RIA procedures but may also be labeled antibody in ELISA procedures (Fig 8–7). The most common tracers are ^{125}I and ^{3}H. Most steroids are still labeled internally with ^{3}H. These steroids are chemically identical with the unlabeled hormone but require more time to count accurately than ^{125}I and may reduce the sensitivity of the assay because of low specific activity. More commonly, ^{125}I is employed as the tracer in peptide, protein, and increasingly in steroid hormone assays. Because of high specific activity, counting times are reduced and assay sensitivity improved. The possible disadvantage is that the tracer hormone may react differently than unlabeled hormone in the assay. This will be discussed in more detail in a later section.

Nonisotopic tracers are becoming more common (Table 8–1). They are usually employed in assays that involve a solid phase to which the binding agent has been attached. The tracer is on another antibody. The primary advantage of these "sandwich" assays is the elimination of the separation step and radiation hazard because these

TABLE 8–1. EXAMPLES OF COMPOUNDS USED FOR NONRADIOLABELING OF TRACERS

Compound	Reaction
Horseradish peroxidase	Colorimetric
Alkaline phosphatase	Colorimetric
Glucose oxidase	Colorimetric
Malate dehydrogenase	Colorimetric
Fluorescein	Fluorescence
Rhodamine	Fluorescence
Umbelliferone	Fluorescence
Luciferase	Bioluminescence
Luminol	Chemiluminescence
Acridinium	Chemiluminescence
Europium	Time-resolved fluorescence

tracers are measured by their colorimetric, fluorescent, or luminescent properties. It should be pointed out that the actual radiation hazard with BAs can be easily overexaggerated. The amount of isotope in a typical assay would cause no significant radiation effect. By comparison, some substrates used in ELISA assays may present potential health risks themselves. The topics of both nonisotopic and isotopic tracers have been reviewed in detail elsewhere.[20]

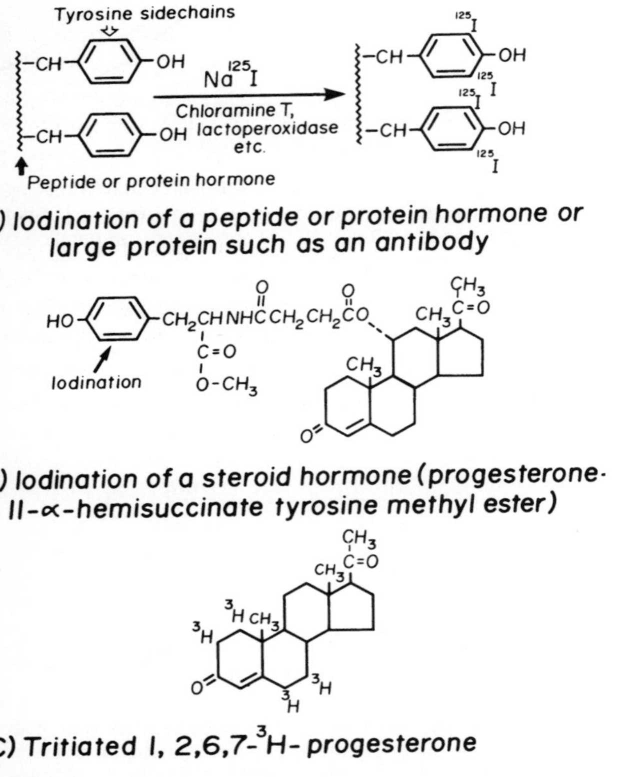

Reference Preparations

Of crucial importance to any assay is a supply of highly purified hormone for use as a reference standard and for labeling purposes. With steroid assays, this has not been a problem but the same has not been true for peptide and protein hormones. The World Health Organization (WHO) and the National Institutes of Health (NIH) have both maintained programs through which purified hormones can be obtained. However, supplies are limited and, as a result, partially purified materials must often be prepared by investigators or commercial vendors. These preparations are then calibrated against the WHO and NIH materials. Because of interlaboratory differences, the reported values from various sources often show considerable variability.

The subject of assay standardization and reference preparations in general has been reviewed innumerable times. To better comprehend the problems associated with reference materials, it is necessary to review some of the older articles and follow the development of such programs. For this purpose, the reader is referred to the literature.[26–29]

For practical purposes and to best utilize laboratory results, ignore variability in laboratory data as the result of calibration error or use of standards with widely disparate potencies but be aware of the reference laboratories' normal ranges. If samples are sent to several laboratories for analysis, there is no way to guarantee comparable or relevant data over time. By identifying the reference standard in each laboratory, published conversion factors can be ap-

(A) Iodination of a peptide or protein hormone or large protein such as an antibody

(B) Iodination of a steroid hormone (progesterone-11-α-hemisuccinate tyrosine methyl ester)

(C) Tritiated I, 2,6,7-^{3}H- progesterone

Figure 8–7. Examples of radiolabeled tracers commonly used in binding assays.

help in the diagnosis of hirsutism and androgen-excess syndromes. The role of testosterone that is loosely bound to albumin is unknown but may well represent additional bioactive steroid.[53–56]

Other Steroid Hormone Assays

Progesterone, 17-hydroxyprogesterone, dehydroepian-drosterone sulfate, androstenedione, and urinary assays for estrone glucuronide and pregnanediol glucuronide are also assayed routinely in reproductive biology clinical laboratories. These assays present no special problems.

QUALITY CONTROL

The primary purpose of any laboratory is to provide a reliable service. The following paragraphs discuss some of the ways this is done. The importance of thorough and constant monitoring of every assay should be obvious simply for the sake of providing accurate and reliable data, but as regulating agencies become increasingly involved through the Federal Clinical Laboratory Improvement Act of 1988 (CLIA '88), these monitoring requirements are rapidly becoming mandatory functions of everyday life in the laboratory. The following are both practical and reasonable ways to approach quality control and meet the regulatory requirements.

Most quality control programs emphasize the tracking of assay reliability by calculating CVs on control samples within and between each assay. Before even running the first assay, there are other requirements to be met and measured on a daily basis. Records must be maintained on all refrigerators and freezers used to store samples and reagents. Daily temperatures are recorded for these and all water baths used during assays. All pipettors should be calibrated quarterly and the accuracy of the rpm gauge confirmed every 6 mo for all centrifuges. All equipment used for actual assay measurement, ie, scintillation and gamma counters, spectrophotometers, and other automated equipment including tube and plate washers, must be calibrated on each day of use. These are minimal requirements for laboratory certification.

Accurate tracking of samples is important in providing a reliable laboratory service. Licensing agencies require a paper trail for every sample from entry into the laboratory to records of the assay performed to reporting the results. These records must be maintained on file for at least 2 yr.

There are three areas relative to actual assays that go into a comprehensive QC program. These involve, first, the design features of the assay itself, its validation, and recording of assay characteristics associated with the standard curve; second, internal QC samples are introduced into each assay and measures of reliability on individual sample results determined; third, participation in external QC programs are mandated by certifying agencies.

The validation of the assay itself has already been discussed. It is important that specificity has been determined and parallel dose–response curves demonstrated. Assuming the assay has been reliably validated (in light of reported performance of many commercially available assays, this is not a matter to be ignored), there are standard curve data that should be recorded on each assay to ensure proper performance.

By means of standard data reduction packages available in most laboratories, standard curve data are linearized by logit-log transformation. Values for the slope and intercept of the curve are available, as are values for 20, 50, and 80 percent displacement of the labeled tracer. Limits should be set for precision of data points on the standard curve (usually less than 10 percent CV) and the B_0, the value upon which the standard curve is based, should be determined and judged reliable. All these measures can then be plotted on Levey–Jennings graphs for easy inspection of day-to-day assay performance (Fig 8–10). The most informative of these characteristics is probably B_0. Widely variable B_0 values may indicate deterioration of the tracer or binding agent. High blanks or nonspecific binding values are also indicative of tracer problems.

It is commonplace to see commercial kits or protocols that limit the number of standard points in an assay or reduce the number of replicates. This makes no sense, for in return for a small savings in the cost of a few tubes, the ability to ensure production of a good standard curve may be lost. If anything, B_0 should be determined at least in duplicate (many laboratories will use three, four, or

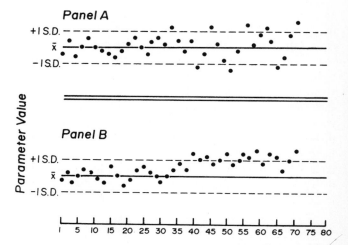

Figure 8–10. Levey–Jennings plot of a QC value (ie, slope of standard curve, B_0, or internal control sample) determined in multiple assays over time. **A.** Example of a loss in precision as judged by increased random error. **B.** Upward shift in values over time.

five tubes for B_0 determination), as should all standard points, of which four to six should be used. Two-site assays may be designed with a zero and a single calibrator only. While the argument can be made that with the high manufacturing standards of today's assays this is satisfactory, if that single point is out of control, the entire assay must be rejected. A few additional standard curve points might well have proven the single calibrator to be an outlier.

Internal QC samples are the mainstay of every QC program. Every assay should have at least two such samples, probably a high and a low pool. These pools can be obtained commercially or prepared from laboratory specimens. They are aliquoted and frozen so that fresh samples can be assayed daily. Enough pool should be available for at least 1 yr so that a long-term record can be established. Another excellent internal control sample is to include a sample from a previous assay.

All these data points can be plotted on Levey–Jennings graphs for visual inspection. Once a continuous record has been obtained for 10 or more assays, the mean and confidence limits can be calculated so that by simple visual inspection it can be determined if the QC samples fall within established cutoffs, usually ±2 SD from the mean. Another important QC monitoring scheme within each assay is the precision of each sample measurement. This can be done only if the sample was run at least in duplicate. Again, the CV can be calculated and it should be less than 10 percent. Many assays are run today as singlecates. While it may be possible to demonstrate that overall precision in the assay is excellent when singlecates are used (mean CV less than 10 percent), there is no way to know that an individual sample has actually been measured within established precision limits.

The final QC requirement is external. Licensing agencies require that each laboratory participate in a proficiency testing program. This is usually the College of American Pathologists Proficiency Program, but others may be acceptable to the licensing authorities depending upon the state in which you reside. Typically, a set of samples is sent quarterly for assay under normal laboratory conditions. Performance is graded by comparison to other laboratories using the same diagnostic kits when possible. According to the latest CLIA regulations, satisfactory performance on these samples is becoming increasingly stringent, and failure on a very limited number of proficiency samples could result in penalties, including closing of the laboratory and loss of certification.

CONCLUSION

The prevailing attitude toward the assay of hormones is of acceptance, compromise, and passivity. We accept the word of commercial vendors that their assays are thoroughly validated and capable of producing precise and accurate results. Yet, five estradiol diagnostic kits gave five unique answers and even disagreed when standards from one assay were run in another system. We compromise accuracy for economy by accepting the argument that a particular procedure is so repeatable that as few as one calibrator and a zero can constitute a reliable standard curve (it will at least be a straight line) and that samples can be run as singlecates in the assay. Indeed, if in any assay in which samples are run in duplicate even one sample is observed to have an unacceptable CV, then why should anything less be expected when samples are run as singlecates?

As with many things, the "old days" seem to have been simpler. No one can argue that the introduction of BAs heralded the greatest advances in reproductive biology seen yet. But, we also are now aware of the existence of pre- and prohormones, heterogeneity of hormones, and the ability of endocrine glands to secrete hormone from time to time with variable biologic activity but no change in binding characteristics observable in existing BAs. It is also probable that some forms of loosely bound circulating steroids may be bioactive, as well as the free forms.

Given this arena in which to work, the techniques available to laboratories are fundamentally inadequate. Specificity, sensitivity, and interpretation of assay results still remain major problems. The clinician needs to be as knowledgeable as possible of assay shortcomings to be better equipped to interpret patient data diagnostically. Communication between clinicians and laboratorians is becoming increasingly important as analytic techniques continue to develop.

The newest generation of automated instruments can pipette the sample, add all reagents, make appropriate dilutions, and print the result in a reportable form. But the fact still remains that the basis of most of these assays is still a binding agent, usually an antibody, and the assay requires all of the same care and upkeep pertinent to any other BA.

REFERENCES

1. Behrman HR. The history of hormone assays. In: Albertson BD, Haseltine FP, eds. *Non-Radiometric Assays: Technology and Application in Polypeptide and Steroid Hormone Detection.* New York, N.Y., Alan R. Liss, 1988: 1–14

2. Gold JJ. Endocrine laboratory procedures and available tests. In: Gold JJ, ed. *Gynecologic Endocrinology.* 2nd ed. Hagerstown, Md., Harper and Row, 1975: 647–667

3. Yalow RS, Berson SA. Assay of plasma insulin in human subjects by immunological methods. *Nature.* 184:1648, 1959

4. Ekins RP. The estimation of thyroxine in human plasma by an electrophoretic technique. *Clin Chem Acta.* 5:453, 1960

5. Robinson GA, Hill HAO, Philo RD, eds. Bioelectrochemical enzyme immunoassay of human choriogonadotropin with magnetic electrodes. *Clin Chem.* 31:1449, 1985

6. Cantor HC, Padmanabhan V, Favreau PA, Midgley AR Jr. Use of a newly designed microperfusion system with amperometric sensors for near-continuous on-line monitoring of hormone secretion. I. Correlation with the luteinizing hormone secretory response to gonadotropin-releasing hormone. *Endocrinology.* 137:2782, 1996

7. Baker TS. The OVEIA dual analyte assay—A new method for profiling the menstrual cycle. In: Albertson BD, Haseltine FP, eds. *Non-Radiometric Assays: Technology and Application in Polypeptide and Steroid Hormone Detection.* New York, N.Y., Alan R. Liss, 1988:101–118

8. Brown JB, Blackwell LF, Cox RI, et al. Chemical and homogeneous enzyme immunoassay methods for the measurement of estrogens and pregnanediol and their glucuronides in urine. In: Albertson BD, Haseltine FP, eds. *Non-Radiometric Assays: Technology and Application in Polypeptide and Steroid Hormone Detection.* New York, N.Y., Alan R. Liss, 1988:119–138

9. Chappel S. Editorial. Biological to immunological ratios: Reevaluation of a concept. *J Clin Endocrinol Metab.* 70:1494, 1990

10. Van Damme MP, Robertson DM, Diczfalusy E. An improved in vitro bioassay method for measuring luteinizing hormone (LH) activity using mouse Leydig cell preparations. *Acta Endocrinol.* 77:655, 1974

11. Ding YQ, Huhtaniemi I. Human serum LH inhibitor(s): Behaviour and contribution to the in vitro bioassay of LH using dispersed mouse Leydig cells. *Acta Endocrinol.* 121:46, 1989

12. Huhtaniemi IT, Dahl K, Rannikko S, Hsueh AJW. Serum bioactive and immunoreactive follicle-stimulating hormone in prostatic cancer patients during gonadotropin-releasing hormone agonist treatment and after orchidectomy. *J Clin Endocrinol Metab.* 66:308, 1988

13. Jia XC, Hseuh AJW. Granulosa cell aromatase bioassay for follicle stimulating hormone: Validation and application of the method. *Endocrinology.* 119:1570, 1986

14. Jia XC, Kessel B, Yen SSC, et al. Serum bioactive follicle-stimulating hormone during the human menstrual cycle and in hyper- and hypogonadotropic states: Application of a sensitive granulosa cell aromatase bioassay. *J Clin Endocrinol Metab.* 62:1243, 1986

15. Jaakkola T, Ding Y-Q, Kellokumpu-Lehtinen P, et al. The ratios of serum bioactive/immunoreactive luteinizing hormone and follicle-stimulating hormone in various clinical conditions with increased and decreased gonadotropin secretion: Reevaluation by a highly sensitive immunometric assay. *J Clin Endocrinol Metab.* 70:1496, 1990

16. Rebar RW. Practical applications of home diagnostic products: A symposium. *J Reprod Med.* 32(Suppl.), 1987

17. Bahar I. The development of over-the-counter (OTC) assays for pregnanediol-3-glucuronide and estrone-B, D-glucuronide. In: Albertson BD, Haseltine FP, eds. *Non-Radiometric Assays: Technology and Application in Polypeptide and Steroid Hormone Detection.* New York, N.Y., Alan R. Liss, 1988: 139–151

18. Ekins RP. General principles of hormone assay. In: Loraine JA, Bell ET, eds. *Hormone Assays and Their Clinical Application.* London, Churchill Livingstone, 1976: 1–72

19. Campfield LA. Mathematical analysis of competitive protein binding assays. In: Odell WD, Franchimont P, eds. *Principles of Competitive Protein-Binding Assays.* New York, N.Y., John Wiley & Sons, 1983: 125–148

20. Chard T. *An Introduction to Radioimmunoassay and Related Techniques.* New York, N.Y., Elsevier, 1987

21. Milstein C, Kohler G. Cell fusion and the derivation of cell lines producing specific antibody. In: Haber E, Krause RM, eds. *Antibodies in Human Diagnosis and Therapy.* New York, N.Y., Raven Press, 1977: 271

22. Erlanger BF, Borek F, Beiser SM, Lieberman S. Steroid–protein conjugates I. Preparation and characterization of conjugates of bovine serum albumin with testosterone and with cortisone. *J Biol Chem.* 228:713, 1959

23. Lieberman S, Erlanger BF, Beiser SM, Agate FJ. Aspects of steroid chemistry and metabolism. Steroid–protein conjugates: Their chemical, immunochemical and endocrinological properties. *Rec Progr Horm Res.* 15:165, 1959

24. Abraham GE, Grover PK. Covalent linkage of hormonal haptens to protein carriers for use in radioimmunoassay. In: Odell WD, Daughaday WH, eds. *Principles of Competitive Protein-Binding Assays.* Philadelphia, Pa., Lippincott, 1971: 134–140

25. Jaffe BM, Behrman HR. *Methods of Hormone Radioimmunoassay.* 2nd ed. New York, N.Y., Academic Press, 1979

26. Albert A, Rosemberg E, Ross GT, et al. Report of the national pituitary agency collaborative study on the radioimmunoassay of FSH and LH. *J Clin Endocrinol Metab.* 28:1214, 1968

27. Bangham DR, Berryman I, Burger H, et al. An international collaborative study of 69/104, a reference preparation of human pituitary FSH and LH. *J Clin Endocrinol Metab.* 36:647, 1973

28. Canfield RE, Ross GT. A new reference preparation of human chorionic gonadotrophin and its subunits. *Bull World Health Org.* 54:463, 1976

29. Bangham DR. Reference materials and standardization. In: Odell WD, Franchimont P, eds. *Principles of Competitive Protein-Binding Assays.* 2nd ed. New York, N.Y., John Wiley & Sons, 1983: 85–105

30. Aschheim S, Zondek B. Hypophysenvorderlapenhormon und ovarialhormon im harn von schwangeren. *Klin Wehschr.* 6:1322, 1927

31. Wide L, Gemzell CA. An immunological pregnancy test. *Acta Endocrinol.* 35:261, 1960

32. Tyrey L. Laboratory methods for the quantitation of human chorionic gonadotropin. In: Szulman AE, Buchsbaum JH, eds. *Gestational Trophoblastic Disease.* New York, N.Y., Springer-Verlag, 1987: 88–100

33. Midgley AR Jr. Radioimmunoasssay: A method for human chorionic gonadotropin and human luteinizing hormone. *Endocrinology.* 79:10, 1966

34. Vaitukaitis JL, Braunstein GD, Ross GT. A radioimmunoassay which specifically measures human chorionic gonadotropin in the presence of human luteinizing hormone. *Am J Obstet Gynecol.* 113:751, 1972

35. Storring PL, Bangham DR, Cotes PM, et al. The international Reference Preparation of human pituitary luteinizing hormone for immunoassay. *Acta Endocrinol.* 88:250, 1978

36. Storring PL, Zaidi AA, Mistry YG, et al. A comparison of preparations of highly purified human pituitary luteinizing hormone: Differences in the luteinizing hormone potencies as determined by in vivo bioassay and immunoassay. *Acta Endocrinol.* 101:339, 1982

37. Storring PL, Gaines Das RE. The International Standard for Pituitary FSH: Collaborative study of the standard and of four other purified human FSH preparations of differing molecular composition by bioassays, receptor assays and different immunoassay systems. *J Endocrinol.* 123:275, 1989

38. Garrett PE. The enigma of standardization for LH and FSH assays. *J Clin Immunoassay.* 12:18, 1989

39. Stadler U, Rovan E, Aulitzky W, et al. Bioassay for determination of human serum luteinizing hormone (LH): A routine clinical method. *Andrologia.* 21:580, 1989

40. Parker DC, Rossman LG, Vanderlaan EF. Sleep-related, nyctohemeral and briefly episodic variation in human plasma prolactin concentrations. *J Clin Endocrinol Metab.* 36:1119, 1973

41. Ehara Y, Siler T, Vandenberg G, et al. Circulating prolactin levels during the menstrual cycle: Episodic release and diurnal variation. *Am J Obstet Gynecol.* 117:962, 1973

42. Fujimoto VY, Clifton DK, Cohen NL, Soules MR. Variability of serum prolactin and progesterone levels in normal women: The relevance of single hormone measurements in the clinical setting. *Obstet Gynecol.* 76:71, 1990

43. Belgorosky A, Escobar ME, Rivarola MA. Validity of the calculation of non-sex hormone-binding globulin-bound estradiol from total testosterone, total estradiol and sex hormone-binding globulin concentrations in human serum. *J Steroid Biochem.* 28:429, 1987

44. Masters AM, Hahnel R. Investigation of sex-hormone binding globulin interference in direct radioimmunoassays for testosterone and estradiol. *Clin Chem.* 35:979, 1989

45. Thomas CMG, Van den Berg RJ, Segers MFG. Measurement of serum estradiol: Comparison of three "direct" radioimmunoassays and effects of organic solvent extraction. *Clin Chem.* 33:1946, 1987

46. Boots LR. Unpublished results.

47. Ismail AAA, Astley P, Cawood M, et al. Testosterone assays: Guidelines for the provision of a clinical biochemistry service. *Ann Clin Biochem.* 23:135, 1986

48. Wheeler MJ, Shaikh M, Jennings RD. An evaluation of 13 commercial kits for the measurement of testosterone in serum and plasma. *Ann Clin Biochem.* 23:303, 1986

49. Wheeler MF, Lowry C. Warning on serum testosterone measurement. *Lancet.* ii:514, 1987

50. Masters AM, Hahnel R. Investigation of sex-hormone binding globulin interference in direct radioimmunoassays for testosterone and estradiol. *Clin Chem.* 35:979, 1989

51. Pearlman WH. Measurement of testosterone binding sites. Karolinska Symposia on Research Methods in Reproductive Endocrinology, 2nd Symposium, Steroid Assay by Protein Binding, 1979, pp 225–238

52. Ekins R. Measurement of free hormones in blood. *Endocrine Rev.* 11:5, 1990

53. Manni A, Pardridge WM, Cefalu W, et al. Bioavailability of albumin-bound testosterone. *J Clin Endocrinol Metab.* 61:705, 1985

54. Cumming DC, Wall SR. Non-sex hormone-binding globulin-bound testosterone as a marker for hyperandrogenism. *J Clin Endocrinol Metab.* 61:873, 1985

55. Nankin HR, Calkins JH. Decreased bioavailable testosterone in aging normal and impotent men. *J Clin Endocrinol Metab.* 63:1418, 1986

56. Belgorosky A, Rivarola MA. Progressive increase in non-sex hormone-binding globulin-bound testosterone and estradiol from infancy to late prepuberty in girls. *J Clin Endocrinol Metab.* 67:234, 1988

Chapter 9

NEUROENDOCRINOLOGY OF REPRODUCTION

Richard E. Blackwell

In 1932, Hohlweg and Junkmann suggested that a sex center might exist in the brain that would regulate human reproduction.[1] Subsequently, in 1937 Harris electrically stimulated the median eminence of the brain and produced ovulation.[2] In addition, Westman and Jacobsohn in 1937 demonstrated that a section of the pituitary stalk blocked ovulation.[3] Markee et al in 1946 showed that direct stimulation of the pituitary gland failed to duplicate this response.[4] These studies strongly suggested that the brain produced some chemical or chemicals that were secreted into the hypothalamic portal system, traveled to the pituitary gland, and regulated the events of ovulation.

The hypothalamic portal system had been described by Popa and Fielding in 1930.[5] Houssay in 1935 showed that blood flowed from the brain to the pituitary and in 1950 Harris sectioned the hypothalamic portal vessels and produced target end organ atrophy.[6,7] It was not until 1955 that Guillemin and Rosenberg incubated fragments of the hypothalamus in vitro with pituitary tissue and were able to show an increased secretion of the hormone that stimulates the adrenal gland, corticotropin (ACTH).[8] It was postulated that ACTH secretion was controlled by a small polypeptide and it was thought that each of the classic pituitary hormones was controlled by one small protein, thus giving rise to the *one peptide, one hormone hypothesis*. This was confirmed for the reproductive hormones in 1971 and 1972 when Matsuo et al and Burgus et al isolated and analyzed the structure of the gonadotropin-releasing hormone (GnRH).[9,10] Concomitant with these studies, it was demonstrated by Bergland and Page that blood flowed not only from the hypothalamus to the pituitary gland but in a retrograde manner.[11] These studies opened the way for our current understanding of the neurochemical control of the reproductive cycle and the modern concept of hormonal feedback.

ANATOMY OF THE MEDIAN EMINENCE

The hypothalamus is phylogenetically old and found in mammals throughout evolution (Fig 9–1). It weighs approximately 10 g and is located at the base of the brain just above the junction of the optic nerves. The arcuate nucleus is one of the medial hypothalamic nuclei. It lies just above the median eminence and adjacent to the third ventricle. The median eminence, which is in close contact with the arcuate nucleus, is the final common pathway for the neurochemical control of anterior pituitary function. It receives peptidergic neurons that contain releasing and inhibiting factors. The median eminence delivers these hormones to hypothalamic pituitary portal capillaries and these neurochemicals are subsequently transmitted to the anterior pituitary gland, where they act on gonadotropes to release both luteinizing hormone (LH) and follicle-stimulating hormone (FSH).[12] As indicated previously, the portal concept has been expanded to encompass not only retrograde flow from pituitary to hypothalamus but inter- and intralobar flow as well (Fig 9–2). This would seem to suggest that different control mechanisms may be involved in regulating reproduction at the central axis, including short-short feedback loop (the regulation of a releasing factor by itself), short feedback loop (regulation of neurohumoral secretion by a target pituitary trophic hormone), paracrine regulation (the regulation of one cell secretion by an adjacent cell), and autocrine control (the self-regulation of a cell by one of its metabolic by-products). The final residence of the pituitary gonadotropic hormones LH and FSH is the gonadotrope.[13] This is a large cell (15 to 25 µm) that is distributed throughout the pituitary.[14] The pituitary is a bilobe gland made up of an anterior and posterior lobe with an intermediate lobe being distinct in some species. It is connected to the median eminence by the infundibular stalk and pars tuberalis. It

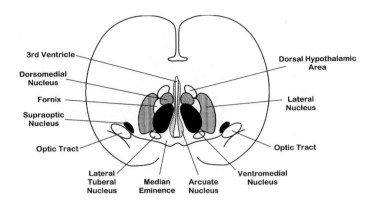

Figure 9–1. Anatomy of the hypothalamic area.

should be recalled that the anterior pituitary is derived from an enfolding of Rathke's pouch and is of epidermal ectoderm origin whereas the posterior pituitary comes from an evagination from the third ventricle and is of neuroectoderm origin. Therefore, communication from the anterior pituitary is primarily vascular whereas communication from brain to posterior pituitary is neural. This is reflected in the histology of these glands in that the anterior pituitary contains three primary cell types (classic) that are distinguished by H&E staining: acidophils, which are found to contain growth hormone, prolactin, and, at times, ACTH; basophils, which contain glycoprotein, LH, FSH, and TSH; and chromophobes, which do not stain.[15] The posterior pituitary histology is

composed primarily of nerve termini and glial tissue. Further examination of anterior pituitary cell types by electron microscopy demonstrates that each trophic hormone is contained in a specific cell type. These cells have different size granules that can be used for identification. However, cell morphology is a dynamic process; eg, lactotropes that contain prolactin can be found in granulated or degranulated states depending on the secretory activity and in fact can vary in size depending on secretory status.[16]

THE ARCUATE NUCLEUS AND THE SECRETION OF GnRH

In 1970, Knobil's group oophorectomized rhesus monkeys and carried out the first close-interval sequential measurement of LH levels. They found that LH was released in hourly pulses, termed circhoral oscillations.[17] Subsequently, it was determined that the arcuate nucleus was the pulse generator for these perturbations in LH secretion.[18,19] Simultaneous with these studies, other laboratories were attempting to isolate a hormone that would release LH and FSH. These were called, respectively, LH/RH by Shalley's group and LRF by Guillemin's group. In 1970, the decapeptide Pyro-Glu-His-Trp-Ser-Tyr-Gly-Leu-Arg-Pro-Gly-amide was isolated and subsequently named GnRH.[20–22] This hormone was shown to trigger ovulation in Innovar-treated rabbits and release LH and FSH in vivo and in vitro in all species tested.[23] Despite extensive investigation, a separate releasing factor for FSH has never been isolated. Therefore, it would appear that GnRH is the major neurochemical controller of gonadotropin secretion. Following isolation of GnRH, Knobil's group electrically destroyed the arcuate nucleus.[24] This produced a fall of LH and FSH to nondetectable levels. They carried out infusion studies, administering synthetic GnRH to rhesus monkeys in variable doses and at variable time

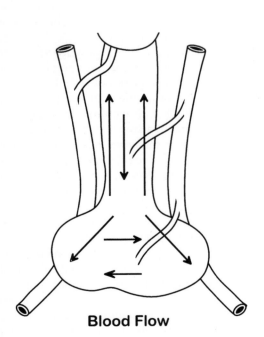

Blood Flow

Figure 9–2. Vascular flow pattern in the anterior pituitary gland and its stalk.

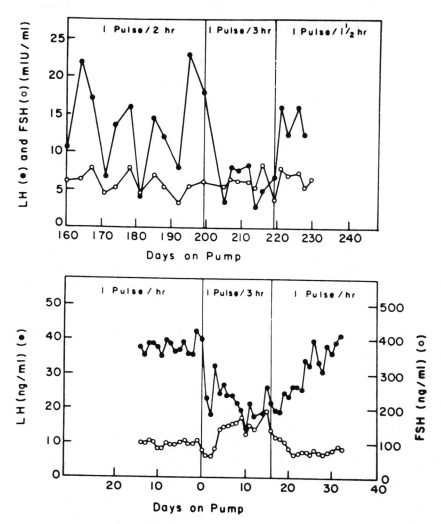

Figure 9–3. Upper panel: serum LH and FSH values during administration of GnRH in a woman with Kallmann's syndrome. Lower panel: changes in LH and FSH secretion with delivery of variable doses of GnRH to primates. *(Reproduced, with permission, from Seibel M, et al.* J Clin Endocrinol Metab. *61:575, 1985.)*

intervals (Fig 9–3). Continuous administration of GnRH resulted in a sustained suppression of gonadotropin level while infusing GnRH at one pulse per hour restored the normal secretory pattern and ultimately produced follicular growth in monkeys.

Simultaneous with these studies, investigations were being carried out in humans, measuring LH and FSH levels over short intervals.[25] FSH secretion was found to rise during the early follicular phase and fall until the time prior to ovulation, whereas LH remained suppressed and rose concomitantly with FSH in the preovulatory period. A change in magnitude of gonadotropin secretion at the time was interpreted as representing an increase in GnRH production. However, the work of Knobil and colleagues clearly demonstrated that administration of a fixed dose of GnRH at hourly intervals could result in the development of the follicle and sub-

sequent ovulation. However, variation of the dose of GnRH administered to primates causes a striking change in the LH/FSH ratio (Fig 9–4). Yen's group showed that exposure to estrogen resulted in increased LH/FSH secretion, not changes in GnRH.[26] After ovulation, LH pulse frequency slows to approximately one per 3-hr interval. Subsequently, with the availability of radioimmunoassays for GnRH, samples were taken from peripheral and portal blood, and it was found that for each hourly LH pulse there is a synchronous pulse of GnRH released. It appears that during the follicular phase of the cycle GnRH is released in a low-amplitude/high-frequency pattern whereas during the luteal phase it is released in a high-amplitude/low frequency pattern.[27] This mechanism has further been elucidated by Knobil and colleagues, who utilized the methods of Hayward to accurately place single tungsten electrodes in the region of

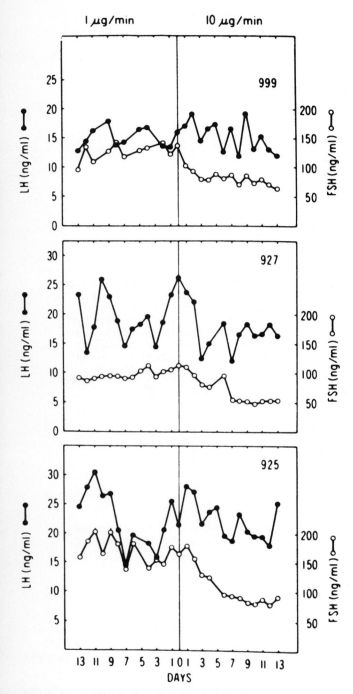

Figure 9–4. Alterations in LH/FSH ratio following an increase in the GnRH dose given intravenously to GnRH-deficient rhesus monkeys every 60 min. *(Reproduced, with permission, from Knobil E, et al. The neuroendocrine control of the menstrual cycle.* Rec Progress Horm Res. *36:53, 1980.)*

the arcuate nucleus of anesthetized rhesus monkeys[28] (Fig 9–5). There was an astonishing increase in multiunit electrical activity that was coupled with each LH pulse measured in peripheral circulation.[29,30]

CONTROL OF GnRH SECRETION

From previous discussions, it is apparent that the pulse frequency of GnRH release is controlled at the level of the arcuate nucleus. Initially, it was thought that a simple push/pull mechanism involving dopamine and norepinephrine controlled the pulse rhythm. Infusion of dopamine had been shown to acutely inhibit LH secretion and following release of inhibin, hypersecretion was demonstrated[31] (Fig 9–6). Interventricular infusion of norepinephrine, on the other hand, stimulates the release of LH in the rat[32] (Fig 9–7). Therefore, it might be envisioned that an interplay between dopamine and norepinephrine could regulate the firing rhythm of GnRH neurons, which would account for the change in pulse frequency of LH secretion seen in peripheral circulation.

The mechanism of the neural control of GnRH appears to be much more complex than a simple push/pull system (Fig 9–8). Neuroanatomic and pharmacologic data suggest that noradrenergic projections of GnRH cell bodies are of major importance. In addition, γ-aminobutyric acid (GABA) interneurons have been shown to express estrogen receptors and are in contact with these adrenergic neurons.[33] They also interface with GnRH dendrites, corticotropin-releasing factor (CRF), and oxytocin-containing projections from the paraventricular nucleus and β-endorphin-containing fibers from the arcuate nucleus.[34–36] Likewise, angiotensin II, neuropeptide Y, neurotensin, opiate peptides, and serotonin have been shown to impinge on GnRH neurons.[37–40] Their activity is a function of estrogen concentrations. These effects are somewhat peculiar in that they do not require a *direct genomic* site of action. For instance, in the absence of estrogen, GnRH nerve terminals in vitro have little capacity to respond to depolarizing stimuli. If castrated animals are pretreated with estradiol and killed and the perfusate contains estradiol concentrations in the nanomolar range, depolarizing capacity is restored. This appears to be a specific effect because inactive stereoisomers are ineffective in restoring the response.[41,42] Progesterone alone is unable to restore depolarizing capacity to GnRH release mechanisms in the absence of estradiol; however, the addition of estrogens to progesterones can modulate the amplitude of the depolarizing-induced response. This may in part account for the synergistic effect of estrogen/progesterone on triggering the LH surge at midcycle.[43]

The mechanism by which dopamine influences GnRH secretion is somewhat different. The tuberoinfundibular track arises within the medial basal hypothalamus and sends projections into the median eminence. These tracks are different from those involved in the synthesis of serotonin and norepinephrine, which are produced in the mesencephalon and lower brain stem. Axons for amines merge into the median forebrain bundle and terminate in the hypothalamus.

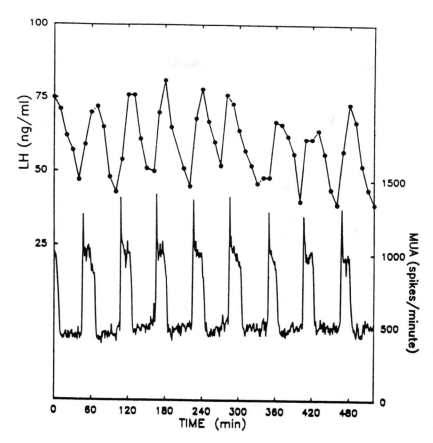

Figure 9–5. GnRH pulse-generator activity monitored by telemetry during the menstrual cycle of a rhesus monkey. *(Reproduced, with permission, from Knobil E. Electrophysiological approaches to the hypothalamic GnRH pulse generator. In: Yen SSC, Vale WW, eds. Neuroendocrine Regulation of Reproduction. Norwell, Mass., Serono Symposia, 1990: 4.)*

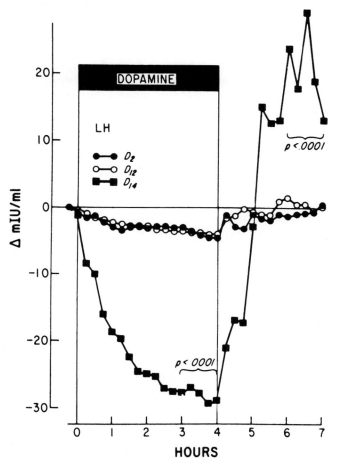

Figure 9–6. Effect of dopamine infusion on LH levels in women. *(Reproduced, with permission, from Judd S, Rakoff J, Yen S, 1978: 494.[31])*

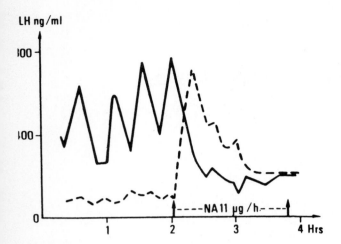

Figure 9–7. Effect of interventricular infusion of noradrenalin on plasma levels in oophorectomized (solid lines) and castrated female rats treated with estradiol (broken lines). *(Reproduced, with permission, from Gallo RV, Drouva SV, 1979: 149.[32])*

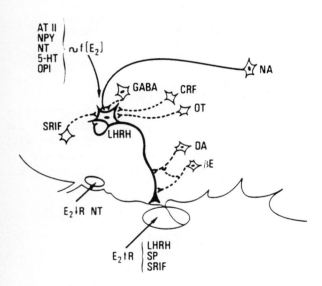

Figure 9–8. Interplay between hypothalamic hormones and sex steroids in the control of neuroendocrine reproductive functions. *(Reproduced, with permission, from Kordon C, Drouva SV. In: Yen SSC, Vale WW, eds. Neuroendocrine Regulation of Reproduction. Norwell, Mass., Serono Symposia: 1990.)*

ENDOGENOUS OPIOID PEPTIDES AND GnRH CONTROL

Opiates are derived from three precursors: pro-opiomelanocortin (POMC), source of the endorphins; proenkephalin-A, source of the enkephalins; and proenkephalin-B (prodynorphin), source of the dynorphins[44]

(Fig 9–9). POMC is synthesized in the anterior and intermediate lobes of the pituitary, the hypothalamus, brain, sympathetic nervous system, placenta, gonads, gastrointestinal tract, and pulmonary system. Under the control of the CRF, POMC is metabolized into ACTH intermediate and β-lipotropin.[45] Subsequently, the ACTH intermediate is metabolized into a 16-K fragment and ACTH, which is composed of 39 amino acids. This is further metabolized into α-MSH, which consists of the first 13 amino acids. β-Lipotropin is subsequently metabolized into β-melanocyte-stimulating hormone (β-MSH), enkephalin, and α, β, and γ endorphins. β-Endorphin is composed of amino acids 61 to 91 and α-endorphin amino acids 61 to 76. β-Endorphin is the major product of POMC metabolism. High levels are found in the arcuate nucleus and medial ventral nucleus. The endorphins serve a wide range of functions including the regulation of temperature, cardiovascular and respiratory system, pain perception, mood, and reproduction. Sex steroids seem to be responsible for POMC gene expression in the hypothalamus; the opioid peptide must act through receptors including μ, κ, δ, ε, and ς.[46] Endorphins act primarily through μ, κ, and ε receptors. Naloxone, a nonspecific receptor antagonist, has been used to study opioid effects in reproduction.[47] Endogenous opiates seem to inhibit GnRH release.[48] LH pulse frequency is directly related to endorphin concentrations, and as endorphin levels rise, LH pulse frequency decreases. Opioid tone is directly linked to estradiol levels, and progesterone seems to have a synergistic effect on this system.[49] Endogenous endorphin levels rise throughout the menstrual cycle and are highest during the late luteal phase. Treatment of women with the opioid antagonist naloxone will increase both the frequency and amplitude of LH pulses in the late luteal phase.[50] Therefore, the endorphins must be added to the groups of transmitters, modulators, and hormones that modify GnRH secretion.

CATECHOL ESTROGENS AND THE REGULATION OF GnRH

Catechol estrogens represent hybrids that contain catechol and estrogen faces (Fig 9–l0). High concentrations of catechol-O-methyltransferase, which catalyzes the reaction norepinephrine to 2-methoxynorepinephrine and estradiol to methoxyestradiol, are located in the hypothalamus. Catechol estrogens have the capacity to bind to either catechol- or estrogen-like receptors. Catechol estrogens inhibit tyrosine hydroxylase, which regulates catecholamine synthesis, and can compete for binding sites on catechol-O-methyltransferase, which regulates both catecholamine and estrogen metabolism.[51] It is appealing

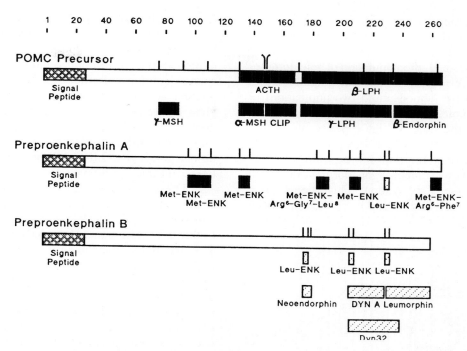

Figure 9–9. Opiate precursors and their metabolism. *(Courtesy of Dr. James Liu.)*

to speculate that this family of compounds might regulate GnRH release. To date, studies in humans have failed to elicit meaningful biologic effects when 2-hydroxyestrone or 2-hydroxyestradiol is administered. Although they function as weak estrogens, this family of compounds is highly unstable and rapidly clears from circulation.

Action of GnRH on the Pituitary

The pituitary contains a heterogeneous population of gonadotropes, some of which contain LH, others FSH, and others both gonadotropins[52] (Fig 9–11). It has been demonstrated that FSH is secreted by primitive gonadotropes prior to the development of the hypothalamic

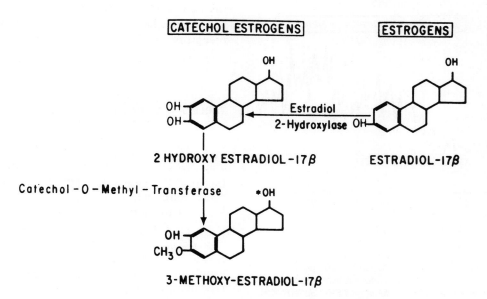

Figure 9–10. Structure of catechol estrogens, their relationships to estrogens, and metabolism.

portal system. Further, in vitro pituitaries release only FSH when treated with GnRH. LH appears only after the establishment of the hypothalamic portal system in vivo.

GnRH interacts with the population of gonadotropes through cell surface receptors. Autoradiographic studies of various tissue have demonstrated two populations of GnRH receptors. One appears to be a high-affinity/low-capacity receptor, the other a high-capacity/low-affinity receptor.[53] GnRH controls the receptor population through autoregulation. Intermittent exposure of a gonadotrope to GnRH will enhance gonadotropin release in response to subsequent stimulation. This phenomenon has been demonstrated in vitro and in vivo and has been called self-priming[54] (Fig 9–11). Conversely, the pituitary

can be desensitized to GnRH by delivery of the molecule to gonadotropes in a chronic or continuous manner. This has been called downregulation and was first demonstrated by Knobil's group, who showed that changing from pulsatile to continuous infusion suppressed gonadotropin levels. Following resumption of pulsatile secretion of GnRH, gonadotropin levels rose to normal 24. Therefore, by altering the frequency and amplitude of GnRH administration, one can either up- or downregulate the GnRH receptor. These findings have been confirmed in humans.[55]

These findings have led to the design of a family of analogs of GnRH that can be used to either downregulate (agonist) or block (antagonist) GnRH receptors (Table 9–1). These molecules have been modified at the 2, 3, and 10 positions to alter their receptor affinity and metabolic clearance rate. They can be used to produce hypogonadotropism and achieve a state of selected hypophysectomy or gonadectomy. It is of interest that antagonists and agonists behave differently in terms of gonadotropin secretion. When gonadotropes are treated with antagonists, native LH and FSH production, as well as α-chain, drops into the hypogonadotropic range.[56] However, when one treats patients with GnRH agonists, α-chain production increases while there is a fall in native gonadotropins, suggesting that while antagonists may work through a classic competitive inhibition mechanism, agonists, while occupying the receptor, do not inactivate it, and the effect of agonists may be at a postreceptor site[57] (Fig 9–12). Originally, it was felt that once receptors were occupied with GnRH analogs they were internalized. Although internalization of receptors occurs with certain molecules such as low-density lipoprotein (LDL) cholesterol, this may not be the case with GnRH analogs. If internalization occurs, perhaps this happens to only the high-affinity/low-capacity receptors.

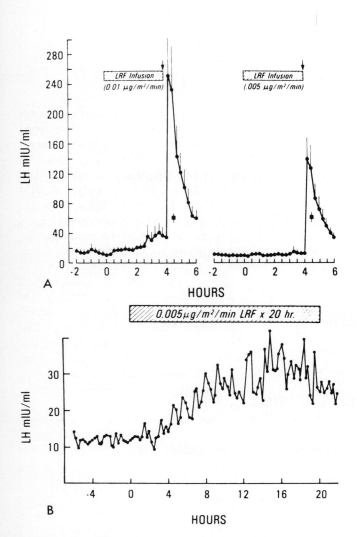

Figure 9–11. Upper panel: Self-timing effect of GnRH. Lower panel: Enhanced LH in response to an infusion of 0.005 µg/M² per minute in the early follicular phase. *(Reproduced, with permission, from Yen SSC. The human menstrual cycle. In: Yen SSC, Jaffe R, eds. Reproductive Endocrinology, Physiology, Pathology and Clinical Management, 2nd ed. Philadelphia, Pa., W. B. Saunders, 1986: 225.)*

TABLE 9–1. COMMERCIALLY AVAILABLE GnRH ANALOGS

Compound	Name	Usual Route of Admin-istration	Dose (mg)	Potency
D-Leu⁶, Pro⁹-HNE	Leuprolide	SC, IM	1.5–1 3.75	15
D-Ser(Bu)⁶, Pro⁹-NHEt	Buserelin	SC, IN	0.2 0.9–1 .2	100
D-His(bz)⁶, Pro⁹-NHEt	Histrelin	SC	0.1	100
D-Trp⁶	Tryptolerin	In polymer	2.4	100
D-[Nal(2)⁶]	Nafarelin	IN	0.4–0.8	200
D-Ser(tBu)⁶, Aza-Gly¹⁰	Goserelin	SC implant	3.6	230

Abbreviations: SC, subcutaneous; IM, intramuscular; IN, intranasal.

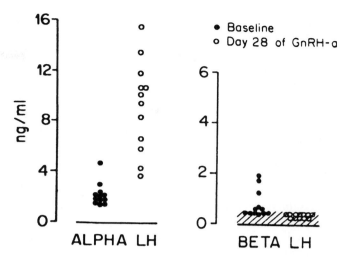

Figure 9–12. Stimulation of LH fragments with reduced bioactivity following GnRH agonist administration in women. *(Reproduced, with permission, from Meldrum DR, et al, 1984: 755.[57])*

One of the factors modulating GnRH receptor populations is estradiol. Numbers of receptors, but not affinity, have been shown to change throughout the estrous cycle in rats. Gonadectomy results in a progressive increase in LH and FSH secretion accompanied by doubling of GnRH receptors in the pituitary within 10 days. The response is blocked by either treatment with a GnRH antagonist, hypothalamic lesion, or sex steroid administration.[58] The action of estrogen may occur at the level of the hypothalamus by altering GnRH secretion; however, sex steroids may have the ability to alter the postreceptor action of GnRH.

EFFECT OF GnRH ON GONADOTROPES

Once GnRH binds to its receptor, many postreceptor events occur that serve as second messages. GnRH action is clearly mediated through a calcium/calmodulin mechanism. This has been demonstrated by the ability of chelating agents such as ethylenediaminetetra-acetic acid (EDTA) to block GnRH-stimulated LH release.[59] The process can be reversed by the addition of calcium chloride.[60] Calcium channel blockers such as verapamil have also been observed to inhibit GnRH-stimulated LH release in vivo and in vitro.[61] Further, agents that increase intercellular calcium levels stimulate LH release without GnRH receptor occupation. Ionophores (ie, compounds that create calcium-specific channels in cell membranes) A23187, X537A, or inomycin stimulate LH release.[62] The effects of ionophores can be blocked by incubation with EGTA (ethylene glycol tetra-acetic acid) and other chelating agents. Likewise, when one incubates liposomes containing calcium or other ions with

pituitary cells, calcium-containing liposomes increase LH secretion whereas other ions do not.[63] These types of studies plus those with calcium ionophores demonstrate the ability of calcium to stimulate LH release in the absence of receptor occupation. Intercellular calcium fluctuations can be measured in response to GnRH using Quin-II, a fluorescent analog of EGTA. Once inside the cell, the methylester form is cleaved and Quin-II binds to calcium, causing a shift in the wavelength of fluorescent emission. Using this technique, a rise in intercellular calcium concentration in gonadotropes will occur within 10 sec following GnRH or agonist treatment.[64] GnRH antagonists, on the other hand, do not provoke an elevation in intercellular calcium. Therefore, it appears that in response to GnRH receptor occupation, mobilization of both intra- and extracellular calcium occurs, resulting in an increase in intracellular calcium levels. Calcium therefore appears to fulfill the requirement of the second messenger for GnRH-stimulating gonadotropin release.

Calmodulin is also involved in the regulation of GnRH-stimulated LH release. Calmodulin is a calcium binder that regulates the activity of various molecules including diesterases, protein kinases, and cytoskeletal proteins. It regulates calcium concentrations by redistribution of the ion from the cytosol to the plasma membrane. This binding occurs in response to GnRH treatment and has been documented by radioimmunoassay.[65] Calmodulin localizes to "GnRH patches" following analog treatment.[66] The activity of calmodulin is inhibited by drugs such as pimozide and chlorpromazine. Agents such as these inhibit LH release stimulated by GnRH or calcium ionophores.[67] Gonadotropes also contain a family of at least five proteins that are involved in the binding of calmodulin.[68] The molecular weights range from 52,000 to 205,000. The presence of EGTA at 1 mmol/L blocks the binding of calmodulin to these proteins. Calcium antagonists such as pimozide also block binding.

Inositol phosphal lipids are linked biologic systems that utilize calcium as a second messenger.[69] GnRH has been shown to increase the rate of conversion of phosphatidic acid to phosphatidylinositol.[70] Further, GnRH stimulates the incorporation of P_{32} into phosphatidic acid and phosphatidylinositol. Calcium-independent phospholipase-C-hydrolysis has been observed in the gonadotrope. This results in the production of inositol l,4,5-triphosphate (IP_3) and diacylglycerol (DAG). IP_3 stimulates the release of calcium stored in nonmitochondrial sites, and DAG can activate protein kinase by altering calcium affinity to the enzyme.[71] The binding of GnRH or an agonist to receptors results in increased production of IP_3s; removal of the agonist from the receptor results in a decreased IP production, and this response can be blocked by the presence of a GnRH antagonist. This would suggest that phosphoinositides break down to DAGs and IP_3s during GnRH-stimulated LH release.[72]

As mentioned earlier, protein kinase C (PKC) activity is increased by the presence of DAG. PKC has been shown to be involved in GnRH receptor upregulation, and GnRH has been shown to activate PKC through the production of DAG. Compounds such as synthetic DAG and phorbol esters can increase LH release from pituitary cell cultures.[73] This action appears to be relatively insensitive to the removal of extracellular calcium by chelation or blockade of calcium channels or inhibition of calmodulin. Thus, the activation of PKC may be independent of calcium. This might suggest that PKC's action occurs subsequent to calcium mobilization or PKC may act by a mechanism different from GnRH. This assumption is favored because PKC inhibitors will suppress phorbol ester-stimulated LH release but not GnRH-stimulated release in two different model systems.

Pituitary Secretions

The glycoproteins LH, FSH, human chorionic gonadotropin (hCG), and thyroid-stimulating hormone (TSH) are composed of α- and β-subunits. The α-subunit is the same for all these glycoproteins, with the β-subunit being specific for each hormone. Therefore, it is responsible for the specificity of biologic effects, and it appears that the concentration of the beta-subunit mRNA is the rate-limiting step in the synthesis of glycoproteins.[74] For instance, it has been shown that GnRH is able to stimulate an increase in LH and β-mRNA concentrations and regulate LH biosynthesis. In addition to regulating biosynthesis, it also stimulates LH release. It is of interest that at low concentrations of GnRH (<1 nmol/L), LH β-mRNA levels are stimulated whereas at higher con-

centrations (>10 ng/ml) a decrease in the expression of LH β-mRNA occurs. Gonadectomy and steroid replacement produce differential changes in subunit mRNA expression in the rat model. Gonadotropin subunit mRNAs are increased at times when LH and FSH secretion is basal, suggesting that gonadotropin secretion and subunit gene expression may be differentially regulated.[75] It should be noted that both the amplitude and frequency of pulsatile GnRH secretion can modify subunit mRNA concentrations and both LH and FSH secretion.[76] This would imply that the pattern of GnRH secretion is responsible for the differential regulation of a gonadotropin subunit expression. Other factors can modify GnRH gene expression. As an example, the GnRH gene contains glucocorticoid regulatory elements, the activation of which in states of hyperadrenalism may be responsible for a menstrual disturbance.[77]

The inhibins and activins, two related gonadal proteins, are found in nearly all FSH- and LH-containing gonadotropes.[78] Biologically active inhibin suppresses FSH release and is a heterodimer consisting of an α-subunit and one or two distinct β-subunits (β-A or β-B). Activin molecules, which stimulate FSH secretion, are a β-dimer (B^A-$B^A$$B^B$-$B^B$). mRNA encoding for each of the inhibin activin subunits has been shown to be expressed in the number of extragonadal tissues including the pituitary and brain.[79] α- and β-B immunoreactivities have been localized to the cytoplasm of gonadotropes. No other cell type displays α- or β-B immunoreactivities; however, β-A subunit is found in nuclei ubiquitously distributed throughout the anterior, intermediate, and posterior lobes. The intensity of α- and β-B subunit staining varies throughout the estrous cycle of the rat. The number and intensity of anterior pituitary cells stained is highest during proestrous and lowest during estrous. Gonadectomy increases the size and number of cells that are fluorescently stained for α- and β-B polypeptides and for FSH and LH as well. Replacement therapy with estradiol benzoate prevents the oophorectomy-induced increases in staining and message levels. The role of activins and inhibin proteins in the pituitary remains to be determined. The gonads supply the vast majority of peripherally circulating inhibins; therefore, the pituitary contributes little to the circulating pool. However, inhibin and activin molecules produced in the pituitary could function as paracrine or autocrine regulators of gonadotropin secretion.

BIOSYNTHESIS AND STORAGE OF GONADOTROPINS

Cytochemistry has demonstrated that LH and FSH are found in single gonadotropes. Other studies have shown that pure FSH- or LH-secreting lines of gonadotropes could be cloned. Gonadotropes are angular cells found throughout the anterior pituitary and contain granules from 275 to 375 nm. The content of LH measured after sudden death in women has shown a decrease in the early follicular phase with a gradual rise at the time of ovulation.[80] After ovulation there is a fall in gonadotropin content and a subsequent rise at the beginning of the next cycle.

Infusion of GnRH in hypogonadotropic men and women shows an initial LH peak at 30 min, followed by a secondary rise at 90 min that continues up to 4 hr. The size of the second peak is augmented by the presence of sex steroids, and these observations suggest the existence of two pools of gonadotropins, one preformed that may be rapidly released, and the second said to exist in "storage."[81] It has been suggested that the earlier released pool might represent the effect of GnRH on the recruitment of granules in the proximity of the gonadotrope membrane. This is compatible with the fact that the release of LH in response to GnRH does not require protein synthesis. The second pool may be prestored or represent hormone synthesis. The size of the reserve pool varies with the cycle and with steroidal exposure, which would be compared with the postmortem hormonal findings.

The biosynthesis of gonadotropins occurs on the ribosome; subsequently, the proteins enter the posttranslational phase. The addition of sugars and transfer of proteins to correct intracellular destinations is completed in Golgi's stacks. These stacks comprise a series of flat and saccular membranous compartments and encompass four histological and functionally distinct regions: *cis-*, medial, *trans-*, and *trans-*Golgi network (TGN). The *cis* network is proximal to the translational elements of the endoplasmic reticulum whereas the TGN is most distal. It has been suggested that proteins are transferred in vesicles between compartments that are not contiguous. It is in the Golgi apparatus that the N-link carbohydrate cores are further modified. Multiple glycosidases digest the high mannose peripheral sugars in the N-link carbohydrate cores. Subsequent addition of distal or terminal sugars occurs by way of glucosyltransferase. The process of carbohydrate maturation occurs in the different Golgi compartments; polypeptides are delivered to their appropriate targets in the *trans-*Golgi, and it is in this area that secretory granules and vesicles are formed.

It is known that α-chain biosynthesis occurs more actively in the pituitary than does β.[82] It is suggested that the concentration of free β-subunit is the rate-limiting factor in the biosynthesis of LH and FSH. A possible mechanism for the union of α- and β-chain may be extrapolated from the choriocarcinoma cell in which α-subunit is synthesized in a ratio of 5:10. αβ-Diamers rapidly form prior to removal of the N-linked high-mannose oligosaccharide.[83] Glycosylation is completed prior to secretion of the whole molecule. The gonadotrope would seem to regulate its biologic output by altering either α- or β-chain synthesis or the coupling process or by reduction of glycosylation, which would increase metabolic clearance.

RECEPTOR PHYSIOLOGY AND NEW ANATOMIC CORRELATIONS

Recently, the human GnRH receptor has been cloned, sequenced, and its expression investigated.[84] The cDNA encodes a protein with a transmembrane topology similar with that of other G-protein coupled, 7-transmembrane receptors. Binding studies of cloned receptors show high affinity and properties similar to native pituitary GnRH receptor. Northern blotting and reverse transcriptase/PCR analysis showed that its messenger RNA is expressed in the pituitary, ovaries, testes, breasts, and prostate, but not in the liver and spleen. The availability of this human GnRH receptor allows comparison with animal models such as the rat, which has shown differences in molecular size by up to 4 kd. This results in differences of a binding affinity for some GnRH antagonists and sensitivity toward monovalent and diavalent cations.

Further, receptors have been isolated in the pituitary and hypothalamus that function in growth hormone release.[85] Secretion of growth hormone is controlled by two hypothalamic hormones: growth hormone-releasing hormone and somatostatin, which function in a push/pull relationship. The synthetic hexapeptide GHRP-6 (HIS-D-TRP-ALA-TRP-D-PHE-/-NH2) appears to stimulate growth hormone release by a pathway that is distinct from growth hormone-releasing hormone, implying the presence of a third receptor.[86] Growth hormone-releasing hormone, a natural 44-amino acid protein isolated from the hypothalamus, does not compete with GHRP-6 for its receptor, nor does the hexapeptide seem to compete with binding for somatostatin receptors. Growth hormone seems to be directly involved in ovulatory regulation, and its releasing hormone, GHRF, given in amenorrheic conditions to patients with lower body mass index, induces a higher response in controlled subjects. This implies a disregulation of growth hormone as well as IgF-1 in weight loss-related amenorrheic conditions.[87]

Other growth-promoting agents, most notably transforming growth factor alpha (TGF-α), a member of the epidermal growth factor family, have been shown to be involved in the developmental regulation of hypothalamic LH/RH release. Both TGF-α and epidermal growth factor (EGF) stimulate LH/RH release, although they do not appear to act directly on LH/RH neurons, as no receptors for these factors have been detected on these cells, at least in vitro. It appears that TGF brings about FSH release by acting through a glial intermediary, and recently hypothalamic astrocytes have been found to respond to TGF-α with the secretion of a neuroactive substance that stimulates the release of LH/RH (GnRH).[88] Another factor that appears to be secreted by the astrocytes is PG2, as immunoneutralization of this molecule appears to block the response. However, other factors yet to be defined appear to be involved in the control.

Nerve growth factors (NGF) belong to a family of protein molecules that are required for the survival and development of neuronal populations, both in the central and peripheral nervous systems. Originally thought to be restricted to the nervous system, NGF molecules appear to have non-neural effects, most notably on the immune and endocrine systems. NGF molecules act through tyrosine kinase receptors (TRK-A), with the induction of the release of inflammatory mediators from mast cells, promotion of differentiation of specific granulocytes, and modulating immune responses by stimulating the growth and differentiation of both B and T lymphocytes. In the endocrine system, NGF has been shown to affect the differentiation of hormone-secreting cells of the pancreas and pituitary mammotropes. Recently, Ojeda's group has found that nerve growth factors participate in the ovulatory cascade by inhibiting gap junctional communications between thecal cells.[89] The sites of interaction appear to be universal as a 13.1-kd protein, cystine-rich neurotropic factor (CRNF), was recently purified from the invertebrate cephalopod mollusk *Lymnaea stagnalis*. This factor interacts with a P75 neurotropin receptor.[90]

Neuroanatomy of reproduction appears to be a dynamic process as Naftolin's group[91] has demonstrated synaptic remodeling in the arcuate nucleus during the estrous cycle. His group demonstrated that this is induced by estrogen and precedes the preovulatory gonadotropin surge in female rats. These types of correlates might well apply to humans, as it has been demonstrated that gonadotropin-releasing hormone gene expression is increased in the medial basal hypothalamus of postmenopausal women using hybridization histochemistry.[92] Further, the expression of γ-amino butyric acid and gonadotropin-releasing hormone has been investigated during neural migration through the olfactory system. It is suggested that GABA is transiently expressed and may directly influence GnRH neural migration and development.[93] This is significant as cases of Kallmann's syndrome, a disorder characterized by anosmia secondary to olfactory bulb dysgenesis and isolated hypogonadotropic hypogonadism secondary to deficiency in hypothalamic secretion of GnRH, show incomplete generation of GnRH neurons when human fetuses are evaluated using immunofluorescence double immuno-staining technique combined with confocal laser scanning microscopy.[94]

It appears that the posterior pituitary gland plays a significant role in the regulation of gonadotropin secretion, at least in vitro. Neuropeptide-Y (NPY) has been shown to increase gonadotropin secretion directly at the level of the anterior pituitary, both in the presence and absence of GnRH. However, high-affinity binding sites have not been localized in the anterior pituitary for NPY, but in the posterior pituitary. Further, removal of the posterior pituitary appears to alter LH secretion in vivo. NPY induces greater LH secretion in the presence of posterior pituitary cells; however, FSH secretion is not affected. GnRH-induced LH secretion also appears to be greater in the presence of posterior pituitary cells; however, GnRH induction of LH secretion is significantly decreased. NPY appears to potentiate GnRH induced LH secretion in anterior pituitary cells cultured in the presence and absence of posterior pituitary cells.[95]

Finally, additional information is available regarding cell-cell communication in the anterior pituitary. Evidence now exists for gap junctional mediated exchanges between endocrine cells and folliculostellate cells. Gap junctions are transmembrane channels that allow cell-cell exchange of cytoplasmic molecules MR <1000. Such components include water, ions, metabolic substrates such as sugars, amino acids, nucleotides, secondary messengers including calcium, and IB3. In the rat model, the introduction of Lucifer yellow, an agent that passes freely through gap junctions, has demonstrated communications between cells containing prolactin, growth hormone, and folliculostellate cells. There appears to be a limited amount of gap junctional communication between LH, TSH, and ACTH-containing cells.[96]

ROLE OF GALANIN AND OTHER NOVEL PEPTIDES IN CONTROL OF GONADOTROPIN SECRETION

Galanin is a 29-amino acid peptide that was isolated from porcine intestines by means of a biochemical assay that could detect C-terminally alpha-amidated polypeptides. The structure of galanin has been derived in several species of mammals as well as nonmammalian vertebrates, and recently galanin has been extracted from the stomach of the amphibian *Rana ridibunda*, indicating that it is conserved throughout evolution. Further, galanin has been demonstrated to be present in a variety of endocrine glands including the pituitary, pancreas, and adrenal medulla, which suggests that it can function as a neurohormone.[97] Recently, in the rat model, a subset of GnRH neurons has been demonstrated to express and synthesize the neuropeptide galanin. The distributions and concentration of this peptide in the GnRH neuron are sexually differentiated, with females having a greater number of GnRH-containing neurons and messenger for galanin than males. Further, estrogen/progestogen induction of the galanin gene in the GnRH neuron occurs at the time of the LH surge and, likewise, it is sexually differentiated during the neonatal period. This suggests that the increase in the galanin gene expression in GnRH neurons could be one of the mechanisms underlying sexual difference in gonadotropin release seen in the rodent.[98] Further, neuropeptide Y (NPY) and galanin, the two most abundant peptides, at least in the rat hypothalamus, have individually been shown to play an excitatory role in the hypothalamic control of the basal and cyclic pituitary release of LH. It has been suggested that both neuropeptide Y and galanin act in concert to generate pulsatile GnRH release.[99]

Another family of peptides, the endothelins (ET1, ET2, and ET3), are biologically active 21-amino acid products that have been isolated from porcine aorta and induce long-acting vasoconstriction. The endothelins are secreted into many biologic fluids including the follicle. Endothelin-1 has been shown to inhibit the gonadotropin-supported accumulation of cyclic adenosine monophosphate and progesterone, and endothelin-1 has also been shown to inhibit morphologic agglutination inhibitor and as a suppressor of premature luteinization. Further, it has been suggested that endothelin-3 has a direct action on GnRH neurons. Recently, it has been demonstrated that the administration of estrogen to adolescent girls with primary amenorrhea reduces endothelin-1 levels in both the hyper- and hypogonadotropic state.[100] Further, other peptides appear to inhibit not only the secretion of LH but prolactin, by acting in the medial basal hypothalamus. Pituitary adenylate cyclase-activating peptide (PACAP) was isolated from ovine hypothalami. Two peptide forms exist, one being 27, the other 38 amino acid. It has been recently demonstrated that this peptide acts in the arcuate nucleus region of the mediobasal hypothalamus to inhibit both LH and prolactin secretion.[101]

In addition, using the immortalized GnRH neuron (GTI-7), which has been shown to express receptors for GnRH, LH, and prolactin, treatment of these cells with hCG causes a dose-dependent increase in cyclase A and P production. This results in an inhibitory action on GnRH pulse release and may be responsible for the initiation of suppression of pituitary LH during early pregnancy via a short feedback mechanism.[102] These feedback loops may be important, as it has been recently demonstrated that the preovulatory LH surge found in sheep depends on GnRH stimulation throughout the entire time course.[103] Further, GnRH has been shown to regulate steroidogenic factor I (SF-1 gene expression) in the rodent pituitary, and pulsatile GnRH stimulates a 51 to 64 percent increase in the message, suggesting that it is a critical component of the stimulation of the gonadotropin subunit transcription.[104]

GONADOTROPIN SURGE ATTENUATING INHIBITING FACTOR (GnSAF/IF)

A variety of nonsteroidal agents have been suggested as inhibitors of gonadotropin secretion. The best known of these agents is inhibin, and it would suggest that these compounds reduce pituitary sensitivity to GnRH, at least in the rodent, and inhibit GnRH-induced LH secretion in vitro as well as the gonadotropin subunit mRNA message. This results in a prevention of GnRH receptor up-regulation and binding. Conversely, in cultured ovine pituitary cells, AIT stimulates GnRH-induced LH secretion and GnRH receptor number. Activins, on the other hand, stimulate LH secretion in the monkey but not the rat. Follistatin binds activin in an inactive form in the ovary, human follicular fluid, peripheral circulation, and pituitary. The presence and expression of follistatin in the pituitary regulates GnRH pulse frequency and may regulate gonadotrope function. A variety of biochemical immunologic studies suggest that GnSAF/IF is a distinct entity from the inhibin family. It appears to be a product of the ovarian follicle, and current evidence suggests that it is a part of the mechanism of ovarian pituitary feedback that regulates the ovarian cycle. It is thought to be secreted in increasing quantities during the first half of the follicular phase; as subdominant follicles regress, the dominant follicle is thought to secrete less of the GnSAF/IF and more estradiol, resulting in the generation of a positive feedback.[105]

ROLE OF NITRIC OXIDE IN REPRODUCTION

Nitric oxide (NO) is synthesized from the amino acid L-arginine. It functions as a biologically active endothelium relaxing factor, a regulator of blood flow, and a pressure mediator. A growing body of evidence suggests that nitric oxide interacts with estrogen to regulate blood flow. Estrogens have been demonstrated to potentiate the endothelium-dependent basal dilation, both in terms of resistance and conductance in arteries. Recently, plasma concentrations of nitric oxide have been demonstrated to be higher in the follicular phase with respect to the secretory phase. The nitric oxide concentration peaks at midcycle.[106] Nitric oxide appears to be able to function as an intracellular second messenger, a local substance for regulation of neighboring cells, a neurotransmitter in the central and peripheral neuron complex, and perhaps a hormone.[107] Recently, it has been suggested that nitric oxide controls the release of GnRH. Experiments carried out by McCann, incubating arcuate nucleus median eminence implants from male rats, showed that sodium nitroprusside, a spontaneous releaser of oxide, increased GnRH in a dose-related fashion.[108]

ROLE OF LEPTINS IN REPRODUCTION

"In vertebrates, and especially among land-dwelling mammals, the ability to store large quantities of energy dense fuel in the form of adipose tissue allows survival during prolonged periods of food deprivation. To maintain such food stores without undergoing continual alterations in its size and shape, an animal needs to achieve a balance between energy, intake, and expenditure."[109] A principal part of this mechanism appears to be mediated by the leptins, a protein product of the obesity gene, which is secreted by adipose tissue into the circulation and is thought to signal the brain regarding the size of fat droplets. The administration of recombinant leptin to mice that are obese because of a genetic defect in leptin secretion results in a reduction in food intake and an increase in locomotor activity along with a reduction in body weight.[110] Further, administration of leptin to prepubertal female mice results in the early onset of reproductive function.[111] As weight increases, there is an increase in leptin levels and the hypothalamus through melinocortinergic neurons exerts a tonic inhibition on feeding behavior. Disruption of this inhibitory signal is an explanation of agouti obesity syndrome.[112]

In cases of weight loss there is a decreased secretion of leptin which affects the hypothalamus via neuropeptide Y (NPY). This response to starvation results in increased food intake, decreased energy expenditure, suppression of reproductive function, decreased temperature, and increased parasympathetic activity. In obese ob/ob mice, deficient for neuropeptide Y, reduced food intake induces sterility and other somatotropic effects, suggesting that neuropeptide Y is the central effector of leptin deficiency.[113] Leptin receptor messenger RNA has been shown to be densely concentrated in the arcuate nucleus, and observation suggests that leptin acts on the rat hypothalamus to alter the expression of key neural peptide genes and implicate leptin in the hypothalamic response to fasting.[114] Further, hypoleptinemia has been demonstrated in women athletes.[115] Leptin has been shown to rise continuously with increasing adiposity with gender, age, and short-term caloric restriction being important secondary to regulators.[116] Further, in vitro leptin has been implicated as a regulator of insulin activity in obese individuals.[117] Finally, closely related to the leptin system is corticotropin-releasing factor, a 41 amino acid peptide widely distributed throughout the brain. CRF has been reported to be involved in the anorectic effects of treadmill running and stress, and is thought to be an important neuroregulator of energy balance.[118] Recently, urocortin, a CRF-related peptide that binds with high affinity to CRF-2 receptor, has been demonstrated to produce a marked suppression of appetite, further suggesting the relationship of stress to the CRF system and appetite regulation.[119]

ESTROGEN AND MENTAL FUNCTION

Estrogen is thought to affect mood and behavior in women. Estrogen significantly increases the density of 5-hydroxytryptamine to A receptors in higher centers. Estrogen is thought to be associated with affective disorders including depression and mania, which is suggested by the fact that during menopause and postnatal depression there is an associated massive drop in plasma estrogens. Estrogen produces a state of mild euphoria and has been implicated in improving memory and cognitive function.[120]

ESTROGEN, PROGESTERONE, AND THE NEUROREGULATION OF VASCULAR REACTIVITY

Cyclic migraine headaches are a common clinical complaint and often occur at the time of ovulation or menstruation. It has been demonstrated that oophorectomy in the rabbit model affects cerebral and coronary artery function in vitro by changing the position of the active link tension curve for pharmacomechanical, but not electromechanical, coupling.[121] Further, 17-β-estradiol affects norepinephrine-induced contractions in omental arteries differently in pregnant and nonpregnant states.[122] Endothelin-1, a 21-amino acid peptide—which is the most powerful vasoconstrictor found, with a potency 100-fold greater than norepinephrine—is increased in states of vascular resistance including pulmonary hypertension, congestive heart failure, cardiac hypertrophy, postischemic renal change, and vasospasm. This system may work in conjunction with estrogen and progesterone, with the former inhibiting voltage-gated calcium channels, the latter stimulating them. The female sex steroids may also influence the sensitivity of contractile proteins depicting vascular contraction and relaxation. This may inhibit the production or effect of endothelin-1, and this balance of vasodilation versus vasoconstriction seems to be mediated through endothelin-derived vascular nitric oxide.[123,124,125] These observations are clinically relevant in that headache is produced by an antidromic release of neurotransmitters, which is thought to initiate a sterile inflammation. This is supported by animal and human studies of trigeminal stimulation. Olesen et al have suggested that nitric oxide may be the causative molecule in migraines. The sphenopalatine ganglion may be an important link with these systems, and in experimental animals a high percentage of nitric oxide synthesized positive cells have been located. These observations have resulted in the use of intranasal lidocaine as a treatment for refractory migraine, and in a randomized double-blind controlled trial, 55 percent of affected individuals received relief within 5 min, and 58 percent had persistent symptom relief for at least 24 hr following administration of the compound.[126]

IMMUNE NEUROENDOCRINE INTERACTIONS

A delicate and complex relationship exists between the immune and neuroendocrine systems. Immune, endocrine, or neural cells can express receptors for cytokines, hormones, neurotransmitters, and neuropeptides. Immune and neuroendocrine products have been shown to coexist in lymphoid, endocrine, and neural tissue. Endocrine and neural mediators can affect the immune system, and immune mediators can affect the endocrine and neural system. Cytokines that can mediate immune neuroendocrine action include the interleukins, interferon, tumor necrosis factor alpha, transforming growth factor beta, macrophage colony stimulating factor, granulocyte colony stimulating factor, granulocyte and macrophage colony stimulating factor, and stem cell factor. Neuroendocrine agents affect the immune mechanism by intermediate metabolism, signal transduction selection, recirculation, homing, traffic, cytokines, cell interactions, antigen presentation, affective mechanisms, and autoregulatory processes. Immune-derived products affect the neuroendocrine system via cytokine and other immune cell-derived products to affect neurotransmitters, neuropeptides, neuronal activity, neuronal growth, differentiation and repair, thermal regulation, food intake, sleep, and behavior. A catalog of these effects can be found in the review by Besedovsky and Delray.[127]

SUMMARY

Over the last 50 yr, investigators have relentlessly evaluated the neuroendocrine control of reproduction. The arcuate nucleus has been defined as the key anatomic and functional component of this system and may be thought of as a pulse generator that serves as the final common regulator of reproduction. Many neurotransmitters influence the activity of the arcuate nucleus including the opioid system, dopamine, norepinephrine, GABA, CRF, oxytocin, angiotensin II, neuropeptide Y, neurotensin, and serotonin. These neurotransmitters cause the arcuate nucleus to release the decapeptide GnRH in a pulsatile manner that corresponds to LH surges seen approximately every 1 to $1^1/_2$-hr interval during the follicular phase and every 3-hr interval during the luteal phase. GnRH is delivered to the median eminence and released from nerve terminals into the hypothalamic portal system and transferred to the anterior pituitary, where it acts on the gonadotrope. Binding of GnRH to its receptor activates a number of second messenger systems including inositol phosphate, cal-

cium and calmodulin, and protein kinase C. This results in the acute release of LH and FSH followed by mobilization of reserve from the storage pool. This process is regulated not only by the magnitude and rate of exposure to GnRH but by feedback from estrogen, progesterone, and inhibin. The final biologic expression of the gonadotrope is regulated by the degree of glycosylation of the glycoproteins and the level of activity of β-chain LH and FSH mRNA.

REFERENCES

1. Hohlweg W, Junkmann K. Die hormonal-nervose regulierung der funktion des hypophysen vorderlappens. *Klin Wochschr.* 11:321, 1932
2. Harris GW. Induction of ovulation in rabbit by electrical stimulation of hypothalamohypophysial mechanism. *Proc Royal Soc (Biol).* 122:374, 1937
3. Westman A, Jacobsohn D. Experimentelle untersuchungen ober die bedeutung des hypohysen-zwischenhirn-systems für die produktion gonadotroper hormone des hypophysenvorderlappens. *Acta Obstet Gynecol Scand.* 17:235, 1937
4. Markee JE, Sawyer CH, Hollinshead WH. Activation of anterior hypophysis by electrical stimulation in rabbit. *Endocrinology.* 38:345, 1946
5. Popa GT, Fielding V. Portal circulation from pituitary to hypothalamic region. *J Anat.* 65:88, 1930
6. Houssay BA, Biasotti A, Sammartino R. Modifications fonctionnelles de l'hypophyse apres les lesions infundibulotuberlennes chez le crapaud. *C.R. Acad Sci (Paris).* 120:725, 1935
7. Harris GW. Destrous rhythm. Pseudopregnancy and pituitary stalk in rat. *J Physiol.* 111:347, 1950
8. Guillemin R, Rosenberg B. Humoral hypothalamic control of anterior pituitary: Study with combined tissue cultures. *Endocrinology.* 57:599, 1955
9. Matsou H, Baba Y, Nair R, et al. Structure of the porcine LH- and FSH-releasing hormone. *Biochem Biophys Res Comm.* 43:1344, 1971
10. Burgus R, et al. Primary structure of the ovine hypothalamic luteinizing hormone-releasing factor (LRF). *Proc Natl Acad Sci USA.* 69:278, 1972
11. Bergland RM, Page RB. Pituitary secretion to the brain; anatomical evidence. *Endocrinology.* 102:1025, 1978
12. Blackwell RE, et al. Concomitant release of FSH and LH induced by native and synthetic LRF. *Am J Physiol.* 244:170, 1973
13. Baker BL, Pierce JG, Cornell JS. The utility of antiserums to the subunits of TSH and LH for immunochemical staining of the rat hypophysis. *Am J Anat.* 135:251, 1972
14. Phifer RF, Midgley AR, Spicer SS. Immunohistologic and histologic evidence that follicle-stimulating hormone and luteinizing hormone are present in the same cell type in the human pars distalis. *J Clin Endocrinol Metab.* 36:125, 1973

15. Duello TM, Ralmi NS. Ultrastructural-immunocytochemical localization of growth hormone and prolactin in human pituitaries. *J Clin Endocrinol Metab*. 49:189, 1979

16. Neill JD, Pan G, Wei N, et al. GnRH receptor regulation. In: Yen SSC, Vale WW, eds. *Neuroendocrine Regulation of Reproduction*. Norwell, Mass., Serono Symposia, 1989: 249–257

17. Deirschke DH, Bhattacharya AN, Atkinson LE, et al. Circhoral oscillations of plasma LH levels in the ovariectomized rhesus monkey. *Endocrinology*. 87:850, 1970

18. Krey LC, Butler WR, Knobil E. Surgical disconnection of the medial basal hypothalamus and pituitary function in the rhesus monkey. I. Gonadotropin secretion. *Endocrinology*. 96:1073, 1975

19. Plant TM, Krey LC, Moossy J, et al. The arcuate nucleus and the control of the gonadotropin and prolactin secretion in the female rhesus monkey *(Macaca mulatta)*. *Endocrinology*. 102:52, 1978

20. Amoss M, Burgus R, Blackwell RE, et al. Purification, amino acid composition and N-terminus of the hypothalamic luteinizing hormone releasing factor (LRF) of ovine origin. *Biochem Biophys Res Comm*. 44:205, 1971

21. Monahan M, Rivier J, Burgus R, et al. Synthese totals per phase solide d'um decapeptide qui stimule las secretion des gonadotropines hypophysailres LH eg FSH. *C.R. Acad Sci (Paris)*. 273:508, 1971

22. Burgus R, Butcher N, Ling N, et al. Structure moleculaire du facteur hypothalaminques (LRF) d'origine ovine controlant la secretion de l'hormone gonadotrop hypophysaire de luteinisation (LH). *C.R. Acad Sci (Paris)*. 273:1611, 1971

23. Amoss MR, Blackwell RE, Guillemin R. Stimulation of ovulation in the rabbit triggered by synthetic LRF. *J Clin Endocrinol Metab*. 39:434, 1972

24. Belchetz PE, et al. Hypophyseal responses to continuous and intermittent delivery of hypothalamic gonadotropin releasing hormone. *Science*. 202:631, 1978

25. Wang CF, Lasley BL, Lein A, et al. The functional changes of the pituitary gonadotrophs during the menstrual cycle. *Clin Endocrinol Metab*. 42:718, 1976

26. Wang CF, Yen SSC. Direct evidence of estrogen modulation of pituitary sensitivity to luteinizing hormone releasing factor during the menstrual cycle. *J Clin Invest*. 55:201, 1975

27. Soules MR, Steiner RA, Cohen NL, et al. Nocturnal slowing of pulsatile luteinizing hormone secretion in women during the follicular phase of the menstrual cycle. *J Clin Endocrinol Metab*. 61:43, 1985

28. Hayward JN. Functional and morphological aspects of hypothalamic neurons. *Physiol Rev*. 57:574, 1977

29. Wilson RC, Kesner JS, Kaufman JM, et al. Central electrophysiologic correlates of luteinizing hormone secretion in the rhesus monkey. *Neuroendocrinology*. 39:256, 1984

30. Silverman AJ, Wilson RC, Kesner JS, et al. Hypothalamic localization of multiunit electrical activity associated with pulsatile LH release in the rhesus monkey. *Neuroendocrinology*. 44:168, 1986

31. Judd S, Rakoff J, Yen S. Inhibition of gonadotropin and prolactin release by dopamine effect of endogenous estradiol levels. *J Clin Endocrinol Metab*. 47:494, 1978

32. Gallo RV, Drouva SV. Effect of intraventricular infusion of catecholamines on luteinizing hormone release in ovariectomized and ovariectomized, steroid-primed rats. *Neuroendocrinology*. 29:149, 1979

33. Jennes L, Beckman W, Stumpf W, et al. Anatomical relationships of serotoninergic and noradrenalinergic projections with the GnRH system in septum and hypothalamus. *Exp Brain Res*. 46:331, 1982

34. Leranth C, Maclusky N, Salamoto H, et al. Glutamic acid decarboxylase-containing axons synapse on LHRH neurons in the rat medial preoptic area. *Neuroendocrinology*. 40:536, 1985

35. Flugge G, Oertel W, Wuttke W. Evidence for estrogen receptive GABAergic neurons in the preoptic/anterior hypothalamic area of the rat brain. *Neuroendocrinology*. 43:1, 1986

36. Swanson LW, Sawchenko PE, Rivier J, et al. Organization of ovine corticotropin-releasing factor immunoreactive cells and fibers in the rat brain: An immunohistochemical study. *Neuroendocrinology*. 38:165, 1983

37. Steele MK, Gallo RV, Ganong WF. Stimulatory or inhibitory effects of angiotensin II upon LH secretion in ovariectomized rats: A function of gonadal steroids. *Neuroendocrinology*. 40:310, 1985

38. Advis J, McCann SM, Negro-Villar A. Evidence that catecholaminergic and peptidergic (luteinizing hormone-releasing hormone) neurons in suprachiasmatic-medial preoptic, medial basal hypothalamus and median eminence are involved in estrogen-negative feedback. *Endocrinology*. 107:892, 1980

39. Bhanot RN, Wilkinson M. Opiatergic control of gonadotropin secretion during puberty in the rat: A neurochemical basis for the hypothalamic "gonadostat." *Endocrinology*. 113:596, 1983

40. Kalra SP, Crowlev WR. Norepinephrine-like effects of neuropeptide Y on LH release in the rat. *Life Sci*. 35:1173, 1984

41. Drouva SV, Laplante E, Kordon C. Effects of ovarian steroids on in vitro release of LHRH from mediobasal hypothalamus. *Neuroendocrinology*. 37:336, 1983

42. Drouva SV, Laplante E, Gautron JP, et al. Effects of 17 beta estradiol on LH-RH release from rat mediobasal hypothalamic slices. *Neuroendocrinology*. 38:152, 1984

43. Hoff et al. Hormonal dynamics at midcycles: A reevaluation. *J Clin Endocrinol Metab*. 57:792, 1983

44. Hughes J, Smith TW, Kosterlitz LH, et al. Identification of two related pentapeptides from the brain with potent opiate agonist activitv. *Nature*. 255:577, 1978

45. Roberts JL, Chen CLC, Ebervine JH, et al. Glucocorticoid regulation of pro-oipiomelanocortin gene expression in rodent pituitary. *Rec Prog Horm Res*. 38:227, 1982

46. Kosterlitz HW, Waterfield AA. In vitro models in the study of structure–activity relationships of narcotic analgesics. *Annu Rev Pharmacol*. 15:29, 1975

47. Rasmussen DD, Liu JH, Yen SSC. Endogenous opioid regulation of GnRH release from the human medio-basal hypothalamus (MBH) in vitro. *J Clin Endocrinol Metab*. 57:881, 1983

48. Reid RL, Hoff JD, Yen SSC, et al. Effects on pituitary hormone secretion and disappearance rates of estrogenous

β_h-endorphin in normal human subjects. *J Clin Endocrinol Metab.* 52:1179, 1981

49. Cetel NS, Quigley ME, Yen SSC. Naloxone-induced prolactin secretion in women: Evidence against a direct prolactin stimulatory effect of endogenous opioids. *J Clin Endocrinol Metab.* 60:191, 1985

50. Quigley ME, Yen SSC. The role of endogenous opiates on LH secretion during the menstrual cycle. *J Clin Endocrinol Metab.* 51:179, 1980

51. Fishman J. The catechol estrogens. *Neuroendocrinology.* 4:363, 1976

52. Phifer RF, Midgley AR Jr, Spicer SS. Immunohistologic and histologic evidence that FSH and LH are present in the same cell type in the human pars distalis. *J Clin Endocrinol Metab.* 36:125, 1973

53. Haour F, Crumeyrolle J, Latouche J, et al. Visualization and characterization of GnRH receptors in animal and human tissues. In: Lunenfeld B, ed. *Gynecological Endocrinology.* Parthenon Publishing, Parkridge, N.J., 1990; 4: 12

54. Hoff JO, Quigley M, Yen SSC. The functional relationship between priming and releasing actions of luteinizing hormone-releasing hormone. *J Clin Endocrinol Metab.* 49:8, 1979

55. Rabin D, McNeil LW. Pituitary and gonadal desensitization after continuous luteinizing hormone releasing-hormone infusion in normal females. *J Clin Endocrinol Metab.* 51:873, 1980

56. Roger M, Lahlou N, Chaussain JL, et al. Secretion patterns of glycoprotein hormone alpha-subunit after GnRH agonist and antagonist administration. In: Lunenfeld B, ed. *Gynecological Endocrinology.* Parthenon Publishing, Parkridge, N.J., 1990; 4: 24

57. Meldrum DR, et al. Stimulation of LH fragments with reduced bioactivity following GnRH agonist administration in women. *J Clin Endocrinol Metab.* 58:755, 1984

58. Frager MS, Pieper DR, Tonetta S, et al. Pituitary gonadotropin-releasing hormone (GnRH) receptors: Effects of castration, steroid replacement and the role of GnRH in modulating receptors in the rat. *J Clin Invest.* 67:615, 1981

59. Hopkins CR, Walker AM. Calcium as a second messenger in the stimulation of luteinizing hormone secretion. *Mol Cell Endocrinol.* 12:189, 1978

60. Stern JE, Conn PM. Perifusion of rat pituitaries; requirements of optimal GnRH-stimulated LH release. *Am J Physiol Endocrinol Metab.* 240:E504, 1981

61. Barbarino A, DeMarinis L. Calcium antagonists and hormone release. II. Effects of verapamil on basal gonadotropin-releasing hormone and thyrotropin-releasing hormone induced pituitary hormone release in normal subjects. *J Clin Endocrinol Metab.* 51:749, 1980

62. Conn PM, Rogers DC. Restoration of responsiveness to gonadotropin releasing hormone (GnRH) in calcium depleted rat pituitary cells. *Life Sci.* 24:2461, 1979

63. Conn PM, Kilpatrick D, Kirshner N. Ionophoretic Ca^{2+} mobilization in rat gonadotropes and bovine adrenomedullary cells. *Cell Calcium.* 1:129, 1980

64. Clapper DA, Conn PM. GnRH stimulation of pituitary gonadotrope cells produce an increase in intracellular calcium. *Biol Reprod.* 32:269, 1985

65. Conn PM, Chafouleas JG, Rogers D, et al. Gonadotropin-releasing hormone stimulates calmodulin redistribution in rat pituitary. *Nature.* 292:264, 1981

66. Jennes L, Bronson D, Stumpf WE, et al. Evidence for an association between calmodulin and membrane patches containing gonadotropin-releasing hormone receptor complexes in cultured gonadotropes. *Cell Tissue Res.* 239:311, 1985

67. Levin RM, Weiss B. Mechanism by which psychotropic drugs inhibit cycle AMP phosphodiesterase. *Mol Pharmacol.* 12:581, 1976

68. Wooge CH, Conn PM. Characterization of calmodulin binding components in the pituitary gonadotrope. *Mol Cell Endocrinol.* 56:41, 1988

69. Mitchell RH, Jafferji SS, Jones LM. The possible involvement of phosphatidylinositol breakdown in the mechanism of stimulus response coupling at receptors which control cell-surface calcium gates: In: Bazin NG, et al, eds. *Function and Biosynthesis of Lipids.* New York, N.Y., Plenum Press, 1977: 447–464

70. Snyder GD, Bleasdale JE. Effect of LHRH on incorporation of [^{32}P]-orthophosphate into phosphatidyl-inositol by dispersed anterior pituitary cells. *Mol Cell Endocrinol.* 28:55, 1982

71. Streb H, Irvine RF, Berridge MJ, et al. Release of Ca^{2+} from a nonmitochondrial intracellular store in pancreatic acinar-cells by inositol-1,4,5,-triphosphate. *Nature.* 306:67, 1983

72. Conn PM, McArdle CA, Andrews WV, et al. The molecular basis of gonadotropin-releasing hormone (GnRH) action in the pituitary gonadotrope. *Biol Reprod.* 36:17, 1987

73. Sharkey NA, Blumberg PM. Kinetic evidence that 1,3-diolein inhibits phorbol ester binding to protein kinase C via a competitive mechanism. *Biochem Biophys Res Comm.* 133:1051, 1985

74. Lalloz MRA, Detta A, Clayton RN. GnRH desensitization preferentially inhibits expression of the LH beta-subunit gene in vivo. *Endocrinology.* 122:1689, 1988

75. Papavasiliou SS, Zmeili S, Herbon L, et al. Alpha and LH beta mRNA of male and female rats after castration: Quantitation using an optimized RNA dot blot hybridization assay. *Endocrinology.* 119:691, 1986

76. Papavasiliou SS, Zmeili SM, Khoury S, et al. GnRH differentially regulates expression of the genes for LH alpha and beta subunits in male rats. *Proc Natl Acad Sci USA.* 83:4026, 1986

77. Radowick S, et al. Structural studies on the human GnRH gene. *Endocrine Soc Program.* 192:200, 1988

78. Roberts VJ, Meunier H, Vaughan J, et al. Production and regulation of inhibin subunits in pituitary gonadotropes. *Endocrinology.* 124:552, 1989

79. Meunier H, Rivier C, Evans RM, et al. Gonadal and extragonadal expression of inhibin α, β_A and β_B subunits in various tissues predicts diverse functions. *Proc Natl Acad Sci USA.* 85:247, 1988

80. Bischoff K, Bettendorf G, Stegner HE. FSH- and LH-gehalt in menschlichen hypophysen wahrend des ovariellen cyclus. *Arch Gynak.* 208:44, 1969

81. Bremner WJ, Paulsen CA. Two pools of luteinizing hormone in the human pituitary: Evidence from constant administration of luteinizing hormone-releasing hormone. *J Clin Endocrinol Metab.* 39:811, 1974

82. Edmonds M, Molitch M, Pierce JG, et al. Secretion of alpha subunits of luteinizing hormone (LH) by the anterior pituitary. *J Clin Endocrinol Metab.* 41:551, 1975

83. Peters BP, Krzesicki RF, Hartle RJ, et al. A kinetic comparison of the processing and secretion of the αβ dimer and the uncombined subunits of chorionic gonadotropin synthesized by human choriocarcinoma cells. *J Biol Chem.* 259:15123, 1984

84. Kakar SS, Musgrove LC, Devor DC, et al. Cloning, sequencing, and expression of human gonadotropin releasing hormone (GnRH) receptor. *Biochem Biophys Res Comm.* Nov 1992, 289

85. Howard AD, Feigliner SC, Cully DF, et al. A receptor in pituitary and hypothalamus that functions in growth hormone release. *Science.* 273:974, 1996

86. Conn PM, Bowers CY. A new receptor for growth hormone-release peptide. *Science.* 273:923, 1996

87. Genazzani AD, Petraglia F, Gastaldi M, et al. Growth hormone (GH)-releasing hormone-induced hypothalamic amenorrhea: Evidence of altered central neuromodulation. *Fertil Steril.* 65:935, 1996

88. Ma YJ, Emde KB, Rage F, et al. Hypothalamic astrocytes respond to transforming growth factor-alpha with the secretion of neuroactive substances that stimulate the release of luteinizing hormone-releasing hormone. *Endocrinology.* 138:19, 1997

89. Mayerhofer A, Dissen GA, Parroff JA, et al. Involvement of nerve growth factor in the ovulatory cascade: trkA receptor activation inhibits gap junctional communication between thecal cells. *Endocrinology.* 137:5662, 1996

90. Fainzilber M, Smit AB, Syed NI, et al. CRNF, a molluscan neurotrophic factor that interacts with the p75 neurotrophin receptor. *Science.* 274:1540, 1996

91. Naftolin F, Mor G, Horvath TL, et al. Synaptic remodeling in the arcuate nucleus during the estrous cycle is induced by estrogen and precedes the preovulatory gonadotropin surge. *Endocrinology.* 137:5576, 1996

92. Rance NE, Uswandi SV. Gonadotropin-releasing hormone gene expression is increased in the medial basal hypothalamus of postmenopausal women. *J Clin Endocrinol Metab.* 81:3540, 1996

93. Tobet SA, Chickering TW, King JC, et al. Expression of γ-aminobutyric acid and gonadotropin-releasing hormone during neuronal migration through the olfactory system. *Endocrinology.* 137:5415, 1996

94. Quinton R, Hasan W, Grant W, et al. Gonadotropin-releasing hormone immunoreactivity in the nasal epithelia of adults with Kallmann's syndrome and isolated hypogonadotropic hypogonadism and in the early midtrimester human fetus. *J Clin Endocrinol Metab.* 82:308, 1997

95. O'Conner JL, Wade MF. Evidence that the posterior pituitary plays a role in neuropeptide Y and luteinizing hormone-releasing hormone-stimulated gonadotropin secretion in vitro. *Soc Exp Biol Med.* 213:59, 1996

96. Morand I, Fonlupt P, Guerrier A, et al. Cell-to-cell communication in the anterior pituitary: Evidence for gap junction-mediated exchanges between endocrine cells and folliculostellate cells. *Endocrinology.* 137:3356, 1996

97. Gasman S, Vaudry H, Cartier F, et al. Localization, identification, and action of galanin in the frog adrenal gland. *Endocrinology.* 137:5311, 1996

98. Finn PD, McFall TB, Clifton DK, et al. Sexual differentiation of galanin gene expression in gonadotropin-releasing hormone neurons. *Endocrinology.* 137:4767, 1996

99. Xu B, Pu S, Kalra S, et al. An interactive physiological role of neuropeptide Y and galanin in pulsatile pituitary luteinizing hormone secretion. *Endocrinology.* 137:5297, 1996

100. Creatsas GC, Malamitsi-Puchner AB, Hassan EA, et al. Endothelin plasma levels in primary amenorrheic adolescents before and after estrogen treatment. *J Soc Gynecol Invest.* 3:330, 1996

101. Anderson ST, Sawangjaroen K, Curlewis JD. Pituitary adenylate cyclase-activating polypeptide acts within the medial basal hypothalamus to inhibit prolactin and luteinizing hormone secretion. *Endocrinology.* 137:3424, 1996

102. Mores N, Krsmanovic LZ, Catt KJ. Activation of LH receptors expressed in GnRH neurons stimulates cyclic AMP production and inhibits pulsatile neuropeptide release. *Endocrinology.* 137:5731, 1996

103. Evans NP, Dahl GE, Caraty A, et al. How much of the gonadotropin-releasing hormone (GnRH) surge is required for generation of the luteinizing hormone surge in the ewe? Duration of the endogenous GnRH signal. *Endocrinology.* 137:4730, 1996

104. Haisenleder DJ, Yasin M, Dalkin AC, et al. GnRH regulates steroidogenic factor-S (SF01) gene expression in rat pituitary. *Endocrinology.* 137:5719, 1996

105. Fowler PA, Templeton A. The nature and function of putative gonadotropin surge-attenuating/inhibiting factor (GnSAF/IF) *Endocr Rev.* 17:103, 1996

106. Cicinelli E, Ignarre LJ, Lograno M, et al. Circulating levels of nitric oxide in fertile women in relation to the menstrual cycle. *Fertil Steril.* 66:1036, 1996

107. Murad F. Signal transduction using nitric oxide and cyclic guanosine monophosphate. *JAMA.* 276:1189, 1996

108. McCann SM, Rettori V. The role of nitric oxide in reproduction. *Soc Exp Biol Med.* 0037:7, 1996

109. Friedman JM. The alphabet of weight control. *Nature.* 385:119, 1997

110. Kohrt WM, Landt M, Birge SJ Jr. Serum leptin levels are reduced in response to exercise training, but not hormone replacement therapy, in older women. *J Clin Endocrinol Metab.* 81:3980, 1996

111. Fan W, Boston BA, Kesterson RA, et al. Role of melanocortinergic neurons in feeding and the agouti obesity syndrome. *Nature.* 385:165, 1997

112. Erickson JC, Hollopeter G, Palmiter RD. Attenuation of the obesity syndrome of ob/ob mice by the loss of neuropeptide Y. *Science.* 274:1704, 1996

113. Gerald C, Walker MW, Criscione L, et al. A receptor subtype involved in neuropeptide-Y-induced food intake. *Nature.* 382:168, 1996

114. Schwartz MW, Seeley RJ, Campfield A, et al. Identification of targets of leptin action in rat hypothalamus. *J Clin Invest.* 98:1101, 1996

115. Laughlin GA, Yen SC. Hypoleptinemia in women athletes: Absence of a diurnal rhythm with amenorrhea. *J Clin Endocrinol Metab.* 82:318, 1997

116. Ostlund RE Jr, Yang JW, Klein S. Relation between plasma leptin concentration and body fat, gender, diet, age, and metabolic covariates. *J Clin Endocrinol Metab.* 81:3909, 1996

117. Cohen B, Novick D, Rubinstein M. Modulation of insulin activities by leptin. *Science.* 274:1185, 1996

118. Richard D, Rivest R, Naimi N, et al. Expression of corticotropin-releasing factor and its receptors in the brain of lean and obese Zucker rats. *Endocrinology.* 137:5786, 1996

119. Spina M, Merlo-Pich E, Chan RKW, et al. Appetite-suppressing effects of urocortin, a CRF-related neuropeptide. *Science.* 273:1561, 1996

120. Fink G, Sumner BEH. Oestrogen and mental state. *Nature.* 383:306, 1996

121. Hansen VB, Skajaa K, Aalkjaer C, et al. The effect of oophorectomy on mechanical properties of rabbit cerebral and coronary isolated small arteries. *Am J Obstet Gynecol.* 175:1272, 1996

122. Belfort MA, Saade GR, Wen TS, et al. The direct action of 17-beta-estradiol in isolated omental artery from nonpregnant and pregnant women is related to calcium antagonism. *J Obstet Gynecol.* 175:1163, 1996

123. Levin ER. Editorial: Endothelin-1, prostaglandin F_{2a}, and the corpus luteum—the crisis of lysis. *Endocrinology.* 137:5189, 1996

124. White MM, Zamudio S, Stevens T, et al. Estrogen, progesterone, and vascular reactivity: Potential cellular mechanisms. *Endocr Rev.* 16:739, 1996

125. Rosenfeld CR, Cox BE, Roy T, et al. Nitric oxide contributes to estrogen-induced vasodilation of the ovine uterine circulation. *J Clin Invest.* 98:2158, 1996

126. Maizels M, Scott B, Cohen W, et al. Intranasal lidocaine for treatment of migraines. *JAMA.* 276:319, 1996

127. Besedovsky HO, Del Rey A. Immune-neuro-endocrine interactions: Facts and hypotheses. *Endocr Rev.* 17:64, 1996

Chapter 10

HORMONAL REGULATION OF BREAST PHYSIOLOGY

Richard E. Blackwell, Scott M. Slayden, and J. Benjamin Younger

In 1765, Haller first concluded that milk was derived from blood. Sir Ashley Cooper first described the physiology of lactogenesis and milk letdown. However, it was not until the 1930s that, through pressure monitoring, milk ejection and milk secretion were shown to be separate events.[1] At about the same time, prolactin was extracted from the human pituitary and was shown to be a distinct hormone.[2] The prevailing philosophy in the 1940s was that estrogen and progesterone were capable of promoting full growth of the mammary gland. It was thought that progesterone produced during pregnancy inhibited lactation, and the fall of this hormone at parturition, accompanied by the rise in circulating prolactin and cortisol, triggered lactation.[3] Although this concept is incorrect, it endured for more than 20 yr and was challenged only when it was discovered that mammary growth could occur in the absence of steroid hormones in adrenalectomized gonadectomized rats that were recipients of pituitary mammotrophic tumor xenografts that secreted prolactin, corticotropin (ACTH), and growth hormone.[4] Subsequently, studies showed that estrogen would stimulate prolactin secretion, and this response could be partially inhibited by progesterone.[5] Recently, it has been proposed that the elevation in progesterone levels during pregnancy prevents the secretion of milk and the withdrawal of the hormone after parturition is in part responsible for the initiation of lactogenesis.[6]

The relationship of hyperprolactinemia to the menstrual cycle was first described separately by Chiari et al and Frommel in 1855 and 1882, respectively.[7,8] Chiari et al described two cases of peurperal atrophy of the uterus associated with persistent lactation following pregnancy. Subsequently, Argonz and Del Castillo described the clinical picture of persistent lactation occurring independent of pregnancy associated with hyposecretion of estrogens.[9] Finally, Forbes et al described the syndrome of galactorrhea, amenorrhea associated with low urinary follicle-stimulating hormone (FSH). This was described in 1954, and approximately 25 percent of the patients studied by Forbes et al were found to have pituitary tumors[10]; although at the time prolactin could not be measured in these tissues, subsequent clinical studies have demonstrated that micro- and macroadenomas of the pituitary are capable of secreting a variety of prolactin molecules that bring about persistent lactation and concomitant menstrual dysfunction.

ANATOMY OF THE MAMMARY GLAND

The mammary gland lies on the pectoralis fascia and the muscles of the chest wall over the anterior rib cage. It is surrounded by fat and encased in skin. The tissue extends into the axilla, forming the tail of Spence. The gland is composed of 12 to 20 glandular lobules surrounded by a ductal system. The ducts are surrounded by both connective and periductal tissue and these are responsive to hormonal stimulation. The lactiferous ducts enlarge as they approach the nipple, which is pigmented and surrounded by the areola. The ductal tissue is lined by epithelial cells. The major functional unit of the breast is the alveolar cell, which is surrounded by the hormonally responsive myoepithelial cells. Milk is produced at the surface of the alveolar cells and extruded by the contraction of the myoepithelial cells under the influence of the octopeptide, oxytocin. Fibrosepta run from the lobules into the superficial fascia, and the suspensory ligaments of Cooper permit mobility of the breast. The principal blood supply of the breast comes from the lateral thoracic and internal thoracic arteries. Arterial supply also comes from the anterior intercostal vessels. The innervation of the breast is chiefly by the intercostal nerves, which carry both sensory and autonomic fibers. The nipples and areolae are innervated by the inferior ramus of the fourth intercostal nerve. Seventy-five percent of the lymphatic drainage of the breast involves the axillary pathways to the pectoral and apical axillary nodes. There is also drainage via the peristernal routes.[11]

EMBRYOLOGY AND HISTOLOGIC DEVELOPMENT OF THE MAMMARY GLAND

The mammary gland is derived from ectoderm and can be identified at 6 wk after fertilization. By 20 wk gestation, 16 to 24 primitive lactiferous ducts have invaded the mesoderm. These components continue to branch and grow into the tissue. Canalization occurs at term. Although the central lactiferous duct is present at birth, the gland does not differentiate until it receives the appropriate hormonal signals much later in life. At the 7-mm embryo stage, the mammary gland forms a mammary crest or milk line that extends along the ventral lateral body wall from the axilla to the inguinal region bilaterally. The caudal epithelium progresses and the crest in the thoracic region thickens to form a primordial mammary bud by the time the embryo reaches the 10- to 12-mm stage. These embryologic origins account for the occasional development of supernumerary nipples and accessory breast tissue.

Mammary tissue remains relatively unresponsive until pregnancy. However, it is responsive to systemic hormone administration during fetal life. It is in the third trimester when fetal prolactin levels increase that terminal differentiation of ductal tissue occurs. This hormonal milieu accounts for the "witches' milk" expressible from the nipples of some normal newborn girls.[12] After birth, these cells revert to a primitive state and the gland remains quiescent until the establishment of ovulatory menstrual cycles, at which time breast development proceeds in the manner described by Marshall and Tanner (see Chap 5). Although the hormonal regulation of mammogenesis is unclear, estrogen in vitro appears to bring about ductal proliferation, although it has little ability to stimulate lobuloalveolar development.[13] In vitro, estrogens do not promote mammary growth. It has been suggested that various epidermal growth factors might participate in this process.[14] Progesterone appears to stimulate lobuloalveolar development in vivo.[15] It should be noted, however, that administration of estrogen and progesterone to hypophysectomized animals fails to promote full mammogenesis.[16] These data would suggest that hormones other then the sex steroids play a role in mammogenesis. As an example, if the pituitary and adrenal glands were removed from oophorectomized rats the addition of estrogen plus corticoids and growth hormone restores full duct growth similar to that seen during puberty.[17]

Before pregnancy, breast lobules consist of ducts lined with epithelium embedded in connective tissue. The majority of tissue in the glands is of connective and adipose type. Their skin contribution forms glandular parenchyma, and a few bud-like sacculations arise from the ducts. The entire gland consists predominantly of lactiferous ducts. The breast, however, undergoes cyclic changes associated with normal ovulation, and premenstrual breasts are engorged probably secondary to tissue edema and hyperemia. Epithelial proliferation is also detectable during the menstrual cycle.[18]

Following conception, the mammary glands undergo remarkable changes in development. Lobuloalveolar elements differentiate during the first trimester. Mammary development can be induced either in vivo or in vitro with placental lactogen or prolactin in the absence of sex hormones.[19] Both placental lactogen and prolactin increase throughout pregnancy, and data suggests that either of these hormones can stimulate complete mammogenesis. The role of estrogen in mammogenesis appears to be secondary as lactation has been reported in pregnancy of women with placental sulfatase deficiencies.[20] Progesterone stimulates lobuloalveolar development and also appears to antagonize the terminal effects induced by prolactin at least in the in vitro model. Cortisol, which potentiates the action of prolactin on mammary differentiation, is unnecessary for either ductal or alveolar proliferation.[21] Insulin and other growth factors stimulate mammogenesis; eg, insulin is required for the survival of postnatal mammary tissue in vitro.[22] Insulin-like molecules such as the insulin-like growth factors may participate in the process as well. It has been suggested that epidermal growth factor is involved in mammogenesis and together with the glucocorticoids facilitates the accumulation of type IV collagen, a component of the basal lamina by which epithelial cells are supported.

CONTROL OF LACTATION

Milk ejection occurs abruptly between the second and fourth days postpartum in the human, although the transition from colostrum production to mature milk secretion is gradual. This may take up to 1 mo to complete and seems to correlate with a fall in plasma progesterone levels and a rise in prolactin level. Twelve wk before parturition, there are marked changes in milk composition (Table 10–1). There is an increased production in lactose, proteins, and immunoglobulins and a decrease in sodium and chloride content. Blood flow increases in the breast and there is an increased utilization of both oxygen and glucose. There is a marked increase in the amount of citrate at about the time of parturition.[23] The composition of milk remains stable until term, best exemplified by the stable production of α-lactalbumin, a milk-specific protein. At parturition, there is a marked fall in placental lactogen production, and progesterone

TABLE 10–1. COMPOSITION OF HUMAN MILK

Major Proteins
α-Lactalbumin (30%)
Lactoferrin (20%)
Casein (40%)
IgA (10%)

Minor Proteins

IgG	
IgM	Enzymes
Albumin	Epidermal growth factor
Bombesin	Folate-binding protein
Calcitonin	Insulin-like growth factor (IGF-I)
Corticosterone-binding protein	Prolactin
	Vitamin B_{12}-binding protein

levels reach nonpregnant levels within several days.[24] Plasma estrogen falls to basal levels in 5 days, whereas prolactin decreases over 14 days.[25] The fall in progesterone seems to be the most important event in the establishment of lactogenesis. Exogenous progesterone prevents lactose and lipid synthesis after oophorectomy in pregnant rats and in sheep.[26] Furthermore, progesterone administration inhibits casein and α-lactalbumin synthesis in vitro.[27]

MAINTENANCE OF LACTATION

Lactation is the product between interaction of numerous hormones (Table 10–2). Removal of the pituitary and adrenal glands in many species terminates milk production.[28] The reinstitution of milk production varies with the type of replacement therapy and the species involved. For instance, in the rabbit and sheep, prolactin is effective alone, whereas in ruminants milk secretion is restored by the addition of sex steroids, thyroxine, growth hormone, and prolactin. In humans, prolactin appears to be the key hormone in the maintenance of lactation, as administration of the dopamine agonist bromocriptine blocks lactogenesis.[29] The role of thyroid hormones in the maintenance of lactation is uncertain. Thyroidectomy inhibits lactation, and replacement therapy with thyroxine increases milk yield. It has also been suggested that there is a synergy between growth hormone and thyroxine that affects milk yield. T3 also apparently acts directly on mammary tissue in vitro to increase its sensitivity to prolactin.[30] Therefore, as can be seen in the human, prolactin is the key hormone in the process of initiation and maintenance of lactation.

BIOLOGY OF PROLACTIN SECRETION

Prolactin is an ancient molecule whose actions involve not only the initiation and maintenance of lactation but free fatty acid metabolism, salt and water metabolism, behavior, etc. Human prolactin was isolated, purified, and shown to be different from human growth hormone, which has a similar structure, in 1970.[31] Specific and sensitive radioimmunoassays were subsequently developed that allowed accurate measurement of prolactin secretion in the early 1970s.[32] Prolactin was found to be a single polypeptide containing 198 amino acid residues with a molecular weight of 22,000. The structure is folded into a globular form with folds being connected by three disulfide bonds. There is great similarity between the structures of human prolactin, human growth hormone, and placental lactogen. The gene for human prolactin was cloned in the early 1980s, and it was believed that this gene was derived from a common somatomammatropic precursor.[33] The prolactin gene is positioned on chromosome 6 and located near the human leukocyte antigen (HLA).[34,35]

There is great heterogeneity of the prolactin molecule. At least five forms have been described (Table 10–3): Little prolactin, molecular weight 22,000, is the monomeric form and has the highest biologic activity; big prolactin, molecular weight 50,000, is a mixture of dimeric and trimeric forms; big-big prolactin weighs approximately 100,000 and has little biologic activity; Iso-B

TABLE 10–2. HORMONAL REGULATION OF THE BREAST

Ductal Growth	Lactogenesis
Cortisol	Prolactin
GH	Insulin
Estrogens	IGF[1]
Alveolar Growth	Cortisol
Estrogen	
Progesterone	
Prolactin	
Cortisol	
GH	

TABLE 10–3. ISOFORMS OF PROLACTIN

Monomeric MW 23,000
Bioactive

Glycosylated (G^1-PRL and G^2-PRL) MW 25,000
↓ Immunoactivity and ↓ bioactivity

Big MW 50,000
Both dimeric and trimeric glycosylated forms can be converted to monomeric form

Big-big MW 100,000
↓ Bioactivity

prolactin has recently been isolated by the isofocusing technique; and glycosylated prolactin has a molecular weight of approximately 25,000.[36–38]

These forms of prolactin reside in the human lactotrope, which is located in the anterior pituitary. The lactotrope may arise from a common stem cell that gives rise to somatotropes and lactotropes. Lactotropes are commonly found in the pituitary and make up at least 20 percent of the cell population. These cells are aggregated mainly in the lateral wings of the bilobe pituitary. The concentration of pituitary prolactin varies considerably, which probably reflects the fact that it is a dynamic hormone being released by such agents as stress, food intake (particularly the amino acid arginine), breast examination, and exercise. In addition, prolactin shows some variation during the menstrual cycle, being highest immediately prior to ovulation in the middle of the luteal phase, and has a diurnal variation.[39] Lactation is also reflected in the variable morphology one sees in lactotropes. This has been studied extensively by Neill's group, using the reverse hemolytic plaque assay.[40] Several populations of cells were described: one that showed little biologic activity and secreted a small amount of prolactin and another that secreted large amounts of prolactin. Increasing dopamine concentrations in vitro was found to progressively decrease the frequency of cells secreting large amounts of prolactin. It is suggested that some lactotropes are more responsive to the inhibitory influences, such as dopamine, than are others. There may, in fact, be some populations that are totally unresponsive to dopamine inhibition.

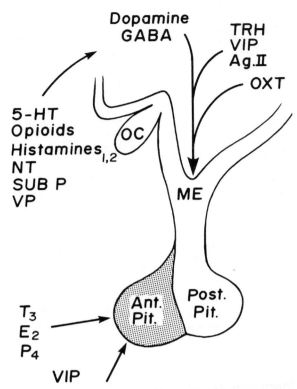

Figure 10–1. Summary of neuropeptides and hormones that control prolactin secretion either through classic endocrine, paracrine, or autocrine mechanisms.

CONTROL OF PROLACTIN SECRETION

Prolactin is unique among the anterior pituitary hormones in that its release is governed primarily by an inhibitory influence from the hypothalamus. This concept arose following the demonstration that persistent prolactin secretion occurred when the pituitary gland was transplanted in vitro to sites removed from the base of the brain, such as the kidney capsule or pneumoderma pouch, or maintained in organ or cell culture.[41] Prolactin-inhibiting factor was thought to be a polypeptide that belongs to the family of neural hormones. However, despite many attempts, no such factor has been isolated from hypothalamic tissue. Instead, prolactin seems to be regulated by a host of chemical signals, both stimulatory and inhibitory (Fig 10–1). The principal inhibitory agent appears to be dopamine.[42] Administration of L-dopa, a metabolic precursor of dopamine, crosses the blood–brain barrier and decreases prolactin secretion within $2\frac{1}{2}$ hr. The recovery phase includes a rebound above basal levels, and this is greater in women than in men. Dopamine inhibits prolactin section promptly in many in vitro and in

vivo model systems[43] (Fig 10–2). Further, in vitro studies in the rat have demonstrated that dopamine produced in the median eminence and secreted into the hypothalamic portal system accounts for most of the inhibition. These conclusions were reached after dopamine was measured in hypothalamic portal blood. Those concentrations were simulated by infusing similar levels of dopamine into animals that had been pretreated with an inhibitor of dopamine synthesis, α-methylparatyrisine. It was shown that 70 percent of prolactin activity could be blocked in these animals and the remaining 30 percent appears to arise from factors produced in the neurohypophysis.[44] Such studies have been confirmed in the monkey model but not in humans. The infusion studies, 0.02 to 8 mg/kg per min, had been carried out in humans for 3 to 4 hr. A dose-related suppression of prolactin occurs. Dopamine is not thought to cross the blood–brain barrier; however, the median eminence and adenonhypophysis lie outside this hypothetical barrier. It is noted that dopamine isolated from stalk portal blood is approximately 0.8 ng/ml, which is eightfold greater than that found in peripheral plasma (rhesus monkey model).

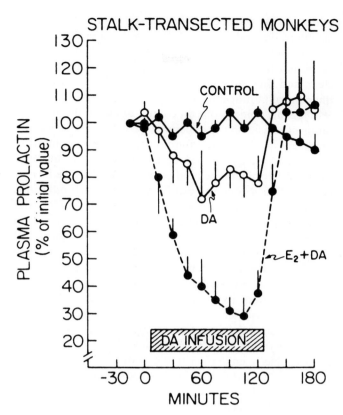

Figure 10–2. Inhibition of plasma prolactin levels by infusion of physiologic levels of dopamine in stalk-transected monkeys. Dopamine infusion rate was 0.1 mg/kg per min. *(Reproduced, with permission, from Neill JD, et al. Regulation of prolactin secretion. In: Blackwell RE, Chang RJ, eds.* Prolactin-Related Disorders, Proceedings of a Symposium. *New York, N.Y., Macmillan Healthcare Information, 1987: 5–14.)*

be secreted into portal blood, and receptors for GABA have been isolated on human lactotropes.[48] It should be noted that the prolactin-inhibitory effect of dopamine, however, is far greater than for GABA, and it has been suggested that these two agents serve different functions with the lactotrope. As an example, dopamine as opposed to GABA induces the storage of newly synthesized prolactin, which may be rapidly released after the withdrawal of dopamine. Although inhibition is the primary mechanism for the control of prolactin secretion, certain pharmacologic agents will produce acute prolactin release. Extensive studies were carried out attempting to isolate a prolactin-releasing factor, but none has been found. However, thyrotropin-releasing hormone (TRH) acutely stimulates the release of prolactin.[49] Further, compounds such as vasoactive intestinal peptide (VIP) and angiotensin II (ANG II) have been shown to stimulate the synthesis and release of prolactin.[50, 51] The injection of hormones such as TRH provokes a concomitant release of thyroid-stimulating hormone (TSH) and this response is modified by the presence of circulating T3 and T4. However, it should be noted that prolactin secretion can occur independent of TSH; eg, there is a short-term release of prolactin after suckling that is not accompanied by an increase in TSH secretion.

VIP purified from porcine duodenum is a 28-amino acid polypeptide found throughout the central nervous

Further evidence for dopamine's being the principal regulator of prolactin secretion comes from stalk-transection and suckling experiments in both monkeys and rats.[45,46] A brief decrease in exogenous dopamine infusion in primates leads to a large increase in prolactin secretion (Fig 10–3). In the rat model, a similar small decrease in hypothalamic secretion could be observed during simulated suckling.

At the cellular level, dopamine appears to act on lactotropes by way of both cyclic adenosine monophosphate (cAMP) and calcium-dependent mechanisms. High-affinity dopamine receptors have been isolated on lactotrope membranes and after establishment of the dopamine receptor complex inhibition of adenylcyclase occurs. This brings about a reduction in cAMP production that results in a decrease in prolactin secretion and an inhibition in prolactin synthesis.[47]

Other agents seem to be involved in the inhibition of prolactin secretion, the most prominent being γ-aminobutyric acid (GABA). GABA has been shown to

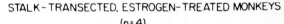

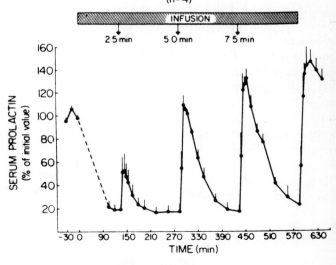

Figure 10–3. Effect of decreases in dopamine infusion on prolactin levels in the monkey. The study was carried out on four stalk-transected female monkeys pretreated with estrogen and infused with dopamine at a rate of 0.1 mg/kg per min. *(Reproduced, with permission, from Frawley LS, Neill JD.* Am J Physiol. *10:E778, 1984.)*

system. This hormone has been measured in hypothalamic blood samples and its release appears to be prostaglandin mediated. VIP may also be produced in the pituitary gland and may serve as an autocrine regulator of prolactin secretion[52] (Fig 10–4). ANG II has also been shown to stimulate prolactin release both in vivo and in vitro. ANG II receptors are found on lactotrope, implying a direct action. ANG II is an octapeptide found throughout the brain and its injection brings about a rapid release of prolactin that is in fact greater than TRH. This effect is blocked by coincubation of the ANG II antagonist saralasin.[53]

Other compounds have been shown to modify prolactin secretion; eg, serotonin causes an increase in prolactin levels, while treatment with the serotonin antagonist cyproheptadine blocks this response.[54] The opioids may also modify prolactin secretion by inhibiting dopamine turnover. Histamine, a hypothalamic neurotransmitter, also stimulates prolactin release by acting on the H_1 receptors. Stimulation of H_2 receptors, however, results in

inhibition of prolactin.[55] Likewise, neurotensin, a tridecapeptide, and substance P, a unidecapeptide, stimulate prolactin secretion. The precise role of any of these neurotransmitters in stimulating prolactin release is unclear, and they may serve little physiological purpose in the control of prolactin secretion.

To this point, prolactin control has been discussed in terms of classic neuroendocrinology, ie, dopamine's being produced in the tuberoinfundibular dopamine neurons of the arcuate nucleus, which delivers the catecholamine to the nerve termini of the median eminence, followed by secretion of these neurotransmitters with the hypothalamic portal system, which transfers them to the lateral lobes of the pituitary gland, where prolactin is inhibited. It would appear, however, that the mechanism for the control of prolactin secretion is much more complicated. First, retrograde flow has been demonstrated in the hypothalamic portal system as described earlier, and prolactin has been shown to affect its own secretion via a short feedback loop.[56] For instance, in the rat it has been shown that interventricular injection of prolactin results in an increased dopamine turnover in the median eminence. A high rate of turnover has been demonstrated during both lactation and pregnancy, and this is decreased by hypophysectomy or treatment with bromocriptine, a dopamine agonist. These data probably account for the observation that autoradiographs of prolactin-secreting tumors have been associated with reduced pituitary prolactin content. In addition, intrahypophyseal mechanisms are involved in the regulation of prolactin secretion. VIP is synthesized in the lactotrope from radiolabeled amino acids and has been shown to markedly stimulate prolactin secretion.[57] A number of reports have appeared, suggesting that gonadotropes may exert regulatory influence on the secretion of prolactin in vivo and in vitro. For instance, synthetic gonadotropin-releasing hormone (GnRH) has been shown to release prolactin in vivo and in vitro using rat superfusion and human pituitary monolayer culture systems. Incubation of GnRH with lactrotropes separated from large gonadotropes fails to increase prolactin secretion, whereas coaggregation of these two cell types restores the stimulatory effect of GnRH on prolactin.[58] Coincubation of a potent GnRH antagonist with native GnRH inhibited the release of prolactin, whereas coincubation of this antagonist with synthetic TRH failed to alter the release of prolactin.[59] Incubation of the α-chain of luteinizing hormone (LH) with fetal rat lactotropes stimulates the differentiation of these cells.[60] The incubation of β-LH or FSH with human pituitary cells in vitro fails to stimulate prolactin secretion; however, coincubation of antiserum to LH and FSH inhibited the GnRH-mediated release of prolactin.[61] In addition, GnRH-associated peptide (GAP), a peptide component of the precursor of GnRH, has been reported to inhibit prolactin secretion in the rodent model.[62]

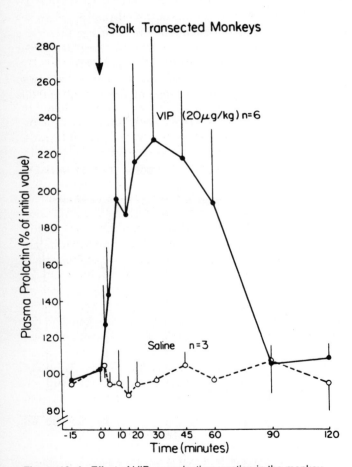

Figure 10–4. Effect of VIP on prolactin secretion in the monkey. The studies were carried out in six stalk-transected monkeys treated intravenously with 20 mg/kg VIP. *(Reproduced, with permission, from Frawley LS, Neill JD. Neuroendocrinology. 33:79, 1981.)*

Further, it is suggested that hypothalamic and sexually dependent diurnal changes in lactotrope proliferation can be induced by short-term estrogen treatment in oophorectomized and cycling rats. Long-term treatment with estradiol for up to 14 days prevents the diurnal change in lactotrope proliferation.[63] Finally, at the subcellular level it has been shown that the withdrawal of dopamine stimulates a rebound secretion of prolactin. Dopamine induces hyperpolarization of the lactotrope membrane. Electrophysiologic studies show that normal lactotropes exhibited a period of decreased calcium action potential firing after dopamine withdrawal and recovery of the resting membrane potential. Secretory rebound of prolactin can be prevented when dopamine is withdrawn in the presence of calcium channel blockers such as verapamil. It has recently been demonstrated that dopamine withdrawal elicits prolonged calcium rise, which supports the prolactin rebound phenomenon.[64] Therefore, prolactin appears to have a complex control mechanism that involves the classic neuroendocrine, paracrine, and autocrine components.

MILK EJECTION

The process of milk ejection involves both a neural and an endocrine arc. Suckling or stimulation of the nipple generates impulses in thoracic nerves 3, 4, and 5 that are transmitted via the spinal cord to the hypothalamus. This results in stimulation of the supraoptic and the paraventricular nuclei, the site of synthesis of the posterior pituitary hormones oxytocin and vasopressin (Fig 10–5). These compounds are released from the posterior pituitary, the median eminence, or into the cerebrospinal fluid. These compounds are carried by their respective neurophysins, which are carrier proteins synthesized as parts of large glycoprotein molecules called propresophysin and prooxyphysin, respectively.[65] These compounds are processed in small biologically active molecules during the

transport process within the axon. Storage of these molecules is carried out in the nerve terminals and they are released following depolarization in the presence of calcium. Subsequently, recycling occurs and retrograde transport up the neurohypophyseal stalk has been demonstrated. Arginine vasopressin is the principal compound involved in water metabolism; oxytocin, an octapeptide isolated by du Vigneaud in 1950, is a hormone that causes milk ejection by action on the myoepithelial cells of the breast.[66] This brings about contraction of these cells with ejection of the milk in the lactiferous ducts. The secretion of oxytocin is controlled by many central neurotransmitters; eg, acetylcholine stimulates both vasopressin and oxytocin via nicotinic cholinergic receptors, and application of acetylcholine to superoptic neurons will increase their firing rate.[67] Adrenergic pathways seem to stimulate oxytocin and vasopressin secretion, whereas β-adrenergic pathways inhibit it.[68] For instance, drugs such as propranolol, a β-adrenergic antagonist, will facilitate milk letdown. The opioid peptides are thought to influence neurohypophyseal hormone secretion at the nerve termini, and drugs such as morphine will decrease urinary flow as the result of an antidiuretic effect.[69] Further, opioids will inhibit oxytocin release by action on the axon terminals. For instance, naloxone, an opioid receptor antagonist, enhances the release of oxytocin.[70] Likewise, ANG II is a potent releaser of vasopressin, and TRH will increase the secretion of both vasopressin and oxytocin.[71,72] Cholecystokinin is found in the posterior pituitary and is markedly decreased by stimuli that effect vasopressin and oxytocin release. It is possible that these hormones may be co-secreted.[73] Finally, estrogen is a potent stimulator of the release of oxytocin carrier protein.[74]

While suckling results in the release of oxytocin, it also causes the release of prolactin (Fig 10–6). Suckling or breast manipulation leads to an elevation in prolactin levels within 40 min, and it should be noted that in lactating women the integrated baseline level of prolactin is elevated.[75] In the rodent model, this response can be mimicked by electrical stimulation of the mammary gland. It should be noted that both growth hormone and cortisol are also increased. The response is greatest in the immediate postpartum period and is attenuated over time. Lidocaine application of the nipple, which blocks nerve conduction, abolishes prolactin release.[76] Further, if two infants suckle simultaneously, the rise in prolactin is amplified. With the initiation of suckling, there is an 8- to 12-hr delay before milk secretion is fully stimulated, and the response seems to be correlated with the frequency and duration of vigorous suckling. There is, however, no correlation between prolactin release and milk yield. As mentioned earlier, suckling of the breast increases intramammary pressure bilaterally, and this is secondary to the action of oxytocin on myoepithelial cells.

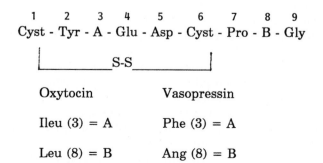

1   2   3   4   5   6   7   8   9

Cyst - Tyr - A - Glu - Asp - Cyst - Pro - B - Gly

|_____S-S_____|

Oxytocin	Vasopressin
Ileu (3) = A	Phe (3) = A
Leu (8) = B	Ang (8) = B

Figure 10–5. Structure of the octapeptides, oxytocin and vasopressin, showing the substitutions at the 3 and 8 positions.

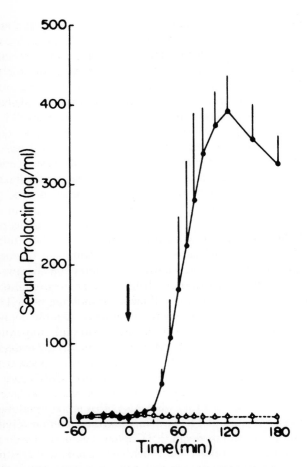

Figure 10–6. Effect of suckling on plasma prolactin levels in unrestrained, unanesthetized female rhesus monkeys. *(Reproduced, with permission, from Neill JD, et al. Regulation of prolactin secretion. In: Blackwell RE, Chang RJ, eds. Prolactin-Related Disorders: Proceedings of a Symposium. New York, N.Y., Macmillan Healthcare Information, 1987:5–14.)*

As stated, about 2 ng oxytocin are released per 2- to 4- sec pulse interval.[77] The synthesis and release of oxytocin are rapid. Ninety minutes after injection of a radioaminoacid into cerebrospinal fluid, radiolabeled oxytocin is released by exocytosis and electrical pulse activity has been measured in oxytocic neurons 5 to 15 sec before milk ejection. The response may be conditioned because the cry of an infant or various other perceptions associated with nursing can trigger activity in the central pathway. Thus, both oxytocin and prolactin are released in the response to suckling, but the patterns of release are different.[78] When nursing women are allowed to hold their infants but not breast-feed, serum prolactin concentrations do not increase despite the occurrence of the milk letdown reflex. Prolactin levels rise only with nursing. The increase in prolactin with nursing apparently is sufficient to

maintain lactogenesis and an adequate milk supply for the next feeding. This accounts for the ability of wet nurses to continue breast-feeding for years, even after menopause, once lactation is established.

Nursing behavior also appears to be effected by a host of hormones. For instance, both progesterone and estradiol are required for lactogenic stimulation of maternal behavior. Further, prolactin seems to have an effect on maternal behavior as well. Recently, placental lactogen-1 extracted from the rat was shown to be similar to rat prolactin in effecting the central lactogenic regulation of maternal behavior.[79]

ASSOCIATION BETWEEN HYPERPROLACTINEMIA AND AMENORRHEA

In 1898, Comte was the first to describe hypertrophy and hyperplasia in the human anterior pituitary during pregnancy.[80] The pituitary increases in size by approximately one third during gestation with hyperplasia of lactotropes being responsible for the majority of this hypertrophy. Pituitary hyperplasia is considered modulated by circulating levels of estrogen; also, it appears that previous pregnancy determines to some degree the size of the pituitaries in that primagravidas have glands averaging 820 mg while those of multigravidas weigh 954 mg.[81,82] Such observations have also been confirmed in animals. As a result of this hyperplasia, basal serum prolactin levels rise throughout normal gestation, attaining a level of 200 to 300 ng/ml at term.[83] Simultaneous with these events, the pituitary gland becomes refractory to exogenous GnRH administration.[84] The basal gonadotropin levels fall precipitously and doses of GnRH as large as 500 mg fail to exhibit any response midgestation.[85] It should be noted that 1 wk following pregnancy there is a blunting of the response of LH and FSH to the administration of 25 mg exogenous GnRH. In addition to these observations, other mechanisms may be involved in the generation of amenorrhea during the lactational state. For instance, prolactin has been shown to increase the turnover of central catecholamines, at least in the rat model, which might result in direct inhibition of GnRH neurons at the level of the arcuate nucleus.[86,87] On the other hand, it has been demonstrated that in some groups of patients hyperprolactinemia resulted in an increased responsiveness of the anterior pituitary to synthetic GnRH administration. Therefore, the pituitary gonadotropin in the nonpregnant state is capable of responding to GnRH in the face of hyperprolactinemia.

The relationship of prolactin to GnRH has been further explored in the rat model. In this species, GnRH has been shown to exert both the stimulatory and an inhibitory influence on prolactin secretion. Using pituitary grafted female rats in diestrous, the administration of GnRH at 60 and 120 min increased mean serum prolactin levels to the absolute amplitude of the hormone peaks and its mean half-life compared with the controls. These animals demonstrated diminished mean serum prolactin levels, absolute pulse amplitude, and frequency of prolactin peaks. These data suggest that GnRH significantly suppresses pulsatile prolactin secretion and that this effect is blunted by exposure to previous elevated circulating prolactin levels.[88] Finally, pulsatile GnRH administration stimulates normal cyclic ovarian function in amenorrheic lactating postpartum women. These results demonstrate that the pituitary gonadotropes and the ovary remain fully responsive to GnRH stimulation in amenorrheic breast-feeding women, and that chronic treatment with pulsatile GnRH can restore cyclic ovarian activity, ovulation, and normal luteal function. This response is as rapid as that seen with hypothalamic amenorrhea. Therefore, it must be concluded that postpartum amenorrhea seems to result entirely from reduced GnRH secretion.[89]

It has been suggested that prolactin can suppress ovarian function by binding to high-affinity prolactin receptors. Such speculation is supported by the finding that in the rat fetus ovarian interstitial cells contained a single class of specific receptors.[90] In this system, prolactin acts as a potent inhibitor of LH-mediated androgen synthesis. Because androgen substrates are derived from the thecal cell, a decrease in this production secondary to hyperprolactinemia could reduce estrogen synthesis. In addition, high-affinity prolactin receptors have been demonstrated on the surface membranes of granulosa cells.[91] These receptors are located near the basal lamina, which contain aromatase enzyme. As FSH induces aromatase enzyme activity in vitro, this effect is blocked by co-incubation of granulosa cells with prolactin in the range of 100 ng/ml. Also, in vivo prolactin blocks aromatase activity in rat preovulatory follicles. Therefore, these observations would suggest that hyperprolactinemia can disrupt the synthesis of androgen precursors and the induction of aromatase enzyme necessary for follicle growth. Although hyperprolactinemia may alter ovarian function in the rodent model, similar evidence in humans is less clear. It has been demonstrated that prolactin is present in the microenvironment of follicles in vitro and in the early follicular phase of the cycle a four- to sixfold increase of prolactin is found in fluid of developing follicles compared to blood. It is of interest that most follicles with a high concentration of prolactin were noted to have very low concentrations of estradiol.[92] Further, in patients with hyperprolactinemia exceeding 100 ng/ml, 100 percent of the follicles in the ovaries were atretic.[93] Finally, high levels of prolactin block basal and

human chorionic gonadotropin-stimulated estrogen synthesis in human follicles in vitro. These observations imply that, in humans, prolactin in excessive amounts such as those found in pregnancy are capable of disrupting normal follicular development.

Likewise, investigations using the MA-10 murine Leydig cell tumor line demonstrate that prolactin has a biphasic effect on Leydig cell steroidogenesis and signal transduction. This implies that the MA-10 cell possesses highly specific and biologically functional prolactin receptors that mediate direct and dose-dependent biphasic effects on hCG-induced progesterone secretion.[94]

RESOLUTION OF LACTATION

The postpartum lactational state is characterized by physiologic hyperprolactinemia that is maintained over a long period of time by discontinuous suckling. The mean levels of prolactin decrease progressively over the weeks despite breast-feeding. Physiologic postpartum hyperprolactinemia is achieved by selectively altering the endogenous secretory rate in each prolactin release episode with no change in the number of bursts of prolactin discharge or prolactin half-life as demonstrated by Nunley et al, using a cluster analysis and multiple parameter deconvolution analysis.[95] It was shown that a 24-hr mean serum prolactin concentration was significantly higher at 3 wk than at 3 mo (113 ± 12 vs 66 ± 15 mg/L), with significantly higher maximal prolactin peak heights (296 ± 36 vs 141 ± 44 mg/L) and peak areas (13 ± 3 vs 4 ± 1 mg/L per min). The half-life of prolactin at 3 wk was 29 ± 2.5 min and 26 ± 3 min at 3 mo. Lewis et al evaluated a large group of Australian women breast-feeding for an extended period of time. These patients had a mean of 322 days of anovulation and 289 days of amenorrhea. Less than 20 percent had ovulated and menstruated by 6 mo postpartum, the longest timed ovulation was 750 days, and the longest menstruation was 698 days.[96]

During pregnancy, gonadotropin secretion is inhibited. There is some evidence to suggest that hypothalamic β-endorphins may be responsible for the inhibition of the GnRH secretion. The inhibitory effect of endogenous opioids appears to increase during the postpartum period and diminish in nonlactating women. In addition, gonadotropin secretion increases, as does the responsiveness of gonadotrope to exogenous stimulation with GnRH. There is an increase in GnRH neuronal activity that has been suggested to resemble the onset of puberty and a reinstitution of sleep-entrained LH pulses between the second and fourth week postpartum, again being reminiscent of the events of menarche.

At the level of the breast, involution of the lactating mammary gland appears to be inhibited by the insulin-like growth factor system when evaluated by a transgenic mouse model, using the whey acetic protein (WAP) gene to direct expression of rat IGF-1 and human IGF binding protein-3 to mammary tissue during late pregnancy and throughout lactation. The level of expression of the transgenic material was seen in lobular alveolar cells evaluated by in situ hybridization. The role of IGF-1 and human IGF binding protein-3 was evaluated in the remodeling of mammary tissue during involution, and when compared to controls. The degree of apoptotic cells was lower in the WAP IGF-1 and the WAP-BP3 expressing mice. This strongly suggests that these factors modulate the involuntary process of the lactating mammary gland.[97]

SUMMARY

Lactation serves two purposes in mammals: (1) to furnish nutrition for the newborn; and (2) to provide natural contraception, which provides a survival advantage for the organism. Further, lactation is composed of two functional units: (1) milk secretion and letdown; and (2) milk ejection. These processes are controlled by a concert of central neurotransmitters acting through both the anterior and posterior pituitary. Prolactin is responsible for milk secretion and is held under tonic inhibition by hypothalamic dopamine. Prolactin, along with the growth hormone insulin, the thyroid hormones, and cortisol, acts on the alveolar unit of the breast to synthesize milk. The synthesized milk is released from the breast by suckling. This establishes a reflex arc that results in the release of oxytocin from the posterior pituitary and subsequently acts on the myoepithelial cells of the breast, resulting in milk ejection.

Elevated levels of prolactin result in amenorrhea secondary to alteration in the central nervous system catecholamine concentrations and by direct inhibitory activity on both the thecal and granulosa cells of the ovary. These mechanisms result in the disruption of folliculogenesis throughout pregnancy. The lactational state is characterized by physiological hyperprolactinemia, maintained by discontinuation of suckling. Mean serum prolactin levels triggered by suckling decreased over time. Fewer than 20 percent of individuals ovulate and menstruate by 6 mo postpartum.

REFERENCES

1. Peterson L.V. Lactation. *Physiol Rev.* 24:340, 1944
2. Riddle O, Bates R, Dykshorn S. The preparation, identification and assay of prolactin-A-hormone of the anterior pituitary. *Am J. Physiol.* 105:191, 1933
3. Meites J, Turner C. Studies concerning the mechanism controlling the initiation of lactation of parturition II: Why lactation is not initiated during pregnancy. *Endocrinology.* 30:719, 1942
4. Clifton K, Furth J. Ducto-alveolar growth in mammary glands of adreno-gonadectomized male rats bearing mammotropic pituitary tumors. *Endocrinology.* 66:893, 1960
5. Chen C, Meites J. Effects of estrogen and progesterone on serum and pituitary levels in ovariectomized rats. *Endocrinology.* 86:503, 1970
6. Kuhn N. Progesterone withdrawal as the lactogenic trigger in the rat. *J Endocrinol.* 44:39, 1969
7. Chiari J, Braun C, Spaeth J. Reporter of two cases of puerperal atrophy of the uterus with amenorrhea and persistent lactation. In: *Klinik der Geburtshilfe und Gynackologie.* Erlangen, Enke, 1855, p 371
8. Frommel R. Über puerperale atrophie des uterus. *Gynakologe.* 7:305, 1982
9. Argonz J, Del Castillo E. A syndrome characterized by estrogenic insufficiency, galactorrhea and decreased urinary gonadotropins. *J Clin Endocrinol Metab.* 13:79, 1953
10. Forbes A, Henneman P, Griswold G, Albright F. Syndrome characterized by galactorrhea, amenorrhea and low urinary FSH: Comparison with acromegaly and normal lactation. *J Clin Endocrinol Metab.* 14:265, 1954
11. Romrell LJ, Bland KI. Anatomy of the breast, axilla, chest wall, and related metastatic sites. In: Bland KI, Copeland EM, eds. *The Breast: Comprehensive Management of Benign and Malignant Diseases.* Philadelphia, Pa., W. B. Saunders, 1987: 17–35
12. Marshall W, Tanner J. Variations in pattern of pubertal changes in girls. *Arch Dis Child.* 63:136, 1969
13. Cowie AT. Backward glances. In: Yokoyama A, Mizuno H, Hagasawa H, eds. *Physiology of Mammary Glands.* Baltimore, Md., University Park Press, 1978: 43
14. Tonelli G, Sorof S. Epidermal growth factor: Requirement for development of cultured mammary glands. *Nature.* 285:250, 1980
15. Ichinose R, Nandi S. Influence of hormones on lobuloalveolar differentiation of mouse mammary glands in vitro. *J Endocrinol.* 35:331, 1996
16. Cowie A, Tindal J, Yokoyama A. The induction of mammary growth in the hypophysectomized goat. *J. Endocrinol.* 34:184, 1966
17. Lyons WR. Hormonal synergism in mammary growth. *Proc Roy Soc Biol.* 149:303, 1958
18. Going JJ, Anderson TJ, Battersby S, et al. Proliferative and secretory activity in human breast during natural and artificial menstrual cycles. *Am J Pathol.*130:193, 1988
19. Talwalker P, Meites T. Mammary lobulo-alveolar growth induced by anterior pituitary hormones in adrenoovariectomized-hypophysectomized rats. *Proc Soc Exp Biol Med.* 107:880, 1961.
20. France J, Seddon R, Liggins G. A study of a pregnancy with low estrogen production due to placental sulfatase deficiency. *J Clin Endocrinol Metab.* 36:19, 1973
21. Topper Y, Freeman C. Multiple hormone interactions in the developmental biology of the mammary gland. *Physiol Rev.* 60:1049, 1980

22. Elias J. Effect of insulin and cortisol on organ cultures of adult mouse mammary gland. *Proc Soc Exp Biol Med.* 101:500, 1959

23. Fleet I, Goode J, Hamon M, et al. Secretory activity of goat mammary glands during pregnancy and the onset of lactation. *J. Physiol.* 251:763, 1975

24. Weiss G, Facog E, O'Byrne E, et al. Secretion of progesterone and relaxin by the human corpus luteum at midpregnancy and at term. *Obstet Gynecol.* 50:679, 1977

25. Martin R, Glass M, Wilson G, Woods K. Human alphalactalbumin and hormonal factors in pregnancy and lactation. *Clin Endocrinol (Oxf).* 13:223, 1980

26. Hartmann P, Trevethan P, Shelton J. Progesterone and oestrogen and the initiation of lactation in ewes. *J Endocrinol.* 59:249, 1973

27. Bruce J, Ramirez V. Site of action of the inhibitory effect of estrogen upon lactation. *Neuroendocrinology.* 6:19, 1978

28. Hearn J. Pituitary inhibition of pregnancy. *Nature.* 241:207, 1973

29. Brun del Re R, del Pozo E, deGrandi P, et al. Prolactin inhibition and suppression of puerperal lactation by a Brergocriptine (CB 154): A comparison with estrogen. *Obstet Gynecol.* 41:884, 1973

30. Vonderhaar BK. Studies on the mechanism by which thyroid hormones enhance alpha-lactalbumin activity in explants from mouse mammary glands. *Endocrinology.* 140:1423, 1977

31. Hwang P, Guyda H, Friesen H. A radioimmunoassay for human prolactin. *Proc Natl Acad Sci USA.* 68:1902, 1971

32. Guyda H, Hwang P, Friesen H. Immunologic evidence for monkey and human prolactin. *J Clin Endocrinol Metab.* 32:120, 1971

33. Truong AT, Duez C, Belayew A, et al. Isolation and characterization of the human prolactin gene. *EMBO J.* 3:429, 1984

34. Goffin V, Shiverick KT, Kelly PA, Martial JA. Sequence-function relationships within the expanding family of prolactin, growth hormone, placental lactogen, and related protein in mammals. *Endocr Rev.* 17:385, 1996

35. Ben-Jonathan N, Mershon JL, Allen DL, Steinmetz RW. Extrapituitary prolactin: Distribution, regulation, functions, and clinical aspects. *Endocr Rev.* 17:639, 1996

36. Suh HK, Frantz AG. Size heterogeneity of human prolactin in plasma and pituitary extracts. *J Clin Endocrinol Metab.* 39:928, 1974

37. Farkouh NH, Packer MG, Frantz AG. Large molecular PRL with reduced receptor activity in human serum: High proportion in basal state and reduced after TSH. *J Clin Endocrinol Metab.* 48:1026, 1979

38. Whitaker PG, Wilcox T, Lind T. Maintained fertility in a patient with hyperprolactinemia due to big-big prolactin. *J. Clin Endocrinol Metab.* 53:863, 1981

39. Blackwell RE. In: Wallach EE, Kempers RD, eds. *Modern Trends in Infertility and Conception Control,* vol 4. *Diagnosis and Management of Prolactinomas.* Chicago, Ill., Year Book Medical Publishers, 1988: 197–208

40. Neill JD, Luque EH, Mulchahey JJ, Nagy G. Regulation of prolactin secretion. In: Blackwell RE, Chang RJ, eds. *Prolactin-Related Disorders.* New York, N.Y., Macmillan Healthcare Information, 1987: 5–14

41. Blackwell RE, Guillemin R. Hypothalamic control of adenohypophyseal secretions. *Annu Rev Physiol.* 35:357, 1973

42. MacLeod RM. Influence of norepinephrine and catecholamine-depleting agents on the synthesis and release of prolactin and growth hormone. *Endocrinology.* 85:916, 1969

43. Leblanc H, Lachelin G, Abu-Fadil S, Yen SSC. Effects of dopamine infusion on pituitary hormone secretion in humans. *J Clin Endocrinol Metab.* 43:669, 1976

44. Gibbs OM, Neill JD. Dopamine levels in hypophyseal stalk blood in the fat are sufficient to inhibit prolactin secretion in vitro. *Endocrinology.* 102:1895, 1978

45. Plotsky PM, deGreef WF, Neill JD. In situ voltametric microelectrodes: Release during simulated suckling. *Brain Res.* 250:251, 1982

46. Plotsky PM, Neill JD. Interactions of dopamine and thyrotropin-releasing hormone in the regulation of prolactin release in lactating rats. *Endocrinology.* 111:168, 1982

47. Schettini G, Cronin MJ, MacLeon, RM. Adenosine 3' 5' monophosphate (cAMP) and calcium-calmodulin interrelation in the control of prolactin secretion: Evidence for dopamine inhibition of cAMP accumulation and prolactin release after calcium mobilization. *Endocrinology.* 112:1801, 1983

48. Grossman A, Delitala G, Yeo T, Besser GM. GABA and muscimol inhibit the release of prolactin from dispersed rat anterior pituitary cells. *Neuroendrocinology.* 32:145, 1981

49. Vale W, Blackwell RE, Grant G, Guillemin R. TRF and thyroid hormones on prolactin secretin by rat pituitary cells in vitro. *Endocrinology.* 93:26, 1973

50. Matsushita N, Kato Y, Shimatsu A, et al. Effects of VIP, TRH, GABA and dopamine on prolactin release from superfused rat anterior pituitary cells. *Life Sci.* 32:1263, 1983

51. Dufy-Barbe L, Rodriguez F, Arsaut J, et al. Angiotensin-II stimulates prolactin release in the rhesus monkey. *Neuroendocrinology.* 35:242, 1982

52. Shimatsu A, Kao Y, Matsushita N, et al. Effect of prostaglandin E on vasoactive intestinal polypeptide release from the hypothalamus and on prolactin secretion from the pituitary in rats. *Endocrinology.* 113:2059, 1983

53. Aguilera G, Hyde CL, Catt KJ. Angiotensin-II receptors and prolactin release in pituitary lactotrophs. *Endocrinology.* 111:1045, 1987

54. Clemons JA, Roush ME, Fuller RW. Evidence that serotonin neurons stimulate secretion of prolactin-releasing factor. *Life Sci.* 22:2209, 1978

55. Knigge U, Dejgaard A, Wollesen F, et al. Histamine regulation of prolactin secretion through H_1-H_2-receptors. *J Clin Endocrinol Metab.* 55:118, 1982

56. Bergland R, Page R. Can the pituitary secrete directly to the brain? (Affirmative anatomical evidence.) *Endocrinology.* 102:1325, 1978

57. Hagen TC, Arnaout MA, Scherzer WJ, et al. Antisera to vasoactive intestinal polypeptide inhibit basal prolactin release from disbursed anterior pituitary cells. *Neuroendocrinology.* 43:641, 1986

58. Denef C, Andries M. Evidence for panacine interaction between gonadotrophs and lactotrophs in pituitary cell aggregates. *Endocrinology.* 112:813, 1983

59. Blackwell RE, Rodgers-Neame NT, Bradley EL, Asch RH. Regulation of human prolactin secretion in gonadotropin releasing hormone in vitro. *Fertil Steril.* 56:26, 1986

60. Begot M, Hemming FJ, DuBois PM. Induction of pituitary lactotrope difference by luteinizing hormone alpha subunit. *Science.* 226:566, 1984

61. Blackwell RE, Garrison PN. Inhibition of prolactin secretion by antiserum to the alpha- and beta-subunits of gonadotropin. *Am J Obstet Gynecol.* 156:863, 1987

62. Nikolics K, Mason AJ, Szonyl E, et al. A prolactin-inhibiting factor within the precursor for human gonadotropin-releasing hormone. *Nature.* 316:511, 1985

63. Hashi A, Mazawa S, Chen SY, et al. Estradiol-induced diurnal changes in lactotroph proliferation and their hypothalamic regulation in ovariectomized rats. *Endocrinology.* 137:3246, 1996

64. Ho MY, Kao JPY, Gregerson KA. Dopamine withdrawal elicits prolonged calcium rise to support prolactin rebound release. *Endocrinology.* 137:3513, 1996

65. Brownstein MJ, Russell JT, Gainter H. Synthesis, transport, and release of posterior pituitary hormones. *Science.* 207:373, 1980

66. du Vigneaud V. Hormones of the posterior pituitary gland: Oxytocin and vasopressin. *Harvey Lect.* 50:1, 1956

67. Poulain DA, Wakerley WB. Electrophysiology of hypothalamic magnocellular neurones secreting oxytocin and vasopressin. *Neuroscience.* 7:773, 1982

68. Jijima K, Ogawa T. An HRP study on cell types and their regional topography within the locus coeruleus innervating the supraoptic nucleus of the rat. *Acta Histochem.* 67:127, 1980

69. Clarke G, Wood P, Merrick L, Lincoln DW. Opiate inhibition of peptide release from the neurohumoral terminals of hypothalamic neurones. *Nature.* 282:746, 1979

70. Bicknell RJ, Leng G. Endogenous opiates regulate oxytocin but not vasopressin secretion from the neurohypophysis. *Nature.* 298:161, 1982

71. Sladek CD, Joynt RJ. Role of angiotensin in the osmotic control of vasopressin release by the organ-cultured rat hypothalamo-neurohypophyseal system. *Endocrinology.* 106:173, 1980

72. Weitzman RE, Firemark HM, Glatz TH, Fisher DA. Thyrotropin-releasing hormone stimulates release of arginine vasopressin and oxytocin in vivo. *Endocrinology.* 104:904, 1979

73. Beinfeld MC, Meyer DK, Brownstein MJ. Cholecystokinin octapeptide in the rat hypothalamo-neurohypophyseal system. *Nature.* 288:376, 1980

74. Amico JA, Seif SM, Robinson AG. Oxytocin in human plasma: Correlation with neurophysin and stimulation with estrogen. *J. Clin Endocrinol Metab.* 52:988, 1981

75. Howie P, McNeilly A, McArdle T, et al. The relationship between suckling-induced prolactin response and lactogenesis. *J Clin Endocrinol Metab.* 50:670, 1980

76. Tyson J. Nursing and prolactin secretion: Principal determinants in the mediation of puerperal infertility. In: Crosignani P, Robyn C, eds. *Prolactin and Human Reproduction.* New York, N.Y., Academic Press, 1977: 97

77. Lincoln O, Wakerley J. Electrophysiological evidence of the activation of supraoptic neuronics during the release of oxytocin. *J Physiol (Lond).* 242:533, 1974

78. Brands C, Rozenberg S, Meuris S. Advances in physiology of human lactation. In Angeli A, Bradlow H, Dogliotti L, eds. Endocrinology of the breast. *Ann NY Acad Sci.* 464:66, 1986

79. Bridges RS, Robertson MC, Shiu RP, et al. Central lactogenic regulation of maternal behavior in rats: Steroid dependence, hormone specificity, and behavioral potencies of rat prolactin and rat placental lactogen I. *Endocrinology.* 138:756, 1997

80. Comte L. Contribution a l'etude de l'hypophyse humaine. These de doctorat, Lausanne, 1898

81. Furth J, Clifton KG, Gadsen EL, Buffett RF. Dependent and autonomous mammotrophic pituitary tumors in rats: Their somatic features. *Cancer Res.* 18:608, 1956

82. Erdheim J, Stumme E. Uber der schwanger-schaftsveranderung de hypophyse. *Zeigler's Beitr Path Anat.* 46:1, 1909

83. Biswas S, Rodeck CH. Plasma prolactin levels during pregnancy, *Br J Obstet Gynaecol.* 83:683, 1976

84. Reyes FI, Winter JSD, Faiman C. Pituitary gonadotropin function during human pregnancy: Serum FSH and LH levels before and after LHRH administration. *J Clin Endocrinol Metab.* 42:590, 1976

85. Jeppsson S, Rannevik G, Kullander S. Studies on the decreased gonadotropin response after administration of LH/FSH-releasing hormone during pregnancy and the puerperium. *Am J Obstet Gynecol.* 120:1029, 1974

86. Fuxe KK, Anderson T, Hoxfelt LF, et al. Prolactin–monoamine interaction in rat brain and their importance in regulation of LH and prolactin secretion. In: Robyn C, Harter M, eds. *Progress in Prolactin Physiology and Pathology.* Amsterdam, Elsevier/North Holland, 1978: 95

87. Gudelsky GA, Porter JC. Release of dopamine from tuberoinfundibular neurons into pituitary stalk blood after prolactin or haloperidol administration. *Endocrinology.* 106:526, 1980

88. Lafuente A, Marco J, Esquifino AI. Effects of luteinizing hormone-releasing hormone on pulsatile prolactin secretion in adult hyperprolactinemic female rats. *Soc Exp Biol Med.* 211:251, 1996

89. Zinman MJ, Cartledge T, Tomai T, et al. Pulsatile GnRH stimulates normal cyclic ovarian function in amenorrheic lactating postpartum women. *J Clin Endocrinol Metab.* 80:2088, 1995

90. Magoffin DA, Erickson GF. Prolactin inhibition of LH stimulated androgen synthesis in ovarian interstitial cells cultured in defined medium: Mechanisms of action. *Endocrinology.* 111:2001, 1982

91. Ben-David M, Schenker JG. Human ovarian receptors to human prolactin: Implications in infertility. *Fertil Steril.* 38:182, 1982

92. McNatty KP, Sawers RS, McNeilly AS. A possible role for prolactin in control of steroid secretion by the human graafian follicle. *Nature.* 250:653, 1974

93. McNatty KP. Relationship between plasma prolocatin and the endocrine microenvironment of the developing human antral follicle. *Fertil Steril.* 32:433, 1979

94. Weiss-Messer E, Ber R, Barkey RJ. Prolactin and MA-10 Leydig cell steroidogenesis: Biphasic effects of prolactin and signal transduction. *Endocrinology.* 137:5509, 1996

95. Nunley WC, Urban RJ, Kitchin JD, et al. Dynamics of pulsatile prolactin release during the postpartum lactational period. *J Clin Endocrinol Metab.* 72:287, 1991

96. Lewis PR, Brown JB, Renfree MB, Short RV. The resumption of ovulation and menstruation in a well-nourished population of women breastfeeding for an extended period of time. *Fertil Steril.* 55:529, 1991

97. Neuenschwander S, Schwartz A, Wood TL, et al. Involution of the lactating mammary gland is inhibited by the IGF system in a transgenic mouse model. *J Clin Invest.* 97:2225, 1996

Chapter 11

THE OVARY

Bruce R. Carr

The ovaries serve as the source of ova and the hormones that regulate female sexual function. The rapid growth of a single follicle that will become dominant and eventually ovulate and the consistent regularity of this process for an average of 38 yr is truly a remarkable phenomenon. The cyclic nature of the female reproductive process is dependent upon the ability of the ovary to change in both structure and function. The complex compartmentalization in the ovary that allows follicular growth is regulated by both endocrine and local factors produced within the ovary. Estrogens and progestins, the principal steroid hormones secreted by the ovary, promote growth and differentiation of the uterus, fallopian tubes, and vagina, as well as other signs of sexual maturation. Alteration in this complex process can result in disorders of the ovary, as well as the development of sexual precocity, disorders of the menstrual cycle, androgen excess, and infertility. As a consequence of aging, the majority of remaining follicles undergo atresia such that by age 50 few follicles remain. Estrogen levels then decline, resulting in atrophy and regression of secondary sexual characteristics and the onset of menopause.

FETAL OVARY EMBRYOGENESIS

The development of the gonads takes place early in fetal life. While sexual differences between fetuses are not seen until development of the gonads, the genetic sex is determined at conception. The bipotential gonadal analgen, which gives rise to either the ovary or testis, can be identified in human embryos within 1 mo of conception.[1] Three principal cell types play key roles in the developing ovary: (1) coelomic epithelial cells, which are derived from the gonadal ridge and later differentiate into the granulosa cells; (2) mesenchymal cells of the gonadal ridge, which give rise to the ovarian stroma; and (3) primordial germ cells, which arise from the endoderm of the yolk sac and differentiate into ova.

During the third week of gestation, the primordial germ cells arise, as previously stated, in the yolk sac at the caudal end of the ovary. During the sixth week, the primordial germ cells migrate into the underlying mesenchyme and become incorporated into the primary sex cords. Primordial cell migration can be traced by cytochemical techniques due to their high alkaline phosphatase activity. The mechanisms that control the ameboid movement of primordial cells to the gonadal ridge are still being investigated; however, chemotactic substances secreted by the gonadal anlagen are thought to play a role in regulating the migratory process.[2] During migration, the continued replication of the germ cells acts to amplify the original number of cells from the yolk sac. In the human embryo, approximately 1000 germ cells are present at 5 wk that by 8 wk may be increased to 600,000 cells.[3]

The sex of the migrating primordial cells can often be predicted by the status of the sex chromatin. Specifically in female germ cells, one X chromosome is inactivated during migration to the gonadal ridge.[4] As proposed by Lyon,[5] a dose compensation by X chromosome inactivation prevents aneuploidy. Two X chromosomes are required for normal development of the ovary. In individuals with a 45,X karyotype, initial ovarian development occurs with primordial germ cells appearing in the gonad, but follicular development is reduced and the rate of atresia is accelerated so that only a fibrous streak remains at the time of birth.[6]

Histologic recognition of the ovary cannot be made until 10 to 11 wk of fetal life, whereas the fetal testis is distinguishable somewhat earlier. After the primordial cells reach the fetal gonad, they continue to proliferate by successive mitotic division (Fig 11–1). The ovary will contain a finite number of germ cells, a maximal number of 6 to 7 million oogonia being reached by the twentieth wk of gestation.[3] Follicular maturation is continuous following midgestation and progresses through the antrum stage. Afterward, a majority of the germ cells are lost by the process known as atresia such that only 1 million remain at birth.[7]

During early fetal development, the ovary is in close proximity to the mesonephros (a temporary functioning kidney). The mesonephros influences both testicular and

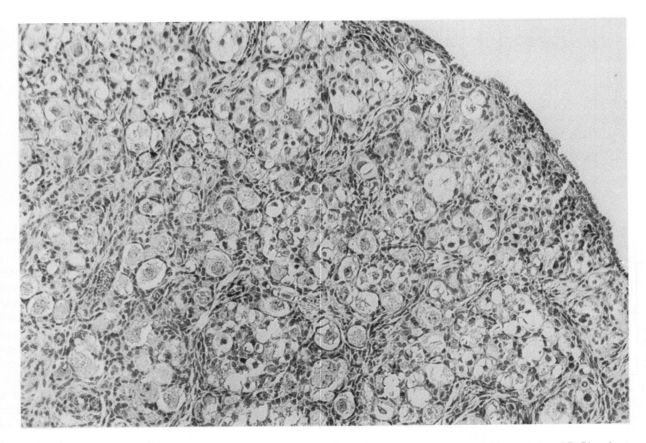

Figure 11–1. Histologic section of an ovary from a 16-wk human fetus. *(Reproduced, with permission, from Carr BR. Disorders of the ovary and female reproductive tract. In: Wilson JD, Foster DW, eds.* William's Textbook of Endocrinology, *8th ed. Philadelphia, Pa., W. B. Saunders, 1992:733–798.)*

ovarian differentiation and is required for the completion of ovarian development.[8] The ovarian–mesonephros association is retained during early ovarian differentiation, with the mesonephros tissue regressing slowly. In the human, the ovary is invaded by mesonephric cells that form the medulla and force the germ cells to occupy the ovarian cortex. The oogonia continue to undergo mitosis until they enter meiosis, whereafter they are converted to primary oocytes, which begins as early as the twelfth wk of gestation.[9] The primary oocytes initiate meiosis, but meiosis is arrested in the diplotene or resting stage of the first meiotic division and remains there until the onset of ovulation at puberty, where the first meiotic phase is completed (Fig 11–2).

The second meiotic phase will be initiated following fertilization by spermatozoa. The arrestation of meoisis appears to be controlled by substances produced locally in the ovary. Meiosis-preventing substance (MPS), also known as oocyte maturation inhibitor (OMI), is produced by granulosa cells and arrests the oocyte in the diplotene stage.[10] After the primary oocyte is arrested at the diplotene stage of meiosis, it is surrounded by a layer of primitive granulosa cells giving rise to the primordial follicle, the morphologic

marker of fetal ovarian differentiation. A basement membrane is formed that separates the primordial follicle from the surrounding stroma. Later, meiosis is triggered to continue by meiosis-inducing substance (MIS).[11]

The conversion of oogonia into primary oocytes and subsequent formation of primordial follicles is continued until 6 mo after birth. Oocytes that are not incorporated into follicles undergo degeneration, which explains why the majority of oocytes have disappeared by birth. The primordial follicles are first located at the inner part of the cortex near the medulla. At approximately 20 wk of fetal life, the follicles begin to grow under the influence of gonadotropins. The need for gonadotropic influence for normal development of the ovary is suggested by the reduced follicular development seen in both the anencephalic human fetus and in monkeys following fetal hypophysectomy.[12] The primordial follicle is first surrounded by layers of granulosa cells giving rise to the development of primary follicles. By the seventh mo of gestation, follicle maturation reaches the antrum stage, and is located at the outer part of the cortex.

The early human ovary, by the eighth wk of gestation, has the capacity to produce estrogens from androgens, but

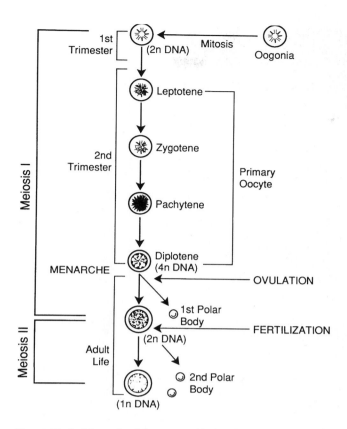

Figure 11–2. Life cycle of the oocyte. During the first trimester of fetal life, the oogonium undergoes mitosis. During the second trimester, meiosis I is initiated but arrested at the diplotene stage (4n DNA). Following menarche, at the time of ovulation, meiosis resumes in one ovum with the formation of the first polar body (2n DNA). Meiosis II is initiated at the time of fertilization and completed with the formation of the second polar body (1n DNA). Fusing with the male pronucleus restores the nuclear content to 2n DNA. *(Reproduced, with permission, from Carr BR. Disorders of the ovary and female reproductive tract. In: Wilson JD, Foster DW, eds.* William's Textbook of Endocrinology, *8th ed. Philadelphia, Pa., W. B. Saunders, 1992: 733–798.)*

produces only small amounts of steroids when examined in vitro.[13] Luteinizing hormone (LH)/human chorionic gonadotropin (hCG) binding sites are not detected in human fetal ovaries, and LH, follicle-stimulating hormone (FSH), and hCG do not stimulate steroidogenesis in vitro, suggesting that steroidogenic enzyme expression at this stage of development is independent of gonadotropin control.[14] Even though the human fetal ovaries possess the enzymes required for steroidogenesis, as demonstrated using isolated cells in vitro, there is no evidence that fetal ovaries secrete significant quantities of steroid hormones in vivo.[15]

The primitive form of the genital ducts, namely, the Wolffian ducts (male) and the Müllerian ducts (female), do not arise simultaneously. The Wolffian duct develops first from the mesonephros and in the fetus destined to be a female may participate in the formation of the Müllerian ducts. The loss of the Wolffian duct is due to

the lack of locally produced androgen. While degeneration of the Wolffian duct begins soon after appearance of the ovary, it is not completed until the beginning of the third trimester of pregnancy.[16] In the female, the Müllerian duct gives rise to the fallopian tubes, uterus, and the upper one third of the vagina. By 10 wk, the uterus has differentiated into an upper part, the corpus, and the lower part, the cervix. Although the cervix and corpus are initially the same length, the cervix is two thirds of the total length by birth. The development of the Müllerian duct is independent of the gonad or hormonal secretion because it develops normally in fetuses without gonads.[11]

CHILDHOOD AND PREMENARCHEAL OVARY

The mean ovarian weight increases from 250 mg at birth to reach a mean weight of approximately 4000 mg by menarche. The increase in size and weight of the ovaries are due to an increase in the amount of stroma, size of follicles, and number of follicles that occurs due to the continuing growth of the ovary.[17] The final maturation of the ovarian follicles occurs during puberty in response to increasing levels of gonadotropins. The two major hormones responsible for follicular development and the initiation of ovulation are FSH and LH.

There are significant variations in the levels of gonadotropin during the different stages of life in women (Fig 11–3). Indeed, the hypothalamus, pituitary, and ovary of the fetus, newborn, and prepubertal child are functional and capable of secreting hormones. During the second trimester of fetal development, the plasma levels of gonadotropins rise to levels similar to those observed in menopause.[18] This peak in fetal gonadotropin levels is associated with maximal development of follicles. In addition, during the second trimester of pregnancy the hypothalamic–pituitary axis (gonadostat) undergoes maturation and becomes more sensitive to the high levels of circulating steroid hormones, namely, estrogen and progesterone, which are secreted by the placenta.[19,20] These steroids cause gonadotropins to fall to low levels prior to birth. Following birth, the levels of gonadotropins rise abruptly due to separation from the placenta, which results in a decrease in estrogen and progestogen levels and loss of negative feedback.[21] The elevated levels of gonadotropins in the newborn persist for the first few months of life, declining to low levels by 1 to 3 yr of life.[21] An explanation for the low gonadotropin levels during childhood years is the increased sensitivity of the hypothalamic–pituitary axis to circulating low levels of gonadal steroids.[20] In addition, evidence obtained from normal children suggests that the prepubertal hypothalamic axis is much more sensitive to estrogen treatment than the adult feedback mechanism.[22] There appears also to be an intrinsic role of the central nervous system

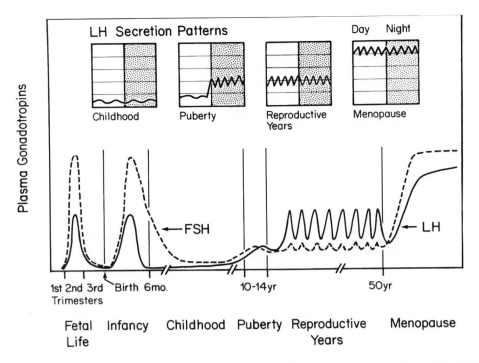

Figure 11–3. Pattern of gonadotropin secretion during different stages of life in women. Abbreviations: FSH, follicle stimulating hormone; LH, luteinizing hormone. The secretory patterns of LH during the waking hours (clear area) and night (stippled area) for each stage are indicated in the upper inserts. *(Reproduced, with permission, from Carr BR, Wilson JD. Disorders of the ovary and female reproductive tract. In: Wilson JD, Braunwald E, Isselbacher KJ, et al, eds. Harrison's Principles of Internal Medicine, 12th ed. New York, N.Y., McGraw-Hill, 1991: 1776–1795.)*

(CNS) in decreasing gonadotropin levels.[20] This is suggested by the fall in gonadotropins that occurs in the absence of a gonad or in children with gonadal dysgenesis between ages 5 and 11.[23] The ability of gonadotropin-releasing hormone (GnRH) (also known as LH-releasing hormone [LHRH]) to stimulate the level of gonadotropins in agonadal children suggests that a central nonsteroidal substance is acting to inhibit the hypothalamic axis.[24] However, no physiologic inhibitors of GnRH secretion have been identified in humans or primates.

Although basal gonadotropin secretion in prepubertal females is diminished, small pulses are detected at 2- to 3-hr intervals.[25] During puberty, the pituitary becomes more sensitive to infusions of LHRH, and the LH and FSH response to LHRH increases in an age-dependent manner. The progression into puberty appears to be preceded by three major developments: (1) adrenarche (onset of adrenal androgen secretion); (2) decreased sensitivity of the hypothalamic–pituitary axis; and (3) gonadarche, the increased release of LHRH from the medial basal hypothalamus, leading to increased pituitary gonadotropin release and estrogen secretion by the ovary.

The increase in secretion of adrenal androgens occurs prior to significant quantitative and qualitative alterations in gonadotropin secretion. The levels of androstenedione, dehydroepiandrosterone, and dehydroepiandrosterone sul-

fate increase in children beginning at approximately 6 to 8 yr of age. A decline in the expression of 3β-hydroxysteroid dehydrogenase in the reticularis zone of the human adrenal occurs after age 5, which may explain in part the rise in adrenal androgen levels.[26] This increased activity and secretion by the adrenal cortex is termed adrenarche and is thought to be primarily under the control of corticotropin (ACTH) secretion. A variety of other peptide and protein hormones have been proposed as alternative adrenal androgen-stimulating factors involved in the initiation of adrenarche but conclusive evidence for such a hormone does not currently exist.[27] Adrenal androgens (preandrogens) actually have little androgenic effect until they are converted to more potent androgens (true androgens) in peripheral or target tissues. True androgens (testosterone and dihydrotestosterone) can then exert biologic effects in target tissues that express androgen receptors. Adrenal androgens and their metabolites may be responsible for the initial growth spurt and development of axillary and pubic hair. Because of the close association of the onset of adrenarche and gonadarche, some believe adrenarche is an important initiating event in the increased secretion of LHRH and gonadotropin by the hypothalamic–pituitary axis. However, there is considerable evidence that the controlling mechanisms that initiate and regulate adrenarche and gonadarche are independent. In girls with hypothalamic amenorrhea, such as Kallmann syndrome (olfactogenital dysplasia), or in hypergonadotropic hypogonadism (gonadal dysgenesis), adrenarche occurs in the absence of gonadarche. Premature pubarche (also called premature adrenarche) with premature development of pubic and axillary hair before age 8 is not associated with premature gonadarche. In children with absence of adrenarche due to adrenal hypofunction (Addison disease), gonadarche still occurs.[20]

Factors that regulate the onset of gonadarche and increased secretion of LH and FSH are complex but are believed to be initiated by a decreased responsiveness of the CNS–hypothalamic–pituitary axis to circulating levels of steroid hormones. Other potential initiators of puberty include loss of neuronal inhibition or increase of neuronal stimulation by neurotransmitters. One of the first signs of increased pubertal gonadotropin release is a sleep-associated surge of LH release[28] (Fig 11–3). Similar sleep-related LH pulses are also reported to occur in children with idiopathic precocious puberty, agonadal subjects during the return of elevation of gonadotropins after age 11, and women with anorexia nervosa during stages of recovery.[29] An increased secretion of estrogen occurs, leading to a positive feedback in LH secretion and eventually to ovulation and then menarche.

Several lines of evidence suggest that the attainment of a pulsatile secretion of LHRH is critical for the initiation of puberty. In rhesus monkeys where the hypothalamus has been destroyed, gonadotropin hormones decline. If these monkeys are treated with pulsatile LHRH given at hourly intervals, LH and FSH pulsatile secretion is reestablished.[30] In addition, infantile female rhesus monkeys treated with pulsatile injections of LHRH undergo pubertal maturation.[30] In women at puberty, an increase in pulse frequency and amplitude of LH release occurs. The infusion of pulsatile LHRH will initiate puberty in women with sexual infantilism (Kallmann syndrome).[31] Finally, the administration of LHRH analogs causes regression of pubertal changes in girls with isosexual precocious puberty.[32,33]

The changes in FSH, inhibin, LH, and estrogen levels during puberty in females are illustrated in Figure 11–4. The levels of FSH rise early in puberty while those of LH lag behind, rising later.[34] Prior to puberty the ratio of FSH/LH is >1, and at the end of puberty is reversed (ie, FSH/LH <1) until menopause, when the FSH/LH ratio is again >1. The level of estradiol (more than 90 percent derived from the ovary) increases progressively throughout puberty, apparently following the increase in serum FSH levels. The level of bioactive LH is greater during early puberty than is immunologic LH. This discrepancy may be due to alterations in the amount of glycosylation of LH that alter immunoreactivity.[35] In addition to ovarian feedback on the hypothalamus and pituitary by steroid hormones, ovarian-derived peptide factors

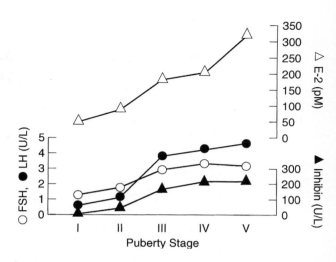

Figure 11–4. The mean serum FSH, inhibin, LH, and estradiol (E₂) levels during the stages of puberty in girls. *(Adapted in part, with permission, from Burger HG, et al, Serum inhibin concentrations rise throughout normal male and female puberty. J Clin Endocrinol Metab. 67:689, 1988.)*

such as inhibin also appear to be involved in regulating gonadotropin levels. Recently, it has been reported that serum inhibin levels increase and parallel FSH levels during puberty in girls (Fig 11–4).[36] Inhibin is secreted in two forms, A and B, each with a molecular weight of 32,000. It is postulated that FSH stimulates granulosa cells to secrete inhibin and that the levels rise until adulthood, at which time the inhibin–FSH negative feedback relationship is established (described later).

The development of female secondary sexual characteristics occurs at puberty as the result of increased release of estradiol. The rise in estrogen levels is responsible for the initiation of accelerated growth (growth spurt) and female secondary characteristics, ie, development of breasts, maturation of the female internal and external genitalia, and female habitus. Androgens derived from the ovary (and, to a lesser degree, adrenal androgens) regulate axillary and pubic hair development. The age of initiation of puberty, as well as the rate of progression, will vary within the population (see Chap 5). Most girls start with breast development between ages 10 and 11, followed by the development of pubic and axillary hair. A growth spurt ensues and a peak growth rate is attained at a median age of 11.4 yr. In part, the increase in height and growth during puberty is regulated by hormonal changes that include growth hormone, insulin-like growth factor-I (IGF-I), and estrogen. Growth hormone stimulates production of IGF-I, particularly within the liver. IGF-I levels increase progressively during puberty. The increase in IGF-I is mediated indirectly by an increase in sex steroids, which are believed to stimulate an increased secretion of growth hormone.[37] If, on the other hand, IGF-I levels do not rise, a growth spurt does not occur, as demonstrated by African pygmies.[38]

The culmination of puberty is the onset of regular, spontaneous, predictable, cyclic ovulatory menses. The age of menarche is variable and determined in part by socioeconomics as well as genetic factors, general health, nutrition, geography, and altitude.[20,39] In the United States, the mean age of menarche has decreased at a rate of 3 to 4 mo per decade over the last 100 yr and is now 12.7 yr, a decrease believed due primarily to improved nutrition.[40] Frisch and colleagues analyzed growth and development of 169 girls. They observed that at a mean or "critical" body weight of 48 kg, menarche occurred.[40,41] However, other investigators as well as Frisch proposed that additional factors are also important in determining the onset of menarche and the maintenance of ovulatory menses. These include: percent of body fat, percent of body water, ratio of lean to fat, and lean body mass, as well as body "shape." Obese girls with a body weight 20 to 30 percent above ideal experience earlier menarche than do women with normal weight. In contrast, women with decreased body fat associated with participation in certain sports or ballet, malnutrition, and chronic debilitating diseases commonly experience delayed menarche. Although the theory of "critical" body weight is still speculative and controversial, the theory of a metabolic signal related to body composition appears to be an important factor in the maturation or activation of the hypothalamic LHRH pulse generator[20] (see Chap 5).

OVARY OF THE REPRODUCTIVE YEARS

Structure of the Adult Ovary

Adult human ovaries are oval with the following dimensions: length, 2 to 5 cm; width, 1.5 to 3 cm; thickness, 0.5 to 1.5 cm. The weight of each ovary of normal women during the reproductive years is 5 to 10 g, average 7 g. The ovaries lie in approximation with the posterior and lateral pelvic wall and are attached to the posterior surface of the broad ligament by a peritoneal fold named the mesovarian. Blood vessels, nerves, and lymphatics tra-

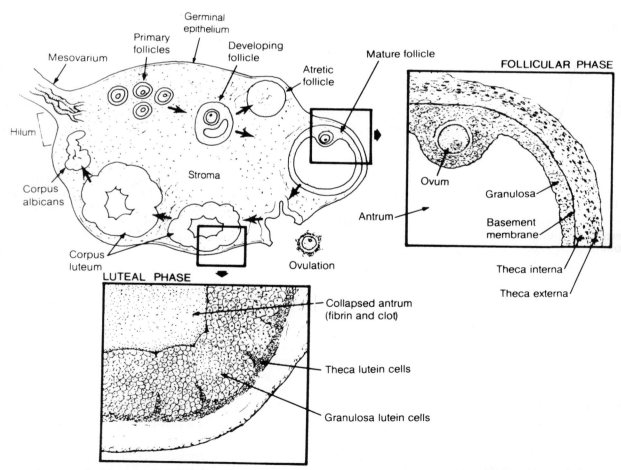

Figure 11–5. Developmental changes in the adult ovary during a complete menstrual cycle. *(Reproduced, with permission, from Carr BR, Wilson JD. Disorders of the ovary and female reproductive tract. In: Wilson JD, Braunwald E, Isselbacher KJ, et al, eds.* Harrison's Principles of Internal Medicine, *12th ed. New York, N.Y., McGraw-Hill, 1991: 1776–1795.)*

verse the mesovarian and enter the ovary at its hilum.[42] The ovary is comprised of three distinct regions: an outer cortex containing the ovarian follicles, a central medulla consisting of ovarian stroma, and an inner hilum around the area of attachment of the ovary to the mesovarian. The components and function of the adult ovary are illustrated schematically in Figure 11–5.

Follicles. Follicles are embedded in the connective tissue of the ovarian cortex and are either inactive or growing.[43] The majority of follicles are inactive throughout the reproductive life of women and are termed primordial follicles (Fig 11–6). In each cycle, several primordial follicles initiate growth and undergo significant changes in size, structure, and function. The growing follicles are divided into five stages: primary, secondary, tertiary, graafian, and atretic. The first three stages of growth can occur in the absence of

gonadotropin secretion and thus appear to be under intraovarian control.[44] However, for a follicle to enter the tertiary stage there is a dependence upon gonadotropin secretion.

During each cycle, an ovum is selected from the pool of primordial follicles. Primordial follicles are composed of a single layer of granulosa cells and a single immature oocyte arrested in the diplotene stage of the first meiotic division. These follicles are separated from the surrounding stroma by a thin basal lamina (basement membrane). The oocyte is surrounded by a single layer of spindle-shaped cells with cytoplasmic processes that reach the basal lamina, providing a route for transfer of nutrients. Because of the basal lamina, the oocyte and granulosa cells do not have a blood supply and thus exist in a microenvironment without direct contact with other cells.

One of the first signs of follicular recruitment is a change in the spindle-shaped cells that surround the follicle.

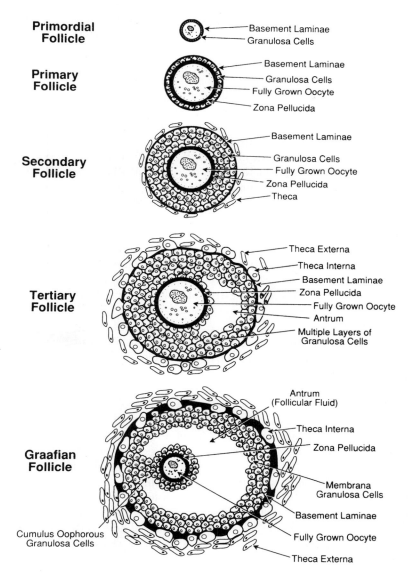

Figure 11–6. Structure and classification of the ovarian follicle during growth and development. *(Adapted in part, with permission, from Erickson GF, Magoffin DA, Dyer CA, Hofeditz C. The ovarian androgen cells: A review of structure/function relationships. Endocrine Rev. 6:371, 1985.)*

These cells become cuboidal and undergo successive mitotic division, giving rise to a multilayered stratum granulosa or zona granulosa. In addition, the oocyte enlarges and secretes a mucoid substance containing glycoproteins that surrounds the oocyte. This substance is called the zona pellucida and can be seen to separate the granulosa cells from the oocyte (see Chap 1). These changes represent the differentiation of the primordial follicle into a primary follicle (Fig 11–6).

A secondary follicle results from the proliferation of granulosa cells, development of the theca, and the completion of the oocyte growth. The proliferation of granulosa cells is associated with the differentiation of stroma cells outside the basal lamina. These cells become arranged in concentric perifollicular layers and constitute the theca (Fig 11–6). The theca interna are the cells adjacent to the basal lamina. The theca cells that merge with the surrounding stroma are named the theca externa. During the development of the secondary follicle, the follicle acquires an independent blood supply that consists of arterioles that terminate at the basal lamina in a capillary bed. The granulosa cells and oocyte remain avascular because the blood supply does not penetrate the basement membrane. One distinct morphologic feature of the granulosa cells, called the Call–Exner bodies, appears during the development of the secondary follicle. Little is known about how they form or their physiologic importance.

Formation of the tertiary follicle is associated with further hypertrophy of the theca and the appearance of a fluid-filled space among the granulosa cells named the antrum (Fig 11–6). This fluid consists of a plasma filtrate and the secretory products of granulosa cells, some of which are found in concentrations greater than those in peripheral blood.[45] Associated with the continuing hypertrophy of the granulosa and theca cells is the development of specialized contacts between cells known as gap junctions.[46] Gap junctions allow small molecules to pass from one cell to another, allowing for cell-to-cell communication and synchronized coordination of ovarian function.

FSH stimulates the tertiary follicle to rapidly increase in size and form the mature or graafian follicle (Fig 11–6). During this stage, the granulosa and oocyte are still contained within the basal lamina and remain devoid of direct vascularization. The antral fluid increases in volume and the oocyte, surrounded by an accumulation of granulosa cells called the cumulus oophorus, occupies a polar position within the follicle. At this stage of development, the mature graafian follicle is ready to release the ova during a process called ovulation.

Follicles that progress beyond primordial follicles will either develop into a dominant mature graafian follicle destined to ovulate or degenerate through a process called atresia. As a result of atresia, the oocyte and granulosa cells within the basal lamina are replaced by fibrous tissue. The theca cells, in contrast to the cells within the basal lamina, do not die but return to the pool of cells consisting of ovarian interstitial or stromal cells.[42] Atresia is generally thought to occur secondary to the absence of certain hormones or growth factors that were formed by the mature dominant follicle. It is now confirmed that atresia of follicles is an apoptotic process or programmed cell death.[47]

Ovum. Oocyte growth continues and meiosis is completed in the mature graafian follicle. The oocyte during this period increases in diameter from 20 to 120 μmol/L. In addition, there is an accumulation of nutritional, as well as genetic, information that will be required by the developing zygote following fertilization. Oocyte growth is linear until the follicle reaches the tertiary stage and then ceases to grow further.[48]

Granulosa cells play an integral role in the growth of the oocyte.[48] The oocyte is surrounded by a group of granulosa cells called the corona radiata that interact with the oocyte by gap junctions. The zona pellucida (consisting of three glycoproteins) forms between the corona radiata and the oocyte during formation of the primary follicle and exhibits a variety of biologic functions including receptors for sperm and blockage of polyspermy and improves the ability of the embryo to move freely in the fallopian tube on its passage to the uterus (see Chap 1).[49]

The resumption of meiosis occurs following the preovulatory surge of LH (Fig 11–2). The ability of oocytes of mature follicles to undergo meiosis when placed in culture supports the hypothesis of an in vivo inhibitory influence for meiosis prior to ovulation. The resumption of meiosis in the mature oocyte is characterized by loss of the nuclear or germinal membrane, condensation of chromatin, separation of homologous chromosomes, and arrest at metaphase II. Meiosis is completed with the release of the second polar body at the time of fertilization. High concentrations of estradiol in follicular fluid are required for normal meiotic maturation.[50]

Stroma. The ovarian stroma consists of three specific cell types: contractile cells; connective tissue cells, which function to give structural support; and interstitial cells. The interstitial cells secrete sex steroid hormones (principally androgens) and undergo morphologic changes in response to LH and hCG.[45] Interstitial cells are derived from mesenchymal cells of the ovarian stroma.[51] The human ovary contains four major categories of interstitial cells: (1) primary interstitial; (2) secondary interstitial; (3) thecal interstitial; and (4) hilus cells.

The primary interstitial cells are the first interstitial cells to develop in the ovary and are identifiable only between 12 to 20 wk of fetal life.[52] These cells resemble premature Leydig cells of the fetal testis and have an ultrastructural appearance of steroid-secreting cells. Secondary interstitial cells are derived from the thecal cells of atretic follicles that undergo hypertrophy.[53] These large epithelial cells maintain the active steroidogenic features of thecal interstitial cells from which they are derived and retain their responsiveness to LH. However, as opposed to thecal interstitial cells, secondary interstitial cells are innervated and respond to catecholamines that stimulate structural changes and hormone secretion.[54]

Thecal interstitial cells are present in all tertiary follicles and represent the most widely studied interstitial cell type. Thecal interstitial cells develop from mesenchymal cells that differentiate when secondary follicles form. Thecal interstitial cells develop LH receptors and are the site of androgen secretion.[54] Cell transformation from mesenchymal cells is influenced locally by the secondary follicle and appears to be under control of gonadotropin stimulation.[55] During development, these cells markedly increase in size and develop ultrastructural changes char-

acteristic of steroid-secreting cells. Thecal interstitial cells give rise to secondary interstitial cells following follicular atresia as stated earlier.

The hilum of the ovary contains a specific type of interstitial cell known as the hilus cell. These cells contain crystalloids of Reinke and are virtually indistinguishable morphologically from Leydig cells of the testes.[56] Hyperplastic or neoplastic changes in hilus cells occasionally result in virilization associated with excessive amounts of testosterone secretion. Indeed, normal hilus cells have been shown to synthesize and secrete testosterone in response to LH.[53] The function of hilus cells is unclear but because of their close association with nerve fibers and blood vessels they may influence ovarian function.

Corpus Luteum. The mature corpus luteum (yellow body) develops from a mature graafian follicle following ovulation (Figs 11–5 and 11–7). A series of biochemical

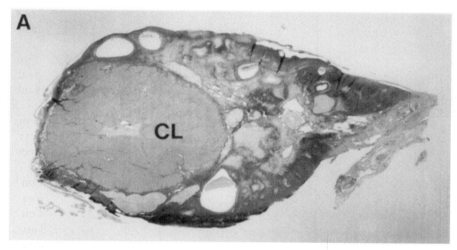

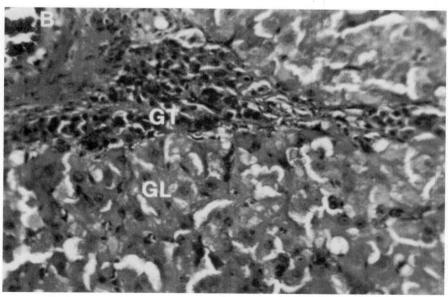

Figure 11–7. A. Photomicrograph of a human corpus luteum (CL). **B.** The larger, pale-staining granulosa-lutein cells (GL) can readily be distinguished from the smaller, dark-staining theca-lutein cells (TL). *(Reproduced, with permission, from Carr BR. Disorders of the ovary and female reproductive tract. In: Wilson JD, Foster DW, eds.* William's Textbook of Endocrinology, *8th ed. Philadelphia, Pa., W. B. Saunders, 1992: 733–798.)*

and morphologic changes, known as luteinization, occur in the cells of the granulosa and theca interna at the time of the preovulatory surge of LH. These cells undergo hypertrophy and exhibit increased nuclear activity under the influence of LH.[57] The basement membrane separating the granulosa from the theca breaks down after ovulation has occurred. Thereafter, vascularization of the granulosa cells occurs from invading blood vessels and capillaries leading to formation of the corpus luteum. The events leading to the development of the corpus luteum have been well described.[58] First, proliferation of the granulosa cells occurs during the day after ovulation. Capillary invasion of the granulosa cells begins on day 2 following ovulation and reaches the central cavity by day 4. Hemorrhage into the cavity can occur on any day, and fibroblasts appear in the central cavity by day 5. The center of the mature corpus luteum, the antrum, is filled with a fibrin clot. Maximal capillary enlargement or dilation is attained by days 7 to 8 at a time that corresponds to maximal progesterone secretion (up to 40 mg/day).[59] The cells that comprise the corpus luteum are derived from cells that compose the follicle, namely, the granulosa and theca. The granulosa cells enlarge and are called granulosa-lutein cells while smaller cells called theca-lutein cells develop from theca cells. In addition, the so-called K cells are found scattered throughout the corpus luteum and are believed to represent macrophages.[60]

In the absence of pregnancy, the corpus luteum undergoes degeneration. This process is called luteolysis and is first apparent by the eighth day following ovulation. During luteolysis, the granulosa-lutein cells shrink and the theca cells appear more prominent.[61] Later, both cells undergo cell death, possibly involving the process of apoptosis. The remaining corpus luteum consists of dense connective tissue called the corpus albicans.

Ovarian Physiology

Hypothalamic–Pituitary–Ovarian Axis. The hypothalamus plays a critical role in the complex interplay that allows reproductive function in women (Fig 11–8).[62] The hypothalamus communicates with the pituitary by a portal vascular system. The primary direction of blood flow is from the hypothalamus to the pituitary. This vascular system thus acts as a conduit for the hormones released from the hypothalamus that can control pituitary function. Interruption of this hypothalamic–pituitary connection leads to a decline in gonadotropin levels and eventually to atrophy of the ovaries and a decline in ovarian hormone secretion. Evidence also suggests that a retrograde flow occurs in the portal vessels, providing a short feedback loop of the pituitary on hypothalamic function.[63]

LHRH, a decapeptide, is the principal hypothalamic releasing factor that regulates reproductive func-

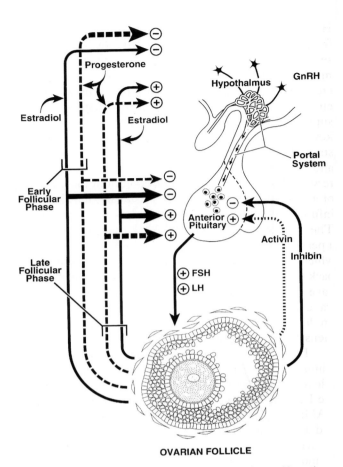

Figure 11–8. The regulation of feedback mechanisms of hypothalamic–pituitary–ovarian axis. (—, estradiol; --- progesterone.) Primary action (large arrow), secondary action (small arrow).

tion. It was originally proposed that separate releasing hormones existed for LH and FSH; evidence now supports the view that there is only one GnRH, LHRH. Moreover, LHRH analogs modulate both LH and FSH but neither selectively.[64] The variations in response of LH and FSH following LHRH infusions are believed to be due to the feedback exerted by ovarian hormones on the hypothalamic–pituitary axis. The release of LHRH by the hypothalamus is influenced by neurons from other regions of the brain whose terminals end in the arcuate nucleus.[30] Neurotransmitters such as epinephrine and norepinephrine increase LHRH release whereas dopamine and serotonin, as well as endogenous opioid peptides, inhibit LHRH release.[65] A variety of other hormones, in particular gut-related peptide hormones, also modulate LHRH release.[65]

The half-life of LHRH is 2 to 4 min, and metabolic clearance of LHRH averages approximately 800 L/m² per day.[66] Because LH and FSH are secreted in pulsatile bursts, it follows that LHRH release is also pulsatile.[30]

Hypothalamic–pituitary portal venous blood collected from monkeys and sheep demonstrates that LHRH is secreted in a pulsatile fashion at frequencies of 70 to 90 min.[67,68] Investigators have shown that the pulsatile secretion pattern of LHRH is a prerequisite for normal secretion of pituitary gonadotropins.[30] This concept is supported by experimental evidence in the rhesus monkey by stimulating gonadotropin secretion following destruction of the arcuate nucleus. The reactivation of LH and FSH release requires that LHRH be infused at intervals of approximately 1 hr. Infusion of LHRH pulses of a lesser or greater frequency or following continuous infusion failed to stimulate the release of LH and FSH.[69] The pulsatile release of LHRH is required but plays only a permissive role in the midcycle surge of gonadotropins, which is regulated primarily by ovarian hormone feedback at the level of the pituitary.[70] These observations have been confirmed in humans. The pulsatile administration of LHRH to women with LHRH deficiency reproduces the hormonal changes observed during the menstrual cycle, resulting in ovulation and pregnancy.[71]

LHRH acts on the gonadotropes of the pituitary to stimulate the release of LH and FSH. LHRH stimulates release of gonadotropins following high-affinity binding to the LHRH receptor via cyclic adenosine monophosphate (cAMP)-independent pathways that requires calcium and activation of protein kinase C.[72,73] LHRH regulates (1) synthesis and storage of gonadotropins; (2) activation or movement of gonadotropins from reserve to a pool ready for secretion; and (3) immediate release of gonadotropins. LH, FSH, thyroid-stimulating hormone (TSH), and hCG are glycoproteins composed of two polypeptide chains named α and β. There appears to be a single gene for the expression of the α-subunit that is similar for all glycoproteins and contains 92 amino acids.[74] The β-chains for each glycoprotein hormone are unique and provide specific biologic activity for each hormone. The α- and β-subunits must combine for full expression of biologic activity.[75] The largest of these hormones is hCG, which is similar to LH except for an additional 30 amino acid residues and a large carbohydrate moiety at the carboxyl end.[75] The half-life of β-hCG is the longest, followed by FSH and then LH, and is determined in part by the higher sialic acid content of the two former hormones.[76]

Three types of secretory patterns can be distinguished due to the variations and frequency of gonadotropin release: "Trigintan" or "circatrigintan" are low-frequency changes during the normal menstrual cycle occurring every 30 days.[77] "Diurnal" are intermittent frequency changes in gonadotropin secretion that recur every 24 hr. These changes are minimal in adult women but are marked during sleep in girls at the initiation of puberty as discussed previously.[28] "Circhoral" are high-frequency changes in gonadotropin secretion characterized by pulses of gonadotropins at approximately every hour.[30]

Follicle growth, ovulation, and maintenance of the corpus luteum are regulated by the coordinated secretion of FSH and LH. As discussed previously, the release of FSH and LH requires continuous pulsatile release of LHRH from the hypothalamus. In addition, the release of LH and FSH is affected both positively and negatively by estrogen and progesterone, and at least two gonadal protein hormones also modulate FSH release. Whether estrogen and progesterone stimulate or inhibit gonadotropin release depends upon the level of exposure and duration of the steroid.[78]

Ovarian steroid and peptide hormones can exert a negative feedback on both the hypothalamus and pituitary (Fig 11–8). A decline in ovarian hormone secretion during menopause or following castration causes increased secretion of LH and FSH. The negative feedback exerted by estrogen on the pituitary appears to be dependent upon the concentration of estrogen.[79] Progesterone inhibits FSH and LH at high concentrations and primarily at the level of the hypothalamus.[80] Both inhibin and follistatin selectively inhibit FSH secretion[62] (see Chap 9).

Gonadal steroid and peptide hormones are also able to exert positive effects on gonadotropin secretion (Fig 11–8). This positive feedback is important in the regulation of the LH surge required to induce ovulation and is regulated by a sharply rising level of estrogen in the late proliferative phase (see Chap 12). There are two requirements for the positive effect of estrogen on production of LH: (1) an estradiol concentration of over 200 pg/ml; and (2) a sustained level of estradiol for at least 48 to 50 hr.[81–83] Progesterone is also responsible for the midcycle FSH surge.[81] Progesterone at low concentrations will stimulate LH release but only after previous exposure to estrogen.[78] In addition, granulosa cell secretion of activin stimulates FSH release (Fig 11–8).[62]

Ovarian Hormones

Steroid Hormones

PROGESTOGENS. The principal progestogens are 21-carbon steroids (see Fig 11–9) and include pregnenolone, progesterone, and 17α-hydroxyprogesterone. Pregnenolone has little biologic activity but is important as the precursor of all steroid hormones. Progesterone is the principal secretory steroid of the corpus luteum and is responsible for induction of secretory activity and decidual development in the endometrium of the estrogen-primed uterus. Progesterone is required for the implantation of the fertilized ovum and maintenance of pregnancy. Progesterone also inhibits uterine contractions, increases the

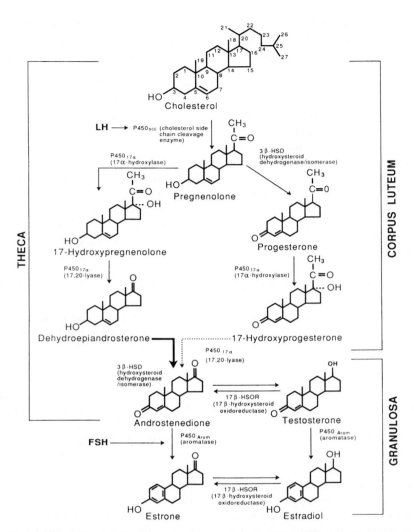

Figure 11–9. Principal pathways of steroid hormone biosynthesis in the human ovary. Although each cell type of the ovary contains the complete enzyme complement required for the formation of estradiol from cholesterol, the amounts of the various enzymes and consequently the predominant hormones formed differ among the cell types. The major enzyme complement for the corpus luteum, theca, and granulosa cells are shown by the brackets; as a consequence, these cells produce predominantly progesterone and 17-hydroxyprogesterone (corpus luteum); androgen (theca); and estrogen (granulosa). The major sites of action of LH and FSH in mediating this pathway are shown by the horizontal arrows. The dotted line emphasizes that the metabolism of 17-hydroxyprogesterone is limited in the human ovary. *(Reproduced, with permission, from Carr BR. Disorders of the ovary and female reproductive tract. In: Wilson JD, Foster DW, eds.* William's Textbook of Endocrinology, *8th ed. Philadelphia, Pa., W. B. Saunders, 1992: 733–798.)*

viscosity of cervical mucus, promotes glandular development of the breast, and increases basal body temperature. 17α-Hydroxyprogesterone is also secreted by the corpus luteum but has little biologic activity.[84]

ESTROGENS. Estrogens are 18-carbon steroids characterized by the presence of an aromatic A ring, a phenolic hydroxyl group at C-3, and either a hydroxyl group (estradiol) or a ketone group (estrone) (see Fig 11–9). The principal and most potent estrogen secreted by the ovary is 17β-estradiol. Although estrone is also secreted by the ovary, the principal source of estrone is from the extraglandular

conversion of circulating androstenedione.[85] Estriol (16-hydroxyestradiol) is the most abundant estrogen in urine and arises from hepatic metabolism of estrone and estradiol. Obesity and hypothyroidism are associated with an increase in estriol formation.[86] Catechol estrogens are formed by hydroxylation of estrogens at the C-2 or C-4 position. The physiologic role of catechol estrogen is unclear at present; however, low body weight and hypothyroidism are associated with increased formation of catechol estrogen.[87] Estrogens, through activation of their receptor, promote development of the secondary sexual characteristics of women and promote uterine growth, thickening of the vaginal mucosa, thinning of the cervical mucus, and development of the ductal system of the breast.[84]

ANDROGENS. The ovary (principally thecal cells) secretes a variety of 19-carbon steroids including dihydroepiandrosterone, androstenedione, testosterone, and dihydrotestosterone. The principal 19-carbon steroid secreted by thecal cells is androstenedione (see Fig 11–9). Part of the androstenedione is released into plasma and the remainder converted to estrone by the granulosa cells. In addition, androstenedione can be converted to estrone or testosterone in peripheral tissues. Only testosterone and dihydrotestosterone are true androgens capable of high-affinity binding to the androgen receptor. Thus, the ability to convert androstenedione to active sex steroids is critical for activation of target tissues' androgen receptors. Excessive production of 19-carbon steroids by the ovary or adrenal can cause sexual ambiguity in the newborn and hirsutism or virilization in women.

Steroid Hormone Biosynthesis. Steroids formed by the ovary, as well as other steroid-producing organs, are derived from cholesterol. There are several sources of cholesterol that can provide the ovary with substrate for steroidogenesis. These include (1) plasma lipoprotein cholesterol; (2) cholesterol synthesized de novo within the ovary; and (3) cholesterol from stores of cholesterol esters within lipid droplets. Considerable evidence suggests that the primary source of cholesterol utilized by the ovary is derived from the uptake of lipoprotein cholesterol.[88,89] In the human ovary, low-density lipoprotein (LDL) cholesterol is the principal source of cholesterol utilized for steroidogenesis.[88] LH stimulates the activity of adenylate cyclase, increasing cAMP production, which serves as a second messenger to increase LDL receptor mRNA and the binding and uptake of LDL cholesterol, as well as the formation of cholesterol esters.[88,89] cAMP-activated steroidogenic acute regulatory (StAR) protein increases the intracellular transport of cholesterol to the inner mitochondria membrane.[90] The conversion of cholesterol to pregnenolone within the mitochondria is the rate-limiting step in ovarian steroidogenesis and is catalyzed by the cholesterol side-chain cleavage enzyme complex consisting of cytochrome P_{450} side-chain cleavage (P_{450SCC}), adrenodoxin, and flavoprotein.[91]

The granulosa, theca, and corpus luteum cells possess the complete enzymatic complement required for steroid hormone formation. The preferred pathway of steroid synthesis in the human corpus luteum is the Δ^4 pathway, which involves the conversion of pregnenolone to progesterone (see Fig 11–9). Recent studies suggest that in the human ovarian follicle the Δ^5 pathway is the preferred pathway for the formation of androgens and estrogens because theca cells of the human ovary metabolize 17α-hydroxypregnenolone to a greater extent than 17α-hydroxyprogesterone.[92] However, the predominant steroid secreted differs among each of these cell types so that the corpus luteum forms progesterone and 17α-hydroxyprogesterone, whereas the theca and stromal cells secrete androgen and the granulosa cells secrete predominantly estrogen. The determination of which steroid is secreted by each cell type includes the level of gonadotropin and gonadotropin receptors; the activity, amount, and expression of steroidogenic enzymes; and the vascularity and availability of LDL cholesterol. Evidence suggests that the rate of steroid production during the menstrual cycle is related to the amount of follicular and luteal cell content of five key steroid-metabolizing enzymes: P_{450SCC}, 3β-hydroxysteroid dehydrogenase (3β-HSD), 17α-hydroxylase cytochrome P_{450} ($P_{45017\alpha}$), aromatase P_{450} ($P_{450AROM}$), and 17β-hydroxysteroid dehydrogenase (17β-HSD), type 1.[93–95] These enzymes are responsible for the conversion of cholesterol to pregnenolone, pregnenolone to progesterone, pregnenolone and progesterone to androgens, androgens to estrogens, and estrone to estradiol (Figs 11–10 and 11–11). LH acts acutely to regulate the first step in steroid hormone biosynthesis by regulating the conversion of cholesterol to pregnenolone, and FSH acts to increase the conversion of androgens to estrogens. Chronically, these hormones act to regulate the expression of the necessary steroid-metabolizing enzymes. Recently, the immunohistochemical localization, in situ hybridization, and expression of mRNA species encoding P_{450SCC}, 3β-HSD, $P_{45017\alpha}$, $P_{450AROM}$, and 17β-HSD type 1 have been determined in human follicles and corpora lutea throughout the menstrual cycle (Fig 11–10).[93–95] The expression of P_{450SCC} mRNA is present in most stages of follicular development and located in both granulosa and theca interna cells of the follicle. There is a marked increase in the expression of P_{450SCC} mRNA in corpora lutea in both the theca-lutein and granulosa-lutein cells as localized by immunohistochemistry. There is little expression of 3β-HSD mRNA in the follicle, whereas there is marked expression of 3β-HSD in corpora lutea. The increase in 3β-HSD and P_{450SCC} in the corpus luteum is consistent with the enormous increase in the secretion of progesterone during the luteal phase of the cycle. The pattern of expression of $P_{45017\alpha}$ is similar in follicles and corpora lutea (Fig 11–10). $P_{45017\alpha}$ can be localized only in the theca interna cells of the follicle and the theca-lutein cells of the corpus luteum but is virtually absent from granulosa and granulosa-lutein cells. The expression of $P_{450AROM}$ is seen only in mature follicles and is localized in granulosa cells, consistent with the marked rise in estrogen biosynthesis prior to ovulation. $P_{450AROM}$ mRNA is

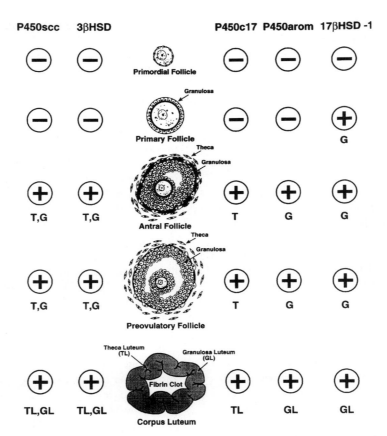

Figure 11–10. Expression and localization of key enzymes involved in ovarian steroidogenesis. P_{450scc} (cholesterol side-chain cleavage enzyme) 3βHSD (3 beta-hydroxysteroid dehydrogenase), P_{450c17} (177-hydroxylase), $P_{450AROM}$ (aromatase), 17β-HSD-1, 17-beta hydroxysteroid dehydrogenase type 1. (–, absent; +, present; T, theca cell; G, granulosa cell.) (*Reproduced, with permission, from Carr BR, Disorders of the Ovary and Female Reproductive Tract. In: Wilson JD, Foster DW, eds.* Williams Textbook of Endocrinology. *Philadelphia, Pa: W. B. Saunders Co. In press.*)

greatest in corpora lutea and localized in granulosa-lutein cells (Fig 11–10). 17β-HSD type 1 is localized in granulosa cells and converts estrone to estradiol (Fig 11–10). The results of studies on the expression of the mRNA encoding the various steroidogenic enzymes are consistent with previous reports of enzymatic activity in human ovaries.[94] The amount of immunoreactive $P_{450AROM}$ and mRNA was also shown to be stimulated by FSH in human granulosa cells.[96] These observations help explain the rationale for the predominance of estrogen secreted by granulosa cells and the corpus luteum, the secretion of androgens by the theca, and secretion of progesterone by both types of corpus luteum cells of the ovary. The reports of the steroidogenic capacities of isolated granulosa and theca cells led to the two cell–two gonadotropin theory (Fig 11–11), which states that the theca cells produce C_{19} steroids in response to LH (predominantly androstenedione) and that FSH stimulates granulosa cells to aromatize the preformed androstenedione to produce estrone. The final step involves 17β-HSD type 1, which converts estrone to estradiol.[97]

The availability of LDL cholesterol also plays a regulatory role in the levels of steroid hormones secreted in the various cell types of the human ovary. The granulosa cells of the follicle are avascular and devoid of a blood supply as discussed previously. The granulosa cells do not have ready access to plasma LDL and because of its large molecular weight only very low levels of LDL are found in follicular fluid bathing granulosa cells[88,98] (Fig 11–12). Thus, the granulosa cells have limited ability to form progesterone in large quantities characteristic of the luteal phase. Following ovulation, extensive vascularization of the follicle takes place, providing increased amounts of cholesterol to the luteinized granulosa cells. The increased availability of LDL to the granulosa-lutein cells now provides the ability for these cells to secrete increased quantities of progesterone during the luteal phase of the menstrual cycle (see Chap 12). Corpus luteum tissue treated with hCG stimulates progesterone secretion in vitro, as well as the number of LDL binding sites.[99] In addition, women with abetalipoproteinemia who have low levels of LDL cholesterol have extremely

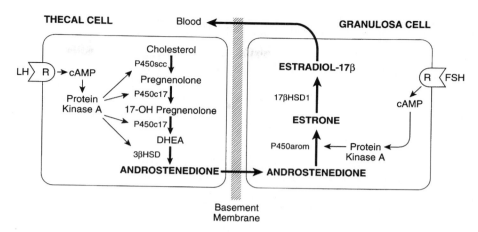

Figure 11–11. The principal pathways of human ovarian steroidogenesis and the two cell–two gonadotropin hypothesis. (See Fig 11–10 for abbreviations.) (*Reproduced, with permission, from Carr BR, Disorders of the Ovary and Female Reproductive Tract. In: Wilson JD, Foster DW, eds.* Williams Textbook of Endocrinology. *Philadelphia, Pa: W. B. Saunders Co. In press.*)

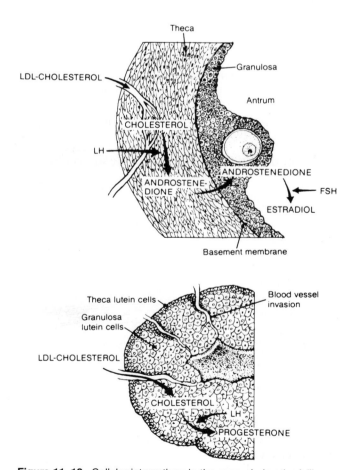

Figure 11–12. Cellular interactions in the ovary during the follicular phase (top) and luteal phase (bottom). (LDL, low-density lipoprotein; FSH, follicle-stimulating hormone; LH, luteinizing hormone.) (*Reproduced, with permission, from Carr BR, MacDonald PC, Simpson ER, The role of lipoproteins in the regulation of progesterone secretion by the human corpus luteum. Fertil Steril. 38:303, 1982.*)

low levels of progesterone secretion during the luteal phase.[100]

Regulation of Ovarian Steroidogenesis by Gonadotropins. FSH and LH are required for estrogen synthesis, and the amount of estrogen produced depends upon the relative exposure of each gonadotropin. FSH receptors are present exclusively on the granulosa cell.[101] FSH also stimulates the activity of aromatase and the mRNA for $P_{450AROM}$ in granulosa cells that convert androgens produced by the theca cells into estrogens as discussed previously. Enhanced secretion of estradiol causes an increase in the activation and number of estradiol receptors, which cause further proliferation of granulosa cells and follicular growth.[101] In the mature follicle, FSH in concert with estradiol causes an increase in LH receptors on granulosa cells. LH acts to augment progesterone secretion by granulosa cells, which stimulates FSH release at midcycle. The binding of gonadotropin to their respective plasma membrane receptors stimulates secretion of adenylate cyclase (Fig 11–11). Following ovulation, the number of LH receptors in the lutein cells increases and the FSH receptor numbers and FSH responses decrease.[101] Taken together, these observations emphasize the important roles of autocrine and paracrine actions of steroids and the two-cell gonadotropin hypothesis discussed earlier.

Extragonadal Steroidogenesis. The application of isotopic dilution methods has provided insight into the complexity of the processes involved in understanding the secretion rate (SR), production rate (PR), and the metabolic clearance rate (MCR) of steroid hormones. The concept of extragonadal hormone formulation utilizing the following principles has clarified the regulation of plasma

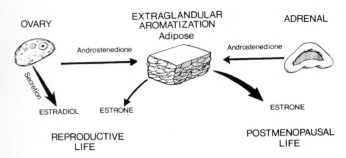

Figure 11–13. Various sources of circulating estrogens in women during reproductive and postmenopausal life. *(Adapted, with permission, from Carr BR, MacDonald PC. Estrogen treatment of postmenopausal women. In: Stollerman GH, ed.* Advances in Internal Medicine, *vol 28. Chicago, Ill., Year Book Medical Publishers, 1983: 491–508.)*

levels of steroid hormones in women, particularly of plasma estrogens[102,103] (Fig 11–13). The amount of hormone released by an endocrine gland into the circulation per unit of time is the SR. Steroid hormones may also be derived from the extragonadal or peripheral conversion of a precursor steroid that may be secreted by the original or by another endocrine gland. The PR of a hormone is the rate at which a hormone enters the circulation and is determined by the SR plus hormone formation at extraglandular sites. If a hormone is derived exclusively via glandular secretion, the SR and PR are equal. However, when the hormone is formed from peripheral conversion as well as from secretion the PR will be greater than the SR. The MCR is the volume of blood per unit of time that is irreversibly cleared of a hormone. The blood PR of a hormone equals the MCR multiplied by the concentration of the hormone in blood (PR = MCR × C).

The SR and PR of steroid hormones can be determined by a variety of techniques.[104,105] The most common technique involves the intravenous infusion of a radiolabeled hormone until a constant level of this hormone is attained in blood. The PR or the total entry of this hormone into the circulation can be calculated from the specific activity of the hormone in plasma. In the instance in which a steroid hormone is derived from more than one precursor steroid, infusion of each of these radiolabeled hormones makes it possible to calculate their relative contributions to the blood PR of the hormone.[102] The plasma concentrations, PR, MCR, and SR of ovarian steroid hormones in normal women are presented in Table 11–1.

The origin of plasma estrogens has been clarified using these methods as discussed previously. In normal women of reproductive age, the vast majority of plasma estradiol is derived by direct secretion from the ovary. There is little, if any, estradiol formed from testosterone by extraglandular conversion. On the other hand, little estrone

TABLE 11–1. CONCENTRATION, METABOLIC CLEARANCE RATES (MCR), PRODUCTION RATES (PR), AND OVARIAN SECRETION RATES (SR) OF STEROIDS IN BLOOD

Compound	MCR of Compound in Peripheral Plasma (L/day)	Phase of Menstrual Cycle	Concentration in Plasma		PR of Circulating Compound (mg/day)	SR by Both Ovaries (mg/day)
			nmol/L	(μg/dl)		
Estradiol	1350	Early follicular	0.2	(0.006)	0.081	0.07
		Late follicular	1.2–2.6	(0.033–0.070)	0.445–0.945	0.4–0.8
		Midluteal	0.7	(0.020)	0.270	0.25
Estrone	2210	Early follicular	0.18	(0.005)	0.110	0.08
		Late follicular	0.5–1.1	(0.015–0.030)	0.331–0.662	0.25–0.50
		Midluteal	0.4	(0.011)	0.243	0.16
Progesterone	2200	Follicular	3.0	(0.095)	2.1	1.5
		Luteal	36	(1.13)	25.0	24.0
20α-Hydroxyprogesterone	2300	Follicular	1.5	(0.05)	1.1	0.8
		Luteal	7.5	(0.25)	5.8	3.3
17-Hydroxyprogesterone	2000	Early follicular	0.9	(0.03)	0.6	0–0.3
		Late follicular	6	(0.20)	4.0	3–4
		Midluteal	6	(0.20)	4.0	3–4
Androstenedione	2010		5.6	(0.159)	3.2	0.8–1.6
Testosterone	690		1.3	(0.038)	0.26	
Dehydroepiandrosterone	1640		17	(0.490)	8.0	0.3–3

(Reproduced, with permission, from Tagatz GE, Gurpide E. Hormone secretion by the normal human ovary. In: Greep RP, Astwood EB, eds. Handbook of Physiology, Section 7: Endocrinology, Vol II, Part 1. *American Physiological Society. Baltimore, Md., Williams and Wilkins, 1973: 603–613.)*

is formed by direct ovarian secretion, and most estrone circulating in plasma originates from extraglandular conversion from androstenedione and to a minor extent from estradiol (Fig 11–13).[103] The primary site of extraglandular aromatization of androstenedione to estrone occurs in adipose tissue and is influenced by age, liver function, and thyroid dysfunction.[84]

The importance of the extragonadal formation and the prohormone concept of estrogen formation is highlighted by a variety of clinical conditions. The amount of extraglandular hormone production of estrogen can increase to a level that can interfere with the normal feedback mechanisms and produce disturbances of the ovarian cycle. The formation of estrogens by the placenta during pregnancy is dependent entirely upon 19-carbon steroids (prohormones) secreted by the fetal adrenal gland and to a lesser extent the maternal adrenal[105] (see Chap 2). In nonpregnant premenopausal women, estrone is formed by androstenedione secreted by the ovary and adrenal. In menopausal women, the ovarian contribution of prohormone (androstenedione) is negligible, but these women still have considerable estrone circulating in blood formed by extraglandular conversion of androstenedione secreted by the adrenals. An increase in estrogen formation occurs with aging and obesity that can yield enough estrogen to produce endometrial hyperplasia and bleeding.[84] Similar findings can occur in premenopausal women with polycystic ovarian disease or ovarian tumors associated with increased secretion of androstenedione.

Ovarian Steroid Hormone Transport. Most steroid secreted by the ovary and peripheral tissues is bound to plasma proteins. The bulk of steroid hormones are bound to albumin or specific globulins (>97 to 98 percent). For example, the majority of testosterone is bound to sex hormone-binding globulin (SHBG) and to a lesser degree to albumin. Estradiol exhibits a lower binding affinity to SHBG than does testosterone; thus, the majority of estradiol is bound to serum albumin (60 percent) while 38 percent is bound to SHBG and 2 to 3 percent is free.[106] It is assumed that the protein-bound hormone is "inactive" and that only the "free" hormone is active and directly available to enter target tissues, but recent evidence suggests that the transport of steroid hormones could be more complex.[107–109]

SHBG, a β-globulin, is formed by the liver and has a molecular weight of about 95,000. It has a high affinity (10^{-9} mol/L) and low binding capacity (one binding site per molecule).[110] Dihydrotestosterone followed by testosterone has the highest binding affinity for SHBG, whereas estradiol has one third the affinity of dihydrotestosterone to SHBG. In contrast, dehydroepiandrosterone (DHEA) and progesterone have negligible affinity to SHBG. The MCR of sex steroids is inversely related to the affinity to SHBG

and thus alterations in the concentration of SHBG influence sex steroid metabolism and target tissue action.[110] The level of SHBG and thus the level of "free" hormone may be altered by a variety of clinical conditions. Levels of SHBG are increased by estrogens (pregnancy and oral contraceptive pills) and thyroid hormones (hyperthyroidism) but lowered by androgens, hypothyroidism, and obesity.[111] Also, women have double the concentration of SHBG compared to men, which appears to be due to the higher estrogen levels observed in women.

Mechanisms of Steroid Hormone Action. The concentration of steroid hormones in the circulation is low and for target cells to respond, specific steroid receptors are required for steroid hormone action. Steroid hormones have low molecular weights and because of their hydrophobic nature enter cells by diffusion, although carrier-mediated transport may occur. The affinity, specificity, and concentration of steroid receptors in target cells allow a low concentration of steroid hormones to produce biologic responses. Estrogen can enter any cell, but only in specific target tissues, such as the uterus, is estrogen action observed due to the presence of estrogen receptors.[112] In contrast, in most cells estrogens are not able to manifest a response due to the lack of estrogen receptor expression.

Two theories have been proposed to explain the mechanism by which steroids cause intracellular response.[113] The original receptor or translocation model requires the receptor hormone complex to be translocated from the cytoplasm to the nucleus to interact with DNA. This translocation is followed by a transformation or conformational change of the hormone-receptor complex that binds to DNA and alters gene transcription and the production of mRNA. This concept was based upon the observation that unoccupied receptors were found in the cytosol and that following exposure to steroid hormones the receptor was translocated to the nucleus with loss of receptors from the cytosol. Although this concept is still held by some, the finding of cytosolic receptors was based upon methods that produced artifactual results.[113] Recently, through the utilization of monoclonal antibodies, it was discovered that steroid receptors are localized exclusively in the nucleus.[114,115] This has led to a new concept known as the nuclear localization model.[113] This concept is based upon two principles, namely, that the steroid receptor is a nuclear protein (occupied or unoccupied) and that the receptor is immobilized by association with elements within the nucleus. In the nuclear localization model, steroid hormones diffuse across the cell membrane and enter the nucleus and become associated with a nuclear steroid receptor. The nuclear steroid receptor consists of a number of units: a steroid hormone binding domain (carboxy terminus), a DNA binding domain, a hinge region, and a transcription activation functional domain at the nitrogen terminus. Active transformation occurs after nuclear binding and involves a conformational change in the receptor and the activated steroid–nuclear receptor complex. This complex then interacts with specific DNA sequences known as steroid response elements (SREs).[115] Next, interaction of the nuclear hormone–receptor complex with DNA leads to synthesis of mRNA and finally protein synthesis in the cytoplasm, which causes specific cellular responses.

Steroid receptors for estrogen, progesterone, glucocorticoids, and androgens have been cloned and sequenced. The unoccupied estrogen receptor is located loosely bound in the nucleus as a monomer. Following exposure to estrogen, activation of the receptor involves the formation of a dimer.[116] Following activation of the estrogen receptor by estrogen, a further increase in affinity for estrogen in other nuclear binding sites occurs, named cooperatively. This phenomenon allows for an increase in biologic response to estrogen in response to small changes in hormone concentration and is greater for 17β-estradiol than for estrone.[113] The positive cooperativity for estradiol leads to longer duration of action due to increased affinity for the estrogen receptor. Estrogens also stimulate the expression of new estrogen receptors that are synthesized in the cytoplasm and rapidly transferred to the nucleus. This process, called receptor replenishment, further increases the biologic actions of estrogen. Following gene activation by the estrogen–receptor complex, the receptor converts from a high-affinity site to a dissociated form with lower affinity and decreased binding capacity.[113] These aspects of the estrogen receptor help explain clinical response to pharmacologic agents and other hormones. For example, although estradiol stimulates cooperativity and receptor replenishment, progesterone and clomiphene citrate block

these processes, leading to a reduction in cellular biologic response to estrogens.[117]

Nonsteroidal Hormones and Growth Factors of the Ovary. A variety of nonsteroidal hormones and growth factors are produced by the ovary and appear to modulate local steroidogenesis via autocrine and paracrine mechanisms. In addition, some of these factors may influence hypothalamic and pituitary secretion of gonadotropin via an endocrine mechanism (for review, see references 118–133). A list of nonsteroidal hormones and their proposed functions is presented in Table 11–2. The recognition that only one follicle is destined to ovulate and that the rest are destined to undergo atresia supports the view of a complex intraovarian regulation of follicle growth of a single follicle and inhibition of growth of the remaining follicles. Some of these nonsteroid factors, as well as steroids produced by the dominant follicle, may play a role in local regulation of follicular growth.[118–133]

MENOPAUSAL OVARY

Successive cycles of ovulation and atresia deplete the ovarian content of its follicles (Fig 11–14). This leads to menopause, the final episode of menstrual bleeding in women. The median age of menopause is 50 to 51 yr.[134] The term menopause commonly refers to the period of the climacteric encompassing the transition between the reproductive years up to and beyond the last episode of menstrual bleeding. The predominant event during menopause is the cessation of cyclic ovarian function, which in turn affects various endocrine, somatic, and psychological changes (see also Chaps 37 and 38).

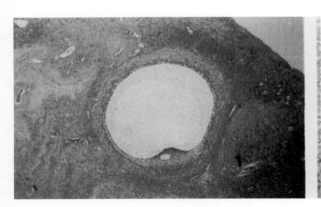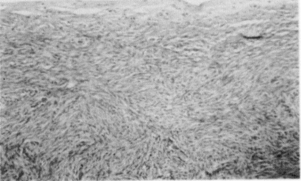

Figure 11–14. Left panel: Photomicrograph of histologic section of an ovary obtained from a woman during reproductive life. Note the large graafian follicle with single ovum in the center of the photograph and a group of primary follicles in the upper right corner (× 33). Right panel: Ovary obtained from a postmenopausal woman. Note the absence of germ cells and prominent ovarian stroma (× 132). *(Reproduced, with permission, from Carr BR, MacDonald PC. The menopause and beyond. In: Andres R, Bierman EL, Hazzard WR, eds. Principles of Geriatric Medicine. New York, N.Y., McGraw-Hill, 1985: 325–336.)*

TABLE 11–2. NONSTEROIDAL FACTORS PRODUCED BY THE OVARY THAT MAY REGULATE ENDOCRINE-AUTOCRINE OR PARACRINE REGULATION OF OVARIAN FUNCTION

Nonsteroidal Factor	Proposed Function
Activin	Stimulates FSH release, inhibits P450c17 in theca, increases granulosa LH receptors
Adenosine	Regulation of atresia, maintenance of corpus luteum, regulation of oocyte maturation
Angiogenic factors	Neovascularization of corpus luteum
Catecholamines	Modify steroidogenesis
Cytokines	Modify steroidogenesis
Eicosanoids	Ovulation, corpus luteum regulation
Follicular-regulating protein (FRP)	Atresia, aromatase inhibitor, inhibition of FSH action
Follistatin	Suppresses FSH release
FSH binding inhibitor (FSH BI)	Inhibits binding of FSH to receptor, atresia
γ-Aminobutyric acid (GABA)	Unknown, modulation of ovarian function?
GnRH-like peptides	Stimulatory and inhibitory actins on FSH and LH, regulation of atresia
Growth factors	
Epidermal growth factor (EFG)	Mitogenic-granulosa, inhibits steroidogenesis, atresia
Fibroblast growth factor (FGF)	Mitogenic, inhibits steroidogenesis, atresia
Insulin-like growth factors (IFGs)	Mitogenic, stimulates steroidogenesis, modulate corpus luteum
Growth hormone	
Growth hormone releasing hormone	
IGF-1, IGF 2	
IGF-binding proteins	
Platelet-derived growth factor (PDGF)	Unknown, enhances steroidogenesis?
Transforming growth factors (TGFs)	
TGF-α	Growth regulation, inhibits steroidogenesis
TGF-β	Stimulates FSH release, stimulates steroidogenesis-granulosa, inhibits steroidogenesis-theca, inhibits granulosa cell growth
Inhibin	Inhibits FSH release, increases P450cc in theca
LH binding inhibitor (LH BI)	Inhibits binding of LH to receptor, atresia
Luteinization inhibitor	Inhibits corpus luteum development and function
Antimüllerian hormone	Inhibits oocyte maturation
Oocyte maturation inhibitor (OMI)	Inhibits meiosis
Oxytocin (corpus luteum)	Modulates progesterone secretion, regulates life span of corpus luteum
Pro-opiomelanocortin (POMC)-derived peptides	Unknown
Relaxin	Remodeling of reproductive tract, modulates corpus luteum
Renin-angiotensin	Ovulation, regulation of steroidogenesis (rat), no receptors or action in human granulosa
Substance P	Regulation of ovarian blood flow
Tissue-type plasminogen activator (tPA)	Ovulation, atresia
Vascular endothelial growth factor	Angiogenesis
Vasoactive intestinal peptide	Stimulates steroidogenesis
Vasopressin	Unknown

(Reproduced, with permission, from Carr BR. Disorders of the ovary and the female reproductive tract. In: Wilson JD, Foster DW, eds. William's Textbook of Endocrinology, *8th ed. Philadelphia, Pa., W. B. Saunders, 1992: 733–798.)*

The average age of menopause has remained constant, suggesting that menopause age is unrelated to the onset of menarche, socioeconomic conditions, race, parity, height, or weight.[135] However, menopause may occur earlier in women who smoke.[136] Since the life expectancy of women extends 30 yr beyond menopause and occupies one third of the life of women, the medical and economic impact of these changes is significant.

During menopause, the continuous loss of ovarian follicles results in a decrease in estrogen secretion. The ovary of postmenopausal women is reduced in size, weighing less than 2.5 g, and is wrinkled or prune-like in appearance. Furthermore, the loss of ova and follicles results in a reduction of the cortical area. Rarely, a few immature follicles undergoing maturation or atresia may be seen at the corticomedullary junction for up to 5 yr or more after the last menses.[137] The most striking changes of the postmenopausal ovary occur as the stroma becomes hyperplastic and dominates the ovary. The interstitial and hilar cells are readily apparent in ovaries from postmenopausal women. Virilizing syndromes secondary to hilar cell hyperplasia and neoplasia are more common after menopause.[138]

A reduction in the responsiveness of the ovary to gonadotropins is apparent several years prior to the cessation of menstruation. Compared to younger women, FSH and LH levels are elevated in perimenopausal women still experiencing follicular growth and ovulatory menstrual cycles. Following cessation of follicular development, a decrease in 17β-estradiol and inhibin secretion occurs, two factors responsible for negative feedback to the hypothalamus and pituitary. The absence of the negative feedback mechanism allows gonadotropin levels to rise with an FSH, rising earlier and to a greater extent than LH. Two possible explanations for the difference in gonadotropin levels exist. First, the decrease in inhibin levels may be responsible for higher FSH levels or, second, the greater sialic acid content of FSH may decrease its clearance rate.[76] Intravenous infusion of LHRH in postmenopausal women elicits an exaggerated increase in the release of both FSH and LH, similar to women with other forms of ovarian failure.[139] Some investigators report that the concentration of gonadotropins remains elevated after age 60, but others report a downward trend during later decades of life.[139,140]

In contrast to gonadotropins, the mean levels of ovarian steroid hormones decrease from premenopause to postmenopause. Prior to menopause, plasma androstenedione is derived equally from both the adrenal and ovary, but after menopause the ovarian contribution is minimal and plasma androstenedione levels fall by 50 percent.[141] As discussed previously, circulatory estrogens in premenopausal ovulating women are derived from two sources. Greater than 60 percent of estrogen is produced by direct ovarian secretion as estradiol; the remainder is estrone, derived from the extraglandular conversion of androstenedione.[85] After menopause, the ovarian estrogen contribution from both sources is reduced and the extraglandular formation of estrone from adrenal androstenedione secretion predominates (Fig 11–13). As expected, removal of the ovaries in postmenopausal women does not result in a significant decline in estrogen or androstenedione levels.[141] Because adipose tissue is a major site of extraglandular estrogen production, estrogen levels in obese postmenopausal women may equal or surpass those in premenopausal women.[142,143] Here, the predominant form of estrogen in postmenopausal women is estrone rather than estradiol.

The decrease in estrogen formation triggers vasomotor instability (hot flash), atrophy of the urogenital epithelium, a reduction in size of reproductive organs and breasts, an increased risk of cardiovascular disease, and osteoporosis.[144-148] Hot flashes are characterized by periods of warmth and heat followed by profuse sweating. The frequency, duration, and intensity of vasomotor symptoms vary but in the majority of women they begin to subside 2 to 5 yr following menopause.[149] The pathogenesis of the hot flash or flush is complex and appears to involve catecholamines, prostaglandins, endorphins, and other neuropeptides following the cessation of estrogen secretion.[150]

There is a close temporal relationship between estrogen deprivation and the development of osteoporosis. Loss of bone, both trabecular and cortical, due to osteoporosis may result in mechanical fragility and fracture. Following menopause, bone loss proceeds at a rate of 1 to 2 percent each year.[151] By age 80, women have lost 50 percent of their bone mass. It has been estimated that 25 percent of women sustain a vertebral or hip fracture between the ages of 60 and 90.[152] Such fractures are a major cause of mortality and morbidity. A number of factors influence the development of osteoporosis including diet, activity, smoking, general health, and, most importantly, estrogen deprivation.[153-155]

The principal cause of death in postmenopausal women is cardiovascular disease.[156] Studies comparing postmenopausal women to premenopausal controls indicate that postmenopausal women are at greater risk for cardiovascular disease.[157] Lower high-density lipoprotein and higher LDL cholesterol levels are present in postmenopausal women. Likewise, women who undergo oophorectomy and are not treated with estrogen have an increased risk of cardiovascular disease.[158] Growing evidence supports the use of estrogen replacement therapy in reducing the risk of death from cardiovascular disease (see Chap 38).

REFERENCES

1. Gillman J. The development of the gonads in man, with a consideration of the whole fetal endocrines and the histogenesis of ovarian tumors. *Contrib Embryol Carneg Inst Wash.* 32:67, 1948

2. Kuwana T, Maeda-Suga H, Fujimoto T. Attraction of chick primordial germ cells by gonadal anlage *in vitro*. *Anat Rec.* 215:403, 1986

3. Baker TG. A quantitative and cytological study of germ cells in the human ovaries. *Proc Roy Soc London (B).* 158:417, 1963

4. Ohno S, Klinger HP, Atkin WB. Human oogenesis. *Cytogenetics.* 1:42, 1962

5. Lyon MF. Gene action in the X-chromosome of the mouse (*Mus musculus*). *Nature.* 190:372, 1961

6. Singh RP, Carr DH. The anatomy and histology of XO human embryos and fetuses. *Anat Rec.* 155:369, 1966

7. Peters H, Byskov AG, Grinsted J. Follicular growth in fetal and prepubertal ovaries in humans and other primates. *Clin Endocrinol Metab.* 7:469, 1978

8. Wartenberg H. Development of the early human ovary and the role of the mesonephros in the differentiation of the cortex. *Anat Embryol.* 165:253, 1982

9. Baker TG, Franchi LL. The fine structure of oogonia and oocytes in human ovaries. *J Cell Sci.* 2:213, 1967

10. Tsafriri A, Dekel N, Bar-Ami S. The role of oocyte maturation inhibitor in follicular regulation of oocyte maturation. *J Reprod Fertil.* 64:541, 1982

11. Byskov AG, Hoyer PE. Embryology of mammalian gonads and ducts. In: Knobil E, Neill JD, eds. *The Physiology of Reproduction*, 2nd ed. New York, N.Y., Raven Press, 1994; 1: 487–540

12. Guylas BJ, Hodgen GD, Tullner WW, Ross GT. Effects of fetal and maternal hypophysectomy on endocrine organs and body weight in infant monkey (*Macaca mulatta*) with particular emphasis on oogenesis. *Biol Reprod.* 16:216, 1977

13. Jungman RA, Schweppe JS. Biosynthesis of steroids and steroids from acetate-^{14}C by human fetal ovaries. *J Clin Endocrinol Metab.* 28:1599, 1968

14. Molsberry RL, Carr BR, Mendelson CR, Simpson ER. Human chorionic gonadotropin binding to human fetal testes as a function of gestational age. *J Clin Endocrinol Metab.* 55:791, 1982

15. Miller W. Molecular biology of steroid hormone synthesis. *Endocrine Rev.* 9:295, 1988

16. O'Rahilly R. The embryology and anatomy of the uterus. In: Norris HJ, Hertig AT, Abell MR, eds. *The Uterus.* Baltimore, Md., Williams and Wilkins, 1973: 17–39

17. Peters H, McNatty KP. *The Ovary.* Los Angeles, Calif., University of California Press, 1980: 12–34

18. Faiman C, Winter JSD, Reyes FI. Patterns of gonadotropins and gonadal steroids throughout life. *Clin Obstet Gynecol.* 3:467, 1976

19. Kaplan SL, Grumbach MM, Aubert ML. The ontogenesis of pituitary hormones and hypothalamic factors in the human fetus: Maturation of the central nervous system regulation of anterior pituitary function. *Rec Prog Horm Res.* 32:161, 1976

20. Styne DM, Grumbach MM. Disorders of puberty in the male and female. In: Yen SSC, Jaffe RB, eds. *Reproductive Endocrinology,* 3rd ed. Philadelphia, Pa., W. B. Saunders, 1991: 511–554

21. Winter JSD, Hughes IA, Reyes FI, Faiman C. Pituitary–gonadal steroid concentrations in man from birth to two years of age. *J Clin Endocrinol Metab.* 42:679, 1976

22. Yanovski JA, Cutler GB. The reproductive Axis pubertal activation. In: Adashi EY, Rock JA, Rosenwaks Z, eds. *Reproductive Endocrinology, Surgery, and Technology.* Philadelphia, Pa., Lippincott-Raven, 1996: 76–101

23. Conte FA, Grumbach MM, Kaplan SL. A diphasic pattern of gonadotropin secretion in patients with the syndrome of gonadal dysgenesis. *J Clin Endocrinol Metab.* 40:670, 1975

24. Roth JC, Kelch RP, Kaplan SL, Grumbach MM. FSH and LH response to luteinizing hormone-releasing factor in prepubertal and pubertal children, adult males and patients with hypogonadotropic and hypergonadotropic hypogonadism. *J Clin Endocrinol Metab.* 37:680, 1973

25. Jakacki RI, Kelch RP, Sauder SE, et al. Pulsatile secretion of luteinizing hormone in children. *J Clin Endocrinol Metab.* 55:453, 1982

26. Gell JS, Atkins B, Margraf L, et al. Adrenarche is associated with alterations in adrenal reticularis expression of 3β-hydroxy steroid dehydrogenase. *J Soc Gynecol Invest.* 13(suppl.):104(A), 1996

27. Parker L, Odell WD. Control of adrenal androgen secretion. *Endocrine Rev.* 1:392, 1980

28. Boyer RM, Rosenfeld RS, Kaplan S, et al. Simultaneous augmentation secretion of luteinizing hormone and testosterone during sleep. *J Clin Invest.* 54:609, 1974

29. Kapen S, Boyer RM, Hellman L, Weitzman ED. Twenty-four-hour patterns of luteinizing hormone secretion in humans: Ontogenic and sexual considerations. *Prog Brain Res.* 42:103, 1975

30. Knobil E. The neuroendocrine control of the menstrual cycle. *Rec Prog Horm Res.* 36:53, 1980

31. Crowley WF, McArthur JW. Stimulation of the normal menstrual cycle in Kallmann's syndrome by pulsatile administration of luteinizing hormone-releasing hormone (LHRH). *J Clin Endocrinol Metab.* 51:173, 1980

32. Crowley WJ Jr, Comite F, Vale W, et al. Therapeutic use of pituitary desensitization with a long-acting LHRH agonist: A potential new treatment for idiopathic precocious puberty. *J Clin Endocrinol Metab.* 52:370, 1981

33. Mansfield MJ, Beardsworth DE, Loughlin JS, et al. Long-term treatment of central precocious puberty with a long-acting analogue of luteinizing hormone-releasing hormone. *N Engl J Med.* 309:1286, 1983

34. Winter JSD, Faiman C, Reyes FI, Hobson WC. Gonadotropins and steroid hormones in the blood and urine of prepubertal girls and other primates. *Clin Endocrinol Metab.* 7:513, 1978

35. Burstein S, Schoff-Blass E, Blass J, Rosenfeld RL. Changing ratio of bioactive to immunoactive LH through puberty. *J Clin Endocrinol Metab.* 61:508, 1985

36. Burger HG, McLachlan RI, Bangah M, et al. Serum inhibin concentrations rise throughout normal male and female puberty. *J Clin Endocrinol Metab.* 67:689, 1988

37. Mansfield MJ, Rudlin CR, Crigler JF, et al. Changes in growth and serum growth hormone and plasma somatomedin-C levels during suppression of gonadal sex steroid secretion in girls with central precocious puberty. *J Clin Endocrinol Metab.* 66:3, 1988

38. Merimee TJ, Zapf J, Hewlett B, Cavalli-Sforz LL. Insulin-like growth factors in pygmies. *N Engl J Med.* 316:906, 1987

39. Marshall WA, Tanner JM. Variations in pattern of pubertal changes in girls. *Arch Dis Child.* 44:291, 1969

40. Frisch RE, McArthur JW. Menstrual cycles: Fatness as a determinant of minimum weight for height necessary for their maintenance at onset. *Science.* 185:949, 1974

41. Frisch RE. Fatness, puberty, menstrual periodicity and fertility. In: Vaitukaitis JL, ed. *Clinical Reproductive Neuroendocrinology.* New York, N.Y., Elsevier Biomedical, 1982: 105–135

42. Woodburne RT. *Essentials of Human Anatomy.* New York, N.Y., Oxford University Press, 1965: 527–528

43. Franchi LL, Mandl AM, Zuckerman S. The development of the ovary and the process of oogenesis. In: Zuckerman S, Mandl AM, Eckstein P, eds. *The Ovary.* London, U.K., Academic Press, 1961: 1–88

44. Eshkol A, Lunenfeld B, Peters H. Ovarian development in infant mice: Dependence on gonadotropic hormones. In: Butt WR, Crooke AC, Ryle M, eds. *Gonadotropins and Ovarian Development.* London, U.K., E. and S. Livingstone, 1970: 249–258

45. Adashi EY. Endocrinology of the ovary. *Hum Reprod.* 9:815, 1994

46. Albertini DF, Anderson E. The appearance and structure of intracellular connections during the ontogeny of the

rabbit ovarian follicle with particular reference to gap junctions. *J Cell Biol.* 63:234, 1974

47. Tilly JL, Kowalski KJ, Johnson AL, et al. Involvement of apoptosis in ovarian follicular atresia and postovulatory regression. *Endocrinology.* 132:294, 1993

48. Eppig JJ. A comparison between oocyte growth in ooculture with granulosa cells and oocytes with granulosa cell–oocyte junctional contact maintained in vitro. *J Exp Zool.* 209:345, 1979

49. Bleil JD, Wassermann PM. Structure and function of the zona pellucida: Identification and characterization of the proteins of the mouse oocyte's zona pellucida. *Dev Biol.* 76:185, 1980

50. Erickson GF. The ovary: Basic principles and concepts. A. Physiology. In: Felig P, Baxter JD, Broders AG, Frohman LA, eds. *Endocrinology and Metabolism,* 3rd ed. New York, N.Y., McGraw-Hill, 1995: 973–1015

51. Erickson FG, Magoffen D, Dyer CA, Hofeditz C. The ovarian androgen producing cells: A review of structure/function relationships. *Endocrine Rev.* 6:371, 1985

52. Gondos B, Hobel CG. Interstitial cells in the human fetal ovary. *Endocrinology.* 93:736, 1976

53. Dawson AB, McCabe M. The interstitial tissue of the ovary in infantile and juvenile rats. *J Morphol.* 88:543, 1951

54. Dyer CA, Erickson FG. Norepinephrine amplifies hCG-stimulated androgen biosynthesis by ovarian thecal-interstitial cells. *Endocrinology.* 116:1645, 1985

55. Eshkal A, Lunenfeld B. Gonadotropic regulation of ovarian development in mice during infancy. In: Saxena BB, Gandy HM, Billing CG, eds. *Gonadotropins.* New York, N.Y., Wiley, 1972: 335–346

56. Upadhyay S, Zamboni L. Ectopic germ cells: Natural model for the study of germ cell sexual differentiation. *Proc Natl Acad Sci USA.* 79:6584, 1982

57. Patton PE, Stouffer RL. Current understanding of the corpus luteum in women and sub-human primates. *Clin Obstet Gynecol.* 34:127, 1991

58. Corner GW Jr. Histological dating of human corpus luteum of menstruation. *Am J Anat.* 98:377, 1956

59. Gillim SW, Christensen AK, McLennon CE. Fine structure of the human menstrual corpus luteum at its stage of maximum secretory activity. *Am J Anat.* 126:409, 1970

60. Ohara A, Mori T, Taii S, Ban C, Narimoto K. Functional differentiation in steroidogenesis of two types of luteal cells isolated from mature human corpora lutea of menstrual cycle. *J Clin Endocrinol Metab.* 65:1192, 1987

61. Juengel JL, Garverick HA, Johnson AL, et al. Apoptosis during luteal cell regression in cattle. *Endocrinology.* 132:249, 1993

62. Ying SY. Inhibins, activins, and follistatins: Gonadal proteins modulating the secretion of follicle-stimulating hormone. *Endocrine Rev.* 9:267, 1988

63. Oliver C, Mical RS, Porter JC. Hypothalamic–pituitary vasculature: Evidence for retrograde blood flow in the pituitary stalk. *Endocrinology.* 101:598, 1977

64. Conn PM, Crowley WF Jr. Gonadotropin-releasing hormone and its analogs. *N Engl J Med.* 342:93, 1991

65. Marshall JC. Regulation of gonadotropin secretion. In: DeGroot LJ, ed. *Endocrinology.* Philadelphia, Pa., W. B. Saunders, 1989: 1903–1914

66. Huseman CA, Kelch RP. Gonadotropin response and metabolism of synthetic gonadotropin-releasing hormone (GnRH) during constant infusion of GnRH in men and boys with delayed adolescence. *J Clin Endocrinol Metab.* 47:1325, 1978

67. Carmel PW, Araki S, Ferin M. Pituitary stalk portal blood collection in rhesus monkeys: Evidence for pulsatile release of gonadotropin releasing hormone (GnRH). *Endocrinology.* 99:243, 1976

68. Clarke IJ, Cummins JT. The temporal relationship between gonadotropin releasing hormone (GnRH) and luteinizing hormone (LH) secretion in ovariectomized ewes. *Endocrinology.* 111:1737, 1982

69. Belchitz PE, Plant TM, Nakai Y, et al. Hypophyseal responses to continuous and intermittent delivery of hypothalamic gonadotropin-releasing hormone. *Science.* 202:631, 1978

70. Knobil E, Plant TM, Wildt TL, et al. Control of the rhesus monkey menstrual cycle: Permissive role of hypothalamic gonadotropin releasing hormone. *Science.* 207:1371, 1980

71. Leyendecker G, Wildt TL, Hansmen M. Pregnancies following chronic intermittent pulsatile administration of GnRH. *J Clin Endocrinol Metab.* 51:1214, 1980

72. Conn PM. The molecular basis of gonadotropin-releasing hormone action. *Endocrine Rev.* 7:3, 1986

73. Grant G, Vale W, Rivier J. Pituitary binding sites for H^3 labeled LRF. *Biochem Biophys Res Comm.* 50:771, 1973

74. Fiddes JC, Talmadge K. Structure, expression, and evolution of the genes for human glycoprotein hormones. *Rec Prog Horm Res.* 40:43, 1984

75. Vaitukaitis JL, Ross GT, Bourstein GD, Rayford PL. Gonadotropins and their subunits: Basic and clinical studies. *Rec Prog Horm Res.* 32:289, 1976

76. Kholer PO, Ross GT, Odell WD. Metabolic clearance and production rates of human luteinizing hormone in pre- and postmenopausal women. *J Clin Invest.* 47:38, 1968

77. Yen SSC, Rebar RW. Endocrine rhythms in gonadotropins and ovarian steroids with reference to reproductive processes. In: Kreiger DT, ed. *Endocrine Rhythms.* New York, N.Y., Raven Press, 1979: 259–298

78. Fink G. Gonadotropin secretion and its control. In: Knobil E, Neill JD, eds. *The Physiology of Reproduction.* New York, N.Y., Raven Press, 1988; 1: 1349–1377

79. Chappel SC, Resko JA, Norman RL, Spies HG. Studies on rhesus monkeys on the site where estrogen inhibits gonadotropins: Delivery of 17β-estradiol to the hypothalamus and pituitary gland. *J Clin Endocrinol Metab.* 52:1, 1981

80. Wildt TL, Hutchinson JS, Marshall G, et al. On the site of action of progesterone in the blockade of the estradiol-induced gonadotropin discharge in the rhesus monkey. *Endocrinology.* 109:1293, 1981

81. Batista MC, Cartledge TP, Zellmer W, et al. Evidence for a critical role of progesterone in the regulation of the midcycle surge and ovulation. *J Clin Endocrinol Metab.* 74:565, 1992

82. Filcori M, Santoro N, Merriam GR, Crowley WF Jr. Characterization of the physiological pattern of episodic gonadotropin secretion throughout the human menstrual cycle. *J Clin Endocrinol Metab.* 62:1136, 1986

83. Liu JH, Yen SSC. Induction of midcycle gonadotropin surge by ovarian steroids in women: A critical evaluation. *J Clin Endocrinol Metab.* 57:797, 1983

84. Lipsett M. Steroid hormones. In: Yes SSC, Jaffe RB, eds. *Reproductive Endocrinology*, 2nd ed. Philadelphia, Pa., W. B. Saunders, 1986: 140–153

85. Siiteri PK, MacDonald PC. Role of extraglandular estrogen in human endocrinology. In: Greep RO, Astwood EF, eds. *Handbook of Physiology*, Section 7, *Endocrinology*. Baltimore, Md., Williams and Wilkins, 1973: 615–630

86. Fishman J, Hellman L, Zumoff B, Gallager TF. Influence of thyroid hormone on estrogen metabolism in man. *J Clin Endocrinol Metab*. 22:389, 1962

87. Merriam GR, Lipssett MB. *Catechol Estrogens*. New York, N.Y., Raven Press, 1983

88. Carr BR, MacDonald PC, Simpson ER. The role of lipoproteins in the regulation of progesterone secretion by the human corpus luteum. *Fertil Steril*. 38:303, 1982

89. Gwynne JT, Strauss JF. The role of lipoproteins in steroidogenesis and cholesterol metabolism in steroidogenic glands. *Endocrine Rev*. 3:299, 1982

90. Clark BJ, Soo SC, Caron KM. Hormonal and developmental regulation of the steroidogenic acute regulatory protein. *Mol Endocrinol*. 9:1346, 1995

91. Waterman MR, Simpson ER. Regulation of the biosynthesis of cytochrome P-450 involved in steroid hormone synthesis. *Mol Cell Endocrinol*. 39:81, 1985

92. McAllister JM, Kerin JFP, Trant JM, et al. Regulation of cholesterol side-chain cleavage and 17α-hydroxylase/lyase activities in proliferating human theca interna cells in long-term monolayer culture. *Endocrinology*. 125:1959, 1989

93. Doody KJ, Lorence MC, Mason IJ, Simpson ER. Expression of messenger ribonucleic acid species encoding steroidogenic enzymes in human follicles and corpora lutea throughout the menstrual cycle. *J Clin Endocrinol Metab*. 70:1041, 1990

94. Suzuki T, Sasono H, Tamura M, et al. Temporal and spatial localization of steroidogenic enzymes in premenopausal human ovaries: In situ hybridization and immunohistochemical study. *Mol Cell Endocrinol*. 97:135, 1993

95. Zhang Y, Word A, Fesmire S, et al. Human ovarian expression of 17β-hydroxysteroid dehydrogenase types 1, 2, and 3. *J Clin Endocrinol Metab*. 81:3594, 1996

96. Steinkampf MP, Mendelson CR, Simpson ER. Effects of epidermal growth factor and insulin-like growth factor I on the levels of mRNA encoding aromatase cytochrome P-450 of human ovarian granulosa cells. *Mol Cell Endocrinol*. 59:93, 1988

97. McNatty KP, Makris A, DeGrazia C, et al. The production of progesterone, androgens, and estrogens by granulosa cells, theca tissue and stroma tissue from human ovaries in vitro. *J Clin Endocrinol Metab*. 49:687, 1979

98. Carr BR, Sadler RK, Rochelle DB, et al. Plasma lipoprotein regulation of progesterone biosynthesis by human corpus luteum tissue in organ culture. *J Clin Endocrinol Metab*. 52:875, 1981

99. Ohashi M, Carr BR, Simpson ER. Lipoprotein binding sites in human corpus luteum membrane fractions. *Endocrinology*. 110:1477, 1982

100. Illingworth DR, Corbin DK, Kemp ED, Keenan EJ. Hormone changes during the menstrual cycle in abetalipoproteinemia: Reduced luteal phase progesterone in a patient with homozygous hypobetalipoproteinemia. *Proc Natl Acad Sci USA*. 79:6685, 1982

101. Hsueh AJW, Adashi EY, Jones PBC, Welsh TH Jr. Hormonal regulation of the differentiation of culture ovarian granulosa cells. *Endocrine Rev*. 5:76, 1984

102. Baird DT, Horton R, Longcope C, Tait JF. Steroid dynamics under steady state conditions. *Rec Prog Horm Res*. 25:611, 1969

103. Baird DT, Horton R, Longcope C, Tait JF. Steroid prehormones. *Perspect Biol Med*. 11:384, 1968

104. Tait JF. Review: The use of isotopic steroids for the measurement of production rates *in vivo*. *J Clin Endocrinol Metab*. 23:1285, 1963

105. Siiteri PK, MacDonald PC. Placental estrogen biosynthesis during human pregnancy. *J Clin Endocrinol Metab*. 26:751, 1966

106. Rosner W. Sex steroid transport: Binding proteins. In: Adashi EY, Rock JA, Rosenwaks Z. *Reproductive Endocrinology, Surgery, and Technology*. Philadelphia, Pa., Lippincott-Raven, 1996: 605–626

107. Mendel CM. The free hormone hypothesis: Distinction from the free hormone transport hypothesis. *J Androl*. 13:107, 1992

108. Ekins R. The free hormone concept. In: Hennemann G, ed. *Thyroid Hormone Metabolism*. New York, N.Y., Marcel Dekker, 1986: 77–106

109. Pardridge WM, Landaw EM. Tracer kinetic model of blood–brain barrier transport of plasma protein-bound ligands: Empiric testing of the free hormone hypothesis. *J Clin Invest*. 74:745, 1984

110. Iqbal MJ, Johnson MW. Purification and characterization of human sex hormone-binding globulin. *J Steroid Biochem*. 10:535, 1979

111. Anderson DC. Sex hormone-binding globulin. *Clin Endocrinol (Oxf)*. 3:69, 1974

112. Barnea A, Gorsic J. Estrogen-induced protein: Time course of synthesis. *Biochemistry*. 9:1899, 1970

113. Clark JH, Shailaja KM. Actions of ovarian steroid hormones. In: Knobil E, Neill JD, eds. *The Physiology of Reproduction*, 2nd ed. New York, N.Y., Raven Press, 1994: 1011–1059

114. Welshoun WV, Lieberman MS, Gorski J. Nuclear localization of unoccupied estrogen receptors. *Nature*. 307:745, 1984

115. Simpson ER, Mendelson CR. The molecular basis of hormone action. In: Carr BR, Blackwell RE, eds. *Textbook of Reproductive Medicine*. Norwalk, Conn., Appleton and Lange, 1993: 121–140

116. Scholl S, Lippman ME. The estrogen receptor in MCF-7 cells: Evidence from dense amino acid labeling for rapid turnover and a dimeric model of activated nucleic acid receptor. *Endocrinology*. 115:1295, 1984

117. DeSombre ER, Kuivanen PC. Progestin modulation of estrogen-dependent marker protein synthesis in the endometrium. *Sem Oncol*. XII/1(suppl. 1):6, 1985

118. Adashi EY. The ovarian follicle: Life cycle of a pelvic clock. In: Adashi EY, Rock JA, Rosenwaks Z, eds. *Reproductive Endocrinology, Surgery, and Technology*. Philadelphia, Pa., Lippincott-Raven, 1996: 211–234

119. Adashi EY, Leung PCK, eds. *The Ovary.* New York, N.Y., Raven Press, 1993: 1–687

120. Tsafriri A, Adashi EY. Local nonsteroidal regulators of ovarian function. In: Knobil E, Neill JD, eds. *The Physiology of Reproduction*, 2nd ed. New York, N.Y., Raven Press, 1994; 1:861–1009

121. Sawetawan C, Carr BR, McGee E, et al. Inhibin and activin differentially regulate androgen production and 17α-hydroxylase expression in human ovarian thecal-like tumor cells. *J Endocrinol.* 148:213, 1996

122. Koos RD. Potential relevance of angiogenic factors to ovarian physiology. *Sem Rep Endocrinol.* 7:29, 1989

123. Fukuoka M, Yasuda K, Emi N, et al. Cytokine modulation of progesterone and estradiol secretion in cultures of luteinized human granulosa cells. *J Clin Endrocrinol Metab.* 75:254, 1992

124. Li CH, Ramasharma K, Yamashiro D, Chung D. Gonadotropin-releasing peptide from human follicular fluid: Isolation, characterization and chemical synthesis. *Proc Natl Acad Sci USA.* 84:959, 1987

125. Giudice LC. Insulin-like growth factors and ovarian follicular development. *Endocr Rev.* 13:641, 1992

126. McGee E, Sawetawan C, Bird I, et al. The effect of insulin and insulin-like growth factors on the expression of steroidogenic enzymes in a human ovarian theca-like tumor model. *Fertil Steril.* 65:87, 1996

127. Carr BR, McGee EA, Sawetawan C, et al. The effect of transforming growth factor beta on steroidogenesis and expression of key steroidogenic enzymes using a human ovarian theca-like tumor model. *Am J Obstet Gynecol.* 174:1109, 1996

128. Ueno S, Takahashi M, Manganaro TF, et al. Cellular localization of Müllerian inhibiting substance in the developing rat ovary. *Endocrinology.* 124:1000, 1989

129. Khan-Dawood FS, Goldsmith LT, Weiss G, Dawood MY. Human corpus luteum secretion of relaxin, oxytocin and progesterone. *J Clin Endocrinol Metab.* 68:627, 1989

130. Sherwood OD. Relaxin. In: Knobil E, Neill JD, eds. *The Physiology of Reproduction*, 2nd ed. New York, N.Y., Raven Press, 1994; 1:861–1009

131. Lightman A, Palumbo A, DeCherney AH, Naftolin F. The ovarian renin–angiotensin system. *Sem Rep Endocrinol.* 7:79, 1989

132. Rainey WE, Bird IM, Byrd W, Carr BR. Effect of angiotensin II on human luteinized granulosa cells. *Fertil Steril.* 59:143, 1993

133. Trzeciak WH, Ahmed CE, Simpson ER, Ojeda SR. Vasoactive intestinal peptide induces the synthesis of the cholesterol side-chain cleavage enzyme complex in cultured rat ovarian granulosa cells. *Proc Natl Acad Sci USA.* 83:7490, 1986

134. *A Statistical Portrait of Women in the U.S.* Publication 58, Current Population Report, Special Studies Series. Washington, D.C., U.S. Department of Commerce, Bureau of the Census, 1976: 23

135. Utian WH. *Menopause in Modern Perspective.* New York, N.Y., Appleton-Century-Crofts, 1980

136. Linquist O, Bengtsson C. Menopausal age in relation to smoking. *Acta Med Scand.* 205:73, 1979

137. Sauramo H. Histology, histopathology and function of the senile ovary. *Ann Chir Gynaecol Fenn.* 4(suppl.):1, 1952

138. Nagamani M, Stuart CA, Doherty NG. Increased steroid production by ovarian stromal tissue of postmenopausal women with endometrial cancer. *J Clin Endocrinol Metab.* 74:172, 1992

139. Scaglia H, Medina M, Pinto-Ferriera AL, et al. Pituitary LH and FSH secretion and responsiveness in women of old age. *Acta Endocrinol (Kbh).* 81:673, 1976

140. Chakravarti S, Collins WP, Forecast JD, et al. Hormonal profiles after the menopause. *Br Med J.* 2:784, 1976

141. Judd JL. Hormonal dynamics associated with the menopause. *Clin Obstet Gynecol.* 19:775, 1976

142. Edman CD, MacDonald PC. Effect of obesity on conversion of plasma androstenedione to estrone in ovulatory and anovulatory young women. *Am J Obstet Gynecol.* 130:456, 1978

143. Hemsell DL, Grodin JM, Brenner PF, et al. Plasma precursors of estrogen II. Correlation of the extent of conversion of plasma androstenedione to estrone with age. *J Clin Endocrinol Metab.* 38:476, 1974

144. Tataryn IV, Lomax P, Bajorek JG, et al. Postmenopausal hot flushes: A disorder of thermoregulation. *Maturitas.* 2:101, 1980

145. Walsh BW, Schiff I. Physiology of the climacteric. In: Carr BR, Blackwell RE, eds. *Textbook of Reproductive Medicine.* Norwalk, Ct., Appleton-Lange, 1993: 587–600

146. Brincat M, Moniz CJ, Studd JWW, et al. The long term effects of the menopause and of administration of sex hormones on skin collagen and skin thickness. *Br J Obstet Gynaecol.* 92:256, 1985

147. Weiss NS, Ure CL, Ballard JH, et al. Decreased risk of fractures of the hip and lower forearm with postmenopausal use of oestrogen. *N Engl J Med.* 303:1195, 1980

148. Barrett-Connor E, Brown WV, Turner J, et al. Heart disease risk factors and hormone use in postmenopausal women. *JAMA.* 241:2167, 1979

149. Jaszmann L, Van Lith ND, Zoat JCA. The perimenopausal symptoms. *Med Gynecol Sociol.* 4:268, 1969

150. Meldrum DR. The pathophysiology of postmenopausal symptoms. *Sem Reprod Endocrinol.* 1:11, 1983

151. Riggs BL, Wahner HW, Melton LJ III, et al. Rates of bone loss in the appendicular and axial skeletons of women. *J Clin Invest.* 77:1487, 1986

152. Alderman BW, Weiss NS, Daling JR, et al. Reproductive history and postmenopausal risk of hip and forearm fracture. *Am J Epidemiol.* 124:262, 1986

153. Beals RK. Survival following hip fracture: Long term follow-up of 607 patients. *J Chronic Dis.* 25:235, 1972

154. Nilas L, Christianson C. Bone mass and its relationship to age and the menopause. *J Clin Endocrinol Metab.* 65:697, 1987

155. Lindsay R, Herrington BS. Estrogens and osteoporosis. *Sem Reprod Endocrinol.* 1:55, 1983

156. Henderson BE, Ross RK, Paganini-Hill A, Mack TM. Estrogen use and cardiovascular disease. *Am J Obstet Gynecol.* 154:1181, 1986

157. Matthews KA, Meilahn E. Kuller LH, et al. Menopause and risk factors for coronary heart disease. *N Engl J Med.* 321:641, 1989

158. Colditz GA, Willett WC, Stampfer MJ, et al. Menopause and the risk of coronary heart disease in women. *N Engl J Med.* 316:1105, 1987

Chapter 12

THE NORMAL MENSTRUAL CYCLE

The Coordinated Events of the Hypothalamic–Pituitary–Ovarian Axis and the Female Reproductive Tract

Bruce R. Carr

Spontaneous, cyclic, predictable, and regular menstruation are the hallmarks of ovulatory menstrual cycles. Ovulatory menstrual cycles result from carefully regulated interactions of the hypothalamus, pituitary, ovaries, and female genital tract. The menstrual cycle can be divided into two phases: a follicular or proliferative phase and a luteal or secretory phase (Fig 12–1).

Menstrual cycle length is determined from the first day of the onset of menstrual bleeding until the onset of menstruation in the subsequent cycle. The median length of the menstrual cycle in reproductive age women is 28 days and the range is 25 to 30 days.[1–3] The length of the menstrual cycle varies most at the extremes of reproductive life, namely, following menarche and preceding menopause (Fig 12–2). Immediately after menarche, menstrual cycles are often prolonged and unpredictable due to poor or defective follicular development and often result in anovulatory or luteal deficient cycles.[4, 5] Likewise, just prior to the onset of menopause menstrual cycles are anovulatory and prolonged and unpredictable.[6] The least variability of menstrual cycle length is found between ages 20 to 30. Most studies comparing the relative length of the follicular and luteal phases have found that the length of the luteal phase is remarkably constant and lasts 13 to 14 days.[3] The length of the follicular phase may vary from 10 to 16 days, which explains the variation in the length of normal menstrual cycles (see Fig 12–3).

PHASES OF THE NORMAL MENSTRUAL CYCLE

Follicular Phase

The first phase of follicular growth or folliculogenesis is initiated during the last few days of the luteal phase of the preceding menstrual cycle and ends with ovulation. Near the end of the previous luteal phase, plasma progesterone and estrogen levels decline due to demise of the corpus luteum, and a rise in follicle-stimulating hormone (FSH) levels occurs[7–8] (Fig 12–1). FSH initiates the recruitment of follicles of which one will release an ovum at the time of ovulation. In primates, the follicle destined to ovulate most often occurs in the ovary that is contralateral to the ovary containing the corpus luteum.[8] However, evidence from ultrasonographic investigations of women suggests that ovulation occurs randomly in consecutive cycles, not preferentially to the contralateral ovary.[9]

During the midfollicular phase, follicle development continues but FSH levels begin to decline due to the negative feedback of estrogens and inhibin secreted by the developing follicle.[10–12] In response to a decline in FSH together with the proposed effects of various protein and steroid hormones secreted by the theca and granulosa cells of the growing follicle (see Chap 11), the development of adjacent follicles is inhibited. In preparation of the development of a single dominant follicle, three stages have been described (Fig 12–4).[7] The

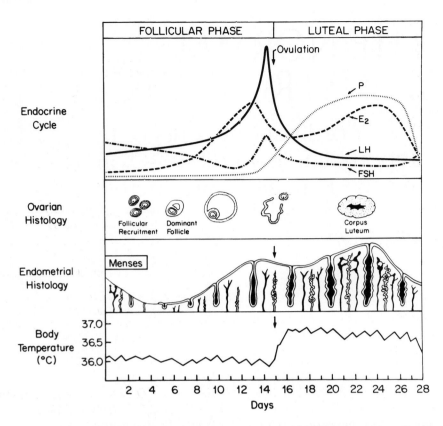

Figure 12–1. Hormonal, ovarian, endometrial, and basal body temperature changes and relationship throughout the normal menstrual cycle. *(Reproduced, with permission, from Carr BR, Wilson JD. In: Wilson JD, Braunwald E, Isselbacher KJ, et al, eds. 1991: 1776.[73])*

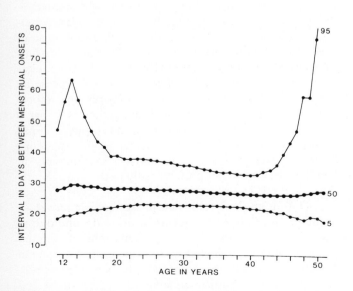

Figure 12–2. Menstrual cycle length in relation to age. The median and 5th and 95th percentiles are indicated. *(Data reproduced from Treloar AE, Boynton BE, Behn BG, et al, 1967:77[1] as adapted by Baird DT. Amenorrhea, anovulation and dysfunctional uterine bleeding. In: Degroot LJ, ed. Endocrinology. Philadelphia, Pa., W.B. Saunders, 1989: 1950–1968.)*

first is recruitment. A cohort of follicles are recruited from a pool of nonproliferating follicles in response to FSH.[9] This process occurs during days 1 to 4 of the menstrual cycle. Once this stage is attained, the recruited follicles must either ovulate or undergo atresia.[7] The second stage is selection, wherein one follicle from those initially recruited is selected to eventually ovulate. The selection stage occurs between days 5 and 7 of the cycle. The third and final stage of folliculogenesis is named dominance, wherein the selected dominant follicle continues to grow and further suppresses maturation of other ovarian follicles. The dominant stage occurs between days 8 and 12 of the cycle and ends with ovulation (days 13 to 15).

During the follicular phase, estrogen levels rise and parallel the growth of the follicle and the number of granulosa cells (Figs 12–1 and 12–4). FSH receptors are located exclusively on granulosa cells (see Chap 11). The increased levels of immunoreactive FSH seen in the late luteal phase of the previous cycle and the subsequent early follicular phase, as well as increased levels of bioactive FSH during the early to midfollicular phase, leads to an increase in the number of FSH receptors and consequently, an increase in estradiol formation by granulosa cells.[13] The observed increase in total FSH receptors is

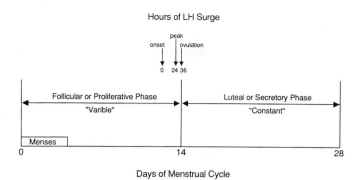

Figure 12–3. Relationship of the LH surge and menstrual cycle length. *(Modified, with permission, from Yen SSC. The human menstrual cycle. In: Yen SSC, Jaffe RB, eds.* Reproductive Endocrinology, *2nd ed. Philadelphia, Pa., W.B. Saunders, 1986: 203.)*

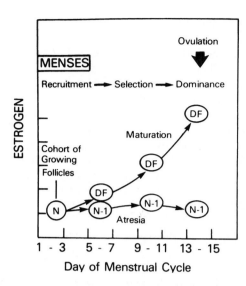

Figure 12–4. Time course for the recruitment, selection, and ovulation of the dominant ovarian follicle (DF) with onset of atresia among other follicles of the cohort (N1). *(Reproduced, with permission, from Hodgen GD, 1982: 281.[7])*

due to an increase in number of granulosa cells rather than an increase in FSH receptors per cell. Each granulosa cell contains about 1500 FSH receptors per cell by the selection stage of folliculogenesis and remains constant throughout the remainder of the follicular phase.[14] FSH also induces aromatase and estradiol secretion that leads to an increase in the number of estradiol receptors.[14] FSH in the presence of estradiol induces the formation of luteinizing hormone (LH) receptors on granulosa cells.[15,16] After LH receptors develop, the preovulatory granulosa cells begin to secrete limited quantities of progesterone and 17-hydroxyprogesterone.[17] In addition to the positive feedback of estrogen on LH levels, the preovulatory secretion of progesterone is believed to exert a positive feedback on estrogen-primed pituitary to further augment LH release.[18] LH also stimulates theca cells to secrete androgens that are passed to adjacent granulosa cells, where they are aromatized to estrogens to further increase estrogen formation by the dominant follicle.

Preantral and small antral follicles secrete small amounts of estrogen and greater amounts of androgen.[19] This occurs because of the presence of the enzyme 5α-reductase in these smaller follicles, which converts testosterone to dihydrotestosterone (DHT), which inhibits aromatase. In contrast, large antral follicles, and in particular the dominant graafian follicle, express large quantities of aromatase and secrete more estrogen. Thus, the balance of androgens and estrogens in the microenvironment of the ovary may be instrumental in the selection of the dominant follicle and the regression of other smaller follicles.[17]

The regulation of steroidogenesis by granulosa cells is further influenced by a variety of hormones and other substances found in follicular fluid bathing the granulosa cells (Table 12–1). The concentration of ovarian steroids in follicular fluid exceeds by manyfold the concentration

TABLE 12–1.   SUBSTANCES FOUND IN FOLLICULAR FLUID

Plasma proteins

Steroid-binding proteins

Enzymes
  Side-chain cleavage enzyme
  3β-Hydroxysteroid dehydrogenase
  17α-Hydroxylase
  C_{17-20} Lyase
  17β-Hydroxysteroid dehydrogenase
  20α-Hydroxysteroid dehydrogenase
  Aromatase
  Plasminogen (proteases)

Micropolysaccharides (proteoglycans)
  Hyaluronic acid
  Chondroitin sulfate acid
  Heparin sulfate

Steroids
  Estrogens
  Androgens
  Progestins

Pituitary hormones
  Follicle-stimulating hormone
  Luteinizing hormone
  Prolactin
  Oxytocin
  Vasopressin

Nonsteroidal ovarian factors
  Inhibin
  Follicular protein (aromatase inhibitor)
  Oocyte meiosis inhibitor
  Luteinization inhibitor
  Luteinization stimulator

(Reproduced, with permission, from Yen SSC. The human menstrual cycle. In: Yen SSC, Jaffe RD, eds. Reproductive Endocrinology. *Philadelphia, Pa., W. B. Saunders, 1986: 208.)*

of that in blood. On the basis of antral follicular fluid concentration of steroids, two populations of antral follicles have been identified. In large follicles (>8 mm in diameter), follicular fluid concentrations of FSH, estrogens, and progesterone levels are high. In small follicles, the concentrations of androgens in follicular fluid are greater but estrogen levels are less than from large follicles. Prolactin levels also vary in follicular fluid and are high in small follicles and less in large, estrogen–progesterone-dominant follicles. These observations further support the hypothesis of microenvironmental influences on follicular growth by the concentrations of hormones in the follicular fluid.[20–24]

As mentioned previously, there are differences in gonadotropin levels during the follicular phase. FSH levels, which are elevated during the early part of the follicular phase, decline until ovulation occurs. In contrast, LH levels are low in the first part of the follicular phase but due to increasing estrogen secretion by the growing follicle and a positive feedback mechanism begin to increase by the midfollicular phase. In response to a single as well as second bolus injection of LH-releasing hormone (LHRH), LH secretion is markedly increased from the early until the late follicular phase. This self-priming action of LHRH is an example of the positive feedback on the enhancement of LH release from the pituitary by LHRH.[25]

The frequency of spontaneous LH pulses also varies during the menstrual cycle. In the early part of the cycle, LH pulses are of constant amplitude and occur at frequencies of 60 to 90 min. During the late follicular phase, just prior to the midcycle surge of LH, LH pulse frequency increases whereas LH pulse amplitude does not increase until following ovulation.[26]

Ovulation

Prior to ovulation, estrogen secretion by the preovulatory follicle increases dramatically and initiates the LH surge. LH in turn initiates the process of luteinization of the granulosa cells and progesterone secretion, which appears to trigger the midcycle surge of FSH. Thirty-four to 36 hr after onset of the LH surge, ovulation occurs with release of the ovum from the follicle (see Fig 12–3).[27] The exact peak of LH secretion is difficult to determine but averages 10 to 16 hr prior to ovulation.[28] The LH surge also initiates the resumption of meiosis followed by release of the first polar body. LH also induces an increase in cyclic adenosine monophosphate (cAMP) in the granulosa cell that stimulates luteinization and an increase in progesterone secretion.[29] Spontaneous luteinization may occur in the absence of LH when granulosa cells are removed from the follicle and cultured. This has led to the hypothesis that some factor or factors (see Chap 11) act to prevent premature follicular luteinization.[30]

Prior to ovulation, extensive vascularization of the follicle develops. A small protrusion of the follicular wall called the stigma appears and represents the location where rupture occurs with release of the oocyte–cumulus complex. The release of the ovum has been photographed and lasts only a few minutes.[31] The exact mechanism of the process of follicular rupture in humans is unknown. cAMP and progesterone are believed to activate proteolytic enzymes such as collagenase or plasmin that cause digestion of collagen in the follicular wall, leading to distensibility and thinning of the wall prior to ovum release.[32,33] Follicular pressure does not increase prior to follicular rupture.[31,32] In certain animal species, tissue plasminogen activator is stimulated by gonadotropins that increase the concentration of plasmin. Plasmin stimulates collagenase activity, which thins and weakens the follicular wall as discussed previously.[33] In addition, in rats treated with antibodies to tissue plasminogen activator and α_2-antiplasmin, human chorionic gonadotropin (hCG)-stimulated ovulation is inhibited.[34] However, in human follicular fluid, plasminogen activator does not increase in mature preovulatory follicles.[35]

Certain prostaglandins (E and F series) and HETES (hydroxyeicosatetraeonic and methyl esters) reach a peak concentration in follicular fluid just prior to ovulation.[36] Prostaglandins have been proposed to be involved in the rupture of the follicle, possibly by stimulation of smooth muscle contractions, thereby aiding the extrusion of the oocyte–cumulus mass.[37] In some cycles the ovum is not released, which has given rise to the concept of the luteinized unruptured follicle syndrome (LUFS), but this process appears to occur equally often in fertile as well as infertile women. However, women treated with high doses of prostaglandin synthetase inhibitors such as indomethacin may develop luteinized unruptured follicles.[38–40] Women who are seeking fertility are advised to avoid the use of drugs that inhibit prostaglandin synthesis at midcycle just prior to ovulation.

Just prior to the LH peak, estradiol levels in plasma fall precipitously (see Fig 12–5). This fall may be due to downregulation of LH on LH receptors or direct inhibiting action of increasing progesterone secretion on granulosa cell growth.[27] An alternative explanation to the fall in estrogen secretion by the ovary prior to ovulation may be secondary to a decline in androgen substrate because aromatase levels in the ovary are high at this time (see Chap 11).[17] The peak of FSH that occurs at midcycle and is thought to be stimulated by progesterone has been proposed to influence a variety of functions including stimulation of plasminogen activator and increase in granulosa cell LH receptors.[17] The fall in LH following ovulation is thought to be secondary to the loss of positive feedback due to a decline in estrogen levels or depletion of LH content of the pituitary.

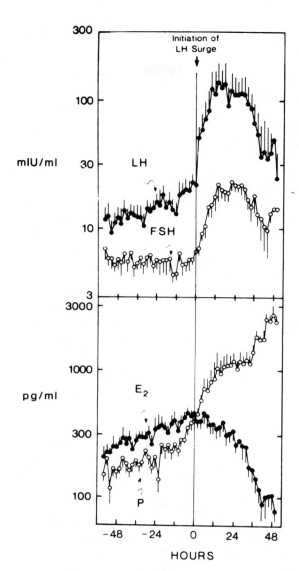

Figure 12–5. Changes in gonadotropins and ovarian steroids at midcycle, just prior to ovulation. The initiation of LH surge is at time 0. Abbreviations: E₂, estrogen; P, progesterone *(Reproduced, with permission, from Hoff JD, Quigley ME, Yen SSC, 1983: 792.²⁷)*

Luteal Phase

Following ovulation, the follicle undergoes marked changes in structure and function. When the process of luteinization is completed, the corpus luteum is established. The purpose of the corpus luteum is to secrete progesterone and ready the estrogen-primed endometrium for acceptance of a fertilized ovum and in maintenance of early pregnancy. The establishment of a vascular supply to the corpus luteum occurs in response to the secretion of angiogenic factors secreted by the granulosa and theca cells.[41] The first few days following ovulation, the granulosa-lutein cells enlarge and are surrounded by the newly formed theca-lutein cells. At the time of peak vascularization of the

corpus luteum, maximal secretion of progesterone occurs (see Fig 12–1). In the absence of conception, the corpus luteum undergoes luteolysis and remains as a fibrous scar, the corpus albicans.

The pattern of secretion of hormones by corpus luteum during the luteal phase is depicted in Figures 12–1 and 12–6. Following ovulation, estrogen levels fall followed by a secondary rise during the midluteal phase, followed by a second decline near the end of the late luteal phase. The rise of estradiol parallels the pattern of progesterone and 17α-hydroxyprogesterone levels. Studies of ovarian venous blood indicate that the corpus luteum is the site of steroid secretion by the ovary during the luteal phase.[42] During the follicular phase, the levels of inhibin remain fairly constant (Fig 12–6). Within 2 to 3 days of ovulation, there is a peak in inhibin levels coincident with the LH and FSH surge, followed by a brief fall and a marked rise in concentrations during the luteal phase.[11,43,44] The corpus luteum is the source of elevated inhibin during the luteal phase. The fall in inhibin levels at the end of the luteal phase is associated with a rise in FSH levels (Fig 12–6).

The mechanisms of the control of the rate of steroid secretion by the corpus luteum in women is determined in part by: (1) gonadotropin LH secretory pattern and LH receptors; (2) the amount of various enzymes regulating steroid hormone formation; (3) the number of granulosa cells formed by the follicle during the follicular phase; (4) the amount of cholesterol substrate (low-density lipoprotein [LDL] cholesterol); and (5) the secretion of other hormones by the corpus luteum by autocrine or paracrine action (see Chap 11).

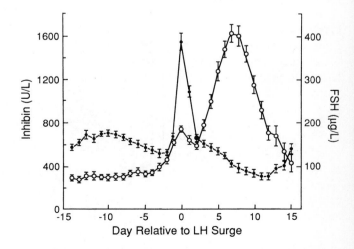

Figure 12–6. Serum levels of inhibin and FSH during the normal menstrual cycle. Day of LH surge = 0. Key: (○), inhibin; (●), FSH. *(Adapted, with permission, from McLachlan RI, Cohen NL, Dahl KD, et al. Serum inhibin in normal women: Relationship with sex steroid and gonadotropin levels. Clin Endocrinol. 32:39, 1980.)*

LH is the primary luteotropic agent in women and was established in hypophysectomized women.[45] In these women, following induction of ovulation the length of the luteal phase and the amount of progesterone secreted was dependent upon repeated injections of LH. LH or hCG administration during the luteal phase of normal women can extend the functional life span of the corpus luteum and the secretion of progesterone up to 2 additional wk.[46] Progesterone secretion during the luteal phase is episodic and progesterone peaks have been reported to correlate with pulses of LH secretion (Fig 12–7).[47]

In addition, evidence suggests that gonadotropin levels during the follicular phase influence the corpus luteum and luteal phase length. This is supported by the observation that the frequency and amplitude of LH secretion during the follicular phase regulate subsequent luteal phase function and length.[48] Similarly, a reduction in FSH during the follicular phase is associated with a shortened luteal phase, smaller corpora lutea, and reduced responsiveness of dispersed corpus luteum cells in vitro.[49] The administration of LHRH analogs during either the follicular or luteal phase likewise reduces the life span of the corpus luteum.[50,51] A decline in LH concentration, pulse frequency, or amplitude during the luteal phase reduces the length of the luteal phase and progesterone secretion.[52] The corpus luteum of primates may recover from a transient withdrawal of LH, but this depends upon the age of the corpus luteum.[53] LH/hCG receptors have also been measured in ovaries obtained from women. The total and unoccupied LH/hCG receptor concentrations parallel progesterone secretion during the luteal phase.[54] Likewise, the basal activity of adenylate cyclase and the response to sodium fluoride (NaF) and forskolin by luteal membrane preparations also parallel progesterone secretion during the luteal phase in women.[55]

The role of luteotropic factors other than LH in women is not clear. Prolactin is not luteotropic in women as in the rat, but defective luteal function may exist when prolactin levels are suppressed in women treated with 2-bromo-α-ergocriptine or in the presence of elevated levels of prolactin.[56,57] Prostaglandin E_2 has been shown to be luteotropic in isolated human corpus luteum cells and stimulates cAMP and progesterone secretion.[58] Relaxin, inhibin, and oxytocin, which are secreted by the human corpus luteum and may modulate corpus luteum function, do not appear to play a role in the maintenance of early pregnancy because agonadal women treated with estrogen and progesterone alone in association with

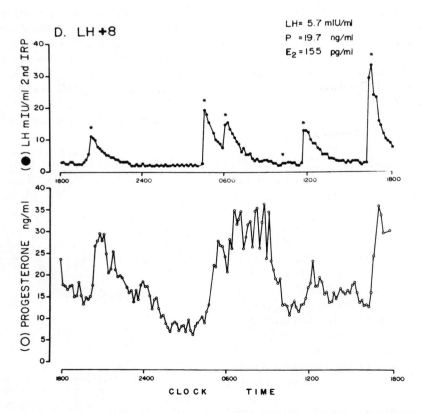

Figure 12–7. Episodic secretion of LH (top) and progesterone (bottom) during the luteal phase of a woman. Abbreviations: LH, luteinizing hormone; P, progesterone; E_2, estradiol; LH + 8, LH surge plus 8 days. *(Reproduced, with permission, from Filicori M, Butler JP, Crowley WF Jr, 1984: 1638.[47])*

donor embryo transfer have carried pregnancies to term.[59,60]

Corpus luteum function begins to rapidly decline 9 to 11 days following ovulation, a process known as luteolysis, but the mechanism of regulation of luteolysis in women remains unclear. Prostaglandin $F_{2\alpha}$ ($PGF_{2\alpha}$) appears to be luteolytic in nonhuman primates and women.[61,62] Likewise, evidence supports the hypothesis that exogenous estrogens are luteolytic in women and primates.[63,64] However, these studies are clouded by the evidence that antiestrogens and aromatase inhibitors fail to increase the length of the luteal phase and corpus luteum function in nonhuman primates.[65] Oxytocin and vasopressin secreted by the corpus luteum may be luteolytic by modulating corpus luteum function by autocrine or paracrine mechanisms.[56,66] Evidence also supports the view that LH induces downregulation of its own receptor, which declines at the end of the luteal phase.

During the normal menstrual cycle, gonadotropins, inhibin, estrogen, and progesterone undergo marked fluctuations as described. However, there are minimal fluctuations other than small peaks near midcycle for androgens and pituitary hormones other than gonadotropins during the menstrual cycle.[67–73] Plasma levels of deoxycorticosterone (DOC) increase during the luteal phase and this is believed to be due to extra-adrenal 21-hydroxylation of progesterone.[74,75]

EFFECT OF HORMONES ON THE FEMALE REPRODUCTIVE TRACT DURING THE MENSTRUAL CYCLE

The interrelationships of the hypothalamic–pituitary–ovarian axis give rise to fluctuations in estrogen and progesterone that produce striking effects on the tissues of the reproductive tract. The most characterized alterations occur in the endometrium. The changes in endometrial histology throughout the menstrual cycle are such that dating of the endometrium is possible (Fig 12–8).[76]

The proliferative phase is less precisely dated and consists of growth of the endometrium up to 5 mm thickness. During the proliferative phase, the glands are narrow and tubular, and mitosis and pseudostratification are present. Two days after ovulation (cycle day 16), glycogen accumulates in the basal portion of the glandular epithelium. The nuclei appear to be displaced to the midportion of the cells, resulting in a pseudostratified configuration. In tissues fixed with formalin, glycogen is solubilized, leaving large vacuoles in the base of the cells. The development of subnuclear vacuolation of the glandular epithelium is evidence that a functional, progesterone-producing corpus luteum has been formed. By day 17, the glands are visibly more tortuous and dilated. On day 18, the vacuoles in the

epithelium are smaller and often located along the nuclei and glycogen is now apparent in the apex of the cells. Intraluminal secretion is present and pseudostratification and vacuolation have nearly disappeared by day 19. On cycle days 21 and 22, the endometrial stroma become edematous. By day 23, stromal cells surrounding the spiral arterioles enlarge and mitoses are visible. Day 24 is characterized by predecidual changes in the stromal cells around the spiral arterioles and increased mitoses. By day 25, predecidual changes in the stromal cells begin under the surface epithelium. By day 27, the upper half of the endometrial stroma is a solid sheet of well-developed decidualized cells. Differentiation of the decidua is accompanied by a marked increase in lymphocytic infiltration and menstruation begins on day 28.

The breakdown of the endometrium occurs in cycles where conception fails to occur and corpus luteum function ceases with a resulting decrease of estrogen and progesterone levels. These hormonal changes induce three endometrial events: vascular alterations, loss of tissue, and menstruation. In association with shrinkage of the height of the endometrium, a concomitant decrease in blood flow of the spiral vessels and vasodilation ensues. The spiral vessels feeding the endometrium undergo rhythmic cycles of vasoconstriction and vasodilation. This results in necrosis of the blood vessels and eventually to endometrial ischemia and cell death.[77,78] Menstruation follows and consists of blood and desquamation of superficial endometrial tissues. Menstrual flow lasts 4 to 6 days and the average amount of blood lost is 30 ml/cycle.[79] By the midfollicular phase, estrogen secretion by the ovarian follicles increases and induces endometrial healing. Vasoconstriction occurs and platelets and clot formation develop over the denuded endometrial vessels.[80]

The development of necrosis and vasospasm of the spiral vessels is thought to be due to prostaglandins. Prostaglandins are present in large quantities in secretory endometrium and menstrual blood.[81–83] The infusion of $PGF_{2\alpha}$ to women during the luteal phase will induce endometrial necrosis and subsequent bleeding.[84] Prostaglandin release is believed to be secondary to a disruption of the lysosomal membranes in the endometrial cell.[84] This is followed by the liberation of phospholipids and subsequent synthesis of $PGF_{2\alpha}$. Interestingly, the use of PG synthetase inhibitors decreases the amount of menstrual bleeding in normal women and women using contraceptive devices. The inability of menstrual blood to coagulate is thought to be due to the presence of fibrinolytic activity.[85]

The levels of steroid receptors for estrogen and progesterone vary markedly during the menstrual cycle. Estrogen receptor content of the endometrium is high during the proliferative phase and declines in the secretory phase due to the action of progesterone formed by the corpus luteum.[86] Because estrogen not only stimulates

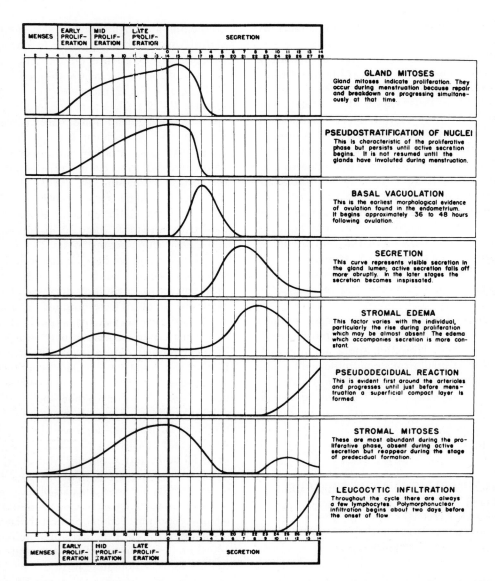

Figure 12–8. Dating of the endometrium. *(Reproduced, with permission, from Noyes RW, Hertig AW, Rock J, 1950: 3.[76])*

the formation of estrogen receptors but also progesterone receptors, the content of progesterone receptors increases during the late proliferative phase, peaks at ovulation, and declines less rapidly than the estrogen receptors during the secretory phase.

In addition to steroid receptors, the activities of endometrial steroidogenic enzymes also vary during the menstrual cycle, particularly the activity of 17β-hydroxysteroid oxidoreductase (17β-HSOR). 17β-HSOR stimulates the conversion of the potent estrogen, 17β-estradiol, to the less potent estrogen, estrone. The activity of 17β-HSOR is enhanced during the secretory phase, resulting in a decline of the endometrial content of estradiol and increase in the content of estrone.[87] Thus, by progesterone's inhibitory action on the estrogen receptor and its stimulatory action on

17β-HSOR the effect of estrogen action on secretory endometrium is diminished.

The endocervical glands undergo cyclic changes that are more similar to the changes in vaginal epithelium than in the endometrium. Following the menses, the amount of mucus secreted by the endocervical gland is limited and viscous. The quantity of mucus increases up to 30-fold in response to increasing levels of estrogen secreted by the follicle during the latter half of the follicular phase. The quality of endocervical mucus also changes and becomes watery and elastic. A fine thread of mucus can be demonstrated by stretching a drop of secretion (spinnbarkeit). Also, a characteristic ferning or palm-leaf arborization can be demonstrated in mucus dried on a microscope slide. Progesterone secretion during the luteal phase reverses the effects of estrogen on the cervical mucus.

Vaginal epithelial cells are also influenced by cyclic changes in estrogen and progesterone levels. In the early follicular phase, exfoliated vaginal epithelial cells are basophilic and contain vesicular nuclei. When estrogen levels increase in the latter half of the follicular phase, vaginal epithelial cells become acidophilic with pyknotic nuclei. During the luteal phase with increasing levels of progesterone, the percentage of acidophilic cells decreases and the number of leukocytes increase. A number of indices to characterize vaginal cytology are also available (see Chap 14).

REFERENCES

1. Treloar AE, Boynton BE, Behn BG, Brown RW. Variations of the human menstrual cycle throughout reproductive life. *Int J Fertil.* 12:77, 1967

2. Ferin M, Jewelewicz R, Warren M. *The Menstrual Cycle.* New York, Oxford University Press, 1993

3. Presser HB. Temporal data relating to the human menstrual cycle. In: Ferin M, Halber F, Richart RM, et al, eds. *Biorhythms and Human Reproduction.* London, U.K., John Wiley & Sons, 1974: 145–160

4. Apter D, Raisanen I, Ylostalo P, Vihko R. Follicular growth in relation to serum hormonal patterns in adolescence compared with adult menstrual cycles. *Fertil Steril.* 47:82, 1987

5. Fraser IS, Michie EA, Wide L, Baird DT. Pituitary gonadotropin and ovarian function in adolescent dysfunctional uterine bleeding. *J Clin Endocrinol Metab.* 37:407, 1973

6. Sherman BM, West JH, Korenman SG. The menopausal tradition: Analysis of LH, FSH, estradiol, and progesterone concentrations during menstrual cycles of older women. *J Clin Endocrinol Metab.* 42:629, 1976

7. Hodgen GD. The dominant ovarian follicle. *Fertil Steril.* 38:281, 1982

8. Goodman AL, Hodgen GD. The ovarian triad of the primate menstrual cycle. *Rec Prog Horm Res.* 39:1, 1983

9. Baird DT. A model for follicular selection and ovulation: Lessons from superovulation. *J Steroid Biochem.* 27:15, 1987

10. Mais V, Cetel NS, Muse KN, et al. Hormonal dynamics during luteal-follicular transition. *J Clin Endocrinol Metab.* 64:1109, 1987

11. McNeilly AS, Tsonis CG, Baird DT. Inhibin. *Human Reprod.* 3:45, 1988

12. Franchimont P, Hazee-Hagelstein MT, Jaspar JM, et al. Inhibin and related peptides: Mechanisms of action and regulation of secretion. *J Steroid Biochem.* 32:193, 1989

13. Dorrington JH, Armstrong DT. Effects of FSH on gonadal functions. *Rec Prog Horm Res.* 39:301, 1979

14. Nimrod A, Erickson GF, Ryan KJ. A specific FSH receptor in rat granulosa cells: Properties of binding *in vitro*. *Endocrinology.* 98:56, 1976

15. Zeleznik AJ, Midgley AR Jr, Reichert LE Jr. Granulosa cell maturation in the rat: Increased binding of human chorionic gonadotropin following treatment with follicle-stimulating hormone in vivo. *Endocrinology.* 95:818, 1974

16. Erickson GF, Wang C, Hsueh AJW. FSH induction of functional LH receptors in granulosa cells cultured in a chemically defined medium. *Nature.* 279:336, 1979

17. Baird DT. The ovarian cycle. In: Hillier SG, ed. *Ovarian Endocrinology.* Oxford, U.K., Blackwell Scientific Publications, 1991: 1–24

18. Fink G. Gonadotropin secretion and its control. In: Knobil E, Neill JD, eds. *The Physiology of Reproduction.* New York, N.Y., Raven Press, 1988; 1: 1349–1377

19. McNatty KP, Makris A, Reinhold VN, et al. Metabolism of androstenedione by human ovarian tissue in vitro with particular reference to reductase and aromatase activity. *Steroids.* 34:429, 1979

20. McNatty KP. Cyclic changes in antral fluid hormone concentrations in humans. *J Clin Endocrinol Metab.* 7:577, 1978

21. McNatty KP, Smith DM, Makris A, et al. The microenvironment of the human antral follicle: Interrelationships among the steroid levels in antral fluid, the population of granulosa cells, and the status of oocyte in vivo and in vitro. *J Clin Endocrinol Metab.* 49:851, 1979

22. Sanyal MK, Berger MJ, Thompson IE, et al. Development of graafian follicles in adult human ovary. I. Correlation of estrogen and progesterone concentration in antral fluid with growth of follicles. *J Clin Endocrinol Metab.* 38:828, 1974

23. Brailly S, Gourgeon A, Milgrom E, et al. Androgens and progestins in human ovarian follicle. Differences in the evolution of preovulatory, healthy nonovulatory and atretic follicles. *J Clin Endocrinol Metab.* 53:128, 1981

24. Bomsel-Helmreich O. The preovulatory human oocyte and its microenvironment. In: Beier HM, Lindner HR, eds. *Fertilization of the Human Egg In Vitro.* Berlin, Springer-Verlag, 1983: 10–34

25. Wang CF, Lasley BL, Lein A, Yen SSC. The functional changes of the pituitary gonadotropins during the menstrual cycle. *J Clin Endocrinol Metab.* 42:718, 1976

26. Ream N, Saunder SE, Kelch RP, Marshall JC. Pulsatile gonadotropin secretion during the menstrual cycle: Evidence for altered frequency of gonadotropin-releasing hormone secretion. *J Clin Endocrinol Metab.* 59:328, 1984

27. Hoff JD, Quigley ME, Yen SSC. Hormonal dynamics at midcycle: A re-evaluation. *J Clin Endocrinol Metab.* 57:792, 1983

28. Brown JB, Gronow M. Endocrinology of ovulation prediction. In: Sherman RP, ed. *Clinical Reproductive Endocrinology.* Edinburgh, Churchill Livingstone, 1985: 165–184

29. Weiss TJ, Seamark RF, McIntosh JEA, Moor RM. Cyclic AMP in sheep ovarian follicles: Site of production and response to gonadotropins. *J Reprod Fertil.* 46:347, 1976

30. Channing CP, Schaerf FW, Anderson LD, Tsafriri A. Ovarian follicular and luteal physiology. In: Greep RO, ed. *International Review of Physiology*, Vol 22. Baltimore, Md., University Park Press, 1980: 117–201

31. Lipner H, Espey LL. Mechanism of mammalian ovulation. In: Knobil E, Neill JD, eds. *The Physiology of Reproduction*, 2nd ed. New York, N.Y., Raven Press, 1994; 1: 725–780

32. Espey LL. Ovarian proteolytic enzymes and ovulation. *Biol Reprod.* 10:216, 1974

33. Beers WH. Follicular plasminogen and plasminogen activator and the effect of plasmin on ovarian follicular wall. *Cell.* 6:379, 1975

34. Tsafriri A, Bicsak TA, Cajander SB, et al. Suppression of ovulation rate by antibodies to tissue-type plasminogen activator and α_2-antiplasmin. *Endocrinology.* 124:415, 1989

35. Jones PBC, Vernon MW, Muse KN, Curry TE Jr. Plasminogen activator and plasminogen activator inhibitor in human preovulatory follicular fluid. *J Clin Endocrinol Metab.* 68:1039, 1989

36. Tsafriri A, Chun SY. Ovulation. In: Adashi EY, Rock JA, Rosenwaks Z, eds. *Reproductive Endocrinology, Surgery, and Technology.* Philadelphia, Lippincott-Raven, 1966: 236–249

37. Yoshimura Y, Wallach EE. Studies on the mechanisms of mammalian ovulation. *Fertil Steril.* 47:22, 1987

38. Doody KJ, Carr BR. Diagnosis and treatment of luteal dysfunction. In: Hillier SG, ed. *Ovarian Endocrinology.* Oxford, U.K., Blackwell Scientific Publications, 1991: 260–318

39. Killick S, Elstein M. Pharmacologic production of luteinized unruptured follicles by prostaglandin synthetase inhibitors. *Fertil Steril.* 47:773, 1987

40. Murdoch WJ, Cavender JL. Effect of indomethacin on the vascular architecture of preovulatory ovine follicles: Possible implication in the luteinized unruptured follicle syndrome. *Fertil Steril.* 51:153, 1989

41. Koss RD. Potential relevance of angiogenic factors to ovarian physiology. *Sem Rep Endocrinol.* 7:29, 1989

42. Niswender GD, Nett TM. The corpus luteum and its control. In: Knobil E, Neill JD, eds. *The Physiology of Reproduction,* 2nd ed. New York, N.Y., Raven Press, 1994; 1: 781–816

43. Reddi K, Wickings EJ, McNeilly AS, et al. Circulating bioactive follicle stimulating hormone and immunoreactive inhibin during the human menstrual cycle. *Clin Endocrinol.* 33:547, 1990

44. Roseff SJ, Bongah ML, Kettel M, et al. Dynamic changes in circulating inhibin levels during the luteal-follicular transition of the human menstrual cycle. *J Clin Endocrinol Metab.* 69:1033, 1989

45. Vande Wiele RL, Bogumil J, Dyrenfurth I, et al. Mechanisms regulating the menstrual cycle in women. *Rec Prog Horm Res.* 26:63, 1970

46. Segaloff A, Sternberg WH, Gaskill CJ. Effects of luteotrophic doses of chorionic gonadotropin in women. *J Clin Endocrinol Metab.* 11:936, 1951

47. Filicori M, Butler JP, Crowley WF Jr. Neuroendocrine regulation of the corpus luteum in the human. *J Clin Invest.* 73:1638, 1984

48. McNeely MJ, Soules MR. The diagnosis of luteal phase deficiency. *Fertil Steril.* 50:1, 1988

49. Stouffer RL, Hodgen GD. Induction of luteal phase defects in rhesus monkeys by follicular fluid administration at the onset of the menstrual cycle. *J Clin Endocrinol Metab.* 51:669, 1980

50. Sheehan KL, Casper RF, Yen SSC. Luteal phase defects induced by an agonist of luteinizing hormone releasing factor: A model for fertility control. *Science.* 215:170, 1982

51. Keyes PL, Wiltbank MC. Endocrine regulation of the corpus luteum. *Annu Rev Physiol.* 50:465, 1988

52. Cooke ID. The corpus luteum. *Human Reprod.* 3:153, 1988

53. Hutchison JS, Zeleznik AJ. The corpus luteum of the primate menstrual cycle is capable of recovering from a transient withdrawal of pituitary gonadotropin support. *Endocrinology.* 117:1043, 1985

54. Yeko TR, Khan-Dawood FS, Dawood MY. Human corpus luteum: Luteinizing hormone and chorionic gonadotropin receptors during the menstrual cycle. *J Clin Endocrinol Metab.* 68:529, 1989

55. Rojas FJ, Moretti-Rojas I, Balmaceda JP, Asch RH. Regulation of gonadotropin-stimulable adenyl cyclase of the primate corpus luteum. *J Steroid Biochem.* 32:175, 1989

56. Auletta FJ, Flint APF. Mechanisms controlling corpus luteum function in sheep, cows, nonhuman primates, and women especially in relation to the time of luteolysis. *Endocrine Rev.* 9:88, 1988

57. Schulz KD, Geiger W, Del Poso E, Kunzig HJ. Pattern of sexual steroids, prolactin and gonadotropic hormones during prolactin inhibition in normally cycling women. *Am J Obstet Gynecol.* 132:561, 1978

58. Hahlin M, Dennefors B, Johanson C, Hamberger L. Luteotropic effects of prostaglandin E_2 on the human corpus luteum of the menstrual cycle and early pregnancy. *J Clin Endocrinol Metab.* 66:909, 1988

59. Hodgen GD. Surrogate embryo transfer combined with estrogen–progesterone therapy in monkeys: Implantation, gestation and delivery without ovaries. *JAMA.* 250:2167, 1983

60. Lutjen P, Trounson A, Leeton J, et al. The establishment and maintenance of pregnancy using in vitro fertilization and embryo donation in a patient with primary ovarian failure. *Nature.* 307:174, 1984

61. Auletta FJ. The role of prostaglandin $F_{2\alpha}$ in human luteolysis. Contemp *Obstet Gynecol.* 30:119, 1987

62. Wentz AC, Jones GS. Transient luteolytic effect of prostaglandin $F_{2\alpha}$ in the human. *Obstet Gynecol.* 42:172, 1973

63. Schoonmaker JN, Bergman KS, Steiner RA, Karsch FJ. Estradiol-induced luteal regression in the rhesus monkey: Evidence of an extra-ovarian site of action. *Endocrinology.* 110:1708, 1984

64. Gore BA, CaIdwell BV, Speroff L. Estrogen-induced human luteolysis. *J Clin Endocrinol Metab.* 36:615, 1973

65. Ellinwood WE, Resko JA. Effect of inhibition of estrogen synthesis during the luteal phase on function of the corpus luteum in rhesus monkeys. *Biol Reprod.* 28:636, 1983

66. Khan-Dawood FS, Huang JC, Dawood MY. Baboon corpus luteum oxytocin: An intragonadal peptide modulator on luteal function. *Am J Obstet Gynecol.* 158:882, 1988

67. Givens JR, Andersen RN, Ragland JB, et al. Adrenal function in hirsutism. I. Diurnal change and response of plasma androstenedione, testosterone, 17-hydroxyprogesterone, cortisol, LH and FSH to dexamethasone and 1/2 unit of ACTH. *J Clin Endocrinol Metab.* 40:988, 1975

68. Judd HL, Yen SSC. Serum androstenedione and testosterone levels during the menstrual cycle. *J Clin Endocrinol Metab.* 36:475, 1973

69. Abraham GE, Chakmakjian AH. Serum steroid levels during the menstrual cycle in a bilaterally adrenalectomized woman. *J Clin Endocrinol Metab.* 37:581, 1973

70. Dyrenfurth I, Jewelewica R, Warren M, et al. Temporal relationships of hormonal variables in the menstrual cycle. In: Ferin M, Halberg F, Richart RM, et al, eds. *Biorhythms and Reproduction.* New York, N.Y., John Wiley & Sons, 1974:171–201

71. Genazzani AR, Lemarchand-Beraud TH, Aubert ML, Felber JP. Pattern of plasma ACTH, hGH and cortisol during menstrual cycle. *J Clin Endocrinol Metab.* 41:431, 1975

72. Carr BR, Parker CR Jr, Madden JD, et al. Plasma levels of adrenocorticotropin (ACTH) and cortisol in women receiving oral contraceptive treatment. *J Clin Endocrinol Metab.* 49:346, 1979

73. Carr BR, Wilson JD. Disorders of the ovary and female reproductive tract. In: Wilson JD, Braunwald E, Isselbacher KJ, et al, eds. *Harrison's Principles of Internal Medicine*, 12th ed. New York, N.Y., McGraw-Hill, 1991: 1776–1795

74. Casey ML, Macdonald PC. Extraadrenal formation of a mineralocorticosteroid: Deoxycorticosterone and deoxycorticosterone sulfate biosynthesis and metabolism. *Endocrine Rev.* 3:396, 1982

75. Parker CR Jr, Winkel CA, Rush AJ, et al. Plasma concentrations of 11-deoxycorticosterone in women during the menstrual cycle. *Obstet Gynecol.* 58:26, 1981

76. Noyes RW, Hertig AW, Rock J. Dating the endometrial biopsy. *Fertil Steril.* 1:3, 1950

77. Sixma JJ, Cristiens GCML, Hospels AS. The sequence of hemostatic events in the endometrium during normal menstruation. In: Dicefalusy E, Fraser IS, Webb FTG, eds. *WHO Symposium on Steroid Contraception and Endometrial Bleeding.* Washington, WHO (World Health Organization). 1980:86

78. Wilborn WH, Flowers CE Jr. Cellular mechanisms for endometrial conservation during menstrual bleeding. *Sem Reprod Endocrinol.* 2:307, 1984

79. Hallberg L, Hogdahl A, Nilsson L, Rybo G. Menstrual blood loss—A population study. *Acta Obstet Gynecol Scand.* 45:320, 1966

80. Edman CD. The effects of steroids on the endometrium. *Sem Reprod Endocrinol.* 1:79, 1983

81. Pickles VR, Hall WJ, Best FA, Smith GN. Prostaglandins in endometrium and menstrual fluid from normal and dysmenorrheic subjects. *J Obstet Gynecol. Br Commonw.* 72:185, 1965

82. Willman EA, Collins WP, Clayton SG. Studies in the involvement of prostaglandins in uterine symptomatology and pathology. *Br J Obstet Gynaecol.* 83:337, 1976

83. Schwarz BE. The production and biologic effects of uterine prostaglandins. *Sem Reprod Endocrinol.* 1:189, 1983

84. Turksoy RN, Safaii HS. Immediate effect of prostaglandin $F_{2\alpha}$ during the luteal phase of the menstrual cycle. *Fertil Steril.* 26:634, 1975

85. Todd AS. Localization of fibrinolytic activity in tissues. *Br Med Bull.* 20:210, 1964

86. Lessey BA, Killam AP, Metzger DA, et al. Immunohistochemical analysis of human uterine estrogen and progesterone receptors throughout the menstrual cycle. *J Clin Endocrinol Metab.* 67:334, 1988

87. Tseng L, Masella J. Cyclic changes of estradiol metabolic enzymes in human endometrium during the menstrual cycle. In: Kimball FA, ed. *The Endometrium.* New York, N.Y., SP Medical and Scientific Books, 1980: 211–226

Chapter 13

THE PHYSIOLOGY OF THE TESTIS AND MALE REPRODUCTIVE TRACT AND DISORDERS OF TESTICULAR FUNCTION

James E. Griffin

The testes produce sperm and the hormones that regulate male sexual function under complex feedback control by the hypothalamic–pituitary system. Testosterone, the major hormone secreted, serves as a circulating prohormone for two other classes of steroid hormones, 5α-reduced androgens and estrogens, which mediate most of the cellular actions of testosterone. Testicular hormones are responsible for the induction of male phenotype during embryogenesis. At puberty, testicular hormones mediate the changes of sexual maturation. As a consequence, abnormalities of testicular function cause different clinical consequences depending upon the phase of life in which they develop, from early gestation through old age.

EMBRYOGENESIS

The gene (or genes) that control testicular differentiation is located on the Y chromosome. Analyses of individuals with structural abnormalities of the Y chromosome and others with gonadal sex discordant with chromosomal sex indicate that the *SRY* (sex-determining region Y chromosome) gene on the short arm of the Y encodes a transcription regulatory factor responsible for testicular development.[1]

The mechanism by which the testis-determining gene(s) of the Y chromosome dictates testicular development is not known, but at a minimum three principal cell types are involved in formation of the testes: (1) germ cells derived from primitive ectodermal cells of the inner cell mass and initially identifiable in the endoderm of the yolk sac; (2) supporting cells derived from the coelomic epithelium of the gonadal ridge that differentiate into the Sertoli cells; and (3) stromal (interstitial) cells derived from the mesenchyme of the gonadal ridge.

The primordial germ cells migrate by amoeboid movement from the gut endoderm through the mesentery, eventually reaching the gonadal ridges.[2] After reaching the gonadal ridge, the germ cells, together with adhering epithelial cells, infiltrate the underlying mesenchyme. This process is identical in male and female embryos and culminates in the formation of the gonadal blastema containing the three basic cell types by 5 to 6 wk of gestation. Sexual dimorphism of the human gonad first becomes apparent with the appearance of seminiferous cords in the fetal testis between 6 and 7 wk of gestation. Histologic development of the testis is largely complete by the end of the third month, whereas descent of the testis from the abdominal cavity to the scrotum occurs during the latter two thirds of gestation. The forces that regulate testicular descent are poorly understood.

At the time of endocrine differentiation of the gonad (the eighth wk), the testis and mesonephros are anatomically adjacent to the kidney and are attached to the posterior abdominal wall by a broad peritoneal fold. As the mesonephros degenerates, the cranial portion of this fold disappears, but the caudal portion persists as a narrow ligament that is continuous with a band of mesenchyme extending into the genital swellings. This mesenchymal band, the gubernaculum, anchors the fetal testes to the inguinal region. During the third month of gestation, a herniation of the coelomic cavity, termed the processus vaginalis, forms through the ventral abdominal wall along the course of each gubernaculum. Enlargement of the processus vaginalis causes the formation of the inguinal canals. In the human embryo, the actual movement of the testes from the abdominal cavity through the inguinal canal and into the scrotum usually occurs during the seventh month.

A minimum of three factors are believed to participate in testicular descent: Müllerian-inhibiting substance, intra-abdominal pressure, and androgen. Degeneration of the proximal portion of the peritoneal fold may be controlled by Müllerian-inhibiting substance, a peptide hormone formed in the seminiferous tubules; some subjects with persistent Müllerian duct syndrome, thought to be due to deficient formation or action of Müllerian inhibiting substance, have testes located high in the retroperitoneal space.[3] Conditions associated with impaired development of intra-abdominal pressure, such as congenital defects in the abdominal musculature, also are commonly associated with cryptorchidism. Finally, androgens are believed to play a role in testicular descent because about half of subjects with severe androgen resistance, such as the testicular feminization syndrome, have intra-abdominal testes usually located near the inguinal rings.[4]

For an overall description of normal sexual differentiation of the Wolffian and Müllerian ducts, the formation of the external genitalia, and the hormonal control of these processes, see Chapter 6. In brief, in regard to male development Müllerian duct regression is the initial event in the virilization of the male urogenital tract starting at 7 to 8 wk of gestation. Wolffian duct development follows shortly after Müllerian regression begins. Mesonephric tubules adjacent to the testes lose their primitive glomeruli and establish contact with the developing rete and spermatogenic tubules to form the efferent ducts of the testis (Fig 13–1). The portion of Wolffian duct immediately distal to the efferent ducts becomes elongated and convoluted to form the epididymis. The central portion of the Wolffian duct develops thick muscular walls to become the vas deferens. At about the thirteenth wk of gestation, the seminal vesicles begin to develop as buds from the lower portions of the Wolffian ducts. The terminal portions of the ducts between the developing seminal vesicles and the urethra become the ejaculatory ducts and ampullae of the vas deferens. Differentiation of the Wolffian ducts is largely complete by the end of the first trimester.

The prostate develops from the pelvic portion of the urogenital sinuses at about 10 wk of gestation. Beginning in the ninth wk and continuing through the

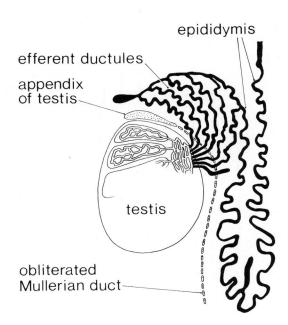

Figure 13–1. Relationship of the upper Wolffian duct-derived structures to the testis and fate of the Müllerian duct. *(Adapted, with permission, from Arey LB. Developmental Anatomy. A Textbook and Laboratory Manual of Embryology, 7th ed. Philadelphia, Pa., W. B. Saunders, 1965: 325.)*

twelfth wk of gestation, the external genitalia of the male develop. The genital swellings enlarge and migrate posteriorly to form the scrotum. The genital folds fuse over the urethral groove to form the penile urethra. The formation of the male genital tract is largely complete by 13 wk of gestation. The mechanisms for the developmental change are complex, involving mesenchyme–epithelial interaction and the effects of two hormones secreted by the fetal testis, Müllerian-inhibiting substance and testosterone.[5] Testosterone mediates Wolffian development directly whereas dihydrotestosterone formed from testosterone at its site of action is responsible for development of the prostate and external genitalia.

During the last two trimesters of gestation, descent of the testes (discussed earlier) and growth of the external genitalia occur.

STRUCTURE OF THE TESTES AND REPRODUCTIVE TRACT

The testes contain two functional units: a network of tubules for the production and transport of sperm to the excretory–ejaculatory ducts and a system of interstitial or Leydig cells that contain the enzymes for the production of androgens. As illustrated in Figure 13–2, spermatogenic tubules are composed of germ and Sertoli cells. Tight junctions between the Sertoli cells at a site between the spermatogonia and the primary spermatocyte form a diffusion barrier that divides the testis into two functional compartments, the basal and the adluminal. The barrier between these two compartments has limited permeability to macromolecules, analogous to the blood–brain barrier and other epithelial barriers.[6] The basal compartment consists of the Leydig cells; the boundary tissue of the tubule, including peritubular myoid cells; and the outer layers of the tubules containing the spermatogonia. The adluminal compartment contains the inner two thirds of the tubules, including primary spermatocytes and more advanced stages of spermatogenesis.

The base of the Sertoli cell is situated adjacent to the outer basement membrane of the spermatogenic tubule,

while the inner portion consists of a progressively arborized cytoplasm containing large gaps or lacunae. The mechanism by which the spermatogonia pass through the tight junctional complexes between the Sertoli cell as they begin spermatogenesis is not known. The cytoplasm of the Sertoli cell encompasses the differentiating spermatocytes and spermatids so that spermatogenesis takes place within a network of Sertoli cell cytoplasm.

The lipid droplets within Leydig cells are responsible for the characteristic foamy appearance of the cytoplasm and contain mainly esterified cholesterol, derived in part from circulating lipoproteins and in part from cholesterol synthesized locally within the endoplasmic reticulum. This pool of esterified cholesterol serves as a reservoir of substrate for testosterone synthesis.[7] Following hydrolysis of the cholesterol ester, free cholesterol moves to mitochondria for side-chain cleavage of cholesterol to pregnenolone.

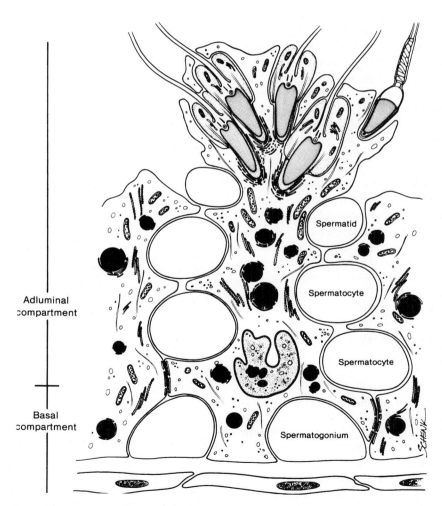

Figure 13–2. Diagram of Sertoli cell showing the relationship between Sertoli cell cytoplasm and developing spermatocytes. *(Reproduced, with permission, from Griffin JE, Wilson JD. Disorders of the testes and male reproductive tract. In: Wilson JD, Foster DW, eds.* Williams Textbook of Endocrinology, *7th ed. Philadelphia, Pa., W. B. Saunders, 1985: 259-311)*

Pregnenolone in turn is converted in the endoplasmic reticulum to testosterone. The amount of testosterone stored within the Leydig cell is small because the newly synthesized testosterone diffuses promptly into the plasma.

The seminiferous tubules empty into a network of ducts termed the rete testes. Sperm are then transported into a single duct, the epididymis. Anatomically, the epididymis can be divided into the caput, corpus, and cauda regions. The caput epididymis consists of 8 to 12 ductuli efferentes that have a larger lumen tapering to a narrower diameter at the junction of the ductus epididymides. The diameter then remains constant through the corpus, or body, of the epididymis. In the cauda epididymis, the diameter of the duct enlarges substantially and the lumen acquires an irregular shape. The entire epididymal length is 5 to 6 m. The epithelium exhibits regional differences of ciliated and nonciliated cells with evidence for a blood–epididymis barrier.[8]

The vas deferens is a tubular structure about 30 to 35 cm in length beginning at the cauda epididymis and terminating in the ejaculatory duct near the prostate. In cross section, there is a middle circular muscle layer surrounded by inner and outer longitudinal muscle layers. The pseudostratified epithelium lining the lumen of the vas deferens is composed of basal cells and three types of tall, thin, columnar cells, all three of which have cilia.

The normal adult prostate weighs about 20 g. The gland is composed of alveoli that are lined with tall, columnar, secretory epithelial cells. The acini of these alveoli drain into the floor and lateral surfaces of the posterior urethra. The alveoli and the ducts draining them are embedded with a stroma of fibromuscular tissue. The seminal vesicles are paired pouches 4 to 5 cm long that join the ampulla of the distal vas deferens to form the ejaculatory ducts. The seminal vesicles are composed of tubular alveoli containing viscous secretions. The ejaculatory ducts pass through the prostate and terminate within the prostatic urethra.

HYPOTHALAMIC–PITUITARY–TESTICULAR AXIS

The hypothalamus is anatomically linked to the pituitary both by a portal vascular system and by neural pathways (Fig 13–3). The portal vascular system provides a mechanism for the delivery of releasing hormones from the brain to the pituitary and thus provides the major pathway by which the brain controls anterior pituitary function. The preoptic area and the medial basal region of the hypothalamus (and particularly the arcuate nucleus) contain important centers for control of gonadotropin secretion. Peptidergic neurons in this region secrete luteinizing hormone-releasing hormone (LHRH, also called

gonadotropin-releasing hormone [GnRH]).[9] Neurons from other regions of the brain terminate in this area and influence LHRH synthesis and release via catecholaminergic, dopaminergic, and endorphin-related mechanisms.[10] There are excitatory noradrenergic influences, but dopamine is thought to play only a minor role. The opioid peptide involved in the endorphin-related mechanisms appears to be β-endorphin, which exerts an inhibitory role in the control of gonadotropin secretion.[10]

LHRH is a decapeptide that is widely distributed in the central nervous system and in other tissues as well. However, a physiologic role for LHRH in sites other than the pituitary has not been established. The primary pituitary hormones that regulate the testes are luteinizing hormone (LH) and follicle-stimulating hormone (FSH). Both hormones were named on the basis of their

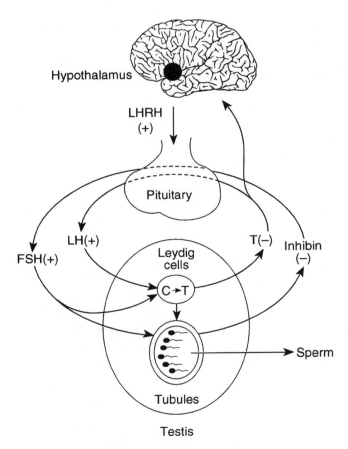

Figure 13–3. Hypothalamic–pituitary–testicular axis. Schematic diagram to indicate feedback relationship of testosterone and inhibin produced by the testes on gonadotropin secretion by the hypothalamic–pituitary complex, and site of action of FSH and LH on the testis. Abbreviations: C, cholesterol; T, testosterone; FSH, follicle-stimulating hormone; LH, luteinizing hormone; LHRH, LH-releasing hormone. *(Reproduced, with permission, from Griffin JE, Wilson JD. The testes. In: Bondy PK, Rosenberg, LE, eds. Metabolic Control and Disease, 8th ed. Philadelphia, Pa., W. B. Saunders, 1980:1535-1578)*

function in females before their equal importance in men was recognized. LH and FSH are secreted by the same basophilic cells in the pituitary. LH and FSH are glycoproteins composed of two polypeptide chains designated α and β. The α-subunit is identical; the distinct immunologic and functional characteristics are determined by unique β-subunits.

LHRH interacts with high-affinity cell surface receptor sites on the plasma membrane of pituitary gonadotrophs. It stimulates acutely the release of both LH and FSH by a calcium-dependent mechanism that is independent of cyclic adenosine monophosphate (cAMP).[11] Diacylglycerols may serve as amplifiers of the calcium-mediated signal.[11] It is generally assumed that LHRH has a long-term effect on the regulation of gonadotropin synthesis as well. The amount of LH and FSH released in response to LHRH depends upon age and hormonal status. Prior to puberty, the secretion of FSH in response to LHRH is greater than that of LH.

LH interacts with specific high-affinity cell surface receptors on the plasma membrane of Leydig cells.[12] The binding of LH to its receptor stimulates the membrane-bound adenylate cyclase that catalyzes the formation of cAMP (see Chap 7). The release of cAMP into the cytoplasm is followed by binding of cAMP to the regulatory subunit of a protein kinase, dissociation of the regulatory subunit, and consequent activation of the catalytic subunit of the enzyme. Activation of the Leydig cell protein kinase, operating through unidentified intermediate steps, eventually results in stimulation of the conversion of cholesterol to pregnenolone. This in turn enhances the synthesis of testosterone. The rate of testosterone synthesis correlates more closely with the degree of occupancy of the regulatory subunits of the protein kinase by cAMP than with the total amount of cAMP in the cells.

The epithelium of the seminiferous tubule is the primary site of action of FSH. In the Sertoli cell, FSH binding has been localized by autoradiography to the basal aspect of the cell.[13] The initial biochemical events following the binding of FSH to its receptor are similar to those for LH. The intracellular messenger is cAMP, and adenylate cyclase activity is stimulated when seminiferous tubules are incubated with FSH in vitro. In Sertoli cells, the elevation of cAMP following FSH binding activates cAMP-dependent protein kinase and stimulates RNA and protein synthesis, including the synthesis of androgen-binding protein (ABP)[14] and the aromatase enzyme complex that converts testosterone to estradiol. The precise role of FSH in the control of spermatogenesis remains uncertain.

The secretion of LHRH into the hypophyseal portal system is episodic, and the episodic release of LHRH results in turn in episodic secretion of both immunoreac-

tive and bioactive LH. The secretory pulses of LH in adult men occur at a frequency of 8 to 14 pulses per 24 hr and vary greatly in magnitude[15] (Fig 13–4). Pulsatile secretion of FSH is temporally coupled to LH pulses but is less in amplitude.

The rate of secretion of LH is controlled by the action of gonadal steroids on the hypothalamus and pituitary. The control of LH in men operates primarily by negative feedback because normal levels of gonadal steroids inhibit secretion. Both testosterone and estradiol can inhibit LH secretion. Testosterone can be converted to estradiol in the brain and the pituitary, but the two hormones are thought to act independently. Testosterone, or its metabolites, acts on the central nervous system to slow the hypothalamic pulse generator and consequently decreases the frequency of LH pulsatile release.[16] Endogenous opiates have a role in the negative feedback actions of androgen and estrogen on pulsatile LH secretion in men.[17] In studies of the infusion of the nonaromatizable androgen 5α-dihydrotestosterone into normal men, selective inhibition of LH pulse frequency by the androgen was blocked by the coadministration of the opiate receptor antagonist naltrexone.[17] Acute infusions of estradiol also lower LH levels associated with an increased frequency and decreased amplitude of the LH pulses.[18] The fact that dihydrotestosterone, which cannot be converted to estrogen, exerts negative feedback on LH secretion indicates that testosterone does not require aromatization to inhibit LH secretion.[18] Testosterone also appears to have a negative feedback action on LH secretion directly at the pituitary level because LHRH-deficient patients given pulsatile LHRH infusions have a decrease in mean LH levels and LH pulse amplitude when exogenous testosterone is administered.[19]

The negative feedback inhibition of testicular hormones on FSH secretion involves both gonadal peptide and steroid hormones. Serum FSH concentrations increase in proportion to the loss of germinal elements in the testis whereas LH levels change little if at all. Inhibin, a peptide inhibitor of pituitary FSH that is secreted by Sertoli cells, is a glycoprotein consisting of two disulphide-linked subunits.[20] Because the β-subunit can exist in two forms, there are two forms of inhibin, inhibin A and inhibin B. The sequence of inhibin is partially homologous to transforming growth factor β and to Müllerian-inhibiting substance. An in vivo study of the relative roles of FSH and androgen (as stimulated locally in the testes by LH) in the control of inhibin secretion in normal men concluded that both FSH and androgen are necessary for normal inhibin production.[21]

A primate model has been useful in defining the relative importance of inhibin and gonadal steroids in physiologic feedback control of FSH secretion. In a hypophysiotrophic clamp preparation, in which episodic

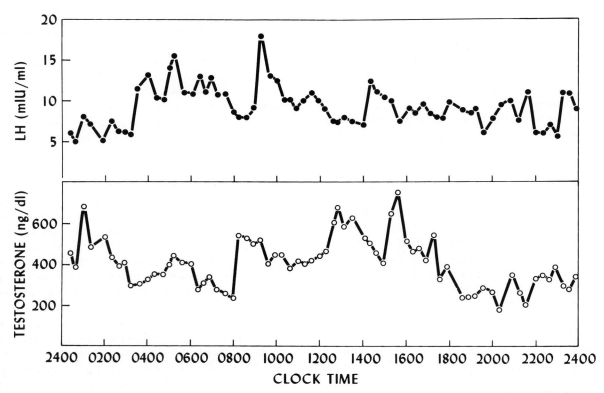

Figure 13–4. Twenty-four-hour pattern of serum LH and testosterone in a 21-year-old normal man sampled every 20 min. *(Courtesy of RM Boyar. Reproduced, with permission, from Griffin JE, Wilson JD. The testes. In: Bondy PK, Rosenberg LE, eds.* Metabolic Control and Disease, *8th ed. Philadelphia, Pa., W. B. Saunders, 1980: 1535-1578)*

gonadotropin secretion was maintained by a chronic, un-changing, intermittent LHRH infusion, replacement of inhibin after castration maintained control of FSH secretion in the absence of testosterone.[22]

ANDROGEN SYNTHESIS, TRANSPORT, METABOLISM, AND ACTION

The pathway by which testosterone is *synthesized* in the testis and the conversion of testosterone to active metabolites is shown schematically in Figure 13–5. As stated above, cholesterol, the precursor steroid, can either be synthesized de novo from acetyl CoA or derived from the plasma pool by receptor-mediated endocytosis of low-density lipoprotein (LDL). In the human testis, both sources are quantitatively important.[23]

Five enzymatic processes are involved in the conversion of cholesterol to testosterone: cholesterol side-chain cleavage enzyme ($P_{450_{SCC}}$), 3β-hydroxysteroid dehydrogenase/isomerase (3β-HSD), 17α-hydroxylase ($P_{450_{17\alpha}}$), 17,20-lyase ($P_{450_{17\alpha}}$), and 17β-hydroxysteroid oxidoreductase (17β-HSOR). The initial reaction in the process involves the side-chain cleavage of cholesterol by $P_{450_{SCC}}$ in mitochondria to form pregnenolone, and is the rate-limiting reaction in testosterone synthesis under regulatory control of LH. The remaining four reactions in the pathway of testosterone synthesis are located in the microsomes. The 3β-HSD complex oxidizes the A ring of the steroid to the Δ^4-3-keto configuration. Both 17α-hydroxylase and 17,20-lyase activities are present in $P_{450_{17\alpha}}$.[24] Although testosterone is the major secretory product, some of the precursors in the pathway, as well as dihydrotestosterone and estradiol, are also directly secreted by the testis. The major sites of formation of dihydrotestosterone and estradiol are androgen target tissues and adipose tissue, respectively (see below). Concentrations of testosterone in testicular lymph and testicular venous blood are similar; however, because of its greater flow the major route for testosterone secretion is via the spermatic venous blood. About 25 μg testosterone are present in the normal testes so that the total hormone content must turn over more that 200 times each day to provide the average of 5 to 10 mg secreted daily.

In addition to stimulation by gonadotropin, Leydig cell function is also under paracrine control within the

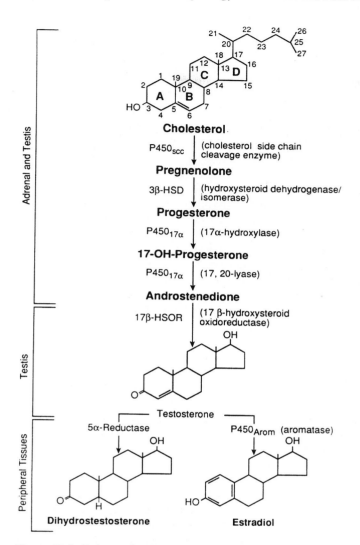

Figure 13–5. Pathway of testosterone formation in the testis and conversion of testosterone to active metabolites in peripheral tissues.

testis. Insulin-like growth factor I augments gonadotropin-stimulated testosterone production by cultured rat Leydig cells by interacting with a specific receptor on Leydig cells.[25] Transforming growth factor-β, epidermal growth factor, transforming growth factor-α, and fibroblast growth factor may also have paracrine effects on Leydig cell function.[26]

Testosterone is *transported* in the plasma largely bound to plasma proteins. The major binding molecules are albumin and testosterone-binding globulin (TeBG, also called sex steroid hormone binding globulin [SHBG]). TeBG, a β-globulin composed of nonidentical subunits, has a molecular weight of about 95,000 and contains about 30 percent carbohydrate.

In the blood of normal men, about 2 percent of testosterone is free (unbound), 44 percent is bound to TeBG, and 54 percent is bound to albumin and other pro-

teins.[27] Albumin has about 1000-fold lower affinity for testosterone than does TeBG but the concentration of albumin is so much higher than that of TeBG that the binding capacity is similar. The proportion of testosterone bound to TeBG in serum is proportional to the TeBG concentration. For many years, the free fraction was regarded as the biologically active portion available for entry into cells and receptor interaction. It is now clear that dissociation of protein-bound testosterone can occur within a capillary bed so that the active fraction can be larger than the free fraction measured under equilibrium conditions in vitro.[28] In studies of tissue delivery in vivo, nearly all of the albumin-bound testosterone is available for tissue uptake. Thus, the bioavailable circulating testosterone in normal men is about half the total (or equal to the free plus albumin bound). Estradiol appears to bind differently to TeBG than does testosterone, as a consequence of which there is increased availability of TeBG-bound estradiol to tissues. The reason for these differences of testosterone and estradiol binding to what is thought to be a single competitive binding site on TeBG is thought to be the presence of multiple isoforms of TeBG in serum.[29]

The concentration of TeBG in plasma is regulated by several hormones. The level in men is one third to one half that in women, and concentrations in hypogonadal men are elevated above those of normal men. Decreased TeBG levels occur in hypothyroidism, and thyroid hormone excess increases TeBG levels, possibly because of increased estrogen formation. In men who have an intact hypothalamic–pituitary–testis axis, alterations in TeBG levels have little effect on androgen physiology in the steady state; for example, increase in plasma TeBG is followed by temporary decreases in the free (active) plasma testosterone and an increased rate of testosterone synthesis until the normal free (active) component is reconstituted. In contrast, changes in the plasma levels of binding proteins have profound consequences when the levels of bioavailable hormone are not tightly regulated. The level of plasma estradiol in men is probably determined by the amount of androgen available as substrate for estrogen formation and by the amount of aromatase activity in extraglandular sites and thus is not regulated directly by usual feedback mechanisms. Because TeBG binds estradiol less avidly than testosterone or dihydrotestosterone, increases in TeBG amplify the amount of estradiol cleared by liver relative to the amount of testosterone; eg, increases in TeBG cause decreased hepatic clearance of testosterone but have little effect on the hepatic clearance of estradiol. Thus, even in normal men, changes in TeBG levels can cause alteration in the ratios of androgens to estrogens that persist even when androgen levels themselves are not permanently altered.

An important feature of the *metabolism* of testosterone, noted above, is that it serves as a circulating precursor, or prohormone, for the formation of two types of active metabolites, which in turn mediate many of the physiologic phenomena involved in androgen action (Fig 13–5). On the one hand, testosterone can undergo irreversible reduction to 5α-reduced steroids, principally dihydrotestosterone, that are thought to mediate many of the differentiative, growth-promoting, and functional aspects of male sexual differentiation and virilization.[30] Alternatively, circulating androgens can be aromatized to estrogens in the extraglandular tissues of both sexes. These estrogens in some instances act in concert with androgens to influence physiologic processes but also may exert independent effects on cellular function and even have effects opposite those of androgens. Thus, the physiologic actions of testosterone are the result of the combined effects of testosterone itself plus those of estrogen and the active androgen metabolites of the parent molecule. Circulating dihydrotestosterone is thought to be formed principally in the androgen target tissues themselves.[30] Aromatization takes place in many tissues, the most significant of which is probably adipose tissue.

5α-Reductase accepts a number of Δ^4-3-ketosteroids as substrate and requires NADPH as cofactor. The reaction is not reversible under physiologic conditions. There are two separate isozymes: steroid 5α-reductase 1 and 2.[31] Enzyme 2 is expressed in the male urogenital tract, genital skin, and liver. Enzyme 1 is expressed in liver and nongenital skin. Enzyme 2 is defective in subjects with 5α-reductase deficiency. In normal men, about 6 to 8 percent of the total testosterone produced is metabolized to dihydrotestosterone by 5α-reductase. 5α-Dihydrotestosterone is the principal intracellular androgen and is about twice as potent as testosterone in most bioassay systems.[30]

The aromatization of androgens to estrogens in the testis and in extraglandular tissues of men is catalyzed by the same $P_{450_{Arom}}$ complex present in placenta and ovary. Estrogen formation involves sequential hydroxylation, oxidation, and removal of the C-19 carbon and aromatization of the A ring of the steroid. Human aromatase is a microsomal enzyme, $P_{450_{Arom}}$, coded by a gene with nine coding exons. Tissue-specific expression is determined by tissue-specific promotors.[32] The rate of overall aromatase in nongonadal tissue does not appear to be influenced by gonadotropins but rises with advancing age.

Current concepts of androgen *action* in target cells are summarized in Figure 13–6. Major functions include regulation of gonadotropin secretion by the hypothalamic–pituitary system, initiation and maintenance of spermatogenesis, formation of the male phenotype during sexual differentiation, and promotion of sexual maturation at puberty.[30] Inside the cell, testosterone and dihydrotestosterone bind to the same high-affinity androgen receptor protein. The androgen receptor appears to be primarily in the nucleus in the unbound state. Following hormone binding, the hormone–receptor complexes undergo a transformation reaction in which they acquire an increased affinity for nuclear components. The hormone–receptor complexes interact with acceptor sites in nuclei to effect a biologic response. Although the nature and number of the acceptor sites within chromatin are not known, presumably the receptor complexes interact with specific DNA sequences upstream from androgen-regulated genes to result in increased transcription and subsequent appearance of mRNA. Estradiol, as discussed above, may be either secreted directly by the testis or formed in peripheral tissues. The mechanisms by which estrogens augment or block androgen action are not fully understood.

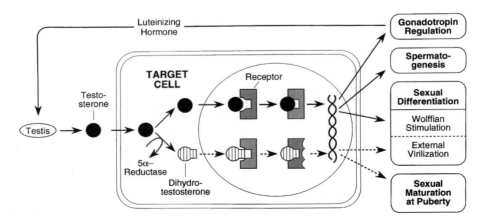

Figure13–6. Normal androgen physiology. Testosterone, secreted by the testis, binds to the androgen receptor in a target cell, either directly or after conversion to dihydrotestosterone. Dihydrotestosterone binds more tightly than testosterone, and the complex of dihydrotestosterone and the androgen receptor can bind more efficiently to the chromatin. The major actions of androgens, shown on the right, are mediated by testosterone (solid lines) or by dihydrotestosterone (broken lines). *(Reproduced, with permission, from Griffen JE. Androgen resistance—the clinical and molecular spectrum. N Engl J Med. 326:611, 1992.)*

Based upon studies in humans and animals, it appears that the testosterone–receptor complex is responsible for gonadotropin regulation and the virilization of the Wolffian ducts during sexual differentiation, and is probably responsible for the characteristic male muscle development and stimulation of spermatogenesis, whereas the dihydrotestosterone–receptor complex is responsible for external virilization during embryogenesis and for most male secondary sexual characteristics of the adult.[30] Androgen receptor concentrations are highest in the accessory organs of male reproduction that depend upon androgens for their growth. Other tissues such as skeletal muscle, liver, and heart have smaller amounts of the receptor. In the testis, androgen receptors are present both in isolated Sertoli cells and in interstitial cells. Whether the presence of androgen receptors identifies a tissue as androgen responsive is not clear, although androgen receptors are present in greater numbers in tissues known to respond to androgen. Single gene mutations in humans and animals indicate that a single androgen receptor binds both testosterone and dihydrotestosterone and that the receptor protein is coded by a locus on the X chromosome.[33] The cDNA encoding the human androgen receptor has been cloned and predicts a protein of 917 amino acids with a mass of about 99 kD.[34] Dihydrotestosterone formation appears to be required for normal androgen action even though there is only a single receptor. In the case of the human androgen receptor, a partial explanation for this requirement of dihydrotestosterone may be the severalfold greater affinity of the receptor for dihydrotestosterone than for testosterone and the more rapid

dissociation rate of the testosterone–receptor complex. Thus, a difference in the interaction of the two hormones with the androgen receptor may serve as an amplifying mechanism for androgen action in certain target tissues (reviewed in reference 33).

SPERM FORMATION, TRANSPORT, AND HORMONAL CONTROL

After the migration of the germ cells to the gonadal ridges, the total number of germ cells is approximately 3×10^5 per gonad. This number increases by the time of puberty and the net result is the *formation* of approximately 2×10^8 sperm each day. As illustrated in Figure 13–7, after puberty each spermatogonium undergoing differentiation gives rise to 16 primary spermatocytes, each of which then enters meiosis and gives rise to 4 spermatids and ultimately 4 spermatozoa. Thus, 64 spermatozoa can develop from each spermatogonium. Because half of potential sperm production is lost during meiosis, the actual number of spermatogonia that begin this process is close to 3 million per day.[35] Contiguous groups of spermatogonia undertake the process simultaneously, resulting in certain typical cellular associations in seminiferous tubules.

The transformation of the human spermatid into a spermatozoon consists of a coordinated reorganization of nucleus and cytoplasm and development of a flagellum. The nucleus comes to occupy an eccentric position adjacent to the cranial pole of the spermatid, separated from it by an acrosomal cap. The cilial structure that

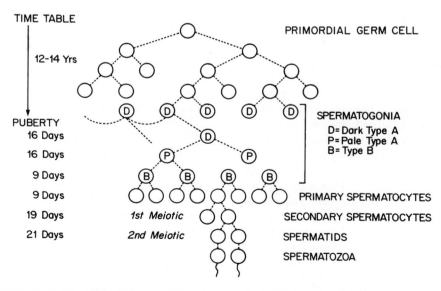

Figure 13–7. Cell divisions during spermatogenesis. *(Reproduced, with permission, from Griffin JE, Wilson JD. Disorders of the testes and male reproductive tract. In: Wilson JD, Foster DW, eds. Williams Textbook of Endocrinology, 7th ed. Philadelphia, Pa., W. B. Saunders, 1985: 259-311)*

serves as the core of the sperm tail consists of nine outer fibers and two inner fibers. The mitochondria form a helix around the cilia in the middle piece, and the terminal region of the tail consists of the axial filament surrounded by the cell membrane after loss of most of the cytoplasm.

Sperm formation takes approximately 70 days, and *transport* of the sperm through the epididymis to the ejaculatory duct requires an additional 12 to 21 days. When sperm leave the testes, they are relatively immature and have a poor capacity to fertilize. During passage through the epididymis, maturation is evidenced by the development of the capacity for sustained motility, modification of the structural state of the nuclear chromatin and the tail organelles, and loss of the remnant of spermatid cytoplasm.[36] The epididymis also serves as a reservoir for sperm. After transport of the sperm and secretory products of the testis and epididymis through the vas deferens, the fluid reaching the ejaculatory ducts is enriched by the secretions from the seminal vesicles. The seminal vesicles are the source of seminal fluid fructose and prostaglandins and contribute about 60 percent of the total volume of the seminal fluid. Approximately 20 percent of the total seminal fluid volume is derived from prostatic secretions added to the semen when the ejaculatory ducts terminate in the prostatic urethra. The prostatic fluid is the source of seminal fluid spermine, citric acid, zinc, and acid phosphatase. Final acquisition of the capacity of the sperm to fertilize is poorly understood, but completion of the process may take place in the female genital tract.

The *hormonal control* of spermatogenesis involves both LH and FSH. FSH appears to act directly on the spermatogenic tubule whereas LH influences spermatogenesis indirectly by its enhancement of testosterone synthesis in the adjacent Leydig cells. Testosterone interacts with androgen receptors in the adjacent Sertoli cells to activate specific genes necessary for the differentiation process. There is increasing evidence for the importance of a number of paracrine factors in the control of spermatogenesis.[37] Following hypophysectomy in the adult, no spermatocytes are formed. Spermatogenesis can be restored or initiated by treatment with FSH (human menopausal gonadotropin) plus human chorionic gonadotropin (hCG), and once restored spermatogenesis can be maintained by hCG alone. This might seem to imply that FSH is required only for initiation of spermatogenesis but not its maintenance. However, in otherwise normal men in whom FSH is selectively suppressed by the sequential administration of exogenous testosterone followed by hCG, FSH administration is necessary for quantitatively normal spermatogenesis.[38] Thus, it is likely that both FSH and LH play a significant role in normal control of sperm formation.

PHASES OF NORMAL TESTICULAR FUNCTION

The phases of normal testicular function can be related to changes in the plasma testosterone. During embryogenesis, testosterone levels increase in the late first trimester, associated with male sexual differentiation (see Chap 6). In the first 6 mo of life, the testosterone level rises to about half of adult levels before falling back to low levels before age 1 yr. The concentration then remains low, but higher in boys than in girls, until the onset of puberty, when the concentration again increases in boys, reaching adult levels by age 17 or thereabout. Plasma concentrations remain more or less constant in the adult until late middle age and then decline somewhat during the later decades of life.

Puberty

In the prepubertal years, plasma levels of gonadotropins and gonadal steroids are low. The secretion of adrenal androgens, dehydroepiandrosterone, dehydroepiandrosterone sulfate, and androstenedione, starts to increase in boys as early as 6 or 7, several yr prior to maturation of the hypothalamic–pituitary–gonadal axis. The secretion of these androgens is probably under the control of corticotropin (ACTH) and appears to be independent of activation of the pituitary–gonadal axis.[39] Maturation of adrenal androgen secretion is termed adrenarche. In part, the prepubertal growth spurt and the early development of axillary and pubic hair are mediated by these adrenal androgens, which are believed to bind to the androgen receptor only after conversion to testosterone and/or dihydrotestosterone in target tissues.

Prior to the onset of puberty, the low levels of plasma gonadotropin are under feedback control by the small amounts of androgen secreted by the testes, as evidenced by the fact that castration at this time results in a rise in plasma gonadotropins. The degree of elevation of gonadotropins in the absence of gonadal feedback is less during late childhood years than at other times, suggesting that more than extreme sensitivity of the hypothalamic–pituitary system to feedback inhibition is involved in the low gonadotropin levels of normal prepubertal boys (see Chap 5).

The sequence of pubertal maturation has been well characterized. Its onset in boys is heralded by sleep-associated surges in LH secretion.[40] Later in puberty, the increased plasma gonadotropin levels become sustained throughout the day, as do the resulting increases in plasma testosterone. The rise in gonadotropin secretion is believed to be the consequence both of an increase in LHRH secretion and an increased sensitivity of the pituitary to LHRH.[41] Plasma levels of bioactive LH increase even more than those of the immunoreactive hormone.[42]

The overall changes in gonadotropin and steroid hormone levels in plasma are compatible with the concept that with maturation the hypothalamic–pituitary system becomes less sensitive to feedback inhibition by circulating androgens, resulting in a higher mean plasma androgen concentration. As discussed above, endogenous opiates may be involved in the negative feedback inhibition of gonadal steroids on the hypothalamic–pituitary system.[17] Studies of prepubertal and pubertal boys suggest that the development and/or maturation of the opioid control of LH secretion is temporally related with the onset of puberty.[43] How this maturational change in the hypothalamic–pituitary system is accomplished is unclear, but it appears to be triggered by the attainment of a critical body mass and/or percent body fat.[44]

The changes in the testes at puberty include the maturation of Leydig cells and the initiation of spermatogenesis. The anatomic changes characteristic of puberty are a result of testosterone secretion. Usually, the first sign of male puberty is testis enlargement with some reddening and wrinkling of the scrotal skin. Pubic hair growth begins first at the base of the penis. On average, this initiation of pubertal development occurs between ages 11 and 12, but occasionally begins as early as age 9 or as late as age 13 or 14. About 1 yr after the onset of testis growth, the penis begins to increase in size. The prostate, seminal vesicles, and epididymis increase in size over a period of several years. Characteristic hair growth includes development of mustache and beard, regression of the scalp line, appearance of body and extremity hair, and extension of pubic hair upward into the upper pubic triangle. The larynx enlarges and the vocal cords become thickened, resulting in a lower pitch of the voice. There is an enhanced rate of linear growth, resulting in a height spurt somewhat later in puberty to a rate of about 3 in per yr. At this time, the androgen-sensitive muscles of the pectoral region and the shoulder also increase in their characteristic male pattern, the hematocrit increases, and libido and sexual potency develop. These various maturation processes take place over about 4 yr and reach some normal limit for the individual based upon genetic and nutritional factors (see Chap 5).

Adulthood

On average, puberty is largely completed and reproductive capacity matures between the ages of 16 and 19. Most anatomic changes are also completed by this time. However, androgen-mediated hair growth is usually not maximal until the middle to late twenties.

Some effects of androgen such as the development of the larynx are permanent and do not reverse if androgen production decreases. Other effects of androgen such as the enhancement of erythropoietin production and hemoglobin levels reverse with androgen deprivation. Beard growth slows but rarely stops following postpubertal an-

drogen deficiency. Postpubertal androgen deficiency results in a negative nitrogen balance; the probable sites of loss include the secretory tissues of the male urogenital tract and, to some extent, other androgen target tissues such as muscle. Androgen replacement to hypogonadal men restores both nitrogen balance and the secretory capacity of the epididymis, seminal vesicles, and prostate as well.[45] Complete androgen deficiency is followed by a progressive decline in male sexual drive so that only rare subjects are able to have intercourse after a few years. In such individuals, physiologic androgen replacement results in a rapid and predictable restoration of male sexual activity.

At the completion of puberty, plasma testosterone levels have attained the adult male level of 10 to 35 nmol/L (300 to 1000 ng/dl), sperm production has reached a steady level, and plasma concentrations of gonadotropins are in the adult range (see below). Thus, the mature set for the feedback regulatory system described in Figure 13–3 has been established and is sustained in the normal man for approximately 40 yr. Even under the best circumstances the system can be perturbed, usually temporarily, by a variety of influences both at the level of the testis and of the hypothalamic–pituitary system.

CLINICAL AND LABORATORY ASSESSMENT

History and Physical Examination

The assessment of androgen status should include inquiry about developmental abnormalities at birth (eg, hypospadias, microphallus, and/or cryptorchidism), sexual maturation at puberty, rate of beard growth, and current libido, sexual function, strength, and energy. Inadequate Leydig cell function of androgen action during embryogenesis may manifest itself by the presence of hypospadias, cryptorchidism, or microphallus. If Leydig cell failure occurs prior to puberty, sexual maturation will not occur and the individual will develop the clinical features termed eunuchoidism, including an infantile amount and distribution of body hair, poor development of skeletal muscles, and failure of closure of the epiphyses so that the arm span is more than 2 in greater than height and the lower body segment (heel to pubic) more than 2 in longer than the upper body segment (pubic to crown). Detection of Leydig cell failure beginning after puberty requires a high index of suspicion and, usually, appropriate laboratory assessment. One reason is that the complaint of decreased sexual function is a relatively common one among adult men. In one large study of over 1000 men in a medical outpatient clinic, about one third claimed impotence whereas an abnormality of the hypothalamic–pituitary–testicular axis was present in only about one fifth of the impotent group.[46] The second reason is that when Leydig cell failure is severe certain functions that required androgens for initiation continue unabated, and those functions that eventually regress may do so slowly. The frequency of shaving may not decrease for many months or even years because of the slow decline in rate of beard growth once established.

The prepubertal testis measures about 2 cm in length and increases in size to a range of 3.5 to 5.5 cm in length in the normal adult. When damage to the seminiferous tubules occurs before puberty, the testes are small and firm. Following postpubertal damage, the testes are typically small and soft. Considerable testicular damage must occur before overall size is decreased below the lower limits of normal. Breast enlargement is a consistent feature of feminizing states in men and may be an early sign of androgen deficiency.

Assessment of Gonadotropins, Androgens, and Inhibin

Because of pulsatile secretion of LH and testosterone and the need to interpret each hormone in light of the other, it is usually appropriate to measure gonadotropins and testosterone in a pool formed by combining equal quantities of blood obtained from three or four samples at 15- to 20-min intervals.[15,47] In this way, only a single pooled sample of serum is submitted to the laboratory and the "averaging" of values is accomplished prior to assay. The usual assay for LH is an immunoassay. The usual normal range of plasma LH in adult men is 1.3 to 13 U/L using the appropriate standard. Dual-site immunometric assays have largely replaced competitive radioimmunoassays. Bioactive LH can be assessed by rat interstitial cell assay and may be detectable at times when the immunoreactive LH is undetectable.[48] FSH is usually measured by immunoassay with the appropriate standard. The usual normal range in adult men is 0.9 to 15 U/L. Pulsatile secretion is less pronounced for FSH. Plasma testosterone is also measured by immunoassay. The normal range in adult men is 10 to 35 nmol/L (300 to 1000 ng/dl). Free testosterone concentrations can be measured by equilibrium dialysis, but a more accurate assessment of available testosterone in vivo can be obtained by measuring the non-TeBG-bound fraction (or free plus albumin-bound fraction) (see above). At the time of puberty, random daytime levels of plasma testosterone show a gradual increase that correlates roughly with the stages of puberty. In young men the plasma testosterone level is higher in the morning than in the late afternoon, and it is preferable to measure testosterone levels in the morning. Dihydrotestosterone can also be measured by immunoassay. In normal young men, the plasma concentration averages about 10 percent of the testosterone value. Inhibin B, measured by a two-site immunoassay, appears to be the physiologically important form of inhibin in men.[49] A close negative correlation exists between inhibin B and

FSH concentrations in men with abnormalities of seminiferous tubule function.

Leydig cell function may be assessed before puberty by measuring response of plasma testosterone to gonadotropin stimulation as an index of Leydig cell reserve. Normal prepubertal boys respond to 3 to 5 days of injection of 1000 to 2000 IU hCG with an increase of plasma testosterone to about 7 nmol/L (200 ng/dl); the magnitude of the response increases with the initiation of puberty and peaks in early puberty.[50]

In certain circumstances, the response of plasma LH to administration of LHRH is measured to assess the functional integrity of the hypothalamic–pituitary–Leydig cell axis. The responsiveness of the pituitary to LHRH changes at the time of puberty. Prior to puberty, quantitative responses of LH and FSH are similar. With pubertal development, the LH response to acute administration of LHRH increases while the FSH response remains the same. The amount of LH released following acute administration of LHRH probably reflects the amount of stored hormone in the pituitary. When 100 µg LHRH are given subcutaneously or intravenously to normal men, there is, on average, a four- to five-fold increase in LH with the peak level at 30 min.[51] However, the range of response is broad, with some normal men having less than a doubling of LH levels. In general, the peak LH following a single LHRH injection correlates with the basal levels. In patients with primary testicular failure, measurement of basal LH is usually sufficient and measurement of LHRH response adds little to aid the diagnosis.[52] Men who have pituitary or hypothalamic disease may have either a normal or an abnormal LH response to an acute dose of LHRH. Therefore, a normal response is of no diagnostic value in determining the presence or absence of disease or in distinguishing hypothalamic from pituitary disease. A subnormal response is of value in determining that an abnormality exists, even though the site is not determined.

Semen Analysis and Testicular Biopsy

Routine evaluation of the seminal fluid assesses parameters that do not necessarily reflect the functional capacity of the sperm. Although methods to measure sperm penetration of bovine cervical mucus and zona-free hamster ova have been developed, they are not part of the usual evaluation. Seminal fluid should be obtained by masturbation into a clean glass or plastic container. The volume of the normal ejaculate is 2 to 6 ml. The specimen should be analyzed within 1 hr. Estimation of motility is made by examining a drop of undiluted seminal fluid and recording the percentage of motile forms. The quality of motility can be graded 1 to 3. Spermatozoa with grade 3 motility tend to move rapidly across the field, spermatozoa with grade 2 motility move aimlessly, and spermatozoa with grade 1 motility have only a beating tail but do not change position. Normally, 60 percent or more of the sperm should be motile with an average quality of motility of grade 2.5 or more. Sperm density may be determined by diluting seminal fluid 20-fold with an appropriate solution and counting in a hemocytometer or using an electronic particle counter. The normal value is usually considered greater than 20 million/ml with total sperm per ejaculate of greater than 60 million.

After the first 2 days, daily sperm output is relatively constant in normal men who ejaculate daily.[53] The daily sperm output is calculated from the total sperm in the ejaculate divided by the number of days since the previous ejaculation. Counts in the first 2 days are variable and not closely related to the output during subsequent days because of differences in extragonadal sperm reserves.[53] In addition to the problem of variable reserves of sperm in the male excretory ducts, random sampling of sperm density is complicated by effects of factors such as hot baths, acute febrile illnesses, and unknown medications. The net result is that it is difficult to define the minimally adequate ejaculate.[54] Ordinarily, three ejaculates are required to establish inadequacy of sperm number or cytology, and as many as six or more estimates may be necessary for valid assessment if the initial ejaculates are of equivocal quality.[54]

Seminal cytology is a useful index of fertility. Normal spermatozoa have symmetrically oval heads, midpieces that are slightly larger at the proximal ends and that are symmetrically inserted into the head, and tails that are 7 to 15 times longer than the head. Some abnormal spermatozoa are present in all semen. The best correlations between histologic abnormalities and infertility occur when a single anomaly is found in a large percentage of the sample.

It is generally believed that 60 percent or more of the spermatozoa should have a normal morphology.[54] For research purposes, the details of sperm structure can be studied by electron microscopy. Such studies are particularly useful in identifying specific abnormalities in immotile sperm. However, care must be exercised in defining defects in axonemal ultrastructure because there is considerable heterogeneity among normal men.[55]

Testicular biopsy is useful in some men with oligospermia and azoospermia both as an aid in diagnosis and a guide to treatment (see Chap 28). The most clearcut indication is in that group of infertile men in whom the possibility of ductal obstruction is suggested by the finding of azoospermia and normal plasma FSH levels.

ABNORMALITIES OF TESTICULAR FUNCTION

Abnormalities of testicular function have different consequences depending upon the phase of sexual life in which they first become manifest. The clinical disorders of the testis can be classified as abnormalities of fetal development, puberty, adult life, and senescence. Some aspects of the classification are arbitrary; eg, the Klinefelter syndrome is a disorder of chromosomal sex but is not usually clinically apparent until after the time of expected puberty.

The disorders of the fetal testis resulting in abnormal sexual development are considered in Chapter 6. This chapter will discuss briefly those disorders of puberty associated with sexual precocity (see also Chap 5) and focus mainly on the abnormalities of testicular function in adulthood. Because disorders of deficient or incomplete pubertal development are often present in adults, such conditions as isolated gonadotropin deficiency and Klinefelter syndrome will be discussed in the latter section.

Sexual Precocity

Those disorders in which the developing sexual characteristics are appropriate for the phenotype, ie, virilization in boys, are termed isosexual precocity. Heterosexual precocity refers to feminizing syndromes in boys.

Sexual development before age 9 in boys is generally considered abnormal. *True precocious puberty* or complete isosexual precocity occurs when both premature virilization and spermatogenesis take place; *precocious pseudopuberty* or incomplete isosexual precocity refers to virilization in the absence of spermatogenesis, indicating that androgen formation is not the result of premature activation of the hypothalamic–pituitary system.[56] This distinction is blurred in practice because true virilizing syndromes may cause activation of gonadotropin secretion secondarily and thus be followed by development spermatogenesis. Furthermore, local androgen production in the testis, as in Leydig cell tumors, can cause local areas of spermatogenesis around the tumor and thus cause limited sperm production. Virilization syndromes in which the hypothalamic–pituitary system is appropriate for age are more common in boys than are disorders in which there is a premature activation of the hypothalamic–pituitary system.

Virilizing syndromes can result from Leydig cell tumors, hCG-secreting tumors, adrenal tumors, congenital adrenal hyperplasia, primary cortisol resistance, androgen administration, or Leydig cell hyperplasia. In all these situations, serum testosterone is inappropriately elevated for the age. Leydig cell tumors are rare in children but should be suspected in men when the testes are asymmetrical in size. Virilizing adrenal tumors secrete large amounts of adrenal androgen (mainly androstenedione and dehydroepiandrosterone). Congenital adrenal hyperplasia is usually due to 21-hydroxylase deficiency and leads to elevated 17-hydroxyprogesterone levels and as a consequence elevated androgen levels (see Chap 6).

Primary cortisol resistance results in increased ACTH levels with resultant increased adrenal androgen production.[57] Gonadotropin-independent sexual precocity in boys may occur as a result of autonomous Leydig cell hyperplasia in the absence of Leydig cell tumor formation.[58] The disorder is caused by activating mutations in the LH receptor leading to constituitive stimulation of adenylyl cyclase.[58] Testosterone levels are often elevated to the adult male range, but immunoreactive and bioactive LH levels and the response to LHRH are prepubertal.[58]

Premature activation of the hypothalamic–pituitary system may be "idiopathic" or due to central nervous system tumors, infections, or injuries. Such early hypothalamic–pituitary activation typically is associated with a normal pubertal pattern of sleep-associated LH release, elevated bioactive LH, and enhanced response to LHRH. Because the diagnosis of idiopathic true precocious puberty is one of exclusion, rare patients later prove to have been misclassified and to have an identified central nervous system abnormality.

Management of sexual precocity due to steroid- or gonadotropin-producing tumors, congenital adrenal hyperplasia, or an identified CNS abnormality is that appropriate for the primary disease. Leydig cell hyperplasia has been treated with agents to block androgen action and estrogen formation.[59] Idiopathic true precocious puberty and true precocious puberty due to inoperable central nervous system lesions are treated with LHRH analog therapy.[60]

Feminizing syndromes in boys may result from absolute or relative increases in estrogen due to a variety of causes.[61]

Adulthood

Adult abnormalities of testicular function can be due to hypothalamic–pituitary defects, testicular disorders, or abnormalities in sperm transport. Most such abnormalities are manifested by both underandrogenization and infertility (Table 13–1), but some exhibit isolated infertility (see Chap 28). Defective Leydig cell function usually causes infertility because spermatogenesis is dependent upon normal androgen formation and action. Even partial decreases in testosterone production can cause infertility. Therefore, although the evaluation of the infertile man differs from that of the man who also has evidence of underandrogenization, it is essential to exclude the presence of subtle Leydig cell dysfunction in every man with infertility.

Disorders of the hypothalamus and pituitary can impair secretion of gonadotropins and consequently cause decreased androgen production and defective spermatogenesis either as an isolated defect or as part of more complex pituitary insufficiency. Thus, destructive lesions of the pituitary such as infarction, pituitary macroadenomas, metastatic or suprasellar tumors, infections, or granulomatous processes can result in *panhypopituitarism* and lead to a secondary testicular defect.

Primary *isolated gonadotropin deficiency* (the Kallmann syndrome) occurs in both sporadic and familial forms. The incidence of the disorder has not been established, but in most centers it is second only to the Klinefelter syndrome as a cause of hypogonadism in men. The disorder was originally described as a familial syndrome associated with anosmia. The term Kallmann syndrome is now used to refer to both the sporadic and familial forms with and without anosmia. Affected individuals can sometimes be ascertained in childhood because of the presence of microphallus and/or cryptorchidism. Most affected individuals are ascertained because of a failure to undergo puberty. A subset of subjects, particularly familial cases, have associated congenital defects, commonly anomalies involving the midline facial and head structures, and partial deficiencies of other pituitary hormones.[62] At the opposite end of the spectrum, less severely affected subjects have only partial defects in FSH and/or LH. The pattern of inheritance in most families is compatible either with X-linkage or with autosomal transmission with primary manifestations in males. Half or more patients have a negative family history, suggesting that new mutations may be common. The underlying defect is at the hypothalamic level. After repetitive treatment with LHRH for 5 days or longer, plasma gonadotropins rise to the normal range in most Kallmann subjects but not in individuals with panhypopituitarism. The X-linked form has been related to a gene that predicts a protein with homology to neural-cell adhesion molecules.[63] Crowley and colleagues established that the disor-

TABLE 13–1. CAUSES OF INFERTILITY WITH UNDERANDROGENIZATION IN ADULT MEN

Site of Defect/Type	Disorder
Hypothalmic–Pituitary	Panhypopituitarism; isolated gonadotropin deficiency; Cushing syndrome
Testicular	
Developmental–structural	Klinefelter syndrome; XX male syndrome
Acquired	Viral orchitis; trauma; radiation; drugs, autoimmunity; granulomatous processes
Associated with systemic diseases	Liver disease; renal failure; sickle cell disease; immune disease; neurologic disease; other major illnesses
Androgen receptor	Androgen resistance syndromes

(Adapted, with permission, from Griffin JE, Wilson JD. Disorders of the testes and male reproductive tract. In: Wilson JD, Foster DW, eds. Williams Textbook of Endocrinology, 7th ed. Philadelphia, Pa., W. B. Saunders, 1985: 259-311)

der encompasses defects in the pulsatile release of LHRH including total absence of LH secretion, defects in the amplitude and frequency of LH secretion, and altered bioactivity of the gonadotropin released.[64]

Three forms of therapy can be used for isolated gonadotropin deficiency: androgen replacement to virilize, gonadotropin therapy to induce fertility, and administration of LHRH analogs to replace the deficit in the most physiologic way possible. In the infant or young child with microphallus, the administration of testosterone for limited periods (3 mo) may cause enlargement of the penis to the normal range without affecting linear growth or causing other significant virilizing signs.[65] In the older child or adult, long-acting testosterone esters are administered parenterally as in other forms of hypogonadism. Administration of hCG long term also causes serum testosterone to increase to normal adult male levels, but in subjects with severe (prepubertal) hypogonadotropic hypogonadism, induction of fertility usually requires administration of FSH in the form of human menopausal gonadotropin in addition to hCG.[66] The response to gonadotropin therapy in this disorder is not influenced by prior testosterone therapy.[67] Once normal sperm count is achieved, it may be maintained by hCG. In occasional patients with partial defects in gonadotropin secretion, spermatogenesis can be promoted by testosterone therapy alone.[68] Long-term administration of LHRH in a pulsatile manner to men with hypogonadotropic hypogonadism results in the achievement of normal plasma testosterone, normal pulsatile secretion of LH, normal mean levels of plasma LH and FSH, and, in most, mature sperm in the ejaculate.[69]

Acquired gonadotropin deficiency can be caused by factors other than hypothalamic or pituitary pathology. For example, elevated plasma cortisol levels, as in *Cushing syndrome,* can depress LH secretion independent of a space-occupying lesion of the pituitary.[70] The serum LH in these men, as in other forms of secondary testicular dysfunction, is usually in the normal range and only occasionally decreased. However, it is inappropriately low for the depressed serum testosterone. Even when Cushing syndrome is associated with a pituitary adenoma, ie, Cushing's disease, the hypogonadotropic hypogonadism appears to be secondary to the hypercortisolism because treatment by bilateral adrenalectomy or mitotane results in return of testosterone levels to normal.[70] Chronic administration of exogenous glucocorticoids can also lower testosterone levels by inhibiting LHRH secretion.[71]

Hyperprolactinemia is also a cause of secondary testicular dysfunction. Hyperprolactinemia can be produced by either microadenomas or macroadenomas of the pituitary. Macroadenomas may give rise to hyperprolactinemia because of either direct secretion by the tumor (prolactino-

mas) or interference with the delivery of normal inhibitory influences from the hypothalamus to the pituitary by mass effect of a nonsecretory tumor. Hypogonadism can result from hyperprolactinemia itself, diminished gonadotropin secretion because of destruction of the normal pituitary, or a combination of these effects. Prolactin excess by itself can cause both underandrogenization and infertility and lead to impotence.[72] It probably causes hypogonadism by impairing LHRH release. Impotence associated with hyperprolactinemia is not always the consequence of a decreased serum testosterone level. Some hyperprolactinemic men given testosterone replacement do not have return of potency until the prolactin levels are corrected by administration of bromocriptine.[73] In part because of delays in seeking evaluation, men with prolactin-secreting pituitary adenomas usually have macroadenomas at the time of diagnosis.[72,73] Bromocriptine is the preferred treatment.[74]

Idiopathic *hemochromatosis* cause iron deposition in the pituitary and testes, and about half of affected men have hypogonadism, usually accompanied by testicular atrophy. The abnormalities of testicular function in this disorder may in part result from the associated liver disease and occasionally from a primary testicular abnormality, but most testicular dysfunction is due to hypogonadotropic hypogonadism.[75] Acquired transfusional iron overload can cause similar abnormalities of the pituitary–testicular axis.[76] The hypogonadism secondary to hemochromatosis can be corrected by iron depletion therapy is some men.[77]

In several other conditions, testosterone levels may be decreased in association with normal LH levels and the mechanism is less clear. Men with massive obesity have decreased TeBG and decreased levels of total and bioavailable testosterone that return toward normal with weight loss.[78] Some men with seizures of temporal lobe origin also have hormonal findings consistent with hypogonadotropic hypogonadism.[79] Finally, hypogonadotropic hypogonadism may occur as an apparently acquired idiopathic disorder.[80]

Abnormalities of testicular function in the adult with the defect at the level of the testis can be grouped into several categories: developmental and structural defects of the testes, acquired testicular defects, abnormalities associated with systemic or neurologic diseases, and androgen resistance.

The most common developmental defect of the testis is *Klinefelter syndrome* (see also Chap 6). The disorder is characterized by small, firm testes, varying degrees of impaired sexual maturation, azoospermia, gynecomastia, and elevated gonadotropins. The underlying defect is the presence of an extra X chromosome, the common karyotype being either 47,XXY (the classic form) or 46,XY/47,XXY (the mosaic form).[81] The incidence is approximately 1 in 500 males. The diagnosis is usually made after the time of expected puberty, when the disorder is manifested by gynecomastia and/or underandrogenization

TABLE 13–2. CHARACTERISTICS OF MEN WITH CLASSIC VERSUS MOSAIC KLINEFELTER SYNDROME

	47,XXY (%)	46,XY/47,XXY (%)
Abnormal testicular histology	100	94[a]
Decreased length of testis	99	73[a]
Azoospermia	93	50[a]
Decreased testosterone	79	33
Decreased facial hair	77	64
Increased gonadotropins	75	33[a]
Decreased sexual function	68	56
Gynecomastia	55	33[a]
Decreased axillary hair	49	46
Decreased length of penis	41	21

Based upon 518 XXY men and 51 XY/XXY men.
[a]Significantly different at $P < .05$ or better.
(Adapted, with permission, from Gordon DL, Krmpotic E, Thomas W, et al. Pathologic testicular findings in Klinefelter's syndrome. 47,XXY vs. 46,XY/47,XXY. Arch Intern Med. 130:726, 1972.)

(Table 13–2). Damage to the seminiferous tubules and azoospermia are consistent features of the 47,XXY variety. The small, firm testes are characteristically less than 2.0 cm and always less than 3.5 cm in length. Typical histological changes in the testes include hyalinization of the tubules, absence of spermatogenesis, and apparent increase in the number of Leydig cells.

The increased mean body height in the disorder is the result of an increased lower body segment, a feature present prior to puberty.[82] Obesity and varicose veins occur in one third to one half of subjects, and mild mental deficiency and/or social maladjustment,[83] subtle abnormalities of thyroid function, diabetes mellitus, and restrictive pulmonary disease are more common than in the general population. Most individuals have a male psychosexual orientation and function sexually as men.

46,XY/47,XXY mosaicism is the cause of about 10 percent of Klinefelter syndrome, as estimated by chromosomal karyotypes on peripheral blood leukocytes. The true prevalence may be underestimated because chromosomal mosaicism can be present in the testes in subjects in whom the karyotype in peripheral leukocytes is normal.[81] As summarized in Table 13–2, the clinical manifestations of the mosaic form are usually less severe than the 47,XXY variety and the testes may be normal in size.[81] The endocrine abnormalities are also less severe, and gynecomastia and azoospermia are less common. In some individuals, the diagnosis may not be suspected because of the minor degree of the associated abnormalities.

Characteristic endocrine changes include elevation of plasma FSH and LH. FSH shows the best discrimination, and little overlap occurs with normals. In the late teen years, the plasma testosterone concentration may be normal.[84] By the mid-20s the plasma testosterone aver-

ages half normal but the range of values is broad and overlaps the normal range.[84] Mean plasma estradiol levels are elevated.[85] After the age of expected puberty, the increase in plasma gonadotropins following administration of LHRH is exaggerated and the normal feedback inhibition of testosterone on pituitary LH secretion is diminished.[86] Older patients with untreated Klinefelter syndrome may have enlarged or abnormal sella turcicas, presumably secondary to the persistent lack of gonadal steroid feedback and hyperplasia of gonadotrophs.[87] Underandrogenized patients may benefit from supplemental androgen, but such treatment may paradoxically worsen the gynecomastia, presumably by providing increased androgen substrate for the conversion to estrogens in the peripheral tissues. Following administration of testosterone, plasma LH returns to normal but usually only after several months.

The XX *male syndrome* is a variant of Klinefelter syndrome. The incidence of a 46,XX karyotype in phenotypic males is approximately 1 in 20,000 to 24,000 male births.[88] Over 150 XX males have been described. The findings resemble those in Klinefelter syndrome: The testes are small and firm, generally less than 2 cm in length; gynecomastia is usual; the penis is normal to small in size; azoospermia and hyalinization of the seminiferous tubules are present. Affected individuals have male psychosexual identification and absence of female internal genitalia. Mean plasma testosterone is low while plasma estradiol and gonadotropins are high.[89] Affected individuals differ from typical Klinefelter patients in that average height is less than in normal men, the incidence of mental deficiency is not increased, and hypospadias is common.[90]

Four theories have been proposed to explain the pathogenesis of this disorder: (1) mosaicism in some tissues for a Y-containing cell line or early loss of a Y chromosome; (2) an autosomal gene mutation; (3) interchange of a Y-chromosomal gene with the X chromosome; and (4) deletion or inactivation of X-chromosomal gene(s) that normally suppress testis development. Mosaicism has not been documented and no clear-cut evidence has been provided for an autosomal gene mutation. More than half of XX males whose DNA was probed with Y chromosome DNA fragments containing the testis-determining factor did contain Y-related DNA.[91] Thus, the majority appear to have the Y-linked testis determining factor, presumably by transfer of a critical fragment of the Y chromosome to the X chromosome.

A common cause of acquired testicular failure in the adult is *viral orchitis*. Mumps virus is the most common viral agent, although others act in a similar fashion.[92] Orchitis is a common complication of mumps, occurring in as many as one fourth of adult men with the disease.[93] In about two thirds of the cases, it is unilateral. After the acute inflammatory phase, the testis gradually decreases in size and may return to normal size and function or undergo atrophy. The histologic appearance of the atrophic testis includes progressive tubular sclerosis and hyalinization, sometimes not dissimilar to that in the Klinefelter syndrome. The degree of atrophy is not necessarily proportional to the severity of the orchitis. It is usually apparent within 1 to 6 mo after the orchitis subsides, but the full extent of the damage may not be evident until 10 yr later. Atrophy occurs in approximately one third of men who develop orchitis and is bilateral in about one tenth. The initial treatment of mumps orchitis is bedrest and scrotal support. If severe pain is present, the administration of prednisone often results in prompt defervescence and reduction of testicular swelling and pain.

Trauma is a cause of testicular atrophy in the adult; the exposed position of the testis in the scrotum renders it uniquely susceptible to both thermal and physical damage. Both spermatogenesis and testosterone production are sensitive to *radiation;* the diminished secretion of testosterone appears to be a consequence of diminished testicular blood flow.[94] Although doses of radiation as low as 0.2 Gy (20 rads) result in temporary increases of both LH and FSH levels and damage to spermatogonia, permanent decrease in testosterone production is uncommon. However, one tenth of patients receiving approximately 8 Gy (800 rad) of scattered radiation to the testes during childhood and most boys receiving 24 to 30 Gy (2400 to 3000 rads) of direct testicular radiation for acute lymphoblastic leukemia[95] have permanently low plasma testosterone levels.

Drugs can cause underandrogenization and infertility in several ways: direct inhibition of testosterone synthesis, blockade of the peripheral actions of androgen, or enhancement of estrogen levels. Certain drugs have multiple effects. Two drugs that in high doses block testosterone synthesis are spironolactone and cyproterone, both of which interfere with the late reactions in testosterone biosynthesis.[96] Spironolactone appears to impair 17α-hydroxylase and 17,20-lyase activities.[96] Plasma testosterone levels do not change appreciably, however, during usual therapeutic regimens. The antifungal agent ketoconazole blocks testosterone synthesis also by inhibiting the 17,20-lyase and the 17α-hydroxylase reactions.[97] The decrease in testosterone following a single dose of ketoconazole is transient with the nadir occurring 4 to 8 hr after administration and returning to baseline by 24 hr as ketoconazole concentrations fall. However, with doses of ketoconazole greater than 400 mg/day depression of plasma testosterone levels may be sustained.[98] Impairment of libido is common in men with epilepsy. This may be partly a consequence of medication.[99] Enzyme-inducing antiepileptic drugs such as phenytoin and carbamazepine lower bioactive

testosterone and raise LH levels. The effect is more pronounced with multiple drug regimens. Valproic acid does not appear to have as severe an adverse effect in this regard.[99]

Independent of its effects on the liver, ethanol ingestion reduces testosterone levels both acutely and chronically.[100] This action is the result of inhibition of testosterone synthesis. In men without liver disease given 40 percent of food intake as alcohol, a 25 to 50 percent decrease in the plasma testosterone levels and testosterone production rate is demonstrable within 5 days after starting and lasts for as long as 3 wk.[101] The fact that the lower testosterone levels in most men given alcohol are not accompanied by appropriate elevations of plasma LH suggests that hypothalamic–pituitary function is also impaired.[100,101]

Combination chemotherapy for acute leukemia, Hodgkin's disease, and other malignancies may impair Leydig cell function.[102] In pubertal boys, this is manifested by decreased serum testosterone, elevated LH, and marked gynecomastia. In adult men, testosterone levels do not decline and the impaired Leydig cell function is only detectable by an exaggerated LH response to LHRH stimulation. This toxic effect on the Leydig cell seems to be produced primarily by alkylating agents such as cyclophosphamide. Plasma testosterone levels may be low in men taking large amounts of marijuana, heroin, or methadone.[103,104] In general, elevations of plasma LH do not occur, suggesting a hypothalamic–pituitary abnormality, as well as a testicular effect. Elevated plasma estradiol levels and decreased plasma testosterone levels may occur in men taking digitalis preparations, the mechanism of the effect being unclear.[105] Drugs can interfere with gonadotropin production either as the result of a direct inhibition, as in medroxyprogesterone acetate administration,[106] or as a secondary consequence of enhanced prolactin secretion.[107] Medroxyprogesterone acetate also seems to decrease testosterone secretion at the testicular level.[108]

Several drugs inhibit androgen action by competition at the receptor level. Although spironolactone can inhibit testosterone synthesis, in the usual dosage regimens it primarily acts by antagonizing androgen binding to the androgen receptor, leading to gynecomastia and impotence.[96] A commonly administered drug that is an androgen antagonist is cimetidine. Gynecomastia can occur in men treated with the drug, and decreased sperm density and elevated basal testosterone levels are accompanied by a slight diminution of the LH response to LHRH.[109] Ranitidine appears to be a less potent antiandrogen.[110]

Prolonged exposure of men to *lead* as an environmental toxin appears to result in a direct testicular toxicity with an impaired pituitary response, as indicated by slight LH elevation.[111] Testicular failure can occur as part of a generalized *autoimmune* disorder in which multiple primary endocrine deficiencies coexist and in which circulating antibodies to the basement membrane of the testes can be documented.[112] The testis can also be a site of involvement in *granulomatous disease.* Testicular atrophy occurs in 10 to 20 percent of men with lepromatous leprosy.[113] Destruction of the testis is less common in other types of systemic granulomatous disease.

Abnormalities of the hypothalamic–pituitary–testicular axis occur in a number of systemic diseases. Given the chronic ill health and generalized wasting that may occur with these disorders, it is often difficult to distinguish effects specifically due to the underlying condition (eg, renal failure) from those attributable to malnutrition. About half of men with *renal failure* on dialysis experience decreased libido and impotence, complaints associated with impairments both in spermatogenesis and testosterone biosynthesis. Plasma testosterone is decreased and plasma LH and FSH are increased, indicating a defect at the testicular level.[114] Following dialysis, plasma testosterone and testosterone production rates improve but usually not to the normal range. The etiology of the testicular abnormalities in renal failure is not well understood. Zinc deficiency may be a contributing factor. Uremic men have abnormal zinc metabolism and may be zinc deficient despite dialysis. In one study, oral zinc therapy led to a return of plasma testosterone to normal with lowering of LH and FSH levels and an improvement in libido and potency.[115] Hyperprolactinemia occurs in one fourth of men on chronic dialysis, and treatment with bromocriptine to lower prolactin may raise testosterone levels and restore potency in some individuals.[116] Successful renal transplantation is associated with return of testosterone and prolactin to normal and partial reduction of LH and FSH levels.

The effects of *cirrhosis of the liver* on testicular function occur independent of the direct toxic effects of ethanol. Gynecomastia and testicular atrophy are present in half of men with cirrhosis, and three fourths are impotent.[117] Extraglandular conversion of androgens, primarily adrenal androgens, to estradiol and estrone is increased about threefold, presumably because of decreased hepatic extraction of androgens.[118] Basal plasma levels of LH and FSH range from normal to moderately elevated.[117] Modest elevation of basal LH and FSH levels coupled with the lack of hyperresponsiveness to LHRH suggest that the hypothalamic–pituitary response to the diminished testosterone levels is blunted.[119] The reason for impairment of testosterone production and hypothalamic–pituitary response is uncertain. Elevated estrogen levels could cause both defects. The reversibility of the gonadal changes in cirrhosis cannot be assessed as in renal failure. Testosterone therapy has been tried.[120] Although estradiol levels increased (in direct correlation with the severity of the cirrhosis) after administration of testosterone enanthate, the estrogen:androgen ratio became normal. Men with alcoholic cirrhosis may have spontaneous recovery of sexual function when they abstain from alcohol despite the persistence of liver abnormalities.[121] However, those with testicular atrophy are less likely to experience improvement in sexual function with abstinence from alcohol.[121]

Boys with *sickle cell anemia* have impaired skeletal and sexual maturation in adolescence.[122] Furthermore, in 32 adult men with sickle cell anemia, secondary sexual characteristics were abnormal in all but 2 and testicular atrophy was noted in about one third.[122] Abnormalities in Leydig cell function, frequently accompanied by decreased sperm counts, occur in a variety of chronic systemic diseases including protein calorie *malnutrition,*[123] advanced *Hodgkin's disease* and cancer before chemotherapy,[124] *cystic fibrosis,*[125] and *amyloidosis.*[126] Except for amyloidosis, in which the abnormalities seem to be limited to the testis, all these disorders cause a lowered plasma testosterone coupled with normal to increased plasma LH, suggesting combined hypothalamic–pituitary and testicular defects. Because the mean plasma TeBG is elevated, the decrease in available testosterone may be even greater than indicated by the total level.[127] The above pattern of changes in testosterone and LH may be nonspecific effects of illness because similar changes in plasma testosterone and LH occur following *surgery, myocardial infarction,* and *severe burns.*

Immune disease may be associated with testicular dysfunction. Half of men with AIDS have low testosterone levels, usually without appropriate elevation of plasma LH.[128] It is unclear how much the low testosterone contributes to the wasting. Men with rheumatoid arthritis may have low testosterone levels associated with low-dose prednisone therapy.[129]

Neurologic disease can cause testicular abnormalities. Men with myotonic dystrophy usually have small testes, low plasma testosterone levels, and elevated plasma LH and FSH levels.[130] Although the effects are variable, depending upon the exact nature of the defect, spinal cord lesions that result in quadriplegia or paraplegia initially cause diminished plasma testosterone levels that generally return toward normal, but defective spermatogenesis appears to persist.[131]

Men with trisomy 21 have impairment of both germinal and Leydig cell function. Plasma FSH and LH are elevated.[132]

A limited form of *androgen resistance* results in underandrogenization and infertility in men who have normal development of the external genitalia.[133] An even less severe manifestation of androgen resistance due to an androgen receptor defect has been observed in men who have gynecomastia and undervirilization associated with fertility in some affected family members.[134]

HORMONAL THERAPY

Androgens

Effective androgen therapy requires administration either in a slowly absorbed from of testosterone (dermal patches or micronized oral preparation) or chemically modified analogs. Such chemical modifications either retard the rate of absorption or catabolism so as to maintain effective blood levels or enhance the androgenic potency of each molecule so that hormonal effects can be achieved at a lower plasma level of the drug. Three general types of modifications of testosterone are clinically useful: esterification of the 17β-hydroxyl group; alkylation at the 17α-position; and modification of the A, B, or C rings, particularly substitutions at the 2, 9, and 11 carbons (Fig 13–8). Most agents actually contain combinations of ring structure alterations and either 17α-alkylation or esterification of the 17β-hydroxyl. Esterification decreases the polarity of the steroid, makes it more soluble in the fat vehicles used for injection, and hence slows release of the injected steroid into the circula-

tion. Testosterone cypionate or enanthate is the most common treatment for male hypogonadism.[45,86,135] The esters must be hydrolyzed before the hormone acts so that effectiveness of therapy can be monitored by measuring the plasma level of testosterone following administration. Most esters cannot be administered by mouth and must be injected. Testosterone undecanoate can be given by mouth because it is absorbed via the lymphatic system into the systemic circulation, and physiological blood levels of testosterone can be achieved at doses of approximately 120 mg/day.[136] Because of rapid turnover in plasma, however, testosterone undecanoate must be administered twice daily.

17α-Alkylated androgens, such as methyltestosterone and methandrostenolone, are effective when given by mouth because alkylated steroids are absorbed into the portal circulation but slowly catabolized by the liver and reach the systemic circulation in effective amounts. For this reason, 17α-methyl or ethyl substitution is a common feature of most orally active androgens. Because all

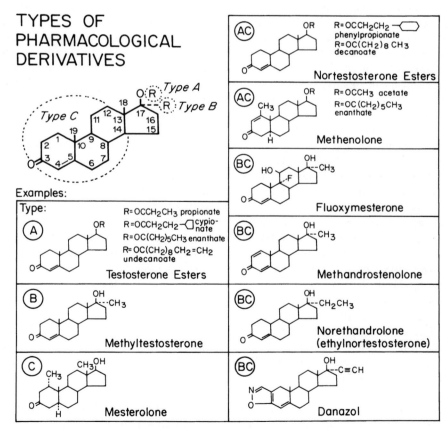

Figure 13–8. Some of the androgen preparations available for clinical use, classified into three types. Type A derivatives are esterified in the 17β-position. Type B steroids have alkyl groups in a 17α-position. Type C derivatives include a variety of additional alterations of ring structure that enhance activity, impede catabolism, or influence both functions. Most androgen preparations involve combinations of Type AC or BC changes. *(Reproduced, with permission, from Griffin JE, Wilson JD. Disorders of the testes and male reproductive tract. In: Wilson JD, Foster DW, eds.* Williams Textbook of Endocrinology, *7th ed. Philadelphia, Pa., W. B. Saunders, 1985: 259-311)*

17α-alkylated steroids may cause abnormalities of liver function, these steroids are not recommended.[45]

Other alterations of the ring structure have been adopted empirically; in some instances, the effect is to slow the rate of inactivation, while in others the alteration enhances the potency of a given molecule or alters its metabolism. As is true for 17-alkylated steroids, androgens with ring alterations are usually not converted to testosterone in vivo and hence specific assays for each must be utilized to monitor blood levels. Because most steroids with altered ring structures also contain 17α-substitutions, they also have the same deleterious effects on liver function as methyltestosterone and thus have little clinical usefulness.

The use of a transdermal therapeutic preparations of testosterone in which testosterone patches are applied each day makes it possible to sustain serum testosterone levels in the normal male range.[137–139] These systems thus offer advantages over other modalities for administering testosterone in that they simultaneously replace the missing molecule specifically and avoid the necessity for parenteral administration. There are two kinds of patches, a scrotal and a non-scrotal patch. A single scrotal patch is applied in the morning,[137,138] or two non-scrotal patches are applied at bedtime.[139] In each instance higher serum testosterone levels are achieved in the morning.

Other means of administering testosterone, such as subcutaneous implantation of silastic capsules, oral testosterone in microparticulate form, topical creams, rectal suppositories, or nasal drops, all have limited practicality.

The aim of androgen therapy in hypogonadal men is to restore or bring to normal male secondary sexual characteristics (beard, body hair, external genitalia) and male sexual behavior and promote normal male somatic development (hemoglobin, voice, muscle mass, nitrogen balance, and epiphyseal closure). Because a reliable assay for plasma testosterone is widely available for monitoring therapy, the treatment of androgen deficiency is straightforward and almost universally successful. The parenteral administration of a long-acting testosterone ester such as 100 to 300 mg testosterone enanthate at 1- to 3-wk intervals results in a sustained increase in plasma testosterone to the normal male range or slightly above.[45,86,135] The usual replacement regimen is 200 mg every 2 wk.[135] Similar effects are obtained with percutaneous administration of testosterone.[138,139] In most subjects, such regimens suppress plasma LH and maintain serum testosterone within the normal range.[135] If the hypogonadism is primary and of long duration (as in Klinefelter syndrome), suppression of plasma LH to the normal range may not occur for many weeks if at all.[86] There is considerable variability in the relation between plasma testosterone and male sexual behavior, but resumption of normal sexual activity is usual following adequate replacement.[140] The major effects of androgen appear to be on libido[141] and frequency of erections.[142] Androgen therapy does not ordinarily restore spermatogenesis to normal in hypogonadal states, but the volume of the ejaculate, which is derived largely from the prostate and seminal vesicles, and other secondary sex characteristics return to normal.

In men of all ages in whom hypogonadism develops prior to expected puberty (such as subjects with isolated gonadotropin deficiency), it is appropriate to bring plasma testosterone into the adult range slowly. When therapy is begun at the time of expected puberty in such patients, the normal events of male puberty proceed in the usual fashion and require several years for completion. Intermittent androgen therapy is sometimes administered to prepubertal hypogonadal boys with microphallus to stimulate the growth of the external genitalia into the normal range.[65] If patients are monitored closely and androgen is given only for short periods, such therapy probably has no adverse effects on somatic growth. In boys of pubertal age with either gonadotropin deficiency or primary testicular deficiency, the initial administration of small doses of testosterone esters followed by a gradual increase to doses of 100 to 150 mg/m[2] of surface area per mo results in the development of a normal pubertal growth spurt. The usual practice is to institute androgen therapy in hypogonadal boys between the ages of 12 and 14 yr depending upon their subjective need for sexual development. Testosterone exerts its full action only in the presence of a balanced hormonal environment and, particularly, in the presence of adequate levels of growth hormone.[143] Testosterone may enhance growth in pubertal boys by enhancing the secretion of growth hormone and insulin-like growth factor I.[144]

Because androgens have significant effects on muscle mass and body weight when administered to hypogonadal men, it was initially assumed that androgens in pharmacologic amounts could promote growth of muscle mass above the levels produced by normal testicular secretion. Because the anabolic and androgenic actions of androgens were believed to be distinct and independent hormone actions, a concerted effort was made to devise pure "anabolic" steroids that have no androgenic effects. In fact, however, androgenic and anabolic effects do not result from different actions of the same hormone but represent the same action in different tissues. All anabolic agents tested in man so far are also androgens.

The use of androgens by athletes in the belief that athletic performance will be improved constitutes a widespread form of drug abuse. The abuse of these substances at all levels of athletic competition from high school to professional has become widespread despite the absence until recently of evidence that such agents have a positive effect and with disregard of the adverse effects of the drugs.[145] Indeed, in many appropriately controlled studies it was not possible to show that these agents cause an increase in muscle bulk, strength, or athletic performance,[145] and when effects on strength have been reported it was not clear that such effects necessarily result in improved performance. It is true, however, that many published trials of efficacy involve administration of drugs at smaller doses than are actually taken by many athletes. However, Bhasin and colleagues have shown that administration of 600 mg of testosterone esters weekly, especially when combined with strength training, increases fat-free mass and muscle size and strength.[146]

Some *side effects* of androgens result from physiological actions of the hormones (via the androgen receptor) but occur in an inappropriate setting. For example, the virilizing actions are desirable in hypogonadal men but undesirable in young boys. In some older hypogonadal men, administration of androgens may cause previously unrecognized prostate cancer to become clinically apparent. Other side effects are the results of actions of androgen metabolites, and, because different androgens are metabolized differently, the side effects vary. Testosterone can be metabolized to estrogens and may cause feminizing as well as virilizing effects.

Side effects of androgen therapy can also result from actions of the steroid derivatives that have no relation to the androgenic actions of these compounds. These latter effects constitute the true complications of androgen therapy. Some degree of sodium retention is a common consequence of therapy with androgens, but the amount of retained sodium is usually minor. However, in patients with underlying heart disease or renal failure the degree of sodium retention may be sufficient to produce edema. 17α-Alkylated androgens impair liver function, as evidenced by frequent elevation of plasma alkaline phosphatase and conjugated bilirubin during therapy.[45] The most serious complication of oral androgens is the development of peliosis hepatis (blood-filled cysts in the liver) or hepatoma.[45] 17α-Alkylated androgens cause striking reductions in serum high-density lipoprotein cholesterol levels.[147] Such unfavorable changes in the plasma lipoproteins were not seen in men given high-dose parenteral testosterone ester therapy.[147] Sleep apnea has been reported in occasional men given pharmacologic amounts of testosterone esters.[148]

Gonadotropin Therapy

Gonadotropin treatment can establish or restore fertility in men who have gonadotropin deficiency either as an isolated disorder or as part of more extensive anterior pituitary failure. Because men with hypogonadotropic hypogonadism may become resistant to gonadotropins after long-term treatment (presumably as the result of the development of neutralizing antibodies), the customary strategy is to treat such subjects initially with testosterone esters or transdermal preparations as described above and reserve gonadotropin therapy until fertility is desired. Prior androgen therapy does not impair subsequent gonadotropin induction of spermatogenesis in subjects with hypogonadotropic hypogonadism.[67]

Two gonadotropin preparations are available: human menopausal gonadotropins (hMG) and hCG. The usual preparation of hMG (menotropin), purified from the urine of postmenopausal women, contains 75 IU FSH and 75 IU LH per vial. hCG is available from several sources in vials containing 5000 to 20,000 IU. hCG is devoid of FSH activity and resembles LH in its ability to stimulate Leydig cells. Because of the expense of hMG, treatment is usually begun with hCG alone, and hMG is added later to stimulate the FSH-dependent stages of spermatoid development. A high ratio of LH/FSH activity and a long duration of treatment (3 to 6 mo) are necessary to bring about the maturation of prepubertal testis.[149] In men with hypogonadotropic hypogonadism, the dose of chorionic gonadotropin required to maintain a normal plasma testosterone varies from 1000 to 6000 IU weekly.[149] Most treatment regimens for the induction of spermatogenesis involve starting with doses of 2000 IU three or more times a week until most of the clinical parameters including normal male plasma testosterone indicate an optimal effect. During initial treatment, testis size may reach only 8 ml. Menotropin is then added, with as little as 12.5 IU FSH and 12.5 IU LH being required three times a week to complete the development of spermatogenesis and cause further growth of the testes.

LHRH

LHRH agonists can produce diametrically opposite effects depending upon the mode of administration. When administered in a pulsatile fashion that approximates the physiologic secretory pattern, such therapy results in enhancement of gonadotropin secretion. In contrast, tonic administration of the same agonist inhibits gonadotropin secretion and causes a physiologic (reversible) castration. Agonistic effects have proven of benefit: In isolated gonadotropin deficiency, LHRH is the most "physiologic" treatment. Induction of puberty can be accomplished by long-term pulsatile administration of low-dose LHRH using a portable infusion pump; normal levels of plasma testosterone, LH, and FSH can be attained over 3 mo of therapy with 25 ng LHRH (gonadorelin) per kg body weight administered subcutaneously every 2 hr.[64] However, the achievement of adult levels of spermatogenesis may require high dosages.[64] Whether pulsatile LHRH therapy will prove to have advantages over gonadotropin therapy in men with hypogonadotropic hypogonadism is uncertain. In one study, LHRH therapy was more effective than gonadotropin therapy in stimulating testicular growth but not in increasing sperm count.[150]

REFERENCES

1. Sinclair AH, Berta P, Palmer MS, et al. A gene from the human sex-determining region encodes a protein with homology to a conserved DNA-binding motif. *Nature.* 346:240, 1990
2. Peters H. Migration of gonocytes into the mammalian gonad and their differentiation. *Philos Trans Roy Soc Lond (Biol).* 259:91, 1970
3. Guerrier D, Tran D, VanderWinden JM, et al. The persistent Müllerian duct syndrome: A molecular approach. *J Clin Endocrinol Metab.* 68:46, 1989
4. Hauser GA. Testicular feminization. In: Overzier C, ed. *Intersexuality.* London, U.K., Academic Press, 1963: 255–297
5. George FW, Wilson JD. Embryology of the genital tract. In: Walsh PC, Retik AB, Stamey TA, Vaughan ED Jr, eds. *Campbell's Urology,* 6th ed. Philadelphia, Pa., W. B. Saunders, 1992: 1496–1508
6. Neaves WB. The blood–testis barrier. In: Johnson AD, Gomes WR, eds. *The Testis.* New York, N.Y., Academic Press, 1977: 125–161
7. Freeman DA. Cyclic-AMP mediated modification of cholesterol traffic in Leydig tumor cells. *J Biol Chem.* 262:13061, 1987
8. Turner TT. On the epididymis and its function. *Invest Urol.* 16:311, 1979
9. Silverman AJ, Krey LC, Zimmerman EA. A comparative study of the luteinizing hormone releasing hormone (LHRH) neuronal networks in mammals. *Biol Reprod.* 20:98, 1979
10. Veldhuis JD, Rogol AD, Johnson ML, et al. Endogenous opiates modulate the pulsatile secretion of biologically active luteinizing hormone in man. *J Clin Invest.* 72:2031, 1983
11. Conn PM. The molecular basis of gonadotropin-releasing hormone action. *Endocrine Rev.* 7:3, 1986
12. Dufau ML, Catt KJ. Gonadotropin receptors and regulation of steroidogenesis in the testis and ovary. *Vitam Horm.* 36:461, 1978
13. Wahlström T, Huhtaniemi I, Hovatta O, et al. Localization of luteinizing hormone, follicle-stimulating hormone, prolactin, and their receptors in human and rat testis using immunohistochemistry and radioreceptor assay. *J Clin Endocrinol Metab.* 57:825, 1983
14. Means AR, Fakunding JL, Huckins C, et al. Follicle-stimulating hormone, the Sertoli cell, and spermatogenesis. *Recent Prog Horm Res.* 32:477, 1976
15. Santen RJ, Bardin CW. Episodic luteinizing hormone secretion in man: Pulse analysis, clinical interpretation, physiologic mechanisms. *J Clin Invest.* 53:2617, 1973
16. Matsumoto AM, Bremner WJ. Modulation of pulsatile gonadotropin secretion by testosterone in man. *J Clin Endocrinol Metab.* 58:609, 1984
17. Veldhuis JD, Rogol AD, Samojlik E, et al. Role of endogenous opiates in the expression of negative feedback actions of androgen and estrogen on pulsatile properties of luteinizing hormone secretion in man. *J Clin Invest.* 74:47, 1984
18. Santen RJ. Is aromatization of testosterone to estradiol required for inhibition of luteinizing hormone secretion in men? *J Clin Invest.* 56:1555, 1975
19. Sheckter CB, Matsumoto AM, Bremner WJ. Testosterone administration inhibits gonadotropin secretion by an effect directly on the human pituitary. *J Clin Endocrinol Metab.* 68:397, 1989
20. Robertson DM, McLachlan RI, Burger HG, et al. Inhibin-related proteins in the male. In: Burger H, de Kretser D, eds. *The Testis,* 2nd ed. New York, N.Y., Raven Press, 1989: 231–254
21. McLachlan RI, Matsumoto AM, Burger HG, et al. Relative roles of follicle-stimulating hormone and luteinizing hormone in the control of inhibin secretion in normal men. *J Clin Invest.* 82:880, 1988
22. Majumdar SS, Mikuma N, Iswad PC, et al. Replacement with recombinant human inhibin immediately after orchidectomy in the hypophysiotropically clamped male rhesus monkey (*Macaca mulatta*) maintains follicle-stimulating hormone (FSH) secretion and FSH beta messenger ribonucleic acid levels at precastration values. *Endocrinology.* 136:1969, 1995
23. Carr BR, Parker CR Jr, Ohashi M, et al. Regulation of human fetal testicular secretion of testosterone: Low-density lipoprotein-cholesterol and cholesterol synthesized de novo as steroid precursor. *Am J Obstet Gynecol.* 146:241, 1983
24. Miller WL. Molecular biology of steroid hormone synthesis. *Endocrine Rev.* 9:295, 1988
25. Kasson BG, Hsueh AJW. Insulin-like growth factor-I augments gonadotropin-stimulated androgen biosynthesis by cultured rat testicular cells. *Mol Cell Endocrinol.* 52:27, 1987
26. Saez JM. Leydig cells: Endocrine, paracrine, and autocrine regulation. *Endocrine Rev.* 15:574, 1994
27. Dunn JF, Nisula BC, Rodbard D. Transport of steroid hormones: Binding of 21 endogenous steroids to both testosterone-binding globulin and corticosteroid-binding globulin in human plasma. *J Clin Endocrinol Metab.* 53:58, 1981
28. Pardridge WM, Landaw EM. Testosterone transport in brain: Primary role of plasma protein-bound hormone. *Am J Physiol.* 249:E534, 1985
29. Terasaka T, Nowlin DM, Pardridge WM. Differential binding of testosterone and estradiol to isoforms of sex hormone-binding globulin: Selective alteration of estradiol binding in cirrhosis. *J Clin Endocrinol Metab.* 67:639, 1988
30. Wilson JD. Metabolism of testicular androgens. In: Greep RO, Astwood EB, eds. *Handbook of Physiology. Section 7. Endocrinology. Vol V, Male Reproductive System.* Washington, D.C., American Physiological Society, 1975: 491–508
31. Russell DW, Wilson JD. Steroid 5α-Reductase: Two genes/two enzymes. *Annu Rev Biochem.* 63:25, 1994

32. Mahendroo MS, Mendelson CR, Simpson ER. Tissue-specific and hormonally controlled alternative promoters regulate aromatase cytochrome P450 gene expression in human adipose tissue. *J Biol Chem.* 268:19463, 1993

33. Griffin JE, McPhaul MJ, Russel DW, Wilson JD. The androgen resistance syndromes: Steroid 5α-reductase 2 deficiency, testicular feminization, and related disorders. In: Scriver CR, Beaudet AL, Sly WS, Valle D, eds. *The Metabolic and Molecular Bases of Inherited Disease,* 7th ed. New York, McGraw-Hill, 1995; 2:2967–2998

34. Tilley WD, Marcelli M, Wilson JD, et al. Characterization and expression of a cDNA encoding the human androgen receptor. *Proc Natl Acad Sci USA.* 86:327, 1989

35. Johnson L, Petty CS, Neaves WB. Further quantification of human spermatogenesis. Germ cell loss during post-prophase of meiosis and its relationship to daily sperm production. *Biol Reprod.* 29:207, 1983

36. Hinrichsen MJ, Blaquier JA. Evidence supporting the existence of sperm maturation in the human epididymis. *J Reprod Fertil.* 60:291, 1980

37. Pescovitz OH, Srivastava CH, Breyer PR, Monts BA. Paracrine control of spermatogenesis. *Trends Endocrinol Metab.* 5:126, 1994

38. Matsumoto AM, Karpas AE, Bremner WJ. Chronic human chorionic gonadotropin administration in normal men: Evidence that follicle-stimulating hormone is necessary for the maintenance of quantitatively normal spermatogenesis in man. *J Clin Endocrinol Metab.* 62:1184, 1986

39. Wierman ME, Beardsworth DE, Crawford JD, et al. Adrenarche and skeletal maturation during luteinizing hormone releasing hormone analogue suppression of gonadarche. *J Clin Invest.* 77:121, 1986

40. Boyar RM, Rosenfeld RS, Kapen S, et al. Human puberty: Simultaneous augmented secretion of luteinizing hormone and testosterone during sleep. *J Clin Invest.* 54:609, 1974

41. Ducharme JR, Collu R. Pubertal development: Normal, precocious and delayed. *Clin Endocrinol Metab.* 11:57, 1982

42. Lucky AW, Rich BH, Rosenfield RL, et al. LH bioactivity increases more that immunoreactivity during puberty. *J Pediatr.* 97:205, 1980

43. Mauras N, Veldhuis JD, Rogol AD. Role of endogenous opiates in pubertal maturation: Opposing actions of naltrexone in prepubertal and late pubertal boys. *J Clin Endocrinol Metab.* 62:1256, 1986

44. Katz SH, Hediger ML, Zemel BS, et al. Adrenal androgens, body fat and advanced skeletal age in puberty: New evidence for the relations of adrenarche and gonadarche in males. *Human Biol.* 57:401, 1985

45. Wilson JD, Griffin JE. The use and misuse of androgens. *Metabolism.* 29:1278, 1980

46. Slag MF, Morley JE, Elson MK, et al. Impotence in medical clinical outpatients. *JAMA.* 249:1735, 1983

47. Goldzieher JW, Dozier TS, Smith KD, et al. Improving the diagnostic reliability of rapidly fluctuating plasma hormone levels by optimized multiple-sampling techniques. *J Clin Endocrinol Metab.* 43:824, 1976

48. Rich BH, Rosenfield RL, Moll GW Jr, et al. Bioactive luteinizing hormone pituitary reserves during normal and abnormal male puberty. *J Clin Endocrinol Metab.* 55:140, 1982

49. Illingworth PJ, Groome NP, Byrd W, et al. Inhibin-B: A likely candidate for the physiologically important form of inhibin in men. *J Clin Endocrinol Metab.* 81:1321, 1996

50. Toublanc JE, Canlorbe P, Job JC. Evaluation of Leydig-cell function in normal prepubertal and pubertal boys. *J Steroid Biochem.* 6:95, 1975

51. Wollesen F, Swerdloff RS, Odell WD. LH and FSH responses to luteinizing-releasing hormone in normal, adult, human males. *Metabolism.* 28:845, 1976

52. Harman SM, Tsitouras PD, Costa PT, et al. Evaluation of pituitary gonadotropic function in men: Value of luteinizing hormone-releasing hormone response versus basal luteinizing hormone level for discrimination of diagnosis. *J Clin Endocrinol Metab.* 54:196, 1982

53. Johnson L. A re-evaluation of daily sperm output of men. *Fertil Steril.* 37:811, 1982

54. Sherins RJ, Brightwell D, Sternthal PM. Longitudinal analysis of semen of fertile and infertile men. In: Troen P, Nankin HR, eds. *The Testis in Normal and Infertile Men.* New York, N.Y., Raven Press, 1977: 473–488

55. Wilton LJ, Teichtahl H, Temple-Smith PD, et al. Structural heterogeneity of the axonemes of respiratory cilia and sperm flagella in normal men. *J Clin Invest.* 75:825, 1985

56. Styne DM, Grumbach MM. Puberty in the male and female; its physiology and disorders. In: SSC Yen, RB Jaffe, eds. *Reproductive Endocrinology,* 2nd ed. Philadelphia, Pa., W. B. Saunders, 1986: 313–394

57. Malchoff CD, Javier EC, Malchoff DM, et al. Primary cortisol resistance presenting as isosexual precocity. *J Clin Endocrinol Metab.* 70:503, 1990

58. Shenker A, Laue L, Kosugi S, et al. A constituitively activating mutation of the luteinizing hormone receptor in familial male precocious puberty. *Nature.* 365:652, 1993

59. Laue L, Kenigsberg D, Pescovitz OH, et al. Treatment of familial male precocious puberty with spironolactone and testolactone. *N Engl J Med.* 320:496, 1989

60. Mansfield MJ, Beardsworth DE, Loughlin JS, et al. Long-term treatment of central precocious puberty with a long-acting analogue of luteinizing hormone-releasing hormone. *N Engl J Med.* 309:1286, 1983

61. Wilson JD, Aiman J, MacDonald PC. The pathogenesis of gynecomastia. In: Stollerman GH, ed. *Advances in Internal Medicine.* Chicago, Ill., Year Book Medical Publishers, 1980; 5: 1–32

62. Lieblich JM, Rogol AD, White BJ, et al. Syndrome of anosmia with hypogonadotropic hypogonadism (Kallmann syndrome). Clinical and laboratory studies in 23 cases. *Am J Med.* 73:506, 1982

63. Franco B, Guioli S, Pragliola A, et al. A gene deleted in Kallmann's syndrome shares homology with neural cell adhesion and axonal path-finding molecules. *Nature.* 353:529, 1991

64. Santoro N, Filicori M, Crowley WF Jr. Hypogonadotropic disorders in men and women: Diagnosis and therapy with pulsatile gonadotropin-releasing hormone. *Endocrine Rev.* 7:11, 1986

65. Burstein S, Grumbach MM, Kaplan SL. Early determination of androgen-responsiveness is important in the management of microphallus. *Lancet*. 2:983, 1979

66. Finkel DM, Phillips JL, Snyder PJ. Stimulation of spermatogenesis by gonadotropins in men with hypogonadotropic hypogonadism. *N Engl J Med*. 313:651, 1985

67. Ley SB, Leonard JM. Male hypogonadotropic hypogonadism: Factors influencing response to human chorionic gonadotropin and human menopausal gonadotropin, including prior exogenous androgens. *J Clin Endocrinol Metab*. 61:746, 1985

68. Rowe RC, Schroeder M-L, et al. Testosterone-induced fertility in a patient with previously untreated Kallmann's syndrome. *Fertil Steril*. 40:400, 1983

69. Spratt DI, Finkelstein JS, Odea LSTL, et al. Long-term administration of gonadotropin-releasing hormone in men with idiopathic hypogonadotropic hypogonadism. *Ann Intern Med*. 105:848, 1986

70. McKenna TJ, Lorber D, Lacroix A, et al. Testicular activity in Cushing's disease. *Acta Endocrinol*. 91:501, 1979

71. MacAdams MR, White RH, Chipps BE. Reduction of serum testosterone levels during chronic glucocorticoid therapy. *Ann Intern Med*. 104:648, 1986

72. Carter JN, Tyson JE, Tolis G, et al. Prolactin-secreting tumors and hypogonadism in 22 men. *N Engl J Med*. 299:847, 1978

73. Franks S, Jacobs HS, Marti N, et al. Hyperprolactinaemia and impotence. *Clin Endocrinol*. 8:277, 1978

74. Prescott RWG, Johnston DG, Kendall-Taylor P, et al. Hyperprolactinaemia in men—Response to bromocriptine therapy. *Lancet*. 1:245, 1982

75. Charbonnel B, Chupin M, Le Grand A, et al. Pituitary function in idiopathic haemochromatosis: Hormonal study in 36 male patients. *Acta Endocrinol*. 98:178, 1981

76. Schafer AI, Cheron RG, Dluhy R, et al. Clinical consequence of acquired transfusional iron overload in adults. *N Engl J Med*. 304:319, 1981

77. Kelly TM, Edwards CQ, Meikle AW, et al. Hypogonadism in hemochromatosis: Reversal with iron depletion. *Ann Intern Med*. 101:629, 1984

78. Strain GW, Zumoff B, Miller LK, et al. Effect of massive weight loss on hypothalamic–pituitary–gonadal function in obese men. *J Clin Endocrinol Metab*. 66:1019, 1988

79. Herzog AG, Seibel MM, Schomer DL, et al. Reproductive endocrine disorders in men with partial seizures of temporal lobe origin. *Arch Neurol*. 43:347, 1986

80. Korenman SG, Stanik-avis S, Mooradian A, et al. Evidence for a high prevalence of hypogonadotropic hypogonadism. *Clin Res*. 35:182A, 1987

81. Gordon DL, Krmpotic E, Thomas W, et al. Pathologic testicular findings in Klinefelter's syndrome. 47,XXY vs 46,XY/47,XXY. *Arch Intern Med*. 130:726, 1972

82. Schibler D, Brook CGD, Kind HP, et al. Growth and body proportions in 54 boys and men with Klinefelter's syndrome. *Helv Paediatr Acta*. 29:325, 1974

83. Nielsen J, Pelsen B. Follow-up 20 years later of 34 Klinefelter males with karyotype 47,XXY and 16 hypogonadal males with karyotype 46,XY. *Human Genet*. 77:188, 1987

84. Gabrilove JL, Frieberg EK, Nicholis GL. Testicular function in Klinefelter's syndrome. *J Urol*. 124:825, 1980

85. Wang C, Baker HWG, Burger HG, et al. Hormonal studies in Klinefelter's syndrome. *Clin Endocrinol*. 4:399, 1975

86. Caminos-Torres R, Ma L, Snyder PJ. Testosterone-induced inhibition of the LH and FSH responses to gonadotropin-releasing hormone occurs slowly. *J Clin Endocrinol Metab*. 44:1142, 1977

87. Samaan NA, Stepanas AV, Danziger J, et al. Reactive pituitary abnormalities in patients with Klinefelter's and Turner's syndromes. *Arch Intern Med*. 139:198, 1979

88. de la Chapelle A. Analytic review: Nature and origin of males with XX sex chromosomes. *Am J Human Genet*. 24:71, 1972

89. Schweikert HU, Weissbach L, Leyendecker G, et al. Clinical, endocrinological, and cytological characterization of two 46,XX males. *J Clin Endocrinol Metab*. 54:745, 1982

90. Roe TF, Alfi OS. Ambiguous genitalia in XX male children: Report of two infants. *Pediatrics*. 60:55, 1977

91. Muller U, Dunlon T, Schmid M, et al. Deletion mapping of the testis determining locus with DNA probes in 46XX males and in 46XY and 46X (dic) (Y) females. *Nucl Acid Res*. 14:6489, 1986

92. Riggs S, Sandord JP. Viral orchitis. *N Engl J Med*. 266:990, 1962

93. Adamopoulos DA, Lawrence DM, Vassilopoulos P, et al. Pituitary testicular interrelationships in mumps orchitis and other viral infections. *Br Med J*. 1:1177, 1978

94. Wang J, Galil KAA, Setchell BP. Changes in testicular blood flow and testosterone production during aspermatogenesis after irradiation. *J Endocrinol*. 98:35, 1983

95. Brauner R, Czernichow P, Cramer P, et al. Leydig cell function in children after direct testicular irradiation for acute lymphoblastic leukemia. *N Engl J Med*. 309:25, 1983

96. Loriaux DL, Menard R, Taylor A, et al. Spironolactone and endocrine dysfunction. *Ann Intern Med*. 85:630, 1976

97. Rajfer J, Sikka SC, Rivera F, et al. Mechanism of inhibition of human testicular steroidogenesis by oral ketoconazole. *J Clin Endocrinol Metab*. 63:1193, 1986

98. Pont A, Graybill JR, Craven PC, et al. High-dose ketoconazole therapy and adrenal and testicular function in humans. *Arch Intern Med*. 144:2150, 1984

99. Macphee GJA, Larkin JG, Butler E, et al. Circulating hormones and pituitary responsiveness in young epileptic men receiving long-term antiepileptic medication. *Epilepsia*. 29:468, 1988

100. Cicero TJ. Alcohol-induced deficits in the hypothalamic–pituitary–luteinizing hormone axis in the male. *Alcoholism* (*NY*). 6:207, 1982

101. Gordon GG, Altman K, Southern AL, et al. Effect of alcohol (ethanol) administration on sex-hormone metabolism in normal men. *N Engl J Med*. 295:793, 1976

102. Whitehead E, Shalet M, Blackledge G, et al. The effects of Hodgkin's disease and combination chemotherapy on gonadal function of the adult male. *Cancer*. 49:418, 1982

103. Kolodny RC, Masters WH, Kolodner RM, et al. Depression of plasma testosterone levels after chronic intensive marihuana use. *N Engl J Med*. 290:872, 1974

104. Wang C, Chan V, Yeung RTT. The effect of heroin addiction on pituitary–testicular function. *Clin Endocrinol*. 9:455, 1978

105. Stoffer SS, Mynes KM, Jiang N-S, et al. Digoxin and abnormal serum hormone levels. *JAMA*. 255:1643, 1973

106. Blumer D, Migeon C. Hormone and hormonal agents in the treatment of aggression. *J Nerv Ment Dis*. 160:127, 1975

107. Bixler EO, Santen RJ, Kales A, et al. Inverse effects of thioridazine (Mellaril) on serum prolactin and testosterone concentrations in normal men. In: Troen P, Nankin HR, eds. *The Testis in Normal and Infertile Men*. New York, N.Y., Raven Press, 1977: 403–408

108. Rosenthal SM, Grumbach MM. Gonadotropin-independent familial sexual precocity with premature Leydig and germinal cell maturation (familial testotoxicosis): Effects of a potent luteinizing hormone-releasing factor agonist and medroxyprogesterone acetate therapy in four cases. *J Clin Endocrinol Metab*. 57:571, 1983

109. Van Thiel DH, Gavaler JS, Smith WI Jr, et al. Hypothalamic–pituitary–gonadal dysfunction in men using cimetidine. *N Engl J Med*. 300:1012, 1979

110. Peden NR, Boyd EJS, Browning MCK, et al. Effects of two histamine H$_2$-receptor blocking drugs on basal levels of gonadotrophins, prolactin, testosterone and oestradiol-17β during treatment of duodenal ulcer in male patients. *Acta Endocrinol*. 96:564, 1981

111. Rodamilans M, Osaba MJM, To-Figueras J, et al. Lead toxicity on endocrine testicular function in an occupationally exposed population. *Human Toxicol*. 7:125, 1988

112. Elder M, Maclaren N, Riley W. Gonadal autoantibodies in patients with hypogonadism and/or Addison's disease. *J Clin Endocrinol Metab*. 52:1137, 1981

113. Morley JE, Distiller LA, Sagel J, et al. Hormonal changes associated with testicular atrophy and gynaecomastia in patients with leprosy. *Clin Endocrinol*. 6:299, 1977

114. Lim VS, Fang VS. Gonadal dysfunction in uremic men. A study of the hypothalamic–pituitary–testicular axis before and after renal transplantation. *Am J Med*. 58:655, 1975

115. Mahajan SK, Abbasi AA, Prasad AS, et al. Effect on oral zinc therapy on gonadal function in hemodialysis patients. *Ann Intern Med*. 97:357, 1982

116. Vircburger MI, Prelevic GM, Peric LA, et al. Testosterone levels after bromocriptine treatment in patients undergoing long-term hemodialysis. *J Androl*. 6:113, 1985

117. Baker HWG, Burger HG, de Kretser DM, et al. A study of the endocrine manifestations of hepatic cirrhosis. *Q J Med*. 45:145, 1976

118. Gordon GG, Olivo J, Rafii F, et al. Conversion of androgens to estrogens in cirrhosis of the liver. *J Clin Endocrinol Metab*. 40:1018, 1975

119. Distiller LA, Sagel J, Dubowitz B, et al. Pituitary–gonadal function in men with alcoholic cirrhosis of the liver. *Horm Metab Res*. 8:461, 1976

120. Kley HK, Strohmeyer G, Krüskemper HL. Effect of testosterone application on hormone concentrations of androgens and estrogens in male patients with cirrhosis of the liver. *Gastroenterology*. 76:235, 1979

121. Van Thiel DH, Gavaler JS, Sanghvi A. Recovery of sexual function in abstinent alcoholic men. *Gastroenterology*. 84:677, 1982

122. Abbasi AA, Prasad AS, Ortega J, et al. Gonadal function abnormalities in sickle cell anemia. Studies in adult male patients. *Ann Intern Med*. 85:601, 1976

123. Smith SR, Chhetri MK, Johanson AJ, et al. The pituitary–gonadal axis in men with protein-calorie malnutrition. *J Clin Endocrinol Metab*. 41:60, 1975

124. Chlebowski RT, Heber D. Hypogonadism in male patients with metastatic cancer prior to chemotherapy. *Cancer Res*. 42:2495, 1982

125. Landon C, Rosenfeld RG. Short stature and pubertal delay in male adolescents with cystic fibrosis. *Am J Dis Child*. 138:388, 1984

126. Handelsman DJ, Yue DK, Turtle JR. Hypogonadism and massive testicular infiltration due to amyloidosis. *J Urol*. 129:610, 1983

127. Goussis OS, Pardridge WM, Judd HL. Critical illness and low testosterone: Effects of human serum on testosterone transport into rat brain and liver. *J Clin Endocrinol Metab*. 56:710, 1983

128. Poretsky L, Can S, Zumoff B. Testicular dysfunction in human immunodeficiency virus-infected men. *Metabolism*. 44:946, 1995

129. Martens HF, Sheets PK, Tenover JS, et al. Decreased testosterone levels in men with rheumatoid arthritis: Effect of low dose prednisone therapy. *J Rheumatol*. 21:1427, 1994

130. Takeda R, Ueda M. Pituitary–gonadal function in male patients with myotonic dystrophy-serum luteinizing hormone, follicle stimulating hormone and testosterone levels and histological damage of the testis. *Acta Endocrinol*. 84:382, 1977

131. Cortes-Gallegos V, Castaneda G, Alonso R, et al. Diurnal variations of pituitary and testicular hormones in paraplegic men. *Arch Androl*. 8:221, 1982

132. Hasen J, Boyar RM, Shapiro LR. Gonadal function in trisomy 21. *Horm Res*. 12:345, 1980

133. Aiman J, Griffin JE, Gazak JM, et al. Androgen insensitivity as a cause of infertility in otherwise normal men. *N Engl J Med*. 330:223, 1979

134. Grino PB, Griffin JE, Cushard WG, et al. A mutation of the androgen receptor associated with partial androgen resistance, familial gynecomastia, and fertility. *J Clin Endocrinol Metab*. 66:754, 1988

135. Snyder PJ, Lawrence DA. Treatment of male hypogonadism with testosterone enanthate. *J Clin Endocrinol Metab*. 51:1335, 1980

136. Davidson DW, O'Carroll R, Bancroft J. Increasing circulating androgens with oral testosterone undecanoate in eugonadal men. *J Steroid Biochem*. 26:713, 1987

137. Findlay JC, Place VA, Snyder PJ. Transdermal delivery of testosterone. *J Clin Endocrinol Metab*. 64:266, 1987

138. Korenman SG, Viosca S, Garza D, et al. Androgen therapy of hypogonadal men with transscrotal testosterone systems. *Am J Med*. 83:471, 1987

139. Meikle AW, Mazer NA, Moellmer JF, et al. Enhanced transdermal delivery of testosterone across nonscrotal skin produces physiological concentrations of testosterone and its metabolites in hypogonadal men. *J Clin Endocrinol Metab*. 74:623, 1992

140. Davidson JM, Camargo CA, Smith ER. Effects of androgen on sexual behavior in hypogonadal men. *J Clin Endocrinol Metab.* 48:955, 1979

141. Kwan M, Greenleaf WJ, Mann J, et al. The nature of androgen action on male sexuality: A combined laboratory–self-report study on hypogonadal men. *J Clin Endocrinol Metab.* 57:557, 1983

142. O'Carroll R, Shapiro C, Bancroft J. Androgens, behaviour and nocturnal erection in hypogonadal men: The effects of varying the replacement dose. *Clin Endocrinol.* 23:527, 1985

143. Tanner JM, Whitehouse RH, Hughes PCR, et al. Relative importance of growth hormone and sex steroids for the growth at puberty of trunk length, limb length, and muscle width in growth hormone-deficient children. *J Pediatr.* 89:1000, 1976

144. Ulloa-Aguirre A, Blizzard RM, Garcia-Rubi E, et al. Testosterone and oxandrolone, a nonaromatizable androgen, specifically amplify the mass and rate of growth hormone (GH) secreted per burst without altering GH secretory burst duration or frequency of the GH half-life. *J Clin Endocrinol Metab.* 71:846, 1990

145. Wilson JD. Androgen abuse by athletes. *Endocrine Rev.* 9:181, 1988

146. Bhasin S, Storer TW, Berman N, et al. The effects of supraphysiologic doses of testosterone on muscle size and strength in normal men. *N Engl J Med.* 335:1, 1996

147. Thompson PD, Cullinane EM, Sady SP, et al. Contrasting effects of testosterone and stanozolol on serum lipoprotein levels. *JAMA.* 261:1165, 1989

148. Matsumoto AM, Sandblom RE, Schoene RB, et al. Testosterone replacement in hypogonadal men: Effects on obstructive sleep apnea, respiratory drives, and sleep. *Clin Endocrinol.* 22:713, 1985

149. Rosemberg E. Gonadotropin therapy of male infertility. In: Hafez ESE, ed. *Human Semen and Fertility Regulation in Men.* St Louis, Mo., CV Mosby, 1976: 464–475

150. Liu L, Chaudhari N, Corle D, et al. Comparison of pulsatile subcutaneous gonadotropin-releasing hormone and exogenous gonadotropins in the treatment of men with isolated hypogonadotropic hypogonadism. *Fertil Steril.* 49:302, 1988

Chapter 14

ASSESSMENT OF THE FEMALE PATIENT

Robert W. Rebar

The clinical evaluation of the female patient with reproductive dysfunction is simplified by the fact that the patient serves as her own bioassay. In general, the appearance of the patient is influenced most by her age at the onset of the disorder. Somatic and/or sexual growth and development may be accelerated by increased secretion of growth hormone, thyroid hormone, androgens, or estrogens prepubertally. Growth may be retarded by excessive endogenous or exogenous glucocorticoids or diminished growth hormone or thyroid hormone secretion.

From a practical standpoint, the gynecologist and reproductive endocrinologist almost always evaluate the patient with absent or irregular menses. For this purpose, amenorrhea may be defined as the absence of menstruation for 3 or more mo in women of reproductive age with past menses or failure to menstruate by the age of 16 yr in girls who have never menstruated. Infrequent and irregular menses occurring at intervals of perhaps 40 or more days may also be indicative of anovulation; thus, individuals with oligomenorrhea should be evaluated identically to those with amenorrhea. It is important to remember that amenorrhea is not a disease itself but only a sign of any of a number of disorders involving any of several organ systems. As such, in the presence of an intact genital outflow tract, amenorrhea indicates failure of the hypothalamic–pituitary–ovarian axis to interact to induce cyclic changes in the endometrium resulting in menses.

In viewing the patient as a bioassay subject, breast development indicates exposure to biologically active estrogens, and pubic and axillary hair indicate exposure to biologically active androgens. Thus, the evaluation of the amenorrheic woman should include an assessment of pubertal development as initially delineated by Marshall and Tanner (Fig 14–1).[1] In assessing puberty, it is important to determine whether the patient's development is or was normal for her age and whether the breasts and pubic hair have developed at normal rates in unison and in proper relation to the pubertal growth spurt and menarche.

HISTORY: EVIDENCE OF ENDOCRINE ABNORMALITIES

The aim of the history is to obtain information regarding the biologic effects of the various hormones. The history is obviously developed around the chief complaint, but the patient commonly presents with altered sexual development or reproductive or sexual dysfunction.

Information about early growth and development and about pubertal milestones should be obtained carefully. It may be helpful to obtain some information from the mothers of younger women. To help individual women remember their age at menarche, it may be useful to ask them to recall exactly what they were doing and where they were when their first menstrual period began.

Alterations in sexual development will present as sexual precocity, heterosexual development at the usual age of puberty, delayed puberty, or what can be considered asynchronous pubertal development.

Precocious development is present if a girl begins to show pubertal changes before age 8. Sexual precocity can result from any of several disorders that ultimately lead to an increase in sex steroids.[2] In girls, increased estrogen secretion for age results in isosexual precocity (consistent with the sex of the individual), while increased androgen production for age results in heterosexual precocity (consistent with the opposite sex).

It is important to distinguish true precocious puberty from precocious thelarche, which is characterized by breast development only and may result from transient elevations in circulating estradiol,[3] and from precocious adrenarche, characterized by isolated development of sexual hair, most commonly pubic, and increased

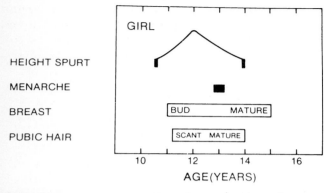

Figure 14–1. Schematic sequence of events at puberty. An average girl is represented. There is a wide range of ages over which these changes can occur normally. *(Adapted, with permission, from Marshall WA, Tanner JM, 1969: 291.[1])*

secretion of weakly androgenic adrenal steroids.[3] In both of the latter disorders, true pubertal maturation occurs at the normal age. Because either early breast development or the precocious appearance of pubic or axillary hair may herald true precocious puberty, affected children must be questioned carefully and followed longitudinally over time.

The history of girls with precocious puberty may provide clues regarding the etiology. Behavioral changes or symptoms suggestive of epilepsy may be the only symptoms of a central nervous system lesion; conversely, a number of pituitary hormone abnormalities may be apparent.[2,3] For example, several reports have documented that at least some hypothalamic hamartomas apparently produce gonadotropin-releasing hormone (GnRH), leading to a premature increase in the pituitary secretion of gonadotropins.[2] The patient should be questioned for symptoms of thyroid hormone deficiency because of the association between hypothyroidism and precocious puberty.[2,3] Any history of ingestion of drugs containing estrogen also should be elicited.

Heterosexual changes, regardless of the age at which they first become apparent, should be considered evidence of increased biologically active androgen in the genetic female or, much more rarely, signs of a disorder of sexual differentiation. Any consideration of the evaluation of ambiguous genitalia in the newborn is beyond the scope of this chapter. Regardless of the age of the patient, however, the existence of any signs and symptoms of androgen excess, including any history of acne, hirsutism, temporal balding, alterations in body contour and muscle mass, and voice change, should be sought. When hirsutism alone begins together with normal development of secondary sexual characteristics, polycystic ovary syndrome (PCO) or so-called "idiopathic" hirsutism are most likely. The onset of hirsutism or virilization at any other age raises the possibility of an androgen-

secreting neoplasm or Cushing syndrome. In general, amenorrhea or oligomenorrhea occurs earlier in hirsute patients with ovarian disorders than in those with adrenal disease. Some individuals with nonclassical forms of congenital adrenal hyperplasia (CAH) may develop severe hirsutism and acne at puberty.[4] In such individuals, a history of similarly hirsute relatives may be present. Virilization at puberty also may suggest incomplete androgen insensitivity in individuals with appropriate physical findings, including varying degrees of phallic enlargement and labioscrotal fusion, a vagina-like perineal orifice, some breast development, and undescended testes.[5]

Puberty should be considered delayed in girls who have not developed any secondary sex characteristics by age 13, who have not experienced menarche by age 16, or in whom more than 5 yr have passed from the onset of breast development without menarche. Typically, individuals with delayed puberty present with primary amenorrhea, but they may have been prescribed oral contraceptive agents as teenagers because of failure to begin menstruating. Thus, affected women may seek aid when amenorrhea is present again after discontinuation of exogenous steroids. Because errors in gender assignment may not be recognized until sexual infantilism is obvious at the usual age of puberty, chromosomal evaluation is frequently indicated.

Any history of interruption in the orderly progression of pubertal changes suggests a central nervous system lesion but also is observed in young women treated with chemotherapeutic agents and/or radiation for any of a number of childhood malignancies.[6]

Asynchronous pubertal development, with breast development in the absence of pubic and axillary hair, is typical of complete androgen insensitivity (ie, testicular feminization) and indicates the need for chromosomal evaluation.[5] The normal onset and progression of pubertal changes in the absence of menarche may indicate Müllerian aplasia, which should be apparent on physical examination.

Any association of amenorrhea with other events should be determined. It is particularly important to ask the patient about her lifestyle and diet and exercise patterns, as well as any changes in weight. Individuals should be questioned about bulimia and use of laxatives. Any history of environmental and/or psychological "stresses" should be elicited. Hypothalamic forms of amenorrhea are especially common in educated "overachievers." Use of recreational drugs, especially narcotics, also can lead to amenorrhea. Complaints of symptoms typical of estrogen deficiency, including dyspareunia, atrophic vaginitis, vasomotor instability, and emotional lability, should suggest amenorrhea of central origin with low concentrations of circulating gonadotropins or ovarian failure with elevated gonadotropins.

The woman with altered reproductive function may fail to note other obvious symptoms suggestive of a systemic illness or an endocrinopathy. The patient should be questioned about the presence of headaches, fatigue, palpitations, nervousness, altered libido, polyphagia or anorexia, polydipsia, and polyuria. Sexual dysfunction can be one symptom of panhypopituitarism; the patient may also have symptoms characteristic of thyroid or adrenal insufficiency, growth hormone excess or deficiency, or even diabetes insipidus. In addition, it is important to exclude pregnancy as the cause of the amenorrhea at the outset. Evaluation of past reproductive history, sexual activity, and contraceptive practices should provide information regarding the likelihood of pregnancy. The reproductive history may suggest the possibility of Sheehan syndrome of postpartum pituitary necrosis if menses did not resume following a delivery complicated by unusual hemorrhage. In such cases, evidence of thyroid and adrenal insufficiency may be present as well. Any history of dilatation and curettage, postpartum endometritis, or disseminated tuberculosis with absent to scanty menses should suggest the possibility of Asherman syndrome of intrauterine synechiae.

All amenorrheic women should be questioned about the presence of galactorrhea.[7] Women with galactorrhea frequently give a history of drug ingestion, particularly of any of several psychotropic agents, antihypertensive medications, or oral contraceptive agents, or may present with evidence of hypothyroidism. A history of excessive nipple stimulation or chest wall disease should be sought, as should signs and symptoms such as headache and visual disturbances, which are consistent with a prolactin-secreting pituitary tumor.

Careful attention to the family history also may be revealing. The association of a familial history of midline facial defects, including cleft lip and palate, color blindness, and anosmia with Kallmann syndrome, is well known,[8] as is the familial nature of thyroid dysfunction and the background of patients with multiple endocrine dysfunction characterized by hypoparathyroidism, Addison's disease, mucocutaneous candidiasis, and ovarian failure.[9]

THE PHYSICAL EXAMINATION: A SEARCH FOR MANIFESTATIONS OF ENDOCRINE ABNORMALITIES

The physical examination provides the observant clinician the opportunity to discover the manifestations of alterations in hormonal milieu. Careful clinical assessment often makes the diagnosis apparent, reducing the need for extensive laboratory testing.

Although the gynecologic endocrinologist may be tempted to focus on the pelvic examination, to do so would be to miss many opportunities to arrive at correct diagnoses clinically. Recognizing that the entire examination is important, special attention should be paid to: (1) body dimensions and habitus; (2) the distribution and extent of body hair; (3) breast development and secretions; and, lastly, (4) the external and internal genitalia.

Height and weight and skeletal proportions (where appropriate) should be measured carefully and recorded. Because growth rates in children are important in diagnosing various endocrine disorders, it is important to obtain historical data and plot the data on any of several charts relating height and weight to age and showing normal findings. For example, sexual precocity, because of increased estrogen and/or androgen production, induces early growth and epiphyseal closure. Thus, sexually precocious individuals may be tall for their age early in childhood but then become short adults. The earlier the sexual precocity begins, the greater the stunting in growth. Short stature is also seen in patients with panhypopituitarism, whereas individuals with acromegaly in childhood develop giantism. Patients with Turner syndrome are commonly under 5 ft tall.

To determine body dimensions, the distance from the top of the symphysis pubis to the floor can be measured (ie, lower body segment). The upper segment length is then calculated by subtracting the lower segment length from the patient's height. The ratio of upper to lower segment length is about 1.7:1 at birth, reaches equality by 10 yr of age because the legs grow more quickly than the trunk, and remains about 1:1 thereafter. Measurement of the arm span with the arms outstretched horizontally is also helpful. In normal adults, the span is within 2 in of the height, whereas in eunuchoid individuals both the span and lower segment are increased in length because of delayed epiphyseal closure in the absence of sex steroids. (One simple way to determine the difference between height and arm span is to mark the height on the wall. Then, have the patient spread her arms horizontally, bend at the waist to one side, and touch the floor with the fingertips of one hand. Mark the wall at the fingertips of the other hand. The difference between the two marks should be less than 2 in.) Also, eg, hypothyroid dwarfs typically have infantile body proportions. In chondrodystrophies, infantile body proportions are present as well. In hypopituitary and other types of dwarfs, the skeletal proportions typically become more mature as the patients age.

To assess habitus, the patient should be examined fully undressed. Although inspection is simple, it is commonly overlooked. To obtain the patient's confidence and cooperation, it may be important to ask the patient to stand unclothed at the end of the examination. If possible, it is good practice to photograph any patient whose development is incomplete or whose appearance appears abnormal at the time of the initial examination (Fig 14–2).

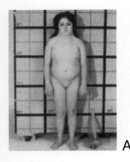

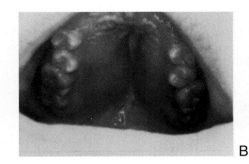

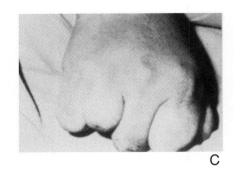

A   B   C

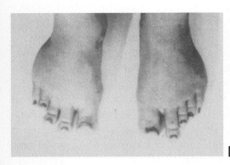

D

Figure 14–2. The unusual but typical habitus of a 16-year-old woman with 45,X gonadal dysgenesis has been recorded photographically in **A** while a number of her unusual features are shown in **B** through **D**. This patient presented with a webbed neck, a shield-like chest with inverted nipples, short stature, and sexual infantilism **(A)**. Although she had a thoracotomy for surgical repair of coarctation of the aorta at a younger age, no other diagnosis was made, no doubt because of failure to consider her habitus. The unusual palate **(B),** short fourth metacarpal **(C),** and short fourth metatarsals with dysplastic toenails **(D)** are also shown.

The general habitus and distribution of fat should be evaluated carefully. For example, the appearance of the individual with Cushing syndrome, with her centripetal obesity, plethoric "moon facies," and supraclavicular fat pad and "buffalo hump," is generally obvious. Primary hypoadrenalism is associated with increased brown pigmentation of the skin and mucous membranes, particularly over pressure points, in scars, in body folds, on the areolae, and in the creases of the palms because of the increased melanocyte-stimulating activity associated with increased corticotropin (ACTH) secretion. Body hair may be decreased, and the patient may appear asthenic as well. Disorders of the thyroid gland may be apparent. In the adult, myxedema results in a puffy face, thickening of the lips and tongue, and roughening and thickening of the skin. The thyrotoxic woman appears nervous and tremulous and has fine, moist skin. The eyes may be protuberant in Graves' disease. Thyroid enlargement or nodules may be apparent on inspection or palpation.

The quality of the skin should be evaluated for dryness or oiliness, pigmentary changes, striae, easy bruisability, and other characteristics of thyroid and adrenocortical dysfunction. Individuals with panhypopituitarism have so-called "alabaster" skin that is pallid, hairless, smooth, and dry. If the hypopituitarism begins in childhood, short stature with sexual infantilism will result.

The distribution, quality, and quantity of body hair should be evaluated while considering the background of the patient. True hirsutism, an increase in sexually stimulated terminal hair, especially in the midline on the face, chest, back, and abdomen, must be distinguished from hypertrichosis, an increased quantity of nonsexually-stimulated terminal hair on the extremities, head, and back. Women of Mediterranean descent typically have more body hair than do those of Asian heritage.

Methods of quantifying hirsutism are many. Most commonly used in research studies are modifications of the method of Ferriman and Gallwey,[10] in which a numerical value for the quantity of hair in each of several body areas is given and all such values are then added. Also utilized has been the measurement of the thickness of individual hairs with an ocular micrometer.[11] For the clinician, the most practical approach may be that suggested by Bardin and Lipsett[12]: Only facial hair is graded, giving a rating of 1+ each for excess terminal hair on the chin, upper lip, or sideburn area and 4+ for a full beard. Photographs are also quite valuable and can be shown to the patient during treatment so she can readily see any change over time (Fig 14–3).

Careful examination of the breasts is warranted in all women. The breasts are exquisitely sensitive to a number of hormones and even change perceptibly throughout each menstrual cycle. The Tanner stage of development should be recorded.[1] An effort should be made to express any secretions from the nipples by applying pressure to all sections of each breast beginning lateral to the nipple and working toward the nipple while the patient is seated. Secretions should be examined as wet mounts, searching for the presence of perfectly round, thick-walled fat

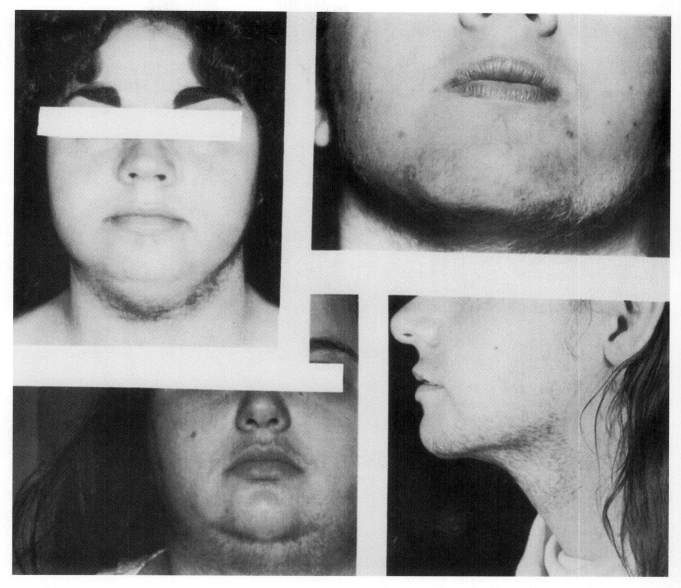

Figure 14–3. Photographs of four women presenting with facial hirsutism, all of whom were shown to have polycystic ovary syndrome. The two on the left also were markedly obese and had glucose intolerance, hyperuricemia, and acanthosis nigricans. The value of documenting the extent of hirsutism is apparent.

globules of varying size indicative of galactorrhea (Fig 14–4).

The external and internal female genitalia are the most sensitive indicators of sex steroid concentrations in a woman's body. Because the sensitivity of the genitalia to androgens decreases in time from the early stages of fetal development to adulthood, the extent of any virilization can help in establishing the diagnosis. The most profound changes—labial fusion or marked clitoral enlargement with or without formation of a penile urethra—are typically observed in individuals exposed to increased quantities of androgens during the first 3 mo of gestation. Such alterations can occur in patients with CAH, her-

maphroditism, and drug-induced virilization. Clitoromegaly beginning postnatally requires extremely high levels of androgens. In the absence of exogenous androgen ingestion, the occurrence of postnatal clitoromegaly strongly suggests existence of an androgen-secreting neoplasm. However, it is always important to exclude excessive masturbation as the cause of the clitoromegaly. In general, the clitoris is considered enlarged when it measures 1 cm or more in diameter at the base; its length is unimportant in determining if clitoromegaly is present. A clitoral index, defined as the product of the sagittal and transverse diameters of the glans at its base, is abnormal if it is greater than 35 mm.[2,13]

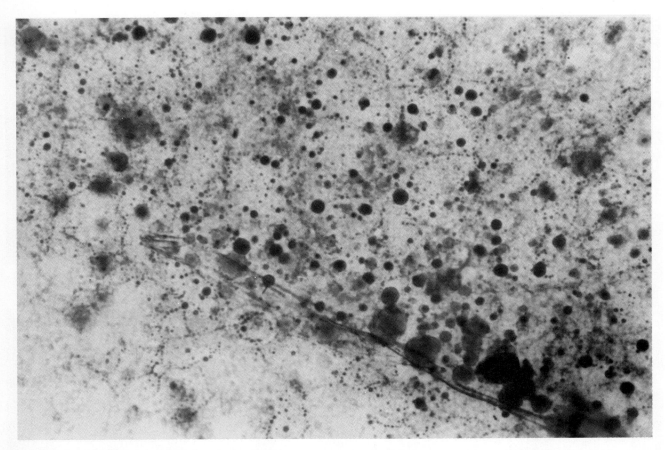

Figure 14–4. Perfectly round, thick-walled fat globules of varying size are characteristic of galactorrhea when the breast secretion is viewed as a wet preparation microscopically (×88). For purposes of photography, oil red 0 stain was added to the specimen, accounting for the dark nature of the fat droplets. *(Reproduced, with permission, from Rebar RW. In: Becker KL, et al, eds, 1995: 880.[36])*

The remainder of the external genitalia should be examined and Tanner staging determined.[1] Then, the internal genitalia should be examined. Overt Müllerian duct anomalies, including imperforate hymen, vaginal and uterine aplasia, and vaginal septa, should be apparent on inspection even if the exact diagnosis is difficult to establish. Inspection of the cervical mucus and vaginal mucosa is very important. Estrogen-stimulated vaginal mucosa is a dull, gray-pink with thick rugations and copious secretions; in the absence of estrogen, the mucosa is thin, poorly rugated, and shiny red with few secretions. Hormone-induced changes in the vaginal epithelium and cervical mucus are particularly helpful to the clinician in the assessment of estrogenic activity in the patient.

Both proliferation and maturation of the cells of the vaginal epithelium are influenced by estrogens and progestins.[14] The cells of this epithelium, consisting of mature *superficial* squamous epithelial cells with pyknotic nuclei, *intermediate* squamous epithelial cells with vesicular nuclei, and small, round *parabasal* cells with large vesicular nuclei, are commonly shed in the vaginal secretions as they are replaced. In general, the usefulness of the vaginal smear in the amenorrheic woman is as an indication of endogenous estrogen secretion. Several indices have been developed in an effort to quantitate the degree of estrogen stimulation (Fig 14–5). Parabasal cells predominate in individuals with estrogen deficiency and may be found normally prepubertally and postmenopausally. Estrogen increases the number of cornified superficial cells. Under the influence of progesterone in the luteal phase of the menstrual cycle, the percentage of cornified cells decreases while the number of precornified, intermediate cells increases. The observation that the epithelium of the lower urinary tract is similarly influenced by steroids was used in the past in examining the cells of the urinary sediment from children suspected of developing increased estrogen levels prematurely.

Typically, estrogens stimulate secretion of thin, watery cervical mucus, while progesterone inhibits the secretory activity of the cervical glands.[15] Under the influence of estrogen, the elasticity, or spinnbarkeit, of the mucus increases and "palm leaf" arborization or ferning becomes

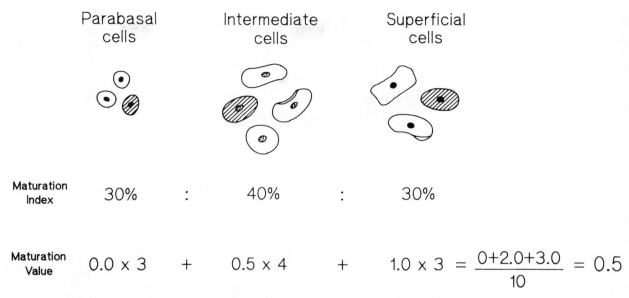

Parabasal cells		Intermediate cells		Superficial cells

Maturation Index	30%	:	40%	:	30%

$$\text{Maturation Value} \quad 0.0 \times 3 \quad + \quad 0.5 \times 4 \quad + \quad 1.0 \times 3 = \frac{0 + 2.0 + 3.0}{10} = 0.5$$

Figure 14–5. Commonly used indices quantifying vaginal cytology. In this idealized representation, the small cells are parabasal. The lined cells stain eosinophilic, and the clear cells stain cyanophilic. The maturation index (MI) represents the relationship, in terms of percentage, among parabasal, intermediate, and superficial cells. The maturation value (MV) assigns values to each cell type, with parabasal cells receiving 0.0, intermediate cells given 0.5, and superficial cells 1.0. The number of each cell type counted is then multiplied by the appropriate value and the total number divided by the number of cells counted. The higher the value, the greater the effect of estrogen (maximum of 1.0). *(Reproduced, with permission, from Rebar, RW. In: Yen SSC, Jaffe RB, eds, 1991: 838.[37])*

prominent. This ferning pattern may be observed simply by spreading cervical mucus collected from the cervical os thickly on a glass slide, allowing it to dry completely for at least 15 min, and then examining the specimen microscopically under low power (Fig 14–6).

INDIRECT EVALUATION OF HORMONE ACTION

Progestin-Induced Withdrawal Bleeding

It is customary to administer either an orally active (medroxyprogesterone acetate, 5 to 10 mg/day for 5 to 10 days) or intramuscular (progesterone in oil, 50 to 100 mg) progestin to amenorrheic women when they first present for evaluation to determine if the endometrium is intact and has been stimulated by estrogen. Estrogen-primed endometrium is typically shed following administration of a progestin and is presumptive evidence of some functioning of the hypothalamic–pituitary–ovarian axis.

Although generally a reasonable "bioassay" of endogenous estrogen production, patient compliance is always uncertain with oral preparations that must be ingested at specified intervals, and variable absorption of any injected preparation is always possible. Moreover, the careful examiner can almost always predict whether bleeding will result. In addition, almost 50 percent of individuals with ovarian "failure" will withdraw to pro-

gestin despite widespread beliefs that such should not be the case.[16] Thus, the value of this clinical test is not as great as presumed.

Evaluation of "Bone Age"

Radiographs of epiphyseal centers should be obtained in patients with disorders of growth and development to provide an objective estimate of the hormonal effects on bone maturation. Classically, "bone age" is estimated by comparing x-rays of the nondominant hand and wrist with films from normal children at different ages as depicted in an atlas.[17]

A number of childhood endocrinopathies affect bone maturation. In hypothyroidism, bone age is retarded more than height age. In Cushing syndrome, growth retardation with accelerated skeletal maturation results. Congenital adrenal hyperplasia and sexual precocity typically result in short stature, but accelerated linear growth and skeletal maturation often are seen in the prepubertal years. An increased growth rate and advanced bone age are common in hyperthyroid children as well. Hypopituitarism beginning before puberty leads to progressive retardation of epiphyseal development. In fact, in individuals with intact growth hormone secretion, hypogonadism from any cause can lead to increased linear growth with delayed fusion.

Clinically, the bone age can be used to predict final adult height using the Bayley–Pinneau tables.[18] Ultimate

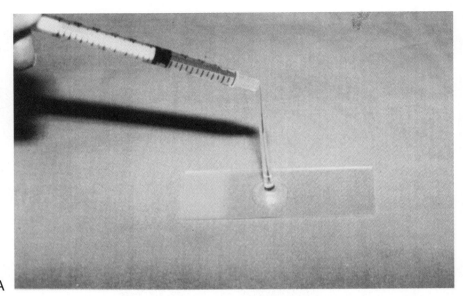

A

B

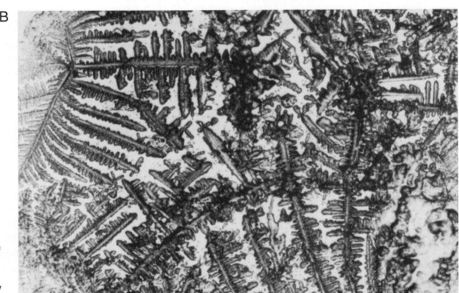

Figure 14–6. A. Demonstration of spinnbarkeit in cervical mucus. **B.** Palm leaf arborization or ferning, indicative of an estrogenic effect, present on a dried sample of cervical mucus examined microscopically (×88). *(**A** courtesy of William Bates.)*

height in adolescents with altered growth and development is a most important concern. The predictions can be used as aids in evaluating efficacy of therapy in individuals with accelerated bone age. Individuals with delayed puberty and retarded bone age can be advised how much further growth is anticipated with pubertal maturation.

Assessment of Bone Density

Recognition that gonadal steroids and prolactin influence bone density indicates the need for measuring this parameter in individuals presenting with hypoestrogenic forms of amenorrhea and hyperprolactinemia. Fortunately, methods for estimation of bone density now exist that are relatively simple and accurate and involve little

radiation exposure. In general, either the distal radius, lumbar spine, or proximal femur is evaluated. Because trabecular bone is more hormonally responsive than cortical bone and because vertebral bodies contain predominantly trabecular bone, the lumbar spine's density is evaluated most commonly.[19] Because vertebral fractures occur relatively early in individuals suffering from osteoporosis, such measurements are of clinical value.

The newest approach to estimating bone density is dual-energy x-ray absorptiometry (DEXA). In this method, x-rays are used to estimate bone density, typically of the lumbar spine. In this, as in other methods, the amount of radiation blocked from passing through a particular bony area is measured and compared to known standards. The bone mineral content is then calculated and expressed as bone mineral per square centimeter scanned. These methods all depend upon careful positioning of the bone site examined during sequential testing. Time required for DEXA is perhaps 5 min, and radiation exposure is less than that for a chest roentgenogram. In dual-energy photon absorptiometry (DPA), a radioisotope of gadolinium, which emits photons at two energy levels, is passed through the individual at the level of the lumbar spine to estimate bone density. Although radiation exposure is also minimal, each study takes perhaps 30 min and reproducibility is not as great as with DEXA. Single-energy photon absorptiometry measures bone mineral content in the appendicular skeleton, usually the radius. This method is simple, rapid, noninvasive, and relatively inexpensive and involves only a small amount of radiation exposure (2 to 5 mrad) to the forearm only. This method appears useful largely for screening large populations of women to identify those who merit further study. Quantitative computed tomography of the spine is less often used to measure bone mineral content because it involves significant radiation exposure and is both costly and time consuming. Other methods, such as total body neutron activation analysis, are used largely as research tools.

LABORATORY EVALUATION: SELECTION OF THE APPROPRIATE TESTS

Evaluation of Amenorrhea

After the appropriate clinical assessment of the amenorrheic woman, measurements of at least basal circulating concentrations of follicle-stimulating hormone (FSH), prolactin (PRL), and thyroid-stimulating hormone (TSH) are warranted to confirm the clinical impression (Fig 14–7).

Increased serum TSH levels of greater than 5 µU/ml with or without hyperprolactinemia indicate primary hypothyroidism (Fig 14–8). It is the increased secretion of thyrotropin-releasing hormone (TRH) that occurs in this disorder that stimulates increased secretion of prolactin, as well as of TSH, in some affected women. Mild primary hypothyroidism, characterized by TSH levels near the upper and tetraiodothyronine (T_4) levels near the bottom of their normal ranges, respectively, may be associated with ovulatory disturbances.[20] Women with hypothyroidism typically resume ovulation with thyroid hormone replacement.

If the initial prolactin measurement is elevated (>20 mg/ml), it should be repeated because prolactin secretion is increased by so many nonspecific stimuli, including sleep, stress, and food ingestion (Fig 14–9). If thyroid hormone determinations are normal and prolactin measurements are repeatedly elevated, then further evaluation is warranted to rule out a prolactin-secreting pituitary tumor. Basal prolactin levels should be determined in all amenorrheic women because they are elevated more than one third of the time.[7]

Elevated serum FSH levels (typically >30 mIU/ml) imply ovarian failure. Chromosomal evaluation is warranted in young women with elevated FSH concentrations because of the frequency of karyotypic abnormalities in individuals with gonadal failure. Gonadectomy is warranted in any patient found to have

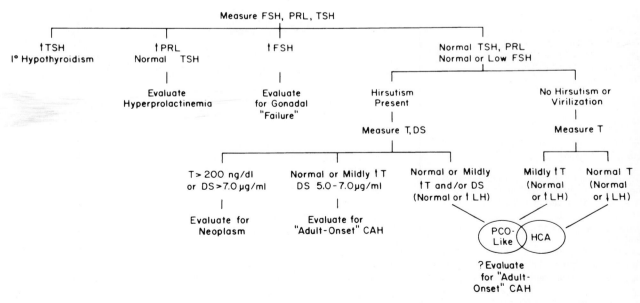

Figure 14–7. Flow diagram for the evaluation of amenorrhea. Such a scheme is an adjunct to the clinical evaluation of the patient (see text). *(Reproduced, with permission, from Rebar, RW. In: Wyngaarden JB, Smith LH Jr, eds, 1992: 1367.*[38]*)*

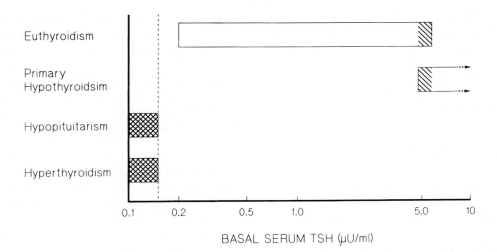

Figure 14–8. Ranges of basal TSH concentrations in various clinical states plotted on a logarithmic scale. The dotted line represents the limits of assay sensitivity. The shaded areas indicate that values in both hypopituitarism and hyperthyroidism are typically undetectable. Note the overlap between euthyroidism and primary hypothyroidism, which can be resolved by TRH testing. Hypothyroid individuals have large responses to exogenous TRH. In primary hypothyroidism, concentrations of TSH may be greater than 100 μU/ml in some individuals, as suggested by the arrows indicating that the upper limit of the range is not shown. *(Reproduced, with permission, from Rebar RW. In Yen SSC, Jaffe RB, eds, 1991: 859.[37])*

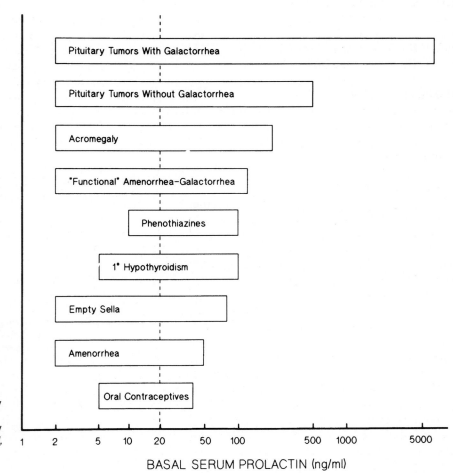

Figure 14–9. Schematic representation of the ranges of basal serum prolactin concentrations observed in various clinical states plotted on a logarithmic scale. The dotted line at 20 ng/ml indicates the upper limit of the normal range in many laboratories. Values less than 2 ng/ml are generally undetectable. Measured values may differ significantly depending upon the laboratory and assay system employed. *(Reproduced, with permission, from Rebar RW. In: Yen SSC, Jaffe RB, eds, 1991: 862.[37])*

a portion of a Y chromosome because of the malignant potential of such gonads.[21] FSH concentrations often begin to rise before the onset of the menopause early in the climacteric.

If prolactin, TSH, and FSH concentrations are either normal or low, then further evaluation should be based upon the clinical findings. The major distinction is between chronic anovulation due to hypothalamic–pituitary dysfunction and anovulation secondary to inappropriate steroid feedback (ie, polycystic ovary [PCO]-like disorders). Circulating thyroid hormone levels should be determined if there is evidence of hyperthyroidism and TSH levels are low. In anovulatory women who are well estrogenized and who do not have obvious "hypothalamic" amenorrhea, the measurement of total circulating testosterone is appropriate. Not all hyperandrogenic women are hirsute because there may be relative insensitivity of hair follicles to androgen in some women. Circulating levels of LH also may aid in distinguishing PCO from hypothalamic–pituitary dysfunction or failure. LH levels and the ratio of LH to FSH tend to be increased in PCO.[22] Levels of both LH and FSH tend to be normal or perhaps slightly reduced in women with hypothalamic–pituitary dysfunction. As represented by the overlapping circles in Figure 14–7, there is some overlap in laboratory values of gonadotropins in women with PCO-like disorders compared to values in those with hypothalamic chronic anovulation.

Radiographic studies of the sella turcica are indicated in all amenorrheic women in whom both LH and FSH levels are low (<10 mIU/ml) to exclude either a pituitary or hypothalamic lesion even if prolactin levels are not increased. It is also apparent that testing of adrenal and thyroid function is indicated whenever panhypopituitarism is suspected.

Evaluation of Hirsutism

The evaluation of the hirsute woman, whether amenorrheic or not, is controversial. As is true for the amenorrheic individual, the most logical approach in evaluating the hirsute woman is to formulate a presumptive diagnosis based upon the clinical findings and then confirm or disprove this diagnosis by using selective laboratory testing.

It is essential to rule out the serious causes of hirsutism, including Cushing syndrome, congenital adrenal hyperplasia, and adrenal and ovarian neoplasms. Most of the time these disorders can be excluded during the examination. A single random blood sample for measurement of serum testosterone (T) and dehydroepiandrosterone sulfate (DHEAS) levels should be obtained from all women with hirsutism. If the serum testosterone level is markedly elevated, generally greater than 200 ng/dl, then the possibility of an ovarian androgen-producing neoplasm must be entertained. If the serum DS level is more than twice normal, generally greater than 7.0 µg/ml, then

the possibility of an adrenal neoplasm must be considered. Computed tomography scanning or magnetic resonance imaging will identify almost all adrenal tumors. Most virilizing ovarian tumors can be visualized by pelvic ultrasonography. Percutaneous venous catheterization of the ovarian and adrenal blood vessels with selective measurement of androgens from each site is now needed rarely to localize a neoplasm before surgery.

There is no need for extensive testing if neither T nor DS is markedly elevated. Biologically active free testosterone need not be measured in the hirsute woman: It is obvious from the examination that biologically active androgen is increased. The only question is whether or not the increased androgen is produced by a neoplasm or an enzymatic defect. Yet, some clinicians measure free T, arguing that it is a more sensitive indicator of increased androgen production and action. Similarly, some physicians recommend measuring 3α-androstanediol glucuronide levels as a marker of androgen action in peripheral tissues such as skin.[23] Once more, the measurement of this hormone seems unnecessary: If neither T nor DS is elevated, there must be increased androgen action in the periphery.

Some clinicians also advocate measurements of 17-hydroxyprogesterone in all hirsute women. Although measurement of this hormone is essential to diagnose congenital adrenal hyperplasia due to 21-hydroxylase deficiency, the low incidence of this disorder in most populations (estimated at perhaps 1 to 5 percent of hirsute women) should obviate the need to measure 17-hydroxyprogesterone in all hirsute women.[24,25] Measurement of this hormone in women with features of "nonclassical" CAH, including severe hirsutism beginning at puberty, shorter height than other family members, defeminization with flattening of the breasts, increased DS levels between 5.0 and 7.0 µg/ml, or those with a strong family history of hirsutism, is warranted (Fig 14–10). Most patients with 21-hydroxylase deficiency have levels of at least 1000 ng/dl. However, basal levels of 17-hydroxyprogesterone may be normal (typically less than 200 ng/dl) in nonclassical CAH, and ACTH testing is indicated in individuals suspected of having this disorder. For women with cyclic menses, it is also important to remember to measure 17-hydroxyprogesterone only in the follicular phase because levels normally increase at midcycle and in the luteal phase.

Evaluation of Adrenocortical Hyperfunction

Some individuals with hirsutism may appear to have Cushing syndrome. The diagnosis of this syndrome is not difficult clinically in individuals with obvious signs but can be quite difficult early in the disease process (Fig 14–11). In general, menstrual disturbances begin late in the disease process and the hirsutism is not as severe as it is in women with androgen-producing tumors. The

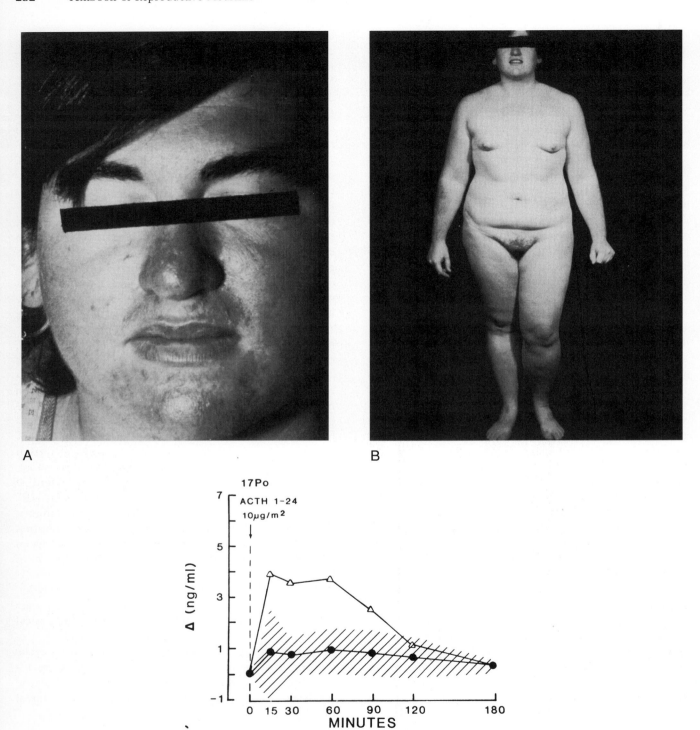

Figure 14–10. This 19-year-old nulligravid individual presented with oligomenorrhea and hirsutism beginning at puberty. Menarche had occurred at age 13. Her facial hirsutism and oily skin are apparent in **A.** Defeminization with flattening of her breasts is apparent in **B.** Despite these findings, androgen levels were just above the limits of the normal range. ACTH testing in this patient, with 10 μg/m² ACTH 1-24 given as an intravenous bolus following dexamethasone suppression, yielded an increase (Δ) in 17-hydroxyprogesterone (17Po) that was greater than two standard deviations (shaded area) of the increase observed in normal women tested in the early follicular phase of the menstrual cycle **(C).** The patient's responses are depicted by the open triangles and the mean of the responses of the normal women by the closed circles. ACTH was administered at time 0. *(Reproduced, with permission, from Kustin J, Rebar RW, 1986: 522.[39])*

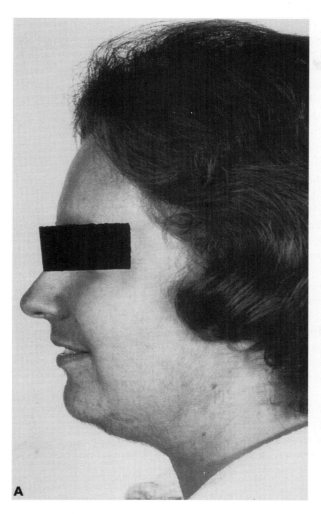
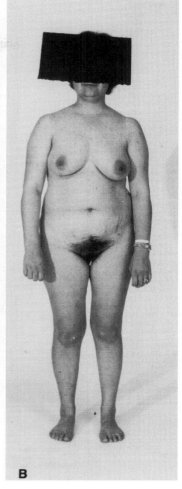
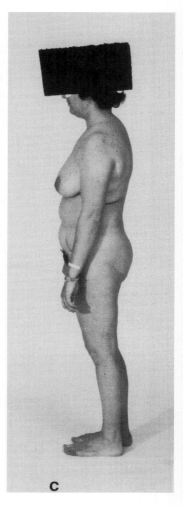

Figure 14–11. Views of a 33-year-old gravida 3 para 3 individual with documented Cushing's disease. She noted a 30-lb weight gain, weakness, and increasing hirsutism over the preceding year. Amenorrhea began approximately 4 mo before presentation. Her blood pressure was 140/98. Facial hirsutism and plethora are apparent in **A**. Centripetal obesity, a "buffalo hump," and pigmented striae can be seen in **B** and **C**.

laboratory diagnosis of Cushing syndrome is difficult and includes urinary measurements of free cortisol or cortisol metabolites and dexamethasone suppression tests, as well as ACTH levels before and following CRH infusion[26–29] (see Chap 18).

Evaluation of Anterior Pituitary Function

Only rarely must the reproductive endocrinologist assess anterior pituitary function. Such evaluation is required in individuals with prolactin-secreting neoplasms greater than 1 cm (so-called macroadenomas), individuals with sexual infantilism as a result of hypothalamic–pituitary dysfunction, and individuals with any size pituitary tumor not secreting prolactin.

Basal levels of thyroid hormone and cortisol often help identify patients with hypothyroidism and hypoadrenalism. Basal cortisol levels may be in the normal range, however, in individuals unable to respond adequately to stressful stimuli. Because of the profound effect of abnormal thyroid function on urinary steroid excretion, the patient must be euthyroid at the time of testing. Although hypoadrenalism may be partial or complete, or acute or chronic, it is subtle abnormalities in patients with proven or suspected pituitary tumor that present the typical problem.

Two practical screening tests exist. In the simpler test, synthetic ACTH 1-24 is rapidly injected intravenously as a 250-µg bolus. Blood samples for cortisol are obtained prior to ACTH administration and 60 and 120 min following injection. Although results vary among laboratories, if plasma cortisol increases by more than 7 µg/dl or to levels greater than 20 µg/dl, hypoadrenalism does not exist.[30] The second screening test involves the serial collection of 24-hr urine specimens for 17-hydroxycorticosteroids and creatinine.

Values of 2.0 mg/g creatinine per 24 hr or less strongly suggest hypoadrenalism.

Several other tests to evaluate adrenocortical reserve have been proposed. The use of synthetic corticotropin-releasing hormone has not proved to be of great value in discriminating between secondary adrenocortical insufficiency of hypothalamic and pituitary origin. Moreover, individual responses are sufficiently variable so as to make interpretation of an "adequate" normal increase in cortisol levels difficult. Indeed, insulin-induced hypoglycemia, which should normally result in increased cortisol levels 40 to 60 min after intravenous injection of 0.1 U/kg body weight of regular insulin, may be the most reliable method for assessing the integrity of the hypothalamic–pituitary–adrenal axis.[31] If blood glucose levels fall by 50 percent or more or to levels less than 40 mg/dl, then plasma cortisol levels should increase 7 μg/dl or to a value of greater than 20 μg/dl in normal individuals. Hypoglycemic side effects are common, and the test may be dangerous in a number of clinical conditions. It should be conducted only in the presence of a medical attendant and should be terminated promptly by administration of intravenous glucose if the patient loses consciousness or complains of palpitations.

It is important to remember that cortisol responses to stress can be evaluated in patients taking dexamethasone. Thus, the insulin tolerance test can be used to evaluate adrenocortical reserve in patients receiving steroids. In a patient acutely ill with hypotension, anorexia, weight loss, and weakness, therapy for Addison's disease can be instituted promptly. A sample for measurement of plasma cortisol should be obtained and 4 mg dexamethasone given immediately. The patient can then be tested later with insulin or with prolonged 48-hr infusion of ACTH.[30]

Although individuals with hypopituitarism may have diminished growth hormone (GH) secretion, the assessment of GH is generally undertaken only in individuals with short stature. Two simple screening tests for GH deficiency are useful.[32] A blood sample obtained 60 to 120 min after the onset of sleep should reveal increased GH levels. Alternatively, a blood sample obtained after approximately 20 min of vigorous exercise should show elevated levels of GH as well, especially in children.

Serum levels of somatomedin C (also known as insulin-like growth factor I [IGF-I]) may also help diagnose GH deficiency.[33] Individuals with GH deficiency have low serum concentrations of somatomedin C. However, the range of values in normal individuals is so wide as to make interpretation difficult in some cases.

If a clinical diagnosis of GH deficiency is strongly suspected or if screening tests fail to elicit significant release of GH (as frequently occurs) or both, then further tests of GH secretion are necessary.[34] The most effective

of these tests is insulin-induced hypoglycemia. When combined sequentially with arginine, the test appears to be approximately 95 percent effective in detecting individuals with GH deficiency. The usefulness of synthetic growth hormone-releasing hormone (GHRH) as a substitute for other provocative stimuli may be limited. Individuals with hereditary GH deficiency may have significant increases in serum GH levels after a single intravenous bolus of GHRH, indicating a hypothalamic defect as the cause of the GH deficiency. Thus, GHRH cannot be used to confirm GH deficiency from any cause. Moreover, individuals with chronic GH deficiency have reduced quantities of GH present within their pituitary glands such that there will be diminished or absent responses to GHRH even if the pituitary is intrinsically normal. Lastly, responses of GH to GHRH are quite variable. Despite such limitations, an increase in GH in response to any stimulus eliminates the diagnosis of GH deficiency.

It is also important to recognize that GH release is inhibited by a number of conditions. These include obesity, Cushing syndrome, and administration of corticosteroids and tranquilizers. In males, responses to arginine are increased by pretreatment with estrogen.

In general, any GH determination greater than 10 ng/ml or any response greater than 5 ng/ml following any stimulus is sufficient to rule out GH deficiency. However, rare abnormalities in somatomedins in the presence of normal or elevated GH secretion have been documented in some individuals with short stature.

Evaluation of Posterior Pituitary Function

Although the posterior pituitary gland, or neurohypophysis, secretes both oxytocin and vasopressin (also known as antidiuretic hormone [ADH]), no disease has ever been associated with oxytocin excess or deficiency. In contrast, both vasopressin excess (termed inappropriate secretion of ADH) and vasopressin deficiency (known as diabetes insipidus) are well-established disorders.

Diabetes insipidus is characterized by polyuria (of 2.5 L or more every 24 hr) and polydipsia. Fluid restriction produces insatiable thirst and dehydration. Because normal glucocorticoid is necessary to excrete a water load, it is necessary to evaluate adrenocortical function and institute any necessary replacement therapy before testing a patient for the possibility of diabetes insipidus.

In the majority of cases, diabetes insipidus will be suspected in individuals with evidence of hypothalamic or anterior pituitary dysfunction or following hypophysectomy. In many cases, the diagnosis is obvious on history alone. If diabetes insipidus exists, failure to treat with exogenous preparations of vasopressin can lead to permanent renal damage. Recognition of partial defects and confirmation of causes of complete diabetes insipidus are best accomplished by use of the dehydration test.[35] Urine osmolality and weight are followed during a period of enforced water deprivation until urine osmolality does not increase further. Normal individuals increase their urine osmolality above their plasma osmolality; in addition, there is no further increase after dehydration upon injection of exogenous vasopressin. Patients with overt diabetes insipidus are generally unable to concentrate urine to greater than the plasma osmolality and increase their urine osmolality by more than 50 percent following vasopressin. Patients with partial diabetes insipidus are often able to concentrate urine to above the plasma osmolality but show a rise in urine osmolality of more than 9 percent after vasopressin administration. Although hypertonic saline also may be infused to test for diabetes insipidus, this test is far more dangerous because it may precipitate seizures. In the future, immunoassay of plasma vasopressin after osmotic stimulation by fluid deprivation or infusion of hypertonic saline may prove to be of diagnostic value.

The syndrome of inappropriate ADH secretion may occur in patients with hypothalamic or pituitary tumors and must be distinguished from acute adrenocortical insufficiency. Although strict limitation of fluid intake will correct all the physiological disturbances of this syndrome despite persistent ADH secretion, glucocorticoids are essential for treatment of adrenal failure.

Radiographic Assessment of the Sella Turcica

Although x-rays of the sella turcica are warranted whenever a hypothalamic or pituitary lesion is suspected, how extensive the evaluation should be is controversial. It is well recognized that pituitary microadenomas can exist in patients with normal lateral and anteroposterior screening views of the sella turcica. Consequently, some clinicians recommend detailed studies in all patients with possible lesions, while others utilize screening views unless the possibility of a neoplasm is high.

Two types of studies are commonly utilized to assess the sellar region in detail: computed tomography (CT) and magnetic resonance imaging (MRI) (Fig 14–12). X-ray polytomography, pneumoencephalography, and carotid arteriography are now seldom utilized.

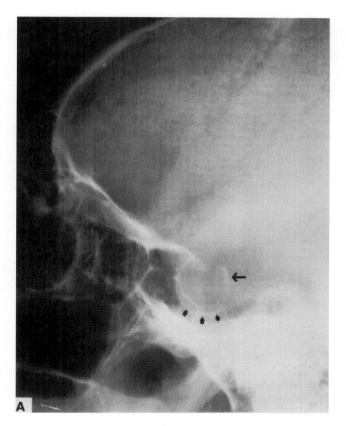

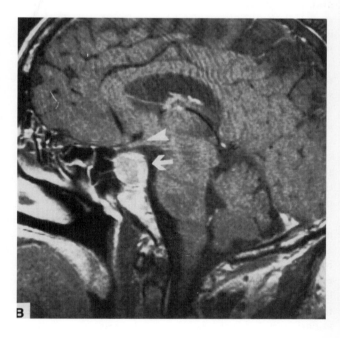

Figure 14–12. Selected views in a 39-year-old woman with a probable nonsecreting neoplasm who presented with amenorrhea–galactorrhea and had prolactin levels of approximately 50 ng/ml. Some of the views suggest the mild hyperprolactinemia is due to stalk compression. **A.** Lateral skull film showing ballooning of the sella turcica with a thin double floor (small black arrows) and erosion of the clinoid processes posteriorly (large black arrow). **B.** Sagittal view of MRI with contrast material showing the large pituitary tumor (white arrow) and the optic chiasm (white arrowhead). *(Reproduced, with permission, from Rebar RW. In: Yen SSC, Jaffe RB, eds, 1991: 849.[37])*

In CT scanning, coronal images perpendicular to the sellar floor are best for identifying normal and abnormal structures in the sellar region. Intravenous injection of contrast material may aid in identifying pituitary adenomas because they opacify less than normal glandular tissue. Intrathecal injection of a contrast agent may help diagnose an empty sella or help define a suspected suprasellar cystic mass.

MRI appears to be at least as effective as CT in visualizing pituitary lesions and does not expose the patient to radiation. Except when cost is a consideration, MRI has become the method of choice for evaluating the sellar and juxtasellar structures. The pituitary stalk, tuber cinereum, and optic chiasm are especially well visualized with MRI. Injected contrast material may further enhance detail.

It is critical to realize that normal anatomic variations (particularly on screening x-rays) may suggest that a pituitary tumor exists even when one does not. Radiographic findings must be interpreted while considering the clinical presentation of the patient. Views of the sella may reveal a double floor, erosion of the posterior clinoid processes, enlargement, ballooning, or suprasellar extension. Calcification may also be seen, most commonly as a result of a craniopharyngioma and less frequently in tuberculous meningitis or in some other disorder.

Controversy also exists over how frequently patients treated and/or monitored for hypothalamic–pituitary lesions should be evaluated radiographically. It is well known that pituitary tumors increase slowly in size. MRI allows the sella to be evaluated without exposing the patient to radiation. However, there is probably little need to evaluate the sella more often than once each year. In addition, endocrine testing is generally more sensitive than radiographic studies in documenting changes in hypothalamic–pituitary function.

In any individual with a large lesion in the hypothalamic–pituitary region, formal visual field testing is also warranted. Proximity of the optic chiasm to the pituitary gland makes the presence of bitemporal hemianopsia the most common abnormality in patients with large lesions. The visual fields also probably should be tested whenever radiographs of the sella are being obtained in individuals with known lesions who are being followed medically.

REFERENCES

1. Marshall WA, Tanner JM. Variations in patterns of pubertal changes in girls. *Arch Dis Child.* 44:291, 1969
2. Kaplan SL, Grumbach MM. Pathogenesis of sexual precocity. In: Grumbach MM, Sizonenko PC, Aubert ML, eds. *Control of the Onset of Puberty.* Baltimore, Md., Williams and Wilkins, 1990: 620–668
3. Rosen D, Kelch RP. Precocious and delayed puberty. In: Becker KL, et al, eds. *Principles and Practice of Endocrinology and Metabolism,* 2nd ed. Philadelphia, Pa., J. B. Lippincott, 1995: 830–842
4. Speiser PW. Congenital adrenal hyperplasia. In: Becker KL, et al, eds. *Principles and Practice of Endocrinology and Metabolism,* 2nd ed. Philadelphia, Pa., J. B. Lippincott, 1995: 686–695
5. Simpson JL, Rebar RW. Normal and abnormal sexual differentiation and development. In: Becker KL, et al, eds. *Principles and Practice of Endocrinology and Metabolism,* 2nd ed. Philadelphia, Pa., J. B. Lippincott, 1995: 788–821
6. Damewood MD, Grochow LB. Prospects for fertility after chemotherapy or radiation for neoplastic disease. *Fertil Steril.* 45:443, 1986
7. Blackwell RE. Hyperprolactinemia. Evaluation and management. *Endocrinol Metab Clin North Am.* 21:105, 1992
8. Santen RJ, Paulsen CA. Hypogonadotropic eunuchoidism. I. Clinical study of the mode of inheritance. *J Clin Endocrinol Metab.* 36:47, 1973
9. Spinner MW, Blizzard RM, Childs B. Clinical and genetic heterogeneity in idiopathic Addison's disease and hypoparathyroidism. *J Clin Endocrinol Metab.* 28:795, 1968
10. Ferriman D, Gallwey JD. Clinical assessment of body hair growth in women. *J Clin Endocrinol Metab.* 21:1440, 1961
11. Cumming DC, Yang JC, Rebar RW, Yen SSC. Treatment of hirsutism with spironolactone. *JAMA.* 247:1295, 1982
12. Bardin CW, Lipsett MB. Testosterone and androstenedione blood production rates in normal women and women with idiopathic hirsutism or polycystic ovaries. *J Clin Invest.* 46:891, 1967
13. Tagatz GE, Kopher RA, Nagel TC, Okagaki T. The clitoral index: A bioassay of androgenic stimulation. *Obstet Gynecol.* 54:562, 1979
14. Rakoff AE. Hormonal cytology in gynecology. *Clin Obstet Gynecol.* 4:1045, 1961
15. MacDonald RR. Cyclic changes in cervical mucus. *J Obstet Gynaecol Br Commonw.* 76:1090, 1969
16. Rebar RW, Connolly HV. Clinical features of young women with hypergonadotropic amenorrhea. *Fertil Steril.* 53:804, 1990
17. Greulich WW, Pyle SI. *Radiographic Atlas of Skeletal Development of the Hand and Wrist,* 2nd ed. London, U.K., Oxford University Press, 1959
18. Bayley N, Pinneau SR. Tables for predicting adult height from skeletal age: Revised for use with the Greulich–Pyle hand standards. *J Pediatr.* 40:423, 1952
19. Chestnut CH. Bone imaging techniques. In: Becker KL, et al, eds. *Principles and Practice of Endocrinology and Metabolism,* 2nd ed. Philadelphia, Pa., J. B. Lippincott, 1995: 508–512
20. Miller MM, Rebar RW. Successful treatment of infertility with thyroid replacement in a clinically euthyroid patient with galactorrhea-amenorrhea syndrome. *Clin Decisions Obstet Gynecol.* 1:1, 1987
21. Manuel M, Katayama KP, Jones HW Jr. The age of occurrence of gonadal tumors in intersex patients with a Y chromosome. *Am J Obstet Gynecol.* 124:293, 1976
22. Rebar RW, Judd HL, Yen SSC, et al. Characterization of the inappropriate gonadotropin secretion in polycystic ovary syndrome. *J Clin Invest.* 57:1320, 1976

23. Horton R, Hawks D, Lobo R. 3α, 17β-Andostanediol glucuronide in plasma. A marker of androgen action in idiopathic hirsutism. *J Clin Invest.* 69:1203, 1982

24. Lobo RA, Goebelsmann U. Adult manifestation of congenital adrenal hyperplasia due to incomplete 21-hydroxylase deficiency mimicking polycystic ovarian disease. *Am J Obstet Gynecol.* 138:720, 1980

25. Chrousos GP, Loriaux DL, Mann DL, Cutler GB Jr. Late-onset 21-hydroxylase deficiency mimicking idiopathic hirsutism or polycystic ovarian disease. *Ann Intern Med.* 96:143, 1982

26. New MI. Congenital virilizing adrenal hyperplasia. In: Adashi EY, Rock JA, Rosenwaks Z, eds. *Reproductive Endocrinology, Surgery and Technology.* Philadelphia, Pa., Lippincott-Raven, 1996: 1555–1570

27. Liddle GW. Tests of pituitary adrenal suppressibility in the diagnosis of Cushing's syndrome. *J Clin Endocrinol Metab.* 20:1539, 1960

28. Besser GM. ACTH and MSH assays and their clinical application. *Clin Endocrinol.* 2:175, 1973

29. Chrousos GP, Schulte HM, Oldfield EH, et al. The corticotropin-releasing factor stimulation test: An aid in the evaluation of patients with Cushing's syndrome. *N Engl J Med.* 310:622, 1984

30. Melby JC. Assessment of adrenocortical function. *N Engl J Med.* 285:735, 1971

31. Jacobs HS, Nabarro JDN. Tests of hypothalamic–pituitary–adrenal function in man. *Q J Med.* 38:475, 1969

32. Eddy RL, Gilliland PF, Ibarra JD Jr, et al. Human growth hormone release: Comparison of provocative test procedures. *Am J Med.* 56:179, 1974

33. Juul A, Bang P, Hertel NT, et al. Serum insulin-like growth factor-1 in 1030 healthy children, adolescents and adults: Relation to age, sex, stage of puberty, testicular size, and body mass index. *J Clin Endocrinol Metab.* 78:744, 1994

34. Merimee TJ, Grant MG. Growth hormone and its disorders. In: Becker KL, et al, eds. *Principles and Practice of Endocrinology and Metabolism,* 2nd ed. Philadelphia, Pa., J. B. Lippincott, 1995: 129–140

35. Miller M, Dalakos T, Moses AM, et al. Recognition of partial defects in antidiuretic hormone. *Ann Intern Med.* 73:721 1970

36. Rebar RW. Disorders of menstruation, ovulation and sexual response. In: Becker KL, et al, eds. *Principles and Practice of Endocrinology and Metabolism,* 2nd ed. Philadelphia, Pa., J. B. Lippincott, 1995: 880–890

37. Rebar RW. Practical evaluation of hormonal status. In: Yen SSC, Jaffe RB, eds. *Reproductive Endocrinology, Physiology, Pathophysiology and Clinical Management,* 3rd ed. Philadelphia, Pa., W. B. Saunders, 1991: 830–886

38. Rebar RW. The ovaries. In: Wyngaarden JB, Smith LH Jr, eds. *Cecil Textbook of Medicine,* 19th ed. Philadelphia, Pa., W. B. Saunders, 1992: 1355–1376

39. Kustin J, Rebar RW. Hirsutism in young adolescent girls. *Pediatr Ann.* 15:522, 1986

ANOVULATION OF CNS ORIGIN

Anatomic Causes

Chapter 15

R. Jeffrey Chang, Eric S. Knockenhauer, Scott M. Slayder, and Richard E. Blackwell

Anatomic lesions within the central nervous system (CNS) that lead to menstrual disturbances include both structural abnormalities as well as functional disruption of the hypothalamus, pituitary gland, and pituitary stalk (infundibulum). The mechanism by which these processes impair gonadotrope production and secretion may arise primarily, secondarily, or as a combination of both. Prime examples of the latter are large functional pituitary tumors. The purpose of this chapter is to discuss central anatomic causes of anovulation and their diagnosis and management.

HYPOTHALAMIC LESIONS

Tumors

The craniopharyngioma is generally manifested in childhood and adolescence. About one third of cases are discovered in the adult. This lesion arises from remnants of Rathke's pouch and is composed of stratified squamous epithelium.[1] It is to be distinguished from Rathke's cleft cyst, which, in addition to squamous elements, also contains cuboidal and columnar epithelial cells.[2] The craniopharyngioma is believed to have originated from epithelial cell rests carried with Rathke's pouch into the neural stalk to form the pars tuberalis. In humans, the pars tuberalis is a thin layer of cells that cover the anterior aspect of the infundibulum (Fig 15–1). These tumors are well encapsulated and may be solid or contain multiloculated cysts composed of dark fluid, in which cholesterol crystals may be found. Not uncommonly, the size of the lesion may reach 8 to 10 cm in diameter. The pattern of growth is aggressive, extending into the optic chiasm, hypothalamus, and third ventricle.[3] Most lesions exist as

suprasellar tumors. In more than one half of cases, a portion of the neoplasm is calcified, which facilitates the diagnosis. Craniopharyngiomas have not been shown to produce any hormone substance. In children, the most common presenting complaints are headaches, vomiting, visual loss, lack of growth, and diabetes insipidus. In adults, diabetes insipidus, visual field loss, dementia, and hypogonadism are most common. The diagnosis is suggested by the clinical presentation and modern imaging techniques of either computed tomography (CT) or magnetic resonance imaging (MRI). Primary therapy consists of surgical resection of tumor, which may not be completely achieved due to the location and size of the tumor.[4] Drainage of cystic lesions is appropriate. Total excision of tumor is associated with extremely low recurrence rates.[5] If complete removal cannot be effected,

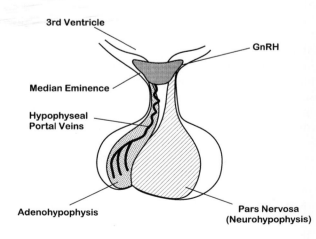

Figure 15–1. Anatomy of the hypothalamic–pituitary system.

then postoperative radiation is indicated, which decreases the rate of tumor recurrence.

A rare class of neoplasms are tumors of the pineal gland, which represent less than 1 percent of intracranial lesions. These tumors are generally encountered in males and can cause hypothalamic hypopituitarism. Originally termed a pinealoma in reference to the pineal parenchymal cell, most of the cellular elements reflect undifferentiated germ cells.[6] Thus, a more appropriate designation for this tumor is the germinoma. Because the histologic appearance bears little, if any, resemblance to pineal parenchyma cells, it has been theorized that during early embryologic development, yolk sac germ cells that migrate to the genital ridge may wander to sites from which the pineal and other organs develop.[7] This explanation would account for atypical sites of the "ectopic pinealoma." Other types of germ cell tumors, such as gliomas (astrocytomas, etc), endodermal sinus tumors, choriocarcinomas, and teratomas, may also exhibit similar migrational behavior and present as tumors of the pineal gland and anterior mediastinum.[8] Commonly, the pineal germinoma infiltrates the third ventricle and floor of the hypothalamus to produce diabetes insipidus, hypogonadism, and optic atrophy. In extending to the third ventricle, these tumors can destroy the hypothalamus by compressive effect. Occasionally, the lesion will grow into the sella turcica to mimic an intrasellar tumor.[9] The diagnosis is achieved by recognition of a central process leading to hypopituitarism and identification of a mass lesion on MRI. Imaging may be facilitated by calcification of the pineal gland. Treatment considerations include surgery and radiation therapy. In many instances, by the time clinical symptoms emerge, the tumor is inoperable or only partially resectable. Fortunately, the germinoma is radiosensitive and has a good record of response to radiation therapy.[10]

The occurrence of other tumors in this category is not confined to the region of the pineal gland and may arise de novo in the hypothalamus. Gliomas (astrocytomas) are most common and damage surrounding structures by their compressive effect. An exceedingly rare tumor of the hypothalamus is the endodermal sinus tumor. Usually, this neoplasm is found in the gonads or reproductive tract of young children and infants. In a few cases, it has been found in the region of the pineal gland.[11] This yolk-sac-derived carcinoma has been described as having a honeycomb consistency and is highly vascular. Production of α-fetoprotein is characteristic for this tumor and metastases to other parts of the CNS are common. The endodermal sinus tumor is highly malignant and almost uniformly fatal. The rapid pattern of growth often precludes operative consideration and radiation therapy is ineffectual. Chemotherapy has been posed as an alternative treatment, although long-term survival rates have been discouraging.

Metastatic tumors to the hypothalamus are similar to those that spread to the pituitary and primarily include carcinoma of the breast and lung. If substantial tumor growth occurs, hypothalamic function may be totally lost, with resulting hypopituitarism, hypogonadism, and diabetes insipidus.

Infiltrative Diseases

Infiltrative diseases of the hypothalamus are uncommon and may display a wide variety of clinical presentation depending upon the nature and extent of the disorder. For instance, in Hand–Schüller–Christian disease, a granulomatous process of unknown etiology, there can be a solitary lesion or multiple nodules. Hand–Schüller–Christian disease, Letterer–Siwe disease, and eosinophilic granuloma comprise the forms of the histiocytosis X.[12] All these conditions share similar cytologic findings and probably should be considered a single entity with varying degrees of clinical presentation. While capable of spread to the pituitary gland, in most cases the hypothalamus or stalk is compromised. The lesion in the basal hypothalamus typically consists of a localized granulomatous defect, poorly or well circumscribed in nodular form, appearing histiocytic with eosinophilic elements.[13] Infiltrative damage to the tuber cinereum and hypothalamus produces diabetes insipidus, the most frequent endocrine manifestation.[14] This symptom may emerge only in partial form early in the course of disease in the absence of other signs. Other endocrine abnormalities include impaired growth, hypogonadism, and partial or complete hypopituitarism. Nonendocrine features that commonly result from the granulomatous process are lytic bone lesions and exophthalmos caused by a retrobulbar infiltration of granulomatous tissue. The diagnosis may be difficult relevant to the unpredictable onset of symptoms and the multiple organ involvement. Absence of a mass lesion in the hypothalamus decreases the value of imaging methodologies. A tissue or bone biopsy is the most reliable test.[15] Treatment of this condition has involved a steroid administration and chemotherapy with alkylating agents.[16] The latter has proven to provide good long-term relief.

Another granulomatous process that may cause hypothalamic damage and anovulation is sarcoidosis. The etiology of sarcoidosis is unknown. The disease may be relatively benign and self-limiting or steadily progressive. Evidence of central nervous system involvement is uncommon. In patients who exhibit hypothalamic disease, the most incriminating symptomatology is panhypopituitarism.[17] Other features of hypothalamic impairment include somnambulance and hyperphagia. In comparison, the pituitary gland seems to be more vulnerable to the granulomatous process, with diabetes insipidus being the most prevalent sign. The infundibulum is particularly affected, which probably reflects its anatomic relationship to the basilar meninges. An inflammatory reaction creates a basilar meningitis that extends upward toward the hypothalamus along perivascular cuffs.[18] All degrees of pituitary insufficiency have been found varying from panhypopituitarism to focal mild dysfunction. The extent of sarcoidosis in the CNS is not limited to the hypothalamus and pituitary, as infiltrative nodules have been noted along the base of the brain, inflicting damage to cranial nerves.[19] Given the disseminated granulomatous nature of sarcoidosis, it should not be surprising that consideration of tuberculosis must be included in the differential diagnosis. Treatment is limited to use of corticosteroids to reduce inflammatory responses associated with this condition.

Vascular Disease

Aneurysms may impact on the hypothalamus, as well as on the pituitary gland. Most aneurysms arise from the internal carotid artery, and the infraclinoid segment of the vessel is the most frequent site of origin.[20] The anterior cerebral, posterior communicating, or basilar arteries are rarely involved. Rupture of either anterior or posterior communicating aneurysms causes hypothalamic ischemia, giving rise to focal areas of necrosis and hemorrhage. Microhemorrhages have been noted in the paraventricular and supraoptic nuclei that were totally obliterated if the hemorrhages coalesce.[21] Thus, substantial damage to hypothalamic tissue may result from aneurysm rupture and bleeding.

Hypothalamic Trauma

An unusual cause of hypogonadotropic hypogonadism is radiation-induced hypothalamic damage. Unlike the pituitary, the hypothalamus is relatively radiosensitive, and conventional radiation therapy for CNS malignancy, nasopharyngeal carcinoma, and carcinoma of the maxillary sinus may result in hypothalamic dysfunction. It has been estimated that the maximum tolerable dose of ionizing radiation by the hypothalamus is 4,500 rad.[22] Beyond this amount, gross tissue necrosis is likely. For example, repeated courses of radiotherapy as in the treatment of resistant growth hormone-producing pituitary adenomas may cause hypothalamic radiation necrosis. In these patients, hypopituitarism is characterized by suppressed circulating levels of anterior pituitary hormones with the exception of prolactin, which is mildly elevated.

Traumatic injury to the pituitary stalk has been described for some victims of head-on collisions. The associated whiplash effect may sever the infundibulum and separate hypothalamic regulation of both anterior and posterior pituitary function. There is loss of anterior pituitary hormone production, and diabetes insipidus is common. Serum prolactin levels are acutely and temporarily elevated. Eventual reduction of prolactin secretion over time suggests that a trophic influence from the

hypothalamus is necessary to maintain lactotroph production of prolactin. Additional consequences of stalk transection include hypotension and hypovolemia, which may predispose to hypothalamic ischemia. Treatment is usually directed toward hormone replacement for specific organ systems.

PITUITARY LESIONS

Tumors

Pituitary tumors occur with relative frequency ranging from 10 to 23 percent within the general population.[23,24] These figures are based upon findings at autopsy and as a result include small, even microscopic, lesions. Understandably, a significant number of cases were asymptomatic. Clinically, pituitary tumors are the most common cause of pituitary dysfunction and represent 10 percent of all intracranial neoplasms. The pathophysiologic impact of these tumors is dictated by (1) size and direction of spread and (2) functional hormone status.

The pituitary gland is a $10 \times 15 \times 5$-mm globular structure with a weight of approximately 0.5 g. It is connected to the base of the brain by the pituitary stalk. The gland is nestled in the sella turcica and therefore bordered anteriorly, inferiorly, and posteriorly by bone. The lateral border primarily consists of the cavernous sinus, including cranial nerves III, IV, and VI and the first division of cranial nerve V, and a portion of the internal carotid artery. Superiorly, the gland is separated from the hypothalamus, optic chiasm, and other cranial structures by a condensation of the dura, the sellar diaphragm. The pituitary is organized into an anterior (adenohypophysis), intermediate, and posterior (neurohypophysis) lobe, which arise from two ectodermal primordia (Fig 15–1). One primordium represents an active proliferation of cells from the anterior wall of Rathke's pouch, which is formed by evagination of the embryonic pharyngeal roof. This process leads to the formation of the anterior lobe. Cells of the posterior wall of Rathke's pouch give rise to the intermediate lobe. However, in humans these cells are inactive and thus the intermediate lobe is small and poorly defined. The pars tuberalis is a thin layer of cells also derived from Rathke's pouch that overlie the anterior surface of the pituitary stalk. The second primordium is an outgrowth from the diencephalic portion of the neural tube. It extends ventrally to attach and become the posterior lobe of the pituitary. This neuroectodermal derivative is also responsible for the development of the pituitary stalk and median eminence.

The cellular composition of the pituitary contains both functional and nonfunctional elements. Immunohistochemistry and electron microscopy have demonstrated distinct and specific cell types within the anterior pituitary that are responsible for synthesis and release of particular peptide hormones. These cells also appear to cluster and localize in particular regions (Fig 15–2).[25] For instance, lactotropes, which are responsible for the production of prolactin, are located in the lateral portions of the anterior pituitary. Adjacent to the lactotropes are somatotrophic cells, which give rise to growth hormone. There are reasons to suspect that these cell types may share a common origin. First, both are in close anatomic approximation. Second, prolactin and growth hormone exhibit close structural similarities.[26] Third, patients with growth hormone-secreting tumors often have associated hyperprolactinemia. Despite these observations, the precise derivative or functional relationship between lactotropic and somatotropic cells is unknown. Pituitary thyrotropes are situated in the midportion of the anterior pituitary. Similarly, corticotropin (ACTH)-producing cells are also concentrated in the central part of the gland. Within the same area are likely located melanocyte stimulating hormone (MSH)-secreting cells. That ACTH and MSH have similar amino acid sequences suggests derivation from a common cell. Recent studies have shown that during pituitary organogenesis there is a progressive differentiation of distinct pituitary specific cell lineages from a common primordium involving a series of developmental decisions and inductive interactions. Targeted gene disruption in the mouse shows that Lhx3, Lim homeobox gene expressed in the pituitary throughout development, is essential for differentiation and proliferation of pituitary cell lineages. Mice homozygous for the Lhx3 mutation show formation of Rathke's pouch but failure of growth and differentiation.[27] Moreover, a distinct melanotropic cell in humans has not been demonstrated. The gonadotrope is distributed throughout the anterior pituitary. Secretion of luteinizing hormone (LH) and follicle-stimulating hormone (FSH) probably occurs from a single gonadotropic cell, although specific and separate LH- and FSH-secreting cells may exist. Approximately 25 percent of cells of the anterior pituitary are nonsecretory based upon the failure to demonstrate secretory granules.[28]

In the posterior pituitary are contained the terminal portions of axons that transport oxytocin and vasopressin from the hypothalamus. These peptides are synthesized by supraoptic and paraventricular nuclei, whose axons also terminate in the median eminence and pituitary stalk.

Classification of Adenohypophyseal Neoplasms

Recently the World Health Organization (WHO) has proposed a classification of adenohypophyseal neoplasms using a five-tiered scheme. The classification system is based on clinical and biochemical results, imaging, operative findings, histology, immunocytochemistry, and electron microscopic studies.[29] Further, the expression of epidermal growth factor and its receptor (EGF-R) in human pituitary adenomas have been shown to correlate with tumor aggressiveness. The overexpression of EGF-R in recurrent somatotroph adenomas and aggressive silent subtype-3 adenomas suggests a selective mechanism for the EGF/EGF-R family in the growth of aggressive pituitary tumors.[30] Likewise, allelic deletions in pituitary adenomas have been described that reflect aggressive biologic activity and have potential value as a prognostic marker. Therefore, these types of growth factor studies may be incorporated into a tumor classification system in the future and may prove useful in predicting tumor aggressiveness.[31]

Nonfunctional Tumors. Pituitary tumors that do not exhibit hormone activity tend to display a slow course of growth. They have been called *null cell*-type tumors. Progressive tumor enlargement will eventually lead to compression of adjacent pituitary tissue and impingement upon surrounding structures and cause clinical symptomatology. In most instances, symptoms are recognized only after significant extrasellar expansion has occurred. A common early sign of suprasellar tumor growth is visual impairment, which results from compression of the optic chiasm.[32] Initially, there is loss of vision in the superior temporal quadrants bilaterally. Subsequently, the inferior quadrants are effected with the development of bitemporal hemianopsia. During this process, visual acuity may become impaired. If unattended, this condition could progress to optic atrophy and blindness (Fig 15–3). It should be noted that the pattern of visual field loss may not always be uniform due to the variation in the anatomic relationship between the optic chiasm and the

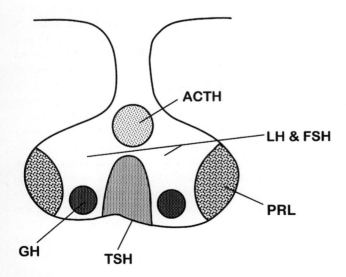

Figure 15–2. Localization of peptide hormones within the anterior pituitary gland.

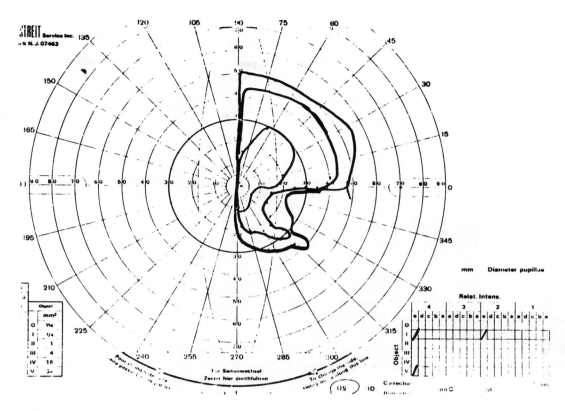

Figure 15–3. Visual field deficit in one eye of a patient with a large prolactinoma. Note the extremely limited field of vision encircled by the indicated border. In the opposite eye (visual field not shown), the patient had lost total vision. *(Reproduced, with permission, from Blackwell RE, 1985:5.[46])*

pituitary gland or possible eccentric location of suprasellar tumor extension. Visual problems also may occur due to lateral tumor extension into the cavernous sinus, which contains cranial nerves III, IV, and VI. Sufficient compression of these nerves may cause extraocular palsy with diplopia and visual blurring.

One of the most common symptoms associated with large pituitary neoplasms is headache. In general, there is no characteristic pattern because the frequency, location, and intensity of pain vary widely. In those patients with small pituitary tumors, headache is uncommon. If present, the cause is unlikely to be a result of tumor size. The mechanism for headache as related to a pituitary tumor has not been elucidated. Infarction of a pituitary tumor or hemorrhage into the lesion may cause the acute onset of severe headache and rapid visual loss.[33] These symptoms result from the sudden expansion of intrasellar contents. Subsequently, pituitary insufficiency may ensue with the development of hypotension and hyperthermia. Finally, there occur mental deterioration, coma, and death.

Uncommonly, large pituitary tumors may extend into the hypothalamus to cause diabetes insipidus and irregularities of sleep, temperature, and appetite. Infrasellar extension into the sphenoid sinus is problem-

atic due to the possibility of spontaneous cerebrospinal fluid leakage.

Intrinsic damage to the pituitary by a large tumor implies destruction of functional cells by compression. The result often is hypopituitarism. Amenorrhea is present in about 5 percent of women with nonfunctional pituitary tumors. Given the dispersed location of gonadotropes within the pituitary, substantial cell destruction is implied and consistent with low serum LH and FSH levels noted in these patients. Thus, hypogonadotropic hypogonadism should always warrant consideration of a pituitary tumor. Growth hormone deficiency is not clinically manifest in adults. Destruction of thyrotropes and adrenocorticotropes causes deficient thyroid-stimulating hormone (TSH) and ACTH secretion, which lead to secondary hypothyroidism and hypoadrenalism, respectively.

Diagnosis of a pituitary tumor, whether functional or nonfunctional, is based primarily upon radiological imaging. This is best achieved by CT or MRI. Each technique has proven satisfactory in the detection of small neoplasms, as well as delineation of rather large tumors (Fig 15–4). High-resolution CT is usually conducted with intravenous contrast medium, which permits identification of soft tissue. The sensitivity of

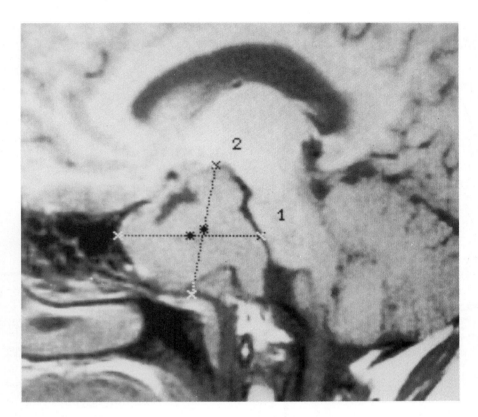

Figure 15—4. Demonstration of a large pituitary macroadenoma by MRI.

this method enables recognition of neoplasms as small as 2 mm in diameter. Most tumors appear as low-density lesions. Occasionally, hyperdense or isodense lesions are encountered and may pose a diagnostic uncertainty in the case of small tumors. In some instances, complete imaging of a large extrasellar mass may require cisternography with intrathecal contrast media. The technique of MRI provides equivalent if not greater detection capabilities compared to that of CT. It is rapidly becoming the method of choice. In contrast to CT, MRI does not require a contrast medium, which may provoke an allergic reaction, nor does it utilize ionizing radiation. Both techniques offer the advantage of differentiating an empty sella from that containing a solid pituitary tumor. In addition, visualization of the internal carotid arteries and their branches may allow for detection of an aneurysm or other vascular lesions.

Despite the utility of MRI, many individuals have problems with claustrophobia and are unable to be constrained in the MRI tube. Further, there is a considerable cost differential between MRI and CT scanning, with MRI being approximately three to four times as expensive. Considering that both of these techniques have a resolution of approximately 2 mm, it would seem prudent to consider using the less expensive technique in

this era of managed care. Further, radiographic imaging was greatly overutilized in the 1970s and 1980s as experience was gained regarding the natural history of pituitary tumors. The current state of knowledge regarding these lesions would seem to speak for less frequent radiographic imaging, and therefore the radiation exposure by CT scanning is probably negligible.

It is worth mentioning the inclusion of plane cone-down views of the sella turcica in the spectrum of imaging techniques used to identify pituitary tumors. In the specific instance of amenorrhea where there is an extremely low risk of a pituitary lesion, ie, exercise amenorrhea, a plane cone-down view may be helpful in detecting extrasellar expansion of a large neoplasm. Failure to detect a nonfunctional microadenoma by this method is high but has far less clinical significance.

Visual field examination is a useful and convenient technique because it can be performed informally by gross confrontation or formally by a number of methods including Goldman perimetry. However, by the time a field defect becomes detectable, considerable tumor growth and irreparable damage may have already occurred.

The management of nonfunctional tumors consists of surgical resection, irradiation therapy, or a combination of both. A consideration of surgery is predicated on the size, shape, and location of the tumor. Most non-functional neoplasms are large and exhibit extrasellar extension at the time of diagnosis. As a result, in these patients, as well as in those with dumbbell-shaped tumors, an intracranial operative approach usually is necessary. Complete extirpation of a tumor may be compromised if direct involvement of surrounding vital structures exceeds technical feasibility.

If the tumor exhibits minimal suprasellar extension, is infrasellar in growth, or is confined to the sella, then transnasal or transsphenoidal microdissection may be utilized. The incidence of complications associated with this approach is lower than that accompanying craniotomy.[34] The most frequent complication is transient diabetes insipidus. Serious postoperative morbidity, such as bleeding and cerebrospinal fluid leakage, may require reoperation.

The role of radiation therapy is generally directed toward management of large pituitary tumors. Commonly, it is used in conjunction with incomplete surgical resection. In selected cases where tumor size and location preclude adequate operative techniques, radiation may be considered primarily. The preferred method is heavy-particle irradiation because of its intensity and ability to target small areas within the body. The major complication of radiation therapy is hypopituitarism.

An unusual finding at transsphenoidal surgery is the patient whose mass represents a parasellar tumor. These individuals may present with signs of anterior pituitary failure, hyperprolactinemia, or visual abnormalities. Cranial neuropathy and diabetes insipidus are also encountered and are often clues to the nonpituitary nature of these lesions.[35]

Functional Tumors

Prolactinomas. Prolactin-secreting pituitary tumors represent the most common functional neoplasm of the pituitary gland.[36] Typically, these lesions are detected in women during their childbearing years because disruption of ovulatory function is a manifestation of prolactin excess. The natural progression of tumor growth appears to be slow and gradual. However, in isolated cases rapid enlargement has been reported. This is particularly true of young women in whom a large neoplasm was discovered soon after menarche or even prior to initiation of menses.[37] Because the tumor manifests itself during the reproductive years, it is tempting to implicate sex steroids in the tumorigenic process. Moreover, it is well known that lactotropes increase in both size and number during pregnancy to cause physiologic pituitary enlargement.[38] Infrequently, this physiologic expansion may be so great as to prove symptomatic and mimic the exis-

tence of a pituitary tumor. It has been difficult to account for the apparent accelerated growth pattern as the factors that promote prolactinoma formation remain elusive. Nonfunctional tumors may simulate a prolactinoma by impinging upon the pituitary stalk to cause hyperprolactinemia. Stalk compression interrupts the normal inhibitory control of prolactin secretion by reducing or eliminating the transport of hypothalamic dopamine. Often, the location of the tumor may not be intrasellar. Parasellar lesions or actual stalk tumors can precipitate the hyperprolactinemic state.

The clinical presentation of a prolactinoma relates to cellular function with excessive production of prolactin and cellular growth as reflected by progressive neoplastic enlargement. As the primary stimulating factor of lactogenesis during pregnancy, prolactin when produced in excessive amounts may induce lactation in both men and nongravid women. In women, the major clinical consequence of hyperprolactinemia is ovulatory disruption as hypothalamic–pituitary–ovarian function has proven to be sensitive to even mild elevations of circulating prolactin levels. Therefore, the classical features of prolactinoma are galactorrhea and/or oligoamenorrhea. The precise incidence of hyperprolactinemia in amenorrheic women without galactorrhea is unknown. However, it would appear to be far less than the 20 percent frequency originally reported in these patients.[39] The finding of galactorrhea in women with normal ovulatory function is poorly correlated with increased prolactin levels. As a result, this symptom alone cannot be used as a reliable clinical marker for hyperprolactinemia. Often, a history of physiologic or pharmacologic stimulation of lactotroph prolactin production can be elicited.[40] The presence of both galactorrhea and amenorrhea warrants strong consideration of abnormal prolactin secretion. In these patients, hyperprolactinemia is commonly associated with a prolactinoma.[41]

The mechanism of hyperprolactinemic anovulation involves inhibition of gonadotropin secretion. It has been well documented that in hyperprolactinemic women pulsatile release of LH and FSH is attenuated, leading to inadequate ovarian stimulation.[42] However, serum concentrations of these peptide hormones may continue to remain in the normal range. The suppression of gonadotropin secretion is probably secondary to decreased gonadotropin-releasing hormone (GnRH) release. It has been proposed that abnormally elevated circulating prolactin levels signal an increase in hypothalamic dopamine via a short loop feedback system (Fig 15–5).[43] The increased production of dopamine inhibits the release of GnRH, which leads to decreased gonadotropin secretion and resultant anovulation. This concept is supported by studies that demonstrate restoration of normal pulsatile

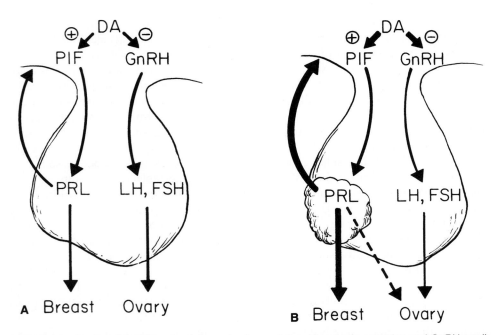

Figure 15–5. A. Conceptualized model of the role of dopamine in regulation of prolactin secretion and GnRH-mediated gonadotropin release in normal women. **B.** In the presence of hyperprolactinemia (prolactinoma), a short loop feedback effect increases dopamine production in the hypothalamus, which inhibits GnRH activity and leads to gonadotropin suppression.

gonadotropin release upon elimination of hyperprolactinemia following extirpative surgery or administration of bromocriptine (Fig 15–6).[44]

A second mechanism for anovulation in prolactinoma patients is the sheer destruction of gonadotropes within the pituitary by virtue of the compressive effects of neoplastic enlargement. Because gonadotropes are distributed throughout the gland, any lesion sufficiently large so as to directly eliminate gonadotrope activity most likely would compromise other anterior pituitary hormone function as well. Indeed, extremely large prolactinomas can be associated with destruction of thyrotropes and adrenocorticotropes, leading to secondary hypothyroidism and hypoadrenalism, respectively. The operative removal of tumor or administration of bromocriptine does not restore gonadotropin secretion in these cases.

The diagnosis of a prolactin-secreting pituitary tumor is based upon the serum prolactin concentration and the radiologic appearance of the pituitary gland. Most laboratories report an upper range of normal prolactin values at 20 to 30 ng/ml. At least two determinations above the normal range are necessary to establish hyperprolactinemia. Consideration of potential pharmacologic and physiologic stimulation, such as exercise, food ingestion, and sleep, should be made to avoid possible false positive results (Fig 15–7). For instance, blood should be drawn in the morning after an overnight fast and well removed from awakening or just before lunch provided there has not been a midmorning snack.

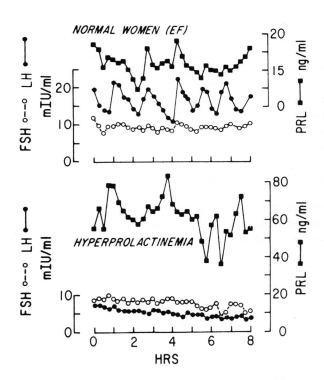

Figure 15–6. Absence of pulsatile fluctuation of LH and FSH associated with elevated serum levels of prolactin (PRL) in a patient with a microprolactinoma (lower panel). A representative pattern of LH, FSH, and PRL in normal women during the early follicular phase of the menstrual cycle (upper panel). *(Reproduced, with permission, from Rakoff J, Yen SSC. In: Yen SSC, Jaffe RB, eds.* Reproductive Endocrinology: Physiology, Pathophysiology and Clinical Management. *Philadelphia, Pa., W. B. Saunders, 1978: 356.)*

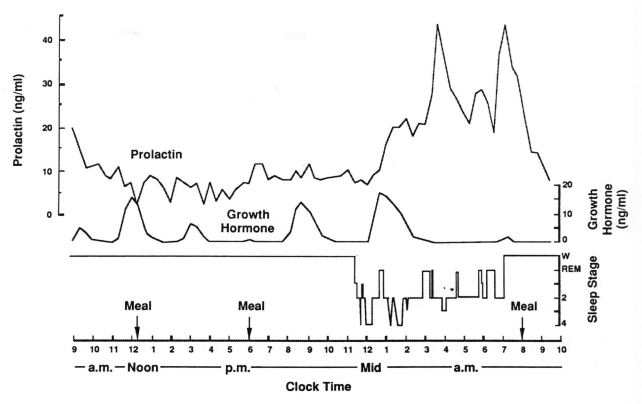

Figure 15–7. Serum prolactin and growth hormone secretion patterns during a 24-hr period. Note elevation of prolactin during sleep. *(Reproduced, with permission, from Sassin JF. Human prolactin: 24 hour pattern with increased release during sleep. Science. 177:1205, 1972.)*

Because galactorrhea and amenorrhea may occur in patients with primary hypothyroidism, a serum thyroxine and TSH determination is necessary in all suspected cases. The results will also allow for the detection of compensated hypothyroidism, in which thyroxine levels are normal and TSH levels elevated.

The value of anterior pituitary function tests in the diagnosis of prolactinomas is limited.[45] This is especially true of women with microprolactinomas who otherwise demonstrate normal anterior pituitary hormone function. Tests of pituitary reserve are helpful in determining the extent of functional compromise in patients with large macroadenomas where there is question of hypopituitarism.

The patient with hyperprolactinemia warrants radiologic evaluation of the pituitary gland. There are varying opinions as to when to perform this procedure based upon the circulating concentration of prolactin. Because mild increases in prolactin may accompany nonfunctional tumors that impact on the pituitary stalk or large tumors that might contain a small focus of lactotrope hyperplasia, it is recommended that at least a baseline radiologic assessment be performed in these patients. A prolactin level greater than 100 ng/ml indicates a need for pituitary imaging. Comparison of circulating prolactin values to

the likelihood of a prolactinemia has revealed that levels greater than 50 ng/ml are associated with a 20 percent frequency; up to 100 ng/ml a 50 percent frequency; and concentrations above 100 ng/ml almost uniformly a demonstrable tumor.[46]

The role of visual field examination is primarily to monitor potential tumor expansion. In patients with microadenomas, visual testing is not absolutely necessary. In contrast, surveillance of large macroadenomas may be facilitated by the performance of visual field testing by gross confrontation and if indicated formal Goldman perimetry.

The clinical management of prolactinomas consists of surgery, medical therapy, or observation. Small microadenomas are amenable to medical treatment using dopamine agonists. Selected cases may be managed expectantly. Bromocriptine has proven extremely effective in normalizing prolactin levels and inducing regular ovulation. The latter benefit is important to women desirous of pregnancy. The drug has a rapid onset of action in that a marked decline in serum prolactin ensues within hours following oral ingestion of a single 2.5-mg tablet (Fig 15–8).[47] The duration of action is approximately 10 to 12 hr, which explains the recommended twice-daily administration. A number of studies have

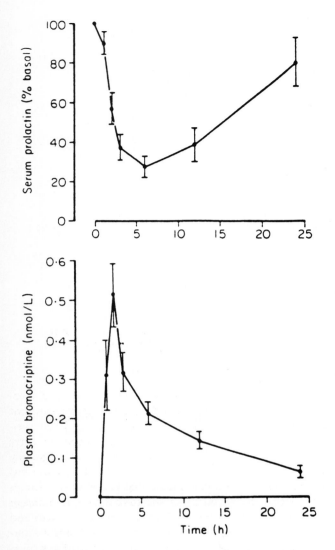

Figure 15–8. Mean ± serum prolactin and plasma bromocriptine concentrations in hyperprolactinemia patients given 2.5 mg bromocriptine orally (n = 8). Pretreatment prolactin levels were 240 to 196,000 mU/L. *(Reproduced, with permission, from Bevan JS, Baldwin D, Burke CW. Sensitive and specific bromocriptine radioimmunoassay with iodine label: Measurement of bromocriptine in human plasma. Ann Clin Biochem. 23:686, 1986.)*

demonstrated a resumption of ovulatory function in approximately 80 to 90 percent of cases. Similar relief has been noted in regard to cessation of lactation. The most frequent side effect includes nausea, occasional vomiting, light-headedness, and nasal stuffiness. Gastric intolerance may be obviated by vaginal administration of the drug.[48]

It has not been established that bromocriptine is curative. Nevertheless, isolated case reports have documented permanent resolution of hyperprolactinemia and disappearance of tumor following protracted therapy. Consideration of this rare outcome may be implemented by cessation of medical therapy after 1 to 2 yr and monitoring ovulatory regularity, serum prolactin levels, and, if indicated, repeat MRI.

Some patients cannot or choose not to institute bromocriptine treatment. An option to manage these patients expectantly is possible, but an awareness of estrogen status is implicit. Most patients with hyperprolactinemic amenorrhea exhibit hypoestrogenism. As a result, the risk of calcium loss from bone is increased in addition to any possible direct effect of hyperprolactinemia on bone demineralization.[49] Thus, consideration of hormone replacement must be entertained. To date, there are no data as to whether current recommended doses of hormone replacement therapy stimulate growth of a prolactinoma. Obviously, this course of management demands careful follow-up. If the patient exhibits anovulation of a lesser degree such that serum estrogen levels are normal, then a potential problem of unopposed estrogen effect on endometrial growth exists. In such cases, intermittent progestin therapy must be a minimal recommendation.

The treatment of large prolactinomas is somewhat more complex than that of microadenomas and may involve surgery, irradiation, bromocriptine, or a combination of these modalities. Transsphenoidal resection has been applied to macroprolactinomas with discouraging results as failure rates have been reported to be as high as 70 percent (Fig 15–9).[50] Lack of success is related to tumor size, as a direct correlation has been established between operative failure and increased size of the lesion. A similar poor surgical outcome exists in patients with prolactin levels greater than 200 ng/ml compared to more favorable results in patients with lower circulating levels.

As previously indicated, radiation therapy has been employed as primary treatment or in combination with surgery. The latter is particularly true when complete resection of tumor is not possible. Primary therapy utilizing dopamine agonist has been associated with substantial decrease in tumor size.[51] In patients with macroprolactinomas, bromocriptine administration resulted in a greater than 50 percent size reduction in two thirds of cases and complete restoration of normal pituitary size in one third (Table 15–1). Correlation of long-term medical treatment has been weighed against the possible complete eradication of disease by surgery. As such, bromocriptine has been used as a preoperative adjunct to facilitate tumor removal. The benefit of this therapeutic regimen has not been established.

PROLACTINOMAS AND PREGNANCY. The physiologic impact of gestation on the pituitary is primarily reflected by changes in the lactotrope. With advancement of pregnancy, rising levels of serum estradiol induce lactotrope hyperplasia and hypertrophy.[38] As a result, the normal pi-

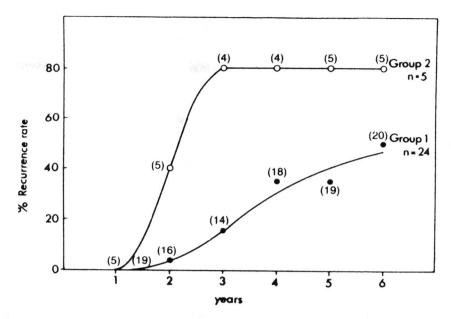

Figure 15–9. Cumulative recurrence rates in patients with microprolactinomas (group1) or macroprolactinomas (group 2) after normalization of serum prolactin following successful surgery. Figures in parentheses indicate numbers of patients seen at each yearly interval. *(Reproduced, with permission, from Serri O, Basio E, Beauregard H, et al, 1983:280.[50])*

tuitary gland may increase in size by as much as twofold or approximately 2 cm. This physiological enlargement has been associated with clinical symptomatology, the most common being visual field loss. Because maximal estrogen production occurs in late pregnancy, problems related to pituitary size emerge at this time. In general, expectant therapy is indicated. Following delivery, estrogen and placental steroid production decline dramatically and all symptoms resolve spontaneously.

Patients with intrasellar microadenomas are at minimal risk for complications during pregnancy. Less than 7 percent of reported cases have demonstrated clinical evidence of tumor enlargement and most of these have been minor.[52] On rare occasion, a significant increase in tumor size may lead to visual compromise or diabetes insipidus. In these situations, reassessment of tumor

TABLE 15–1. REDUCTION OF TUMOR SIZE AND NORMALIZATION OF ELEVATED PROLACTIN LEVELS IN PATIENTS WITH MACROPROLACTINOMAS TREATED WITH BROMOCRIPTINE FOR 12 MO

	Number of Patients	Tumor Reduction >50%	Tumor Reduction 50%	Tumor Reduction 10–25%	Prolactin to Normal Levels
Men	11	7	1	1	6
Women	16	6	4	6	12
Total	27	13	5	9	18

(Reproduced, with permission, from Molitch ME, Elton RE, Blackwell RE, et al, 1985:698.[51])

growth is necessary. If bromocriptine was employed to restore ovulation with a resultant pregnancy, then treatment should be discontinued once pregnancy has been confirmed. Exposure of a fetus to bromocriptine in early pregnancy during ovulation induction or in late pregnancy in an attempt to treat progressive tumor enlargement has not been associated with any teratogenic effects.[53] Long-term follow-up of infants exposed to bromocriptine during conception of gestation demonstrates normal growth and development.[54] Patients who do not experience tumor-related problems should be allowed to breast-feed postpartum. Although most pregnancies are totally uncomplicated, patients should be well informed of their diagnosis and reminded of potential complications.

Monitoring patients with microprolactinomas in pregnancy consists of careful inquiry about headache symptomatology and visual field examination. Severe and persistent headache may reflect tumor enlargement or infarction and requires further evaluation. Visual field examination by gross confrontation is adequate as a screening test. A suspicious or abnormal result warrants formal assessment such as Goldman perimetry. Measurement of serum prolactin levels to monitor tumor growth during pregnancy has not proven helpful and probably should not be utilized.

In contrast to women with intrasellar lesions, patients with macroadenomas are at significant risk for complications during pregnancy with a reported incidence of 17 percent in untreated cases.[52] The appearance of clinical symptoms may emerge at any time throughout gestation. The predominant complaint is headache, nausea, and vomiting. Often, it is difficult to discern whether these symptoms are related primarily to the pregnancy or the tumor. In patients with large neoplasms, the onset of visual field compromise or acuity loss is problematic in that substantial tumor enlargement may have already occurred. Impingement on the optic chiasm or nerve, if untreated, could lead to optic atrophy and blindness. Immediate therapeutic intervention is necessary, utilizing either medical or surgical modalities.

Some patients with macroadenomas who become pregnant following primary bromocriptine therapy experience significant side effects related to tumor enlargement. Commonly, reinstitution of drug reverses the clinical symptomatology for as long as treatment persists.[55] The impressive clinical response to bromocriptine during pregnancy may be anticipated if a similar response has been documented in the nongravid state. A significant reduction in tumor size prior to conception would seemingly suggest a favorable response to the reinstitution of bromocriptine in cases of symptomatic tumor enlargement. On the other hand, some patients with macroadenomas and hyperprolactinemia may not harbor prolactin-secreting tumors and not respond to medical therapy.[56] Thus, to employ bromocriptine as primary treatment for infertility in women with macroadenomas, evidence of tumor regression on drug should be demonstrated before contemplating conception.

ATYPICAL PROLACTINOMAS. In rare instances, prolactin-secreting pituitary tumors do not conform to the well-established behavior of prolactinomas. Recognition of these lesions is important because their clinical course may deviate substantially from that which is expected and pose serious risk to the patient. A notable group of patients in this category are those in whom the levels of prolactin, as well as size of tumor, failed to respond predictably to administration of bromocriptine.[57] Eight patients with prolactin-secreting adenomas and serum prolactin levels between 206 and 1100 ng/ml were administered bromocriptine in daily doses of 15 to 30 mg for at least 3 mo. None of the patients exhibited normalization of prolactin levels in response to treatment. Following an initial mean decrease of prolactin, increasing amounts of bromocriptine failed to achieve further suppression and in half of the patients a paradoxical elevation was observed that appeared to correlate to the dose of drug. Four of the eight patients sustained progressive tumor growth during treatment. In vitro cell culture studies revealed that tumor tissue from these patients was less sensitive to the inhibitory effects of bromocriptine compared to adenoma cells from normally responsive patients. Further examination utilizing binding studies demonstrated a significant decrease of the dopaminergic D_2 receptor in the tumor tissue of resistant patients (Fig 15–10). Thus, an alteration in the dopamine regulatory mechanism was attributed to a lack of the D_2 receptor or represented a postreceptor defect. The prognosis in these patients is problematic as reflected by the limited clinical experience. After repeated transfrontal surgery and radiation therapy, two patients developed invasive spread to the brain and died. One patient was cured by combined treatment. In the remaining five treated initially with operative removal of tumor and the reinstitution of bromocriptine therapy, three have had no further tumor enlargement whereas two have demonstrated growth of their lesions.

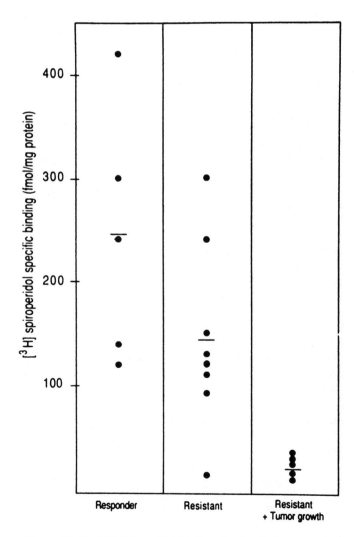

Figure 15–10. [³H] Spiroperidol binding site density in bromocriptine responsive and resistant groups of prolactinomas. Each point represents one patient. Horizontal lines indicate mean values in each group. *(Reproduced, with permission, from Pellegrini I, Rasolonjanahary R, Gunz G, et al. Resistance to bromocriptine in prolactinomas. J Clin Endocrinol Metab. 69:500, 1989.)*

Another group of patients with pituitary tumors and hyperprolactinemia bears discussion because misinterpretation of the diagnosis may lead to inappropriate treatment. Silent subtype 3 pituitary adenomas are uncommon and can be diagnosed only by electron microscopy.[58] The tumor is composed of cells unrelated to those normally known to occur in the pituitary. However, a small portion of these cells display multiple immunoreactivities to some pituitary hormones such as derivatives of pro-opiomelanocortin, growth hormone, thyrotropin, and prolactin. Clinically, it is believed that these lesions are aggressive in their growth as all described patients have been found to harbor macroadenomas at the time of diagnosis. The most common presenting symptoms are galactorrhea, amenorrhea, headache, or visual disturbances. Serum prolactin levels are mildly elevated and have not been reported to exceed 200 ng/ml. The lack of correlation between tumor size and circulating prolactin is a clue to the diagnosis. Another important distinguishing characteristic is that suppression of prolactin level is not accompanied by commensurate reduction in tumor size following administration of bromocriptine. Thus, close observation of tumor responsiveness is mandatory despite normalization of prolactin, cessation of galactorrhea, and a resumption of menses. Recurrence of tumor appears to be common after operative removal, which makes adjunctive radiation therapy a serious consideration. This therapeutic option is reasonable because patients have remained asymptomatic for up to 9 yr following postoperative irradiation.

Growth Hormone-Secreting Pituitary Tumors. Amenorrhea is a common accompaniment of growth hormone-secreting tumors that have achieved a size sufficient to destroy most gonadotropes. Theoretically, this phenomenon is a late-occurring feature of the neoplasm. Characteristically, the increased production of growth hormone produces insidious clinical alterations, which may not be realized until overt acromegalic changes are noted in the face and extremities.[59] Stimulation of bone growth with soft tissue proliferation results in enlargement of the nose, jaw, and supraorbital ridges. Overgrowth of bone and soft tissue about the joints leads to deformity of the hands and feet. The tongue may enlarge, causing difficulty with speech, and spacing between teeth may widen. Due to fibrous tissue growth, carpal tunnel syndrome occasionally develops with weakness and parathesias of the hands. Vocal cord thickening may lead to a deepening of the voice. Epidermal reaction to increased serum growth hormone levels includes excessive sweating and sebum production. Thickening of the skin also occurs and is an early but extremely subtle sign of growth hormone hypersecretion.

Beyond the problem of anovulation are far more serious consequences posed by this functional neoplasm.[60]

Growth hormone excess and acromegaly are associated with significant mortality from cardiovascular, cerebrovascular, and respiratory disease, which is twice that of the normal population. Hypertension is encountered in one fourth of patients and obesity is found in one half. Cardiac, hepatic, and renal enlargement are common. Visual disturbances secondary to chiasmal compression were found to occur frequently in earlier reported studies. With an increased awareness of disease and better methods of detection, the incidence of visual defects currently is approximately 20 percent.[61]

The diagnosis of a growth hormone-secreting pituitary tumor is based upon the serum growth hormone level, response to an oral glucose load, and pituitary imaging. The fasting serum growth hormone concentration should be less than 5 ng/ml. Physiological factors that tend to increase growth hormone values are stress and exercise. Circulating levels beyond 10 ng/ml are definitely abnormal and warrant further evaluation. The growth hormone response to hyperglycemia is examined after a standard glucose (100 g) tolerance test.[62] In normal individuals, serum growth hormone levels are suppressed to less than 2 ng/ml following glucose ingestion. Failure to do so indicates the diagnosis.

Treatment of this tumor involves eradication of tissue mass and reduction of elevated growth hormone levels. Both surgery and irradiation have proved satisfactory.[63,64] Failure to remove all tumor tissue or tumor that is inaccessible or inoperable usually requires adjunctive or primary radiation therapy. Unfortunately, amenorrhea due to hypogonadism resulting from radiation exposure to the hypothalamus or pituitary occurs in about 50 percent of cases.[65] Persistence of growth hormone hypersecretion has prompted the use of bromocriptine with good results in a number of cases.[66] It is unclear whether bromocriptine has a direct impact on tumor growth. Somatostatin analogs have been employed to treat acromegaly, with some patients exhibiting a significant reduction in circulating growth hormone levels.[67] A decrease in tumor size has also been reported, although further study is necessary to establish efficacy in a large number of patients.[68] Failure to respond to either bromocriptine or somatostatin analogue may warrant consideration of combined therapy.

Recent information demonstrated the expression of three somatostatin receptor subtypes in pituitary adenomas. There appears to be a preferential expression in the mammosomatotropic lineage of SSTR5, yet there are three somatostatin receptor subtypes: SSTR3, SSTR4, and SSTR5.[69]

Further, a $G_s\alpha$ mutation has been described in codon 201 in children with pituitary adenomas causing gigantism. This has also been demonstrated in individuals with the McCune–Albright syndrome.[70]

Further, recent studies have demonstrated that Prophet Pit-1 homeodomain factor is defective in Ames dwarfism. Studies of Sornson suggest that there is a cascade of tissue-specific regulators that are responsible for the determination and differentiation of specific cell lineages in pituitary organogenesis. Deficiencies in the cascade could express pituitary pathology.[71]

Data have been presented that suggest that glucocorticoids have an inhibitory effect on hypothalamic somatostatin growth hormone-releasing hormone and growth hormone receptor messenger RNA expression. These results suggest an inhibitory growth hormone-mediated effect of steroids on somatostatin messenger RNA levels in the periventricular nucleus and a direct inhibitory effect of steroids on GHRH neurons in the arcuate nucleus.[72] Finally, it has been demonstrated that galanin with its co-transmitter GHRH is a target for growth hormone action. Galanin may play a role in the feedback control of growth hormone secretion by exerting a direct effect on somatostatin neurons.[73]

ACTH-Secreting Pituitary Tumors. Pituitary tumors that produce excess amounts of ACTH (Cushing's disease) are responsible for adrenal hyperplasia and hypercortisolism (Cushing syndrome). Up to 75 percent of patients with Cushing syndrome experience irregular menstruation or amenorrhea. Destruction of gonadotrophs may be attributed to a huge neoplasm, but ACTH-producing tumors are generally small (less than 1 cm). Therefore, anovulation is likely due to hypercortisolism itself or to hormones produced in excess, such as androgens, during the process of steroidogenesis. The precise mechanism is not understood. Other symptoms of cortisol excess are discussed in another chapter (see Chap 18).

Cushing syndrome is suspected following an abnormal response to overnight dexamethasone suppression or increased 24-hr urinary excretion of cortisol. Both are excellent screening tests. Administration of dexamethasone, 1 mg, before bedtime normally results in a reduction of serum cortisol the following morning to less than 25 µg/100 ml. Values greater than 10 µg/100 ml indicate the need to perform a formal low-dose–high-dose dexamethasone suppression test. The diagnosis of Cushing's disease is established by non-suppressibility of cortisol following low-dose dexamethasone administration and partial suppression in response to high-dose dexamethasone. Plasma ACTH levels may be normal or elevated. Radiological imaging confirms the presence of a tumor. Recently, a new method of detection has been developed that potentially may be the optimum procedure to identify excess pituitary ACTH production.[74] Simultaneous bilateral sampling of the inferior petrosal sinuses has demonstrated a high degree of sensitivity and specificity in the diagnosis of an ACTH-producing pituitary tumor.[75] Adjunctive use of corticotropin-releasing hormone may

further detect a pituitary lesion. This procedure appears to have its greatest utility in patients who exhibit a pituitary tumor by dynamic testing but fail to demonstrate a lesion by radiology imaging.

Because ACTH-secreting pituitary tumors tend to be small at the time of diagnosis, their management is amenable to selective removal by transsphenoidal microdissection. Radiation therapy is usually not a mode of primary treatment but may be used, if necessary, as a therapeutic adjunct.

Recently, Estrada et al exposed 30 adult patients to pituitary radiation with persistent or recurrent Cushing's disease after unsuccessful transsphenoidal surgery. Eighty-two percent of the patients had remission during a median follow-up of 42 months; none of the patients had a relapse of Cushing's disease after remission was achieved.[76] Failure to resolve adrenocorticotropin-secreting adenomas may have to do with the method used in evaluating the tumor. The recent findings of Wilson's group suggests that venous angiography is needed to interpret inferior petrosal sinus and cavernous sinus sampling data when attempting to lateralize the adenoma. Radiography is useful in understanding the venous drainage pattern, and it is thought to be essential to correctly interpret the venous sampling data and warrant positions that lateralization data may be incorrect or unreliable.[77] Further, it has been demonstrated that corticotroph macroadenomas have impaired processing of pro-opiomelanocortin. The variations in clinical symptoms seen in patients with corticotroph adenomas may be attributable to differences in biologic potency between ACTH precursors and ACTH.[78] The mechanism causing this discordance is not clear, although it has been shown that CRH induces activation of a cation current that plays an important role in CRH-induced calcium increase and subsequent ACTH secretion.[79]

Gonadotropin-Secreting Pituitary Tumors. It has been generally considered that gonadotropin-secreting pituitary tumors are exceedingly rare, occurring primarily in men.[80] Moreover, in the few reported cases hypogonadism was not a consistent clinical feature. In a recent study, it has been demonstrated that these lesions are not uncommon and may comprise the majority of nonfunctional tumors in women.[81] In patients described, all had macroadenomas and were postmenopausal. With the exception of elevated serum FSH and LH levels, basal pituitary hormone values were in the normal range. In response to the administration of TRH, significant increases of FSH, LH, LHβ- (LHβ), and α-subunit were noted in some, but not all, instances. The most consistent response was that of LHβ, which occurred in 11 of 16 women. These data were supported by in vitro culture studies and are similar to a number of cases previously reported. Recently Klibanski's group has demonstrated endogenous GnRH gene expression in human pituitary adenomas. The presence of both GnRH and GnRH receptors suggest that GnRH may be a paracrine/autocrine regulator of cell function in the pituitary, and may affect gonadotropic tumor hormone phenotype.[82] Thus, it would appear that the vast majority of functionless neoplasms in women are actually capable of hormone production and derived from gonadotropic cells.

If hypogonadism is not observed in men with gonadotropin-secreting tumors, then in premenopausal patients this neoplasm may prove difficult to diagnose in the absence of clinical signs related to tumor size. In the postmenopausal woman, detection of such lesions is problematic in that the diagnosis would be made only after symptomatic enlargement of a macroadenoma.

Thyrotropin-Secreting Pituitary Tumors. TSH-secreting pituitary tumors are associated with central hyperthyroidism and primary hypothyroidism. The TSH-secreting pituitary adenoma is a rare cause of hyperthyroidism. Their diagnosis is facilitated by the introduction of ultrasensitive TSH immunoassays as well as free thyroid hormone assays that are not obscured by abnormal serum transport proteins. The availability of such tools should aid in early recognition of the tumors and prevent misdiagnosis and treatment. No single diagnostic test is pathopneumonic of the disease, but an elevation in the α-subunit level, elevation in serum sex hormone-binding globulin, absent or impaired TSH response to TRH, and T3 suppression test are useful markers in diagnosing TSH-secreting tumors. The majority of the tumors are small, approximately 3 mm, and therefore may be detected by either CT scanning or MRI. These tumors are generally treated surgically, with radiation therapy used for failure.[83]

Causes of Pituitary Tumors

The cause of a pituitary tumor formation is unclear. There are occurrences being attributed to multiple mechanisms including changes in hypothalamic pituitary vascular supply, alteration of cellular genetics, disregulation of dopamine receptors, disregulation of dopamine metabolism, or malfunction of growth factors or hormonal expression. Page and Bergland demonstrated that the hypothalamus sends a blood supply to the pituitary. This tends to be a bilateral system with numerous intercommunications, and speculation appeared that perhaps atheromatous changes in the vascular supply could account for a differential gradient and delivery of dopamine to the lateral wings of the pituitary, therefore giving rise to the opportunity for hyperplasia and perhaps tumor formation. Recently, morphologic evidence has been presented that arteries exist in human prolactinomas.[84] These may be congenital or developed during tumor formation, and the presence of arterial blood supply in the

anterior pituitary results in escape of that area from normal hypothalamic regulation.

Signal transduction has been found to be defective in a number of types of adenomas.[85] For instance, prolactinomas have been identified which have no dopamine receptors on their surface. D_2 receptors have been described on prolactin-secreting adenomas that maintain their receptor effect or coupling. However, recently dopamine binding has been demonstrated in growth hormone-secreting adenomas, yet dopamine fails to exert an inhibitory activity on adenyl cyclase, indicating a failure of signal transduction.

Further, it has been suggested that inactivation of an oncogene on chromosome 11 is an important and possible early event in the development of four major types of pituitary adenomas. Mutations have been described in GPT binding protein ($G_s\alpha$) in tumors that primarily secrete growth hormone. Further, tumors have been described with multiple autosomal losses. Likewise, T53 and RASG mutations are common events in the pathogenesis of both acromegaly and nonsecreting tumors. Klibanski et al have evaluated 79 tumors and found no RASG mutations identified in either prolactinomas or pituitary carcinomas. Pituitary adenomas also show no loss of heterozygosity at the retinoblastoma gene locus. Finally, an uncoupling of β-subunit gene expression in protein biosynthesis has been described as the setting of ongoing subunit biosynthesis, suggesting a potential mechanism for unbalanced synthesis secretion of free α-subunits.[86–91]

Another intriguing possible cause of prolactinomas involves the secretion of dopamine. Removal of prolactinomas still results in defective regulation of prolactin secretion, and persistent rapid growth hormone pulsatility has been described after removal of growth hormone-secreting pituitary tumors. Further, patients have been described bearing prolactin-secreting adenomas that were responsive to the prolactin inhibiting properties of indirectly acting dopamine agonists. Further, Crosignani et al have postulated a common central defect in hyperprolactinemic patients with or without radiologic signs of pituitary tumors. This hypothesis is supported by dopamine infusion studies in patients with hyperprolactinemia showing normal prolactin suppressibility but abnormal dopamine metabolism. These studies receive minimal support from the observation that cell culture alters the hormonal responsiveness of rat pituitary tumor to dynamic hormonal stimulation. Currently, an altered balance between thyrotropin-releasing hormone and dopamine has been detected in prolactinomas and other pituitary tumors as compared to normal pituitary glands.[92–99] Estrogen receptor expression has been demonstrated in human pituitaries and in macroadenomas. Estrogen receptor expression is present in 2.3 percent of growth hormone, 50 percent of prolactin, 70 percent of FSH, 83 percent of LH, 4 percent of TSH, and 1 percent of ACTH-positive tumors.[100] The estrogen receptor-positive tumors may represent a subset whose growth and secretory profile can be influenced by gonadal steroids. Further, using in situ hybridization techniques, nine lactotropic adenomas have been treated with bromocriptine, and hybridization signals weaken, suggesting suppression of the estrogen receptor gene.[101] Further, men treated with testosterone have been documented to have an exacerbation of their prolactin-secreting tumor despite continued treatment with bromocriptine therapy.[102] The hypothesis would be that the testosterone anaptate is aromatized to estradiol, which would directly stimulate lactotrophs. Finally, various growth factors have been shown to influence prolactin secretion.[103,104] Fibroblastic growth factor stimulates prolactin from human anterior pituitary cell adenomas but does not appear to affect cell proliferation. On the other hand, transforming growth factors alpha and beta are potent and effective inhibitors of prolactin tumor secretion when evaluated in JH4 lines. Therefore, all of these lines of evidence would seem to suggest that vascular, dopaminergic, genetic receptor, and growth factor mechanisms may be involved in the expression of adenomas. On the other hand, it also might suggest that pituitary adenomas may arrive by different pathophysiologic pathways.

SUMMARY

Tumors of the central nervous system often present with headache, ovulatory dysfunction, disorders of growth, or lactation. The most common tumor is of the prolactinoma type, which is diagnosed with multiple serum prolactin levels, followed by computed axial tomography or magnetic resonance imaging. Lesions are generally categorized as microadenomas, that is, less than 10 mm; or macroadenomas, greater than 10 mm. Visual field disturbances do not occur unless the tumor escapes the sella turcica. Many tumors are endocrine inactive (null cell type), yet influence the secretion of pituitary tropic hormones through disturbance of vascular supply, growth factors, or other mechanisms. Pituitary tumors other than those that secrete prolactin are frequently treated surgically, and at times in conjunction with radiation therapy. Prolactinomas are primarily treated with medical therapy using dopamine agonists, with surgery reserved for refractory cases.

REFERENCES

1. Banna M. Craniopharyngioma: Based on 160 cases. *Br J Radiol.* 49:206, 1976
2. Ringel SP, Bailey OT. Rathke's cleft cyst. *J Neurol Neurosurg Psych.* 35:693, 1972
3. Petito CK, DeGirolami U, Earle KM. Craniopharyngiomas, a clinical review and pathological review. *Cancer.* 37:1944, 1976
4. Hoff JT, Patterson RH Jr. Craniopharyngiomas in children and adults. *J Neurosurg.* 36:299, 1972
5. Matson DD, Crigler JF Jr. Management of craniopharyngiomas in childhood. *J Neurosurg.* 30:377, 1969
6. Reiter RJ. Comparative physiology: Pineal gland. *Annu Rev Physiol.* 35:305, 1973
7. Russell DS. The pinealoma: Its relationship to teratoma. *J Pathol Bacteriol.* 56:145, 1945
8. Scully RE. Discussion in case records of the Massachusetts General Hospital. *N Engl J Med.* 284:1427, 1971
9. De Girolami U, Schmidek H. Clinicopathological study of 53 tumors of the pineal region. *J Neurosurg.* 39:455, 1973
10. Bradfield JS, Perez CA. Pineal tumors and ectopic pinealomas, analysis of treatment and failures. *Radiology.* 103:399,1972
11. Bestle J. Extragonadal endodermal sinus tumors originating in the region of the pineal gland. *Acta Pathol Microbiol Scand.* 74:214, 1968
12. Vogel JM, Vogel P. Idiopathic histiocytosis: A discussion of eosinophilic granuloma, the Hand–Schüller–Christian syndrome and Letterer–Siwe syndrome. *Sem Hematol.* 9:349, 1972
13. Avery ME, McAfee JG, Guild HG. The cause and prognosis of reticuloendotheliosis (eosinophilic granuloma, Schüller–Christian disease and Letterer–Siwe disease). *Am J Med.* 22:636, 1957
14. Olin P. Growth hormone response to insulin induced hypoglycemia in a boy with diabetes insipidus and short stature before and after treatment with vasopressin. *Acta Paediatr Scand.* 59:343, 1970
15. Braunstein GD, Kohler PO. Pituitary function in Hand–Schüller–Christian disease; evidence for deficient growth hormone release in patients with short stature. *N Engl J Med.* 286:1225, 1972
16. Dargeon HW. Considerations in the treatment of reticuloendotheliosis. *Am J Roentgenol.* 93:521, 1965
17. Colover J. Sarcoidosis with involvement of the nervous system. *Brain.* 71:451, 1948
18. Plair CM, Perry S. Hypothalamic–pituitary sarcoidosis. *Arch Pathol.* 24:527, 1962
19. Askanazy CL. Sarcoidosis of the central nervous system. *J Neuropath Exp Neurol.* 11:392, 1952
20. White JC. Aneurysms mistaken for hypophyseal tumors. *J Clin Neurosurg.* 10:244, 1964
21. Crompton MR. Hypothalamic lesions following the rupture of cerebral berry aneurysms. *Brain.* 86:301, 1963
22. Peck FC, McGovern ER. Radiation necrosis of the brain in acromegaly. *Neurosurgery.* 25:536, 1966
23. Costello RT. Subclinical adenoma of the pituitary gland. *Am J Pathol.* 12:205, 1936
24. Burrow GN, Wortzman G, Rewcastle NB, et al. Microadenomas of the pituitary and abnormal sellar tomograms in an unselected autopsy series. *N Engl J Med.* 304:156, 1981
25. Hardy J. Transsphenoidal surgery of hypersecreting pituitary tumors. In: Kohler PO, Ross GT, eds. *Diagnosis and*

Treatment of Pituitary Tumors. New York, N.Y., Elsevier, 1973: 179–198

26. Shome B, Parlow AF. Human pituitary prolactin (hPRL): The entire linear amino acid sequence. *J Clin Endocrinol Metab.* 45:1112, 1977

27. Sheng HZ, Zhadanov AB, Mosinger B Jr, et al. Specification of pituitary cell lineages by the LIM homeobox gene Lhx3. *Science.* 272:1004, 1996

28. Kovacs K, Horvath E. Pathology of pituitary tumors. *Endocrinol Metab Clin N Am.* 16:529, 1987

29. Kovacs K, Scheithauer BW, Horvath E, Lloyd RV. The World Health Organization classification of adenohypophyseal neoplasms. *Cancer.* 78:502, 1996

30. LeRiche VK, Asa SL, Ezzat S. Epidermal growth factor and its receptor (EGF-R) in human pituitary adenomas: EGF-R correlates with tumor aggressiveness. *JCE&M.* 81:656, 1996

31. Bates AS, Farrell WE, Bicknell J, et al. Allelic deletion in pituitary adenomas reflects aggressive biological activity and has potential value as a prognostic marker. *JCE&M.* 82:818, 1997

32. Hollenhorst RW, Younge BR. Ocular manifestations produced by adenomas of the pituitary gland: Analysis of 1,000 cases. In: Kohler PO, Ross GT, eds. *Diagnosis and Treatment of Pituitary Tumors.* New York, N. Y., Elsevier, 1973: 53–68

33. Rovit L, Fein JM. Pituitary apoplexy: A review and reappraisal. *J Neurosurg.* 37:280, 1972

34. MacCarty CS, Hanson EJ Jr, Randall RV, Scanlon PW. Indications for and results of surgical treatment of pituitary tumors by the transfrontal approach. In: Kohler PO, Ross GT, eds. *Diagnosis and Treatment of Pituitary Tumors.* New York, N.Y., Elsevier, 1973: 139–145

35. Freda PU, Warklaw SL, Post KD. Unusual causes of sellar/parasellar masses in a large transsphenoidal surgical series. *JCE&M.* 81:3455, 1996

36. Molitch ME. Pathologic hyperprolactinemia. *Endocrinol Metab Clin North Am.* 21:877, 1992

37. Blackwell RE, Younger BJ. Long-term medical therapy and followup of pediatric-adolescent patients with prolactin-secreting macroadenomas. *Fertil Steril.* 45:713, 1986

38. Goluboff LG, Ezrin C. Effect of pregnancy on the somatotroph and the prolactin cell of the human adenohypophysis. *J Clin Endocrinol Metab.* 19:1533, 1969

39. Jacobs HS. Prolactin and amenorrhea. *N Engl J Med.* 295:954, 1976

40. Chang RJ. Hyperprolactinemia and menstrual dysfunction. *Clin Obstet Gynecol.* 26:736, 1983

41. Keye WK, Changs RJ, Wilson CB, Jaffe RB. Prolactin secreting pituitary adenomas: III, frequency and diagnosis in amenorrhea-galactorrhea. *JAMA.* 244:1329, 1980

42. Boyar RM, Kapen S, Finklestein JW, et al. Hypothalamic–pituitary function in diverse hyperprolactinemic states. *J Clin Invest.* 53:1588, 1974

43. Quigley ME, Judd SJ, Gilliland GB, et al. Effects of a dopamine antagonist on the release of gonadotropin and prolactin in normal women and women with hyperprolactinemic anovulation. *J Clin Endocrinol Metab.* 48:718, 1979

44. Quigley ME, Judd SJ, Gilliland GB, et al. Functional studies of dopamine control of prolactin secretion in normal women and women with hyperprolactinemic pituitary microadenoma. *J Clin Endocrinol Metab.* 50:949, 1980

45. Chang RJ, Keye WR Jr, Monroe SE, et al. Prolactin secreting pituitary adenomas in women. IV. Pituitary function in amenorrhea associated with normal or abnormal serum prolactin and sellar polytomography. *J Clin Endocrinol Metab.* 51:830, 1980

46. Blackwell RE. Diagnosis and management of prolactinomas. *Fertil Steril.* 43:5, 1985

47. Cragun JR, Chang RJ. Treatment of hyperprolactinemia: Bromocriptine. In: Barbieri RL, Schiff I, eds. *Reproductive Endocrine Therapeutics.* New York, N.Y., Alan R. Liss, 1988: 83–99

48. Kletzky OA, Vermesh M. Effectiveness of vaginal bromocriptine in treating women with hyperprolactinemia. *Fertil Steril.* 51:269, 1989

49. Klibanski A, Greenspan SL. Increase in bone mass after treatment of hyperprolactinemic amenorrhea. *N Engl J Med.* 315:542,1986

50. Serri O, Basio E, Beauregard H, et al. Recurrence of hyperprolactinemia after selective transsphenoidal adenomectomy in women with prolactinoma. *N Engl J Med.* 309:280, 1983

51. Molitch ME, Elton RL, Blackwell RE, et al. Bromocriptine as primary therapy for prolactin-secreting macroadenomas: Results of a prospective multicenter study. *J Clin Endocrinol Metab.* 60:698, 1985

52. Melmed S, Braunstein GD, Chang RJ, et al. Pituitary tumor secreting growth hormone and prolactin. *Ann Int Med.* 105:238, 1986

53. Turkalj I, Braun P, Krupp P. Surveillance of bromocriptine in pregnancy. *JAMA.* 247:1589, 1982

54. Weiss MH, Teal J, Gott P, et al. Natural history of microprolactinomas: Six-year follow-up. *Neurosurgery.* 12:180, 1983

55. Konopka P, Raymond JP, Meceron RE, et al. Continuous administration of bromocriptine in the prevention of neurologic complications in pregnant women with prolactinomas. *Am J Obstet Gynecol.* 146:935,1983

56. Boulanger CM, Mashchak CA, Chang RJ. Lack of tumor reduction hyperprolactinemic women with extrasellar macroadenomas treated with bromocriptine. *Fertil Steril.* 44:532, 1985

57. Pellegrini I, Rasolonjanahary R, Gunz G, et al. Resistance to bromocriptine in prolactinomas. *J Clin Endocrinol Metab.* 69:500, 1989

58. Horvath E, Kovacs K, Smyth HS, et al. A novel type of pituitary adenoma: Morphological features and clinical correlations. *J Clin Endocrinol Metab.* 66:1111, 1988

59. Melmed S. Acromegaly. *N Engl J Med.* 322:966, 1990

60. Smallridge RC, Rajfer S, Davia J, et al. Acromegaly and the heart. *Am J Med.* 66:22, 1979

61. Wilson CB, Dempsey LC. Transsphenoidal microsurgical removal of 250 pituitary adenomas. *J Neurosurg.* 48:13, 1978

62. Klibanski A, Zervas NT. Diagnosis and management of hormone-secreting pituitary adenomas. *N Engl J Med.* 324:822, 1991

63. Ross DA, Wilson CB. Results of transsphenoidal microsurgery for growth-hormone secreting pituitary adenomas in a series of 214 patients. *J Neurosurg.* 68:854, 1988

64. Kliman B, Kjellberg RN, Swisher B, et al. Long-term effects of proton beam therapy for acromegaly. In: Robbins RJ, Melmed S, eds. *Acromegaly: A Century of Scientific and Clinical Progress.* New York, N.Y., Plenum Press, 1987

65. Snyder PJ, Fowble BF, Schatz NJ, et al. Hypopituitarism following radiation therapy of pituitary adenomas. *Am J Med.* 81:457, 1986

66. Wass JAH, Thorner MD, Morris DV, et al. Long-term treatment of acromegaly with bromocriptine. *Br Med J.* 1:875, 1977

67. Lamberts SWJ. The role of somatostatin in the regulation of anterior pituitary hormone secretion and the use of its analogs in the treatment of human pituitary tumors. *Endocrine Rev.* 9:417, 1988

68. Barkan AL, Lloyd RV, Chandler WF, et al. Preoperative treatment of acromegaly with long-acting somatostatin analog SMs 201-995: Shrinkage of invasive pituitary macroadenomas and improved surgical remission rate. *J Clin Endocrinol Metab.* 67:1040, 1988

69. Greenman Y, Melmed S. Expression of three somatostatin receptor subtypes in pituitary adenomas: Evidence for preferential SSTR5 expression in the mammosomatotroph lineage. *JCE&M.* 79:724, 1994

70. Dotsch J, Kiess W, Hanze J, et al. $G_s\alpha$ mutation at codon 201 in pituitary adenomas causing gigantism in a 6-year-old boy with McCune–Albright syndrome. *JCE&M.* 81:3839, 1996

71. Somson MW, Wu W, Dasen JS, et al. Pituitary lineage determination by the prophet of Pit-1 homeodomain factor defective in Ames dwarfism. *Nature.* 384:327, 1996

72. Senaris RM, Lago F, Coya R, et al. Regulation of hypothalamic somatostatin, growth hormone-releasing hormone, and growth hormone receptor messenger ribonucleic acid by glucocorticoids. *Endocrinology.* 137:5236, 1996

73. Chan YY, Grafstein-Dunn E, Delemarre-Van de Walal HA, et al. The role of galanin and its receptor in the feedback regulation of growth hormone secretion. *Endocrinology.* 137:5303, 1996

74. Doppman JL, Oldfield E, Krudy AG, et al. Petrosal sinus sampling for Cushing syndrome: Anatomical and technical considerations: Work in progress. *Radiology.* 150:99, 1984

75. Oldfield EH, Chrousos GP, Schulte HM, et al. Preoperative lateralization of ACTH-secreting pituitary microadenomas by bilateral and simultaneous inferior petrosal venous sinus sampling. *N Engl J Med.* 312:100, 1985

76. Estrada J, Boronat M, Melgo M, et al. The long-term outcome of pituitary irradiation after unsuccessful transsphenoidal surgery in Cushing's disease. *N Engl J Med.* 336:172, 1997

77. Mamelak AN, Down CF, Tyrrell JB, et al. Venous angiography is needed to interpret inferior petrosal sinus and cavernous sinus sampling data for lateralizing adrenocorticotropin-secreting adenomas. *JCE&M.* 81:475, 1996

78. Gibson S, Ray DW, Crosby SR, et al. Impaired processing of proopiomelanocortin in corticotroph macroadenomas. *JCE&M.* 81:497, 1996

79. Takano K, Yasufuki-Takano J, Teramoto A, Fujita T. Corticotropin-releasing hormone excites adrenocorticotropin-secreting human pituitary adenoma cells by activating a nonselective cation current. *J Clin Invest.* 98:2033, 1996

80. Snyder PJ. Gonadotroph cell adenomas of the pituitary. *Endocr Rev.* 6:552, 1985

81. Daneshdoost L, Gennarelli TA, Hildegarde M, et al. Recognition of gonadotroph adenomas in women. *N Engl J Med.* 324:589, 1991

82. Miller GM, Alexander JM, Klibanski A. Gonadotropin-releasing hormone messenger RNA expression in gonadotroph tumors and normal human pituitary. *JCE&M.* 81:80, 1996

83. Beck-Peccoz P, Brucker-Davis F, Persani L, et al. Thyrotropin-secreting pituitary tumors. *Endocr Rev.* 17:610, 1996

84. Schechter J, Goldsmith P, Wilson C, et al. Morphological evidence for the presence of arteries to human prolactinomas. *JCE&M.* 67:713, 1988

85. Spada A, Basset M, Reza-Elahi F, et al. Differential transduction of dopamine signal in different subtypes of human growth hormone-secreting adenomas. *JCE&M.* 78:411, 1994

86. Roman SH, Goldstein M, Kourides IA, et al. The luteinizing hormone-releasing hormone (LHRH) agonist [D-Trp[6]-Pro[9]-NEt] LHRH increased rather than lower LH and α-subunit levels in a patient with an LH-secreting pituitary tumor. *JCE&M.* 58:313, 1984

87. Rubio MA, Cabranes JA, Schally AV, et al. Prolactin-lowering effect of luteinizing hormone-releasing hormone agonist administration in prolactinoma patients. *JCE&M.* 69:444, 1989

88. Hammond E, Griffin J, Odell WD. A chorionic gonadotropin-secreting human pituitary cell. *JCE&M.* 72:747, 1991

89. Samuels MH, Henry P, Kleinschmidt-Demasters BK, et al. Pulsatile glycoprotein hormone secretion in glycoprotein-producing pituitary tumors. *JCE&M.* 73:1281, 1991

90. Paoletti AM, Depau GF, Mais V, et al. Effectiveness of cabergoline in reducing follicle-stimulating hormone and prolactin hypersecretion from pituitary macroadenoma in an infertile woman. *Fertil Steril.* 62:822, 1994

91. Comtois R, Bouchard J, Robert F. Hypersecretion of gonadotropin by a pituitary adenoma: Pituitary dynamic studies and treatment with bromocriptine in one patient. *Fertil Steril.* 52:569, 1989

92. Kwekkeboon DJ, de Jong FH, Lamberts SWJ. Gonadotropin release by clinically nonfunctioning and gonadotroph pituitary adenomas in vivo and in vitro: Relation to sex and effects of thyrotropin-releasing hormone, gonadotropin-releasing hormone, and bromocriptine. *JCE&M.* 68:1128, 1987

93. Crosignani PG, Ferrari C, Malinverni A, et al. Effect of central nervous system dopaminergic activation on prolactin secretion in man: Evidence for common central defect in hyperprolactinemic patients with and without radiological signs of pituitary tumors. *J Clin Endocrinol Metab* 51:1068, 1980

94. Genazzani AR, de Leo V, Murru S, et al. Dynamic tests of prolactin secretion in hyperprolactinemic states:

Carbidopa-L-Dopa and indirectly acting dopamine agonists. *J Clin Endocrinol Metab* 54:428, 1982

95. Melmed S, Carlson HE, Briggs J, et al. Cell culture alters the hormonal response of rat pituitary tumors to dynamic stimulation. *Endocrinology* 107:789, 1980

96. Camanni F, Ghigo E, Ciccarelli E, et al. Defective regulation of prolactin secretion after succesful removal of prolactinomas. *J Clin Endocrinol Metab* 57:1270, 1983

97. Ho PJ, Jaffe CA, Friberg RD, et al. Persistence of rapid growth hormones (GH) pulsatility after successful removal of GH-producing pituitary tumors. *J Clin Endocrinol Metab* 78:1403, 1994

98. Ho KY, Smythe GA, Duncan M, et al. Dopamine infusion studies in patients with pathological hyperprolactinemia: Evidence of normal prolactin suppressibility but abnormal dopamine metabolism. *J Clin Endocrinol Metab* 58:128, 1984

99. Le Dafniet M, Blumberg-Tick J, Gozlan H, et al. Altered balance between thyrotropin-releasing hormone and dopamine in prolactinomas and other pituitary tumors compared to normal pituitaries. *J Clin Endocrinol Metab* 69:267, 1989

100. Friend KE, Chiou K, Lopes MBS, et al. Estrogen receptor expression in human pituitary: Correlation with immunohistochemistry in normal tissue, and immunohistochemistry and morphology in macroadenomas. *J Clin Endocrinol Metab* 78:1497, 1994

101. Stefaneanu L, Kovacs K, Horvath E, et al. In situ hybridization study of estrogen receptor messenger ribonucleic acid in human adenohypophysial cells and pituitary adenomas. *J Clin Endocrinol Metab* 78:83, 1994

102. Prior JC, Cox TA, Fairholm D, et al. Testosterone-related exacerbation of a prolactin-producing macroadenoma: Possible role for estrogen. *J Clin Endocrinol Metab* 64:291, 1987

103. Ramsdel JS. Transforming growth factor-α and -β are potent and effective inhibitors of GH_4 pituitary tumor cell proliferation. *Endocrinology* 128:1981, 1991

104. Atkin SL, Landolt AM, Jeffreys RV, et al. Basic fibroblastic growth factor stimulates prolactin secretion from human anterior pituitary adenomas without affecting adenoma cell proliferation. *J Clin Endocrinol Metab* 77:831, 1993

Chapter 16

ANOVULATION OF CNS ORIGIN

Functional and Miscellaneous Causes

James H. Liu

Through the pioneering work from the laboratories of Schally, Guillemin, and Knobil, it is now well established that pulsatile secretion of gonadotropin-releasing hormone (GnRH) from the hypothalamus is directly responsible for the activation and maintenance of pituitary gonadotropin secretion. It is the interaction of the hypothalamic–pituitary–ovarian (HPO) compartments that is responsible for pubertal development and initiation of the menstrual cycle. Disruption of this process at either the hypothalamic, pituitary, or ovarian level can lead to reproductive dysfunction. The focus of this chapter will be to review functional and organic disorders arising from the central nervous system that can disrupt GnRH and gonadotropin secretion from the H-P axis leading to anovulation.

In the human, the GnRH neuronal system has been localized to the medial basal hypothalamus, principally the arcuate nucleus (Fig 16–1), which contains the highest concentration of GnRH neurons.[1,2] GnRH neuronal cell bodies project to and terminate in the median eminence.[3] This area is well supplied by the pituitary portal capillary bed, which is lined by fenestrated endothelium and is considered to be outside the blood–brain barrier. These portal vessels are also capable of carrying secretions from the pituitary towards the brain.[4] Physiologic studies indicate that these GnRH neurons depolarize and release GnRH in a synchronous fashion at a critical frequency between 60 to 120 min in the primate.[5–7] When the frequency is shifted from this range, pituitary gonadotropin release is altered and there is disruption of the menstrual cycle. In addition to GnRH neurons, other neuronal networks are localized to the arcuate nucleus. These neurotransmitter systems include neurons that contain β-endorphin, dopamine, and norepinephrine. Each neuronal system appears to have synaptic contacts

or interneuronal connections with GnRH neurons within the arcuate nucleus. Thus, these neurotransmitter networks can play a modulatory role on GnRH neurosecretion. For example, stimulation of the noradrenergic system appears to enhance GnRH neuronal activity, while activation of the opioidergic system appears to inhibit GnRH activity.[8,9]

Disorders of the CNS associated anovulation can be categorized into those disorders that are associated with normal neuroanatomic findings and characterized by alteration in lifestyle factors such as nutritional deprivation, excessive exercise, and psychogenic stress; and those neuroendocrine abnormalities that are associated with organic disease such as isolated gonadotropin deficiency, Sheehan's syndrome, pituitary apoplexy, head trauma, and radiation effects (Table 16–1).[10] Irrespective of the etiology, the final common pathway appears to be the disruption of episodic GnRH secretion resulting in ovulatory dysfunction. These major disorders will be discussed in this chapter.

FUNCTIONAL CAUSES OF HYPOTHALAMIC AMENORRHEA

Functional anovulation that is associated with hypoestrogenism, normal or low levels of gonadotropins, and psychogenic factors was first described by Klinefelter, Albright, and Griswold in 1943.[11] These investigators were the first to introduce the term "hypothalamic hypoestrogenism." They postulated that this type of disorder was caused by the "failure of the hypothalamic–pituitary nervous pathways to release luteinizing hormone from the anterior pituitary.[11] Over the past 10 years, many clinical studies have confirmed this notion.[12–14] In general, these

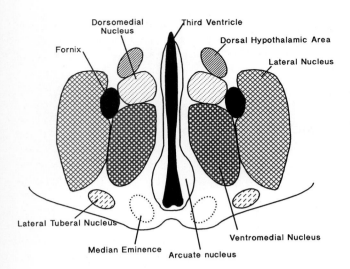

Figure 16–1. Coronal view of the neuroanatomic relationships between the arcuate nucleus, median eminence, third ventricle, and other hypothalamic nuclei.

TABLE 16–1. CLASSIFICATION OF ANOVULATION CAUSED BY THE CNS HYPOTHALAMIC-PITUITARY SYSTEM

Functional Hypothalamic Anovulation
- Psychogenic or stress factors
- Nutritional factors
- Exercise-related factors

Physiologic Anovulation
- Prepubertal phase
- Postpartum phase

Pharmacologic-Induced Anovulation
- Dopaminergic antagonist
- Opiate agonist

Psychiatric-Associated Disorders
- Anorexia nervosa
- Pseudocyesis

Organic Defects of the Hypothalamic–Pituitary Unit
- Isolated gonadotropin deficiency
- Kallmann syndrome
- Pituitary tumors
- Sheehan syndrome
- Pituitary apoplexy/aneurysm
- Empty sella syndrome
- Head trauma
- Inappropriate prolactin secretion
- Infection (human immunodeficiency virus, tuberculosis)
- Postirradiation effects

(Reproduced, with permission, from Liu JH, 1990.[109])

studies show that the common underlying defect is an alteration in the pulsatile secretion of GnRH-luteinizing hormone (LH). A more detailed evaluation of patients presenting with this type of disorder has revealed that environmental factors such as malnutrition or caloric restriction, psychogenic depression or stress, excessive energy expenditure due to exercise, or combinations of these factors have preceded the onset of functional hypothalamic amenorrhea. Unfortunately, because our current culture emphasizes a lifestyle that includes a youthful appearance, slenderness, altered nutritional patterns, and exercise, the incidence of hypothalamic amenorrhea continues to increase.

Clinical and Biochemical Features of Hypothalamic Amenorrhea

Functional hypothalamic amenorrhea (HA) can be defined as the absence of menstrual cycles for more than 6 mo without evidence of anatomic or organic abnormalities. It must be emphasized that functional hypothalamic amenorrhea is considered a diagnosis of exclusion. There are other more serious organic disorders that can mimic HA (eg, isolated gonadotropin deficiency; Table 16–1). Therefore, a careful and complete diagnostic evaluation should be performed in patients before this diagnosis can be established.

Most individuals with this disorder have a prior history of a normal onset of menarche with regular menstrual cycles between 26 and 35 days in duration. A typical profile of these women shows that they are highly motivated, intelligent, involved in high-stress occupations, and usually are thin or of normal body weight (Table 16–2). A careful, structured interview may reveal a variety of emotional crises or stressful events (eg, di-

vorce, death of a friend) preceding the onset of amenorrhea. During the interview, additional environmental and interpersonal factors may become evident including academic pressure, social maladjustment, and psychosexual problems. The evaluation should also review the patient's current lifestyle including dietary habits, type and intensity of exercise, and the use of sedatives and hypnotics.

A thorough physical examination should be performed to exclude galactorrhea, thyroid enlargement, and evidence of excessive androgen secretion (eg, hirsutism). These women should have normal secondary sexual characteristics. On pelvic examination, there may be thinning of the vaginal mucosa, scant or absent cervical mucus, and a normal size or small uterus. Despite findings of hypoestrogenic changes in the genital tract, these patients do not usually complain of hot flashes.

Initial laboratory testing should include LH, FSH, prolactin (PRL), and TSH. In general, most of the other

TABLE 16–2. CLINICAL FEATURES OF WOMEN WITH PSYCHOGENIC HYPOTHALAMIC AMENORRHEA

Single marital status
Involved in professional occupations or highly intelligent
Obsessive–compulsive habits
History of significant stressful life events
Tendency to consume sedatives or hypnotic drugs
Normal or slightly underweight
History of prior menstrual irregularities
History of sexual abuse

TABLE 16–3. SERUM HORMONAL PARAMETERS IN FUNCTIONAL HYPOTHALAMIC AMENORRHEA

	Hypothalamic Amenorrhea	Early Follicular Phase
LH (IU/L)	8.5 ± 1.1[a]	11.6 ± 1.2
FSH (IU/L)	9.3 ± 0.5[a]	12.1 ± 1.0
PRL (μg/L)	12.2 ± 0.8[b]	17.1 ± 1.4
TSH (μU/L)	1.05 ± 0.33	1.33 ± 0.26
GH (μg/L)	6.7 ± 1.3	4.2 ± 0.7
Estradiol (pmol/L)	142 ± 15	156 ± 10
ACTH (pmol/L)	1.2 ± 0.2	1.3 ± 0.2
Cortisol (nmol/L)	230 ± 10[b]	170 ± 10
Testosterone (nmol/L)	1.1 ± 0.2	0.9 ± 0.1
T3 (nmol/L)	1.19 ± 0.07[a]	1.48 ± 0.09
T4 (nmol/L)	59.2 ± 4.4[a]	79.8 ± 5.1

[a] $P < .05$
[b] $P < .01$

(Data derived from Berga et al, 1989,[16] and Suh et al, 1988.[32])

pituitary hormones appear to be in the normal range (Table 16–3). The progestin challenge test (medroxyprogesterone acetate 10 mg for 7 to 10 days) will show an absence of withdrawal uterine bleeding in most patients. This confirms that there is scant or absent estrogenic effect in the endometrium, because circulating estradiol levels are typically in the low or early follicular phase range (Table 16–3). To exclude an occult pituitary lesion, it would be prudent to perform radiographic imaging (computerized tomography or magnetic resonance imaging) of the sella turcica and adjacent structures.

GnRH-LH Secretion in Hypothalamic Amenorrhea

The major defect in patients with functional HA is a failure of the H-P axis to increase gonadotropin output in the presence of severe hypoestrogenism. There is now convincing evidence by several research groups that there is a slowing in the frequency of pulsatile GnRH-LH secretion which is the basic underlying cause of decreased ovarian function in women with HA.[14–16] In these studies, frequent peripheral blood samples (every 5 to 20 min) are obtained to quantitate the episodic secretion of LH to provide an indirect assessment of endogenous GnRH secretion. These studies make the assumption that only GnRH is capable of stimulating pituitary LH secretion and that there is a close correlation between GnRH and LH secretion, as demonstrated previously in several animal models.[17,18]

Examples of the types of LH secretory patterns are shown in Figure 16–2A to C. There is considerable variability in the amplitude and frequency of pulsatile LH secretion. Compared with the follicular phase of the menstrual cycle (Fig 16–2D), these LH secretory patterns are characterized by abnormalities in LH frequency, amplitude, and in some cases, a regression to a

pubertal pattern.[14,15] These LH patterns also suggest that GnRH pulsatile secretion is not altered to the same degree in each individual. During the recovery phase of HA, a reversal of the GnRH-LH secretory pattern is often present, characterized by a sleep-associated increase in LH amplitude (Fig 16–2C).

The pituitary gland's ability to synthesize and release LH and FSH does not appear to be compromised in patients with HA. GnRH stimulation tests show a variable response in HA and LH and FSH responses can be absent, normal, or supranormal.[12,19] With intravenous pulsatile GnRH administration, normal levels of LH and FSH can be restored. The normal positive LH feedback response to estrogen appears blunted or absent in these patients. Taken together, it appears that pituitary sensitivity is not impaired and the deficiency in gonadotropin secretion is due to a relative deficiency in endogenous GnRH secretion.

Role of Opioidergic, Dopaminergic, and Excitatory Amino Acids on GnRH Secretion

Several major neurotransmitter systems that secrete norepinephrine, dopamine, and serotonin have been shown to modulate GnRH or LH release in animal studies.[20] The disruption of normal menstrual cycles in patients on phenothiazines (dopamine antagonists), sedatives, antidepressants, and stimulants provides circumstantial evidence that interference with these neuronal systems can alter GnRH release in the human. From these observations, it appears that activation of the noradrenergic neurons principally stimulates release of GnRH,[7,21] while dopaminergic and serotonergic neurons can stimulate or inhibit GnRH-LH secretion.[20,22–24]

Recently, excitatory amino acids such as aspartate and glutamate have been localized in large concentrations in presynaptic locations of hypothalamus nucleus such as the arcuate nucleus,[25] which has been implicated in a regulatory role for GnRH secretion in monkeys primarily during puberty.[26] Because of obvious experimental limitations in the human, it is difficult to directly ascertain which neurotransmitter systems are involved in the suppression of gonadotropin secretion. Most studies have utilized administration of a variety of neuropharmacologic agents as probes to determine if GnRH-LH secretion can be normalized. Using this indirect approach, Quigley and coworkers administered the dopamine receptor antagonist metaclopramide to patients with HA to block the action of dopamine.[27] Following metaclopramide injection, there was a prompt increase in LH secretion. Studies such as these suggest that, in some patients with hypothalamic amenorrhea, there is enhanced dopaminergic activity.

The endogenous opioid peptides are another neurotransmitter system that has known inhibitory effects on GnRH secretion.[28,29] Three major classes of opioidergic

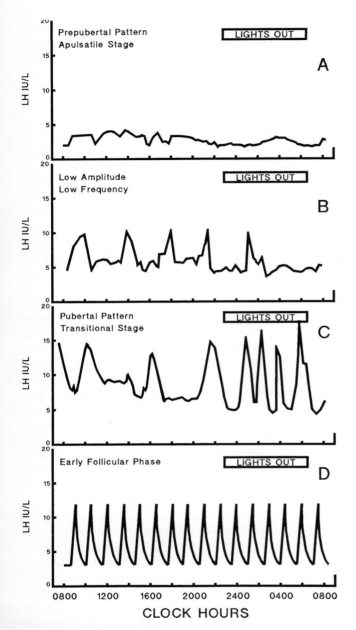

Figure 16–2. Examples of the varying pulsatile pattern of LH secretion in women with hypothalamic amenorrhea and during the early follicular phase of the menstrual cycle. *(Modified, with permission, from Liu, 1990.[109])*

TABLE 16–4. OTHER NEUROENDOCRINE ABNORMALITIES IN HYPOTHALAMIC AMENORRHEA

Increased amplitude and duration of nocturnal melatonin secretion
Increased nocturnal secretion of growth hormone
Increased daytime cortisol secretion
Decreased 24-hr PRL secretion with exaggerated nocturnal elevation
Blunted elevation in PRL, ACTH, and cortisol during the noon meal
Elevation of CRH levels in cerebral spinal fluid

(Modified, with permission, from Liu, 1990.[109])

are found in the GI tract, placenta, adrenal medulla, and brain, the highest concentrations are found in the hypothalamus and pituitary gland.

The inhibitory effects of opiate peptides on GnRH and LH secretion can be demonstrated in several ways. Injection of morphine, a potent opiate agonist, will rapidly reduce depolarization of GnRH neurons and reduce LH secretion.[8,9] In individuals with HA, blockade of endogenous opiate receptors by the antagonist naloxone causes an increase in the frequency and amplitude of pulsatile LH release.[27,30] If the activity of the opiate system is blocked by long-term treatment with the opiate receptor antagonist naltrexone in HA patients, there is a resumption of gonadotropin secretion and a return of ovulatory function in some patients.[31] Collectively, these studies suggest that there is an overall increase in endogenous opiate activity, which can reduce pulsatile GnRH secretion in HA. Because the dopaminergic and opioidergic neuronal systems are also involved in hypothalamic and suprahypothalamic function including temperature regulation, pain perception, and mood, and regulate other hypothalamic hormones, it is not surprising that the secretion of other hormones such as growth hormone, prolactin, ACTH, cortisol, and melatonin is altered in women with hypothalamic amenorrhea (Tables 16–3 and 16–4).[19,32]

Stress and Reproductive Dysfunction

Chronic exposure to stress has been reported to disrupt reproductive function in both animal species and humans.[11,13,33] According to Selye's original observations, the stress response is characterized by activation of the hypophyseal–adrenocortical axis.[34] In women with HA, there is evidence that suggests that "stressors" such as exercise or psychogenic stress can chronically activate the hypothalamic–pituitary–adrenal (HPA) axis. These women have significant elevations in daytime cortisol levels, a delay or absent response in ACTH, cortisol secretion during the noon meal, and a blunted pituitary response to corticotropin-releasing hormone (CRH).[19,32] On a neuroendocrine basis, the stress response is associated with an increased secretion of CRH, ACTH, cortisol, PRL, oxytocin, vasopressin, epinephrine, and norephinephrine.[35]

peptides have been identified: endorphins, enkephalins, and dynorphins. Each group of peptides is derived from a larger precursor protein, which is enzymatically cleaved to yield smaller biologically active peptides. For example, pro-opiomelanocortin is the precursor peptide for the opiate peptides β-endorphin, β-lipotropin, α-MSH, and corticotropin (ACTH). Met-enkephalin, leu-enkephalin, and the dynorphins are derived from proenkephalin A and proenkephalin B, respectively. Although opiate peptides

Potential Mechanism(s) for Hypothalamic Amenorrhea

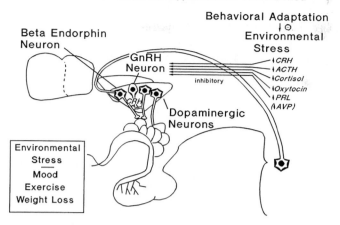

Figure 16–3. Proposed mechanisms by which environmental stressors activate stress response hormones that can directly inhibit GnRH neurons, or active the opioidergic system to indirectly inhibit GnRH neuronal activity.

These effects on the reproductive axis by the HPA axis appear to be mediated at several levels, and are summarized in Figure 16–3. In rats and monkeys, CRH administration has been shown to inhibit GnRH-LH secretion in vivo[36–38] and in vitro[29] at the hypothalamic level. This inhibitory effect can be prevented by the co-administration of a CRH receptor antagonist or reversed by the opiate receptor antagonist naloxone, which suggests that the action of CRH is mediated in part by activation of the opioidergic system. In addition, another stress hormone, oxytocin, can also inhibit hypothalamic GnRH secretion.[39] At the pituitary level the administration of ACTH can suppress pituitary response to GnRH in vitro[40,41] and in vivo.[42] Thus, chronic activation of the HPA axis appears to be the functional neuroendocrine link between environmental stresses and the induction of ovulatory dysfunction and amenorrhea.

Management of Hypothalamic Amenorrhea

Because of the functional nature of HA, the clinical evaluation should focus on a carefully conducted interview that examines lifestyle variables and interpersonal relationships. Significant organic disease (eg, hyperprolactinemia, hypothalamic lesions, partial hypopituitarism) must be excluded. For many patients, spontaneous recovery of menstrual function will take place after a modification of lifestyle, psychological guidance, or accommodation to environmental stress.[13] For this reason, individualized and expectant management should be the initial approach. For individuals who remain amenorrheic, periodic assessment of reproductive status (every 4 to 6 mo) would be prudent.

For those women with persistent anovulation greater than 1 yr, a major concern is the long-term effect of hypoestrogenism, especially on bone metabolism. Presently, there is very little epidemiologic information with regard to fracture risks and benefits of hormone replacement in this group of women.[43–45] Based on studies in reproductive-aged women who have been ovariectomized or who have undergone treatment with GnRH agonist for endometriosis, bone density would be expected to decrease between 7 and 10 percent during the first 3 yr of amenorrhea.[46] Because these patients are often reluctant to take medications, serial bone density studies such as dual-energy x-ray absorptiometry (DEXA) of the lumbar vertebrae (Ll–L4) may be necessary to convince them of the necessity to begin estrogen replacement therapy.[47] The minimal estrogen replacement doses necessary to conserve bone density (0.625 mg of conjugated estrogen or 1 mg micronized estradiol) have been established primarily in menopausal women. Estrogen therapy should be used in combination with a progestin for 12 to 14 days to ensure that the endometrium is shed regularly and adequately (see Chap 38).

For women who desire fertility, a trial of clomiphene citrate is indicated. Because clomiphene citrate can exert weak estrogenic properties in a hypoestrogenic environment,[48] lower doses of clomiphene (25 mg/day for 5 days) should be used initially. In some patients, higher doses of clomiphene (>100 mg/day) may exert a paradoxic effect and suppress the H-P axis. In women failing to respond to clomiphene, the most physiologic approach is ovulation induction with pulsatile GnRH. Because the primary underlying defect in hypothalamic amenorrhea is decreased endogenous GnRH secretion, this approach could be viewed as a form of "physiologic" replacement therapy. For women with HA, a starting intravenous dose of GnRH of 5 μg/90 min has been shown to be effective.[49,50] Monitoring of serum estradiol levels or follicular development can be minimized because ovarian follicular response and gonadotropin output mimic the natural menstrual cycle (Fig 16–4). In these patients, the corpus luteum function can be supported by either continuation of pulsatile GnRH or human chorionic gonadotropin, 1500 units intramuscularly every 3 days for four doses. Using the intravenous mode of GnRH treatment in HA patients, ovulation rates of approximately 90 percent, conception rates up to 30 percent per ovulatory cycle, and hyperstimulation rates of less than 1 percent have been reported.[51–53]

Anorexia Nervosa and Bulimia

Anorexia nervosa is a psychosomatic disorder characterized by the triad of extreme weight loss (weight decrease of greater than 25 percent of original body

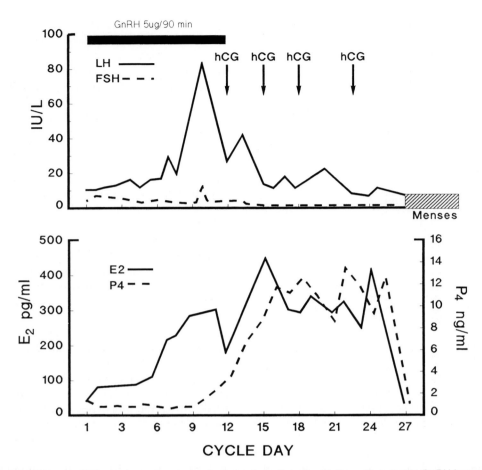

Figure 16–4. LH, FSH, estradiol, and progesterone levels during induction of ovulation with pulsatile GnRH in a patient with hypothalamic amenorrhea. For luteal phase support, human chorionic gonadotropin (hCG) 1500 units intramuscularly, is administered every 3 days for four doses. *(Modified, with permission, from Liu, 1990.[109])*

weight), body-image disturbance, and an intense fear of becoming obese.[54] Bulimia is a related disorder characterized by alternating episodes of consumption of large quantities of food over a short time interval (binge eating) followed by periods of food restriction, self-induced vomiting, or excessive use of laxatives or diuretics.[55] Approximately 90 to 95 percent of anorectic and bulimic patients are female. Demographically, these patients tend to be Caucasians and are from middle-class or upper-middle-class families. The incidence of anorexia has been estimated to range from 0.64 per 100,000 to 1.12 per 100,000.[56,57] Bulimic behavior appears much more prevalent, with an estimated incidence of 4.5 to 18 percent among high school and college students. Clinical symptoms of bulimia nervosa as defined by DSM-IV criteria occur much less frequently and are present in approximately 1 to 2 percent of the female population.[58] Anorexia patients are usually between 12 yr of age and the mid-30s, with a bimodal age of onset at 13 to 14 yr and 17 to 18 yr. Bulimia usually begins at a later age between 17 and 25 yr. Mortality associated with

anorexia nervosa has been reported to be as high as 9 percent. Generally, this is secondary to cardiac arrhythmia, which may be precipitated by diminished heart muscle mass and associated electrolyte abnormalities.[59,60] In addition, suicide has been reported in 2 to 5 percent of patients with chronic anorexia nervosa.[61] Thus, it is important for the clinician to screen for early signs of this disorder so that appropriate intervention and treatment can be instituted.

The clinical manifestations of anorexia nervosa and bulimia are shown in Tables 16–5 and 16–6. From a neuroendocrine perspective, gonadotropin secretion in anorectics exhibit a prepubertal pattern (Figs 16–2A, B) that is similar to other forms of severe hypothalamic amenorrhea. Anorectic patients with intermediate degrees of weight recovery can display transitional patterns of LH secretion and may have normal or supranormal responses to GnRH. Unfortunately, despite restoration to normal body weight, anovulation can persist in up to 50 percent of anorectic patients. As in other forms of hypothalamic amenorrhea, both anorectic and bulimic pa-

TABLE 16–5. CLINICAL FEATURES OF ANOREXIA NERVOSA

Amenorrhea
Constipation, decreased gastric emptying
Preoccupation with handling of food
Bulimic behavior
Hypothermia with defective thermoregulation
Mild bradycardia, cardiac arrhythmia
Hypotension
Hypokalemia secondary to diuretic or laxative abuse
Coarse, dry skin
Soft, lanugo-type hair
Increased serum beta-carotene levels
Hyperactivity
Distortion of body self-image
Obsessive compulsive personality
Increased incidence of past sexual abuse
Osteopenia
Elevated hepatic enzymes
Anemia, leukopenia

TABLE 16–6. CLINICAL MANIFESTATIONS OF BULIMIA

Menstrual irregularities
Parotid gland enlargement
Acute gastric dilatation or rupture
Esophageal rupture
Hypokalemia
Ipecac poisoning
Aspiration pneumonia
Dental enamel erosion

tients exhibit hyperactivation of the HPA axis. Although the diurnal variation is maintained, there is a persistent hypersecretion of cortisol throughout the day (Fig 16–5).[62] Despite the increased cortisol production, peripheral effects of hypercortisolism are not present due to reduced cellular glucocorticoid receptors.[63] The decrease in glucocorticoid receptors may also provide an explanation for the incomplete suppression of the pituitary–adrenal axis by dexamethasone.[64] Pituitary responses to CRH are blunted in both anorectics and bulimics, suggesting that the hypercortisolism in these patients reflects a defect at or above the hypothalamus.[65] Adrenal DHEA secretion is also significantly reduced and is similar if not identical to prepubertal concentrations in anorectic patients (Fig 16–5).

To maintain homeostasis during this interval of reduced caloric intake, basal metabolism is decreased because peripheral conversion of thyroxine to triiodothyronine is decreased. Instead, thyroxine is converted via an alternative pathway to reverse triiodothyronine, a relative inactive isoform. This shift in thyroid function resembles that seen in severely ill patients and during starvation.[67] Anorectics also have partial diabetes insipidus and are unable to appropriately concentrate urine due to the impaired secretion of vasopressin.[68] Other clinical and endocrine manifestations are listed in Table 16–7.

As with other forms of hypothalamic amenorrhea, patients with anorexia nervosa have evidence for increased central opioid activity. Cerebrospinal fluid β-endorphin levels are elevated in severe anorectics.[69] During the recovery phase, LH is released in response to administration of the opiate receptor antagonist naloxone.[70] Even more intriguing is the link between opioids and control of appetite. Administration of β-endorphin intraventricularly into the hypothalamus stimulates eating behavior,[71] while naloxone suppresses feeding behavior in obese patients.[71,72] These observations collectively suggest that increased endogenous opiate activity may modulate abnormal eating behavior.[73]

Treatment modalities for anorexia nervosa and bulimia have low success rates and remain a therapeutic

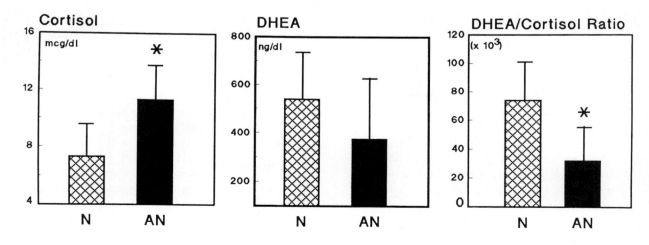

Figure 16–5. Comparison of the 24-hr mean levels ± SD of cortisol, DHEA, and DHEA/cortisol ratio in women with anorexia nervosa and normal eumenorrheic women. *(Data from Zumoff et al, 1983.[66])*

TABLE 16–7. NEUROENDOCRINE ABNORMALITIES IN ANOREXIA NERVOSA

Decrease in GnRH-LH pulse frequency and amplitude
Low serum LH and FSH levels
Increased ACTH secretion
Impaired ACTH response to CRH stimulation test
Increased urinary free cortisol
Resistance to dexamethasone suppression
Low or normal serum PRL levels
Impaired TSH response to TRH
Low or normal TSH levels associated with normal T_4
Low T_3 associated with high reverse T_3
Partial diabetes insipidus
Elevated resting GH
Decrease in IGF-1 levels

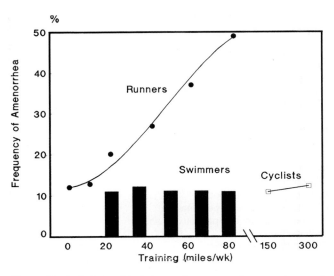

Figure 16–6. Relationship between frequency of amenorrhea and training intensity in women athletes participating in three aerobic type sports. *(Modified from Sanborn et al, 1982.[10])*

challenge. The most accepted approaches include individual psychotherapy, group therapy, and behavior modification.[74,75] At the present time, there are no large control studies that compare the efficacy of these treatments. Psychiatric consultation and follow-up is indicated in all patients with eating disorders to assist in differential diagnosis and treatment planning. A team of clinicians including a psychiatrist and a general medicine specialist with special expertise in eating disorders would be desirable. In those patients who weigh less than 75 percent of their ideal body weight, aggressive in-hospital treatment is recommended. Despite a return to normal weight, up to 50 percent of patients will have persistent amenorrhea. Significant clinical consequences of anorexia nervosa include estrogen deficiency, associated osteoporosis,[76,77] and generalized effects of malnutrition. For these individuals, estrogen replacement therapy is definitely indicated.

Exercise-Induced Hypothalamic Amenorrhea

With the increasing numbers of women participating in sports, it has become apparent that regular strenuous exercise can lead to menstrual disturbances, a delay in menarche, luteal phase dysfunction, and secondary amenorrhea. In ballet dancers, the pubertal progression and onset of menarche has been reported to be delayed in up to 30 percent of girls and occurs at a mean age of 15 yr. Advancement of pubertal stages seems to coincide with times of prolonged rest or following recovery from an injury.[78–80]

The incidence of menstrual dysfunction seems to vary depending on the type of sports. The psychological stress of competition may play a contributory role because the incidence of amenorrhea is higher in competitive athletes. Activities associated with an increased frequency of reproductive dysfunction are those that favor a slimmer, lower body weight physique and include middle and long distance running, gymnastics, and ballet dancing (Fig 16–6). In runners, the frequency of amenor-

rhea approaches 50 percent for those who run more than 70 miles per wk.[10] In contrast, competitive cyclists have much lower rates of amenorrhea (10 to 12 percent) despite a doubling of their training mileage. In competitive swimmers, 82 percent had menstrual irregularities after menarche with a longer duration of irregular cycles.[81] The overall incidence of amenorrhea tends to increase as athletes lose body weight or experience a decrease in total body fat (Fig 16–7). Observations such as these have led Frisch and others to postulate that there is a critical threshold in body fat composition that is required for normal menstrual function.[82]

Bullen and co-workers were able to experimentally induce menstrual dysfunction by the imposition of strenuous aerobic exercise (running 4 to 10 miles/day) combined with caloric restriction in untrained women.[83] In runners, a variety of menstrual abnormalities have been described[19] including luteal phase dysfunction,[84] a loss of the midcycle LH surge,[19] prolonged menstrual cycles,[19] altered patterns of gonadotropin secretion,[84,85] and amenorrhea.[83] These progressive changes reflect the spectrum of abnormalities that can be expected in athletic women who exercise to a significant degree.

Like anorexia nervosa, it is well known that acute exercise activates the HPA axis.[86] Carefully designed studies in trained women runners also suggest that the HPA activity can be chronically elevated. In these athletes, there is evidence for persistent, mild hypercortisolism and a blunted pituitary response to CRH. Because elevations in central CRH or peripheral cortisol levels can disrupt pulsatile LH secretion,[33] one might speculate that the severity of menstrual abnormalities may reflect

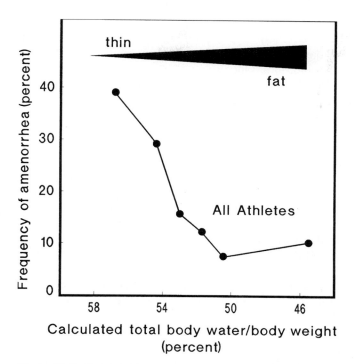

Figure 16–7. Relationship between frequency of amenorrhea and percent calculated water weight in women athletes. *(Modified from Sanborn et al, 1982.[10])*

the degree to which the HPA axis is activated by exercise in athletic women (see Fig 16–3).

Plasma met-enkephalin and β-endorphin levels have been observed to increase before and after strenuous exercise.[87] Such an increase in endogenous opioid release may account for the "runner's high" that is described by some exercise enthusiasts.[88] Whether central opioidergic activity is also elevated and can contribute to the reduction in GnRH-LH secretion in women with exercise-related amenorrhea remains to be demonstrated.

Treatment of amenorrhea should focus on counseling the patient to decrease her exercise level, alter the type and duration of exercise, and to gain weight.[89] Significant osteopenia usually affecting trabecular bone has been reported in amenorrheic athletes.[44] The loss in bone density is secondary to chronic hypoestrogenism, and apparently nullifies the beneficial effects of weight-bearing types of exercise in strengthening and remodeling bone.[90] Amenorrheic athletes remain at risk for stress fractures, especially in the weight-bearing areas such as the lower extremities. If lifestyle changes are not feasible, serious consideration should be given to starting these individuals on long-term hormone replacement.

Pseudocyesis

Pseudocyesis represents a classic example of a psychoneuroendocrine disorder that disrupts the menstrual cycle. This term was introduced by John Good and is derived from the Greek terms (*pseudes,* "false," and *kyesis,* "pregnancy"). This disorder has also been called "imaginary or phantom" pregnancy and is characterized by subjective symptoms of pregnancy including amenorrhea or oligomenorrhea, morning sickness, an increase in abdominal girth secondary to fat deposition or accumulation of intestinal gas, enlargement of the breasts, pigmentation and increases in the nipple areolae, galactorrhea, and softening of the cervix with congestion.[91] These patients also have hormonal abnormalities including hypersecretion of PRL, increased LH levels, and reduced FSH levels.[92]

The psychogenic nature of this disorder becomes obvious when there is a spontaneous resolution of this process at the time the diagnosis is revealed to the patient. These patients should be under the care of a psychiatrist because there are often underlying emotional problems or a significant depression that can lead to suicidal attempts.

MISCELLANEOUS CAUSES OF HYPOTHALAMIC AND PITUITARY CHRONIC HYPOFUNCTION

Isolated Gonadotropin Deficiency

One disorder that shares many of the biochemical features with functional hypothalamic amenorrhea is Kallmann syndrome or isolated gonadotropin deficiency (IGD). IGD is characterized by a decrease or absence of secretion of endogenous GnRH, leading to hypogonadotropic hypogonadism, eunuchoid features, incomplete development of secondary sexual characteristics, primary amenorrhea, and in some cases anosmia.[93,94] This disorder can be inherited as an autosomal dominant pattern. The defect is due to a failure of GnRH neurons to form completely in the medial olfactory placode or to migrate from the olfactory bulb to the medial basal hypothalamus during embryogenesis. In some individuals with this disorder, the anosmia or hypo-osmia is associated with hypoplasia of the olfactory bulbs, which is evident on magnetic resonance scan.[95]

The baseline gonadotropin levels in this disorder are in the low or normal range and are similar to those in patients with other forms of HA. Levels of other pituitary hormones such as GH, TSH, PRL, and ACTH are also in the normal range. Because these patients fail to undergo gonarche and have prepubertal levels of sex steroids during pubertal maturation, closure of the epiphyseal plates of the long bones is delayed, resulting in a eunuchoid habitus (arm span > height). Not uncommonly, patients will be treated with exogenous sex steroids such as birth control pills prior to a complete evaluation. This can induce a partial or even a complete development of the normal female secondary sex characteristics; however, breast development is usually incomplete (Tanner stage III) and will be delayed in comparison to pubic hair development (Tanner stage IV or V). Provocative testing with exogenous GnRH will yield highly variable LH responses (Fig 16–8) dependent on the degree of endogenous GnRH deficiency.[96,97] However, if pulsatile GnRH is given for 7 to 10 days intravenously (priming effect of GnRH), gonadotropin responses will become similar to eumenorrheic women.

The treatment goal of individuals with IGD is to induce the completion of pubertal development and provide continued estrogen replacement until pregnancy is desired. Estrogen treatment should be started at lower doses (100 ng/kg/day of ethinyl estradiol). Patients should be evaluated on a 2- or 3-mo basis to determine the rate

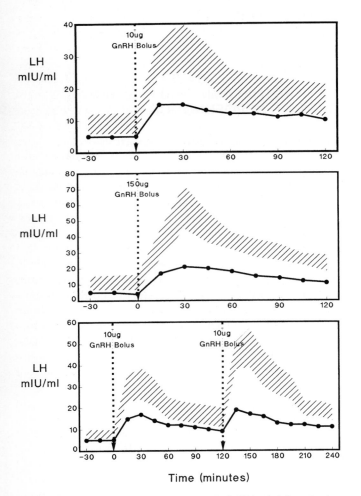

Figure 16–8. LH responses to exogenous GnRH administration in patients with isolated gonadotropin deficiency at two different doses and during two sequential GnRH boluses. The stippled areas represent the 95 percent confidence limit of normal responses. *(Modified from Sanborn et al, 1982.[10])*

of growth and development. The addition of a progestin such as medroxyprogesterone acetate 10 mg/day for 12 days should then be instituted to stabilize and shed the endometrium. Once secondary sexual characteristics are completely developed, maintenance doses of estrogen (2 mg micronized estradiol or 0.625 to 1.25 mg conjugated estrogens given daily) with 12 days of progestin each mo can be utilized. If fertility is desired, ovulation induction with pulsatile GnRH would be the most sensible choice (Fig 16–4). Although human menopausal gonadotropins are equally efficacious, this approach exposes the patient to the unnecessary risk of multiple births and ovarian hyperstimulation syndrome.

Sheehan Syndrome (Postpartum Pituitary Necrosis)

The onset of postpartum pituitary necrosis constitutes a potentially life-threatening endocrine emergency. Autopsy studies of obstetric patients who die between 12 hr and 35 days following delivery reveal that approximately 25 percent are found to have necrosis of the anterior pituitary. The most complete description of this disorder is attributed to Sheehan,[98] although Simmonds was the first to report this condition.

In almost all cases, pituitary necrosis is preceded by a history of massive obstetric hemorrhage characterized by severe circulatory collapse, hypotension, and shock. Since the pituitary gland enlarges during pregnancy, severe hypotension predisposes the pituitary to a greater risk of ischemia. Sheehan hypothesized that hypotension led to an occlusive spasm of the arteries that supply the anterior pituitary and stalk. When arteriospasm subsides, blood flows into the damaged vessels, resulting in further stasis and thrombosis. Autopsy studies often reveal a variable degree of pituitary necrosis.[99] However, the exact pathogenesis remains to be determined.

The spectrum of clinical manifestations can range from partial deficiency of one or two pituitary hormones and accompanied amenorrhea to panhypopituitarism.[100] The posterior pituitary is usually not compromised because its blood supply is less dependent on portal vasculature. Most patients present with an absence of postpartum breast engorgement and failure to lactate due to deficient PRL secretion. More severe damage to the anterior pituitary may result in hypoadrenalism with symptoms of hypotension, nausea, vomiting, lethargy, and asthenia. Later, signs of hypothyroidism may appear with a failure to resume normal menstrual cycles. Because of the variable extent of pituitary necrosis, there are isolated case reports that document return of fertility in several patients.[101]

To evaluate pituitary reserve, provocative testing should be performed utilizing TRH, GnRH, GRH, and CRH.[102] The latter two hypothalamic neuropeptides may not be readily available at all centers. However, pituitary ACTH reserve can be determined with either metyrapone or the insulin tolerance test (see Chaps 14 and 18).

Once the pituitary deficiencies have been characterized, long-term treatment is aimed at replacing the target gland hormones. In the patient presenting with symptoms of severe hypocortisolism, the immediate administration of glucocorticoids is essential. Cortisone acetate 100 mg IM or its equivalent should be used. Once the patient has been stabilized, maintenance doses of cortisone acetate, 15 to 25 mg/day or prednisone 5 mg/day, can be given. During times of increasing metabolic stress (infection, trauma, surgery), a doubling or tripling of the daily dose is indicated.

In patients with hypothyroidism, thyroid hormone replacement should be given as thyroxine (T_4) 50 µg/day, and gradually increased by 50 µg increments at 1 to 3 wk intervals until full replacement doses (0.10 to 0.20 mg) are achieved. Estrogen replacement therapy should be instituted to prevent bone mineral loss and genital atrophy. In women desiring further childbearing, ovulation induction will require human menopausal gonadotropins.

Pituitary Apoplexy

Pituitary apoplexy is a disorder characterized by acute hemorrhagic infarction of the pituitary gland.[103,104] Typically, the patient will complain of a sudden onset of a severe retro-orbital headache, visual and pupillary disturbances, and depressed sensorium, followed by loss of consciousness. These symptoms may simulate other neurologic disorders such as basilar artery occlusion, hypertensive encephalopathy, or cavernous sinus thrombosis. CT or MRI imaging will usually reveal hemorrhagic changes in the pituitary area. In some cases emergency surgical decompression may be required. This disorder seems to occur with greater frequency with GH or ACTH-producing adenomas and other pituitary tumors.[105] Because of the high likelihood of multiple deficits in anterior pituitary function, evaluation of these deficits should be carried out with provocative testing of pituitary function as described in the previous section. Management would be based on the respective pituitary deficiencies.

Posttraumatic Hypopituitarism

Severe head trauma usually as a result of a sudden deceleration of the head in a traffic accident can result in pituitary or hypothalamic damage and a partial or complete transection of the pituitary stalk. There may also be an associated basal skull fracture and a prolonged period of unconsciousness. Although there is usually a delay of months to years from injury to presentation, these individuals will often manifest partial or panhypopituitarism. Diabetes insipidus may be present and PRL levels may

be greatly elevated.[106] The most common initial symptoms are those of hypogonadism, amenorrhea, loss of pubic and axillary hair, anorexia, weight loss, and galactorrhea. In the initial evaluation of these patients, the most important axis to consider is the pituitary–adrenal axis, since glucocorticoid deficiency has potentially fatal consequences. The evaluation and management of these patients are similar to those described for Sheehan syndrome.

Radiation-Induced Hypopituitarism

Patients who have received conventional or supervoltage radiotherapy for head tumors such as craniopharyngiomas, GH adenomas, ACTH-producing adenomas, and nasopharyngeal carcinoma are at increased risk for delayed development of hypopituitarism.[107] Serial endocrine studies suggest that there are differences in pituitary and hypothalamic cell sensitivity to radiation. In most cases, there is a gradual and progressive loss in gonadotropin function followed by corticotropin and thyrotropin function. In one study by Lam and co-workers, impaired gonadotropin secretion was evident in some patients within 1 yr after radiotherapy.[108] Serum PRL levels can become significantly elevated. For this reason, periodic assessment of hypothalamic–pituitary function must be carried out for an indefinite time period. Selective replacement of target tissue hormones such as estrogen, cortisol, and thyroid should be instituted when dynamic pituitary testing reveals a compromise in hypothalamic–pituitary function.

SUMMARY

Because the control of the menstrual cycle resides at the hypothalamic level, it is not surprising that an individual's perception of environmental stressors, a suprahypothalamic process, can lead to functional disruption of reproductive function. Limited studies suggest that these stressors can chronically activate the HPA axis, increase the activity of the endogenous opioidergic system, and ultimately reduce the secretion of GnRH. For individuals with organic central lesions, disruption of pulsatile GnRH secretion either directly or through other mechanism(s) will induce menstrual abnormalities and reproductive dysfunction.[109]

REFERENCES

1. Barry J. Characterization and topography of LHRH neurons in the human brain. *Neurosci Lett.* 3:287, 1976
2. Barry J. Immunofluorescence study for LRF neurons in man. *Cell Tiss Res.* 181:1, 1977

3. King JC, Anthony ELP. LHRH neurons and their projections in humans and other mammals. *Peptides.* 5(suppl.): 195, 1984

4. Bergland RM, Page RB. Can the pituitary secrete directly to the brain? (Affirmative anatomical evidence). *Endocrinology.* 102:1325, 1978

5. Knobil E. Patterns of hormonal signals and action. *N Engl J Med.* 305:1582, 1981

6. Kessner JS, Kaufman J, Wilson RC, et al. On the short-loop feedback regulation of the hypothalamic luteinizing hormone releasing hormone "pulse generator" in the rhesus monkey. *Neuroendocrinology.* 42:109, 1986

7. Wilson RC, Kesner JS, Kaufman JM, et al. Central electrophysiologic correlates of pulsatile luteinizing hormone secretion in the rhesus monkey. *Neuroendocrinology.* 39:256, 1984

8. Kesner JS, Kaufman J, Wilson RC, et al. The effect of morphine on the electrophysiological activity of the hypothalamic luteinizing hormone-releasing hormone pulse generator in the rhesus monkey. *Neuroendocrinology.* 43:686, 1986

9. Williams CL, Nishihara M, Thalabard JC, et al. Duration and frequency of multiunit electrical activity associated with the hypothalamic gonadotropin releasing hormone pulse generator in the rhesus monkey: Differential effects of morphine. *Neuroendocrinology.* 52:225, 1990

10. Sanborn CF, Martin BJ, Wagner WW. Is athletic amenorrhea specific to runners? *Am J Obstet Gynecol.* 143:859, 1982

11. Klinefelter HF Jr, Albright F, Griswold GC. Experience with a quantitative test for normal or decreased amounts of follicle-stimulating hormone in urine in endocrinological diagnosis. *J Clin Endocrinol Metab.* 3:529, 1943

12. Yen SSC, Rebar RW, Vandenberg G. Hypothalamic amenorrhea and hypogonadotropinism: Responses to synthetic LRF. *J Clin Endocrinol Metab.* 36:811, 1973

13. Lachelin GCL, Yen SSC. Hypothalamic chronic anovulation. *Am J Obstet Gynecol.* 130:825, 1978

14. Reame NE, Sauder SE, Case GD, et al. Pulsatile gonadotropin secretion in women with hypothalamic amenorrhea: Evidence that reduced frequency of gonadotropin secretion is the mechanism of persistent anovulation. *J Clin Endocrinol Metab.* 61:851, 1985

15. Khoury KA, Reame NE, Kelch RP, Marshall JC. Diurnal patterns of pulsatile luteinizing hormone secretion in hypothalamic amenorrhea: Reproducibility and responses to opiate blockade and an alpha2-adrenergic agonist. *J Clin Endocrinol Metab.* 64:755, 1987

16. Berga S, Mortola J, Gierton L, et al. Neuroendocrine aberrations in women with functional hypothalamic amenorrhea. *J Clin Endocrinol Metab.* 68:301, 1989

17. Levine JG, Paw KF, Ramirez VD, Jackson GL. Simultaneous measurement of luteinizing-hormone-releasing hormone release in unanesthetized ovariectomized sheep. *Endocrinology.* 111:1449, 1982

18. Clarke IJ, Cummins JT. The temporal relationship between gonadotropin releasing hormone (GnRH) and luteinizing hormone (LH) secretion in ovariectomized ewes. *Endocrinology.* 111:1737, 1982

19. Loucks AB, Mortola JF, Girton L, Yen SSC. Alterations in the hypothalamic–pituitary–ovarian and the hypothalamic–pituitary–adrenal axes in athletic women. *J Clin Endocrinol Metab.* 68:402, 1989

20. Kalra SP, Kalra PS. The neural control of luteinizing hormone secretion in the rat. *Endocr Rev.* 4:311, 1983

21. Kalra SP. Catecholamine involvement in preovulatory LH release: Reassessment of the role of epinephrine. *Neuroendocrinology.* 40:139, 1985

22. Rasmussen DD. The interaction between mediobasohypothalamic dopaminergic and endorphinergic neuronal systems as a key regulator of reproduction: An hypothesis. *J Endocrinol Invest.* 14:323, 1991

23. Rasmussen DD, Liu JH, Wolf PL, Yen SSC. GnRH neurosecretion in the human hypothalamus: In vitro regulation by dopamine. *J Clin Endocrinol Metab.* 62:479, 1986

24. Rasmussen DD, Liu JH, Swartz WH, et al. Human fetal hypothalamic GnRH neurosecretion: Dopaminergic regulation in vitro. *Clin Endocrinol.* 25:127, 1986

25. Brann DW, Mahesh VB. Excitatory amino acids: Function and significance in reproduction and neuroendocrine regulation. *Front Neuroendocrinol.* 15:3, 1994

26. Mitsushima D, Marzban F, Luchansky LL, et al. Role of glutamic acid decarboxylase in the prepubertal inhibition of the luteinizing hormone releasing hormone release in female rhesus monkeys. *J Neurosci.* 16:2563, 1996

27. Quigley ME, Sheehan KL, Casper RF, Yen SSC. Evidence for increased dopaminergic and opioid activity in patients with hypothalamic hypogonadotropic amenorrhea. *J Clin Endocrinol Metab.* 50:949, 1980

28. Ropert JF, Quigley ME, Yen SSC. Endogenous opiates modulate pulsatile luteinizing hormone release in humans. *J Clin Endocrinol Metab.* 52:583, 1981

29. Gambacciani M, Yen SSC, Rasmussen DD. GnRH release from the mediobasal hypothalamus: In vitro inhibition by corticotropin-releasing factor. *Neuroendocrinology.* 43:533, 1986

30. Yen SSC, Quigley ME, Reid RL, et al. Neuroendocrinology of opioid peptides and their role in the control of gonadotropin and prolactin secretion. *Am J Obstet Gynecol.* 152:485, 1985

31. Genazzani AD, Petraglia FP, Gastaldi M, et al. Naltrexone treatment restores menstrual cycles in patients with weight loss-related amenorrhea. *Fertil Steril.* 64:951, 1995

32. Suh BY, Liu JH, Berga SL, et al. Hypercortisolism in patients with functional hypothalamic amenorrhea. *J Clin Endocrinol Metab.* 66:733, 1988

33. Rivier C, Rivier J, Vale W. Stress-induced inhibition of reproductive functions: Role of endogenous corticotropin-releasing factor. *Science.* 231:607, 1986

34. Selye H. The stress syndrome. *Nature.* 138:32, 1936

35. Gibbs DM. Dissociation of oxytocin, vasopressin, and corticotropin secretion during different types of stress. *Life Sci.* 35:487, 1984

36. Rivier C, Vale W. Influence of corticotropin-releasing factor on reproductive function in the rat. *Endocrinology.* 114:914, 1984

37. Petraglia F, Sutton S, Vale W, Plotsky P. Corticotropin-releasing factor decreases plasma luteinizing hormone levels in female rats by inhibiting gonadotropin-releasing hormone

release into hypophysial–portal circulation. *Endocrinology.* 120:1083, 1987

38. Xiao E, Luckhaus J, Niemann W, Ferin M. Acute inhibition of gonadotropin secretion by corticotropin-releasing hormone in the primate: Are the adrenal glands involved? *Endocrinology.* 124:1632, 1989

39. Gambacciani M, Yen SSC, Rasmussen DD. GnRH release from the mediobasal hypothalamus: In vitro regulation by oxytocin. *Neuroendocrinology.* 42:181, 1986

40. Matteri RL, Moberg GP, Watson JG. Adrenocorticotropin-induced changes in ovine pituitary gonadotropin secretion in vitro. *Endocrinology.* 118:2091, 1986

41. Kamel F, Kubajak CL. Modulation of gonadotropin secretion by corticosterone: Interaction with gonadal steroids and mechanism of action. *Endocrinology.* 121:561, 1987

42. Matteri RL, Watson JG, Moberg GP. Stress or acute adrenocorticotrophin treatment suppresses LHRH-induced LH release in the ram. *J Reprod Fert.* 72:385, 1984

43. Prior JC, Vigna YM, Schechter MT, Burgess AE. Spinal bone loss and ovulatory disturbances. *N Engl J Med.* 323:1221, 1990

44. Drinkwater BL, Nilson K, Chestnut CHIII, et al. Bone mineral content of amenorrheic and eumenorrheic athletes. *N Engl J Med.* 311:277, 1984

45. Drinkwater BL, Nilson K, Ott S, Chestnut CH III. Bone mineral density after resumption of menses in amenorrheic athletes. *JAMA.* 256:380, 1986

46. Johansen JS, Riis BJ, Hassager C, et al. The effect of a gonadotropin-releasing hormone agonist analog (nafarelin) on bone metabolism. *J Clin Endocrinol Metab.* 67:701, 1988.

47. Rupich R. New techniques in bone imaging for determination of bone density. *Semin Reprod Endocrinol.* 10:27, 1992

48. Hsueh AJW, Erickson GF, Yen SSC. Sensitisation of pituitary cells to luteinising hormone releasing hormone by clomiphene citrate in vitro. *Nature.* 273:57, 1978

49. Liu JH, Yen SSC. The use of gonadotropin-releasing hormone for the induction of ovulation. *Clin Obstet Gynecol.* 27:975, 1984

50. Martin K, Santoro N, Hall J, et al. Management of ovulatory disorders with pulsatile gonadotropin-releasing hormone. *J Clin Endocrinol Metab.* 71:1081A, 1990

51. Reid RL, Loepold GR, Yen SSC. Induction of ovulation and pregnancy with pulsatile luteinizing hormone-releasing factor: Dosage and mode of delivery. *Fertil Steril.* 36:553, 1981

52. Leyendecker G, Wildt L, Hansmann M. Pregnancies following chronic intermittent (pulsatile) administration of GnRH by means of a portable pump ("zyklomat")—a new approach to the treatment of infertility in hypothalamic amenorrhea. *J Clin Endocrinol Metab.* 51:1214, 1980

53. Santoro N, Elzahr D. Pulsatile gonadotropin-releasing hormone therapy for ovulatory disorders. *Clin Obstet Gynecol.* 36:727, 1993

54. Vigersky RA, Loriaux D, Andersen AE, Lipsett MR. Anorexia nervosa: Behavioral and hypothalamic aspects. *Clin Endocrinol Metab.* 5:517, 1976

55. Pyle RL, Mitchell JE, Eckert ED, et al. The incidence of bulimia in freshman college students. *Int J Eat Disord.* 2:75, 1983

56. Crisp AH, Palmer RL, Kalucy RS. How common is anorexia nervosa? A prevalence study. *Br J Psychiatry.* 128:549, 1976

57. Willis J, Grossmann S. Epidemiology of anorexia nervosa in a defined region of Switzerland. *Am J Psychiatry.* 140:564, 1983

58. Schotte DE, Stunkard MD. Bulimia vs bulimic behaviors on a college campus. *JAMA.* 258:1213, 1987

59. Schwartz DM, Thompson M. Do anorectics get well?: Current research and future needs. *Am J Psychiatry.* 138:319, 1981

60. Patton G. Mortality in eating disorders. *Psychol Med.* 18:947, 1988

61. Swift WJ. The longterm outcome of early onset anorexia nervosa: A critical review. *J Am Acad Child Psychiatry.* 21:38, 1982

62. Boyar RM, Hellman LD, Roffwarg H, et al. Cortisol secretion and metabolism in anorexia nervosa. *N Engl J Med.* 296:190, 1977

63. Kontula K, Anderson LC, Huttumen M, Pelkonen R. Reduced level of cellular glucocorticoid receptors in patients with anorexia nervosa. *Horm Metab Res.* 14:619, 1982

64. Gerner RH, Gwirtsman HE. Abnormalities of dexamethasone suppression test and urinary MHPG in anorexia nervosa. *Am J Psychiatry.* 138:650, 1981

65. Gold PW, Gwirtsman H, Avgerinos PC, et al. Abnormal hypothalamic–pituitary–adrenal function in anorexia nervosa. *N Engl J Med.* 314:1335, 1986

66. Zumoff B, Walsh BT, Katz JL, et al. Subnormal plasma dehydroisoandrosterone to cortisol ratio in anorexia nervosa: A second hormonal parameter of ontogenic regression. *J Clin Endocrinol Metab.* 56:668, 1983

67. Moshang T Jr, Utiger R. Low triiodothyronine euthyroidism in anorexia nervosa. In: Vigersky RA, ed. *Anorexia Nervosa.* New York, Raven Press, 1977: 263–270

68. Gold PW, Kaye W, Robertson GL, Ebert M. Abnormalities in plasma and cerebrospinal fluid arginine vasopressin in patients with anorexia nervosa. *N Engl J Med.* 308:1117, 1983

69. Kaye WH, Gwirtsman HE, George DT, et al. Elevated cerebrospinal fluid levels of immunoreactive corticotropin-releasing hormone in anorexia nervosa: Relation to state of nutrition, adrenal function, and intensity of depression. *J Clin Endocrinol Metab.* 64:203, 1987

70. Baranowska B, Rozbicka G, Jeske W, Abdel-Fattah MH. The role of endogenous opiates in the mechanism of inhibited luteinizing hormone (LH) secretion in women with anorexia nervosa: The effect of naloxone on LH, follicle-stimulating hormone, prolactin, and beta-endorphin secretion. *J Clin Endocrinol Metab.* 59:412, 1984

71. Grandison L, Guidotti A. Stimulation of food intake by muscimol and beta endorphin. *Neuropharmacology.* 16:533, 1977

72. Atkinson RL. Naloxone decreased food intake in obese humans. *J Clin Endocrinol Metab.* 55:196, 1982

73. Morley JE, Levine AS. Stress-induced eating is mediated through endogenous opiates. *Science.* 209:1259, 1980

74. Garner DM, Bemis KM. A cognitive-behavioral approach to anorexia nervosa. *Cognitive Ther Res.* 6:123, 1982

75. Fairburn C. A cognitive behavioural approach to the treatment of bulimia. *Psychol Med.* 11:707, 1981

76. Rigotti NA, Nussbaum SR, Herzog DB, Neer RM. Osteoporosis in women with anorexia nervosa. *N Engl J Med.* 311:1601, 1984

77. Rigotti NA, Neer RM, Skates SJ, et al. The clinical course of osteoporosis in anorexia nervosa: A longitudinal study of cortical bone mass. *JAMA.* 265:1133, 1991

78. Frisch RE, Wyshak G, Vincent L. Delayed menarche and amenorrhea in ballet dancers. *N Engl J Med.* 303:17, 1980

79. Frisch RE, Gotz-Webergen AV, McArthur JW, et al. Delayed menarche and amenorrhea of college athletes in relation to age of onset of training. *JAMA.* 246:1559, 1981

80. Warren MP. Effect of exercise and physical training on menarche. *Semin Reprod Endocrinol.* 3:17, 1985

81. Constantini NW, Warren MP. Menstrual dysfunction in swimmers: A distinct entity. *J Clin Endocrinol Metab.* 80:2740, 1995

82. Frisch RE. Body fat, menarche, and reproductive ability. *Semin Reprod Endocrinol.* 3:45, 1985

83. Bullen BA, Skriinar GS, Beitins IZ, et al. Induction of menstrual disorders by strenuous exercise in untrained women. *N Engl J Med.* 312:1349, 1985

84. Cumming DC, Vickovic MM, Wall SR, Fluker MR. Defects in pulsatile LH release in normal menstruating runners. *J Clin Endocrinol Metab.* 60:810, 1985

85. Veldhuis JD, Evans WS, Demers LM, et al. Altered neuroendocrine regulation of gonadotropin secretion in women distance runners. *J Clin Endocrinol Metab.* 61:557, 1985

86. Villanueva AL, Schlosser C, Hopper B, et al. Increased cortisol production in women runners. *J Clin Endocrinol.* 133:136, 1986

87. Howlett TA, Tomlin S, Hgahfoong L, et al. Release of beta-endorphin and met-enkephalin during exercise in normal women: Response to training. *Br Med J.* 288:1950, 1984

88. Laatikainen T, Virtanen T, Apter D. Plasma immunoreactive beta-endorphin in exercise-associated amenorrhea. *Am J Obstet Gynecol.* 154:94, 1986

89. Stager JM, Ritchie-Flanagan RB, Robertshaw D. Reversibility of amenorrhea in athletes. *N Engl J Med.* 310:51, 1984

90. Fisher EC, Nelson ME, Frontera WR, et al. Bone mineral content and levels of gonadotropins and estrogens in amenorrheic running women. *J Clin Endocrinol Metab.* 62:1232, 1986

91. Brown E, Barglow P. Pseudocyesis: A paradigm of psychophysiological interactions. *Arch Gen Psychiatry.* 24:221, 1964

92. Yen SSC, Rebar RW, Quesenberry W. Pituitary function in pseudocyesis. *J Clin Endocrinol Metab.* 43:132, 1976

93. Kallmann F, Schonfeld WA, Barrera SW. Genetic aspects of primary eunuchoidism. *Am J Ment Defic.* 48:203, 1944

94. Lieblich JM, Rogol AD, White BT, Rosen SW. Syndrome of anosmia with hypogonadotropic hypogonadism (Kallmann's syndrome). *Am J Med.* 73:506, 1981

95. Klingmuller D, Dewes W, Krahe T, et al. Magnetic resonance imaging of the brain in patients with anosmia and hypothalamic hypogonadism (Kallmann's syndrome). *J Clin Endocrinol Metab.* 65:581, 1987

96. Weinstein RL, Reitz RE. Pituitary–testicular responsiveness in male hypogonadotropic hypogonadism. *J Clin Invest.* 53:408, 1974

97. Yeh J, Rebar RW, Liu JH, Yen SSC. Pituitary function in isolated gonadotropin deficiency. *Clin Endocrinol.* 31:375, 1989

98. Sheehan HL. Postpartum necrosis of the anterior pituitary. *J Pathol Bacteriol.* 45:189, 1937

99. Sheehan HL, Davis JC. Pituitary necrosis. *Br Med Bull.* 24:59, 1968

100. Sheehan HL. Atypical hypopituitarism. *Proc Roy Soc Med.* 54:43, 1961

101. Jackson IMD, Whyte WG, Garrey MM. Pituitary function following uncomplicated pregnancy in Sheehan's syndrome. *J Clin Endocrinol Metab.* 209:315, 1969

102. Sheldon WR Jr, DeBold CR, Evans WS, et al. Rapid sequential intravenous administration of four hypothalamic releasing hormones as a combined anterior pituitary function test in normal subjects. *J Clin Endocrinol Metab.* 60:623, 1985

103. Reid RL, Quigley ME, Yen SSC. Pituitary apoplexy: A review. *Arch Neurol.* 42:712, 1985

104. Veldhuis JD, Hammond JM. Endocrine function after spontaneous infarction of the human pituitary: Report, review, and reappraisal. *Endocr Rev.* 1:100, 1980

105. Arisaka O, Hall R, Hughes IA. Spontaneous endocrine cure of gigantism due to pituitary apoplexy. *Br Med J.* 287:1007, 1983

106. Edwards OM, Clark JDA. Post-traumatic hypopituitarism. *Medicine.* 65:281, 1986

107. Lam KSL, Tse VKC, Wang C, et al. Early effects of cranial irradiation on hypothalamic–pituitary function. *J Clin Endocrinol Metab.* 64:418, 1987

108. Feek CM, McLelland J, Seth J. How effective is external pituitary irradiation for growth hormone-secreting pituitary tumors? *Clin Endocrinol.* 20:401, 1984

109. Liu JH. Hypothalamic amenorrhea: Clinical perspectives, pathophysiology, and management. *Am J Obstet Gynecol.* 163:1732, 1990

Chapter 17

THYROID DYSFUNCTION AND OVULATORY DISORDERS

Earl W. Stradtman, Jr.

EVIDENCE THAT THYROID DYSFUNCTION IS ASSOCIATED WITH OVULATION DISORDERS

Normal functioning hypothalamic–pituitary–thyroid and hypothalamic–pituitary–ovarian axes are mutually dependent, and pathologic alterations in either axis can affect the other.[1-3] Extremes of thyroid dysfunction have been associated with ovulatory and menstrual disturbances. Primary hypothyroidism can result in pubertal delay or precocity, ovarian cysts, secondary hyperprolactinemia, or chronic anovulation. Thyroiditis represents part of a spectrum of autoimmune endocrinopathies, which can be associated with ovarian failure. Hyperthyroidism is less common, but can cause pubertal delay or precocity, amenorrhea, or chronic anovulation. Perturbations of thyroid hormone levels can alter production of sex hormone-binding globulin and sex steroid hormone metabolic pathways and clearance rates. This discussion will address the interactions of thyroid hormone production and the hypothalamic–pituitary–ovarian axis in physiologic and pathologic states.

THYROID PHYSIOLOGY

Thyroid Embryologic Development

The thyroid is the first endocrine gland to appear embryologically.[4] Its formation begins about 24 days after fertilization as an anlage from a median endodermal thickening from the floor of the pharynx. It is located caudal to the median tongue bud and is attached to the tongue by the thyroglossal duct. This duct becomes the thyroid diverticulum, which divides into lobes joined by an isthmus. A pyramidal lobe, present in about 50 percent of patients, represents a persistent inferior thyroglossal duct.

At 10 wk gestation epithelial cords divide into cell clusters, forming a monolayer at lumen. At 11 wk colloid follicles appear, signifying the onset of thyroxine production. Thus, maternal exposure to toxic substances, which are actively transported into the fetal thyroid at this gestational age, can ablate it.

Thyroid Hormone Production and Secretion

Iodine Transport and Assimilation. Iodide is actively transported from the serum by the membrane-associated iodide pump, reaching concentrations 20- to 40-fold higher in the follicle cell[5] ("a" in Fig 17–1). Stimulation by thyrotropin (thyroid-stimulating hormone or TSH) may increase the gradient another 20-fold. Follicular free iodide is organically bound within minutes, keeping its concentration low ("b" in Fig 17–1). Little is known about the mechanism of iodide release into the cytoplasm by the pump.

Iodide must be oxidized in order to iodinate tyrosine residues on thyroglobulin. Thyroid peroxidase (TPO), a membrane-bound enzyme, catalyzes the transfer of electrons from I^- to H_2O_2 and the binding of oxidized iodine to tyrosine (Fig 17–2).

Thyroid Hormone Synthesis. Thyroglobulin (Tg) (MW 660,000) is the iodinated polypeptide of the thyroid that is a precursor and reservoir in the biosynthesis of thyroid hormones.[5] Since Tg normally contains only about 2 to 3 iodothyronine sites per molecule, it is unclear why a small number of hormone molecules is produced from such a complex protein.

The Tg gene is a single-copy gene and has been mapped to chromosome 8q (8q 242 to 8q 243). Iodination of tyrosine is a post-translational event, since no transfer

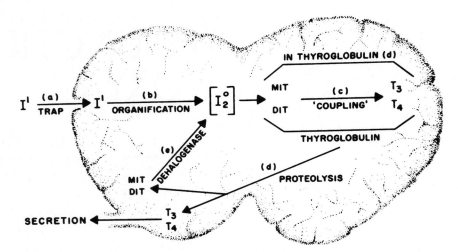

Figure 17–1. Synthetic pathways for thyroid hormones. *(Reproduced, with permission, from Jackson IMD, Cobb WE. In: Kohler PO, ed.* Clinical Endocrinology. *New York, John Wiley and Sons, 1986.)*

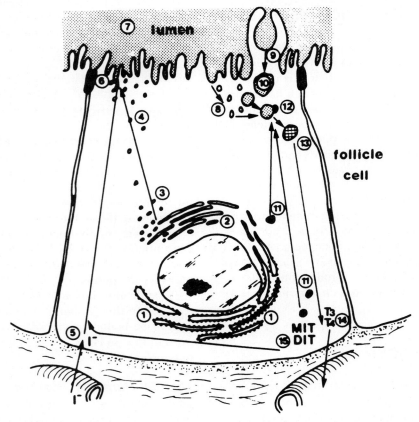

Figure 17–2. Diagrammatic scheme of thyroid hormone formation and secretion. Key: (1) thyroglobulin (Tg) and protein synthesis in the rough endoplasmic reticulum; (2) completion of the Tg carbohydrate units in the smooth endoplasmic reticulum; (3) formation of exocytotic vesicles; (4) transport of exocytotic vesicles with non-iodinated Tg to the apical surface of the follicle cell and into the follicular lumen; (5) iodide transport at the basal cell membrane; (6) iodide oxidation, Tg iodination, and coupling of iodotyrosyl to iodothyronyl residues; (7) storage of iodinated Tg in the follicular lumen; (8) endocytosis by micropinocytosis; (9) endocytosis by macropinocytosis (pseudopods); (10) colloid droplets; (11) lysosomes migrating to the apical pole; (12) fusion of lysosomes with colloid droplets; (13) phagolysosomes with Tg hydrolysis; (14) T_4 and T_3 secretion; (15) MIT and DIT deiodination. *(Reproduced, with permission, from Refetoff S, Larsen PR. Transport, cellular uptake, and metabolism of thyroid hormone. In: DeGroot LJ, ed.* Endocrinology, *2nd ed. Philadelphia, W. B. Saunders, 1989: 525.)*

RNA was found that accepts iodotyrosine. The amino acid sequence for Tg was determined from complementary DNA clones of the mRNA. Its primary structure comprises four major hormone synthetic domains. The most active synthetic site for thyroxine (T_4) is located at the tyrosine near the N-terminus and accounts for about 50 percent of the T_4 produced per molecule of Tg. The three other sites for T_4, one of which is the only site for 3,5,3'-triiodothyronine T_3, are at the C-terminus. The same hormonogenic site can produce thyroxine (T_4) or (T_3) depending on the level of iodine reserve, but the thyroid usually releases T_3 preferentially to T_4. Perhaps location of the synthetic sites of these two important hormones at opposite ends of Tg allows optimal binding of iodine or enzymatic hormone release.

The iodinated tyrosine residues on Tg comprise MIT and DIT, which are coupled by a diphenyl ether linkage (thyronine) to produce T_4 and T_3 ("c" in Fig 17–1). All four species are stored on Tg within the colloid droplets until they are mobilized for secretion.

Iodination and glycosylation are the major post-translational modifications of Tg. N-glycosylation occurs just after Tg synthesis with preassembled oligosaccharides. A monosaccharide transferase finally adds N-acetylglucosamine, galactose, and sialic acid chains.

Secretion of Thyroid Hormone. The fate of Tg from its mobilization from storage in follicular colloid to thyroid hormone secretion is complex (Fig 17–2, steps 8 to 15). Colloid droplets are engulfed by endocytosis at the luminal membrane, the vesicles fuse with and are digested by lysosomes, and Tg is hydrolyzed, releasing thyroid hormones that are secreted into the bloodstream at the basal membrane.

The exact mechanism of secretion of thyroid hormones across the basal membrane into the serum is not known. Lysosomes fuse with the endocytotic vesicles forming phagolysosomes, whose enzymes cleave T_4 from Tg. Enzymatic cleavage of the iodothyronine residues from Tg results in free T_4, T_3, monoiodothyronine

TABLE 17–1. DAILY PRODUCTION RATES AND CONTRIBUTION OF THYROID HORMONES TO TRIIODOTHYRONINES

Thyroid Hormone	Daily production Rate (nmol/24 hr)	Contribution to Serum Triiodothyronines (%)
T_4	110	45–83
T_3	10	15–25
rT_3	3	2.5–20

(Reproduced, with permission, from Refetoff S, Larsen PR. Transport, cellular uptake, and metabolism of thyroid hormone. In: DeGroot LJ, ed. Endocrinology, 2nd ed. Philadelphia, Pa., W. B. Saunders, 1989: 512–530.)

(MIT) and diiodothyronine (DIT), reverse T_3 (rT_3), and iodide ("d" in Fig 17–1). The approximate daily production of thyroid hormones by the thyroid gland is given in Table 17–1. MIT and DIT represent about 80 percent of Tg iodine. Most of the iodide resulting from enzymatic deiodination is recycled for Tg synthesis ("e" in Fig 17–1) and accounts for about 2 to 3 times the amount accumulated from the serum. Tg itself is secreted in small amounts into the serum, from about 5 to 32 ng/ml, though the mechanism is unclear.

TRANSPORT OF THYROID HORMONES AND ACTIONS IN PERIPHERAL TISSUES

Transport of Thyroid Hormones. The majority of thyroid hormone circulates bound to the serum proteins thyroxine-binding globulin (TBG), thyroxine-binding prealbumin (TBPA), and albumin (ALB).[6] Table 17–2 contains estimates of the relative proportions of hormones, free and bound.

The concentration of free hormone is proportional to that of the total hormone and inversely proportional to the sum of the products of the concentrations of the three thyroid hormone binding proteins and their affinity constants. An increase in TBG would bind free T_4, transiently lowering the free serum level, until a rise in TSH could stimulate an increase in T_4, bringing about a new

TABLE 17–2. SERUM DISTRIBUTION OF THYROXINE

Hormone Status	Proportion Total T_4	T_4, T_3 Proportion Total T_3	Binding sites (n)	Half-Life (days)
Free	0.03	0.3	—	—
Thyroxine-binding albumin (TBG)	0.70–0.75	0.70–0.75	1	5
Thyroxine-binding prealbumin (TBPA)	0.20–0.25	0.10	2	2
Albumin (ALB)	0.05–0.10	0.20	5–6	15

(Adapted, with permission, from Refetoff S, Larsen PR. Transport, cellular uptake, and metabolism of thyroid hormone. In: DeGroot LJ, ed. Endocrinology, 2nd ed. Philadelphia, Pa., W. B. Saunders, 1989: 512–530.)

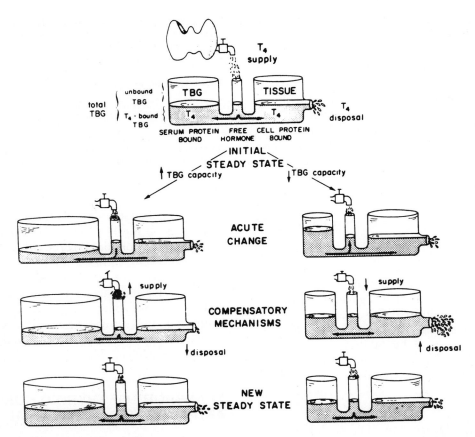

Figure 17–3. Graphic representation of sequence of events following an acute change in serum TBG concentration in a subject with normal regulation of thyroid hormone secretion and metabolism. The communicating vessel principle is used for analogy. The width of the two large vessels represents available T_4-binding sites in serum (TBG) and in peripheral cells (TISSUE), which are partially saturated by T_4 (fluid level). The height of fluid in the small central vessel represents free T_4 concentration in equilibrium with bound T_4 in each of the large vessels. Free T_4 is proportional to the level of saturation of the binding sites in serum (TBG) and in cells (TISSUE). Thyroidal secretion (supply) of T_4 is represented by the input of fluid through the faucet, and hormone metabolism (disposal) by the overspill of the tissue reservoir. *(Reproduced, with permission, from Refetoff S, Larsen PR. Transport, cellular uptake, and metabolism of thyroid hormone. In: DeGroot LJ, ed.* Endocrinology, *2nd ed. Philadelphia, W. B. Saunders, 1989: 545.)*

steady state (Fig 17–3). The role of the thyroid hormone-binding proteins is incompletely understood, but they seem to act as a reservoir of thyroid hormone to maintain serum levels with abrupt changes in thyroid hormone production.

TBG is the major thyroid hormone-binding serum protein with the highest affinity of the major proteins. With normal levels, about one third of TBG is bound to thyroid hormone. Immunologic testing for TBG is replacing the T_3 resin uptake assay. Although specific thyroid hormones bind to specific substituents on TBG, a number of substances, such as diphenylhydantoin and salicylates, can competitively displace the hormones from the binding sites.

The thyroid hormone-binding proteins are produced by the liver, and certain inherited, physiologic, and patho-

physiologic states can alter liver function and TBG concentration. Table 17–3 summarizes conditions that can change TBG concentrations. Similar changes can occur in TBPA and ALB levels, but the effect on serum levels of thyroid hormones is minimal.

Actions of Thyroid Hormones in Peripheral Tissues. Although T_4 is the principal circulating thyroid hormone, T_3 is more potent in peripheral tissues. The thyroid gland produces about 10 percent as much T_3 as T_4, but the major source of tissue T_3 is the monodeiodination of T_4 in the tissues themselves. T_4 (3,5,3',5-tetraiodo-L-thyronine) can undergo monodeiodination at either the 5' (outer) or the 5 (inner) sites, yielding T_3 (3,5,3'-tri-iodo-L-thyronine) or rT_3 (3,3',5'-tri-iodo-L-thyronine), respectively (Fig 17–4).

TABLE 17–3. INHERITED AND ACQUIRED CONDITIONS WHICH CAN ALTER SERUM TBG CONCENTRATION

Condition		Increased TBG	Decreased TBG
Genetic		Inherited TBG excess	Inherited TBG deficiencies (Quantitative, complete or partial; qualitative)
Acquired	Hormonal	Estrogen use (eg, oral contraceptives) or hyperestrogenic states (eg, pregnancy, newborn, tumor)	Androgens or anabolic steroids Glucocorticolism hypercortisolism L-asparaginase
	Drugs	Perphenazine (Trilafon) Heroin and methadone Clofibrate 5-Fluorouracil	
	Diseases	Acute intermittent porphyria Hepatitis Primary biliary cirrhosis Myeloma Collagen diseases Hypogammaglobulinemia Hypothyroidism	Systemic illness Protein–calorie malnutrition or loss states Galactosemia Hepatic cirrhosis Active acromegaly Hyperthyroidism

(Adapted, with permission, from Refetoff S, Larsen PR. Transport, cellular uptake, and metabolism of thyroid hormone. In: DeGroot LJ, ed. Endocrinology, *2nd ed. Philadelphia, Pa., W. B. Saunders, 1989: 512–530.)*

The distribution of T_4 in various organs is as follows: liver and kidney, 31 percent; muscle, brain, and skin, 44 percent; and plasma, 22 percent. T_3 is distributed in the liver (5 percent), plasma (18 percent), and other organs (75 percent).

The actions of unbound thyroid hormones in the target organs seem to depend on active transport and monodeiodination of T_4 to T_3. T_3 is released more rapidly from thyroid hormone binding proteins than T_4, which may explain the higher daily metabolic clearance rate of the former over the latter. T_3 and T_4 can inhibit the transport of each other, but apparently not by competition.

The mechanisms by which thyroid hormones exert their effects are intriguing but not fully understood.[7] For example, it is not clear whether thyroid hormones have ubiquitous, but tissue-specific, effects or whether they affect multiple endocrine systems that in turn affect their target organs. Thyroid hormones affect such processes as gluconeogenesis and lipogenesis; oxygen uptake in heart, liver, and kidney; epidermal derivatives; cholesterol metabolism; the onset of puberty; thermogenesis; and central nervous system development. Thyroid hormones seem to have multiple cellular sites of action: the cell surface, mitochondria, and the nucleus.

T_3 probably modulates the basal metabolic rate, which is manifest by mitochondrial activity and O_2 uptake by tissues. Occupation of nuclear receptors by T_3 is correlated with increased O_2 consumption and mitochondrial enzyme activity. Its role in thermogenesis is unclear and may result from its global effect on metabolic rate.

An analysis of the nuclear actions of thyroid hormone may explain its ubiquitous, yet specific, actions in target tissues. Age and developmental status may also influence thyroid hormone actions. Thyroid hormone action can modulate synthesis of RNA and proteins, in general, or a single protein, in particular. Low concentrations of nuclear receptors have made their isolation and sequencing difficult. Genes encoding for thyroid hormone-receptor proteins have been localized to chromosomes 17 and 3, suggesting different types of receptors. Nuclear receptor concentration may depend upon the metabolic state, such as with fasting, glucocorticoid status, or diabetes mellitus, but apparently not in hypo- or hyperthyroidism. In summary, the cellular effects of thyroid hormone may depend upon the target tissue, the activity of the nuclear receptor, the metabolic state, the age, and the development of the individual.

Metabolism and Excretion of Thyroid Hormones. Up to 38 percent of T_4 is metabolized by monodeiodination to T_3 or rT_3, and about 20 percent is excreted unchanged in the feces. T_3 and rT_3 are further deiodinated at the 3, 3', 5, and 5' sites to yield di- and monoiodothyronines and

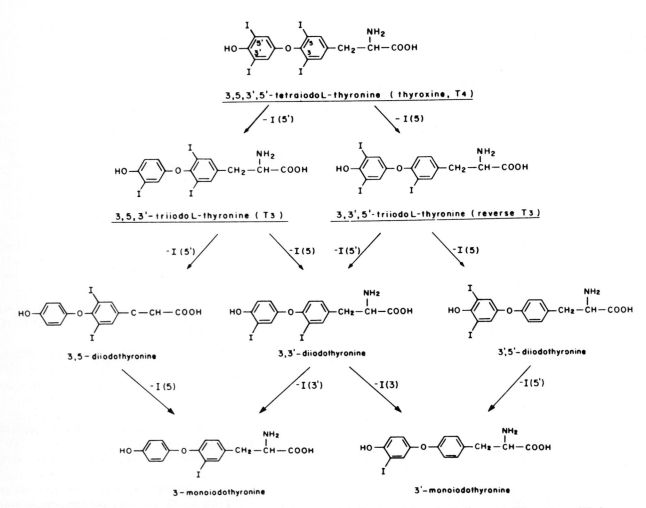

Figure 17–4. Metabolic products resulting from successive monodeiodination of thyroxine in the outer (5') and inner (3') rings. *(Reproduced, with permission, from Refetoff S, Larsen PR. Transport, cellular uptake, and metabolism of thyroid hormone. In: DeGroot LJ, ed. Endocrinology, 2nd ed. Philadelphia, W. B. Saunders, 1989: 550.)*

thyronine (Fig 17–4). Hepatic metabolism of some intermediary forms results in sulfated species, which are usually deiodinated more rapidly than the nonsulfated ones.

Monodeiodination of T_4 occurs by at least three 5'-monodeiodinases, types I, II, and III. The relative activities of types I and II differ according to the target organ: type I in liver and kidney; type II in anterior pituitary, cerebral cortex, brown adipose, and placenta. Type III is present in the central nervous system and deiodinates the inner ring, and it is the only enzyme that has been isolated. Since the brain and pituitary can intracellularly convert T_4 to T_3, the HPT axis can compensate for a decrease in serum T_4 levels by an increase in TSH, while reserves are still available.

Hyperthyroidism leads to increased type I activity in the liver, but not in the kidney, and decreased type II activity. In hypothyroidism, type I activity is about half normal in liver and kidney, but type II increases by 2 to 100 times. These compensations likely accelerate T_3 metabolism in states of excess and maintain T_3 availability to the CNS and pituitary when T_4 is limited. A compensatory decrease in peripheral T_3 production occurs with carbohydrate restriction or starvation, diabetes, the fetal or neonatal period, glucocorticoids, estrogen, and somatostatin. Pharmacologic agents that reduce T_3 conversion include propyl thiouracil, amiodarone, propranolol (β-blockers), prazosin, and oral cholecystographic contrast (iopanoic acid [Telepaque] or ipodic acid [Oragrafin]).

REGULATION OF THYROID HORMONE SECRETION

Hormone synthesis and secretion by the thyroid gland is regulated primarily by TSH from pituitary thyrotropes, although autoregulation contributes to thyroid hormone

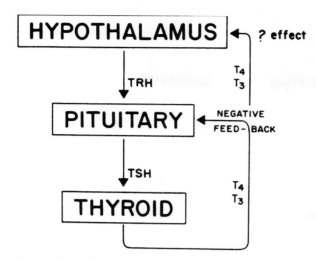

Figure 17–5. Feedback relationships between thyroid hormone, pituitary, and the hypothalamus. *(Reproduced, with permission, from Jackson IMD, Cobb WE. In: Kohler PO, ed.* Clinical Endocrinology. *New York, John Wiley and Sons, 1986.)*

secretion. TSH is subject to positive and negative feedback loops involving mainly thyrotropin-releasing hormone (TRH) and thyroid hormone, respectively (Fig 17–5). A summary of the components of the HPT axis and their interactions follows.

Hypothalamic–Pituitary–Thyroid (HPT) Axis

Hypothalamic Regulation: Thyrotropin-Releasing Hormone.
TRH, the modified tripeptide pyroglutamyl-histidyl-prolinamide (Fig 17–6), was identified and synthesized by Guillemin,[8] Schally,[9] and their respective colleagues. TRH has been detected in various hypothalamic regions, but the major sites of synthesis concerned with TSH regulation seem to be in the periventricular nuclei and in the median eminence–arcuate

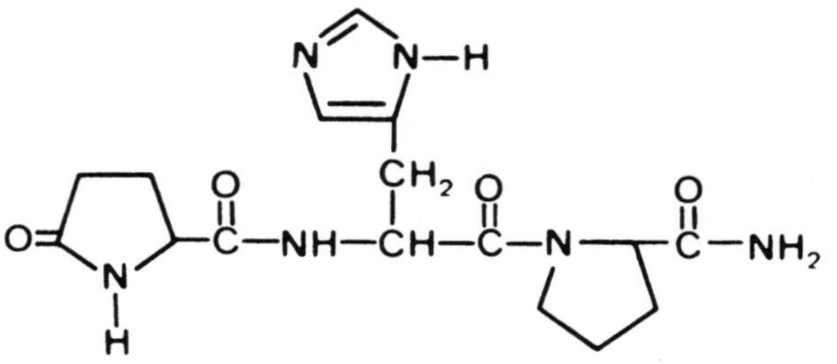

Figure 17–6. Schematic molecular structure of thyrotropin-releasing hormone. *(Reproduced, with permission, from Greenspan FS, Rapoport B. In: Greenspan FS, Forsham PH, eds.* Basic and Clinical Endocrinology. *Los Altos, CA, Lange, 1983: 139.)*

nucleus area. TRH is secreted into the hypophyseal portal system, binds to receptors on anterior pituitary cells, and stimulates TSH synthesis and secretion and prolactin synthesis and release. Although acutely administered boluses of TRH stimulate prolactin, normal physiologic stimuli of prolactin secretion in humans, such as suckling, do not appear to be mediated by TRH. The mechanism by which the binding of TRH to its receptors exerts its effect on the pituitary cells is unclear. TRH binding produces a rapid increase in the action of phospholipase C on phosphatidylinositol and a rise in intracellular calcium, which may activate a C-kinase leading to TSH secretion.[10,11] TRH probably downregulates its receptors on pituitary cells, since repeated boluses result in a decreased release of TSH. However, a constant infusion of TRH produces increased levels of TSH, T_4, and T_3. Given its short half-life of between 2 and 6 min, the measurement of serum TRH and its principal metabolite, cyclo-His-Pro, suggests a peripheral source and metabolism rather than a central one.

TRH is stimulated by norepinephrine and inhibited by somatostatin.[12] Potential in vivo stimulators of TRH include the preoptic region, arginine vasopressin, catecholamines (norepinephrine, epinephrine, and phenylephrine), and endogenous opiates; dopamine is a putative inhibitor. Mechanisms of physiologic regulation are currently undetermined.

TRH seems to exert a permissive role in the regulation of TSH by its tonic stimulation. The finding of secondary hyperprolactinemia in primary hypothyroidism suggests that TRH responds to negative feedback from T_4 and T_3, but their role in TRH regulation has not been established.

Pituitary Regulation: Thyroid-Stimulating Hormone.
Thyroid-stimulating hormone (TSH or thyrotropin) is a 28,000 glycoprotein comprising two subunits, α and β.[12] The peptide portion of the α-subunit is similar to those of luteinizing hormone (LH), follicle-stimulating hormone (FSH), and human chorionic gonadotropin (hCG), but their carbohydrate portions differ. The unique β-subunits confer immunologic and biologic specificity and are transcribed by different regions of messenger RNA. Higher serum concentrations of α-subunit than β-subunit indicate that production of the latter is a rate-limiting step in synthesis of TSH peptide and may play a role in its regulation. After passage from the ribosomes to the rough endoplasmic reticulum, special sequences are cleaved, and glycosylation occurs by addition of preformed oligosaccharides, from which various residues are cleaved, including sialic acid. The importance of glycosylation has not been established. Secretion involves release of TSH and free α- and β-subunits from storage in secretory granules.

TSH synthesis and secretion are maintained by tonic production of TRH and are under negative feedback control by thyroid hormones. TRH stimulates TSH synthesis and release independently of each other and induces cleavage of oligosaccharide residues, perhaps decreasing bioactivity of TSH in tertiary hypothyroidism. The mechanism of suppression of TSH by treatment with exogenous thyroid hormone or in hyperthyroidism is not clear, but may result from decreased transcription of α- and β-subunits or by downregulation of TRH pituitary cell receptors. In hypothyroidism TSH synthesis increases probably because of the loss of thyroid hormone inhibition of TRH and the increased number of thyrotropes.

TSH release appears to be proportional to TRH dose, based on observations from TRH stimulation testing. However, adding thyroid hormone can blunt or abolish the TSH response to TRH. Somatostatin, glucocorticoids, calcium-channel blockers, and dopamine agonists can also blunt the TSH response. T_3 and TSH levels do not correlate as well as T_4 and TSH, probably because most of the pituitary T_3 is derived from intracellular conversion of T_4 to T_3 rather than from serum T_3 directly. Drugs such as iopanoic acid, which inhibit the intrapituitary conversion of T_4 to T_3, demonstrate that unconverted T_4 is insufficient to suppress TSH. In hyperthyroidism, baseline TSH levels are undetectable and do not usually rise with TRH administration.

The normal range for serum levels of TSH can range from 0.35 to 5.5 mU/ml, using a highly sensitive TSH (HSTSH) assay. The daily production rate of TSH is from 40 to 150 mU, the serum half-life is 54 minutes, and the volume of distribution is about 5 to 6 L. In hypothyroid patients serum TSH levels can exceed 1000 μU/ml, with production rates over 4000 mU/day. In thyrotoxic patients serum levels are undetectable and production rates are significantly decreased. Hepatic and renal metabolism prevails, and renal failure can compromise TSH elimination. Several investigators have reported a circadian rhythm but have not yet defined a daily pattern.

Thyroid Gland Regulation: T_4, T_3, rT_3. TSH exerts its effects on thyroid follicle cells by initially binding to membrane receptors. At least two second-messenger systems are operative: the adenylate cyclase–cyclic AMP (cAMP) and the calcium–cyclic GMP (cGMP) systems.[13] Stimulation of adenylate cyclase by the TSH-receptor complex is mediated by the guanine nucleotide regulatory proteins (G proteins), which involves transfer of phosphate GTP and GDP. The activated adenylate cyclase catalyzes the production of cAMP. This second messenger probably activates a phosphokinase that results in increased RNA and protein synthesis, iodide uptake, colloid resorption, and thyroid hormone secretion; and agents that increase cAMP can simulate TSH action.

A second regulatory system of thyroid hormone secretion involves receptor occupation that results in calcium mobilization, protein kinase-C activation, arachidonic acid release, prostaglandin E synthesis, and cGMP production. Muscarinic cholinergic agonists (acetylcholine), α-adrenergic agonists (norephinephrine), prostaglandins F, TRH, and possible somatostatin increase iodine organification and TSH-stimulated thyroid hormone release but do not act by cAMP. The mechanism of action of the calcium–cGMP system in thyroid hormone inhibition is not clear.

Autoregulation of thyroid hormone secretion by excess or deficient iodide is a third pathway and is incompletely understood. Acute increases in serum iodide result in decreased TSH-stimulated cAMP and serum thyroid hormone levels, a process which is independent of iodine organification.[13] The mechanism of inhibition is unknown. Irrespective of the presence of TSH, the block in iodide organification and thyroid hormone secretion in response to excess iodide is called the Wolff–Chaikoff effect. This block may be accentuated in Graves' disease, in Hashimoto's thyroiditis, with impairment of iodide organification, or by pretreatment with TSH, probably because the increased iodide transport results in a greater intracellular iodide level at any serum level. Therefore, the Wolff–Chaikoff effect can be advantageous clinically by using potassium iodide (KI) to suppress excess thyroid hormone secretion, as in Graves' disease.

Thyroid hormones themselves can exert autoregulatory functions. Thyroxine can decrease the ratio of intrathyroid to serum iodide, and T_3 and T_4 can suppress cAMP and its mediated responses in the thyroid.

Although the thyroid gland is innervated with sympathetic and parasympathetic nerve fibers that contribute to thyroid hormone regulation, the physiologic role of the autonomic nervous system in thyroid hormone release has not been determined. Thyroid hormone release has been documented with sympathetic and parasympathetic stimulation, and catecholamines have had stimulatory effects, inhibitory effects, and no effects on release.

INTERACTIONS BETWEEN HYPOTHALAMIC–PITUITARY–THYROID AND HYPOTHALAMIC–PITUITARY–GONADAL AXES

Influence of HPT Axis on Gonadotropins

TRH. Since TRH is found in the median eminence and paraventricular nuclei, as is gonadotropin-releasing hormone (GnRH), the potential exists for hypothalamic interactions between these peptide hormones. The production of these hormones can be altered by similar insults, such as space-occupying hypothalamic lesions. The finding of concomitant hypothalamic hypothyroidism and hypogonadotropic amenorrhea, which does not resolve after thyroid hormone therapy, suggests that common hypothalamic mediators influence TRH and GnRH secretion.

The effect of TRH on FSH and LH secretion is incompletely understood. Mortimer and associates[14] evaluated the responses of FSH and LH, TSH and prolactin, and growth hormone and corticosteroids to GnRH, TRH, and insulin-induced hypoglycemia, respectively, in 12 normal male volunteers. Although no women were studied, each hypothalamic hormone stimulated only its respective pituitary hormone. Specifically, TRH did not cause significant changes in FSH or LH secretion.

Colon et al[15] studied the effect of an intravenous bolus of TRH on FSH and LH secretion in normal ovulatory women. TRH 200 µg administered to 5 ovulatory women in the early follicular (days 3 through 5) and midluteal phases (days 21 through 23) produced a significant increase in LH in both cycle phases but not in FSH. The results suggest that pharmacologic boluses of TRH stimulate LH release in both cycle phases.

Lasso and associates[16] reported the effect of long-term oral TRH on FSH and LH secretion. Although the 6 normally ovulating women who took TRH 60 mg bid for 2 consecutive menstrual cycles had transiently elevated prolactin levels, neither serum FSH nor LH levels changed appreciably. At the tested dose there was no significant interference with ovulatory cycling in these women.

Based on these three studies, TRH boluses at pharmacologic doses may mildly stimulate LH release in ovulatory women, but FSH does not rise significantly. It is unclear whether TRH exerts a permissive effect on gonadotropin secretion.

TSH. Ober[17] reported an 18-year-old postpartum patient with hypopituitarism who maintained normal ovulatory function despite deficiencies in thyroxine, cortisol, and growth hormone. Although hypogonadism often occurs early in hypopituitarism, this patient continued to have regular menses, vaginal estrogenization, and normal FSH levels despite the other hormonal deficiencies. Apparently, deficiencies in TSH and other non-gonadotropic pituitary hormones had no demonstrable effect in the HPO axis in this patient.

In the rare case of pituitary adenomas secreting TSH, Smallridge and Smith[18] found that only 1 of 17 women with elevated TSH secretion sufficient to cause thyrotoxicosis had amenorrhea. Though elevations of thyroid hormones themselves might have altered the menstrual cycling and ovulation disorders other than amenorrhea were not reported, elevated TSH secretion per se may not have a profound effect on gonadotropins.

T₄ or T₃. In general, hypothyroidism results in lower basal levels of FSH and LH than in euthyroid control patients.[19] In hyperthyroidism, basal serum LH and FSH levels are elevated.[20] Distiller and colleagues[21] evaluated FSH and LH responses to intravenous GnRH 100 µg in hyperthyroid and hypothyroid women. In hyperthyroid premenopausal women, FSH and LH responses were similar to euthyroid controls, and in postmenopausal women the LH response was exaggerated, implying normal pituitary gonadotropin reserve. In 2 of 8 hypothyroid women LH responses were blunted in the face of a normal FSH response, suggesting that hypothyroidism may be associated with decreased gonadotropin reserve. Implications of the alterations in thyroid hormone production on the HPO axis will be discussed more thoroughly in the sections on hypothyroidism and hyperthyroidism.

Influence of HPT Axis on Ovarian Steroids

TRH. Lasso and colleagues[16] found that pharmacologic doses of TRH had no significant effect on serum estradiol levels or on luteal length based on basal body temperature charts, pregnanediol excretion, or endometrial biopsies. It may be inferred cautiously that physiologic secretion of TRH would not likely have a significant effect on peripheral estrogen, androgen, or progesterone production. The permissive role of hypothalamic TRH and the role of peripheral TRH on gonadal steroidogenesis are unclear.

TSH. As discussed in the parallel section regarding the effects of TSH on gonadotropins, the deficiency or excess of TSH by itself appears to have little demonstrable effect on ovarian steroidogenesis. Perhaps studying the menstrual cycles in patients with inappropriate secretion of TSH or with thyroid hormone insensitivity may provide clues to the role of elevated TSH on steroidogenesis.

T₄ or T₃. Because hypothyroidism is associated with decreased serum levels of sex hormone-binding globulin (SHBG), serum total estradiol is usually also decreased.[19] Anovulatory hypothyroid patients have progesterone levels below the normal luteal range, as expected. In hyperthyroidism, SHBG[22] and total serum estradiol levels[20] are increased, with free estradiol initially decreased until a new steady state is reached. Parallel changes occur with serum total testosterone levels. Progesterone levels reflect the menstrual cycle status, not the thyroid status: cycling women have luteal progesterone levels similar to euthyroid controls, and anovulatory patients have values below the luteal range. When thyrotoxic women are rendered euthyroid, the sex steroid levels return to the normal ranges. These topics will be expanded in the respective sections under thyroid disorders.

Changes in Menstrual Cycle With Aberrations in Thyroid Disease

Joshi et al[23] studied the menstrual and reproductive histories of 178 women referred for evaluation of thyroid disease, comparing them to 49 healthy controls. Cases were classified as euthyroid, hypothyroid, or hyperthyroid based on history, physical examination, and measurement of serum T_3, T_4, and TSH levels. Only 31.8 percent of hypothyroid and 35.3 percent of hyperthyroid patients had normal menstrual cycles, compared to 56.3 percent of euthyroid and 87.8 percent of control women. Reproductive failure (infertility, pregnancy loss, lactation failure) occurred in 37.5 percent of hypothyroid and 36.5 percent of hyperthyroid patients in contrast to 16.3 percent of euthyroid and 16.7 percent of control women. In 45 percent of cases the menstrual abnormality preceded the clinical findings of thyroid dysfunction by 2 mo to 10 yr. Reproductive failure and lactation failure also preceded the development of thyroid dysfunction or goiter, suggesting that evaluation of these reproductive disorders include obtaining basic thyroid function tests.

Influence of HPO Axis on HPT Axis

GnRH. Mortimer and colleagues[14] conducted pituitary stimulation testing by hypothalamic-releasing hormone administration or by insulin-induced hypoglycemia. They reported that GnRH 100 µg did not acutely affect TSH or prolactin secretion with provocative testing in men, despite an appropriate rise in FSH and LH.

Gonadal Steroids

Gonadal Steroids and the TSH Response to TRH.
Estradiol appears to be a factor in the greater responses women have of TSH to TRH than do men,[24] but studies of pharmacologic doses of estrogen have had conflicting results. However, basal levels of TSH and thyroid hormones appear to have no significant variation with the menstrual cycle.[25,26] Some effects of estrogen on the HPT axis include an increase in rat thyrotrope TRH receptors,[27] reversal of the inhibition of thyroid hormone on the TSH response to TRH, decreased iodide release from the thyroid,[28] and stimulation of TBG production by the liver.

Rutlin and co-workers[29] sought to determine the effect of estrogen on the TSH response to TRH. They performed TRH stimulation tests on normally cycling women without regard to cycle phase, on postmenopausal women before and after treatment for 5 days with 2 mg estradiol valerate, and on men on long-term estrogen therapy. In both groups of women, estrogen had no effect on the basal TSH levels nor on its response to TRH. In the estrogen-treated men, the TRH response was similar to normal men. In these patients estrogen seemed to have no significant influence on the pituitary response to its hypothalamic-releasing hormone. This finding was confirmed in a study that compared TSH and prolactin responses in TRH stimulation testing of healthy euthyroid pre- and postmenopausal women (13 each group).[30] The only difference in the responses in the two groups was a weak decrease in TSH incremental response, which was not statistically significantly different, in the postmenopausal group, which was assumed to be related to hypoestrogenism.

In contrast, Spitz and associates[31,32] and Kohler[32] evaluated the effects of androgen and estrogen treatment on TSH secretion in female and male patients with isolated gonadotropin deficiency. Hypogonadal women had decreased basal TSH levels and responses to TRH. Following treatment with ethinyl estradiol for 3 mo, the TSH response to TRH normalized but the basal TSH remained low. The men had normal TSH basal levels and responses to TRH. HCG therapy elevated serum testosterone and estradiol levels but did not alter the TSH parameters. Treatment of the men with ethinyl estradiol increased the TSH response to TRH. The authors postulated that estrogen may be required for a normal TSH response to TRH in women, but that testosterone may oppose the effect of estrogen on the TSH response in men.

Faglia and colleagues[33] also found that estrogen increased the TSH response to TRH in men treated with estradiol valerate 10 mg for 5 days, but not in treated women. Their results indicate that estrogen is a factor in modulating the pituitary response to TRH.

Sanchez-Franco and associates[34] studied the changes in TSH response to intravenous TRH 200 µg in the follicular (cycle days 7 through 8) and luteal phases (cycle days 21 through 22) of normally cycling women and in men. The TSH response in the follicular phase was significantly greater than in the luteal phase, which itself was not different from the response in men. Considering women as a group, the TSH response at each interval and the overall mean response were greater than those of men. It would be interesting to speculate about the results if each woman was tested in both phases of the same cycle, rather than two different groups in each phase.

Morley et al[35] measured the TSH response to TRH before and after treatment of a group of hypogonadal men treated with a nonaromatizable androgen, compared to a group of eugonadal men. Since androgen therapy significantly decreased the TSH response compared with pretreatment testing, it seems that androgen is in part responsible for the difference in TSH response between men and women.

In summary, most of the data suggest that estrogens increase the thyrotrope response to TRH, whereas androgens decrease it. Interpretation of the studies should be done in light of the types of steroids used, the doses, and the durations.

Testosterone/Androgens. Other than the effect on the TSH response to TRH, androgens appear to have a limited effect on the HPT axis. In normal men the androgen-induced decrease in TBG lowers serum total T_4, but free T_4 levels are normal.[32] Seven clinically and chemically euthyroid women treated with the androgen fluoxymesterone for metastatic breast cancer[36] had reversible decreases in total T_4 and TBG during and after therapy. However, four breast cancer patients with long-standing treated hypothyroidism became clinically hyperthyroid within the first 4 wk of therapy, when the serum free T_4 levels increased and the TSH levels decreased. Thyroid hormone doses had to be decreased by 25 to 50 percent to bring the levels within the normal ranges. This study highlights the need to monitor thyroid hormone levels in patients undergoing androgen treatment and perhaps with significant androgen excess states.

Gonadal Steroids and TBG. As previously discussed, changes in thyroxine binding globulin (TBG) alter measurements of total serum T_4 but do not ultimately affect free T_4 levels[37] in euthyroid patients. Estrogens increase and androgens decrease hepatic production of TBG by a mechanism that is not clear. Assuming a constant affinity of TBG for T_4, an increase in TBG shifts the equilibrium toward increasing T_4 binding, lowering free T_4, increasing TSH, and increasing serum T_4, restoring normal free T_4 levels. Cessation of estrogen administration or initiation of androgen treatment decreases TBG levels more rapidly than T_4 can be metabolized, resulting in a transient elevation of free T_4 and suppression of TSH.

Changes in Thyroid Parameters During the Menstrual Cycle

Perez and associates[25] found no significant differences in serum levels of T_4, T_3, and TSH in the follicular and luteal phases of 17 women (ages 20 to 24) with regular cycles. Rasmussen and colleagues[38] sampled "thyroid hormones," TSH (a high-sensitivity assay), thyroid-binding globulin (TBG), and thyroid volume by ultrasound on cycle days 2, 9, 16, 23, and 2 of 10 women volunteers. They found increases in TSH, TBG, and thyroid volume from cycle days 2 to 23, and concluded that the difference in TBG levels may reflect changes in TSH levels and thyroid volume during the cycle. Although Hegedus et al[26] found a significant difference in mean thyroid volume between the follicular (15.4 cc, day 9) and luteal phases (24.4 cc, day 23), they found no differences in the levels of T_4, T_3, T_3RU, TBG, and TSH between the two phases. They attributed the difference in thyroid volume to differences in vascularity. In summary, thyroid gland volume in the luteal phase appears to be greater than in the follicular phase, but

serum levels of thyroid hormones are probably not significantly different.

The interaction of the HPT axis with the menstrual cycle was studied in women undergoing high-volume athletic training having regular menstrual cycles compared with those having amenorrhea and a control group of cycling sedentary women, matched for factors such as weight, calorie intake, and intensity of exercise. Serum thyroid hormone levels differed between athletes and sedentary women. The amenorrheic athletes had significantly ($P < 0.01$) lower mean serum total and free T_4, total and free T_3, and rT_3 levels compared to the cycling sedentary women, but the cycling athletes differed from the cycling sedentary women only by a lower mean serum total T_4 level. The amenorrheic athletes had significantly lower mean free T_4 ($P < 0.01$), free T_3 ($P < 0.01$), and rT_3 ($P < 0.05$) than cycling athletes. Interestingly, the levels of TBG and SHBG were within the normal ranges in all groups. The TSH response to TRH was blunted in the amenorrheic athletes compared to the cycling athletes but not the cycling sedentary women. In summary, high-volume athletic training resulting in amenorrhea is associated with impairment of the HPT axis despite apparently normal serum TSH levels by a mechanism that is yet to be determined.

The interaction of the HPT axis with changes in the menstrual cycle was also studied in 15 patients with premenstrual syndrome (PMS) and 15 control women.[39] Each woman underwent testing in the follicular and luteal phase of the menstrual cycle. Although the mean serum thyroid hormone levels were not significantly different during either phase of the cycle, the women with PMS showed greater variability of serum TSH, T_3 uptake, total T_4, and free thyroxine index measurements than the control women. The authors concluded that HPT axis abnormalities may contribute to symptoms in some women with PMS.

Interactions of the HPT Axis With Other Endocrine Systems

Glucocorticoids in large doses decrease TSH secretion and its response to TRH, reduce TBG levels, and decrease the peripheral conversion of T_4 to T_3.[40] They increase renal iodide clearance, decrease iodide uptake, and reduce the effect of TSH on the thyroid.

A decreased response of TSH to TRH has been associated with acromegaly and growth hormone repletion in growth hormone-deficient children and may be related to increased somatostatin levels. In about 25 percent of patients with acromegaly, diffuse or nodular thyromegaly has been observed, and although the basal metabolic rates and renal and thyroid clearances of iodide are elevated, these patients are not thyrotoxic. In contrast, patients with GH deficiency show an increased response TSH to TRH compared to normals.

THYROID DYSFUNCTION AND OVULATION DISORDERS

Hypothyroidism

Definition and Epidemiology. Hypothyroidism is the syndrome of decreased production of thyroid hormone with abnormal serum thyroid hormone levels that responds to hormone repletion.[41] Since clinical situations occur in which certain hormone levels only are abnormal, such as with decreased peripheral conversion of T_4 to T_3 in non-thyroidal illness or low total T_4 levels in hypoestrogenic states, this definition emphasizes nonreversible conditions that clinical symptoms or signs have resulted or would be expected to result from decreased hormonal production.

Hypothyroidism occurs more frequently in women than men and in all age groups. Surveys have estimated that 8 to 10 percent of women, as opposed to 1 to 2 percent of men, have subclinical or compensated hypothyroidism, often associated with thyroid autoantibodies. About 0.5 to 1.5 percent of women appear to have clinical hypothyroidism, with up to 4 percent of postmenopausal women affected.

Pathophysiology. Hypothyroidism results from decreased thyroid hormone production, which can be affected from disease in any of the three major components of the HPT axis: hypothalamic, pituitary, or thyroid disease, of which the latter is the most common. When T_4 production by the thyroid is decreased, T_3 production is proportionally less affected. Compensatory TSH secretion has several consequences: the sensitivity of the pituitary to small decreases in serum levels of thyroid hormones may minimize or prevent further decreases or symptoms by stimulating thyroid hypertrophy or hyperplasia, and TSH preferentially stimulates T_3 synthesis compared to T_4 and increases thyroidal T_4 5'-deiodinase activity, actions that increase the relative thyroidal production of T_3 over T_4 and rT_3. Peripheral conversion and local production of T_4 to T_3 are also increased, but the mechanisms are not clear.

Compared with hypothyroid patients, those with non-thyroidal illness, such as calorie deprivation or chronic illness, have adaptive thyroid deficiency, presumably to limit metabolic activity in the face of the demands of illness. Decreased peripheral conversion of T_4 to T_3 is the hallmark finding, but in severe illness TSH, thyroidal T_4 and T_3 production, and serum T_4 levels may also be decreased.

Primary (Thyroidal or Thyroprivic) Hypothyroidism

Deficient thyroid hormone production from intrinsic thyroid disease has been called primary, thyroidal, and thyroprivic hypothyroidism. In general, causes of primary hypothyroidism result from a reduction of thyroid-hormone producing tissue or biosynthetic defects in hormone production.

Reduction of Thyroid Hormone-Producing Tissue. A list follows of the most common causes of hypothyroidism associated with loss of functional tissue. Discussion of the etiologies resulting from direct manipulation of thyroidal tissue will be omitted.

Autoimmune thyroiditis
Ablative radiotherapy of the thyroid gland
Postoperative hypothyroidism
Transient hypothyroidism postinjury
Thyroid dysgenesis
Infiltrative thyroid disease

Autoimmune thyroiditis can occur in transient and chronic forms. The most common setting for transient autoimmune thyroiditis is in the postpartum period; otherwise, the syndrome is rare. In two studies, 3 and 5 percent of women developed transient hypothyroidism within the yr following delivery.[42,43] The onset is usually 3 to 6 mo postpartum, and the syndrome is characterized by thyromegaly and high levels of thyroid microsomal antibodies that spontaneously resolve in a few wk or mo. Affected patients appear to have an increased risk of recurrence with subsequent pregnancies, probably because they have mild autoimmune thyroiditis. The antibody titers usually persist but tend to decrease at the end of gestation and as the symptoms and signs resolve. The risk of developing chronic thyroiditis is probably increased but not proved. The diagnosis may be obscured because depression, fatigue, and other nonspecific symptoms commonly occur postpartum.

Chronic autoimmune thyroiditis is the most common cause of spontaneous hypothyroidism, typically presenting in women in the fourth decade or later and less commonly in men. It is associated with or without a goiter, and the latter form is Hashimoto's thyroiditis. The autoimmunity in both forms is mediated by humoral and cell-mediated processes, most commonly with high titers of antibodies to the thyroid antigens thyroglobulin and thyroid microsomal peroxidase. Since thyroid peroxidase is located on the surface, the autoantibodies probably exert cytotoxic effects. Because thyroglobulin comprises the intrathyroidal colloid, the corresponding antibodies seem to have no adverse effect. Other autoantibodies may result in impaired bonding of TSH to thyroid receptors, inhibition of thyroid adenylate cyclase activity, blocked cAMP mediation of iodine metabolism, and enhancement of thyroid growth.

As noted elsewhere in this chapter, risk factors for chronic autoimmune thyroiditis include female sex and a positive family history. Antithyroglobulin and thyroid microsomal antibodies are present in as many as 50 percent of siblings of patients and less often in other relatives. Various HLA haplotypes, such as HLA-DR3 and -DR5, are associated with certain populations of patients with chronic autoimmune thyroiditis. Since patients and relatives are at risk for other autoimmune endocrine disorders, such as premature ovarian failure, it would be prudent to be alert to symptoms and signs of insufficiencies in other systems.

The prognosis for chronic autoimmune thyroiditis is variable. If no goiter is present, autoantibody titers by themselves do not necessarily predict hypothyroidism. If compensated hypothyroidism is present, then frank hypothyroidism develops at a rate of 5 to 25 percent per yr, and spontaneous resolution is uncommon. In patients with Hashimoto's thyroiditis who are euthyroid initially, most ultimately develop hypothyroidism. Monitoring patients with compensated hypothyroidism closely is important since, although the goiter may resolve as hypothyroidism develops, the path to clinical hypothyroidism is usually inevitable.

Various degrees of thyroid hypoplasia can occur in newborns. One extreme is thyroid agenesis, but about half the patients with hypoplasia have some tissue detectable on thyroid scan, which may occur anywhere along the developmental tract of the thyroid gland. The etiology is not clear, and the role of maternal autoantibodies is unclear because they have been detected at the same rate in euthyroid and hypothyroid babies. Autoantibodies that inhibit TSH binding have been found in transiently hypothyroid children whose mothers have chronic autoimmune thyroiditis.

Other causes of primary hypothyroidism include withdrawal of thyroid hormone therapy in euthyroid patients and infiltrative diseases, such as sarcoidosis, amyloidosis, hemochromatosis, cystinosis, scleroderma, and fibrous invasive thyroiditis.

Defects of Thyroid Hormone Biosynthesis or Metabolism.
Biosynthetic defects of thyroid synthesis can be congenital or acquired. Congenital anomalies include iodide concentrating and organification defects, thyroglobulin synthesis defects, iodotyrosine deiodinase defect, and thyroid insensitivity to TSH. Acquired abnormalities consist of iodide deficiency or excess and prior treatment with antithyroid drugs. Such drugs may not have intended antithyroid activity. Methimazole and propylthiouracil inhibit thyroid hormone secretion, but inadequately monitored use may cause hypothyroidism. Lithium carbonate can induce hypothyroidism by inhibiting thyroid hormone release. Other agents include aminoglutethimide, ethoinamide, sulfonamides, nitroprusside, thiocyanate, and many other chemicals. Medications such as diphenylhydantoin and rifampin can cause an accelerated metabolism of T_4.

Secondary (Pituitary) Hypothyroidism
Any pituitary disease that compromises or destroys the thyrotropes can cause secondary, or pituitary, hypothyroidism. Maintenance of thyroid gland size and hormone production is dependent on TSH. Pituitary causes of hypothyroidism are much less common than primary disease as a cause. Specific etiologies include space-occupying pituitary lesions such as functioning or nonfunctioning macroadenomas, cysts, carotid artery aneurysms, or craniopharyngiomas; infiltrative or other disease processes, such as tuberculosis, hemochromatosis, histiocytosis (Hand–Schüller–Christian disease), the rare entity postpartum pituitary necrosis (Sheehan syndrome), sarcoidosis, autoimmune hypophysitis, or metastatic tumors; trauma, either secondary to head injury or surgical or radiation therapy; and the uncommon inappropriate secretion of TSH, a syndrome of presumed decreased target-organ sensitivity to thyroid hormone action. Rarely, familial TSH deficiency or varying degrees of pituitary hypoplasia may be found. Compensatory thyrotrope hypertrophy and hyperplasia in primary hypothyroidism may produce an apparent pituitary lesion; TSH levels should be markedly elevated and respond to thyroid hormone repletion.

TSH values in patients with pituitary hypothyroidism are either normal, undetectable, or inappropriately low for the serum thyroxine level. A "normal" TSH value may result from an assay that is not linear in the "low end" (as is the HSTSH assay) and cannot discriminate between a low normal and a low value. Since the HSTSH assay is linear below 1 µU/ml, diagnosing central (secondary or tertiary) hypothyroidism is more precise than with older TSH assays.

Tertiary (Hypothalamic) Hypothyroidism
Hypothalamic TRH deficiencies are rare causes of hypothyroidism, are usually more common in children than adults, and may be isolated or one of multiple hypothalamic hormonal insufficiencies. The usual etiologies have similar mechanisms as those in secondary hypothyroidism: space-occupying lesions, such as neoplasms, which obstruct hypophyseal–portal blood flow; infiltrative, infectious, or inflammatory diseases or trauma (therapeutic or nontherapeutic), which destroy the neuroendocrine cells or tracts; or congenital absence. Since somatostatin suppresses TSH secretion, GH-deficient children treated with GH or patients with acromegaly can develop hypothyroidism, likely secondary to increased somatostatin secretion. The increase in CNS dopamine with hyperprolactinemia may suppress TSH, causing decreased T_4 and T_3 serum levels.

Syndromes of Resistance to Thyroid Hormone
Syndromes of resistance to thyroid hormone are characterized by hyposensitivity of target tissues to thyroid

hormone.[44] Patients with generalized resistance to thyroid hormone (GRTH) demonstrate a clinically euthyroid state or transient symptoms of hypothyroidism, thyromegaly, elevated total and free T_4 and T_3 serum levels, inappropriately normal to mildly elevated TSH values, and a failure to respond to T_3 (resistance in peripheral tissues and pituitary). A second form of the disorder has been described, selective pituitary resistance to thyroid hormone (PRTH).[45] In contrast, patients with PRTH appear clinically hyperthyroid. A third syndrome is selective peripheral resistance to thyroid hormone (PerRTH), in which the resistance occurs in the peripheral tissues but not in the pituitary.[46] A patient so described had normal serum thyroid hormone and TSH levels but was clinically hypothyroid and responded to thyroid hormone treatment. In GRTH the resistance appears incomplete because patients are euthyroid or mildly hypothyroid, and TSH levels and the TSH response to TRH are normal to mildly increased. The inheritance pattern appears to be sporadic or autosomal dominant or recessive,[47] and the mechanisms may be heterogeneous, including a

postreceptor defect. Studies are showing that various point mutations in the human T_3 receptor-beta (hTR-beta) gene have been identified. In GRTH the point mutation usually results in an amino acid substitution in or a partial or complete deletion of the T_3-binding domain of the receptor. Whether PRTH is a qualitatively different disorder or a clinical variation is not clear. Since patients have been misdiagnosed as having thyrotoxicosis and treated with thyroid ablation or iatrogenic hypothyroidism, it would be advisable to consider the syndromes of thyroid hormone resistance when the clinical picture is atypical, before embarking on an irreversible treatment.

Hypothyroidism and Reproductive Endocrinology

Sex Hormone-Binding Globulin and Gonadal Steroids. Hypothyroidism results in decreased production of sex hormone-binding globulin (SHBG) (Fig 17–7), with decreased total estradiol[17] but normal free estradiol levels.[48] Secretion and clearance of estradiol is

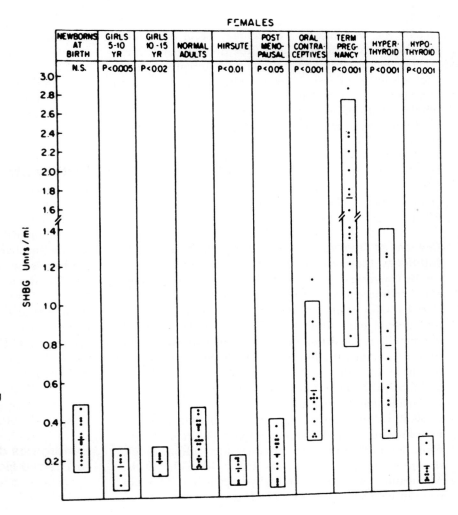

Figure 17–7. Serum sex hormone-binding globulin (SHBG) concentrations in women. *P* values compare the test group with normal adults. (N.S., not significant.) *(Reproduced, with permission, from Tulchinsky D, Chopra IJ. Competitive ligand-binding assay of measurement of sex-hormone-binding globulin [SHBG]. J Clin Endocrinol Metab. 37:877,1973.)*

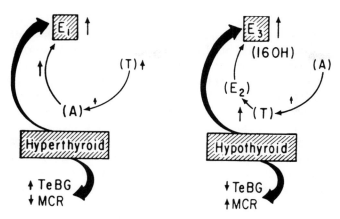

Figure 17–8. Alterations in interconversion and metabolism of androgens and estrogen in hyper- and hypothyroidism. (A, androstenedione; T, testosterone; TeBG, testosterone-estradiol binding globulin; 16-OH, 16-hydroxylation; E_1, estrone; E_2, estradiol, E_3, estriol; MCR, metabolic clearance rate. Arrows indicate increase or decrease.) *(Reproduced, with permission, from Yen SSC. In: Yen SSC, Jaffe RB, eds.* Reproductive Endocrinology: Physiology, Pathophysiology, and Clinical Management, *3rd ed. Philadelphia, W. B. Saunders, 1991: 619.)*

decreased to a proportionally greater degree than progesterone.

The decrease in SHBG production also results in an increase in the metabolic clearance rate (MCR) for testosterone. The MCR for Δ-4-androstenedione does not appear to be altered, but its conversion to testosterone is increased, thus increasing conversion of testosterone to estradiol. The metabolism of estradiol is altered to favor the 16-hydroxylation pathway, producing estriol preferentially to catecholestrogens (Fig 17–8). Increasing the fraction of estrogens may not allow the normal estrogen nadir toward the end of the luteal phase, which increases FSH by negative feedback. If the follicular FSH rise is diminished, inadequate follicle development and oligo-ovulation could result.

Cavaliere et al[49] studied the impact on plasma levels of testosterone and SHBG of treating hyperthyroid and normal control patients with incremental doses of levo-T_4 (L-T_4) (0.2, 0.4 mg for 30 days) and levo-T_3 (L-T_3) (0.05 and 0.2 mg). In the control women a small but significant increase in plasma testosterone occurred with L-T_4 0.4 mg. No significant changes in plasma testosterone levels were observed in hyperthyroid women. SHBG increased in a dose-dependent manner with L-T_4 and L-T_3 in relationship to the serum thyroid hormone levels. Basal plasma SHBG levels were lower in hypothyroid women and increased toward normal with treatment with L-T_4 and L-T_3, although the response to therapy was lower than in the control women. This study indicates that thyroid hormone increases plasma SHBG in normal and hypothyroid women. The

response of serum levels of SHBG to short-term T_3 treatment in patients with GRTH was studied.[50] Basal levels were in the normal range for all patients with GRTH and were not significantly different from normal and hypothyroid patients but were lower than those in thyrotoxic patients. Basal SHBG correlated with FT_4I in normal, hypothyroid, and thyrotoxic patients but not in patients with GRTH. Patients were treated with T_3 at doses of 50, 100, and 200 μg daily for 3 days each and the changes in SHBG were measured. The mean SHBG levels decreased in a dose-response fashion at 50 and 100 μg in patients with GRTH and only increased by 0.7 nmol/L at 200 μg. In comparison, patients with normal tissue responsiveness had dose-dependent increases in levels, the maximum being 16.6 nmol/L at 200 μg/day. This study suggests that although hyperthyroid patients could not always be distinguished from those with GRTH using basal levels of thyroid hormones, SHBG, or the relationship between FT_4I and SHBG, the combination of elevated thyroid hormone levels and the failure of SHBG to rise above basal levels with T_3 treatment for 6 days distinguished 9 of 10 patients with GRTH from thyrotoxic patients, all of whom responded appropriately.

Gonadotropins and Ovulation Disorders. In hypothyroid patients, FSH and LH levels may be increased, normal, or decreased, and the LH surge may be absent. Ovulation disorders may be manifest as a menorrhagia, luteal phase insufficiency, oligo-ovulation, or amenorrhea. Ovarian cysts associated with primary hypothyroidism in infancy or childhood probably are caused by a gonadotropin-like or a direct effect of TRH on GnRH or TRH receptors on the gonadotropes.

Akande[19] compared daily FSH and LH levels in five patients with primary hypothyroidism to euthyroid women. The mean FSH and LH values were significantly lower than controls, and the LH peaks were absent.

Drake and associates[51] performed GnRH stimulation testing on six premenopausal women with primary hypothyroidism. In contrast to the previous study, these women had elevated basal gonadotropins, irrespective of the estradiol level, with normal gonadotropin responses. They concluded that, while hypothyroidism may not alter pituitary responsiveness to GnRH, chronically elevated gonadotropin levels may be a factor in the ovulatory disorders associated with primary hypothyroidism.

Ylostalo et al[52] examined the effect of thyroxine therapy in patients with hypothalamic amenorrhea and low normal thyroid function tests. Within 6 mo of treatment, 59 percent (10/17) of treated patients had at least one regular cycle, compared to 36 percent (4/11) who were untreated. Some of the treated patients had elevated T_4 and free T_4 index levels, but no correlation was made between the thyroid hormone levels and menstrual patterns.

Evers and Rolland[53] reported a 14-yr-old female who had a right ovarian cyst and signs of hypothyroidism and who initially presented with irregular bleeding and galactorrhea at age 8 yr. TSH, FSH, LH, and prolactin were elevated, T_4 was undetectable, and T_3 was low, consistent with primary hypothyroidism. After thyroid hormone repletion with levothyroxine, her symptoms resolved and she developed cyclic menses, the hormonal abnormalities were corrected, and the ovarian cyst regressed. In general, elevated gonadotropins are found when primary hypothyroidism is the etiology of isosexual pseudopuberty.

The etiology of the elevated gonadotropin levels in primary hypothyroidism is unclear. Proximity of the GnRH neurons to the TRH neurons, which are highly stimulated, may result from a lack of specificity on negative feedback. Another theory suggests that an overlap in glycoprotein hormone synthesis occurs, which is supported by evidence that dissimilar FSH and LH release by some authors, the former greater than the latter. The increased production of α-subunits may bind β-subunits of pituitary hormones other than TSH. If interference with GnRH pulsatility by altered TRH or other hypothalamic hormone secretion is significant, then disturbance of the normal negative and positive feedback systems could contribute to anovulation.

Hyperprolactinemia–Galactorrhea. Since primary hypothyroidism may be associated with secondary hyperprolactinemia, patients who would be screened for the latter should also have thyroid function tests performed. As an example, Naguib and associates[54] evaluated 12 patients who presented with infertility, regular menses, and galactorrhea, but who were free of pituitary adenomas. Eight of the 12 had hypothyroidism, hyperprolactinemia, anovulation, and psychological disturbances. A significant proportion of patients in this small series had hyperprolactinemia secondary to primary hypothyroidism.

Subclinical (Compensated) Hypothyroidism. Subclinical or compensated hypothyroidism refers to asymptomatic or minimally symptomatic patients with borderline to elevated levels of TSH or an exaggerated TSH response to a bolus of TRH.[55] Other terms such as potential or early hypothyroidism have been used, but these diagnoses seek to identify patients with laboratory evidence of hypothyroidism with minimal or no symptoms.

Wilansky and Greisman[56] sought to exclude subclinical hypothyroidism with TRH stimulation testing in 67 clinically euthyroid women with menorrhagia, loosely defined as heavy bleeding sufficient to consider surgical therapy. Positive TRH stimulation tests (TSH >30 μIU/ml at 20 or 30 min) were present in 15 of 67 patients (22 percent). Eight of 15 patients (53 percent) who were treated with thyroxine had resolution of menorrhagia within 1 to 3 yr. Since this study did not evaluate the HPO axis, ovulation, or uterine anatomy, it provides no compelling evidence for or mechanism by which subclinical hypothyroidism affects the menstrual cycle.

In a brief communication, Louvet et al[57] reported on 37 of 68 infertile patients from an endemic goiter area with symptoms of mild hypothyroidism. Thirty patients (81 percent) had mild thyromegaly, 11 (30 percent) had decreased serum thyroid hormone levels, and 11 (30 percent) had elevated titers of microsomal antibodies. TRH stimulation in 22 of 37 patients with normal basal values revealed 11 (50 percent) with serum TSH levels greater than two standard deviations from the mean for controls. All 37 were treated with dessicated thyroid extract and had biphasic BBT charts, and 20 of 37 became pregnant.

Kabadi[58] in 1993 followed 30 patients with subclinical hypothyroidism, defined as having normal serum T_4 and T_3 levels with elevated TSH levels on three measurements 2 to 3 wk apart, for 4 to 15 yr with repeat serum levels obtained every 3 to 6 mo. Sixteen patients developed primary hypothyroidism with a progressive rise in TSH levels and decline of T_4 and T_3 levels, with T_4 levels falling below the normal range. Fourteen of 16 hypothyroid patients had known etiologic factors but in 2 none were found. In the remaining 14 patients with subclinical hypothyroidism, the serum TSH elevation persisted following a cyclic pattern. Eleven of the 14 patients had had non-radical surgery or radiation therapy to the neck but in 3 no etiology was found. He concluded that not all patients with subclinical hypothyroidism develop frank hypothyroidism, but two populations emerged: (1) true preclinical hypothyroidism often predicted by a known risk factor and (2) euthyroidism with a "reset thyrostat" that may result from a previous subtle insult to the thyroid gland and probably does not progress to frank hypothyroidism. The main indications for treatment for subclinical or early hypothyroidism are probably thyromegaly or mild symptoms. Some investigators[59] have suggested that treatment with T_4 may be simpler and less expensive than frequent thyroid function testing to detect worsening thyroid failure.

Diagnosis

Hypothyroid patients may have life-threatening symptoms or be asymptomatic. As with other endocrinopathies, vague or nonspecific symptoms with a slow or insidious onset may delay making the diagnosis. Classically, the basal metabolic rate and physical, mental, cardiovascular, gastrointestinal, and neurologic functions are decreased. Typical symptoms, in approximately decreas-

TABLE 17–4. SERUM TOTAL T_4 CONCENTRATION IN NORMAL AND DISEASE STATES

	High	Low	Normal
Thyrotoxic State	Hyperthyroidism (all causes)	Intake of excessive T_3	Low TBG
	Thyroid hormone leak (early subacute thyroiditis, transient thyrotoxicosis)		T_3 toxicosis; more common in iodine-deficient areas
	Excess T_4 (exogenous or ectopic) (thyrotoxicosis factitia, struma ovarii)		Drugs competing with T_4 binding to serum proteins
	Pituitary resistance to thyroid hormone		Hypermetabolism of nonthyroidal origin (Luft's syndrome)
Euthyroid State	High TBG	Low TBG	Normal
	T_4 antibodies	T_4 antibodies	
	T_4-binding albumin variant	Mildly elevated or normal T_3 (T_3 replacement, iodine deficiency, chronic thyroiditis, congenital goiter, treated thyrotoxicosis)	
	Replacement with T_4 only or D-T_4	Drugs competing with T_4 binding to serum proteins	
	Partial peripheral tissue resistance to T_4		
Hypothyroid State	Generalized peripheral tissue resistance to T_4	Thyroid gland failure (primary; secondary, pituitary failure; tertiary, hypothalamic failure)	High TBG

(Adapted, with permission, from Refetoff S. Thyroid function test and effects of drugs on thyroid function. In: DeGroot LJ, ed. Endocrinology, 2nd ed. Philadelphia: W. B. Saunders, 1989: 598.)

ing order of frequency, include dry skin, cold intolerance, hoarseness, weight gain, constipation, decreased sweating, paresthesias, hearing impairment, and weakness. Common signs are coarse skin and hair, slow movements, cold skin, periorbital puffiness, bradycardia, and slow deep-tendon reflex relaxation (Fig 17–9). Myxedema, a hallmark of hypothyroidism, results from the increased synthesis and deposition of glycosaminoglycans, mainly hyaluronic acid, in interstitial tissues. Since hyaluronic acid is polar and hydrophilic, the resulting mucinous edema of the dermis and other organs is likely responsible for much of the dysfunction associated with hypothyroidism. Increases in the skeletal muscle isoenzyme fraction of creatine phosphokinase (CPK) may occur prior to development of clinical symptoms and possibly reflect early myxedema or increased sarcolemmal membrane permeability.

In general, the diagnosis of hyperthyroidism is made on the basis of decreased serum free T_4 (or FT_4I) levels with or without decreased total T_4 (Table 17–4). As noted elsewhere, euthyroid patients may have a decreased total T_4 in the face of decreased TBG. Alternately, total T_4 levels may be in the normal range in hypothyroidism. The T_3RU is usually low, indicating an increased number of occupied T_4-binding sites on TBG (Fig 17–10). Patients with significant nonthyroidal illness usually have similar findings in T_4 values as in hypothyroidism. Serum T_3 levels are often decreased because of its decreased thyroidal production and less T_4 is produced for conversion to T_3. Compensatory TSH secretion increases peripheral metabolism of T_4 to T_3, so about 20 to 30 percent of hypothyroid patients have normal T_3 values. Conversely, low T_3 concentrations can coexist with normal T_4 and TSH levels in patients with nonthyroidal illness or

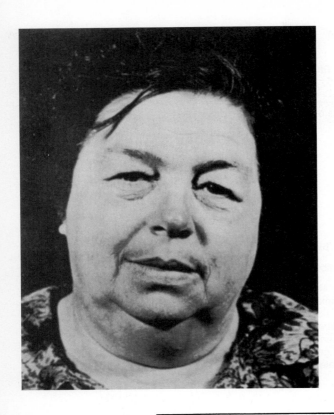

Figure 17–9. Representative facies in hypothyroidism. The woman has moderate periorbital edema, blepharoproptosis, and coarse facial features. *(Reproduced, with permission, from Utiger RD. Hypothyroidism. In: DeGroot LJ, ed. Endocrinology, 2nd ed. Philadelphia, W. B. Saunders, 1989: 709.)*

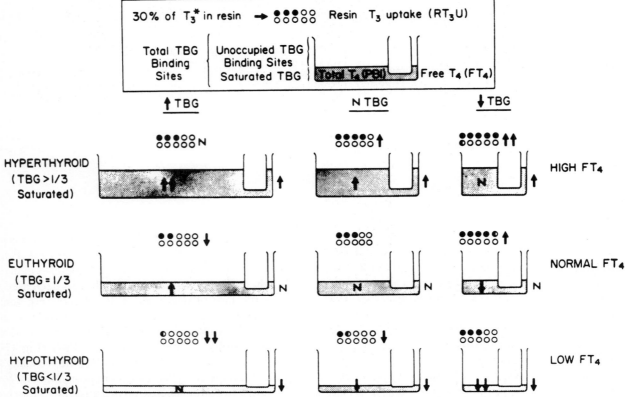

Figure 17–10. Graphic representation of the relationship between the serum total T_4 (TT_4) concentration, the resin T_3 uptake (RT_3U) test, and the free T_4 (FT_4) concentration in various metabolic states and in association with changes of TBG concentration. The principle of communicating vessels is used as analogy. The height of fluid in the small vessel represents the level of FT_4; the total amount of fluid in the large vessel, the TT_4 concentration; and the total volume of the large vessel, the TBG capacity. The RT_3U test result (black dots) is inversely proportional to the unsaturated TBG represented by the unfilled capacity of the large vessel. *(Reproduced, with permission, from Refetoff S. Thyroid function test and effects of drugs on thyroid function. In: DeGroot LJ, ed. Endocrinology, 2nd ed. Philadelphia, W. B. Saunders, 1989: 600.)*

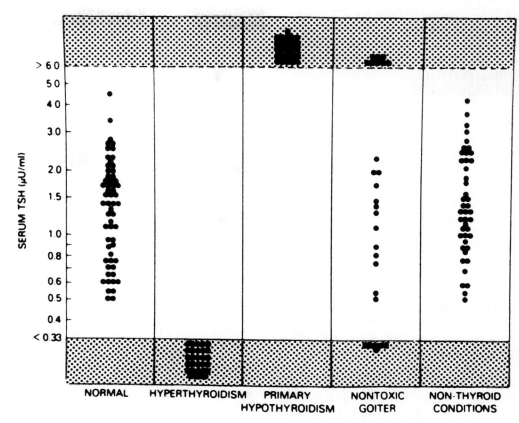

Figure 17–11. Serum thyroid-stimulating hormone (TSH) in thyroid disease. Serum TSH levels were measured by a sensitive assay in normal subjects and in patients with hyperthyroidism, primary hypothyroidism, nontoxic goiter, and various nonthyroid conditions. *(Reproduced, with permission, from Wehman R, Rubenstein HA, Pugeat MM, Nisula BC. Extended clinical utility of a sensitive and reliable radioimmunoassay of thyroid-stimulating hormone. South Med J. 76:971, 1983.)*

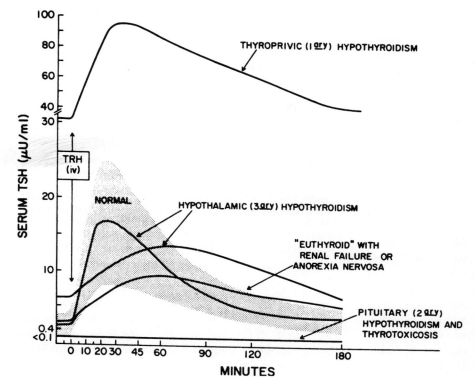

Figure 17–12. TSH responses to a TRH challenge in various thyroid states. Administration of a single intravenous 400-μg bolus of TRH usually produces typical TSH responses depending on the thyroid state of the patient. The normal response is indicated by the shaded area. Data used for this figure were averaged from several studies. *(Reproduced, with permission, from Refetoff S. Thyroid function test and effects of drugs on thyroid function. In: DeGroot LJ, ed. Endocrinology, 2nd ed. Philadelphia, W. B. Saunders, 1989: 618.)*

with some drugs. The measurement of total T_3 in suspected hypothyroidism is not routinely useful. Patients with low total T_3 levels with a normal total T_4 usually have decreased peripheral conversion of T_4 to T_3 from an acute or chronic illness or calorie deprivation. Decreased conversion can occur in as rapidly as 24 to 48 hours.

Measurement of TSH usually discriminates between primary and central (secondary or tertiary) hypothyroidism. In most patients with primary hypothyroidism, TSH levels are elevated above 6 µU/ml (Fig 17–11). In compensated hypothyroidism TSH levels are increased with normal total and free T_4 values. In central disease, TSH levels are normal, low, or undetectable. The combination of a low free T_4 (or FT_4I) with an inappropriately low TSH value indicates central disease until disproved. Screening for hypothyroidism with only a TSH level will usually detect primary disease, the most common form, but omitting a free T_4 or total T_4 could miss central hypothyroidism. A TSH level may not discriminate between secondary and tertiary hypothyroidism, but a HSTSH can at least determine if the value is below normal. As above, in nonthyroidal illness TSH secretion decreases and the serum level may be normal or low as a result. All thyroid function tests should be interpreted in light of the patient's clinical condition to try to differentiate overt hypothyroidism from adaptive thyroid deficiency in nonthyroidal illness.

The TRH stimulation test has been used to attempt to distinguish secondary from tertiary hypothyroidism (Fig 17–12). Although the TSH response to TRH in primary hypothyroidism is proportional to the basal level, the TRH test might be needed only to confirm subclinical hypothyroidism. The classic response of TSH to a bolus of TRH in secondary hypothyroidism is absence, and in tertiary disease a delayed rise of normal magnitude is typical. However, some patients with pituitary disease and nonthyroidal illness may also have delayed responses, so the TRH test may not always be diagnostic.

Nonthyroid laboratory abnormalities in hypothyroidism may include elevated cholesterol, triglycerides, carcinoembryonic antigen, and carotene, and hyperlipidemia may contribute significantly to vascular disease. Angiotensin-converting enzyme may be decreased. Hypothyroidism should be considered when these abnormalities are found unexpectedly.

In summary, the following approach is suggested to evaluate suspected hypothyroidism (Fig 17–13.) First, serum total T_4 or free T_4, T_3RU, and HSTSH should be measured. In otherwise healthy patients, a low T_4 and T_3RU indicate hypothyroidism. These values coupled with a high TSH represent primary hypothyroidism, and a low or normal TSH, central disease. All normal values suggest a euthyroidism, but may not rule out hypothyroidism. In seriously ill patients, normal or low studies are consistent with tertiary disease or adaptive hypothyroidism associated with nonthyroidal illness. Whenever

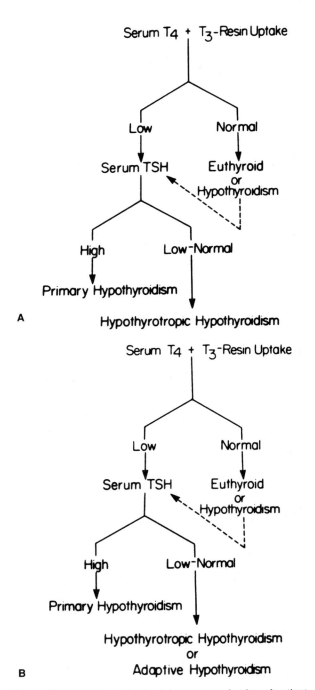

Figure 17–13. Scheme for the laboratory evaluation of patients with suspected hypothyroidism who are otherwise healthy (**A**) or who have serious nonthyroidal illness (**B**). *(Reproduced, with permission, from Utiger RD. Hypothyroidism. In: DeGroot LJ, ed. Endocrinology, 2nd ed. Philadelphia, W. B. Saunders, 1989: 715.)*

central disease is suspected, a search for symptoms or findings of pituitary or hypothalamic disease is indicated. Reverse T_3 (rT_3) is usually decreased in hypothyroidism but increased in nonthyroidal illness, and measurement may assist in the diagnosis.

Therapy

The goal of treatment is clinical and biochemical euthyroidism. Stopping or changing offending medications should be the first step when practical. As long as the hypothyroidism is not considered transient, repletion with thyroxine (T_4) is the method of choice and is usually lifelong. Starting doses range from 0.1 to 0.15 mg (1.0 to 2.0 µg/kg) daily in healthy patients, but 0.25 to 0.05 mg daily in elderly patients or those with cardiovascular disease to avoid precipitating angina pectoris or heart failure. Thyroxine exerts its effects in about 4 to 8 wk, and most signs and symptoms resolve in several mo. Only after reaching the steady state should the dose be adjusted, unless severe manifestations supervene. The doses for normal healthy patients will almost always restore TSH values to normal. The amount of functioning residual thyroid gland tissue may determine the ultimate replacement dose needed. TSH, free T_4, and free T_3 appear to have a diurnal variation with thyroid hormone replacement, a fact that should be considered in monitoring serum levels on therapy.[60] In 11 clinically and biochemically euthyroid treated hypothyroid patients (once-daily morning dose), TSH followed a diurnal rhythm with a peak level at 2330 and trough at 1430 hr. Four patients had TSH trough levels with the normal range but peak levels outside the normal range. Free T_4 and free T_3 levels fell from peak 3 hr after ingestion to nadir just prior to the next dose.

About 80 percent of T_4 is absorbed from the gastrointestinal tract, and such disease may result in malabsorption. An increased dose may be needed in colder climates. In euthyroid-replete patients, serum T_4 and T_3 concentrations are usually normal to mildly elevated. Since simply normal values may be inadequate for replacement, restoration of serum TSH to the normal range is perhaps the best indicator of biochemical euthyroidism. Excessive replacement usually results in a low or undetectable HSTSH level.

Other thyroid hormone preparations are available for replacement therapy and include T_3, combinations of T_3 and T_4, desiccated thyroid, and thyroglobulin. Since T_3 values often vary substantially and T_4 levels are low, treatment with drugs other than T_4 offers no significant benefit and may lead to iatrogenic hyperthyroidism trying to normalize the T_4. Recent studies have reported on the use of T_3 and have shown promise of its efficacy.

Once thyroid hormone therapy has been discontinued in a hypothyroid patient, symptoms take about 3 or 4 wk to recur, and severe symptoms usually appear in about 2 or 3 mo. The peripheral stores of T_4 and its long half-life, which increases with worsening hypothyroidism, are probably a buffer against a more rapid onset and profound decline.

An understanding of changes that occur in nonthyroidal illness and in the perioperative period is important in hypothyroid patients. While serum T_3 decreases in hypothyroid and euthyroid patients, TSH increases in the former usually only in severe disease. When TSH concentrations decrease with fever, or dopamine or glucocorticoid therapy, diagnosis of hypothyroidism may be difficult. The increase of perioperative complications, such as intraoperative hypotension, has been controversial in the literature. Knowledge of the change in metabolism of various medications, such as anesthetics, should guide their use in hypothyroid patients, because of the prolonged metabolism in a number of drugs.

Hyperthyroidism

Definition and Epidemiology.
Hyperthyroidism is the clinical syndrome of increased secretion of thyroid hormones, T_3 and/or T_4, usually with symptoms or physical findings consistent with hyperthyroidism. It is important to distinguish laboratory abnormalities alone from the correlation of abnormal levels and the clinical assessment of the patient's metabolic status. Two types of hyperthyroidism predominate and should be distinguished: toxic nodular goiter (single or multiple adenomata), and toxic diffuse goiter or Graves' disease.[61] Toxic multinodular goiter is probably the result of either multiple hyperfunctioning adenomata or Graves' disease. Less common forms of hyperthyroidism include iatrogenic hyperthyroidism (thyrotoxicosis factitia), functioning metastatic thyroid carcinoma, molar thyrotropin (TSH-like activity secreted from nonendocrine malignant tumors), inappropriate secretion of TSH, struma ovarii, iodide-induced hyperthyroidism and silent thyroiditis, and Hashimoto's thyroiditis.

Toxic Nodular Goiter.
Toxic nodular goiter is an entity that is most common in older patients and would not likely be found in a reproductive-aged woman. The adenomata secrete elevated levels of thyroid hormone, which suppress TSH and the normal surrounding thyroid tissue. Diagnosis is suggested by elevated free T_4, undetectable HSTSH, and uptake of 131-iodine in the nodule(s) on thyroid scanning with decreased uptake in the adjacent tissue. Administration of TSH followed by another scan demonstrates increased uptake in the surrounding tissue that is suppressed but responsive. Treatment is directed toward ablation by 131-iodine or surgery, either of which usually, but not always, leads to hypothyroidism.

Toxic Diffuse Goiter (Graves' Disease).
Graves' disease represents a systemic disease of autoimmunity with variable expression. Multiple lines of evidence suggests a hereditary component: family history of thyroid antibodies, association with other autoimmune diseases, and increases in certain HLA haplotypes (HLA-B8 and

-DR3 in Caucasians, HLA-Bw35 in Japanese, and HLA-Bw46 in Chinese from Singapore).

The pathophysiology of Graves' disease is mediated by an IgG autoantibody known as the long-acting thyroid stimulator (LATS). Two types of assays have been used to characterize the antibodies: the direct stimulation of a thyroid cell preparation and the inhibition of binding of ^{125}I-TSH to its receptor. The antibodies so identified are termed thyroid-stimulating antibody (TSAb) and TSH-binding inhibition (TBI), respectively. The antibody in question should bind to the TSH receptor, inhibit binding of TSH, and stimulate the thyroid. The TSAb assay probably measures an IgG that satisfies these criteria, but the TSI may measure IgG inhibitors of TSH binding that are not stimulatory.

Iatrogenic Hyperthyroidism. With the ease and low cost of thyroid function testing, empiric treatment with thyroid hormone for such symptoms as fatigue, weight loss, or fertility should be avoided. Risks of thyroid hormone excess include thyrotoxicosis with fever, nausea, vomiting, tachycardia, arrhythmias, tremulousness, anxiety, and so forth. Recent evidence indicates that long-term treatment with L-thyroxine can contribute to decreased hip bone density in premenopausal women,[62] but studies have reported conflicting results. In one study, 31 hypothyroid women who had been treated for at least 5 yr were compared to 31 control women without thyroid hormone or bone abnormalities. The T_4-treated women had 12.8 percent less femoral neck and 10.8 percent less trochanter bone density than controls, as assessed by dual-photon absorptiometry (coefficient of variation 1.5 percent). There was no significant difference in lumbar spine bone density between the groups.

In another study,[63] 202 white women taking thyroid hormone were evaluated for clinical characteristics related to bone mineral density (BMD). BMD was measured at L2–L4 (N = 335 in 195 patients), three sites of the hip (N = 247 in 157 patients), and proximal radius (N = 172 in 125 patients). Increasing age and prior thyrotoxicosis adversely affected, and body mass index (BMI) positively affected, spine BMD. Dose of thyroid hormone, duration of treatment, type of thyroid disease, history of thyroidectomy, or serum free thyroxine index did not affect either initial BMI or change in BMD over time. At the hip sites age and a history of prior thyrotoxicosis ($0.05 < P < 0.10$) negatively and BMI positively correlated with BMD. No other clinical parameters correlated with BMD or its change over time. At the proximal radius, age, prior thyrotoxicosis, and dose of thyroid hormone negative affected BMD.

Finally, BMD was evaluated in postmenopausal women with subclinical hypothyroidism treated short-term with levo-thyroxine[64] in a randomized, prospective trial. Seventeen postmenopausal women were randomly assigned to receive either levo-thyroxine or no treatment. The patients in the treatment group did not significantly differ in the mean serum TSH levels but were older (68 ± 7 versus 60 ± 5 yr [$P < 0.02$]). The average levothyroxine dose needed to normalize the serum TSH levels was 0.072 mg (±0.027) daily. At baseline bone density studies did not differ between the groups, and after 14 mo of therapy single-photon absorptiometry of the wrist decreased by 1.8 percent (±3.2) in the untreated group and by 0.5 percent (±4.1) in the treatment group (P = NS). Dual-energy x-ray absorptiometry of the lumbar spine decreased by 0.7 percent (±2.9) in untreated patients compared to an increase of 0.1 percent (±4.75) in treated patients. The authors concluded that unlike the BMD decrease seen in early treatment of overt hypothyroidism, postmenopausal patients potentially symptomatic with subclinical hypothyroidism can be treated short term without significant loss of BMD.

Hyperthyroidism and Reproductive Endocrinology

Sex-Hormone Binding Globulin and Gonadal Steroids. In hyperthyroidism, high levels of T_4 increase hepatic production of SHBG, thus decreasing the metabolic clearance rate (MCR) of androgens and estrogens. However, its effect on estrogen and its metabolism has been controversial. Some investigators have reported normal estrogen concentrations and production rates, and others have found increased total and free estradiol levels with decreased metabolic clearance rates. In general, Akande and Anderson[22] found that SHBG, estradiol, and testosterone levels were markedly elevated in 15 thyrotoxic women. Akande and Hockaday[20] confirmed these steroid findings and noted that the progesterone levels reflected the menstrual, not the thyroid, status. Once treatment rendered the patients euthyroid, all levels became normal.

In men, elevated SHBG levels increase total testosterone but lower its metabolic clearance rate, maintaining a normal production rate. The ratio of estrogens to androgens seems to be increased in hyperthyroid men, because gynecomastia is found frequently. Chopra and Tulchinsky[65] found that unbound serum estradiol levels were increased in hyperthyroid men out of proportion to the rise in SHBG, which correlated with gynecomastia.

Sex steroid metabolism is altered in hyperthyroidism.[66] Hyperthyroidism results in increased serum and an increased conversion of testosterone to Δ-4-androstenedione, both of which are aromatized to increased levels of estradiol and estrone, respectively. The MCR of testosterone is decreased and that of androstenedione is normal, but the production rates are both increased in hyperthyroid women. The two major metabolic pathways for estrogens are 2-hydroxylation and 16-hydroxylation. In hyperthyroidism, increased 2-hydroxylation activity[13] leads to elevated catecholestrogens, 2-hydroxyestradiol, and 2-hydroxyestrone, which are weak estrogen agonists. These metabolites may contribute to negative feedback at the hypothalamus or pituitary predisposing to anovulation. Perhaps these shifts toward increased androgens and catecholestrogens help explain the anovulation and elevated LH values seen in hyperthyroidism. Androgens undergo preferential 5α-reduction rather than 5β, which would increase dihydrotestosterone. Contrast the metabolic products in hypothyroidism in the section above.

Gonadotropins and Ovulation Disorders.
Menstrual cyclicity is altered in hyperthyroidism, often with oligomenorrhea, oligo-ovulation, hypomenorrhea, and decreased fecundity. Thyrotoxic patients may be at risk for spontaneous abortion,[67] but the mechanism is not clear.

Akande and Anderson[22] and Akande and Hockaday[20] found elevated FSH and LH levels in 15 thyrotoxic women. LH and FSH midcycle peaks were present in menstruating patients and controls but were absent in amenorrheic women. Levels normalized with successful treatment. The authors proposed several possible explanations for these changes: (1) the rise in SHBG and decrease in free androgens and estrogens might increase the gonadotropin response by negative feedback at the pituitary, but a new steady state should be reached; (2) although the menstrual irregularity correlated with the severity of thyrotoxicosis, SHBG levels did not; and (3) a reduced effectiveness of estrogen in suppressing LH or GnRH might affect the normal negative and positive feedback perhaps mediated through hypothalamic catecholamine production.

Gonadotropin response to GnRH was studied in 41 women with hyperthyroidism,[68] according to menstrual status: regular menses, hypomenorrhea, and amenorrhea, as well as the phase of menstrual cycle. Compared with normal controls, LH responses to GnRH were increased in hyperthyroid women regardless of cycle phase, but those with regular cycles had more marked responses than those with menstrual disorders. Basal and peak FSH responses were greater in follicular than luteal phase, regardless of menstrual status. Data suggest that high circulating levels of thyroid hormones augment gonadotropin response to GnRH and that increased FSH and LH probably helps maintain cyclicity in hyperthyroidism.

Diagnosis
A characteristic symptom complex helps differentiate Graves' disease from thyrotoxicosis from a toxic adenoma. Because autonomic lability may accompany thyrotoxicosis in Graves' disease, characteristic symptoms include nervousness, tremulousness, heat intolerance, palpitations, and diarrhea to a greater degree than in other types of thyrotoxicosis, and some symptoms persist when euthyroid. Libido may be increased or decreased. Other symptoms of hyperthyroidism are weight loss despite an increased appetite or with anorexia, diaphoresis, dyspnea on exertion, and emotional lability.

Physical findings may include goiter, thyroid nodularity, exophthalmos, periorbital or bulbar inflammation, pretibial myxedema, and acropathy. Ophthalmopathic findings can vary from a stare to blindness from corneal or optic nerve compromise, associated with inflammation (Fig 17–14A). Pretibial myxedema occurs in about 4 percent of patients with Graves' disease and is not limited to the lower extremities (Fig 17–14B). Acropathy refers to soft tissue swelling and subperiosteal new bone formation noted on radiologic examination. Other findings of thyrotoxicosis consist of tachycardia, widened pulse pressure, lid lag, tremors, warm moist skin, changes in skin pigmentation, fine hair texture, onycholysis, a hyperdynamic precordium, cardiac arrhythmias such as atrial fibrillation, and in severe cases, muscle wasting.

In hyperthyroidism, (see Fig 17–11) TSH values are very low or undetectable, except in pituitary-related hyperthyroidism, T_3 is almost always increased but T_4 levels may be high or normal. The increase in total T_3 is disproportionately greater than in T_4 because of greater conversion of T_4 to T_3. In T_3 thyrotoxicosis, total T_3 is usually elevated with normal free T_4 and total T_4 levels. Treated thyrotoxic patients with Graves' disease may have similar values. According to McKenzie and Zakarija,[61] measurement of thyroid uptake of radioiodine routinely in suspected Graves' disease has been supplanted by measuring T_3 and T_4. In silent thyroiditis, it is meaningful since the uptake is virtually absent. TRH-stimulation testing in hyperthyroidism results in no TSH response (see Fig 17–12), but a euthyroid-treated hyperthyroid patient may also have no response. The results should be interpreted in light of the patient's clinical condition. This test can be used in pregnancy to avoid radioiodine, and the physiologic TSH to TRH administration is exaggerated, but an HSTSH assay should almost always confirm hyperthyroidism. A thyroid suppression test can be performed by giving T_3 100 μg daily for 7 days. The total T_4 level should be reduced by at least 50 percent of the baseline value.

Titers of antibody to thyroid microsomal peroxidase (antimicrosomal antibodies) are usually elevated in Graves' disease, but also in other diseases such as Hashimoto's thyroiditis. Antithyroglobulin titers are usually lower in both disease states. The usefulness of antibody testing is limited for this reason and because the levels do not correlate with disease severity or thyroid function. Knowledge of their presence may be important for interpreting thyroid function tests, since they may bind T_3 or T_4.

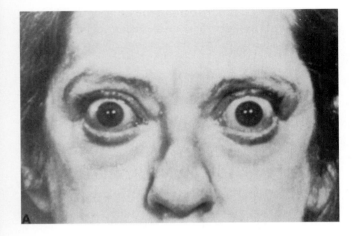

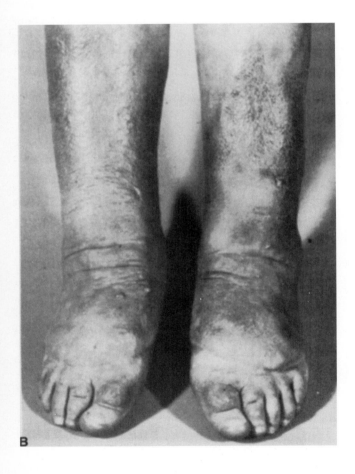

Figure 17–14. A. Photograph of a patient with ophthalmopathy of Graves' disease. Appearance when she was hyperthyroid with bilateral proptosis and moderate inflammatory changes; she was rendered euthyroid by treatment with [131]I. **B.** Photograph of legs of a patient with pretibial myxedema. All changes are characteristically bilateral and usually symmetrical. Extension to the dorsa of the feet is unusual. The shiny appearance of the indurated skin is characteristic. *(Reproduced, with permission, from McKenzie JM, Zakarija M. Hyperthyroidism. In: DeGroot LJ, ed.* Endocrinology, *2nd ed. Philadelphia, W. B. Saunders, 1984: 661, 669.)*

Nonthyroid laboratory abnormalities include elevations in liver function tests, such as transaminases, alkaline phosphatase; megaloblastic or normochromic normocytic anemia, transient or unmasked carbohydrate intolerance, hypercalciuria probably from a direct effect of thyroid hormone on bone resorption, and hypomagnesemia which can stimulate parathyroid hormone release. Autoimmune conditions that have been associated with Graves' disease are antiparietal cell and anti-intrinsic factor antibodies, idiopathic thrombocytopenic purpura, and others.

Therapy

Since the causes and treatment of hyperthyroidism can be extensive, this discussion will be limited to principles of treatment. Five treatment modalities may be used in hyperthyroidism: antithyroid drugs, radioiodine, surgical resection, β-blockade, and sedation. Beta-blockers, such as propranolol, are safer for symptomatic management of mild hyperthyroidism and thyrotoxicosis, because prolonged iodine administration can exacerbate the condition. Iodide can be used preoperatively but may cause hypothyroidism. Preoperative preparation may include treatment with a thionamide (such as propylthiouracil, methimazole, or carbamizole), iodide, and/or propranolol until euthyroid. Indications for surgical therapy depend on the skill of the surgeon balanced against the risks of hypoparathyroidism and recurrent laryngeal nerve damage. The typical therapeutic dose of radioiodine is 6000 to 7000 rads of 131-iodine. Less hypothyroidism may result from smaller doses, but times to remission are usually longer. In general, radioiodine and surgical resection result in hypothyroidism, providing the patient's life expectancy is reasonable. Propylthiouracil works by inhibiting thyroid hormone synthesis and peripheral deiodination to T_3. The relapse rate with thionamide drugs can be significant, but hypothyroidism may be prevented.

LABORATORY EVALUATION OF THYROID HORMONES

Rather than provide an exhaustive listing of thyroid function tests that might be needed by a thyroidologist,[69] this section will deal with well-known assays used initially to diagnose a perturbation of the HPT axis. The practicing physician should have easy access to most of these assays in a local or regional laboratory. This discussion is meant to familiarize the physician with the techniques currently available and with the merits and limitations of the assays.

Thyroid-Stimulating Hormone

The current test of choice for measurement of thyroid-stimulating hormone (TSH) in clinical practice is the immunoradiometric or immunoenzymometric "sandwich" assays, which are the so-called "high-sensitivity" (HSTSH) or "ultra-sensitivity" assays. Previous radioimmunoassays (RIAs) were less specific than current ones largely because of cross-reactivity of the α-subunit of TSH with those of FSH, LH, and hCG. Older RIA kits had normal ranges of less than 0.5 to 6.0 μU/ml, but the normal range of the HSTSH assay is from less than 0.4 to 4.5 μU/ml. Since the minimum detectable level is about 0.01 μU/ml, the HSTSH assay can discriminate a hyperthyroid from a euthyroid state. Figure 17–11 shows HSTSH values in five groups of patients: euthyroid, hyperthyroid, primary hypothyroid, nontoxic goiter, and nonthyroid conditions. Note the clustering of the extreme values of serum TSH in hyperthyroidism (all less than 0.33 μU/ml) and primary hypothyroidism (all greater than 6.0 μU/ml). Klee and Hay[70] analyzed three HSTSH assays and proposed the following criteria for clinical use: (1) the overlap of the assay detection limit and the lower limit of normal should be less than 1 percent, (2) basal TSH measurements should predict the TSH response to TRH stimulation at least 95 percent of the time, and (3) basal TSH measurements should be 95 percent sensitive and 95 percent specific for detecting hyperthyroidism.

Thyroxine-Binding Globulin

In the euthyroid patient, changes in the T_3RU are inversely proportional to the level of thyroxine-binding globulin (TBG). However, an abnormal value of T_3RU may represent an abnormal value of TBG, a hypo- or hyperthyroid state, or drug artifact. The ability to measure TBG directly should provide more specific evaluation of markedly abnormal thyroid functions tests, congenital abnormalities of binding proteins, and discrepant values of T_3RU.

TBG can be measured by estimating the total T_4-binding capacity at saturation or directly by immunoassays. The saturation technique is labor intensive and requires technical expertise. It evaluates the relative binding to the three major thyroid hormone-binding proteins, which are separated by electrophoresis. A simpler method using an anion-exchange resin has been adapted for clinical use. The normal range is 16 to 24 μg of T_4/dl of serum for TBG capacity.

TBG can also be measured clinically by RIA, Laurell's rocket immunoelectrophoresis, radial immunodiffusion, enzyme immunoassay, and a combination of hormone binding to TBG and immunological techniques. Some kits are based on competition between labeled hormone and TBG and the antibody against the hormone; others use antisera against TBG and labeled T_4 or TBG.

Thyroxine

Total T_4. The RIA is one of the most common methods by which total thyroxine (T_4) is measured clinically. All iodide-containing species in serum are measured with this kind of assay. T_4 bound to TBG cannot be measured, since the affinity of T_4 for TBG can be as high as that for the test antiserum. Extraction or competitive displacement of T_4 or inactivation of TBG has been used to free T_4 from TBG for subsequent measurement. The antibodies do not usually bind selectively L- or D-isomers, which is of no clinical consequence.

Free T_4. Less than 1 percent of T_4 is unbound to proteins and is free to bind to receptors and exert its effects in the peripheral tissues. The serum concentration of free T_4 remains constant despite changing levels of serum proteins as long as the HPT axis is intact. Free T_4 levels better reflect the metabolic state of the patient than do those of total T_4.

The most common methods for determining free thyroid hormone concentrations in serum involve measuring dialyzable T_4 and T_3, calculation of free T_4 and T_3 indices, estimation based on TBG levels, calculating the effective T_4 ratio, and direct measurement of the free hormones. The dialyzable free T_4 assay is often impractical because it is time consuming and cumbersome and it requires technical skill.

Free thyroid hormone indices are calculated estimates. We know that free T_4 binds reversibly to unoccupied binding sites on TBG according to a predictable proportion, or association constant. Assuming that the concentration of TBG-bound T_4 can be approximated by the serum total T_4 concentration, then we have the following relationship:

$$FT_4I = \frac{[\text{Total } T_1]\,[\text{Patient's } T_3RU]}{[\text{Mean standard } T_3RU]}$$

FT_4I, the free T_4 index or adjusted total T_4, compares the patient's T_3RU with a population mean with assumed normal TBG concentrations. The FT_4I correlates linearly with the free T_4 values obtained by dialysis (r = 0.99) and with the metabolic status of the patient. Since actual TBG concentrations can be measured by RIA, its use in the calculations of free T_4 is preferable to the T_3RU. The terms "T_7" and "T_{12}" are products of the total T_4 and the RT_3U artificially defined in commercial kits and have different normal ranges from the FT_4I.

The "direct" assays of T_4 and T_3 use an immobilized antibody to T_4 and labeled T_4. The ratio of labeled T_4 bound to the sample TBG and to the immobilized antibody is proportional to the free T_4 level. In a similar two-step assay, the "indirect" free T_4, the amount of labeled T_4 bound to the immobilized antibody, is indirectly proportional to the free T_4 in serum.

If the assay for dialyzable free T_4 (or T_3) is not feasible, reasonable assays of choice would be either the two-step indirect free T_4 or a FT_4I. Direct measurement of TBG is preferable to performing the T_3RU. TSH measurement by a highly sensitive assay is usually inversely proportional to the level of free hormone and should confirm the estimate of free T_4.

Triiodothyronine

The principles by which total and free triiodothyronine (T_3) are measured are similar to those involving T_4. In general, total T_3 concentrations parallel total T_4, but an understanding of physiologic and pathologic changes should avoid misinterpretation of levels. At birth total T_3 is low, but after an acute TSH surge, T_3 levels increase to about twice normal in the first day of life and decrease over the next day or two to a level in the upper limit of the adult normal range for the first yr of life. Total T_3 levels slowly decline with age, but there is no significant difference between the sexes.

Changes in TBG concentrations alter total T_3 levels similarly to T_4, leaving free T_3 normal. T_3 levels themselves are usually not useful in the hypothyroid patient but are most helpful in evaluating suspected hyperthyroidism or discrepancies in other thyroid function tests. The normal range for total T_3 is 80 to 190 ng/dl but may depend on the individual laboratory.

Resin Triiodothyronine (Thyroxine) Uptake

The resin triiodothyronine uptake (RT_3U) or thyroxine uptake (RT_4U) in vitro test is an indirect measurement of serum thyroid hormone protein-binding capacity, which can help determine whether changes in total thyroid hormone levels have resulted from altered protein concentrations in a euthyroid patient, or from hypo- or hyperthyroidism. The resin thyroid hormone uptake (RT_3U) measures the unbound thyroid hormone binding sites on TBG and is an indirect assay of TBG concentration. Drugs, such as salicylate, that inhibit binding of T_4 to TBG, may give a false elevation in T_3RU.

T_3 (or T_4) radiolabeled with iodine competes with a patient's endogenous hormones for the binding sites on TBG. T_3 is usually selected for its preferential binding to TBG with less affinity than T_4. The sample is passed over an anion-exchange resin, which adsorbs the loosely adherent labeled T_3. The radioactivity on the resin is measured, and the percentage of the total amount of labeled hormone added to the sample is the value of the T_3RU.

The amount of label bound to the resin is inversely proportional to the number of unoccupied thyroid hormone binding sites on TBG, which reflects either changes in TBG concentrations, thyroid disease, or drug artifact. Opposing trends in total T_4 and T_3RU usually suggest changes in TBG levels or binding, but parallel trends often indicate hypo- or hyperthyroidism. For example, in hyperthyroidism, thyroid hormones will occupy increased TBG binding sites, allowing less binding of labeled T_3, more label adsorbed to the resin, and increased radioactivity. Decreased serum levels of TBG will give a

similar result. Normal ranges are assay dependent: 25 to 35 percent or 45 to 55 percent. Normalizing the value to a standard control sample eliminates assay dependence, giving a normal ratio of 0.85 to 1.15.

Provocative Testing of Thyroid Hormone Secretion

Thyrotropin-Releasing Hormone Stimulation Test.
Thyrotropin-releasing hormone (TRH) is the primary physiologic stimulus for TSH secretion and is a potent prolactin-releasing hormone. It may stimulate growth hormone (GH) and adrenocorticotropic hormone (ACTH), as well. Serum TRH levels are difficult to measure and to interpret, since TRH secretion into the hypophyseal portal system leads to significant dilution in peripheral serum, TRH has a short half-life, and it is produced peripherally.

In a euthyroid patient injection of a bolus of synthetic TRH results in a rise in TSH, which is inversely proportional to the serum level of free T_4 (see Fig 17–12). Basal TSH levels also correlate with peak levels after stimulation. For example, in primary hypothyroidism, the TSH response is exaggerated, but in hyperthyroidism it is absent. Since a normal test depends on intact TSH reserve, it has been used to help discriminate between pituitary and hypothalamic hypothyroidism, in the diagnosis of mild hypothyroidism, and in confirming mild thyrotoxicosis with normal thyroid function tests.

The reader is referred elsewhere for the details of the protocol.[42] Since the TSH response to TRH is usually greater in the follicular phase of the menstrual cycle and is lowest at 1100, it is customary to standardize the testing to a time of day and a phase of the cycle.

CONCLUSIONS

Abnormalities of thyroid hormone production can disturb ovulation and the menstrual cycle. Ovulation disorders can also affect thyroid hormone metabolism, but a normal hypothalamic–pituitary–thyroid axis can usually compensate with mild disease. Interactions with the hypothalamic–pituitary–ovarian axis can occur among most of the components of the axes, and investigation of thyroid hormone abnormalities should be considered with ovulation or menstrual disorders. The impact of compensated hypothyroidism on ovulation is incompletely understood. Although ovulation induction may be successful in the untreated mildly hypothyroid patient, there is little cost and risk to diagnosis and treatment, and thyroid hormone repletion is reasonable before attempting pregnancy. There is no role for thyroid hormone treatment in euthyroid patients.[71]

Acknowledgment

The author dedicates this chapter to Rod Powers, who provided the illustrations. In his struggle with leukemia, his faith in Christ strengthened him, encouraged others, and allowed him to face death without fear.

REFERENCES

1. Tyler ET. The thyroid myth in infertility. *Fertil Steril.* 4:218, 1953
2. Buxton CL, Herrmann WL. Effect of thyroid hormone on menstrual disorders and sterility. *JAMA.* 155:1035, 1955
3. Neves-e-Castro M, Calhaz-Jorge C, Correia S, et al. In Crosignani PG, Mishell DR, eds. *Ovulation in Humans.* London, 1976: 301
4. Moore KL. *The Developing Human,* 4th ed. Philadelphia, W. B. Saunders, 1998: 184–186
5. Lissitzky S. Physiology of the thyroid. In: DeGroot LJ, ed. *Endocrinology,* 2nd ed. Philadelphia, W. B. Saunders, 1989: 512–522
6. Refetoff S, Larsen PR. Transport, cellular uptake, and metabolism of thyroid hormone. In: DeGroot LJ, ed. *Endocrinology,* 2nd ed. Philadelphia, W. B. Saunders, 1989: 541–561.
7. Lavin TN. Mechanisms of action of thyroid hormone. In: DeGroot LJ, ed. *Endocrinology,* 2nd ed. Philadelphia, W. B. Saunders, 1989: 562–573.
8. Guillemin R, Yamazaki E, Gard DA, et al. In vitro secretion of thyrotropin (TSH): Stimulation by a hypothalamic peptide (TRF). *Endocrinology.* 73:564, 1963
9. Schally AV, Bowers CY. The nature of thyrotropin-releasing hormone (TRH). Proceedings of the Sixth Midwest Conference on the Thyroid and Endocrinology, 1973: 25–63
10. Rececchi MJ, Kolesnick RN, Gershengorn MC. Thyrotropin-releasing hormone stimulates rapid loss of phosphatidylinositol and its conversion to l,2,-diacylglycerol and phosphatidic acid in rat mammotropic pituitary cells: Association with calcium mobilization and prolactin secretion. *J Biol Chem.* 258:227, 1983
11. Brenner-Gati L, Gershengorn MC: Effects of thyrotropin-releasing hormone on phosphoinositides and cytoplasmic free calcium in thyrotropin pituitary cells. *Endocrinology.* 118:163, 1986
12. Sarne DH, DeGroot LJ. Hypothalamic and neuroendocrine regulation of thyroid hormone. In: DeGroot LJ, ed. *Endocrinology,* 2nd ed. Philadelphia, W. B. Saunders, 1989: 574–589
13. Carayon P, Amr S. Mechanisms of thyroid regulation. In: DeGroot LJ, ed. *Endocrinology,* 2nd ed. Philadelphia, W. B. Saunders, 1989: 530–540
14. Mortimer CH, Besser GM, McNeilly AS, et al. Interactions between secretion of the gonadotropins, prolactin, growth hormone, thyrotropin and corticosteroids in man: The effects of LH/FSH-RH, TRH and hypogylcemia alone and in combination. *Clin Endocrinol.* 2:317, 1973
15. Colon JM, Lessing JB, Yavetz C, et al. The effect of thyrotropin-releasing hormone stimulation on the serum levels of gonadotropins in women during the follicular and luteal phases of the menstrual cycle. *Fertil Steril.* 49:809, 1988
16. Lasso P, Zarate A, Soria J, Canales ES. Long-term administration of thyrotropin-releasing hormone and its effects on gonadotropin secretion on eumenorrheic women. *Fertil Steril.* 27:636, 1976
17. Ober KP. Case report: Postpartum hypopituitarism with preservation of the pituitary–ovarian axis. *Am J Med Sci.* 299:257, 1990
18. Smallridge RC, Smith CE. Hyperthyroidism due to thyrotropin-secreting pituitary tumors. *Arch Int Med.* 143:503, 1983
19. Akande EO. Plasma concentrations of gonadotropins, estrogen and progesterone in hypothyroid women. *Br J Obstet Gynecol.* 82:552, 1975
20. Akande EO, Hockaday TDR. Plasma concentrations of gonadotropins, estrogen and progesterone in thyrotoxic women. *Br J Obstet Gynecol.* 82:541, 1975
21. Distiller LA, Sagel J, Morley JE. Assessment of pituitary gonadotropin reserve using luteinizing hormone-releasing hormone (LRH) in states of altered thyroid function. *J Clin Endocrinol Metab.* 40:512, 1975
22. Akande EO, Anderson DC. Role of sex hormone-binding globulin in hormonal changes and amenorrhea in thyrotoxic women. *Br J Obstet Gynecol.* 82:557, 1975
23. Joshi JV, Bhandarkar SD, Chadha M, et al. Menstrual irregularities and lactation failure may precede thyroid dysfunction or goitre. *J Postgrad Med.* 39:137, 1993
24. Sawin CT, Hershman JM, Boyd AE III, et al. The relationship of changes in serum estradiol and progesterone during the menstrual cycle to the thyrotropin and prolactin responses to thyrotropin-releasing hormone. *J Clin Endocrinol Metab.* 47:1296, 1978
25. Perez PR, Lopez JG, Mateos I, et al. Relation of thyroid secretion with the phases of the menstrual cycle. *Rev Clin Espanol.* 163:239, 1981
26. Hegedus L, Karstrup S, Rasmussen N. Evidence of cyclic alterations of thyroid size during the menstrual cycle in healthy women. *Am J Obstet Gynecol.* 155:142, 1986
27. De Lean A, Ferland L, Drouin, J, et al. Modulation of pituitary thyrotropin releasing hormone receptor levels by estrogens and thyroid hormones. *Endocrinology.* 100:1496, 1977
28. Zaninovich AA, Boado R, Ulloa E, et al. Inhibition of thyroidal iodine release in euthyroid subjects. *Acta Endocrinol.* 99:386, 1982
29. Rutlin E, Haug E, Torjesen PA. Serum thyrotropin, prolactin and growth hormone, response to TRH during estrogen treatment. *Acta Endocrinol.* 84:23, 1977
30. Erfurth EM, Ericsson UB. The role of estrogen in the TSH and prolactin responses to thyrotropin-releasing hormone in postmenopausal as compared to premenopausal women. *Horm Metab Res.* 24:528, 1992
31. Spitz IM, Zybler-Aran EA, Trestian S. The thyrotropin (TSH) profile in isolated gonadotropin deficiency: A model to evaluate the effect of sex steroids on TSH secretion. *J Clin Endocrinol Metab.* 57:415, 1983
32. Kohler P. Thyroid function in reproduction. In: Riddick DH, ed. *Reproductive Physiology in Clinical Practice.* New York, Thieme Medical Publishers, 1987: 171–187

33. Faglia G, Beck-Peccoz P, Ferrari C, et al. Enhanced plasma thyrotropin response to thyrotropin-releasing hormone following estradiol administration in man. *Clin Endocrinol.* 2:207, 1973

34. Sanchez-Franco F, Garcia MD, Cacicedo L, et al. Influence of sex phase of the menstrual cycle on thyrotropin (TSH) response to thyrotropin-releasing hormone (TRH). *J Clin Endocrinol Metab.* 37:736, 1973

35. Morley JE, Sawin CT, Carlson HE, et al. The relationship of androgen to the thyrotropin and prolactin responses to thyrotropin-releasing hormone in hypogonadal and normal men. *J Clin Endocrinol Metab.* 55:173, 1981

36. Arafah BM. Decreased levothyroxine requirement in women with hypothyroidism during androgen therapy for breast cancer *Ann Int Med.* 121:247, 1994

37. Wenzel KW. Pharmacological interference with in vitro tests of thyroid function. *Metabolism.* 30:717, 1981

38. Rasmussen NG, Hornnes PJ, Hegedus L, Feldt-Rasmussen U. Serum thyroglobulin during the menstrual cycle, during pregnancy, and post partum. *Acta Endocrinol* (Copenh). 121:168, 1989

39. Girdler SS, Pedersen CA, Light KC. Thyroid axis function during the menstrual cycle in women with premenstrual syndrome. *Psychoneuroendocrinology.* 20:395, 1995

40. Scanlon MF, Hall R. Thyroid-stimulating hormone: Synthesis, control of release, and secretion. In: DeGroot LJ, ed. *Endocrinology,* 2nd ed. Philadelphia, W. B. Saunders, 1989: 377–383

41. Utiger RD. Hypothyroidism. In: DeGroot LJ, ed. *Endocrinology,* 2nd ed. Philadelphia, W. B. Saunders, 1989: 702–721 .

42. Amino N, Iwatani Y, et al. High prevalence of transient postpartum thyrotoxicosis and hypothyroidism. *N Engl J Med.* 306:849, 1982

43. Jansson R, Bernander S, Karlsson A, et al. Autoimmune thyroid dysfunction in the postpartum period. *J Clin Endocrinol Metab.* 58:681, 1984

44. Refetoff S. Resistance to thyroid hormone and its molecular basis. *Acta Paediatrica Japonica.* 36:1, 1994

45. Usala SJ. Resistance to thyroid hormone in children. *Curr Opin Pediatr.* 6:468, 1994

46. McDermott MT, Ridgway EC. Thyroid hormone resistance syndromes *Am J Med.* 94:424, 1993

47. Ryan M, DeGroot LJ. Congenital defects in hormone formation and action. In: DeGroot LJ, ed. *Endocrinology,* 2nd ed. Philadelphia, W. B. Saunders, 1989: 777–795

48. Burrow GN. The thyroid gland and reproduction. In: Yen SSC, Jaffe RB, eds. *Reproductive Endocrinology: Physiology, Pathophysiology, and Clinical Management,* 3rd ed. Philadelphia, W. B. Saunders, 1991: 555–575

49. Cavaliere H, Abelin N, Medeiros-Neto G. Serum levels of total testosterone and sex hormone binding globulin in hypothyroid patients and normal subjects treated with incremental doses of L-T4 or L-T3. *J Androl.* 9:215, 1988

50. Sarne DH, Refetoff S, Rosenfield RL, Farriaux JP. Sex hormone-binding globulin in the diagnosis of peripheral resistance to thyroid hormone: The value of changes after short term triiodothyronine administration. *J Clin Endocrinol Metab.* 66:740, 1988

51. Drake TS, O'Brien WF, Tredway DR. Pituitary response to LHRH in hypothyroid women. *Obstet Gynecol.* 56:488, 1980

52. Ylostalo P, Kujala P, Kontula K. Amenorrhea with low normal thyroid function and thyroxine treatment. *Int J Gynaecol Obstet.* 18:176, 1980

53. Evers JLH, Rolland R. Primary hypothyroidism and ovarian activity evidence for an overlap in the synthesis of pituitary glycoproteins. *Br J Obstet Gynecol.* 88:195, 1981

54. Naguib YA, Darwish NA, Shaarawy M, et al. Endocrinologic and psychological aspects of galactorrhea associated with normal menstrual cycles. *Int J Gynaecol Obstet.* 19:285, 1981

55. Surks MI, Ocampo E. Subclinical thyroid disease. *Am J Med.* 100:217, 1996

56. Wilansky DL, Greisman B. Early hypothyroidism in patients with menorrhagia. *Am J Obstet Gynecol.* 160:673, 1989

57. Louvet JP, Gouarre M, Salandini AM, Boulard CI. Hypothyroidism and anovulation. *Lancet.* 1:1032, 1979. Letter

58. Kabadi UM. Subclinical hypothyroidism. Natural course of the syndrome during a prolonged follow-up study. *Arch Int Med.* 153:957, 1993

59. Utiger RD. Hypothyroidism. In: DeGroot LJ, ed. *Endocrinology,* 2nd ed. Philadelphia, W.B. Saunders, 1989: 716

60. Sturgess I, Thomas SH, Pennell DJ, et al. Diurnal variation in TSH and free thyroid hormones in patients on thyroxine replacement. *Acta Endocrinol.* 121:674, 1989

61. McKenzie JM, Zakarija M. Hyperthyroidism. In: DeGroot LJ, ed. *Endocrinology,* 2nd ed. Philadelphia, W. B. Saunders, 1989: 646–682

62. Paul TL, Kerrigan J, Kelly AM, et al. Long-term L-thyroxine therapy is associated with decreased hip bone density in premenopausal women. *JAMA.* 259:3137, 1988

63. Duncan WE, Chang A, Solomon B, Wartofsky L. Influence of clinical characteristics and parameters associated with thyroid hormone therapy on the bone mineral density of women treated with thyroid hormone. *Thyroid.* 4:183, 1994

64. Ross DS. Bone density is not reduced during short-term administration of levothyroxine to postmenopausal women with subclinical hypothyroidism: A randomized, prospective study. *Am J Med.* 95:385, 1993

65. Chopra IJ, Tulchinsky D. Status of estrogen–androgen balance in hyperthyroid men with Graves' disease. *J Clin Endocrinol Metab.* 38:269, 1974

66. Chopra IJ. Gonadal steroids and gonadotropins in hyperthyroidism. *Med Clin North Am.* 59:1109, 1975

67. Stray-Pedersen B, Stray-Pedersen S. Etiologic factors and subsequent reproductive performance in 195 couples with prior history of habitual abortion. *Am J Obstet Gynecol.* 2:140, 1984

68. Tanaka T, Tamai H, Kuma K, et al. Gonadotropin response to luteinizing hormone releasing hormone in hyperthyroid patients with menstrual disturbances. *Metabolism.* 30:323, 1981

69. Refetoff S. Thyroid function test and effects of drugs on thyroid function. In: DeGroot LJ, ed. *Endocrinology,* 2nd ed. Philadelphia, W. B. Saunders, 1989: 590–639.

70. Klee GG, Hay ID. Sensitive thyrotropin assays: Analytic and clinical performance criteria. *Mayo Clin Proc.* 63:1123, 1988

71. Comninos AC. Thyroid function and therapy in reproductive disturbances. *Obstet Gynecol.* 7:260, 1956

Chapter 18

DISORDERS OF THE ADRENAL CORTEX

Ricardo Azziz

PHYSIOLOGY OF THE ADRENAL CORTEX

Anatomy and Histology

Histologically and functionally, the adrenal cortex is separated into three zones (Fig 18–1).[1,2] The *zona glomerulosa* lies immediately below the adrenocortical capsule. This zone does not constitute a continuous layer, and is composed of U-shaped nests of cells.[3] The zona glomerulosa is primarily involved in the production of the mineralocorticoid, aldosterone. The *zona fasciculata* lies beneath the glomerulosa and consists of columns of lipid-laden cells, containing primarily cholesterol esters, with a large cytoplasm-to-nucleus ratio. The *zona reticularis* lies below the fasciculata, overlying the adrenal medulla. This zone consists of small cells with relatively little lipid-containing cytoplasm, but numerous mitochondria.[3] The fasciculata and reticularis cells appear to be one and the same. Immediately following the acute administration of adrenocorticotropic hormone (ACTH) a rapid decrease in the cytoplasmic lipid volume occurs within the fasciculata cells at the fasciculata–reticular junction.[3] These cells become increasingly compact and mitochondrial laden, leading to the progressive outward expansion of the zona reticularis. Under prolonged ACTH stimulation, few fasciculata cells may be seen.[1] Thus, reticulara are "compacted fasciculata" cells, and the zona fasciculata–reticulara forms a functional continuum. While fasciculata cells serve as a storage site for the cholesterol utilized in steroid biosynthesis, there is minimal storage of the final hormonal product in the adrenal cortex, in contrast to other endocrine glands.[1]

The adrenal is generously perfused, with the adrenal arteries branching into multiple tiny arterioles which dip into the adrenal cortex through the connective tissue capsule.[4] Some of these vessels quickly return to the exterior while others branch and rebranch as they penetrate the cortex, draining into the medullary venules and eventually into the *central adrenal vein*. Multiple intravenous anastomoses are present between the central vein, its branches, and the pericapsular venous system. The extensive and varied sites for blood drainage from the adrenal cortex is one of the factors accounting for the imprecision of central adrenal vein cauterization. Muscle cells appear to envelop the adrenocortical venules as they connect with the larger vessels draining into the central vein.[1,4] Constriction or relaxation of these muscle cuffs may provide a mechanism by which adrenocortical secretion is regulated, without altering the concentration of steroids in the adrenal vein. The endothelium of the adrenocortical vessels appears to be discontinuous, with the subendothelial space often being in direct communication with the vascular lumen.[3] The exact mechanism by which adrenocortical cells secrete their product into the bloodstream is unclear.

Adrenocortical Steroid Biosynthesis

Steroid biosynthesis begins with free cholesterol, which is stored in either free or esterified form within the lipid droplets of adrenocortical (primarily fasciculata) cells. Although cholesterol may be synthesized directly from two carbon acetate molecules, the preferred source appears to be circulating low-density lipoproteins (LDLs).[5] The administration of ACTH stimulates LDL uptake by increasing the number of specific LDL receptors.[6]

The classic two-dimensional scheme for the biosynthesis of the different adrenocortical steroids is depicted in Figure 18–2. In this simplified scheme, one enzyme usually catalyzes the conversion of more than one precursor.[7] The enzymatic events occur sequentially, and usually irreversibly, with the exception of 17β-hydroxysteroid dehydrogenase. The classic scheme presumes that the various

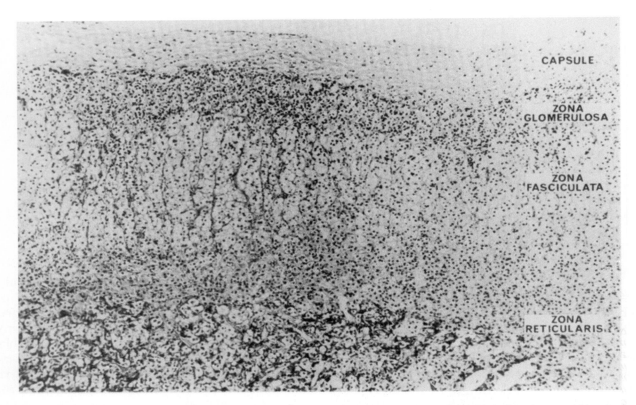

Figure 18–1. Normal human adrenal gland (H&E×60). *(Reprinted, with permission, from Grant JK. An introductory review of adrenocortical steroid biosynthesis. In James VHT, Serio M, Giusti G, Martini L, eds.* The Androgen Function of the Human Adrenal Cortex. *New York, Academic Press, 1978: 1–32.)*

intermediates in the biosynthetic process are stable, isolatable compounds. ACTH acts primarily on the cholesterol side-chain cleavage enzyme system, consisting of the three distinct chemical reactions: 20α-hydroxylation, 22-hydroxylation, and scission of the cholesterol side chain between carbons 20 and 22.[8] Twenty-one carbon (C-21) products include the progestogens (pregnenolone, 17-hydroxypregnenolone, progesterone, and 17-hydroxyprogesterone [17-HP]), the glucocorticoids (cortisol and 11-deoxycortisol or compound 3), and the mineralocorticoids (11-deoxycorticosterone [DOC], corticosterone, and aldosterone). Adrenal androgens (dehydroepiandrosterone [DHEA], androstenedione, androstenediol, and testosterone) are 19-carbon (C-19) steroids, while estrone and estradiol are C-18 products. Inhibitors of steroidogenesis are depicted in Figure 18–3.

More recently, this two-dimensional steroidogenic scheme has been challenged,[9] since it does not take into consideration the fact that many sulfated or lipoidal derivatives of some steroids can be biosynthesized directly from the sulfated or lipoidal derivatives of the precursors. Furthermore, the two-dimensional scheme does not explain the mechanism by which the so-called steroidal intermediates are passed back and forth between the mitochondria and the microsomes, where the various

steroidogenic enzymes required for biosynthesis reside. Lieberman and colleagues have proposed the hypothesis that the processes of steroidogenesis are confined within specific biosynthetic units termed "hormonads."[9] According to this view, each hormonal product is produced within its own hormonad, where all the required enzymes are in close proximity. These enzymes are thought to be arranged in such a way that the various intermediates involved in the conversion of a precursor to product proceed through the biochemical process without leaving this functional unit. The biosynthetic specificity of a hormonad may be regulated by virtue of its affinity for a specific substrate or a specific binding protein, or through the specific arrangement of the enzymes within the unit. As proposed, the hormonad is more a functional than a specific anatomic or morphologic unit. Under this scheme, late, as well as early, steps in the biosynthesis of steroids would be regulated by trophic hormones. This hypothesis also entails the existence of various product-specific isoenzymes that catalyze a single biochemical step, but that superficially appear to be involved in the formation of several hormones. How this proposal meshes with current knowledge concerning the molecular biology of these steroidogenic enzymes is still unknown, since the majority appear to be products of a

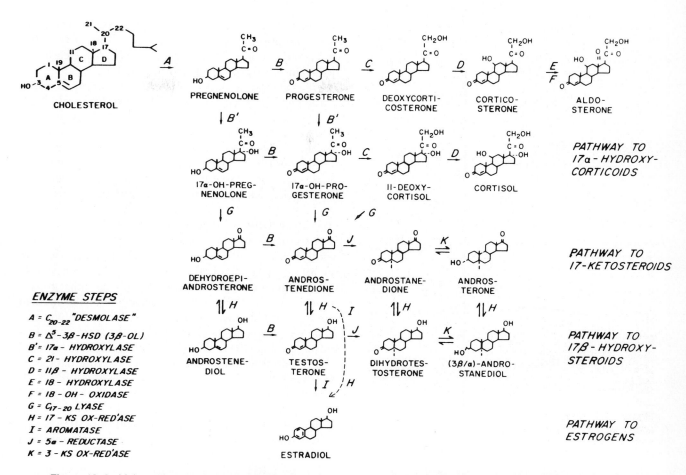

Figure 18–2. Major pathways of steroid biosynthesis from cholesterol. The flow of hormonogenesis is usually to the right and downward. C_{20-22} "Desmolase" (step A) is currently termed the side-chain cleavage enzyme. *(Reprinted,with permission, from Hatch R, Rosenfield RL, Kim MH, Tredway D. Hirsutism: Implications, etiology, and management. Am Obstet Gynecol. 140:815, 1981.)*

single gene. It is possible that these gene products undergo post-transcriptional modification yielding the different isoenzymes involved in the biosynthesis of the different steroidal products.

Molecular Biology of Steroidogenesis

Steroidogenic enzymes of the adrenal cortex can be divided into those that are members of the cytochrome P450 group of oxidases and those that are not.[10] Cytochrome P450 is a generic term for a large number of oxidative enzymes, all of which contain approximately 500 amino acids, a single heme group, and reduce atmospheric oxygen (O_2) with electrons obtained from NADPH. They are termed P450 (pigment 450) because all exhibit a characteristic shift in the Soret absorbance peak, from 420 to 450 nm, upon reduction with carbon monoxide. Most cytochrome P450 enzymes are found in the liver, and in spite of the huge number and variety of substrates metabolized there appear to be less than 200 types. Four distinct P450 enzymes are involved in

adrenocorticalsteroidogenesis.[10] P450scc or the cholesterol side-chain cleavage enzyme (formally termed 20,22-desmolase) is found in the mitochondria of the ovary and adrenal, and uses adrenodoxin reductase as the intermediary to transport the NADPH-yielded electrons. This enzyme is the product of a single, large gene located on chromosome 15.

P450c17 catalyzes both 17α-hydroxylase and 17,20-lyase (formerly termed 17,20-desmolase) activities. It is located in the endoplasmic reticulum (ie, it is microsomal) and uses P450 reductase for electron transfer. 17α-hydroxylation occurs more readily than the 17,20-lyase function, a preference that may be determined by the available concentration of P450 reductase. In general, >5 substrates (ie, containing a double bond between carbons 5 and 6) are preferred. P450c17 is the product of a single gene located on chromosome 10.

P450c21 exhibits 21-hydroxylation activity. This enzyme is present only in the adrenal and is located microsomally. A single, functional gene accompanied by a

NAME	REACTION INHIBITED	FORMULA
Aminoglutethimide	cholesterol side-chain cleavage	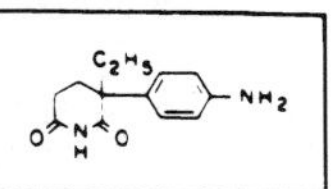 *(structure)*
SU-9055	18-hydroxylation 17 α-hydroxylation	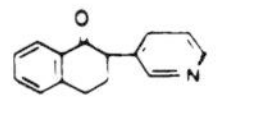 *(structure)*
SU-8000	18-hydroxycorticosterone → aldosterone 17 α-hydroxylation	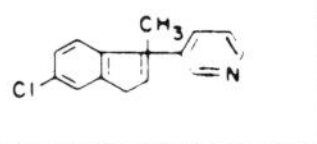 *(structure)*
Cyanoketone	3 β-hydroxysteroid dehydrogenase	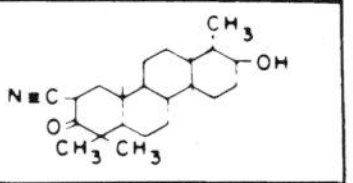 *(structure)*
Metyrapone	11 β-hydroxylation	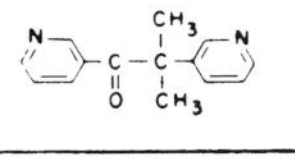 *(structure)*
SKF 12185	11 β-hydroxylation	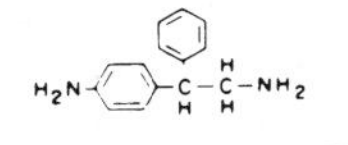 *(structure)*
Mitotane	mitochondrial damage, especially in z. fasciculata and z. reticularis	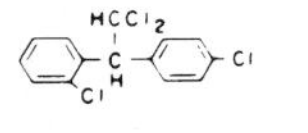 *(structure)*
Amphenone B	cholesterol 20 α-hydroxylase? 17 α, 11 β and 21 hydroxylases?	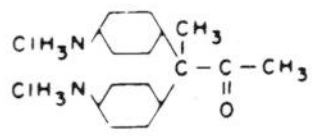 *(structure)*
Trilostane	3 β-hydroxysteroid dehydrogenase	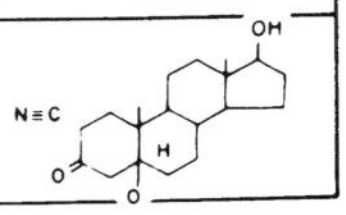 *(structure)*

Figure 18–3. Inhibitors of adrenocortical steroidogenesis, and their sites of action. *(Reprinted, with permission, from Bandy PK. The adrenal cortex. In: Bondy BK, Rosenburg LE, eds.* Metabolic Control and Disease. *Philadelphia, W. B. Saunders, 1980: 1427–1499.)*

pseudogene is located on the short arm of chromosome 6, in close proximity to the human leukocyte antigen (HLA) encoding region. Although extra-adrenal 21-hydroxylase activity has been reported in humans, studies have failed to reveal the presence of messenger RNA for this enzyme in other organs.

P450c11 mediates 11β-hydroxylase, 18-hydroxylase, and 18-oxidase activities, leading to the production of cortisol, corticosterone, and aldosterone. This enzyme is located within the inner membrane of adrenocortical mitochondria and utilizes the adrenodoxin reductase system for electron transfer from NADPH. Two duplicated genes are located on chromosome 8.

Various non-cytochrome P450 steroidogenic enzymes are also involved in adrenocortical biosynthesis.[10] 3β-Hydroxysteroid dehydrogenase appears to be the product of one enzyme, although various isoenzymes are available. 17β-Hydroxysteroid dehydrogenase (or 17-ketosteroid reductase) activity is located in the endoplasmic reticulum and represents the only readily reversible

step of steroidogenesis. Steroid sulfotransferase and sulfatase are also present in the adrenal cortex, with dehydroepiandrosterone sulfotransferase activity appearing to be localized primarily to the reticular zone.

Enzymatic activity appears to be stratified along histologic/functional lines.[2] 17α-Hydroxylase and 17,20-lyase activity are deficient, while 18-hydroxylase and 18-oxidase activities are active, in the zona glomerulosa. Another activity of P450c11, 11β-hydroxylase, is present throughout the adrenal cortex. How these enzymatic activities, often the product of a single gene, are regulated and histologically segregated remains to be determined.

Hypothalamic–Pituitary–Adrenal Axis

Corticotropin-releasing hormone (CRH) is a 41-amino acid peptide found in many cells of the brain (for review, see ref. 11). In the rat brain, CRH is found predominantly in the paraventricular nucleus of the hypothalamus.[12] Axonal processes terminate in the region of the median eminence.[13,14] From here it is released into the hypothalamic portal system to act on the anterior pituitary.[15] It is presumed that CRH, like ACTH and cortisol, is secreted in a pulsatile fashion.[16] There are conflicting data as to whether CRH demonstrates a circadian rhythm,[17,18] although more recent data examining the levels of CRH in the cerebrospinal fluid of normal volunteers suggested this to be the case.[19] The action of CRH is mediated through specific cell membrane receptors and the secondary messengers calcium and cyclic AMP (cAMP).[20] CRH stimulates the pituitary synthesis of pro-opiomelanocortin (POMC), which is then cleared to ACTH, β-lipotropin, and an end-terminal 16K fragment (Fig 18–4). β-Lipotropin is subsequently modified to yield β-endorphin and its metabolic residues α- and γ-endorphin. Administration of CRH also causes all these molecules to be released into the circulation, increasing the production and secretion of ACTH in a dose-dependent fashion.[20] After ovine CRH stimulation, plasma immunoreactive ACTH levels are higher in black versus white women, without a difference in cortisol secretion.[21] This variance in response appears to be primarily due to qualitative differences in the post-CRH immunoreactive ACTH levels, leading to a greater immunoreactive to bioactive ACTH ratio in blacks than whites, without an obvious difference in adrenocortical sensitivity to ACTH.[22]

Adrenocorticotropic hormone is a 39-amino acid peptide, which is released in an episodic fashion and demonstrates a circadian fluctuation. Both ACTH and cortisol pulses occur approximately 12 times in a 24-hr period.[23] It appears that changes in amplitude, but not frequency, of the ACTH pulses give rise to the cortisol circadian rhythm.[24] A sharp increase in the amplitude of the ACTH pulses occurs between the third and fifth hr of sleep, reaching a peak shortly after awakening, in indi-

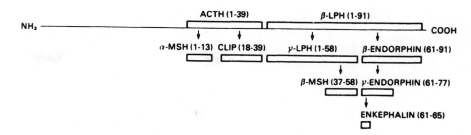

Figure 18–4. Schematic representation of the ACTH/β-lipotropin hormone (β-LPH) precursor molecule (pro-opiomelanocortin or POMC). Arrows represent potential cleavage sites, which may or may not occur in humans, that would yield smaller biologically active peptides. CLIP represents a corticotropin-like intermediate lobe peptide: α-MSH and β-MSH represent α- and β-melanocyte-stimulating hormone, respectively. *(Reprinted, with permission, from Loriaux DL, Cutler Jr GB. Diseases of the adrenal glands. In: Kohler PO, Jordan RM, eds.* Clinical Endocrinology. *New York, John Wiley & Sons, 1986: 167–238.)*

viduals with normal sleep patterns. The nadir is usually between 8:00 and 10:00 PM. The secretion of cortisol mimics the episodic and circadian release of ACTH.[25] The circadian change in adrenocortical activity appears to be, at least in part, the result of a sleep-induced inhibition of the ACTH, and consequently cortisol, response to CRH stimulation.[26] This inhibitory effect appears restricted to the early phases of sleep (slow-wave sleep) and is not present if the subject remains awake. The exact factors determining the changes in pituitary responsiveness during sleep are unclear. The continuous infusion of ovine CRH for 24 hr did not alter the circadian rhythm of ACTH or cortisol.[27] Prolonged (72-hr) pulsatile administration of ovine CRH also did not alter the pulsatility or diurnal rhythm of ACTH or cortisol.[23] From this and other data, it appears that CRH is not the principal determinant of the periodic changes in ACTH and cortisol. Moreover, CRH most likely plays a permissive, rather than a regulatory, role in ACTH release.

ACTH acts directly on the adrenocortical cells through a specific membrane receptor and the secondary messengers cAMP and calcium. ACTH receptors in adrenocortical tissue are present to large excess, and binding of only a small number of these receptors is necessary for maximal steroid production.[28] The response of cortisol to endogenous ACTH stimulation appears to be slightly greater in females than males.[29] Consequently, equivalent daily cortisol secretion is obtained in both sexes, at the expense of a greater ACTH release in men.

Glucocorticoids exert a negative feedback on the secretion of both CRH and ACTH, at the hypothalamic and pituitary level. A diurnal rhythm in the levels of immunoreactive CRH in cerebrospinal fluid is observed negatively mirroring those of cortisol.[19] Alternatively, the inhibitory effect of glucocorticoids on ACTH secretion is relatively complex, depending on the time and duration of exposure.[30] Acute glucocorticoid administration decreases ACTH secretion as long as the circulating concentration of glucocorticoids is rising at a sufficient rate (rate-sensitive feedback). This inhibition is extremely

rapid, and affects ACTH or CRH release but not synthesis. Following a single injection of glucocorticoid, the rate-sensitive or fast phase disappears as soon as the rate of rise in hormone levels drop below a critical point. For a period of time no inhibition in ACTH is evident (intermediate or silent phase). Finally, the slow phase of inhibition affects both secretion and synthesis of ACTH. Usually, exposure to high doses of glucocorticoids for more than 24 hr is required to decrease ACTH synthesis. Overall, the basal ACTH release is less sensitive to the suppressive effects of glucocorticoids than is the response of ACTH to stimulation.

Although normally CRH, and not other POMC products,[31] appears to be the principal determinant of ACTH secretion, other factors play a modulatory role, particularly in response to stress. Insulin-induced hypoglycemia increases ACTH levels above those induced by CRH administration alone.[32] Other factors, including vasopressin, epinephrine, and norepinephrine, may play a role in the elevated ACTH and cortisol levels induced by this stressful stimulus.[33–35] More prolonged stressful situations, such as burns, increase circulating cortisol to levels of approximately 40 to 50 μg/dl.[36] Alternatively, by 3 wk following the burn, circulating dehydroepiandrosterone sulfate (DHEAS) levels decrease to a nadir of approximately 500 ng/ml and remain low for many months thereafter.

The exact mechanism for both the very elevated serum cortisol levels and the prolonged reduction in adrenal androgen production with surgical or other physical stress is unclear. ACTH infusion alone (250 μg over 8 hr) leads to similar rises in circulating cortisol, an increase that nearly doubled by the fourth consecutive day of ACTH infusion.[37] ACTH secretion during surgical and anesthetic stress also appears to be continuous and not pulsatile.[38] Furthermore, several weeks after ablation of the paraventricular nucleus in rats (and depletion of CRH from the median eminence) the response of ACTH to stress is largely restored,[39] suggesting that this response is independent of CRH. Alternatively, in this model the ACTH rise normally seen following adrenal-ectomy remained inhibited, suggesting that the ACTH increase following glucocorticoid deprivation is largely dependent on CRH. Thus, endogenous vasopressin, oxytocin, catecholamines, and other factors appear to act synergistically with CRH to enhance ACTH and cortisol production and secretion,[40,41] particularly during stress.

Secretion and Metabolism of Adrenocortical Steroids

Cortisol. ACTH is the principal determinant of cortisol secretion in humans. As noted, cortisol levels fluctuate in the circulation, more or less paralleling ACTH release (Fig 18–5). The mean circulating concentration at 8:00 in the morning is approximately 13 µg/dl, although it can be as high as 30 µg/dl due to the pulsatile nature of release.[42] Cortisol levels increase at night, from a nadir at approximately 8:00 to 10:00 PM, peaking in the early morning hours (generally 4:00 to 8:00 AM). This so-called nyctohe-

meral rhythm can be shifted if normal sleep time is altered. Cortisol is secreted at a rate of 5 to 28 mg/day, with a mean of approximately 17 mg/day,[42] although more recent estimates suggest that the cortisol production rate is closer to 10 mg/day.[43] The biological half-life of cortisol is 60 to 90 min.[42] The steroid is metabolized by cleavage or oxidation at carbon 20, and reduction of the A ring,[44] with its major metabolites being tetrahydrocortisol, tetrahydrocortisone, cortols, and cortolones, secreted into the urine as glucuronates. A small amount of free cortisol is also excreted through the kidneys, and only a minor amount of cortisol metabolites are excreted by way of the bile.

Under normal conditions approximately 30 percent of cortisol is bound to albumin, 10 to 15 percent is free, and the remaining cortisol is bound to corticosteroid-binding globulin (CBG or transcortin).[45] There appears to be one binding site per molecule of CBG. Since progesterone binds to the same site with approximately three times the affinity of cortisol, significant displacement of the glucocorticoid from CBG can occur in high progesterone states (eg, pregnancy). Normally, this displacement is minimized since progesterone is readily bound by other plasma proteins and the circulating concentration of cortisol is approximately 1000-fold that of progesterone. Furthermore, CBG binding sites are present in large excess, and under basal conditions 70 to 80 percent of circulating CBG is unbound. CBG levels are increased by estrogens and pregnancy, and decrease in the face of androgens. Thus, measurements of total cortisol may not accurately reflect the free fraction.

Mineralocorticoids. Aldosterone is primarily synthesized by the zona glomerulosa, since 18-hydroxysteroid dehydrogenase activity is expressed primarily in these cells. Alternatively, DOC, another potent mineralocorticoid, is synthesized throughout the adrenal cortex and is found predominantly in the zona fasciculata. The production rate of aldosterone is approximately 100 to 150 µg/day.[44]

The secretion of aldosterone appears to be primarily under the control of the renin–angiotensin system (Fig 18–6). The extent of ACTH control over aldosterone secretion remains unclear. The continuous infusion of ACTH initially leads to the rise of both cortisol and aldosterone. As ACTH stimulation continues, cortisol levels are maintained, while aldosterone levels fall and reach preinfusion values approximately 72 hr later.[46] Alternatively, ACTH administered in a pulsatile fashion (0.33 U ACTH over 15 min, every 2 hr) appears to maintain aldosterone secretion at stimulated levels for up to 72 hr.[46] Other factors also play a role in modulating aldosterone secretion, including circulating levels of potassium, sodium, and dopamine.[30]

Renin is an enzyme synthesized by the juxta-glomerular (JG) cells, located within the afferent arteri-

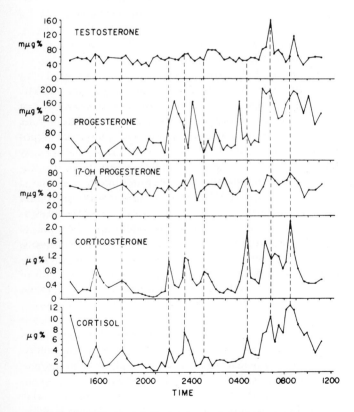

Figure 18–5. Diurnal variation in plasma testosterone, progesterone, 17-hydroxyprogesterone, corticosterone, and cortisol in a 20-year-old, normal, menstruating, preovulatory woman. *(Reprinted, with permission, from West CD, Mahajn DK, Chavre VJ, et al. Simultaneous measurement of multiple plasma steroids by radioimmunoassay demonstrating episodic secretion. J Clin Endocrinol Metab. 36:1230, 1973.)*

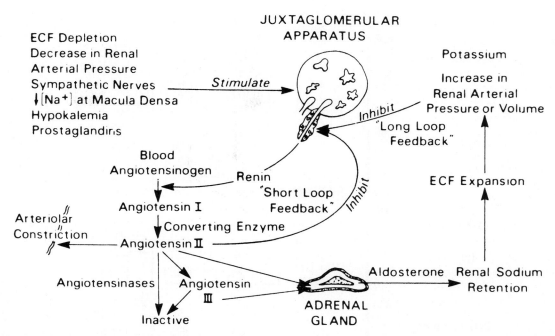

Figure 18–6. Scheme for control of renin secretion. *(Reprinted, with permission, from Tan SY, Mulrow PJ. Aldosterone in hypertension and edema. In: Bondy BK, Rosenburg LE, eds.* Metabolic Control and Disease. *Philadelphia, W. B. Saunders, 1980: 1501–1533.)*

ole adjacent to the initial segment of the distal tubule within the kidneys (Fig 18–6). The release of renin by the JG cells is increased primarily by a drop in the intravascular pressure within the afferent arteriole and a decrease in the concentration of sodium in the tubular fluid. Hypotension alone can stimulate renin release. Other factors may also stimulate renin secretion, including the sympathetic system, prostaglandins, and hypokalemia. Factors that inhibit renin release include volume expansion and increased arteriolar pressure, hypernatremia, prostaglandin synthetase inhibition, hyperkalemia, angiotensin II, vasopressin, and calcium. Circulating renin enzymatically cleaves an α-2-glycoprotein (globulin) synthesized by the liver, the so-called "renin substrate" (Fig 18–6), which causes the decapeptide angiotensin I. The generation of angiotensin I from renin substrate is the technique employed to clinically measure "plasma renin activity" (PRA). Angiotensin I is then converted to angiotensin II, an octapeptide, through the action of the angiotensin-converting enzyme located primarily in the lung. Circulating aminopeptidases convert angiotensin II to angiotensin III, which is subsequently cleaved to inactive peptide fragments. Angiotensin II is a strong pressor agent causing smooth muscle contraction of the vascular bed, and stimulating the synthesis and release of aldosterone. Angiotensin II also stimulates the release of vasopressin. Angiotensin III demonstrates primarily aldosterone-stimulating properties.[30]

Adrenal Androgens. Androgens are secreted by the adrenal cortex and ovaries. Androgens may also be derived (not secreted) from the conversion of other steroids by the liver and some peripheral tissues (eg, adipose tissue, muscle, skin). Principal circulating androgens include testosterone (T) and its metabolite dihydrotestosterone (DHT), androstenedione, and DHEA and its metabolite DHEAS. DHEAS is the most abundant androgen, circulating in a concentration approximately 8000 to 10,000 times that of testosterone. Testosterone and DHT circulate tightly bound to a hepatic α-globulin, sex steroid-binding globulin (TeBG or SHBG) and, to a lesser extent, to albumin. Androstenedione is only weakly bound, while DHEA and DHEAS circulate mostly unbound.[47,48]

A marked increase in serum DHEA and DHEAS concentrations begins at about the age of 5 yr, continuing throughout puberty (Fig 18–7).[42–55] The increased adrenal secretion of androgens and estrogens begins 2 to 3 yr before the onset of puberty and is termed adrenarche. Histopathologically, adrenarche correlates with the appearance of a continuous reticularis zone in the adrenal cortex. Focal development of the reticularis begins at about the age of 5 yr, and by 8 yr it is usually present as a continuous zone.[56] It appears that the relative activity of 3β-hydroxysteroid dehydrogenase decreases, and that of 17,20-lyase and, to a lesser extent, 17-hydroxylase increases during adrenarche. These alterations are not associated with an alteration in circulating cortisol levels,

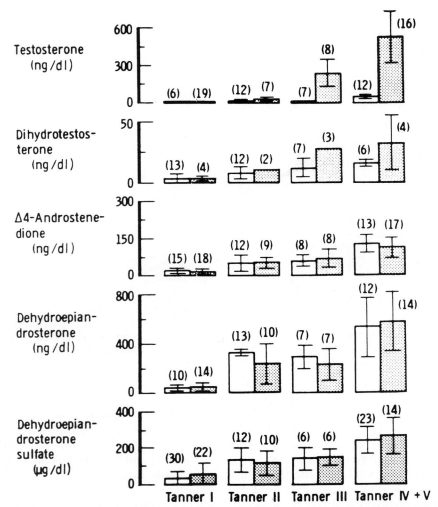

Figure 18–7. Mean (± standard deviation) serum concentrations of testosterone, dihydrotestosterone, Δ4-androstenedione, dehydroepiandrosterone, and dehydroepiandrosterone sulfate in normal boys (speckled bars) and girls (open bars) according to four pubic hair stages (Tanner I, II, III, IV plus V). Testosterone was higher in boys in stages II, III, and IV plus V (*P*<0.001). Dihydrotestosterone was higher in boys in stages III and IV plus V (*P*<0.01). In both sexes differences between stages I and II are significant for all steroids (*P*<0.001). Differences between stages II and III are significant in boys for testosterone (*P*<0.001). Differences between stages III and IV plus V are significant for all steroids, except DHEA, in girls. *(Modified, with permission, from Korth-Schultz S, Levine LS, New MI. Serum androgens in normal prepubertal and pubertal children and in children with precocious adrenarche. J Clin Endocrinol Metab. 42:117, 1976.)*

which remain stable throughout puberty.[56] The pubertal increases in testosterone and androstenedione in girls appear to be mostly due to a higher ovarian production.[51]

The mechanisms responsible for initiating and controlling adrenarche are not clear. Adrenarche appears to occur independently of gonadal maturation.[57] Some investigators have proposed that the development of the continuous reticularis and the changes in adrenocortical biosynthesis at adrenarche are under the control of both ACTH and an unidentified pituitary regulatory factor, termed the adrenal androgen-stimulating hormone (AASH) or cortical androgen-stimulating hormone (CASH).[58,59] Experimental evidence for such a substance rests on the observation that bovine and human pituitary extracts stimulate a greater secretion of DHEA relative to cortisol, from dog and human adrenals in vitro and in vivo.[59] Alternatively, other investigators have suggested that much, if not all, of the changes in adrenal androgen production at puberty can be explained by alterations in the intrinsic adrenocortical hormonal milieu and the progressive development of the reticularis.[60–62] More recently, a fragment of POMC (amino acids 79–96), suggested as the putative AASH, was found not to be effective in primary cultures of fetal adrenal cells.[63] While this does not exclude the possibility that the adrenal cortex may develop receptors for this fragment at a later stage of development, this hypothesis remains to be proven.

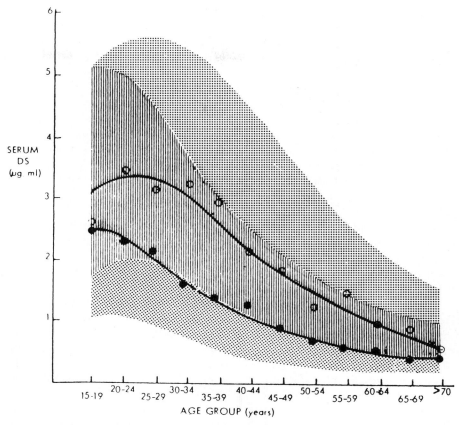

Figure 18–8. Mean serum dehydroepiandrosterone sulfate (DS) in men (open circle) and women (closed circle). Lined areas delineate the region of overlap. *(Reprinted, with permission, from Orentreich N, Brind JL, Rizer RL, Vogelman JH. Age changes and sex differences in serum dehydroepiandrosterone sulfate concentrations throughout adulthood.* J Clin Endocrinol Metab. *59:551, 1984.)*

Following puberty, testosterone originates approximately 25 percent from the ovary, 25 percent from the adrenal, and 50 percent from the peripheral conversion of androstenedione.[64] Testosterone and androstenedione are metabolized to DHT, the most potent of androgens, through the action of the enzyme 5α-reductase, in the liver and skin. Androstenedione is produced equally from the ovary and the adrenal cortex. Approximately 90 percent of DHEA and 98 percent of DHEAS are produced by the adrenal cortex. Circulating DHEA, DHEAS, and androstenedione exhibit a circadian rhythm similar to that of cortisol, with peak serum concentrations in early morning and the nadir in late evening.[65–67] Interestingly, gender appears to have an impact on circulating adrenal androgen concentrations. In individuals under 50 yr of age, DHEA levels are higher in women, without a significant gender difference in circulating DHEAS.[68] Alternatively, after age 50 yr, circulating DHEA levels were similar, but DHEAS levels in women were significantly lower than in men. Consequently, the ratio of DHEAS to DHEA in the circulation is significantly higher at all times in men compared to women, apparently due to differences in DHEA metabolism.[69] Furthermore, in contrast to cortisol, there ap-

pears to a significant degree of individual variability in the secretion of adrenal androgens, basally and in response to ACTH stimulation.[70] In fact, the inter-individual variances appear to persist into menopause.[71] The cause (and effects) of these inter-subject differences in adrenal androgen secretion remains to be determined.

Circulating DHEAS, DHEA, and androstenediol levels begin to decrease at approximately the age of 30 yr (Fig 18–8). This decrease continues linearly until death and is independent of the cessation of ovarian function at menopause.[72] While adrenally secreted androstenedione also decreases during this time period, the drop is less dramatic, beginning later in life and ceasing after age 60 yr. Age-related changes in adrenal androgen levels do not appear to be related to an alteration in the peripheral metabolism of these steroids. Furthermore, the hypothalamic–pituitary–adrenal axis remains relatively unchanged throughout the later reproductive years, and there does not appear to be an impairment in the cortisol secretory response to ACTH with age. Alternatively, the adrenal secretion of >5-steroids in response to ACTH clearly decreases. Overall, adrenopause appears to represent a "reverse adrenarche" (increasing 3β-hydroxysteroid dehydrogenase and decreasing 17,20-lyase activity). The causes and molecular biology of these changes remain to be elucidated.

Actions of Adrenocortical Steroids

Glucocorticoids. These steroids stimulate gluconeogenesis (from which the term "glucocorticoids" originates) (Table 18–1). Following glucocorticoid administration there is an increase in hepatic glucose production, primarily from amino acids derived from muscle catabolism. Glucocorticoids antagonize insulin action, increasing hepatic glycogen deposition and glycosuria, which leads to moderate hyperglycemia when administered pharmacologically. Alternatively, glucocorticoids enhance protein catabolism, inhibit protein synthesis, and induce a negative nitrogen balance. Although centripetal fat deposition is frequently seen in hypercortisolemia, the effect of glucocorticoids on adipocytes is unclear. Glucocorticoids appear to potentiate other lipolytic hormones, particularly catecholamines.[30]

Glucocorticoids decrease the intestinal absorption of calcium, with increased fecal and renal excretion, and antagonize the effects of vitamin D. The net result is a negative calcium balance. Calcium loss, together with a direct inhibitory effect of cortisol on osteocytes, inhibits bone formation, leading to osteoporosis and osteopenia. Cortisol also inhibits the proliferation of fibroblasts, often leading to thinning of the skin (and the formation of purple striae) and a delay in wound healing. Furthermore, growth is inhibited and breakdown stimulated in many other peripheral tissues, including muscle and fat. Glucocorticoids inhibit DNA synthesis in lymphoid tissues, resulting in lymphopenia. Alternatively, glucocorticoids induce neutrophilic leukocytosis, although they decrease the ability of these cells to migrate and act at the site of inflammation. Cortisol also has a stimulatory effect on the central nervous system leading to insomnia, euphoria, and irritability. One should note that many of these actions become manifest only when pharmacologic doses of glucocorticoids are administered.

Mineralocorticoids. Aldosterone acts principally on the kidney to increase the reabsorption of sodium ions from the distal renal tubule, the ascending loop of Henle, and collecting ducts, generally in exchange for potassium and hydrogen ions. Sodium conservation is accompanied by water retention, due to the increased release in vasopressin responding to the increased plasma osmolality.

Adrenal Androgens. Under normal circumstances the exclusive adrenal androgens, DHEA and DHEAS, exert a limited androgenic effect, compared to T and DHT. However, these steroids may serve as precursors for the formation of more potent androgens. The administration of oral DHEA to postmenopausal women was associated with higher circulating testosterone, androstenedione, estradiol, and estrone levels,[73] and the conversion of DHEA and DHEAS to androstenedione and testosterone has been clearly documented.[74,75]

TABLE 18–1. MAIN ACTIONS OF CORTISOL AND SYNTHETIC GLUCOCORTICOIDS

Carbohydrate, protein, and fat metabolism	Enhances gluconeogenesis; peripheral antagonism to insulin like that of growth hormone causes hyperglycemia; if levels in blood are excessive, may lead to diabetes mellitus; causes centripetal distribution of fat, hyperlipemia, and hypercholesterolemia
Anti-inflammatory	Decreases all components of inflammatory response; reduces passage of fluid and cells out of capillaries; reduces fibrous tissue formation
Immunologic	In large doses, causes lysis of lymphocytes and plasma cells with release of antibody; subsequently, antibody levels are lowered
Water metabolism	Enhances water diuresis; prevents shift of water into cells; maintains extracellular fluid volume; antagonizes vasopressin action on renal tubule
Hemopoiesis and hemostasis	Lowers eosinophil and lymphocyte counts; increases neutrophil leukocyte s, red cells, and platelets
Gastrointestinal	Increases gastric acid production; reduces gastric mucus; in excess, may delay healing of peptic ulcers
Cardiovascular	Sensitization of arterioles to the action of noradrenaline, thereby maintaining blood pressure; enhances production of angiotensinogen, which can then increase angiotensin level, which in turn stimulates aldosterone output
Skeletal	Impairs both growth hormone secretion from the pituitary and also its actions on the tissues; impaired formation of cartilage; decreased bone formation and osteoporosis; decreased absorption of calcium from the gut (where cortisol antagonizes action of vitamin D), increased renal excretion of calcium
Neuromuscular	Increased slow-wave activity on EEG; lowers threshold for electrical excitation of brain; both deficiency and excess cause psychiatric disturbances and muscular weakness

(Reproduced, with permission, from Hall R, Anderson J, Smart GA, Besser M. Adrenal. In: Fundamentals of Clinical Endocrinology, 3rd ed. Chicago, Year Book Medical Publishers, 1980: 220.)

Adrenal androgens may play a role in the regulation of insulin action. Mortola and Yen noted that peak insulin levels during 3-hr glucose tolerance testing were higher after 28 days of oral DHEA administration in postmenopausal women.[73] Alternatively, Nestler and colleagues were unable to demonstrate a change in insulin resistance, using the euglycemic insulin clamp technique, in normal men receiving DHEA for 28 days.[76]

The role of adrenal androgens in controlling body weight is also controversial. Weight loss, without a change in caloric intake, has been noted in laboratory rats and dogs. Nestler et al reported that oral DHEA administration for 1 mo was associated with a 30 percent decrease in body fat, without a change in weight, suggesting an associated increase in muscle mass.[76] Alternatively, no change in percent body fat was noted in postmenopausal women receiving the same regimen of DHEA.[73] Furthermore, in another study the same treatment in men was unable to demonstrate a change in lean body mass and energy or protein metabolism.[77]

Adrenal androgens may play a protective role in the development of certain cancers, particularly of the breasts.[78] In addition, low levels of DHEAS are associated with an increased cardiovascular morbidity in men.[79] Adrenal androgens may demonstrate a protective effect against postmenopausal osteoporosis,[80–82] and contribute to epiphyseal maturation during childhood.[83] Finally, it has been suggested that DHEAS may serve as a prehormone for ovarian steroidogenesis.[84] The many potential effects of adrenal androgens have been reviewed,[85,86] but their exact role(s) remain to be fully established.

CUSHING SYNDROME

Cushing syndrome is characterized by an increased secretory rate of cortisol and a loss in the circadian rhythm of this secretion. Simply stated, if there is no evidence of excess glucocorticoid production, there is no evidence of Cushing syndrome. Cushing syndrome is a rare disorder occurring in approximately 1 per 5 million individuals.[87]

Differential Diagnosis

The differential diagnosis of Cushing syndrome is depicted in Table 18–2. The most common cause of Cushing syndrome is iatrogenic. Among reproductive endocrinology patients, mild cushingoid features can occasionally be observed with glucocorticoid treatment, particularly when using dexamethasone. Dexamethasone is a long-acting fluorinated steroid with almost exclusive glucocorticoid properties and with a relative potency of approximately 25 to 30 times that of cortisol. Since there is significant individual variance in the ability to metabolize dexamethasone, in some patients it can accumulate to excess, leading to symptoms. Patients who demon-

TABLE 18–2. DIFFERENTIAL DIAGNOSIS OF CUSHING SYNDROME

Iatrogenic
ACTH Dependent
   Pituitary or Cushing's disease: micro- or macroadenomas, hyperplasia, or pituitary dysfunction
   Ectopic ACTH/CRH-producing tumors
ACTH Independent
   Adrenocortical adenomas
   Adrenal carcinomas
   Micronodular adrenal hyperplasia

strate cushingoid side effects on dexamethasone therapy should have their dose decreased, or be switched to treatment with either prednisone (approximately 4- to 5-fold the potency of cortisol) or hydrocortisone (about the same potency as cortisol).

Pathologic causes of Cushing syndrome can be ACTH dependent or independent. ACTH-dependent causes include pituitary dysfunction, hyperplasia or adenomas, and ectopic ACTH- or CRF-producing tumors. ACTH-independent etiologies, also termed adrenal Cushing syndrome, include adrenal carcinomas, adenomas, and nodular hyperplasia. There is an age and sex predilection for the various forms of Cushing syndrome. Overall, women are affected four times as frequently as men.[88]

ACTH-Dependent Cushing Syndrome

Pituitary Cushing's or Cushing's Disease. Cushing's disease is responsible for 60 to 70 percent of all cases of non-iatrogenic Cushing syndrome.[89–91] Seventy-five percent of pituitary Cushing syndrome cases occur in women, the majority of childbearing age.[92] Two thirds of these are associated with pituitary adenomas, although 10 to 30 percent do not demonstrate any visible pathologic abnormality of the pituitary.[89] These latter cases may represent some form of hypothalamic–pituitary dysfunction or diffuse corticotropic hyperplasia. The majority of pituitary tumors are microadenomas (<10 mm in diameter), while 5 to 10 percent of individuals demonstrate macroadenomas (tumors larger than 10 mm). Only rarely are the tumors large enough to distort the sella turcica.

The exact etiology for the pituitary dysfunction leading to corticotropic hyperfunction and/or adenomas is unclear. Both pituitary and hypothalamic factors have been proposed. Generally, this disorder does not appear to result from the excessive stimulation or secretion of CRH.[17,18,93] The response of CRH to insulin tolerance or metyrapone testing appeared to be deficient, while the response of ACTH to the same stimuli was either normal or exaggerated, in patients with Cushing's disease.[18]

Furthermore, in contrast to normal subjects, the responses of ACTH and cortisol to a 100-µg bolus of ovine CRH in patients with Cushing's disease appeared to be independent of the basal glucocorticoid level.[94] It appears that primary ACTH hypersecretion by pituitary corticotrophes, which are relatively resistant to glucocorticoid suppression while retaining CRH responsivity, gives rise to Cushing disease.[20]

Pituitary or ectopic ACTH-producing causes of Cushing syndrome may occasionally present as an adrenal etiology, since prolonged and excessive ACTH stimulation can lead to macronodular hyperplasia or dysplasia of the adrenal cortex.[95] Following removal of the ACTH-producing source, cortisol production slowly decreases, often taking up to 2 yr to fully normalize, as the nodules slowly atrophy. Because of this slow resolution and the somewhat autonomous nature of these nodules, bilateral adrenalectomy for macronodular hyperplasia may be required.[95]

Ectopic ACTH and CRH Secretion. Ectopic causes of Cushing syndrome account for approximately 5 to 15 percent of all cases, the majority of which are men.[89,91] A number of non-endocrine tumors may secrete ACTH into the circulation, the most common of which is oat cell carcinoma of the lung. The majority of small cell carcinomas of the lung contain ACTH, although it is generally not biologically active,[96] and only 2 percent of patients with lung cancer develop clinical Cushing syndrome.[97] ACTH circulating levels are uniformly above the normal range in these individuals (Fig 18–9).[98] CRH-like activity can frequently be detected in these tumors as well.[85]

Typical Cushing syndrome features are often absent in patients with ectopic ACTH-producing tumors, probably as a consequence of the malnutrition and general wasting resulting from their primary tumor. Imura and colleagues studied 30 patients with ectopic ACTH-producing tumors.[99] None of their 18 lung cancer patients showed signs of Cushing syndrome, while 7 of the remaining 13 patients were cushingoid in appearance, although 2 of these did not demonstrate the centripetal obesity typically seen. CRH-secreting tumors have been reported[100] but are considered rare.

ACTH-independent or Adrenal Cushing Syndrome. Adrenal causes comprise approximately 20 to 25 percent of non-iatrogenic Cushing syndrome.[89–91] The incidence is divided approximately equally between adrenal carcinomas and adenomas. Primary bilateral diffuse micronodular hyperplasia or dysplasia, unrelated to excessive ACTH stimulation, is a rare cause of Cushing syndrome.

Adrenocortical Adenomas. Adrenocortical adenomas are usually unilateral, with an average diameter of 3 cm and

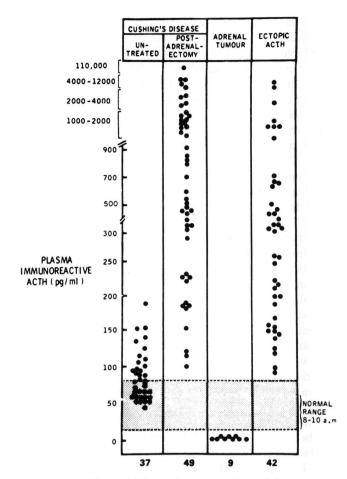

Figure 18–9. Plasma ACTH levels measured by radioimmunoassay in 137 cases of Cushing syndrome. *(Reprinted, with permission, from Besser GM, Edwards CRW. Cushing syndrome. Clin Endocrinol Metab. 1:451, 1972.)*

well-circumscribed borders.[101] However, some adrenal adenomas may attain a large size, particularly those with relatively inefficient steroidogenesis. Adenomas are uniformly independent of endogenous ACTH stimulation, but frequently respond to exogenous ACTH.[101] One should keep in mind that 2 to 9 percent of autopsies in asymptomatic individuals demonstrate adrenocortical nodules or adenomas,[102–104] with an increasing incidence with advancing age. Furthermore, Glazer and colleagues reported the incidental discovery of 14 adrenal masses upon abdominal CT scanning of approximately 2200 patients (0.6 percent), 8 greater than 2 cm.[105] These studies serve to caution against proceeding to radiologic studies of the adrenal in the work-up of Cushing syndrome prior to establishing whether the etiology is ACTH independent or not.

Adrenal Carcinomas. Cushing syndrome in children under the age of 10 is almost always due to adrenal neoplasia,[106,107] and over 65 percent of patients younger than age 15 are found to have adrenal carcinomas.[108] Nevertheless, the average age of patients with hormonally active adrenocortical carcinomas is approximately 45 yr.[109] Seventy percent of adrenal carcinomas demonstrate obvious endocrine function, while only 10 to 15 percent can be considered truly nonfunctional.[110] These tumors are usually greater than 6 cm in diameter by the time they are diagnosed because of their relatively inefficient steroidogenesis compared to normal adrenal tissue.[111] The high adrenal androgen concentrations in these patients generally arise from a relatively greater decrease in 3β-hydroxysteroid dehydrogenase.[112]

Adrenal carcinomas demonstrate an irregular border upon CT scanning. These neoplasms generally produce a variety of adrenocortical products, mostly in low levels, resulting in cushingoid symptoms, virilization, and hypertension (secondary to deoxycorticosterone overproduction).[101,110] Histologic differentiation of the tumor may play a role in the endocrine function. Correlating the histopathology of adrenocortical carcinomas with the presence of endocrine symptoms, none of the patients with anaplastic or poorly differentiated tumors developed virilization or hypertensive symptoms, while 9 of 14 patients with a differentiated neoplasm demonstrated hyperandrogenic symptoms and 5 of 8 hypertension.[109]

Micronodular Adrenal Hyperplasia.

This disorder has also been described as primary adrenocortical nodular dysplasia and occurs predominantly in younger individuals.[30] The hypercortisolemia is usually mild, although osteoporosis occurs frequently. Histopathologically, there are multiple small (<3 mm) black or brown pigmented nodules in both adrenals with atrophy of the intervening adrenal cortex, which pathologically distinguishes this disorder from the adrenal hyperplasia induced by chronic ACTH stimulation.

Clinical Manifestations of Cushing Syndrome.

The signs and symptoms associated with Cushing syndrome can be attributed to either glucocorticoid, mineralocorticoid, or sex steroid action (for review, see ref. 113). The presentation varies somewhat according to the etiology for the Cushing syndrome. The frequency distribution of these clinical features in adults is depicted in Table 18–3. In children the most common presenting features include weight gain, obesity, and facial plethora.[114] Growth retardation was a common feature in those children not fully grown, while 40 percent of children developing the disease in the first decade of life presented with premature sexual development. Alternatively, 3 percent of older children presented with delayed development.

Glucocorticoid Action.

Excess glucocorticoid action is primarily responsible for the typical cushingoid appearance.

There is an increase in centripetal fat, with a yoke-like distribution (Fig 18–10). Vascular fragility leads to easy bruisability, which is one of the earliest signs of this disorder. A puffiness about the face develops ("moon facies"), with a generalized rubor of the cheeks. Mild glucose intolerance is observed, while osteoporosis subsequently leads to kyphosis, vertebral and other fractures, and loss of height. There is a thinning of the skin, with the development of purple striae, particularly about the abdomen. Muscle wasting, with a decrease in extremity muscle mass and generalized weakness, exaggerates the appearance of centripetal obesity. A variety of psychiatric disturbances also may be manifest, including depression and lethargy, with mood swings, irritability, and insomnia.[115] A decrease in the ability to concentrate and recall, and increasing anxiety, also occur, occasionally with the development of paranoia and overt psychosis. The psychiatric symptoms improve as cortisol levels are returned to normal with therapy. Lymphopenia, eosinopenia, and granulocytosis are common, leading to an increased susceptibility to infections.

Mineralocorticoid Action.

Overt alterations in the renin–angiotensin–aldosterone axis have not been reported in Cushing syndrome patients. Nonetheless, an increase in circulating DOC and aldosterone may in part explain the mild to moderate degrees of hypertension present, which may also be accompanied by hypokalemic alkalosis. Hypertension may also, however, be the result of an alteration in vascular reactivity to catecholamines in response to the hypercortisolemia.[116,117] Furthermore, patients with an ectopic-ACTH syndrome often demonstrate significant mineralocorticoid excess and hypokalemic alkalosis, whose cause remains unclear.[118]

Sex-Steroid Action.

Hirsutism is present in 60 to 70 percent of women with Cushing syndrome, and is generally diffuse, mild, and accompanied by varying degrees of hypertrichosis. Hirsutism, with or without menstrual

TABLE 18–3. FREQUENCY OF CLINICAL FEATURES IN CUSHING SYNDROME

Feature	Incidence (%)
Obesity	88–95
Plethora	60–90
Thin skin	80
Diastolic hypertension	76–87
Striae	50
Muscle weakness	60–90
Easy bruisability	42–65
Menstrual disorders	65–85
Hirsutism in women	64–80
Psychiatric problems	42–60
Backache (osteoporosis), edema	40–48

(Adapted, with permission, from Kannan CR, The Adrenal Gland. New York, Plenum Medical Book Co., 1988: 114.)

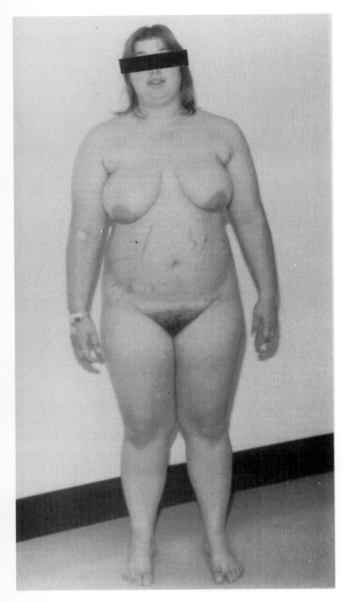

Figure 18–10. Patient with Cushing syndrome secondary to a pituitary microadenoma, who recovered following a transsphenoidal hypophysectomy. *(Courtesy of Robert Kreisberg, M.D., University of Alabama at Birmingham.)*

irregularity, was among the presenting symptoms in 15 of 45 such women, and the only presenting complaint in 11.[88] Menstrual irregularity without overt hirsutism was among the presenting symptoms in 6, and the only symptom in 1 woman. Overall, menstrual irregularities are seen in 80 to 100 percent of women with Cushing syndrome and acne is present in 40 to 50 percent.[89–91]

Contrary to that noted in women, men with Cushing syndrome generally demonstrate lower levels of circulating androgens, usually resulting in varying degrees of im-

potency. In children, reproductive alterations lead to premature or delayed sexual develoment.

Reproductive Endocrinologic Alterations in ACTH-dependent Cushing Syndrome. Cushing's disease and ectopic ACTH/CRH-producing tumors may lead to oligomenorrhea and/or hyperandrogenism in adult women. Ectopic ACTH/CRH-producing tumors are infrequently associated with virilization, since they are rare tumors in females. Imura and colleagues did not note virilization in females with ectopic ACTH-producing neoplasms.[99] However, all patients were of Asian extraction, a population notably resistant to the development of hirsutism.

The exact mechanism for the reproductive endocrinologic abnormalities in Cushing disease is unclear. Circulating testosterone levels are elevated in women with pituitary Cushing's.[119] An adrenal origin was ascribed to the increased androgen level, since (a) dexamethasone caused a parallel decrease in cortisol and testosterone, (b) ACTH stimulation induced an increase in testosterone that was more profound in women with Cushing's disease compared to normals and, (c) bilateral adrenalectomy dramatically decreased circulating testosterone, correcting the oligomenorrhea and hirsutism. Nonetheless, an increase in the adrenal secretion of androgens may not be the only factor accounting for the androgenic symptoms in Cushing's disease. Patients with adrenal adenomas generally demonstrate low levels of adrenal androgens, especially DHEAS.[120] Nonetheless, these women demonstrate a similar frequency of menstrual irregularity, hirsutism, and acne when compared to patients with generalized adrenal hyperplasia (reflecting increased ACTH stimulation).[90] It is possible that an increase in ovarian androgen secretion may in part account for the hyperandrogenism. The role that the increased insulin resistance and gonadotropin abnormalities (discussed later) noted in Cushing syndrome play in promoting ovarian hyperandrogenemia is unknown. Finally, a direct effect of long-term hypercortisolemia on hair growth, particularly that of vellus hairs, cannot be ruled out.

Disturbances in the hypothalamic–pituitary axis may in part explain the ovulatory dysfunction of women with Cushing's disease. In five of six women with Cushing's disease and bilateral adrenal hyperplasia, acute GnRH stimulation did not significantly change circulating LH levels, while an increase in FSH was observed, although somewhat blunted.[121] In two patients with Cushing's disease, Hompes and colleagues reported that the normal LH pulsatility was suppressed prior to therapy, and was restored to normal following transsphenoidal resection of the pituitary adenoma.[122] The decreased response of gonadotropins to endogenous or exogenous GnRH stimulation may be secondary to hypothalamic dysfunction in Cushing's disease. In normal women during the midluteal phase of the menstrual cycle, CRH has been noted to inhibit the release of LH and FSH.[123] This CRH-induced inhibition of gonadotropin secretion appeared to be primarily mediated by endogenous opioid peptides and was not dependent on glucocorticoid levels. However, elevated CRH levels have not been documented in pituitary Cushing's.[17–19] An increase in unopposed estrogen action on the hypothalamic–pituitary axis, resulting from the peripheral conversion of circulating androgens, may play a role.

Reproductive Endocrinologic Alternatives in ACTH-independent Cushing Syndrome.

The incidence of oligomenorrhea and/or hirsutism is as frequent among patients with adrenocortical adenomas as it is among women with Cushing's disease. Many of these adenomas produce primarily cortisol and yet lead to oligomenorrhea and hirsutism/hypertrichosis, suggesting that cortisol may have a direct effect on the hypothalamic–pituitary axis, and on hair growth and differentiation. Hypercortisolemia may have an impact on hair growth via increased ovarian androgen secretion resulting from cortisol-induced oligo-ovulation.

Adrenal carcinomas also frequently demonstrate oligo-ovulation and hirsutism. The frequency with which these symptoms present depends on tumor histopathology. More differentiated tumors tend to produce an increased level of androgens, while less differentiated tumors do not.[109] Overall, adrenocortical neoplasias demonstrate less efficient steroidogenesis than normal adrenocortical tissue. A defect in 11β-hydroxylase activity has been reported in vitro, suggesting that these tumors may demonstrate a reduction in cortisol production relative to other precursors.[124] However, because these tumors are frequently very large, the overall steroid secretion by these neoplasms can be significant.

In the presence of hirsutism and Cushing syndrome, the physician should not be detracted from evaluating the syndrome in proper sequence. However, because in children Cushing syndrome is frequently associated with an adrenal carcinoma, liberal use of adrenal CT scanning is acceptable.

In the absence of cushingoid features, the preoperative diagnosis of an androgen-secreting adrenal neoplasm is difficult. Virilization, particularly of rapid onset, usually suggests an androgen-secreting tumor, although this presentation does not differentiate between an adrenal or ovarian neoplasm. Signs and symptoms of virilization (clitoromegaly, deepening of the voice, and breast atrophy) are encountered with equal frequency in patients with androgen-secreting adrenal adenomas versus adrenal carcinomas.[125] Serum testosterone may be elevated in patients with androgen-secreting tumors, generally above 200 ng/dl.[126,127] However, the use of this

specific cutoff greatly depends on the particular testosterone assay used by each laboratory, and does not allow differentiation between an ovarian or adrenal neoplasm. In fact, recent data suggest that while circulating testosterone may be markedly elevated in some patients with an androgen-secreting adrenal neoplasia, at least 50 percent of these patients will have levels below 200 ng/dl.[128] Furthermore, the majority of patients with circulating testosterone levels above 200 ng/dl do not have a tumor.[129]

Urinary measurements of 17-ketosteroids are usually above normal in patients with adrenal androgen-secreting neoplasms,[125,127] although a number of testosterone-producing adrenocortical adenomas with normal 24-hr urine 17-ketosteroids have been reported.[130,131] It is unclear what percentage of adrenal androgen-secreting carcinomas demonstrate elevated 24-hr urinary 17-ketosteroids.

The level of circulating DHEAS in patients with adrenal pathology has been reported with less frequency. Yeun and colleagues, based on a single case report, suggested that a DHEAS measurement greater than 6600 ng/ml was consistent with the presence of an adrenal tumor.[132] These researchers emphasized the need for serial measurements of serum testosterone and DHEAS, in order for these levels to be useful in the screening of virilizing adrenal neoplasms. However, more recently Derksen and colleagues reported that of 14 androgen-secreting adrenal neoplasms (2 adenomas and 12 carcinomas), less than 50 percent had basal DHEAS values above 7000 ng/dl,[12] consistent with other reports.[133] In addition, testosterone-secreting adenomas with normal DHEAS levels have been reported.[130,131] Finally, Surrey and colleagues noted that the circulating DHEAS level was greater than 7000 ng/ml in one patient with an *ovarian* lipoid cell tumor and *not* in their only patient with an adrenal adenoma.[134] Thus, circulating DHEAS measurements may not be the most useful marker for the screening of androgen-secreting adrenal adenomas, in the absence of clinical evidence of Cushing syndrome.

Suppression and stimulation testing for the detection of androgen-secreting adenomas can be misleading, and have limited value in the screening of hormonally active adrenal or ovarian neoplasms.[128] Since CT scanning is relatively noninvasive and highly sensitive in the detection of adrenal pathology, there is little place today for adrenal vein catheterization in the diagnosis of adrenal neoplasms.

In spite of the high frequency of hirsutism reported among women with Cushing syndrome (approximately 50 to 70 percent), patients with a primary complaint of hirsutism are rarely diagnosed as cushingoid, particularly in a reproductive endocrinologic/gynecologic practice. This is consistent with the vastly greater prevalence of hirsutism,[135–137] compared to that of Cushing syndrome.[87] As illustration, among approximately 700 hyperandrogenic women with whose care the author has been involved, only 1 patient has been diagnosed as suffering from Cushing's disease. However, in another study of 97 hirsute patients clinically suspected of having Cushing syndrome, 2 had Cushing's disease, 1 had an adrenocortical carcinoma, and 7 were suspected of having intermittent Cushing's disease.[138] Screening for Cushing syndrome in hyperandrogenism probably should generally be restricted to overweight individuals, particularly those with recent weight gain, easy bruisability, and generalized weakness, or those with obvious cushingoid features. Nevertheless, in cushingoid patients with rapid or severe virilization, particularly children, liberal use of adrenal CT scanning may be justified for the early detection of an adrenal carcinoma.

Laboratory Evaluation of Cushing Syndrome

The laboratory evaluation of Cushing syndrome involves two phases. The first phase attempts to confirm the diagnosis of hypercortisolemia (Cushing syndrome), and the second aims to establish the etiology and location of the abnormality. The following sections review these steps in the laboratory evaluation of patients suspected of having Cushing syndrome.

Confirming the Diagnosis of Cushing Syndrome.

The first step in the evaluation of Cushing syndrome is establishing whether an increase in cortisol production is truly present in the patient. As previously stated, Cushing syndrome is synonymous with excess cortisol production. Generally, the pulsatile nature of cortisol secretion is retained, although the vast majority of patients demonstrate a loss in the diurnal rhythm of cortisol.[139] Hence, although hypercortisolemia may be obvious in some patients, morning cortisol levels are of limited value in diagnosing Cushing syndrome. Nonetheless, some investigators have suggested that combining the morning values of ACTH and cortisol may allow for greater discrimination between the various adrenocortical disorders.[140] Others have suggested that patients suspected of Cushing syndrome may be screened with a single midnight cortisol level, although the cost-effectiveness of this test is questionable since it requires that patients be hospitalized overnight.[141]

Screening for hypercortisolemia may also be performed using the overnight dexamethasone suppression test, by administering 1 mg of dexamethasone orally at bedtime and measuring the circulating cortisol level in the morning. If the circulating cortisol level is below 5 µg/dl, the patient is considered not to demonstrate excess cortisol production. Although the false negative rate of this test is relatively small (<3 percent), missing an occasional patient with intermittent hypercortisolemia, the false positive rate is significant (up to 30 percent), particularly among patients with endogenous depression or obesity, or who are taking certain drugs that enhance hepatic metabolism (eg, diphenylhydantoin, rifampin).[30,142] Furthermore, given the likelihood of non-suppression in the overnight dexamethasone test in pseudo-Cushing's, and the much higher prevalence of cushingoid obesity relative to Cushing syndrome (600 to 1), the positive predictive value of this test approximates only 0.014.[87] In other words, only 1.4 percent of patients not demonstrating suppression to the test actually will have Cushing syndrome.

A patient demonstrating an abnormal overnight dexamethasone suppression test requires a 24-hr urine free cortisol (UFC) measurement for confirmation of the hypercortisolemia. Alternatively, the 24-hr UFC can be used for the initial screening, and is normally below 100 µg/24 hr. Levels consistently greater than 300 µg/24 hr are practically diagnostic of Cushing syndrome. Alternatively, some patients may require multiple measurements over time in order to establish the diagnosis of hypercortisolemia, since they may suffer from intermittent or periodic Cushing syndrome.[143,144]

If the 24-hr urine cortisol level is elevated, pseudo-Cushing's must be distinguished from true Cushing syndrome. Various alternative approaches have been proposed. Classically, patients proceed to a low-dose dexamethasone suppression test, administering 0.5 mg of dexamethasone orally exactly every 6 hr for 2 days. While the test can be performed on an outpatient basis, it is imperative that the dexamethasone be taken exactly every 6 hr. As originally described, urine is collected for 24 hr during the last day of suppression, and assayed for 17hydroxycorticosteroids (17-OHCS), which normally are below 4 mg/24 hr or 11 µmol/24 hr.[145] Others have suggested measuring UFC on the second day of treatment and considering values above 100 µg/24 hr as abnormal. However, these measures appear to have limited value, with one study reporting a diagnostic accuracy of only 71 percent when either of these measures are used during the low-dose dexamethasone suppression test.[146] Some investigators have suggested substituting the 24-hr urinary measurements for a serum cortisol measurement at 1600 hr during the second day of suppression, which normally should be under 5 µg/dl.[147] Others have proposed measuring serum cortisol on the morning of the third day of the test, exactly 6 hr after the last dose of dexamethasone.[148] The reported true positive rate of this test exceeds 97 percent, while false negatives appear to be rare.[148,149]

It has been suggested that combining dexamethasone suppression with a CRH stimulation test may increase the diagnostic value of the test. Yanovski and colleagues reported that the addition of an acute ovine

CRH stimulation test, performed on the third day of testing 2 hr after the last dose of dexamethasone was taken, increased the diagnostic accuracy of this test for Cushing syndrome to virtually 100 percent.[146] The cutoff value used was a cortisol level below 1.4 μg/dl, 15 min after the administration of CRH. Other investigators suggest the use of the insulin hypoglycemic test to help distinguish patients with depression-induced pseudo-Cushing's, since in these patients the cortisol response to the induced hypoglycemia is usually preserved.[149] However, this test has a significant false positive rate and should not be used as a primary test. The metyrapone stimulation test, although of greater value in diagnosing adrenocortical insufficiency (see below), is not useful in the evaluation of patients with Cushing syndrome.[149] Other tests proposed include stimulation of the hypothalamic–pituitary–adrenal axis (and consequently ACTH and cortisol) with naloxone, lysine or arginine–vasopression, or desmopressin.[141,150,151] However, these methods remain to be validated, and stimulation tests theoretically should be greater than normal only in patients with a cortisol source that is responsive to exogenous stimuli. Finally, distinguishing patients with factitious Cushing syndrome (secondary to the ingestion of exogenous corticosteroids) requires a high degree of suspicion and the use of high-pressure liquid chromatography analysis of urinary steroids.[152]

Overall, if the patient does not demonstrate adequate cortisol suppression following the low-dose dexamethasone test (with or without CRH), she is considered to suffer from Cushing syndrome (hypercortisolemia). At this point one must establish the cause of the abnormality, determining whether the hypercortisolemia is ACTH dependent, and whether it is under hypothalamic–pituitary control.

Establishing the Cause of Cushing Syndrome.
Once an excess production of cortisol is documented, the next step in the evaluation of these patients involves determining whether the hypercortisolemia is ACTH dependent or independent. Subsequently, ACTH-dependent causes must be differentiated into those that remain under hypothalamic–pituitary control and those that do not (ectopic ACTH/CRH-producing tumors).

Traditionally, patients diagnosed as having Cushing syndrome underwent the high-dose dexamethasone suppression test (2 mg of oral dexamethasone q 6 hr for 48 hr) measuring a 24-hr urinary 17-OHCS prior to and during the second day of dexamethasone suppression.[145] More recently, the urinary 17-OHCS test has been replaced by measures of UFC.[153] Patients are hospitalized during the study. Adequate suppression is defined as a decrease in urinary cortisol metabolites to 50 percent or less of the basal value. However, it is important to note that this test was originally designed to distinguish

adrenal tumors from Cushing's disease, prior to the availability of CT or MR imaging. Most adrenal (and ectopic ACTH/CRH-producing) tumors demonstrate inadequate suppression. However, with the availability of ACTH serum measurements and adrenal imaging, this test has been relegated to aiding in discriminating pituitary from ectopic causes of Cushing syndrome, in patients with ACTH-dependent disease.

Current evaluation of patients with Cushing syndrome begins with the measurement of serum ACTH. Patients with ACTH-dependent Cushing's (either ectopic or pituitary) have ACTH levels either in the normal or elevated range, while patients with adrenal tumors generally have suppressed levels (Fig 18–9). Radiologic imaging in those individuals with very low or undetectable ACTH levels will readily confirm the diagnosis of an adrenal neoplasm.

A CT scan of the adrenal, obtained at 0.5-mm intervals, virtually identifies all adrenal adenomas and carcinomas. Rarely, a CT scan will demonstrate grossly normal or slightly hyperplastic adrenals in the face of endocrine evidence for an adrenal cause for the Cushing syndrome, and the diagnosis of primary micronodular hyperplasia should be suspected. It should be noted that premature CT scanning of the adrenal cortex, prior to fully evaluating the hypothalamic–pituitary–adrenal axis, can mislead the physician into assuming a primary adrenal cause for the hypercortisolemia. Approximately 0.16 percent of asymptomatic subjects demonstrate adrenal nodules on CT scanning,[105] and adrenocortical abnormalities are frequently found in patients demonstrating adrenal enzyme deficiencies.[154,155] In the evaluation of Cushing syndrome the adrenal should not be examined radiographically, unless there is first endocrinologic evidence of an adrenal cause for the disorder.

In contrast to the diagnosis of a primary adrenal disorder, differentiating an ectopic from a pituitary source in patients with ACTH-dependent Cushing's is by no means as simple, and remains an area of intense research. A number of factors may increase suspicion for ectopic ACTH or CRH secretion. If a cushingoid patient is known to have cancer, or has clinical features suggestive of disseminated malignancy (eg, pulmonary), an ectopic source is highly probable. Furthermore, persistent hypokalemia in a cushingoid patient is also highly suggestive of an ectopic source. In addition, the highest levels of ACTH are usually found only in patients with an ectopic source. Nonetheless, since ectopic tumors may preferentially secrete "big" ACTH, which may not be detected on routine radioimmunoassays (RIAs) or even the newer immunoradiometric assays (IRMAs) for ACTH, a falsely low level of this hormone may be observed in some patients with an ectopic ACTH-secreting tumor.[149] If suspected, "big" ACTH can be detected using specialized monoclonal antibody-based IRMAs.

In addition to big ACTH, these patients often demonstrate secretion of other tumor secretory products such as calcitonin; gut hormones (eg, vasoactive intestinal peptide or VIP, gastrin-releasing peptide, and gastrin); and oncofetal markers (eg, α-fetoprotein, human chorionic gonadotropin [hCG], and carcinoembryonic antigen [CEA].[156] Finding elevated levels of these markers may suggest an ectopic source of ACTH as the etiology for the Cushing syndrome. Finally, if an ectopic CRH-secreting tumor is suspected, circulating CRH levels should be measured, and under normal circumstances are only detectable in pregnant patients.

Various approaches can be taken to discriminate an ectopic from a pituitary source. Radiologic studies of the pituitary should be performed in order to detect the presence of an ACTH-secreting pituitary tumor, with MR imaging before and after gadolinium enhancement being the preferred method of diagnosis.[149] However, since the majority of ACTH-secreting pituitary tumors are less than 10 mm in diameter (microadenomas), only 50 to 60 percent of patients with Cushing disease can be diagnosed in this fashion.

In patients without an obvious source, the high-dose dexamethasone suppression test has been used to discriminate ectopic from pituitary causes. As interpreted, the results of the test determine whether the source of ACTH is responsive, at least partially, to the negative feedback of glucocorticoids (generally pituitary Cushing's), or not (generally ectopic sources). Approximately 85 to 90 percent of patients with pituitary Cushing syndrome demonstrate suppressibility in response to high-dose glucocorticoid administration, although some ectopic ACTH/CRH-producing tumors may do the same.[156] Alternatively, 10 to 15 percent of Cushing's disease patients do not demonstrate adequate suppression to the high-dose dexamethasone regimen, particularly if they have developed secondary macronodular adrenocortical hyperplasia.

The diagnostic accuracy of the test can be increased by measuring both 17-OHCS and UFC, and requiring a greater than 90 percent and 64 percent suppression for the diagnosis of a pituitary tumor, respectively.[157] More recently, an overnight high-dose dexamethasone suppression test measuring serum cortisol has been proposed in lieu of the 2-day regimen.[158] A baseline serum cortisol is drawn at 0800 hr, 8 mg of dexamethasone is then administered orally at 2300 hr the same day, and the following morning another serum cortisol is drawn. Adequate suppression was reported as a postdexamethasone level 50 percent or less of the basal cortisol. Nonetheless, some investigators have questioned the accuracy of this abbreviated test, at least as originally described.[159]

Patients who demonstrate inadequate suppressibility following high-dose dexamethasone suppression require further testing in order to confirm the diagnosis of an ectopic ACTH/CRH-producing tumor. A complimentary, and possibly alternative, test useful for the diagnosis of an ectopic source of ACTH is acute CRH stimulation. ACTH-secreting pituitary adenomas are assumed to respond to CRH stimulation, while ectopic sources do not. While ovine CRH causes a more prolonged and greater ACTH, and possibly cortisol, secretion, compared to human CRH,[160] the discriminatory value for diagnosing or discriminating the causes of Cushing syndrome appears to be comparable. Simplified criteria for the performance and interpretation of this test have been proposed.[161] Using 1 μg/kg body weight of ovine CRH administered IV, and sampling performed at –5, –1, 15, and 30 min, all patients with an ectopic source were found to have an increase in ACTH levels below 35 percent. An ACTH increase of greater than 100 percent or a cortisol increase of greater than 50 percent virtually eliminates the possibility of an ectopic ACTH syndrome. However, the response could not be used to exclude or include pituitary Cushing's, such that if there were a negative (flat) ACTH response to ovine CRH, the patient would have approximately a 50 percent chance of having either a pituitary tumor or an ectopic ACTH/CRH-producing neoplasm. This probability arises from the fact that while only 10 to 15 percent of pituitary adenomas do not respond to ACTH, they are seven times more common than ectopic ACTH/CRH-producing tumors. Nonetheless, combining the results of the ACTH serum levels, the high-dose dexamethasone suppression and the CRH test may result in a higher degree of certainty regarding the source of the excess ACTH.

In those few patients whose diagnosis remains equivocal, either after high-dose dexamethasone suppression, CRH testing, or both, IPS and peripheral vein sampling can be utilized.[158,162] The IPS receives blood from the pituitary without mixture from other sources, and the ACTH concentration should be greater in this blood than at a peripheral site, particularly in patients with a pituitary adenoma. Both sinuses must be sampled, since each half of the pituitary gland is drained separately. In addition, the pulsatile release of ACTH requires both sinuses to be sampled simultaneously. Overall the procedure is relatively safe. An IPS to peripheral ACTH ratio of 2 or more indicates a pituitary source for the ACTH. An IPS/peripheral gradient below 1.5 generally supports an ectopic cause. More recently, combining CRH stimulation with IPS sampling has resulted in a greater degree of diagnostic accuracy.[163,164] Nonetheless, IPS sampling with CRH stimulation should not be used to attempt to distinguish pseudo-Cushing's from Cushing syndrome, due to its relatively low diagnostic accuracy for distinguishing these two disorders.[165] Finally, lateralization of the pituitary adenoma can be accomplished in many patients with

Cushing's disease by comparing the ACTH values of each IPS sampled simultaneously.

More recently, an alternate algorithm for the evaluation of patients with Cushing syndrome has been proposed, which eliminates the use of the high-dose dexamethasone suppression test.[166] Once circulating ACTH levels suggest ACTH-dependent Cushing's, an acute CRH stimulation test is undertaken. If there is a 50 percent or greater rise in ACTH levels following stimulation, the patient has a 95 percent probability of having Cushing's disease. Under this algorithm, if the patient does not demonstrate an adequate ACTH response following CRH stimulation, one should proceed directly to bilateral inferior petrosal sinus (IPS) sampling, with or without CRH stimulation. The advantage of this approach over the traditional scheme is that hospitalization for the high-dose dexamethasone suppression test is avoided. Furthermore, patients on medications that increase dexamethasone metabolism (eg, phenytoin) may inappropriately not demonstrate adequate suppressibility following high-dose dexamethasone, although this medication should not alter the response to CRH stimulation.

Patients suspected of having ectopic ACTH/CRH-producing tumors should undergo a CT or MR scan of the abdomen (including the adrenals) and lungs. In addition to radiographic studies, these patients should undergo measurement of other tumor secretory products such as calcitonin, VIP, α-fetoprotein, hCG, and CEA. One should remember that many patients with an ectopic source for ACTH will not demonstrate the typical stigmata of Cushing syndrome, in which case evidence of hypercortisolemia should increase the index of suspicion for an ectopic source.

Treatment of Cushing Syndrome

Obviously the treatment of this disorder depends on the specific etiology being addressed.

Cushing's Disease. Contrary to GnRH, continuous long-term exposure to CRH does not desensitize corticotrophin adenoma cells in vitro, and the sensitivity of these cells to the negative feedback of glucocorticoids was not modified by the long-term stimulation of CRH.[167] Furthermore, a continuous intravenous infusion of CRH for 24 hr did not alter the circadian rhythm of ACTH or cortisol.[26] Thus, it is unlikely that long-acting CRH analogs will be useful in the treatment of Cushing's disease.

In the past, patients with pituitary Cushing syndrome were routinely treated by total bilateral adrenalectomy, followed by replacement with gluco- and mineralocorticoids.[89] Operative mortality ranges from 4 to 10 percent. Furthermore, 10 to 20 percent of patients develop a rapid postoperative enlargement in the size of the pituitary tumor, due to the removal of whatever inhibitory effect

adrenocorticoids exerted, resulting in Nelson syndrome. Nelson syndrome is characterized by severe skin hyperpigmentation, markedly elevated ACTH levels, and radiologic evidence of a pituitary adenoma, frequently achieving a large size and exhibiting sellar pressure symptoms. The hyperpigmentation in this syndrome is due to the excessive production of α-, β-, and β-MSH, as well as ACTH and β-lipotropin, all of which have melanocyte-stimulating activity. If untreated, the disorder can lead to progressive blindness due to optic nerve compression. Surgical removal or radiation therapy is the treatment of choice. All patients undergoing bilateral adrenalectomy should have a pituitary CT scan every 6 mo for up to 2 yr following surgery, to detect the development of post-adrenalectomy pituitary enlargement. There are some advantages to bilateral adrenalectomy as primary therapy for pituitary Cushing's. Surgery achieves a rapid remission and is not associated with the possibility of panhypopituitarism.[168] Nonetheless, in view of the not insignificant risk of surgical complications and postoperative Nelson syndrome, today bilateral adrenalectomy is reserved for patients who have failed all other forms of therapy.

High voltage x-ray (cobalt-60) cyclotron radiotherapy to the pituitary has been used as primary therapy.[89] Although only 15 to 25 percent of adults demonstrate total improvement, approximately 80 percent of children respond well. Radiation can be combined with the administration of an adrenolytic drug, or used for recurrent disease (see below).

The treatment of choice today for pituitary Cushing syndrome is surgery, using the transsphenoidal approach and operating microscopes for direct visualization and microdissection of the pituitary tumor.[89] The use of bilateral IPS sampling has added increased direction to the neurosurgeon. Approximately 50 percent of patients with Cushing's disease are candidates for transsphenoidal hypophysectomy, with a 90 to 95 percent remission rate. The mortality ranges from 1 to 2 percent, although there appears to be a 5 to 15 percent morbidity, particularly the development of partial diabetes insipidus.[168,169] Recurrence occurs in between 25 and 35 percent of patients followed for up to 10 yr after surgery,[169,170] in a progressive linear fashion. The risk of recurrence is higher in those patients demonstrating high cortisol levels or a response of cortisol to CRH stimulation following surgery; not requiring long-term glucocorticoid replacement; without a pituitary adenoma on pathologic examination; with severe depression; and based on overall clinical severity.[169,170]

If the pituitary tumor recurs following the initial surgery, a reoperation has a 50 percent chance of definite success, although a very high risk of panhypopituitarism.[171,172] Inhibitors of adrenocortical biosynthesis (Fig 18–3), including ketoconazole, metyrapone, aminoglutethimide, trilostane, and mitotane, have also been used successfully in patients with only partial remission to their therapy. The use of mitotane (o,p'DDD), which in addition to inhibiting steroidogenesis is directly adrenolytic, may be associated with permanent adrenal failure. Other options for recurrent/persistent disease include bilateral adrenalectomy,[168,170] or preferably pituitary irradiation.[173]

Some patients with Cushing's disease may have developed secondary macronodular adrenal hyperplasia, and may demonstrate a slow return of the hypercortisolemia to normal following pituitary surgery. Bilateral adrenalectomy or the use of drugs inhibiting cortisol biosynthesis may be considered in these individuals.

Adrenal Cushing Syndrome. Patients with an adrenal cause for Cushing syndrome should undergo surgery. If a unilateral well-circumscribed adenoma is identified radiologically, removal of the adenoma via a flank approach can be curative. Overall, the long-term prognosis for patients with isolated adrenal adenomas is very good. Alternatively, if the tumor is irregular or large, suggestive of carcinoma, a unilateral adrenalectomy through an abdominal exploratory approach is preferred. Treatment for primary bilateral micronodular hyperplasia (which should not be confused with secondary macronodular adrenal hyperplasia) is bilateral adrenalectomy. As above, all patients undergoing a bilateral adrenalectomy should be followed carefully for any evidence of Nelson syndrome resulting from the growth of a recognized or unrecognized pituitary adenoma. The use of adrenolytic drugs, such as mitotane, can also be used for the treatment of adrenal carcinomas. Unfortunately, patients with adrenal carcinoma usually die within 7 yr, often within a 1 or 2 yr of diagnosis.[101]

Ectopic ACTH/CRH-Producing Neoplasms. Patients with ectopic ACTH/CRH-producing tumors should undergo surgery for their primary neoplasm. If the neoplasm is unable to be completely resected, the use of adrenocortical biosynthesis inhibitors may be considered. The prognosis of ectopic ACTH/CH-producing tumors generally depends on the course of the primary neoplasm.

All patients being treated for Cushing syndrome run the risk of developing adrenal insufficiency. This is particularly notable in patients with a cortisol-producing adenoma in whom the surrounding normal adrenocortical tissue is suppressed and relatively nonfunctional. Temporary or long-term replacement with glucocorticoids and mineralocorticoids must be considered.

ADRENOCORTICAL INSUFFICIENCY

Adrenocortical insufficiency or Addison's disease can be either due to a primary adrenocortical failure, or secondary to insufficient ACTH stimulation. The most common cause of primary adrenal failure is autoimmune adrenalitis.

Infectious diseases, tumorous metastasis, adrenal hemorrhage, and the use of adrenocortical inhibitors can also give rise to primary adrenal insufficiency. Because the adrenals have a large reserve, more than 90 percent of the cortex must be destroyed for patients to become overtly symptomatic.[174] Secondary adrenal insufficiency may be iatrogenic, as in the rapid withdrawal of long-term glucocorticoid administration, or following resection of a benign cortisol-producing or ACTH-producing adrenal or pituitary adenoma, respectively. A pituitary or hypothalamic neoplasm, Sheehan syndrome, and other causes of pituitary failure can also result in insufficient ACTH production and secondary adrenal insufficiency.

Clinical Manifestations

Addison's disease may evolve gradually and insidiously, frequently misleading the clinician. Alternatively, adrenocortical insufficiency may present acutely, in a life-threatening fashion, the so-called Addisonian or adrenal crisis. The most common symptoms of Addison's disease are weight loss, fatigue, and pigmentary changes. Almost 100 percent of patients with Addison's disease demonstrate one or more of these symptoms.[175,176] The hyperpigmentation is usually profound, and involves the extensor surfaces, the lips, buccal mucosa, dental gingival margins, tongue, and skin scars, particularly those acquired after the onset of the disease. The increased pigmentation of skin and mucosal membranes reflects increased levels of MSH, β-lipotropin, and other POMC products with melanocyte-stimulating properties.

Gastrointestinal manifestations are present in over 50 percent of patients with Addison's disease, including lower abdominal cramping, anorexia, vomiting, and diarrhea. Hypotension is present in the majority of patients, and orthostatic hypotension is also common, although less than 20 percent of patients are symptomatic when standing. Contrary to other forms of postural hypotension, postural dizziness in Addison's disease becomes worse as the day progresses. The hypotension is due to mineralocorticoid deficiency resulting in hyponatremia and volume depletion, exacerbated by an abnormally high vasopressin secretion.[177] Hypercalcemia may also be present. Mild to moderate degrees of hypoglycemia, particularly following meals, may be evident due to the loss of the antagonistic effect of glucocorticoids on insulin action. Psychiatric symptoms, including depression, are also common in patients with adrenal failure. Adrenal crisis is characterized by the rapid onset of hypotension, tachycardia, fever, and hypoglycemia, and a progressive deterioration of mental status.

Oligo- or amenorrhea, and impotence are frequently present in patients with adrenocortical insufficiency.[176,178] In some, the menstrual disturbances may be the result of chronic illness, while in other patients autoimmune adrenal failure may be accompanied by gonadal failure. A generalized loss of hair, especially among female patients, is occasionally noted, although less marked than in pan-hypopituitarism (Fig 18–11). The exact mechanism for this is unclear, although it may relate to the decrease in adrenal androgens.

Causes of Adrenocortical Insufficiency

Idiopathic or Autoimmune Adrenalitis. Autoimmune adrenal failure is the most common cause of primary adrenocortical insufficiency, accounting for 60 to 70 percent of such patients (Table 18–4). Autoimmune adrenal failure is more common in females, and affects Caucasians more frequently than Black patients. Previously, this disorder was described as "idiopathic" or "atrophic" Addison's disease. However, two thirds of patients with "idiopathic" adrenal failure demonstrate adrenal antibodies.[179,180] Autoimmune adrenalitis may occur as an isolated event or as part of an autoimmune polyglandular syndrome. There appears to be a familial predisposition, and an association with the inheritance of the HLA antigens B8 and DR3 in white populations.[181]

The course of adrenal failure in autoimmune adrenalitis is usually slow, with a mean duration of approxi-

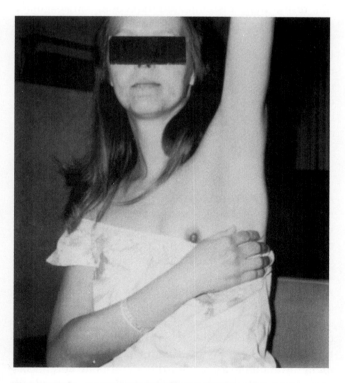

Figure 18–11. Female patient suffering from type II autoimmune adrenal insufficiency (Schmidt syndrome), demonstrating the loss of axillary hair and hyperpigmentation of the areola. While pubic hair was also markedly decreased, there was no scalp hair loss. *(Courtesy of Robert Kreisberg, M.D., University of Alabama at Birmingham.)*

TABLE 18–4. ETIOLOGY OF ADDISON'S DISEASE

I. Autoimmune Adrenalitis

II. Infectious Organisms
Tuberculous
Fungal infections

III. Metastatic Disease
Lung
Breasts
Stomach
Non-Hodgkin's lymphoma

IV. Adrenal Hemorrhage
Waterhouse–Friderichsen syndrome
   Meningococcus
   Pneumococcus
   E coli
   Haemophilus
   DF-2 bacillus
Anticoagulation therapy
Bilateral adrenal vein catheterization

V. Drug-Induced or Related Causes
Withdrawal from steroid therapy
Adrenolytic therapy
   o, p′DDD
   Aminoglutethimide
   Trilostane
Other agents
   Ketoconazole
   Etomidate
   Rifampin
   Cyproterone acetate
   Anticoagulation (coumadin, heparin)

VI. Rare Causes
Acquired immune deficiency syndrome
Sarcoidosis
Amyloidosis

VII. Neonatal Adrenal Insufficiency
Enzymatic blocks in cortisol synthesis
Maternal Cushing syndrome
Adrenal hypoplasia
Adrenal leukodystrophy

(Adapted, with permission, from Kannan CR, The Adrenal Gland. New York, Plenum Medical Book Co., 1988, p 35.)

mately 3 yr. Symptoms may wax and wane, until patients eventually decompensate. The autoimmune destruction is confined to the adrenal cortex and does not involve the medulla. The detection of circulating complement-fixing adrenal antibodies is based on the indirect immunofluorescence technique using unfixed human adrenal tissue. While 70 percent of patients with presumed autoimmune adrenalitis demonstrate these serum antibodies at the time of their diagnosis,[179,180] 1 to 2 percent of patients with other autoimmune endocrine diseases also demonstrate the presence of anti-adrenal antibodies.[180,182,183] Alternatively, the finding of anti-adrenal antibodies in patients asymptomatic for adrenal failure is highly correlated with the subsequent development of the disorder, generally within 4 yr.[182–185]

The most common antigen in autoimmune Addison's disease is the 21-hydroxylase enzyme, with antibodies to this protein present in 64 to 72 percent of patients.[186,187] The region between amino acids 241 and 494 appears to play a critical role in autoantibody binding.[188] In contrast, less than 10 percent of patients' sera contain antibodies directed against the side-chain cleavage and the 17-hydroxylase enzyme. In fact, detection of anti-21-hydroxylase antibodies by a radiobinding assay has the potential of being a simple and sensitive diagnostic test in the evaluation of patients with idiopathic adrenal insufficiency.[189] Nonetheless, although the antibodies against 21-hydroxylase demonstrate an inhibitory effect on the activity of this enzyme in vivo,[190] no such deficiency is able to be observed in vivo.[191]

It appears that the autoantibodies against adrenocortical tissue may also bind to other steroid-producing cells, particularly thyroid, gonadal, or placental tissue. Forty percent of patients with autoimmune Addison's disease have an associated endocrinopathy, usually thyroid disease.[178,181,192] Vitiligo is present in 4 to 6 percent of patients with primary autoimmune adrenal failure.[178,181] Up to 25 percent of patients with idiopathic Addison's disease demonstrate evidence of premature gonadal failure with increased LH and FSH levels.[179,192] The development of gonadal failure may precede or follow adrenal insufficiency, without specific order.[185] Patients with premature ovarian failure in whom adrenocortical antibodies have been identified should be screened regularly for the development of adrenocortical insufficiency. In one series, 1 of 33 patients (7 percent) with premature ovarian failure demonstrated subclinical adrenocortical failure.[193] In general, antibodies directed against either the side-chain cleavage, 21-hydroxylase, or 17-hydroxylase enzymes are not detected in patients with premature ovarian failure, unless accompanied by evidence of adrenal autoimmunity.[187]

Infections. In the past, tuberculosis accounted for up to 70 percent of cases of adrenocortical insufficiency, although it currently is the etiology in only 15 to 20 percent.[176] Extensive damage of the adrenal cortex occurs, including the medulla. Calcification of the gland may be present, and is detectable by CT scanning. Addison's disease can occur during the period of active tuberculosis or many years after the initial event.

Infection with the human immunodeficiency virus (HIV) leading to the acquired immunodeficiency syndrome (AIDS) may also occasionally result in adrenocortical insufficiency.[194] The treatment of opportunistic fungal infections with medications such as ketoconazole, which inhibit adrenocortical biosynthesis, may further compromise adrenal function in patients with disseminated AIDS. Nevertheless, usually only subtle changes in adrenocortical function have been observed, particularly in patients with asymptomatic HIV infection.[195-197] Generally, the adrenocortical profile in AIDS appears to be similar to that of other chronic illnesses, namely an increase in cortisol and a decrease in adrenal androgen secretion.[198] Individuals with AIDS-related complex do not appear to have an overt endocrine deficiency.

Fungal infections, including histoplasmosis, coccidioidomycosis, and blastomycosis, can also result in Addison's disease. Antifungal chemotherapy with ketoconazole can further deteriorate adrenal function, already compromised by the fungal disease, since this drug has adrenolytic properties. Fungal involvement of the adrenal cortex can present as a unilateral adrenal mass, resembling an adrenal neoplasm. As in tuberculosis, the disease may present some time after the initial infection.

Metastatic Lesions. Although the adrenal gland may be involved by tumorous metastasis in approximately 25 percent of patients with a variety of neoplasms, adrenocortical destruction sufficient to induce adrenal insufficiency is rare. The adrenal gland is most commonly involved when the primary tumor is pulmonary, breast, melanoma, or lymphoma.[30]

Adrenal Hemorrhage. Bilateral adrenal hemorrhage can result from disseminated infection, anticoagulant therapy, or trauma. Adrenal hemorrhage associated with fulminant septicemia, also termed the Waterhouse–Friderichsen syndrome, is generally the result of endotoxic septic shock. Over anticoagulation, particularly in older patients with increased capillary fragility and/or during the administration of both coumarin and heparin, can result in acute adrenal hemorrhage and eventual adrenocortical insufficiency. Prompt clinical recognition depends on a high index of suspicion coupled with early CT scanning of the adrenals.

Iatrogenic Adrenocortical Insufficiency. Various medications currently in use can lead to adrenocortical insufficiency, including adrenolytic drugs used for the treatment of Cushing syndrome (Table 18–4). Ketoconazole, a broad-spectrum antifungal drug, also inhibits a variety of cytochrome P450 enzymes and can result in adrenocortical failure. The degree of adrenal insufficiency is dose dependent. The use of the antiandrogen, cyproterone acetate, may also result in adrenal insufficiency. This medication is currently not approved for use in the United States. Rifampin, used for the treatment of tuberculosis, may further deteriorate adrenocortical function already compromised by tuberculosis infection of the adrenal.[30]

Congenital or Familial Causes. A rare cause of adrenal failure in the newborn is X-linked congenital adrenal hypoplasia. Adrenocortical insufficiency may also present in infants with severe deficiencies of 3β-hydroxysteroid dehydrogenase, 21-hydroxylase, or 11-hydroxylase function (ie, congenital adrenal hyperplasia, described later). Neonatal adrenocortical insufficiency may also present in infants born to women receiving very high doses of glucocorticoids during pregnancy and patients with untreated Cushing syndrome. Finally, trauma at delivery, with adrenal hemorrhage, may result in neonatal adrenal insufficiency.

Recently, an autosomal recessive syndrome of familial glucocorticoid deficiency has been reported, in which inherited mutations of the ACTH receptor result in adrenal unresponsiveness to ACTH stimulation.[199] The syndrome is characterized by glucocorticoid deficiency, high plasma ACTH levels, and a normal renin–aldosterone axis. Patients usually present in early childhood with hyperpigmentation, hypoglycemic episodes, failure to thrive, and frequent and severe infections. The associated mortality is high, in excess of 40 percent.

Diagnosis
A high index of suspicion for adrenal insufficiency must exist, since the clinical course of Addison's disease may be prolonged and insidious. Blood chemistries consistent with adrenocortical insufficiency include hyponatremia, hyperkalemia, hypercalcemia, hypoglycemia, and an elevated blood urea nitrogen (BUN) and creatinine. Mild anemia with moderate eosinophilia and lymphocytosis may also be noted. If the initial biochemical screening is normal, but there is a high index of suspicion, repeat testing should be considered.

The measurement of basal serum cortisol levels and/or 24-hr urine for free cortisol or 17-hydroxycorticosteroids are relatively insensitive for the detection of adrenal insufficiency.[140] Generally, the 8:00 AM circulating cortisol level is below μg/dl, although not invariably. A better method of screening for adrenocortical insufficiency is the measurement of serum cortisol following exogenous ACTH stimulation. Since the surviving adrenocortical cells in these patients are assumed to be working at 100 percent capacity, the addition of ACTH results in minimal or no further increase. In normal women, ACTH stimulation causes a marked increase in cortisol levels. Typically, the short (acute or rapid) ACTH stimulation test is used, sampling serum (or plasma) before and 30, 60, and/or 90 min following the intravenous bolus administration of 250 μg of 1-24 ACTH (one ampule of Cortrosyn). While some investigators perform the test in the morning, others prefer to schedule the test in the afternoon, in order to maximize the observable response (since cortisol is at its nadir).[200] The criteria for an adequate response vary, although generally a poststimulation level of 20 or 25 μg/dl is considered normal.[30] Another criterion for normalcy following the short ACTH

test is a doubling of the cortisol level, particularly if it increases at least 10 μg/dl over the baseline level.

One of the more difficult problems in the evaluation of patients with possible adrenocortical insufficiency is the detection of those patients with secondary adrenal failure, and the differentiation between primary and secondary adrenal insufficiency. Both primary adrenal failure and prolonged hypothalamic/pituitary insufficiency may result in a hypoactive ACTH stimulation test, the former due to destruction of the adrenal cortex and the latter due to adrenal atrophy and downregulation of ACTH receptors.[200] However, the basal plasma ACTH level, and the ACTH/cortisol ratio, appear to be useful in differentiating patients with primary adrenal insufficiency from controls or individuals with secondary adrenal failure.[140,201] Furthermore, in general the mineralocorticoid response to the short ACTH test is normal in secondary adrenal failure, while both the cortisol and aldosterone responses are decreased or absent in primary Addison's disease. Aldosterone levels can also be measured during the acute ACTH stimulation test, and normally should increase by an average of 14 ng/dl above the basal level.[202] In fact, the basal plasma renin activity (PRA) to aldosterone ratio may also serve to differentiate patients with primary, but not secondary, adrenocortical insufficiency from normals.[201]

While the short ACTH stimulation test appears to be very effective in detecting primary adrenal failure,[201] such is not the case for patients with secondary adrenal insufficiency.[203,204] Depending on the cutoff cortisol value used (400 nmol/L [15 μg/dl] or 550 nmol/L [20 μg/dl]), between 50 and 100 percent of patients with hypothalamic–pituitary disease will have a normal response to the short ACTH stimulation.[204,205] Tests that may be more sensitive for detecting patients with secondary adrenocortical insufficiency include the low-dose ACTH test, the short metyrapone test, and the insulin stress test. The low-dose ACTH stimulation test was initially reported by Dickenstein and colleagues,[206] and has been found to more sensitive for detecting subtle degrees of adrenal insufficiency.[207–210] The test is performed by sampling before and 20 min after the administration of 0.5 μg/1.73 m^2 of ACTH-(1-24).

Another screen for adrenocortical insufficiency, which has the advantage of providing an assessment of the hypothalamic–pituitary–adrenal axis, is the short metyrapone test. Metyrapone is an inhibitor of 11β-hydroxylase activity, and results in a decrease in cortisol levels and an increase in endogenous ACTH stimulation. The test is performed by administering 30 mg/kg of metyrapone orally at midnight and measuring the levels of cortisol, 11-deoxycortisol, and ACTH at 8:00 AM the following morning.[211] Normally, the rise in 11-deoxycortisol following overnight metyrapone is greater than 60 ng/ml. An adequate ACTH response in the face of an inadequate 11-deoxycortisol rise, suggests primary adrenocortical insufficiency. This test has the disadvantage that measures of aldosterone response cannot be obtained, and that it may aggravate an already compromised adrenocortical function.

Finally, the insulin stress test can be used to screen for subtle adrenocortical deficiencies. The test is performed by administering 0.1 to 0.15 IU insulin/kg body weight intravenously, with blood sampled at 0, 30, 60, 90, and 120 min thereafter for cortisol and ACTH levels.[203] During testing, individuals must develop evidence of hypoglycemic stress, including a glucose level below 40 mg/dl and clinical evidence of a response. However, while this test is more sensitive than the short ACTH test, it is far from perfect, with only between 40 and 60 percent of patients with pituitary tumors demonstrating a subnormal response in cortisol and/or ACTH.[203,212]

The tests mentioned are only used to screen for adrenocortical insufficiency. Confirmation of the diagnosis of primary adrenocortical insufficiency requires a standard ACTH stimulation test. The patient is hospitalized and 24-hr urine 17-OHCS are collected for 2 days. Basal circulating cortisol and ACTH levels are also measured. Forty IU of ACTH are then infused daily over an 8-hr period, for 3 days. Urinary 17-hydroxycorticosteroids and free cortisol and plasma cortisol levels are obtained daily, as well as 2 days following the last ACTH infusion. The total hospitalization time required for this test is 7 days. Normally, the maximum adrenocortical response is observed during the first day of ACTH administration, with the urinary 17-OHCS or urinary free cortisol generally increasing two- to fourfold above baseline. Patients with primary adrenal failure demonstrate a flat response to the test, while patients with "limited reserve" demonstrate a maximal response during the first day of ACTH infusion, after which the magnitude of the response decreases. Patients with secondary adrenocortical insufficiency demonstrate a "stepladder" pattern of increase with the highest responses observed during the second or third day of ACTH stimulation.[30]

Once the diagnosis of adrenal failure is established, CT scanning of the adrenals is used to establish the etiology of primary Addison's disease. The presence of calcifications may suggest tuberculosis, metastasis, or fungal infections. Adrenal hemorrhage or generalized adrenal atrophy may also be observed.

Detection of complement-fixing adrenal antibodies, and/or anti-21-hydroxylase antibodies, can be very helpful in documenting the presence of autoimmune adrenalitis. Furthermore, the presence of these antibodies suggests that screening for other autoimmune endocrine disorders (eg, thyroid, parathyroid, or gonadal failure) is needed.

Treatment

Glucocorticoid and mineralocorticoid replacement is the treatment of choice for Addison's disease. Obviously, therapy for the underlying disease resulting in adrenal failure should be instituted. Approximately 25 to 30 mg of cortisol is secreted daily, which requires replacement in complete adrenocortical insufficiency. Approximately 25 to 35 mg of hydrocortisone is required, since this steroid is only slightly less potent than cortisol (Table 18–5), while 5 to 7.5 mg of prednisone or prednisolone, or 0.5 to 0.75 mg of dexamethasone, is required daily for maintenance replacement. Mineralocorticoid replacement can be provided with the administration of 0.05 to 0.1 mg of 9α-fludrocortisone (fludrocortisone or Florinef) daily. In addition to mineralocorticoid action, this steroid demonstrates some glucocorticoid activity, which should be taken into account when prescribing the hormonal replacement regimen.

Adjustment of the glucocorticoid dose is usually done empirically, depending on the patient's symptomatology. The measurement of a 24-hr urine free cortisol correlates well with clinical symptomatology, but only when hydrocortisone or cortisone acetate are used for glucocorticoid replacement. Dexamethasone, prednisone, and prednisolone are not converted to cortisol and cannot be measured in the urine. Adjustment of the mineralocorticoid dosage is also empiric, but can be aided by the use of electrolyte and plasma renin activity measurements. The dosage of the adrenocortical replacement should be increased temporarily during periods of stress or illness.

Recognition and Management of the Addisonian Crisis

The development of addisonian crisis is a life-threatening situation requiring prompt recognition and therapy. The

TABLE 18–5. DAILY SECRETION RATES OF CORTISOL AND ALDOSTERONE AND RELATIVE POTENCIES OF SYNTHETIC STEROIDS

Steroids	Estimated Potency		Daily Secretion Rate or Maintenance Dose (mg)
	Gluco-corticoid	Mineralo-corticoid	
Cortisol	1.0	0.0015	15–30[a]
Aldosterone	0.1	1.0	0.05–0.2[a]
Fludrocortisone (Florinef)	10.0	0.21	0.1
Cortisone	0.7	0.0012	23–35
Prednisone	4.0	0.002	5–7.5
Dexamethasone (Decadron)	30.0	0	0.5–0.75

[a]Daily secretion rate.
(Reproduced, with permission, from Yen SSC. Chronic anovulation caused by peripheral endocrine disorders. In: Yen SSC, Jaffe RB, eds. Reproductive Endocrinology, 2nd ed. Philadelphia, W. B. Saunders, 1986: 486.)

patient may present with anorexia, complaining of crampy abdominal pain and profuse nausea, vomiting, and diarrhea. A fever may be present, with hypotension, dehydration, and dry skin. Skin and mucosal membrane hyperpigmentation may or may not be present, depending on the rapidity with which the adrenal insufficiency has developed. Laboratory analysis may demonstrate hypoglycemia, hyponatremia, hyperkalemia, acidosis, and elevated BUN and creatinine. Eosinophilia, lymphocytosis, and low plasma cortisol may also be evident.

Immediate recognition and therapy are required to avoid death in these patients. The treatment of addisonian crisis requires the immediate intravenous administration of 100 to 300 mg of hydrocortisone three times daily, with administration of normal saline until adequate urinary flow and blood pressure are maintained. Dextrose or other such carbohydrate solution should be administered to reduce hypoglycemia. The administration of a mineralocorticoid, such as 10 mg of deoxycorticosterone acetate (DOCA) intramuscularly once or twice a day or 0.1 mg fludrocortisone daily, should also be initiated. Following 24 to 48 hr of parenteral therapy, the patient can be slowly switched to oral maintenance. The diagnosis of addisonian crisis should always be entertained if a patient presents in shock with hypoglycemia, hyponatremia, and hypotension.

ADRENOCORTICAL ENZYMATIC DEFICIENCIES

Although an enzymatic block can occur at any site of the steroidogenesis scheme (Fig 18–2), only those at 21-hydroxylase, 11β-hydroxylase, and 3β-hydroxysteroid dehydrogenase result in ovulatory disorders. A deficiency in 17-hydroxylase/17,20-lyase or 17-hydroxysteroid dehydrogenase generally leads to pubertal abnormalities and is discussed in Chapter 5.

Classic Congenital Adrenal Hyperplasia
Also known as the adrenogenital syndrome, classic or congenital adrenal hyperplasia (CAH) is one of the most common autosomal recessive disorders, affecting 1 of every 5000 to 10,000 newborns.[213] The disorder results from the inherited deficiency of any enzyme necessary for the adrenocortical biosynthesis of cortisol. In order to maintain normal cortisol production in face of the enzymatic defect, ACTH levels and adrenocortical activity increase, leading to hyperplasia of the zona reticularis and the excessive accumulation of the enzymatic precursors. The accumulation in the bloodstream of precursors to the affected enzyme, accompanied by a deficiency in cortisol (and sometimes aldosterone) production, results in the signs and symptoms of CAH. These will vary according to the severity and location of the enzymatic block. If the defect is extremely severe (as in the total absence of enzymatic activity), cortisol and aldosterone may not be produced in sufficient quantities to support life with the development of adrenal crisis in the newborn, resulting in death if untreated.[213]

21-Hydroxylase Deficiency. Approximately 90 percent of children suffering from CAH demonstrate a deficiency in 21-hydroxylase function. The accumulation of the enzymatic precursors progesterone, 17-HP, and particularly androstenedione and testosterone, leads to masculinization of the female genitalia in utero. Patients demonstrating inadequate aldosterone production are designated as "salt wasters" (75% of cases). Generally, in these children cortisol is also produced in inadequate amounts. Alternatively, in "simple virilizing" (25% of cases) CAH, cortisol is generally produced in amounts sufficient to sustain life, and androgens accumulate to lesser degrees, producing a less disfiguring genital abnormality in the female fetus. The diagnosis is established by the measurement of basal 17-HP levels usually above 10 ng/ml.[214] The inheritance of CAH appears to be closely linked to the HLA-B47 allele. Multiple abnormalities of the 21-hydroxylase gene have been reported in CAH including deletions, gene conversion, point mutations, and deletion of *both* 21-hydroxylase genes (resulting in severe salt-wasting CAH).

11β-Hydroxylase Deficiency. A less common cause of virilizing adrenal hyperplasia is 11β-hydroxylase deficiency, which accounts for approximately 5 percent of all cases of CAH.[213] In addition to the accumulation of androgens, severe deficiency of 11β-hydroxylase activity can lead to the accumulation of DOC resulting in sodium retention and hypertension. Nevertheless, the clinical picture in 11β-hydroxylase deficient CAH is quite variable.[215] The diagnosis of 11β-hydroxylase deficient CAH can be established by measuring the basal level of 11-deoxycortisol, which usually exceeds 40 ng/ml.

3β-Hydroxysteroid Dehydrogenase Deficiency. An infrequent and usually lethal cause of congenital adrenal hyperplasia is 3β-hydroxysteroid dehydrogenase deficiency, which is diagnosed by extremely high basal levels of 17-hydroxypregnenolone (above 80 ng/ml).[216,217] This disorder leads primarily to the excessive production of the weak androgen, DHEA, and may actually decrease the adrenal and gonadal production of androstenedione and testosterone. There appears to be considerable phenotypic heterogeneity. Thus, males affected with 3β-hydroxysteroid dehydrogenase-deficient CAH may actually demonstrate ambiguous genitalia at birth, due to insufficient androgenic stimulation. A female fetus usually demonstrates only a minimal degree of virilization, if at all. Some individuals may demonstrate salt-wasting, while others are diagnosed only later in life with the appearance of hyperandrogenic signs and symptoms.

Evaluation and Treatment. An electrolyte panel and plasma renin activity level should be obtained in all patients suspected of suffering from CAH. Once the diagnosis is established, replacement with a corticosteroid (with prednisone or hydrocortisone) and, if necessary, mineralocorticoid (with fludrocortisone) is begun (see section on treatment of adrenal insufficiency). In addition to those patients diagnosed with salt-wasting CAH, patients with simple virilizing CAH may also require low doses of mineralocorticoids in the event their basal renin activity measurements are elevated,[218] suggesting that they also have a relative aldosterone deficiency.

Postnatally, untreated males and females with CAH grow more rapidly with advanced epiphyseal maturation, progressive penile or clitoral enlargement, premature adrenarche, hirsutism, and acne. Although they initially may be larger than children of their own age, their earlier epiphyseal closure eventually results in short adult stature. Girls with untreated CAH will develop amenorrhea, acne, hirsutism, and virilization. Amazingly, some lesser affected patients may remain undiagnosed in spite of their progressive masculinization and hirsutism. Fertility is possible and will depend on the degree of genital virilization,[219] which determines the overall coital success following reconstructive surgery,[220] and degree of hyperandrogenemia and oligo-ovulation.

Nonclassic Adrenal Hyperplasia

Adrenal enzyme deficiencies causing hyperandrogenic symptoms some time after birth have been alternatively called late-onset, nonclassic, postpubertal, attenuated, mild, or acquired. Patients previously thought to suffer from the polycystic ovary syndrome (PCOS) and related hyperandrogenic disorders are now being diagnosed as having this genetic disease. By definition, nonclassic adrenal hyperplasia (NCAH) is an autosomal recessive disorder causing symptoms in peri- or postpuberty, and all patients demonstrate a normal female external genitalia. If a child presents with evidence of an adrenal enzyme deficiency and demonstrates virilization of the genitalia, however minor, the disorder is classified as *congenital* or CAH, because the adrenal hyperandrogenemia was present in utero during genital development. Adrenal enzyme deficiencies leading to androgen excess involve either 3β-hydroxysteroid dehydrogenase, 21-hydroxylase, or 11β-hydroxylase.

The most clinically useful test for the diagnosis of adrenocortical enzymatic defects is the adrenal response to acute stimulation with intravenous 1-24 ACTH (Cortrosyn®). In general, the rise in enzymatic precur-

sor(s) and the precursor/product ratio(s) following ACTH stimulation are used to estimate the *relative* enzymatic activity. If the enzyme in question were to be deficient or absent, the rise in precursors or the precursor/product ratio would be excessive. Acute adrenal stimulation with a bolus of either 0.1, 0.25, or 1.0 mg of Cortrosyn intravenously provides equal, reproducible, and maximal adrenal stimulation, regardless of body weight, at least in normal subjects.[221] The use of prestimulation dexamethasone suppression is unnecessary since the peak steroid levels following ACTH administration do not change.

21-Hydroxylase-Deficient NCAH. As for CAH, deficiency of 21-hydroxylase accounts for the vast majority of cases of NCAH. In the United States and United Kingdom, NCAH due to 21-hydroxylase deficiency appears to affect between 1 and 2 percent of hyperandrogenic women, while in Canada, France, Spain, and Italy they account for approximately 5 percent of patients. Among Ashkenazi Jews and some Middle Eastern populations this proportion can be as high as 8 to 10 percent.[222]

Molecular Biology and Genetics of 21-Hydroxylase Deficient NCAH. The 21-hydroxylase gene is located on the short arm of chromosome 6 in the human leukocyte antigen (HLA) region. There are two 21-hydroxylase genes, CYP21 (formerly CYP21B) and CYP21P (formerly CYP21A). Eighty-eight sequence differences between the two genes render CYP21P a nonfunctional pseudogene, such that it is not transcribed in whole into mRNA, and whatever products are transcribed are not translated into a protein. In contrast, CYP21 is actively transcribed and translated into the active enzyme product.

The 21-hydroxylase genes lie in the midst of the HLA complex, between the HLA-B and DR loci. The HLA complex encodes for a large number of leukocyte surface antigens important in human organ transplantation. Because of the close linkage between the 21-hydroxylase genes and specific HLA alleles, HLA-typing has been used in family studies to ascertain the inheritance pattern of the 21-hydroxylase deficiencies. Nonclassic adrenal hyperplasia appears to be linked to HLA-B14 among Ashkenazi Jews, but not some of the other ethnic groups.[223]

Clinically evident deficiency of 21-hydroxylase results from mutations of the CYP21 gene (Table 18–6).[222] Several of these mutations result from unequal crossovers between the CYP21 and the CYP21P genes, which results in large CYP21 gene deletions, or partial conversion of the CYP21 gene to the inactive CYP21P gene. The mutations of CYP21 may yield a variety of phenotypes. For example, the Ile-172 to Arg-172 mutation produces an enzyme with only 1 to 2 percent of normal function, resulting in simple virilizing CAH. Alternatively, the Val-281 to

TABLE 18–6. MUTATIONS OF THE 21-HYDROXYLASE (CYP21) GENE, ENZYMATIC ACTIVITY, AND CLINICAL ASSOCIATION

Normal	Mutation	Location	21-OH Activity[a] (%)	Clinical Association[b]
Val-281	Leu	Exon-7	50	NCAH
Pro-453	Ser	Exon-10	50	NCAH
Pro-30	Leu	Exon-1	50	NCAH
Arg-339	His	Exon-8	50	NCAH
Ile-172	Asn	Exon-4	1–2	SV
Intron-A,C	G	Intron-2	?	SW,SV
8 bp	Deletion	Exon-3	0	SW
Ile-Val-Met	Asn-Glu-Lys	Exon-6	0	SW
Gln-318	Termination	Exon-8	0	SW
Arg-356	Trp	Exon-8	0	SW
Normal	Gene conversion to CYP21P		0	SW
Normal	Large deletion		0	SW

[a]As determined by gene transfection experiments, 21-OH: 21-hydroxylase.
[b]NCAH = non-classic adrenal hyperplasia; SW = salt-wasting congenital adrenal hyperplasia; SV = simple-virilizing congenital adrenal hyperplasia.
(Adapted, with permission, from Azziz R, Dewailly D, Owerbach D. Non-classic adrenal hyperplasia: Current concepts. J Clin Endocrinol Metab. 78:810, 1994.)

Leu-281 mutation produces an enzyme with 20 to 50 percent of normal activity, resulting in a patient with NCAH. Approximately 90 percent of NCAH patients have one or more of the CYP21 mutations noted in Table 18–6. The Leu-281 mutation is the most common, being present in 59.0 percent, while the Ser-453 and Pro-30 mutations are found in 23.1 percent and 10.3 percent of NCAH patients, respectively. While NCAH is considered a homozygous recessive disorder, in most cases the same mutation does not affect both CYP21 alleles. In fact, the majority of patients are "compound heterozygotes," carrying one mild and one severe CYP21 mutation.

Clinical Characteristics. By definition, 21-hydroxylase-deficient NCAH patients do not demonstrate virilization of the external genitalia. Hyperandrogenic symptoms most commonly appear peri- or postpubertally. Androgenic features may be more severe when evident in children with premature adrenarche or even progressive clitoromegaly. Alternatively, adults may first present with a mild form of the disorder. In fact, the clinical presentation cannot be used to distinguish 21-hydroxylase-deficient NCAH patients from those suffering from ovarian hyperandrogenism. Clitoromegaly, male habitus, and temporal baldness are infrequent findings, unless the patient suffers from undiagnosed simple virilizing CAH. While some women may present with no obvious androgenic signs or symptoms, the majority of untreated women with "cryptic" NCAH eventually develop symptoms, if left untreated. In our experience, ovulatory dysfunction is a frequent complaint, with up to 50 percent of patients exhibiting polycystic-appearing ovaries on ultrasonography (Table 18–7).

In males suffering from NCAH, clinical symptoms may never become apparent, although these boys may be shorter than expected with premature facial, pubic, and axillary hair growth.

Biochemically, it is difficult to distinguish NCAH women from other hyperandrogenic or PCOS patients. Circulating testosterone and DHEAS levels are not different from those in patients with ovarian hyperandrogenism (Fig 18–12).[222] In fact, DHEAS levels are often normal in 21-hydroxylase-deficient NCAH, and this steroid should not be used as a marker for this disorder. Although circulating androstenedione is usually higher in NCAH than PCOS patients, overlap between the two populations is too great to allow this hormone to be used as a marker for the disorder. Patients with NCAH do not usually have an abnormally elevated LH/FSH ratio, although neither do many patients with ovarian hyperandrogenism.[224]

In contrast to patients with CAH, the hypothalamic–pituitary–adrenal axis appears to be grossly normal in

TABLE 18–7. CLINICAL FEATURES IN 44 WOMEN WITH 21-HYDROXYLASE-DEFICIENT NONCLASSIC ADRENAL HYPERPLASIA

Clinical Feature	Incidence (%)
Oligomenorrhea	30/44 (68%)
Hirsutism	34/44 (77%)
Ultrasound features of polycystic ovaries	8/22 (36%)
Radiologic adrenal abnormalities[a]	6/15 (40%)

[a]Adrenals studied by either CI or MRI. One patient had a 2 x 3-cm unilateral adenoma. Two others had unilateral, and three bilateral, adrenal hyperplasia.
(Adapted, with permission, from Azziz R, Dewailly D, Owerbach D. Nonclassic adrenal hyperplasia: Current concepts. J Clin Endocrinol Metab. 78:810, 1994.)

NCAH, including its response to corticotropin-releasing hormone.[225,226] Likewise, although patients with NCAH do not usually demonstrate overt signs of mineralocorticoid insufficiency, a subtle defect may be present.[227] However, some patients probably have a mild degree of functional hypocortisolism, and subtle but chronic elevations in ACTH secretion. This is suggested by the presence of radiologic evidence of adrenal hyperplasia and/or adenomas in many NCAH patients (Table 18–7). In contrast, only 0.6 percent of randomly selected patients undergoing CT studies of the upper abdomen demonstrate evidence of an incidental adrenal mass.[105]

Screening for 21-Hydroxylase-Deficient NCAH. Rather than performing an acute ACTH stimulation test on all women suspected of having NCAH, the basal level of 17-HP may be used to screen for these patients. In untreated hyperandrogenic women, Azziz and Zacur have reported that a basal follicular phase 17-HP level of less than 2 ng/ml effectively ruled out 21-hydroxylase-deficient NCAH in hyperandrogenism.[128] Alternatively, hyperandrogenic women with a basal follicular phase 17-HP level above 2 ng/ml merit an ACTH stimulation test to rule out NCAH. In order for this screening test to be most effective, blood for 17-HP measurement should be obtained in the morning and in the follicular phase. In our experience, of patients demonstrating a basal 17-HP level above 2 ng/ml, approximately 10 to 15 percent actually have the disorder upon ACTH testing.

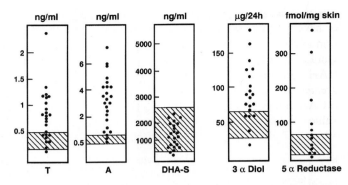

Figure 18–12. Androgen levels in 24 women with 21-hydroxylase-deficient late-onset adrenal hyperplasia. (T = testosterone; A = androstenedione; DHEA-S = dehydroepiandrosterone sulfate; 3αDiol = urinary 3α-androstenediol glucuronide; 5α-reductase = skin capacity for 5α-reduction of T. Hatched areas indicate normal ranges.) *(Reprinted, with permission, from Kuttenn F, Couillin PH, Girard F, et al. Late-onset adrenal hyperplasia in hirsutism.* N Engl J Med. *313:224, 1985.)*

Endocrinologic Diagnosis. In 21-hydroxylase deficiency the precursors considered are 17-HP and/or androstenedione, while the precursor/product ratios include 17-hydroxyprogesterone/11-deoxycortisol. Nevertheless, a single 17-HP level 30 to 90 min post-ACTH administration was found to be the measure most cost effective and simple to interpret (Fig 18–13).[228] Based on patients with an inherited defect of the 21-hydroxylase gene corroborated by mol-

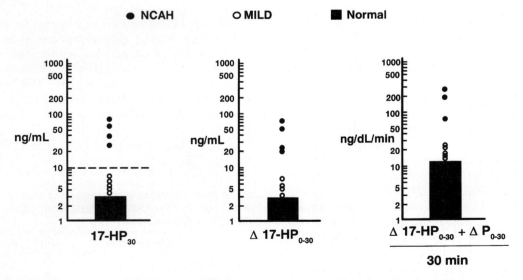

Figure 18–13. From a population of 164 hyperandrogenic patients studied consecutively, all women with abnormal 21-hydroxylase measures after stimulation with 1-24 ACTH are plotted on a logarithmic scale. Measures include the 17-hydroxyprogesterone level 30 min following ACTH administration (17-hydroxyprogesterone$_{30}$), the net increment in 17-hydroxyprogesterone (Δ17-hydroxyprogesterone$_{0-30}$), and the sum of the increments in 17-hydroxyprogesterone and progesterone divided by the stimulation time ([Δ17-hydroxyprogesterone$_{0-30}$ + >P$_{0-30}$]/ 30 min) yielding the rate of rise of these two steroids. The boxed area represents the control response (up to the 95th percentile of normal). (Closed circles = nonclassic adrenal hyperplasia; open circles = patients with a mild exaggeration in their 17-hydroxyprogesterone response to ACTH.) *(Reprinted, with permission, from Azziz and Zacur. 21-Hydroxylase deficiency in female hyperandrogenism: Screening and diagnosis.* J Clin Endocrinol Metab. *69:577, 1989.)*

ecular or family studies, individuals with NCAH are noted to have a 17-HP response to acute adrenocortical stimulation of above l0 ng/ml (Fig 18–14),[224,228,229] although some would argue for a value above 20 ng/ml.[230] Patients with CAH generally demonstrate stimulated 17-HP levels greater than 200 ng/ml. Heterozygotes (carriers) for both NCAH and CAH generally demonstrate stimulated 17-HP values below 10 ng/dl, and often overlapping with the adrenal 17-HP response of the general population.[231]

Treatment and Outcome of 21-Hydroxylase-Deficient Nonclassic Adrenal Hyperplasia.

Glucocorticoid replacement should be implemented as for adrenocortical insufficiency.[232] Normally, between 20 and 25 mg/m^2 of replacement cortisol (or hydrocortisone) is required daily. The average glucocorticoid replacement dose for a normal-sized woman is 25 to 35 mg hydrocortisone/day, 5 to 7.5 mg prednisone/day, or 0.5 to 0.75 mg dexamethasone/day. However, some women may metabolize dexamethasone more slowly and will only require 0.25 mg/day or 0.5 mg/every other day for adequate adrenal suppression. Because of its shorter half-life, prednisone may be easier to

regulate. Treatment with prednisone every other day adequately suppresses adrenal androgen levels, without long-term suppression of the hypothalamic–pituitary–adrenal axis or impairment in cortisol response.

Physicians should not aim to normalize the morning 17-HP plasma level, since adrenal androgens are more sensitive to the suppressive effects of glucocorticoid administration than are C-21 steroids. While circulating DHEAS levels are too easily suppressed, the 17-HP level may never fully normalize in spite of adequate androgen suppression.[233] The androstenedione plasma levels, rather than 17-HP, should be monitored to determine the adequacy of treatment.[232]

When treating hirsutism, anti-androgen therapy, either alone or in combination with glucocorticoids or an oral contraceptive, offers better results than glucocorticoids alone.[232] If patients require control of menstrual function, glucocorticoids alone, oral contraceptives, or a combination, are most useful. Alternatively, treating infertility in these patients requires an understanding of the basis for this difficulty. The main cause of subfertility in women with NCAH is chronic anovulation, secondary to chronic adrenal hyperandrogenism. However, it is probable that long-term elevation of adrenal androgens results in the disruption of the hypothalamic–pituitary–ovarian axis, with development of a PCOS-like phenotype. In fact, polycystic-appearing ovaries may be detected sonographically in up to one third of women with NCAH (Table 18–7). Furthermore, chronic elevations in circulating progesterone and 17-HP levels may also result in inadequate cervical mucus and a persistently atrophic endometrium, in spite of adequate preovulatory estrogen levels and maximal glucocorticoid (and gonadotropic) suppression.

In NCAH patients requiring an improvement in ovulatory function for treatment of infertility, glucocorticoids alone may be sufficient, although additional ovulation induction may also be required. Overall prognosis for fertility in oligo-ovulatory NCAH patients is good and should not be any different from other hyperandrogenic women seeking ovulation induction. In fact, many patients with NCAH become pregnant without requiring treatment.[234]

Management of Pregnancy in NCAH.

While theoretically in utero virilization of children of mothers with NCAH may occur due to transplacental passage of maternal androgens, it is doubtful that the degree of maternal hyperandrogenism associated with this disorder is sufficient to virilize a fetus, in view of the extensive placental aromatase activity present. In utero virilization may also occur due to fetal inheritance of CAH, although this risk appears to be relatively low, between 1.7 and 2.3 per 1000, without knowing the father's carrier status.[222] It can be questioned whether this low risk justifies invasive

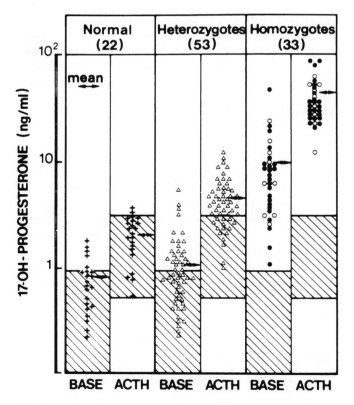

Figure 18–14. Plasma concentrations of 17-hydroxyprogesterone before and after acute ACTH stimulation in patients with nonclassic 21-hydroxylase deficiency and members of their families. (Closed circle = proposit I; open circle = homozygotes; open triangle = heterozygotes + = normals.) *(Reprinted, with permission, from Kuttenn F, Couillin P, Girard F, et al. Non-classic adrenal hyperplasia and hirsutism. N Engl J Med. 313:2224, 1985.)*

prenatal testing, such as amniocentesis to establish sex and intra-amniotic steroid levels. Furthermore, ongoing experience with prenatal dexamethasone therapy in CAH mothers, or those having previously conceived a CAH infant, suggests that the recommended administration of 10 µg/kg may result in significant maternal side effects and complications.[235]

11β-Hydroxylase Deficiency. The prevalence of 11β-hydroxylase deficient NCAH and its diagnostic criteria are less clear. The diagnosis is presumed when the 11-deoxycortisol level or the 11-deoxycortisol/cortisol ratio following acute adrenal stimulation is abnormally high. Some investigators studying small numbers of patients have reported that the frequency of "mild" 11β-hydroxylase deficiency in hyperandrogenism varies from 30 to 87 percent.[236,237] Studying 260 consecutive hyperandrogenic women, we have also observed a high frequency (42.2 percent) of exaggerated responses to adrenal stimulation.[238] However, the higher basal and stimulated 11-deoxycortisol levels were also accompanied by higher basal and stimulated *cortisol* levels. These and other data suggested that the exaggerated 11-deoxycortisol response seen in a large proportion of hyperandrogenic women does *not* reflect 11β-hydroxylase deficiency, and probably represents *adrenocortical hyperactivity*.

The 11β-hydroxylase gene has been localized to the middle of the long arm of chromosome 8, and the disorder is not linked to the human leukocyte antigen (HLA) system. In the absence of a reliable genetic marker, the diagnosis of 11β-hydroxylase deficient NCAH can be presumed only when the 11-deoxycortisol response to ACTH stimulation exceeds a pre-established arbitrary value. Based on the experience with 21-hydroxylase-deficient NCAH, which has been genetically characterized in a more thorough manner, an 11-deoxycortisol response to stimulation of greater than threefold the upper 95th percentile of normal may be selected as consistent with 11β-hydroxylase-deficient NCAH. In our laboratory this represents a poststimulation level of greater than 25 ng/ml. Obligate heterozygotes (carriers) for the congenital form of 11β-hydroxylase adrenal hyperplasia usually demonstrate poststimulation 11-deoxycortisol levels within normal, and always less than 12 ng/ml.[239]

The prevalence of presumed 11β-hydroxylase-deficient NCAH in hyperandrogenism appears to be low.[238,240] Using the diagnostic criteria just given in our population of 260 hyperandrogenic women arising from a large referral area in the Eastern and Southeastern United States, the prevalence of presumed 11β-hydroxylase-deficient NCAH was only 0.8 percent compared to 1.9 percent for the 21-hydroxylase-deficient type.[238] Furthermore, the two patients identified in our study as potentially suffering from 11β-hydroxylase-deficient NCAH have subse-

quently not demonstrated any defects of CYP11 upon molecular analysis.[241]

The clinical variability of 11β-hydroxylase-deficient patients has been well recognized.[215] These patients, as in 21-hydroxylase-deficient NCAH, are clinically indistinguishable from other hyperandrogenic women.[238] The blood pressure in 11β-hydroxylase-deficient NCAH patients ranges from normal to moderately elevated. A pregnancy has been reported in an untreated 11β-hydroxylase-deficient NCAH woman. One of our patients conceived following clomiphene ovulation induction before the diagnosis was established. At present it is not possible to recommend an effective screening method for this rare hyperandrogenic disorder.

3β-Hydroxysteroid-Dehydrogenase Deficient Nonclassic Adrenal Hyperplasia. Various reports have documented the existence of a 3β-hydroxysteroid-dehydrogenase-deficient form of NCAH.[242–244] However, the diagnostic criteria for this disorder are unclear. Some authors presume 3β-hydroxysteroid-dehydrogenase-deficient NCAH simply if the stimulated 17-hydroxypregnenolone is above the normal limit (either mean plus two standard deviations, or the upper 95th percentile).[242] However, if one uses the experience with 21-hydroxylase deficiency as a model, 3β-hydroxysteroid-dehydrogenase-deficient individuals should demonstrate a 17-hydroxypregnenolone stimulated value at least three times the upper normal limit. Each investigator must establish his or her normal standards. In our laboratory the upper 95th percentile for 17-hydroxypregnenolone 60 min post-ACTH administration is 5.0 ng/ml, and the diagnosis of 3β-hydroxysteroid-dehydrogenase-deficient NCAH is presumed only when the stimulated 17-hydroxypregnenolone level is above 15 ng/ml. Using these criteria, we were unable to detect any such patients among 78 consecutively studied hyperandrogenic women.[245] Furthermore, more recent studies of patients presumed to have 3β-hydroxysteroid-dehydrogenase-deficient NCAH reported that the vast majority of these patients had no obvious mutation of their 3β-hydroxysteroid dehydrogenase-II gene.[246,247] Thus, it appears that 3β-hydroxysteroid dehydrogenase deficiency is an infrequent cause of NCAH.

SUMMARY

Disorders of the adrenal cortex relevant to reproduction include pathologic causes of glucocorticoid over- and underproduction, and the adrenal hyperplasias secondary to enzymatic deficiencies. The overproduction of glucocorticoids (Cushing syndrome) is a relatively rare cause of reproductive abnormalities, and can either be ACTH dependent or independent. ACTH-dependent causes include pituitary Cushing's (Cushing's disease), which accounts for 60 to 70 percent of all patients, and ectopic sources of ACTH or, rarely, CRH, accounting for an additional 5 to 15 percent of cases. Adrenal or ACTH-independent causes of glucocorticoid excess comprise approximately 20 to 25 percent of non-iatrogenic Cushing syndrome, with the incidence divided almost equally between adrenal carcinomas and adenomas. Finally, primary bilateral diffuse micronodular hyperplasia or dysplasia, unrelated to excessive ACTH stimulation, is a rare cause of Cushing syndrome. The diagnosis of Cushing syndrome rests on first establishing the actual presence of glucocorticoid excess. Patients can be screened with either an overnight (1 mg) dexamethasone suppression test or a 24-hr urine collection for free cortisol, while morning cortisol levels are of limited value. If results are suspicious or abnormal, the diagnosis of hypercortisolemia is then confirmed by the finding of inadequate cortisol suppression following the low-dose (2 mg/day × 2 days) dexamethasone test, with or without CRH stimulation. The differentiation of adrenal versus ACTH-dependent causes of Cushing's is then made by measuring a basal ACTH level. If ACTH is low or undetectable, then a CT or MR scan of the adrenal is performed. In the event the ACTH level is elevated, exclusion of an ectopic source is required, although the exact approach for establishing this diagnosis is currently somewhat controversial. It generally includes the high-dose dexamethasone test (8 mg/day × 2 days), alone or in combination with an acute CRH stimulation test. Finally, in some patients in whom the diagnosis is still unclear, petrosal sinus sampling combined with CRH stimulation may be useful.

Adrenocortical insufficiency (Addison's disease) can either be due to primary adrenocortical failure or secondary to insufficient ACTH stimulation. The most common cause of primary adrenal failure is autoimmune adrenalitis; while infectious diseases, tumorous metastasis, adrenal hemorrhage, and the use of adrenocortical inhibitors are rare causes. Secondary adrenal insufficiency may be iatrogenic, as in the rapid withdrawal of long-term glucocorticoid administration, or following resection of a benign cortisol-producing or ACTH-producing adrenal or pituitary adenoma, respectively. A pituitary or hypothalamic neoplasm, Sheehan syndrome, and other causes of pituitary failure can also result in insufficient ACTH production and secondary adrenal insufficiency. The detection and diagnosis of Addison's disease greatly depends on a high index of suspicion, since the clinical course may be prolonged and insidious. The measurement of basal serum cortisol levels, and/or 24-hr urine for free cortisol or 17-hydroxycorticosteroids, are relatively insensitive. While the short (maximal or acute) ACTH stimulation test appears to be very effective in detecting primary adrenal failure, such is not the case for patients with secondary adrenal insufficiency. Depending on the cutoff cortisol value used, between 50 and 100 percent of patients with hypothalamic–pituitary disease will have a normal response to the short ACTH stimulation. Secondary adrenal insufficiency may be more readily diagnosed by the low-dose ACTH test, the short metyrapone test, or the insulin stress test. Finally, once the diagnosis of adrenal failure is established, CT or MR scanning of the adrenals is used to exclude a primary adrenal abnormality.

Although enzymatic deficiencies resulting in adrenal hyperplasia can occur at any site of the steroidogenesis scheme, only those at 21-hydroxylase, 11β-hydroxylase, and 3β-hydroxysteroid dehydrogenase result in hyperandrogenic ovulatory disorders. Overall, between 1 and 10 percent of androgen-excess patients are affected with these disorders, depending on geographic or ethnic origin. By far the most common abnormality is that of 21-hydroxylase, accounting for over 90 percent of all cases. Adrenal hyperplasia can be subdivided into classic (congenital) and nonclassic types. Classic adrenal hyperplasia may present in the neonatal period with electrolyte imbalances (salt-wasting type), or solely with virilization, if a female child is affected (simple virilizing type). In fact, 21-hydroxylase-deficient classic adrenal hyperplasia is the most common cause of female pseudohermaphroditism. Alternatively, nonclassic adrenal hyperplasia does not cause genital abnormalities in females, and these patients develop signs and symptoms of androgenization peri- or postpubertally. Overall, reproductive dysfunction secondary to adrenal disorders is relatively rare.

REFERENCES

1. Symington T. The morphology and zoning of the human adrenal cortex. In: Currie AR, Symington T, Grant JK, eds. *The Human Adrenal Cortex*. Baltimore, Williams & Wilkins, 1962: 3–20

2. Long JA. Zonation of the mammalian adrenal cortex. In: Greep RO, Astwood EB, Blaschko H, et al, eds. *Handbook of Physiology*, vol. 7. *Endocrinology, Adrenal Gland*. Baltimore, Williams & Wilkins, 1975: 13–24

3. Luse S. Fine structure of adrenal cortex. In: Eisenstein AB, ed. *The Adrenal Cortex*. Boston, Little, Brown, 1967: 1–59

4. Grant JK. An introductory review of adrenocortical steroid biosynthesis. In: James VHT, Giusti MS, Giusti G, Marini L, eds. *The Endocrine Function of the Human Adrenal Cortex*. New York, Academic Press, 1978: 1–32

5. Brown MS, Covanen PT, Goldstein JL. Receptor-mediated uptake of lipoprotein-cholesterol and its utilization for steroid synthesis in the adrenal cortex. *Recent Prog Horm Res*. 35:215, 1979

6. Faust JR, Goldstein JL, Brown MS. Receptor-mediated uptake of low density lipoprotein and utilization of its cholesterol for steroid synthesis in cultured mouse adrenal cells. *J Biol Chem.* 252:4861, 1977

7. Samuels LT, Nelson DH. Biosynthesis of corticosteroids. In: Greep RO, Astwood EB, Blaschko H, et al, eds. *Handbook of Physiology*, vol. 7. *Endocrinology, Adrenal Gland.* Baltimore, Williams & Wilkins, 1975: 55–68

8. Bell JJ, Harding BW. The acute action of adrenocorticotropic hormone on adrenal steroidogenesis. *Biochim Biophys Acta.* 348:285, 1974

9. Lieberman S, Greenfield NJ, Wolfson A. A heuristic proposal for understanding steroidogenic processes. *Endocr Rev.* 5:128, 1984

10. Miller WL. Molecular biology of steroid hormone synthesis. *Endocr Rev.* 9:295, 1988

11. Orth DN. Corticotropin-releasing hormone in humans. *Endocr Rev.* 13:164, 1992

12. Sawchenko PE, Swanson LW. Localization, colocalization, and plasticity of corticotropin-releasing factor immunoreactivity in rat brain. *Fed Proc.* 44:221, 1985

13. Bloom FE, Battenberg ELF, Rivier J, Vale W. Corticotropin releasing factor (CRF): Immunoreactive neurons and fibers in rat hypothalamus. *Regul Pept.* 4:43, 1982

14. Swanson LW, Sawchenko PE, Rivier J, Vale W. The organization of ovine corticotropin-releasing factor (CRF)-immunoreactive cells and fibers in the rat brain: An immunohistochemical study. *Neuroendocrinology.* 36:165, 1983

15. Plotsky PM, Vale W. Hemorrhage-induced secretion of corticotropin-releasing factor-like immunoreactivity into the rat hypophysial portal circulation and its inhibition by glucocorticoids. *Endocrinology.* 114:164, 1984

16. Avgerinos PC, Schurmeyer TH, Gold PW, et al. Pulsatile administration of human corticotropin-releasing hormone in patients with secondary adrenal insufficiency: Restoration of the normal cortisol secretory pattern. *J Clin Endocrinol Metab.* 62:816, 1986

17. Sasaki A, Sato S, Murakami O, et al. Immunoreactive corticotropin-releasing hormone present in human plasma may be derived from both hypothalamic and extrahypothalamic sources. *J Clin Endocrinol Metab.* 65:176, 1987

18. Suda T, Tomori N, Yajima F, et al. Immunoreactive corticotropin-releasing factor in human plasma. *J Clin Invest.* 76:2026, 1985

19. Kling M, DeBellis M, O'Rourke K, et al. Diurnal variation of cerebrospinal fluid immunoreactive corticotropin-releasing hormone levels in healthy volunteers. *J Clin Endocrinol Metab.* 79:233, 1994

20. Taylor AL, Fishman LM. Medical progress. Corticotropin-releasing hormone. *N Engl J Med.* 319:213, 1988

21. Yanovski JA, Yanovski SZ, Gold PW, Chrousos GP. Differences in the hypothalamic–pituitary–adrenal axis of black and white women. *J Clin Endocrinol Metab.* 77:536, 1993

22. Yanovski JA, et al. Etiology of the differences in corticotropin-releasing hormone-induced adrenocorticotropin secretion of black and white women. *J Clin Endocrinol Metab.* 81:3307, 1996

23. Desir D, Cauter EV, Beyloos M, et al. Prolonged pulsatile administration of ovine corticotropin-releasing hormone in normal man. *J Clin Endocrinol Metab.* 63:1292, 1986

24. Veldhuis JD, Iranmanesh A, Johnson ML, Lizarralde G. Amplitude, but not frequency, modulation of adrenocorticotropin secretory bursts gives rise to the nyctohemeral rhythm of the corticotropic axis in man. *J Clin Endocrinol Metab.* 71:452, 1990

25. Suzuki T. Circadian rhythm of adrenocortical secretory activity. In: Suzuki T, ed. *Physiology of Adrenocortical Secretion.* New York, Karger, 1983: 72–191

26. Spath-Schwalbe E, Ulthgenannt D, Voget G, et al. Corticotropin-releasing hormone-induced adrenocorticotropin and cortisol secretion depends on sleep and wakefulness. *J Clin Endocrinol Metab.* 77:1170, 1993

27. Schulte HM, Chrousos GP, Gold PW, et al. Continuous administration of synthetic ovine corticotropin-releasing factor in man. Physiological and pathophysiological implications. *J Clin Invest.* 75:1781, 1985

28. Catalano RD, Stuve L, Ramachandran J. Characterization of corticotropin receptors in human adrenocortical cells. *J Clin Endocrinol Metab.* 62:300, 1986

29. Roeflsema F, et al. Sex-dependent alteration in cortisol response to endogenous adrenocorticotropin. *J Clin Endocrinol Metab.* 77:234, 1993

30. Kannan CR. The adrenal gland. In: Kannan CR, ed. *Clinical Surveys in Endocrinology.* New York, Plenum, 1988: 2

31. Oelkers W, Boelke T, Bahr V, et al. Dose–response relationships between plasma adrenocorticotropin (ACTH), cortisol, aldosterone, and 18-hydroxycorticosterone after injection of ACTH-(1-39) or human corticotropin-releasing hormone in man. *J Clin Endocrinol Metab.* 66:181, 1988

32. DeCherney GS, DeBold CR, Jackson RV, et al. Effect of ovine corticotropin-releasing hormone administered during insulin-induced hypoglycemia on plasma adrenocorticotropin and cortisol. *J Clin Endocrinol Metab.* 64:1211, 1987

33. Plotsky PM, Bruhn TO, Vale W. Hypophysiotropic regulation of adrenocorticotropin secretion in response to insulin-induced hypoglycemia. *Endocrinology.* 117:323, 1985

34. Watabe T, Tanaka K, Kumagae M, et al. Hormonal responses to insulin-induced hypoglycemia in man. *J Clin Endocrinol Metab.* 65:1187, 1987

35. Tomori N, Suda T, Nakagami Y, et al. Adrenergic modulation of adrenocorticotropin responses to insulin-induced hypoglycemia and corticotropin-releasing hormone. *J Clin Endocrinol Metab.* 68:87, 1989

36. Lephart ED, Baxter CR, Parker, Jr CR. Effect of burn trauma on adrenal and testicular steroid hormone production. *J Clin Endocrinol Metab.* 64:842, 1987

37. Kolanowski J, Pizarro MA, Crabbe J. Potentiation of adrenocortical response upon intermittent stimulation with corticotropin in normal subjects. *J Clin Endocrinol Metab.* 41:453, 1975

38. Udelsman R, Norton JA, Jelenich SE. Responses of the hypothalamic–pituitary–adrenal and renin–angiotensin axes and the sympathetic system during controlled surgical and anesthetic stress. *J Clin Endocrinol Metab.* 64:986, 1987

39. Makara GB. Mechanisms by which stressful stimuli activate the pituitary–adrenal system. *Fed Proc.* 44:149, 1985

40. Antoni FA. Hypothalamic control of adrenocorticotropin secretion: Advances since the discovery of 41-residue corticotropin-releasing factor. *Endocr Rev.* 7:351, 1986

41. Plotsky PM, Cunningham, Jr ET, Widmaier EP. Catecholaminergic modulation of corticotropin-releasing factor and adrenocorticotropin secretion. *Endocr Rev.* 10:437, 1989

42. Nelson DH. Cortisol and the glucocorticoids. In: Smith LH, ed. *The Adrenal Cortex: Physiological Function and Disease.* Vol. 18, *Major Problems in Internal Medicine.* Philadelphia, W. B. Saunders, 1980: 65–88

43. Esteben NV, et al. Daily cortisol production rate in man determined by stable isotope dilution/mass spectrometry. *J Clin Endocrinol Metab.* 71:39, 1991

44. Rosenfeld RS, Fukushima DK, Gallagher TF. Metabolism of adrenal cortical hormones. In: Eisenstein AB, ed. *The Adrenal Cortex.* Boston, Little, Brown, 1967: 103–131

45. Westphal U. Binding of corticosteroids by plasma proteins. In: Greep RO, Astwood EB, Blaschko H, et al, eds. *Handbook of Physiology,* vol. 7. *Endocrinology, Adrenal Gland.* Baltimore, Williams & Wilkins, 1975: 117–125

46. Seely EW, Conlin PR, Brent GA, Dluhy RG. Adrenocorticotropin stimulation of aldosterone: Prolonged continuous versus pulsatile infusion. *J Clin Endocrinol Metab.* 69:1028, 1989

47. Kato T, Horton R. Studies of testosterone binding globulin. *J Clin Endocrinol Metab.* 28:1160, 1968

48. Dunn JF, Nisula BC, Rodbard D. Transport of steroid hormones: Binding of 21 endogenous steroids to both testosterone-binding globulin and corticosteroid-binding globulin in human plasma. *J Clin Endocrinol Metab.* 53:58, 1981

49. Korth-Schutlz S, Levine LS, New MI. Dehydro-epiandrosterone-sulfate (DS) levels, a rapid test for abnormal adrenal androgen secretion. *J Clin Endocrinol Metab.* 42:1005, 1976

50. Collu R, Ducharme R. Role of adrenal steroids in the initiation of pubertal mechanisms. In: James VHT, Giusti MS, Giusti G, Martini L, eds. *The Endocrine Function of the Human Adrenal Cortex. Proceedings of the Serono Symposia,* vol. 18. New York, Academic Press, 1978: 547–559

51. Apter D, Lenko HL, Perheentupa J, et al. Subnormal pubertal increases of serum androgens in Turner's syndrome. *Horm Res.* 16:164, 1982

52. Korth-Schultz S, Levine LS, New MI. Serum androgens in normal prepubertal and pubertal children and in children with precocious adrenarche. *J Clin Endocrinol Metab.* 42:117, 1976

53. De Peretti E, Forest MG. Unconjugated dehydroepiandrosterone plasma levels in normal subjects from birth to adolescence in human: The use of a sensitive radioimmunoassay. *J Clin Endocrinol Metab.* 43:982, 1976

54. Sizonenko PC, Paunier L. Hormonal changes in puberty III: Correlation of plasma dehydroepiandrosterone, testosterone, FSH, and LH with stages of puberty and bone age in normal boys and girls and in patients with Addison's disease or hypogonadism or with premature or late adrenarche. *J Clin Endocrinol Metab.* 41:894, 1975

55. Pintor C, Genazzani AR, Carboni G, et al. Adrenal androgens and pubertal development in physiological and pathological conditions. In: Genazzani AR, et al, eds. *Adrenal Androgens.* New York, Raven Press, 1980: 173–181

56. Dhom G. The prepubertal and pubertal growth of the adrenal (adrenarche). *Beitr Path Bd.* 150:357, 1973

57. Counts DR, Pescovitz OH, Barnes KM, et al. Dissociation of adrenarche and gonadarche in precocious puberty and in isolated hypogonadotropic hypogonadism. *J Clin Endocrinol Metab.* 64:1174, 1987

58. Grumbach MM, Richards GE, Conte FA, Kaplan SL. Clinical disorders of adrenal function and puberty: An assessment of the role of the adrenal cortex in normal and abnormal puberty in man and evidence for an ACTH-like pituitary adrenal androgen stimulating hormone. In: James VHT, Giusti MS, Giusti G, Martini L, eds. *The Endocrine Function of the Human Adrenal Cortex. Proceedings of the Serono Symposia,* vol. 18. New York, Academic Press, 1978: 583–612

59. Parker LN, Odell WD. Control of adrenal androgen secretion. *Endocr Rev.* 1:392, 1980

60. Rich BH, Rosenfield RL, Lucky AW, et al. Adrenarche: Changing adrenal response to adrenocorticotropin. *J Clin Endocrinol Metab.* 52:1129, 1981

61. Dickerman Z, Grant DR, Faiman C, Winter JSD. Intraadrenal steroid concentrations in man: Zonal differences and developmental changes. *J Clin Endocrinol Metab.* 59:1031, 1984

62. Anderson D. The adrenal androgen-stimulated hormone does not exist. *Lancet.* 2:454, 1980

63. Mellon SH, Shively JE, Miller WL. Human proopiomelanocortin-(79-96), a proposed androgen stimulatory hormone, does not affect steroidogenesis in cultured human fetal adrenal cells. *J Clin Endocrinol Metab.* 72:19, 1991

64. James VHT, Goodall A. Androgen production in women. In: Jeffcoate SL, ed. *Androgens and Anti-androgen Therapy.* New York, John Wiley & Sons, 1982: 23–40

65. Rosenfeld RS, Rosenberg BJ, Fukushima DK, Hellman L. 24-Hour secretory pattern of dehydroisoandrosterone and dehydro-isoandrosterone sulfate. *J Clin Endocrinol Metab.* 40:850, 1975

66. Huq MS, Pfaff M, Jespersen D, et al. Concurrence of aldosterone, androgen and cortisol secretion in adrenal venous effluents. *J Clin Endocrinol Metab.* 42:230, 1976

67. Suzuki T. Circadian rhythm of adrenocortical secretory activity. In: Suzuki T, ed. *Physiology of Adrenocortical Secretion,* New York, Karger, 1983: 72–191

68. Zumoff B, Rosenfeld RS, Strain GW, et al. Sex differences in the twenty-four-hour mean plasma concentrations of dehydroisoandrosterone (DHEA) and dehydroisoandrosterone sulfate (DHEAS) and the DHEA to DHEAS ratio in normal adults. *J Clin Endocrinol Metab.* 51:330, 1980

69. Zumoff B, Bradlow HL. Sex difference in the metabolism of dehydroisoandrosterone sulfate. *J Clin Endocrinol Metab.* 51:334, 1980

70. Azziz R, Bradley, Jr EL, Zacur HA, et al. Andrenocortical secretion of dehydroepiandrosterone (DHEA) in healthy women: Variable sensitivity to ACTH. The Endocrine Society, Las Vegas, NV, June 9–12, 1993. no. O-1606

71. Thomas G, Frenoy N, Legrain S, et al. Serum dehydro-epiandrosterone sulfate levels as an individual marker. *J Clin Endocrinol Metab.* 79:1273, 1994

72. Azziz R, Koulianos G. Adrenal androgens and reproductive aging in females. *Semin Reprod Endocrinol.* 9:249, 1991

73. Mortola JF, Yen SSC. The effects of oral dehydroepiandrosterone and endocrine-metabolic parameters in postmenopausal women. *J Clin Endocrinol Metab.* 71:696, 1990

74. MacDonald PC, Chapdelaine A, Gonzalez O, et al. *J Clin Endocrinol.* 25:1557, 1965

75. Mahesh VB, Greenblatt RB. The in vivo conversion of dehydroepiandrosterone and androstenedione to testosterone in the human. *Acta Endocrinol* (Copenh). 41:400, 1962

76. Nestler JE, Barlascini CO, Clore JN, Blackard WG. Dehydroepiandrosterone reduces serum low density lipoprotein levels and body fat but does not alter insulin sensitivity in normal men. *J Clin Endocrinol Metab.* 66:57, 1988

77. Welle S, Jozefowicz, Statt M. Failure of dehydroepiandrosterone to influence energy and protein metabolism in humans. *J Clin Endocrinol Metab.* 71:1259, 1990

78. Bulbrook RD, Hayward JL, Spicer CC. Relation between urinary androgen and corticoid secretion, excretion and subsequent breast cancer. *Lancet.* 2:395, 1975

79. Barrett-Conner E, Khaw KT, Yen SSC. A prospective study dehydroepiandrosterone-sulfate, mortality and cardiovascular disease. *N Engl J Med.* 315:1519, 1986

80. Deutsch S, Benjamin F, Seltzer V, et al. The correlation of serum estrogens and androgens with bone density in the late postmenopause. *Int J Gynecol Obstet.* 25:217, 1987

81. Wild R, Buchanan J, Myers C, Demers L. Declining adrenal androgens: An association with bone loss in aging women. *Proc Soc Exp Biol Med.* 186:355, 1987

82. Wild R, Buchanan J, Myers C, et al. Adrenal androgens sex hormone binding globulin and bone density in osteoporotic menopausal women: Is there a relationship? *Maturitas.* 9:55, 1987

83. Wierman ME, Beardsworth DE, Crawford JD. Adrenarche and skeletal maturation during luteinizing hormone releasing hormone analogue suppression of gonadarche. *J Clin Invest.* 77:121, 1986

84. Haning RV, Austin CW, Carlson IH, et al. Role of dehydroepiandrosterone sulfate as a prehormone for ovarian steroidogenesis. *Obstet Gynecol.* 65:199, 1985

85. Sonka J. Dehydroepiandrosterone: Metabolic effects. *ACTA Univ Carol Med.* 71:9, 1976

86. Parker LN. *Adrenal Androgens in Clinical Medicine.* New York, Academic Press, 1989

87. Kreisberg R. Clinical problem solving. *N Engl J Med.* 330:1295, 1994

88. Ross EJ, Marshall-Jones P, Friedman M. Cushing syndrome: Diagnostic criteria. *QJM* (Oxf). 35:149, 1966

89. Gold EM. The Cushing syndromes: Changing views of diagnosis and treatment. *Ann Intern Med.* 90:829, 1979

90. Ross EJ, Linch DC. Cushing syndrome-killing disease: Discriminatory value of signs and symptoms aiding early diagnosis. *Lancet.* 2:646, 1982

91. Urbanic RC, George JM. Cushing's disease—18 years' experience. *Medicine* (Baltimore). 60:14, 1981

92. Plotz CM, Knowlton AI, Ragan C. The natural history of Cushing syndrome. *Am J Med.* 13:597, 1952

93. Linton EA, McLean C, Kruseman ACN, et al. Direct measurement of human plasma corticotropin-releasing hormone by "two-site" immunoradiometric assay. *J Clin Endocrinol Metab.* 64:1047, 1987

94. Hermus RMM, Pieters GFFM, Pesman GJ, et al. Responsivity of adrenocorticotropin to corticotropin-releasing hormone and lack of suppressibility by dexamethasone are related phenomena in Cushing's disease. *J Clin Endocrinol Metab.* 62:634, 1986

95. Smals AGH, Pieters GFFM, van Haelst UJG, Kloppenborg PWC. Macronodular adrenocortical hyperplasia in long-standing Cushing's disease. *J Clin Endocrinol Metab.* 58:25, 1984

96. Gewirtz G, Yalow S. Ectopic ACTH production in carcinoma of the lung. *J Clin Invest.* 53:1022, 1974

97. Ross EJ. Cancer in the adrenal cortex. *Proc R Soc Med.* 59:335, 1966

98. Ratcliffe JG, Knight RA, Besser GM, et al. Tumor and plasma ACTH concentrations in patients with and without the ectopic ACTH syndrome. *Clin Endocrinol* (Oxf). 1:27, 1972

99. Imura H, Matsukura S, Yamamoto H, et al. Studies on ectopic ACTH-producing tumors, II. Clinical and biochemical features of 30 cases. *Cancer.* 35:1430, 1975

100. Belsky JL, Cuello B, Swanson LW, et al. Cushing syndrome due to ectopic production of corticotropin-releasing factor. *J Clin Endocrinol Metab.* 60:496, 1985

101. Bertagna C, Orth DN. Clinical and laboratory findings and results of therapy in 58 patients with adrenocortical tumors admitted to a single medical center (1951 to 1978). *Am J Med.* 71:855, 1981

102. Commons RR, Callaway CP. Adenomas of the adrenal cortex. *Arch Intern Med.* 81:37, 1948

103. Kokko JP, Brown TC, Berman MM. Adrenal adenoma and hypertension. *Lancet.* 1:468, 1967

104. Hedeland H, Ostberg G, Hokfelt B. On the prevalence of adrenocortical adenomas in an autopsy material in relation to hypertension and diabetes. *Acta Med Scand.* 184:211, 1968

105. Glazer HS, Weyman PJ, Sagel SS, et al. Nonfunctioning adrenal masses: Incidental discovery on computed tomography. *AJR.* 139:81, 1982

106. Hayles AB, Hahn HB, Sprague RG, et al. Hormone-secreting tumors of the adrenal cortex in children. *Pediatrics.* 37:19, 1966

107. Lee PDK, Winter RJ, Green OC. Virilizing adrenocortical tumors in childhood: Eight cases and a review of the literature. *Pediatrics.* 76:437, 1985

108. Gilbert MG, Cleveland WW. Cushing syndrome in infancy. *Pediatrics.* 46:217, 1970

109. Hogan TF, Gilchrist KW, Westring DW, Citrin DL. A clinical and pathological study of adrenocortical carcinoma. *Cancer.* 45:2880, 1980

110. Brennan MF. Adrenocortical carcinoma. *Cancer J Clin.* 37:348, 1987

111. D'Agata R, Malozowski S, Barkan A, et al. Steriod biosynthesis in human adrenal tumors. *Horm Metab Res.* 19:386, 1987

112. Sakai Y, Yanase T, Hara T, et al. Mechanism of abnormal production of adrenal androgens in patients with adrenocortical adenomas and carcinomas. *J Clin Endocrinol Metab.* 78:36, 1994

113. Yanovski JA, Cutler GB Jr. Glucocorticoid action and the clinical features of Cushing syndrome. *Endocrinol Metab Clin North Am.* 23:487, 1994

114. Magiakou MA, et al. Cushing syndrome in children and adolescents. *N Engl J Med.* 331:629, 1994

115. Kelly WF, Kelly MJ, Faragher B. A prospective study of psychiatric and psychological aspects of Cushing syndrome. *Clin Endocrinol* (Oxf). 45:715, 1996

116. Ritchie CM, Hadden DR, Kennedy L, et al. Pathogenesis of hypertension in Cushing's disease. *J Hypertens.* 5(suppl. 5): S497, 1987

117. Grunfield JP. Glucocorticoid in blood pressure regulations. *Horm Metab Res.* 34:111, 1990

118. Stewart PM, Walker BR, Holder G, et al. 11β-hydroxysteroid dehydrogenase activity in Cushing syndrome: Explaining the mineralocorticoid excess state of the ectopic adrenocorticotropin syndrome. *J Clin Endocrinol Metab.* 80:3617, 1995

119. Smals AGH, Kloppenborg PWC, Benraad TJ. Plasma testosterone profiles in Cushing syndrome. *J Clin Endocrinol Metab.* 45:240, 1977

120. Yamaji T, Ishibashi M, Sekihara H, et al. Serum dehydroepiandrosterone sulfate in Cushing syndrome. *J Clin Endocrinol Metab.* 59:1164, 1984

121. Coccuzzi G, Angeli A, Biscocci D, et al. Effect of synthetic luteinizing hormone releasing hormone (LH-RH) on the release of gonadotropins in Cushing's disease. *J Clin Endocrinol Metab.* 40:892, 1975

122. Hompes PGA, Scheele F, Gooren LJG, Schoemaker J. Pulsatile secretory patterns of luteinizing hormone in two patients with secondary amenorrhea suffering from Cushing's disease, before and after transsphenoidal adenectomy. *Fertil Steril.* 57:924, 1992

123. Barbarino A, De Marinis L, Tofani A. Corticotropin-releasing hormone inhibition of gonadotropin release and the effect of opioid blockade. *J Clin Endocrinol Metab.* 68:523, 1989

124. Doerr HG, Sippell WG, Drop SLS, et al. Evidence of 11 beta-hydroxylase deficiency in childhood adrenocortical tumors. *Cancer.* 60:1625, 1987

125. Gabrilove JL, Seman AT, Sabet R, et al. Virilizing adrenal adenoma with studies on the steroid content of the adrenal venous effluent and a review of the literature. *Endocr Rev.* 2:462, 1981

126. Meldrum DR. Testosterone levels and androgen-producing neoplasms. *Am J Obstet Gynecol.* 154:965, 1986

127. Mattox JH, Phelan S. The evaluation of adult females with testosterone producing neoplasms of the adrenal cortex. *Surg Gynecol Obstet.* 164:98, 1987

128. Derksen J, Nagesser SK, Meinders AE, et al. Identification of virilizing adrenal tumors in hirsute women. *N Engl J Med.* 331:968, 1994

129. Friedman CI, Schmidt GE, Kim MH, Powell J. Serum testosterone concentrations in the evaluation of androgen-producing tumors. *Am J Obstet Gynecol.* 153:44, 1985

130. Kaplowitz PB, Mandell J. Virilizing adrenal tumor in a 3-year-old girl: Diagnosis by computed tomographic scan and ultrasound. *Am J Dis Child.* 137:406, 1983

131. Kamilaris TC, DeBold CR, Manolas KJ, et al. Testosterone-secreting adrenal adenoma in a peripubertal girl. *JAMA.* 258:2558, 1987

132. Yuen BH, Moon YS, Mincey EK, Li D. Adrenal and sex steroid hormone production by a virilizing adrenal adenoma and its diagnosis with computerized tomography. *Am J Obstet Gynecol.* 145:164, 1983

133. McKenna TJ, O'Connell Y, Cunningham S, et al. Steroidogenesis in an estrogen-producing adrenal tumor in a young woman: Comparison with steroid profiles associated with cortisol- and androgen-producing tumors. *J Clin Endocrinol Metab.* 70:28, 1990

134. Surrey ES, de Ziegler D, Gambone JC, Judd HL. Preoperative localization of androgen-secreting tumors: Clinical, endocrinologic, and radiologic evaluation of ten patients. *Am J Obstet Gynecol.* 158:1313, 1988

135. Ferriman D, Gallwey JD. Clinical assessment of body hair growth in women. *J Clin Endocrinol.* 21:1440, 1961

136. McKnight E. The prevalence of hirsutism in young women. *Lancet.* 1:410, 1964

137. Hartz AJ, Barboriak PN, Wong A, et al. The association of obesity with infertility and related menstrual abnormalities in women. *Int J Obesity.* 3:57, 1979

138. Bals-Pratsch M, Hanker, Hellhammer DH, et al. Intermittent Cushing's disease in hirsute women. *Horm Metab Res.* 28:105, 1996

139. Fehm HL, Voigt KH. Pathophysiology of Cushing's disease. *Pathobiol Annu.* 9:225, 1979

140. Snow K, Jiang NS, Kao PC, Scheithauer BW. Biochemical evaluation of adrenal dysfunction: The laboratory perspective. *Mayo Clin Proc.* 67:1055, 1992

141. Newell-Price J, et al. A combined test using desmopressin and corticotropin-releasing hormone in the differential diagnosis of Cushing syndrome. *J Clin Endocrinol Metab.* 82:176, 1997

142. Crapo L. Cushing syndrome: A review of diagnostic tests. *Metabolism.* 28:955, 1979

143. Vagnucci AH, Evans E. Cushing's disease with intermittent hypercortisolism. *Am J Med.* 80:83, 1986

144. Sakiyama R., Ashcraft MW, Van Herle AJ. Cyclic Cushing syndrome. *Am J Med.* 77:944, 1984

145. Liddle GW. Tests of pituitary–adrenal suppressibility in the diagnosis of Cushing syndrome. *J Clin Endocrinol Metab.* 20:1539, 1960

146. Yanovski JA, Cutler GB Jr, Chrousos GP, Nieman LK. Corticotropin-releasing hormone stimulation following low-dose dexamethasone administration. *JAMA.* 269:2232, 1993

147. Ashcraft MW, Van Herle AJ, Vener SL, Geffner DL. Serum cortisol levels in Cushing syndrome after low- and high-dose dexamethasone suppression. *Ann Intern Med.* 97:21, 1982

148. Kennedy L, Atkinson AB, Johnston H, et al. Serum cortisol concentrations during low dose dexamethasone suppression test to screen for Cushing syndrome. *Br Med J.* 289:1188, 1984

149. Trainer PJ, Grossman A. The diagnosis and differential diagnosis of Cushing syndrome. *Clin Endocrinol* (Oxf). 34:317, 1991

150. Contreras P, Araya V. Overnight dexamethasone pretreatment improves the performance of the lysine-vasopressin test in the diagnosis of Cushing syndrome. *Clin Endocrinol* (Oxf). 44:703, 1996

151. Jackson RV, Hockings GI, Torpy DJ, et al. New diagnostic tests for Cushing syndrome: Uses of naloxone, vasopressin and alprazolam. *Clin Endocrinol* (Oxf). 23:579, 1996

152. Cizza G, Nieman LK, Doppman JL, et al. Factitious Cushing syndrome. *J Clin Endocrinol Metab.* 81:3573, 1996

153. Flack MR, et al. Urine free cortisol in the high-dose dexamethasone suppression test for the differential diagnosis of the Cushing syndrome. *Ann Int Med.* 116:211, 1992

154. Jaresch S, Schlaghecke R, Jungblut R, et al. Stumme Nebennierentumoren bei Patienten mit Adrenogenital-syndrom. *Clin Wochenschr.* 65:627, 1987

155. Azziz R, Kenney PH. Magnetic resonance imaging of the adrenal gland in women with late-onset adrenal hyperplasia. *Fertil Steril.* 56:142, 1991

156. Wajchenberg BL, et al. Ectopic adrenocorticotropin hormone syndrome. *Endocr Rev.* 15:752, 1994

157. Tsigos C, Chrousos GP. Differential diagnosis and management of Cushing syndrome. *Annu Rev Med.* 47:443, 1996

158. Tyrrell JB, Findling JW, Aron DC, et al. An overnight high-dose dexamethasone suppression test for rapid differential diagnosis of Cushing syndrome. *Ann Intern Med.* 104:180, 1986

159. Dichek HL, Nieman LK, Oldfield EH, et al. A comparison of the standard high dose dexamethasone suppression test and the overnight 8-mg dexamethasone suppression test for the differential diagnosis of adrenocorticotropin-dependent Cushing syndrome. *J Clin Endocrinol Metab.* 78:418, 1994

160. Trainer PJ, et al. A comparison of the effects of human and ovine corticotropin-releasing hormone on the pituitary–adrenal axis. *J Clin Endocrinol Metab.* 80:412, 1995

161. Nieman LK, Oldfield EH, Wesley R, et al. A simplified morning ovine corticotropin-releasing hormone stimulation test for the differential diagnosis of adrenocorticotropin-dependent Cushing syndrome. *J Clin Endocrinol Metab.* 77:1308, 1993

162. Kaye TB, Crapo L. The Cushing syndrome: An update on diagnostic tests. *Ann Intern Med.* 112:434, 1990

163. Tabarin A, et al. Usefulness of the corticotropin-releasing hormone test during bilateral inferior petrosal sinus sampling for the diagnosis of Cushing's disease. *J Clin Endocrinol Metab.* 73:53, 1991

164. Oldfield EH, et al. Petrosal sinus sampling with and without corticotropin-releasing hormone for the differential diagnosis of Cushing syndrome. *N Engl J Med.* 325:897, 1991

165. Yanovski JA, et al. The limited ability of inferior petrosal sinus sampling with corticotropin-releasing hormone to distinguish Cushing's disease from pseudo-Cushing's states or normal physiology. *J Clin Endocrinol Metab.* 77:503, 1993

166. Nieman LK, Chrousos GP, Oldfield EH, et al. The ovine corticotropin-releasing hormone stimulation test and the dexamethasone suppression test in the differential diagnosis of Cushing syndrome. *Ann Intern Med.* 105:862, 1986

167. Grino M, Boudouresque F, Conte-Devolx B, et al. In vitro corticotropin-releasing hormone (CRH) stimulation of adrenocorticotropin release from corticotroph adenoma cells: Effect of prolonged exposure to CRH and its interaction with cortisol. *J Clin Endocrinol Metab.* 66:770, 1988

168. Atkinson AB. The treatment of Cushing syndrome. *Clin Endocrinol* (Oxf). 34:507, 1991

169. Bochicchio D, Losa M, Buchfelder M, et al. Factors influencing the immediate and late outcome of Cushing's disease treated by transsphenoidal surgery: A retrospective study by the European Cushing's Disease Survey Group. *J Clin Endocrinol Metab.* 80:3114, 1995

170. Sonino N, Zielezny M, Fava GA, et al. Risk factors and long-term outcome in pituitary dependent Cushing disease. *J Clin Endocrinol Metab.* 81:2647, 1996

171. Friedman RB, Oldfield EH, Nieman LK, et al. Repeat transsphenoidal surgery for Cushing's disease. *J Neurosurg.* 71:520, 1989

172. Tindall GT, Herring CJ, Clark RV, et al. Cushing's disease: Results of transsphenoidal microsurgery with emphasis on surgical failure. *J Neurosurg.* 72:363, 1990

173. Estrada J, Boronat M, Mielgo M, et al. The long-term outcome of pituitary irradiation after unsuccessful transsphenoidal surgery in Cushing's disease. *N Engl J Med.* 336:172, 1997

174. Brosnan CM, Gowing NFC. Addison's disease. *BMJ.* 312:1085, 1996

175. Nerup J. Addison's disease-clinical studies. A report of 108 cases. *Acta Endocrinol* (Copenh). 76:127, 1974

176. Irvine WJ, Barnes EW. Adrenocortical insufficiency. *Clin Endocrinol Metab.* 1:549, 1972

177. Kamoi K, Tamura T, Tanaka K, et al. Hyponatremia and osmoregulation of thirst and vasopressin secretion in patients with adrenal insufficiency. *J Clin Endocrinol Metab.* 77:1584,1993

178. Nerup J. Addison's disease—A review of some clinical pathological and immunological features. *Dan Med Bull.* 6:201, 1974

179. Irvine WJ. Autoimmunity in endocrine disease. *Proc R Soc Med.* 67:548, 1974

180. Nerup J. Addison's disease—serological studies. *Acta Endocrinol* (Copenh). 76:142, 1974

181. Irvine WJ. Autoimmunity in endocrine disease. In: Greep RO, ed. *Recent Progress in Hormone Research*, vol. 36. New York, Academic Press, 1980: 509–556

182. Scherbaum WA, Berg PA. Development of adrenocortical failure in non-Addisonian patients with antibodies to adrenal cortex. *Clin Endocrinol* (Oxf). 16:345,1982

183. Ketchum CH, Riley WJ, Maclaren NK. Adrenal dysfunction in asymptomatic patients with adrenocortical autoantibodies. *J Clin Endocrinol Metab.* 58:1166, 1984

184. Ahonen P, Miettinen A, Perheentupa J. Adrenal and steroidal cell antibodies in patients with autoimmune polyglandular disease type I and risk of adrenocortical and ovarian failure. *J Clin Endocrinol Metab.* 64:494, 1987

185. Betterle C, Zanette F, Zanchetta R, et al. Complement-fixing adrenal autoantibodies as a marker for predicting onset of idiopathic Addison's disease. *Lancet.* 1:1238, 1983

186. Soderbergh A, et al. Adrenal autoantibodies and organ-specific autoimmunity in patients with Addison's disease. *Clin Endocrinol* (Oxf). 45:453, 1996

187. Chen S, Sawicka J, Betterle C, et al. Autoantibodies to steroidogenic enzymes in autoimmune polyglandular syndrome, Addison's disease, and premature ovarian failure. *J Clin Endocrinol Metab.* 81:1871, 1996

188. Asawa T, Wedlock N, Baumann-Antczak A, et al. Naturally occurring mutations in human steroid 21-hydroxylase influence adrenal autoantibody binding. *J Clin Endocrinol Metab.* 79:372, 1994

189. Falorni A, et al. High diagnostic accuracy for idiopathic Addison's disease with a sensitive radiobinding assay for autoantibodies against recombinant human 21-hydroxylase. *J Clin Endocrinol Metab.* 80:2752, 1995

190. Furmaniak J, Kominami S, Asawa T, et al. Autoimmune Addison's disease—evidence for a role of steroid 21-hydroxylase autoantibodies in adrenal insufficiency. *J Clin Endocrinol Metab.* 79:1517, 1994

191. Boscaro M, et al. Hormonal responses during various phases of autoimmune adrenal failure: No evidence for 21-hydroxylase enzyme activity inhibition in vivo. *J Clin Endocrinol Metab.* 81:2801, 1996

192. Turkington RW, Lebovitz HE. Extra-adrenal endocrine deficiencies in Addison's disease. *Am J Med.* 43:499, 1967

193. Alper MM, Garner PR. Premature ovarian failure: Its relationship to autoimmune disease. *Obstet Gynecol.* 66:27, 1985

194. Tapper ML, Rotterdam HZ, Lerner CW, et al. Adrenal necrosis in the acquired immunodeficiency syndrome. *Ann Intern Med.* 100:239, 1984

195. Oberfield SE, Kairam R, Bakshi S, et al. Steroid response to adrenocorticotropin stimulation in children with human immunodeficiency virus infection. *J Clin Endocrinol Metab.* 70:578, 1990

196. Merenich JA, McDermott MT, Asp AA, et al. Evidence of endocrine involvement early in the course of human immunodeficiency virus infection. *J Clin Endocrinol Metab.* 70:566, 1990

197. Membreno L, Irony I, Dere W, et al. Adrenocortical function in acquired immunodeficiency syndrome. *J Clin Endocrinol Metab.* 65:482, 1987

198. Villette JM, Bourin P, Doinel C, et al. Circadian variations in plasma levels of hypophyseal, adrenocortical and testicular hormones in men infected with human immunodeficiency virus. *J Clin Endocrinol Metab.* 70:572, 1990

199. Weber A, et al. Adrenocorticotropin receptor gene mutations in familial glucocorticoid deficiency: Relationships with clinical features in four families. *J Clin Endocrinol Metab.* 80:65, 1995

200. Oelkers W. Dose–response aspects in the clinical assessment of the hypothalamic–pituitary-adrenal axis, and the low-dose adrenocorticotropin test. *Eur J Endocrinol.* 135:27, 1996

201. Oelkers W, Diederich S, Bohr V. Diagnosis and therapy surveillance in Addison's disease: Rapid adrenocorticotropin (ACTH) test and measurement of plasma ACTH, renin activity, and aldosterone. *J Clin Endocrinol Metab.* 75:259, 1992

202. Dluhy RG, Himathongkam T, Greenfield M. Rapid ACTH test with plasma aldosterone levels. *Ann Intern Med.* 80:893, 1974

203. Ammari F, Issa BG, Millward E, Scanion MF. A comparison between short ACTH and insulin stress tests for assessing hypothalamic–pituitary–adrenal function. *Clin Endocrinol* (Oxf). 44:473, 1996

204. Streeten DHP, Anderson GH Jr, Bonaventura MM. The potential for serious consequences from misinterpreting normal responses to the rapid adrenocorticotropin test. *J Clin Endocrinol Metab.* 81:285, 1996

205. Fiad TM, Kirby JM, Cunningham SK, McKenna TJ. The overnight single-dose. *Clin Endocrinol* (Oxf). 40:603, 1994

206. Dickstein G, Shechner C, Nicholson WE, et al. Adrenocorticotropin stimulation test: Effects of basal cortisol levels, time of day and suggested new sensitive low dose test. *J Clin Endocrinol Metab.* 72:773, 1991

207. Tordjman K, Jaffe A, Grazas N, et al. The role of the low dose (1 µg) adrenocorticotropin test in the evaluation of patients with pituitary disease. *J Clin Endocrinol Metab.* 80:1301, 1995

208. Broide J, Soferman R, Kivity S, et al. Low dose adrenocorticotropin test reveals impaired adrenal function in patients taking inhaled corticosteroid. *J Clin Endocrinol Metab.* 80:1243, 1995

209. Daidoh H, Morita H, Mune T, et al. Responses of plasma adrenocortical steroids to low dose ACTH in normal subjects. *Clin Endocrinol* (Oxf). 43:311, 1995

210. Rasmuson S, Olsson T, Hagg E. A low dose ACTH test to assess the function of the hypothalamic–pituitary–adrenal axis. *Clin Endocrinol* (Oxf). 44:151, 1996

211. Jubiz W, Meikle W, West CD, Tyler FH. Single-dose metyrapone test. *Arch Intern Med.* 125:472, 1970

212. Steiner H, Bahr V, Exner P, Oelkers W. Pituitary function tests: Comparison of ACTH and 11-deoxy-cortisol response in the metyrapone test and with the insulin hypoglycemia test. *Exp Clin Endocrinol Diabetes.* 102:33, 1994

213. New MI, Lavine LS. *Congenital Adrenal Hyperplasia*, New York, Springer-Verlag, 1984

214. Giusti G, Manelli M, Forti G, et al. Plasma steroid values in congenital adrenocortical hyperplasia. In: James VHT, Jiusti MS, Giusti G, Martini L, eds. *The Endocrine Function of the Adrenal Cortex*, vol 18. New York, Academic Press, 1978: 271–287

215. Zachmann M, Tassinari D, Prader A. Clinical and biochemical variability of congenital adrenal hyperplasia due to 11β-hydroxylase deficiency. A study of 25 patients. *J Clin Endocrinol Metab.* 56:222, 1983

216. DePeretti E, Forest MG, Feit JP, David M. Endocrine studies in two children with male pseudohermaphroditism due to 3β-hydroxy (3β-) dehydrogenase defect. In: Genazzani AR, Thijssen JHH, Siiteri PK, eds. *Adrenal Androgens*. New York, Raven Press, 1980

217. Pang S, Lavine LS, Stoner E, et al. Non-salt-losing congenital adrenal hyperplasia due to 3β-hydroxysteroid dehydrogenase deficiency with normal glomerulosa function. *J Clin Endocrinol Metab.* 56:808, 1983

218. Griffiths KD, Anderson JM, Rudd BT, et al. Plasma renin activity in the management of congenital adrenal hyperplasia. *Arch Dis Child.* 59:360, 1984

219. Mulaikal RM, Migeon CJ, Rock JA. Fertility rates in female patients with congenital adrenal hyperplasia due to 21-hydroxylase deficiency. *N Engl J Med.* 316:178, 1987

220. Azziz R, Mulaikal RM, Migeon CJ, et al. Congenital adrenal hyperplasia: Long-term results following vaginal reconstruction. *Fertil Steril.* 46:1011, 1986

221. Azziz R, Bradley E Jr, Huth J, et al. Acute adrenocorticotropin-(1-24) (ACTH) adrenal stimulation in eumenorrheic women: Reproducibility and effect of ACTH dose, subject weight and sampling time. *J Clin Endocrinol Metab.* 70:1273, 1990

222. Azziz R, Dewailly D, Owerback D. Non-classic adrenal hyperplasia: Current concepts. *J Clin Endocrinol Metab.* 78:810, 1994

223. Speiser PW, DuPont B, Rubinstein P, et al. High frequency of nonclassical steroid 21-hydroxylase deficiency. *Am J Hum Genet.* 37:650, 1985

224. Dewailly D, Vantyghem-Haudiquet MC, Sainsard C, et al. Clinical and biological phenotypes in late-onset 21-hydroxylase deficiency. *J Clin Endocrinol Metab.* 63:418, 1986

225. Bouchard P, Kuttenn F, Mowszowicz I, et al. Congenital adrenal hyperplasia due to partial 21-hydroxylase deficiency. A study of five cases. *Acta Endocrinol* (Copenh). 96:107, 1981

226. Feuillan P, Pangs, Schurmeyer T, et al. The hypothalamic–pituitary–adrenal axis in partial (late-onset) 21-hydroxylase deficiency. *J Clin Endocrinol Metab.* 67:154, 1988

227. Kater CR, Biglieri EG, Wajchenberg B. Effects of continued adrenal corticotropin stimulation on the mineralocorticoid hormones in classical and nonclassical symbol virilizing types of 21-hydroxylase deficiency. *J Clin Endocrinol Metab.* 60:1057, 1985

228. Azziz R, Zacur HA. 21-Hydroxylase deficiency in female hyperandrogenism: Screening and diagnosis. *J Clin Endocrinol Metab.* 69:577, 1989

229. Kuttenn F, Couillin P, Girard F, et al. Late-onset adrenal hyperplasia in hirsutism. *N Engl J Med.* 313:224, 1985

230. New MI, Lorenzen F, Lerner DJ, et al. Genotyping steroid 21-hydoxylase deficiency: Hormonal reference data. *J Clin Endocrinol Metab.* 57:320, 1983

231. Knochenhaurer ES, Corte-Rudelli C, Cunningham RD, et al. Carriers of 21-hydroxylase deficiency are not at increased risk for hyperandrogenism. *J Clin Endocrinol Metab.* 82:479, 1997

232. Azziz R. Treatment of non-classic adrenal hyperplasia. In: Bardin CW, et al. *Current Therapy in Endocrinology and Metabolism*, 6th ed. Mosby-Year Book, St. Louis, 1997: 175–178

233. Azziz R, Slayden SM. Mechanisms of steroid excess in 21-hydroxylase deficient non-classic adrenal hyperplasia. *J Soc Gynecol Invest.* 3:297, 1996

234. Feldman S, Billaud L, Thalabard JC, et al. Fertility in women with late-onset adrenal hyperplasia due to 21-hydroxylase deficiency. *J Clin Endocrinol Metab.* 74:635, 1992

235. Pang S, Clark AT, Freeman LC, et al. Maternal side-effects of prenatal dexamethasone therapy for fetal congenital adrenal hyperplasia. *J Clin Endocrinol Metab.* 75:249, 1992

236. Guthrie Jr GP, Wilson EM, Quillen DL, Jawad MJ. Adrenal androgen excess and defective 11β-hydroxylation in women with idiopathic hirsutism. *Arch Intern Med.* 142:729, 1982

237. Gibson M, Lackritz R, Schiff I, Tulchinsky D. Abnormal adrenal responses to adrenocorticotropic hormone in hyperandrogenic women. *Fertil Steril.* 33:43, 1980

238. Azziz R, Boots LR, Parker Jr CR, et al. 11B-hydroxylase deficiency in hyperandrogenism. *Fertil Steril.* 55:733, 1991

239. Pang S, Levine LS, Lorenzen F, et al. Hormonal studies in obligate heterozygotes and siblings of patients with 11β-hydroxylase deficiency congenital adrenal hyperplasia. *J Clin Endocrinol Metab.* 50:586, 1980

240. Carmina E, Malizia G, Pagano M, Janni A. Prevalence of late-onset 11β-hydroxylase deficiency in hirsute patients. *J Endocrinol Invest.* 11:595, 1988

241. Joeher K, Geley S, Strasser-Wozak EMC, et al. CYP11B1 mutations causing nonclassic congenital adrenal hyperplasia due to 11β-hydroxylase deficiency (submitted).

242. Pang S, Lerner AJ, Stoner E, et al. Late-onset adrenal steroid 3β-hydroxysteroid dehydrogenase deficiency, I. A cause of hirsutism in pubertal and postpubertal women. *J Clin Endocrinol Metab.* 60:428, 1985

243. Lobo RA, Goebelsmann U. Evidence for reduced 3β-ol-hydroxysteroid dehydrogenase activity in some hirsute women thought to have polycystic ovary syndrome. *J Clin Endocrinol Metab.* 53:394, 1981

244. Mathieson J, Couzinet B, Wekstein-Noel S, et al. The incidence of late-onset congenital adrenal hyperplasia due to 3β-hydroxysteroid dehydrogenase deficiency among hirsute women. *Clin Endocrinol* (Oxf). 36:383, 1992

245. Azziz R, Bradley Jr EL, Potter HD, Boots LR. 3β-hydroxysteroid dehydrogenase deficiency in hyperandrogenism. *Am J Obstet Gynecol.* 168:889, 1993

246. Zerah M, Rheame E, Mani P, et al. No evidence of mutations in the genes for type I and type II 3β-hydroxysteroid dehydrogenase (3β-HSD) in nonclassic 3β-deficiency. *J Clin Endocrinol Metab.* 79:1811, 1994

247. Sakkal-Alkaddour H, Zhang L, Yang X, et al. Studies of 3 beta-hydroxysteroid dehydrogenase genes in infants and children manifesting premature pubarche and increased adrenocorticotropin-stimulated delta 5-steroid levels. *J Clin Endocrinol Metab.* 81:3961, 1996

Chapter 19

OVARIAN DYSFUNCTION AND ANOVULATION

Machelle M. Seibel

The most common ovarian cause of anovulation is the polycystic ovary syndrome (PCO). PCO represents a self-perpetuating state of chronic anovulation. Classic symptoms have been attributed, but a spectrum of symptomatology, pathology, and laboratory findings is more typically found. This is probably due to the fact that PCO represents a complex ovulatory dysfunction involving the hypothalamus, pituitary, ovaries, adrenal, and peripheral adipose tissues, all contributing to an endocrine imbalance usually associated with oligo-ovulation, hirsutism, and infertility.[1] This chapter will focus on the pathophysiology of PCO and describe its treatment from the perspective of an endocrine disorder.

PREVALENCE OF POLYCYSTIC OVARIES

The prevalence of polycystic ovaries depends in part on the method of diagnosis. When ultrasound inspection of normal volunteers is conducted, PCO is diagnosed in 22 percent of those examined.[2] Polycystic ovaries have also been diagnosed using ultrasound in 85 percent of women with oligomenorrhagia and 95 percent of women with hirsutism. In addition, ultrasound has identified PCO in one third of women with amenorrhea and 75 percent of women with congenital adrenal hyperplasia. Ovarian ultrasound criteria among healthy prepubertal girls has revealed a steadily increasing prevalence of PCO with age, and a 6 percent prevalence of PCO among children 6 yr of age that increased to 25 percent in the teenage years.[3] Studies such as these suggest that PCO is independent of any specific hormone milieu, and in fact should not be diagnosed by ultrasound alone.

HYPOTHALAMIC–PITUITARY RELATIONSHIP

One of the most descriptive endocrine markers associated with PCO is a relative elevation of luteinizing hormone (LH) to follicle-stimulating hormone (FSH). This increased hormonal ratio was initially perceived by many investigators to represent dysfunctional hypothalamic–pituitary regulation of gonadotropins.[4] However, a series of studies demonstrated that this was not an inherent defect but rather a functional derangement. Frequent blood samplings for LH and FSH revealed exaggerated pulse levels of LH in association with low normal levels of FSH.[5] Further additional studies revealed that 17β estradiol (E_2) infusion was capable of negatively inhibiting LH but not FSH. Furthermore, the positive feedback effect of estrogen also appeared intact. Administration of clomiphene citrate elicited an LH rise in PCO patients comparable to those found in normal controls.[1] Further studies did reveal that PCO patients do possess a heightened pituitary responsiveness to gonadotropin-releasing hormone (GnRH). Women with PCO have been found to possess mean LH pulse frequencies indistinguishable from healthy controls. However, the mean LH pulse amplitude in PCO patients (12.2 ± 2.7 mIU/ml) is significantly higher than those identified in the early (6.2 ± 0.8 mIU/ml) or midfollicular (6.4 ± 0.6 mIU/ml) phase. Whether this represents a relative increase in bioactive LH over immunoreactive LH has not been determined.

Several explanations for the relative disparity of LH to FSH have been provided. One of the most intriguing explanations for the inappropriate gonadotropin production found in PCO emanates from a series of studies in the rhesus monkey.[6] Radiofrequency lesions of the arcuate nucleus were performed to eliminate endogenous secretion of GnRH. A series of experiments was then performed in which exogenous GnRH was administered in a variety of frequencies and amplitudes. The administration of GnRH in an appropriate frequency and amplitude resulted in duplication of normal gonadotropin levels for the primate. If GnRH was administered either too frequently or continuously, downregulation occurred and gonadotropin levels fell. Increasing the amplitude of GnRH while maintaining a constant pulse frequency resulted in

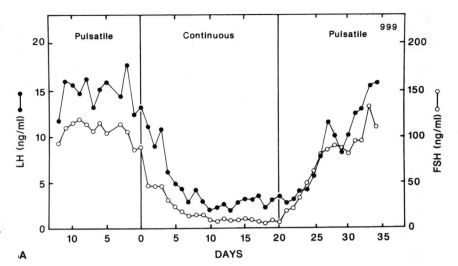

Figure 19–1. A. Effect of pulsatile and continuous GnRH on serum LH and FSH levels. **B.** Increasing the amplitude of GnRH while maintaining a constant pulse frequency reduces FSH levels with little effect on LH. This ratio is similar to those found in PCO patients. *(Reproduced, with permission, from Knobil E, Rec Prog Horm Res. 36:53, 1980.[6])*

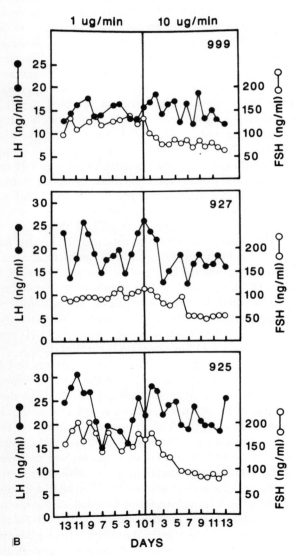

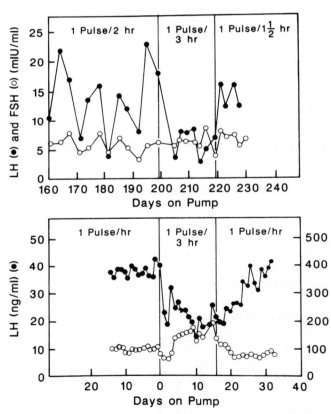

Figure 19–2. Effect of widening the GnRH pulse interval on LH and FSH levels. The upper panel reflects data in a prepubertal patient with Kallmann syndrome. The lower panel is data derived from Knobil's work in the primate. *(Reproduced, with permission, from Seibel MM, et al, J Clin Endocrinol Metab. 61:575, 1985.[7])*

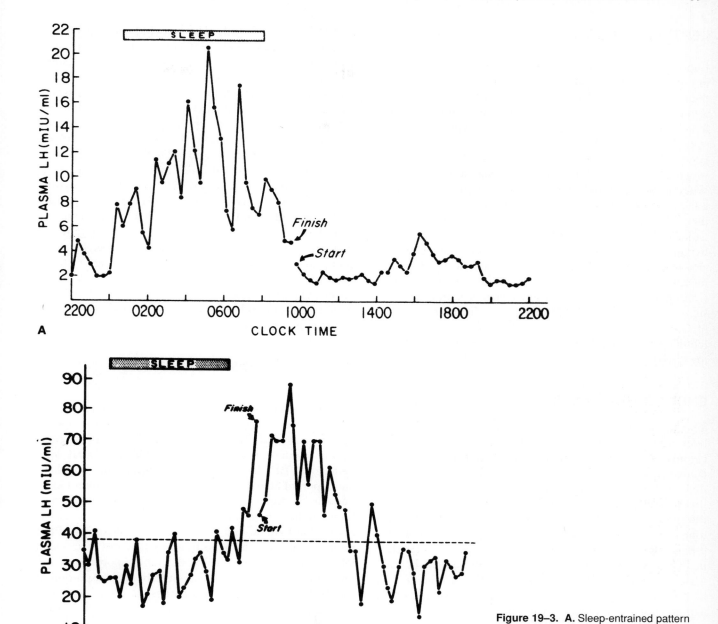

Figure 19–3. A. Sleep-entrained pattern of LH secretion in normal pubertal girls. **B.** Sleep-entrained pattern of LH secretion in pubertal girls found to have PCO. *(Reproduced, with permission, from Zumoff B, Freeman R, Coupey S, et al, N Engl J Med. 61:1206, 1983.[8])*

a reduction of FSH levels with little effect on LH levels (Fig 19–1). This gonadotropin ratio is similar to the one found in patients with PCO. Widening the pulse interval while maintaining GnRH at the same dosage reduced LH levels. Similar studies have been conducted in humans[7] (Fig 19–2).

Further evidence of the hypothalamic–pituitary involvement in the pathophysiology of PCO results from studies of the diurnal variation of LH secretion in pubertal girls. In normal pubertal girls, sleep entrainment of LH is observed, and a nocturnal rise in LH values is identifiable.[8] Conversely, when pubertal girls with PCO were evaluated, sleep entrainment was no longer evident and LH elevations occurred at varying times during the 24 hr of observation (Fig 19–3). Others have shown an increase in both the rate and amplitude of LH pulses.[9] Studies such as these further suggest that PCO is associated with a central disturbance of the frequency and amplitude of GnRH. For this reason, those factors that effect GnRH secretion must also be considered in the pathophysiology of PCO.

LEPTIN AND PCO

Leptin is a protein secreted by adipocytes that is involved in the regulation of food intake. It is believed that one of the primary roles for leptin is to act on the brain as a satiety signal. Because obese individuals are known to have high leptin levels, obesity is interpreted to be a leptin-resistant state. Mice that are homozygous for the "obese" gene are genetically deficient in leptin.[10] These mice are also overweight, infertile, and possess low gonadotropin levels. When these leptin-deficient mice are treated with recombinant leptin, they demonstrate a return of their fertility that cannot be explained by weight reduction. The explanation appears due to an effect of the exogenous leptin on hypothalamic control of gonadotropin secretion. Leptin also inhibits hypothalamic synthesis and release of neuropeptide Y, a substance also known to inhibit GnRH.[11] It is intriguing to postulate that low levels of leptin lead to subnormal gonadotropin secretion through the inhibition of GnRH by neuropeptide Y. Fasting does lower serum leptin levels. Certainly, an association between obesity, eating disorders, leptins, and PCO appears likely.

ENDOGENOUS OPIOIDS IN PCO

The involvement of brain opioid activity in PCO has been inferred on the basis of infusion of the opioid antagonist naloxone.[12] Patients with PCO administered naloxone demonstrate no response of LH.[13] When estradiol levels are taken into account by comparing results of these studies in PCO patients with healthy controls in the midfollicular phase, no differences in central opioid tone have been identified.[14] Furthermore, the infusion of β-endorphins does not suppress the elevated LH levels in PCO,[14] although it is effective in inhibiting LH release in healthy males and females. β-Endorphins have been found to decrease hypothalamic and increase striatal dopamine turnover.[15,16] Enkephalins also have been shown to block dopamine-induced GnRH release from rat medial basal hypothalamus.[17] These findings suggest that there is an interaction among dopamine, opioid, and GnRH secretion or a functional disassociation of the opioid neuronal activity in PCO.

PCO patients have also been found to have elevated peripheral levels of β-endorphin.[18] These levels are even higher in individuals who have increased weight. Other investigators found a naloxone-induced LH release only in oligomenorrheic women with PCO who were overweight but not in those who were of normal weight or in hypogonadotropic women, with the exception of those with prolactin-secreting adenomas.[19] Because β-endorphin and corticotropin (ACTH) are derived from the same precursor, pro-opiomelanocortin (POMC), and it is known that β-endorphin is increased in conditions with increased ACTH production, this may provide an explanation. However, ACTH levels and cortisol production have been found to be normal in PCO.[20] It has been shown that stress can increase peripheral β-endorphin levels and that patients with PCO do have higher levels of psychological stress than ovulatory controls.[21]

In addition, a β-endorphin-like peptide has been identified in the same islet cell clusters that produce insulin.[22] This pancreatic opioid is 2 to 4 times more potent than β-endorphin and 50 times more potent than morphine. Its effects are reversed by naloxone. It is possible that this substance is the source for some of the peripherally elevated opioids identified in PCO. Animal studies have demonstrated both increased pituitary content and circulating levels of β-endorphin in genetically obese mice. Because naloxone inhibits overeating in these mice, it suggests that β-endorphins may play a role in the genesis of obesity. It is also possible that there is an association of β-endorphins, hyperinsulinemia, and obesity that may prove PCO to be a metabolic disorder.

NEUROLOGIC CONSIDERATIONS

Neurological factors may also modulate GnRH and be involved in and therefore contribute to the pathophysiology of PCO. Polycystic ovary syndrome is more common among untreated (30 percent) than treated (13 percent) women with epilepsy.[23] Patients with temporal lobe epilepsy (TLE) have provided an interesting model. In one report of 50 women with TLE, PCO was found in 20 percent of the patients, much more prevalent than is found in the general population.[24] The explanation for this association may be due to the anatomic proximity of the temporal lobe and the hypothalamus. Seizures of temporal lobe origin generally involve the limbic portions of the lobe. The amygdala is an anatomically distinct portion of the limbic structure and has extensive, direct, anatomic connections with the ventromedial and preoptic hypothalamic nuclei, which are involved in GnRH secretion and regulation.[25] Bilateral amygdalectomy in the adult female monkey results in amenorrhea and hypogonadism.[26] Previous studies have described satiety centers for food intake in the ventromedial nucleus.[27] This association could contribute to the obesity often identified in PCO. In addition, elevated levels of β-endorphins, such as those found in PCO, have been shown capable of inducing epileptiform activity in the limbic cortex when injected into the cerebrospinal fluid of rats. This activity occurs at doses that are devoid of analgesic activity, and the epileptiform activity is not associated with behavioral changes. Stimulation of the amygdala has also been shown capable of inducing elevated pituitary and serum LH levels.[28]

Among 30 women with both reproductive endocrine disorders and complex partial seizures with unilateral temporal lobe epileptiform discharges, those with PCO overwhelmingly possessed left-sided discharges (15 versus 1), whereas those with hypogonadotropic hypogonadism had a strong predominance of right-sided discharges (12 versus 2).[29] Studies such as this demonstrating the relationship of laterality of epileptiform discharges with specific endocrine findings may offer insight into the development of PCO. When pulsatile LH secretion is studied in women with epilepsy, untreated women have higher LH pulse frequency than healthy women.[30] Whereas treated women have statistically significantly lower frequencies, temporal epileptiform activity on the left side (the side most associated with PCO) is associated with statistically significantly greater LH pulse frequency than the right.[31]

As will be discussed, patients with polycystic ovary disease often have elevated prolactin levels. Altered concentrations of dopamine and homovanillic acid have been identified in the brains of animals with kindled amygdaloid seizures[32] and in the spinal fluid of patients with TLE. These studies suggest that epileptic discharges in medial temporal limbic structures may modulate hypothalamic dopamine, as well as GnRH, and in some patients contribute to the pathophysiology of PCO.

PROLACTIN AND PCO

There has been a rather long-standing association between galactorrhea, hyperprolactinemia, and PCO. Sommers and Wadman studied pituitary glands from unselected autopsies of 7 of 16 women with bilateral polycystic ovaries and found all 7 to have large numbers of normally granulated basophils collected into hyperplastic nodules.[33] Other reports have associated PCO patients with hyperprolactinemia and pituitary tumors.[34] Some

have felt that the hyperprolactinemia and enhanced prolactin release in PCO simply reflected increased estrogen levels on the dopaminergic system through the peripheral conversion of androgens to estrogens. Such premises have been supported by the findings of exaggerated prolactin responses to thyroid-releasing hormone (TRH) in patients with PCO. Similarly, the administration of the dopamine receptor antagonist metoclopramide has also resulted in elevated prolactin releases in these patients.[35] These types of studies suggest a central deficiency or a defect in the inhibitory influence of hypothalamic dopamine.

Further support of this concept arises from the demonstration of prompt and sustained reduction in circulating LH levels in polycystic ovary patients administered dopamine.[36] Other studies have shown a synchrony between endogenous pulses of LH and prolactin. Furthermore, administration of bromocriptine, a dopamine agonist, decreases both prolactin and the integrated LH secretion of patients with PCO.[37] For this reason, there is a suggestion that replacement of deficient dopamine or its agonist in patients with PCO might provide a therapeutic modality. Results thus far are conflicted.

OVARIAN CONTRIBUTIONS TO PCO

Bilateral polycystic ovaries represent the hallmark of PCO. However, due to the increased resolution of vaginal probe ultrasound transducers some normal ovulatory patients may appear to have PCO in the early follicular phase. Typically, these follicles are 2 to 6 mm in diameter and appear as a string of pearls lying beneath a smooth, glistening capsule (Fig 19–4). Unlike ovulatory patients, the follicle in PCO are generally found to be in varying stages of growth and atresia, with a hyperplastic theca interna, and do not produce a dominant follicle.

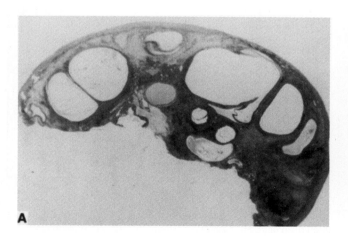
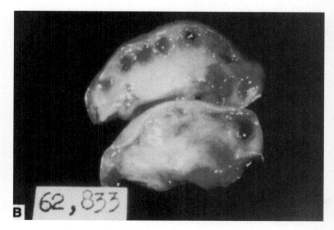

Figure 19–4. A. Microscopic specimen typical of PCO. **B.** Gross specimen typical of PCO. *(Reproduced, with permission, from Seibel MM, 1997.)*

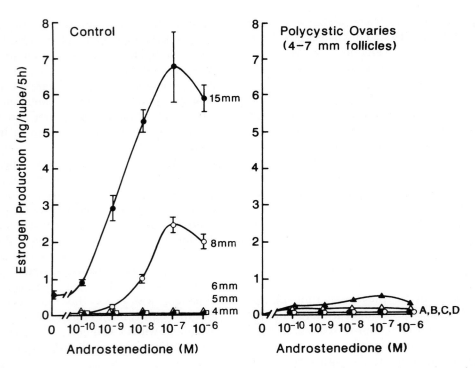

Figure 19–5. Estrogen production from granulosa cells obtained from normal and polycystic ovaries in the presence of an androgen precursor. *(Reproduced, with permission, from Erickson GF, Hsueh AJW, Quigley ME, et al, J Clin Endocrinol Metab. 49:514, 1979.[38])*

Because of this arrested follicular development, patients with polycystic ovary disease were believed to have an inherent defect in ovarian steroidogenesis. That this was not the case was the result of experiments involving the culture of granulosa cells obtained from the follicles of normal and polycystic ovaries.[38] Granulosa cells cultured from normal 8- to 15-mm follicles displayed a dose-related increase in estrogen production when incubated in the presence of the estrogen precursor androstenedione (A). Granulosa cells from follicles derived from polycystic ovaries cultured in the presence of A reveal limited estrogen production (Fig 19–5). However, when the granulosa cells from the polycystic ovary follicles were cultured with androstenedione in the presence of FSH normal amounts of estrogen were produced, suggesting that the granulosa cells were not inherently defective but rather did not possess the enzyme aromatase (Fig 19–6). The addition of LH had little or no effect. These studies suggest that the follicles in polycystic ovary patients are not inherently defective but rather can respond normally in the presence of appropriate gonadotropin secretion or the addition of exogenous FSH. Another ovarian hormone, inhibin, may also be involved in the pathogenesis of PCO. Inhibin has been found to have FSH-suppressing activity and it is present in the follicular fluid of patients with PCO in higher concentrations than in follicular fluid from normal women.[39]

The additive effect of the increased inhibin levels could account for some of the relative reduction of FSH in PCO patients.

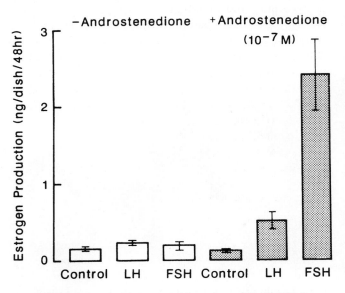

Figure 19–6. FSH corrects the PCO granulosa cell's inability to aromatize estrogen precursors. *(Reproduced, with permission, from Erickson GF, Hsueh AJW, Quigley ME, et al, J Clin Endocrinol Metab. 49:514, 1979.[38])*

THE ROLE OF INSULIN AND INSULIN-LIKE GROWTH FACTORS

The association between insulin and insulin-like growth factors and polycystic ovary disease is now well established.[40] Over the past years, a number of clinical entities have been associated with insulin resistance and ovarian hyperandrogenism. These include: (1) type A insulin resistance, which may be due to either an inherited deficiency of insulin receptors or to postbinding abnormalities in insulin action such as tyrosine kinase activity of the insulin receptor β-subunit; (2) type B insulin resistance due to insulin receptor autoantibodies; (3) lipotrophic diabetes; and (4) PCO. Typically, type A insulin-resistant patients are thin and develop PCO or hyperthecosis during their teenage years, whereas type B insulin-resistant patients are more likely to have evidence of autoimmune disease and manifest type B insulin resistance at an older age. However, it appears that women with PCO possess a specific post-receptor-binding defect in insulin action that prevents the normal insulin-induced tyrosine autophosphorylation to be replaced by phosphorylation of serine.[41] This leads to impairment of insulin signal transduction. This problem may well be genetic in origin, as cells removed for generations from the in vivo environment continue to demonstrate this abnormality.[41]

The insulin resistance associated with PCO may also be due to the obesity often associated with these patients. However, basal insulin levels remain higher in PCO patients than in weight-matched controls.[42] Insulin levels are also elevated in nonobese PCO patients who do not have evidence of acanthosis nigricans.[43,44] There is a strong correlation between fasting insulin levels and the number of menstrual cycles per yr. The interval between menstrual cycles increases as insulin concentration rises.[45] Elevated insulin levels in anovulatory women with PCO have also been associated with reduction of the cardioprotective high density-lipoprotein (HDL) cholesterol.[46] These are important nonreproductive considerations.

In addition, insulin-resistant PCO patients treated with a GnRH agonist to suppress ovarian androgen secretion demonstrate no change in their degree of insulin resistance.[47] For this reason, it appears that the ovarian hyperandrogenism in PCO is unrelated to insulin resistance per se.

Conversely, the role of insulin in the pathophysiology of hyperandrogenism has been strongly suggested by in vivo insulin infusion studies. Whether female patients are obese or nonobese, androstenedione concentrations increase significantly with insulin infusion.[48,49] Testosterone or dehydroepiandrosterone sulfate (DHEAS) production is not augmented.[50] These data corroborate in vitro studies in which insulin potentiates the androgenic activity of porcine theca cells and is synergistic with LH.[51] However, in contrast to the clinical observations in vitro studies suggest that insulin is capable of stimulating androstenedione, testosterone, progesterone, and estradiol in theca cell incubations and androstenedione, testosterone, and dihydrotestosterone (DHT) in stromal incubations.[40] Insulin also stimulates steroidogenesis in porcine and bovine granulosa cells, as well as granulosa cell proliferation in tissue culture.[52]

The mechanism by which this occurs is through specific insulin-binding sites in the ovary. Initial studies demonstrated that polycystic ovary patients had large accumulations of insulin receptors in the stroma.[53] However, normal ovarian tissue also possesses level receptors in the stroma, theca, and granulosa cell layers.[54,55] Because of the structural similarity between insulin and insulin-like growth factor I (IGF-I) and because IGF-I receptors have been identified in both ovarian stroma and purified human granulosa cells, it is possible for both insulin and IGF-I to occupy the respective receptors and stimulate hormone production.[56]

Insulin has been identified in human follicular fluid. Whether it is produced there or simply sequestered there is not known. It is not present in the follicular fluid of all follicles sampled. Insulin has been shown capable of stimulating oocyte maturation in the pig as well as facilitating germinal vesicle breakdown and Rana pipiens.[57] Insulin also correlates with follicular fluid progesterone levels but not with estradiol and androstenedione levels in the human.[58] In addition to the role of insulin in the ovary, a possible central role for insulin in the pathogenesis of PCO has also been suggested. In vitro pituitary cell cultures have shown that GnRH stimulation of LH is enhanced by insulin at physiological concentrations.[59] Circulating insulin has been shown capable of entering the hypothalamus and binding to specific receptors localized to the arcuate nucleus in median eminence.[60,61] Therefore, insulin may effect the pathogenesis of PCO through both central and peripheral mechanisms.

ADRENAL CONTRIBUTION TO PCO

The adrenal gland is a prominent producer of androgens and may be significantly involved in the pathogenesis of some patients with PCO (see Chap 18). Approximately 60 percent of peripheral androstenedione is of adrenal origin, while only 40 percent is derived from the ovaries. In addition, the overwhelming majority of DHEAS is of adrenal origin.

For this reason, congenital or acquired enzyme blocks in the production of androgen steroidogenesis can lead to elevated precursor hormones with androgenizing potential. This may result in hirsutism, acne, oligomenorrhea, infertility, and the appearance of polycystic ovary disease.[62–64] The adrenal gland is regulated through negative feedback between itself and the hypothalamus and pituitary gland. Hypothalamic corticotropin-releasing factor (CRF), a 41-amino acid peptide, is secreted into the hypophyseal portal system. ACTH together with β-lipoprotein (β-LPH) and β-endorphin are derived from a precursor molecule POMC within the corticotroph of anteromedial region of the anterior pituitary gland. Both pituitary ACTH and β-endorphin are released by CRF. In addition, CRF is capable of inhibiting GnRH secretion into the hypophyseal portal circulation.[65] These peptide hormones are difficult to measure because they are located centrally and have an extremely short half-life (less than 10 min).

The association between ACTH and polycystic ovary syndrome has been evaluated. ACTH levels are similar in both normal healthy volunteers and women with PCO,[20] despite the fact that PCO patients have higher levels of LH, DHEAS, DHEA, testosterone, and androstenedione. This implies that adrenal androgen production in PCO patients is due either to altered adrenal responsiveness to ACTH or to factors other than ACTH. Another hormone that may be involved in androgen steroidogenesis among PCO patients is prolactin.[66] Hyperprolactinemic women demonstrate significantly higher levels of DHEAS than normal controls but not testosterone and androstenedione. In addition, treatment of hyperprolactinemia will reduce DHEAS levels. Polycystic ovary patients have been found to commonly possess slightly elevated prolactin levels, as well as elevated levels of DHEAS. Furthermore, in in vitro studies in rats PCO has been induced by the administration of DHEA.[67] Along these lines, patients with TLE provide an interesting group for discussion. Temporal lobe seizures consistently result in the elevation of prolactin whereas seizures not involving those areas do not.[68] Furthermore, the electrical stimulation of the human amygdala, but not sham stimulation, significantly increases serum prolactin.[69] Patients with PCO frequently have DHEAS levels measured as part of their evaluation. Because PCO appears to be overrepresented among women with TLE, it is possible that DHEAS levels may be inadvertently measured in patients receiving antiseizure medications. These medications have been shown to falsely lower DHEAS levels among treated patients with TLE.[70] For this reason, a history of seizure medication must be excluded before interpreting DHEAS levels in this patient population (Fig 19–7).

PERIPHERAL EXTRAGLANDULAR CONTRIBUTIONS TO PCO

Although the overwhelming majority of circulating estrogens originate from glandular secretion, aromatization of androgens to estrogens can occur peripherally in the skin,

brain, and adipose tissue.[71] Because PCO patients are often overweight, and because the level of androgen precursors in this group of patients is abundant, the potential for a relatively large extraglandular contribution of weaker estrogens exists. By far, the largest estrogenic product identified is estrone. When androstenedione is incubated in culture with adipose tissue, only 14 percent of the aromatase activity occurred in the adipocyte; the remaining 86 percent was found to reside in the stromal and vascular fraction of the culture. This information is particularly useful in understanding how relatively thin patients with PCO could possess comparable aromatase activities to those patients who are obese.

Patients with PCO have also been found to have lower levels of sex hormone-binding globulin capacity (SHBG-BC).[72] Because of this, there is a relative abundance of unbound E_2 compared with controls. This hormonal circumstance has been correlated with high LH: FSH ratios in women with PCO. In addition, elevated unbound estradiol has been found to reduce hypothalamic dopamine in experimental animals.[73] Other studies in which estrone benzoate was infused in PCO patients revealed that FSH levels are lowered without altering LH release.[74] Under these sets of conditions, one can postulate a sequence of events that could result in a self-perpetuating hormonal imbalance known as PCO (Fig 19–8).

DIFFERENTIAL DIAGNOSIS

Because PCO is a descriptive term, it is important to exclude more serious clinical entries that could be confused with this diagnosis.[75] Functional disorders of the thyroid (hypothyroidism and hyperthyroidism), adrenal (congenital enzyme deficiencies, acquired androgenic hyperfunction, and Cushing syndrome), and ovary (hyperthecosis and hilus cell hyperplasia) may present with hirsutism simulating PCO. Similarly, neoplastic conditions of the adrenal and ovary, as well as iatrogenic causes such as danazol or nortestosterone derivatives, may also simulate PCO. A number of central nervous system (CNS) diseases have been associated with PCO. Such conditions include destructive CNS lesions and temporal lobe epilepsy.

DIAGNOSTIC APPROACH

Because polycystic ovary disease presents with symptoms of ovulatory disturbances and possibly excessive hirsutism and hyperandrogenism, the principle aim of diagnosis is to establish the presence of a functional versus neoplastic disorder. Usually, this is not difficult based upon history and physical examination. If the symptoms have occurred since menarche in a slow and progressive fashion, the most likely diagnosis is PCO. Conversely, a

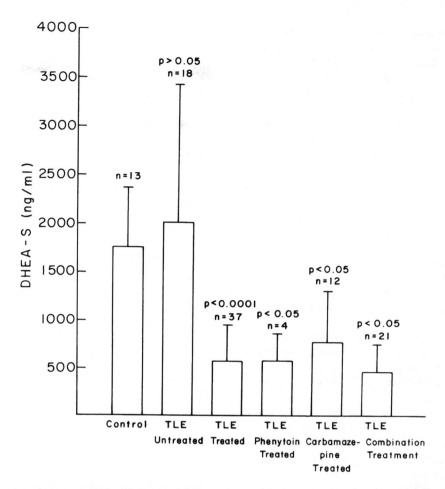

Figure 19–7. Effect of antiseizure medications on serum DHEAS levels. *(Reproduced, with permission, from Levesque LA, Herzog AG, Seibel MM, J Clin Endocrinol Metab. 63:243, 1986.[70])*

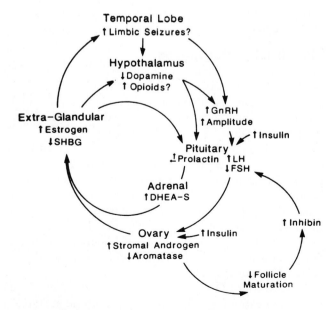

Figure 19–8. Proposed self-perpetuating cycle of PCO. *(Reproduced, with permission, from Seibel MM, 1997.)*

rapid onset of progressive hirsutism and/or masculinization strongly suggests an adrenal or ovarian neoplasm. In particular, symptoms of thyroid disease and Cushing syndrome should be excluded.

In patients with PCO, hirsutism typically is seen on the upper lip and the angle of the jaw with some extension of the sideburns. Presternal hair growth may be noted, as well as some increased evidence of suprapubic hair. The typical triangular female escutcheon is often replaced with a more diamond-shaped male escutcheon. Hair may also grow further down the medial aspects of the leg. Clitoromegaly is seldom observed in women with PCO. Excessive hair that is peripherally located on the arms and legs is usually familial or racially determined.[76] It is important to avoid using labels such as "excess male hormone production" to prevent the patient from feeling less feminine. The most important serum androgens affecting sexual hair growth are plasma free testosterone and DHT. In general, the free (unbound) testosterone concentration is elevated in hirsute women despite the fact that total testosterone concentrations are normal.

This is due to the fact that the excess androgens depress SHBG. Menstrual disturbances are one of the most common symptoms in patients with PCO. It has been suggested[77] that PCO originates before or during the onset of puberty and therefore the abnormal uterine bleeding originates from menarche prior to complete maturation of the hypothalamic–pituitary–ovarian axis. The unopposed circulating estrogens commonly associated with this entity stimulate the cervix and endometrium, which results in thin, watery cervical mucus and dysfunctional uterine bleeding. Unopposed serum estrogens have also resulted in an association of PCO and endometrial carcinoma, the overwhelming majority of which are well-differentiated stage I adenocarcinoma. Therefore, even if PCO patients do not desire conception, they should have withdrawal bleeding or correct their anovulation.

STIMULATION AND SUPPRESSION TESTING

Over the past decades, a number of studies have suggested ovarian stimulation and suppression methods to identify the source of androgen excess in patients with hyperandrogenemia. The majority of clinically used testing surrounding PCO has depended upon androgen suppression using either dexamethasone or adrenal stimulation using ACTH.[78] Both of these types of tests are commonly employed but have limited usefulness because they are not selective. Furthermore, even if a predominantly adrenal or ovarian source is presumed, the treatment frequently is not altered.[64] However, when basal serum levels of testosterone and 17-OHP are greater than 50 percent above the normal limit, ACTH stimulation testing may detect heterozygous or homozygous congenital adrenal hyperplasia. In those instances in which a neoplasia is suggested, either computed tomography or magnetic resonance imaging and/or selective venous catheterization of the adrenals and ovaries may prove useful in localizing a neoplastic source. In general, these tests add little practical usefulness because treatment choices will remain unaltered. The realization that GnRH agonists are capable of suppressing ovarian steroidogenesis (medical oophorectomy) without affecting adrenal hormone production allows for determining if an androgen source is ovarian or adrenal in origin. Studies involving GnRH have shown that the ovary and not the adrenal is the exclusive source of elevated androstenedione and testosterone in PCO patients. Because of this specificity, GnRH agonists may prove helpful in the diagnosis of PCO.

RADIOLOGIC TESTING

The use of ultrasound in the diagnosis of PCO is now a relatively large body of literature. Several patterns have been described based upon the presence of follicular cysts, increased ovarian stroma, and patterns of echogenicity.[2,3,79] Approximately one third of patients with PCO will have ovaries of normal size on ultrasound evaluation. However, ultrasound examination is useful in determining increased numbers of immature follicles ranging from 0.5 to 0.8 cm in diameter. Due to the increasing resolution in vaginal ultrasound probes, a number of patients with normal ovulatory cycles will be observed to possess a suggestion of polycystic ovary syndrome in the early follicular phase. Therefore, a single ultrasound exam cannot be relied on as a determinant of polycystic ovary syndrome.

TREATMENT

Because patients with polycystic ovary syndrome may present with menstrual disturbances, infertility, or hirsutism, therapy must be directed toward the appropriate concern (Fig 19–9). With this in mind, a number of treatment options are currently available.

Weight Loss

Polycystic ovary patients who are capable of reducing their body weight to less than 15 percent above the ideal may realize significant improvement in menstrual abnormalities and hirsutism. The effect of weight loss is a reduction in both hyperinsulinemia and insulin resistance. In addition, gonadotropin and sex steroid secretion may also be corrected. Should the patient's symptoms not respond to weight loss therapy alone, medical management of menstrual disturbances will be more readily corrected in conjunction with weight loss.[80] Few women with PCO and a body mass index (BMI) above 30 kg/m^2 cycle regularly.

Menstrual Disturbances

Polycystic ovary patients with menstrual irregularities who are not interested in conception may best be treated with an estrogen–progestin combined oral contraceptive in an attempt to induce cyclic menses and reduce circulating androgens.[81,82] Serum levels of LH can be completely suppressed within 3 wk of treatment with the 50-μg tablets.[83] Lower-dose oral contraceptives containing 30 to 35 μg ethinyl estradiol may also be used. Because oral contraceptives increase SHBG levels, free testosterone levels are reduced. The oral contraceptives are particularly desirable in those women not seeking pregnancy. In addition, the cyclic bleeding that results from oral contraceptives prevents endometrial hyperplasia and protects against the potential of endometrial carcinoma.

In Europe, Dianette (a tablet that contains 35 μg of ethinyl estradiol and 2 mg of cyproterone acetate) is often used and further supplemented with 50 mg of

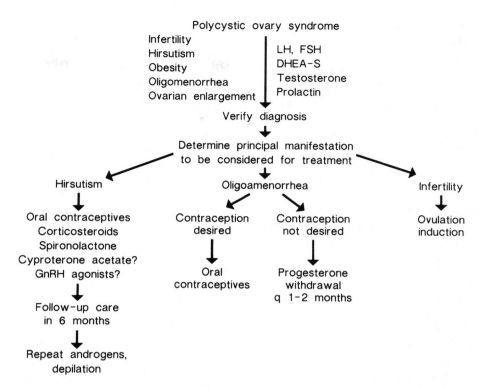

Figure 19–9. Proposed treatment plan for patients with PCO. *(Reproduced, with permission, from Seibel MM, 1997.)*

cyproterone acetate during the first 10 days of each Dianette package.[84]

In those patients who do not desire contraception or do not wish to receive oral contraception, cyclic progestin therapy (medroxyprogesterone acetate 10 mg/day for 10 days each mo) may provide a reasonable alternative.

Should the patient have a diagnosis of adenomatous or atypical adenomatous hyperplasia, careful follow-up evaluation of the endometrium is essential to be certain that these patterns are converted to atrophic endometrium.

Ovulation Induction

Clomiphene Citrate. By far the most prevalent medication used in the induction of ovulation in patients with PCO is clomiphene citrate. Clomiphene citrate is an orally active nonsteroidal weak estrogen distantly related to diethylstilbestrol. Ovulation follows in approximately 80 to 90 percent of cases, of which overall 40 to 50 percent conceive.[85] A negative pregnancy test should be obtained if the patient is amenorrheic. Menses can be induced with medroxyprogesterone acetate 10 mg daily for 5 days and clomiphene initiated in a dose of one half or one tablet daily for 5 days, usually beginning on day 5 of an induced withdrawal bleed. The patient should be asked to maintain a temperature chart and mail it at the onset of flow or 3 wk after the last clomiphene tablet if there is no menstrual flow. If the patient's temperature chart is monophasic, the dosage should be increased by 50 mg daily on days 5 to 9 and the temperature chart again followed. Should this dosage continue to result in a monophasic temperature chart, the daily dosage should again be increased 50 mg for 5 days each mo until ovulation occurs. Although daily dosages up to 250 mg are commonly used, it is the author's tendency not to exceed 150 mg daily as the likelihood of achieving conception above this dose is poor. Patients who do not respond to 150 mg daily of clomiphene are usually best treated with gonadotropins.

For those patients receiving clomiphene citrate who show evidence of follicle development on pelvic ultrasound but do not achieve ovulation, an intramuscular dose of 5000 to 10,000 IU human chorionic gonadotropin (hCG) may be administered to trigger ovulation when the lead follicle is 18 to 20 mm in diameter. However, if hCG is given prematurely, the ovulation frequently will be suboptimal or not occur. Therefore, unless ultrasound is used to monitor the timing of hCG administration, hCG offers little advantage over clomiphene citrate alone.

Patients who are found to have increased levels of DHEAS often respond well to the addition of dexamethasone 0.25 to 0.5 mg at bedtime. Should patients show poor ovulatory response to increasing doses of clomiphene and also have slightly elevated levels of prolactin, the addition of 1.25 to 2.5 mg bromocriptine at bedtime may also be useful in optimizing ovulatory potential. Once again, if these methods are not successful the next choice of treatment would be gonadotropins.

Human Menopausal Gonadotropins/Purified FSH

Both human menopausal gonadotropins (hMG) (Pergonal, Serono Laboratories, Randolph, MA) and purified FSH (Metrodin, Serono Laboratories) have been commonly used preparations in the treatment of PCO. As of April 1997, Metrodin has been replaced with Fertinex urofollitropin (Serono Laboratories), a urinary preparation that involves capture of FSH proteins by use of monoclonal antibodies and a number of high-performance liquid chromatography steps to remove non-FSH proteins. The terminal half-life of Fertinex is 39 to 45 hr, approximately twice that of Metrodin (see Chap 29).[86] Recombinant FSH is also now available in the U.S.

Because patients with PCO have multiple small follicles and an elevated endogenous LH and estrogen level, there is an increased potential risk of ovarian hyperstimulation and multiple births when ovulation induction is required. A number of studies using both these preparations are in the literature. In general, the risk of multiple births and ovarian hyperstimulation are greatest when the dosage of gonadotropins is increased in a rapid step-wise fashion.[86] Conversely, conception rates can be optimized and complication rates minimized by administering gonadotropins in dosages of one to three ampules daily for a duration of 10 to 14 days. It has been the author's preference to favor the use of purified FSH for ovulation induction in PCO patients. It appears that an ovulatory trigger of hCG is necessary to achieve consistent ovulations in this group of patients, although an endogenous LH surge will commonly occur when dosages of one ampule daily are used.

Several investigators have suggested that gonadotropins may be more effective when added to GnRH analogs (GnRHa).[87] The basic premise in this form of treatment is to provide a medical oophorectomy and convert the aberrant type of hypothalamic–pituitary dysfunction in PCO to a more constant hypothalamic amenorrhea-like pattern. Optimum results require that the PCO patient receive the medication until serum estradiol levels are less than 60 pg/ml. The author's experience with this form of treatment has suggested that achieving this goal often requires 3 mo of therapy. Subsequently, ovulation may be induced with either Pergonal or Metrodin. However, in those cases where ovarian hyperstimulation occurs, estradiol levels that would be considered in the safe range in patients not receiving GnRHa may subsequently be associated with

ovarian hyperstimulation in GnRHa gonadotropin-treated PCO patients after receiving hCG. Therefore, measuring serum estradiol levels is no longer as effective a safety precaution when GnRH agonists are used together with gonadotropins. Caution as well as appropriate patient counseling is prudent.

Wedge Resection

The use of wedge resection to treat the ovulatory problems associated with PCO resulted from a clinical observation. PCO patients with bilaterally enlarged ovaries initially thought to be pathological often begin to ovulate following wedge resection performed to establish a diagnosis.[88] However, the significant incidence of postoperative adhesions and the increased number of ovulatory-inducing agents have resulted in wedge resection falling into disfavor. In recent years, several investigators have attempted to use electrocautery or laser vaporization as an endoscopic wedge resection.[83] A three-puncture laparoscopic approach (laparoscope, grasping forceps, and electrocautery or laser probe) is used to create multiple cautery or vaporization points on the ovary. The author's technique has been to use a defocused laser beam on the follicles per se. The follicles are vaporized and the follicular fluid can be seen to escape. The stroma is spared. Often, there is a second layer of small follicles immediately below the more superficial layer. Upon completion of this procedure, the ovary is typically about one third less in diameter, primarily due to loss of follicular fluid. Ovulation will follow in approximately one third of patients. However, this technique does not prevent subsequent adhesions from forming. Should ovulation not follow in a relatively short period, ovulation induction can be performed with any of the medications previously described. Typically, patients who prior to surgery develop multiple follicles will produce only one or two preovulatory size follicles for a number of months postoperatively. This form of treatment should not be used unless medical treatment has proven ineffective. Laparoscopy should be performed to exclude postoperative adhesions if pregnancy does not follow in four to six cycles.

In Vitro Fertilization

In vitro fertilization provides a reasonable form of treatment in polycystic ovary patients with tubal disease. However, ovulatory dysfunction per se should not be an immediate cause for applying in vitro fertilization because cumulative conception rates with ovulation induction alone exceed 60 percent in six ovulatory cycles. Should pregnancy not occur, in vitro fertilization either with or without the use of GnRHa is a viable alternative. However, even if all oocytes are retrieved the risks of ovarian hyperstimulation or multiple birth are not eliminated. Cryopreservation of supernumerary embryos with subsequent transfer may enhance the success rate per retrieval of polycystic ovary patients requiring in vitro fertilization.[89] In the future, in vivo maturation of immature oocytes may also provide a safe application of assisted reproduction in this group of patients.[90]

Hirsutism

A number of medications have been used to treat the hirsutism associated with PCO. In the past, the overwhelmingly most prevalent form of treatment was combined oral contraceptives.[91] Hair growth could be reduced in up to two thirds of hirsute patients.[81] The oral contraceptive chosen should suppress LH levels into the normal range. Complete androgen suppression requires approximately 3 wk of treatment with 15 g ethinyl estradiol or mestranol equivalent.

The patient should be advised that she may not appreciate a clinical change for as long as 6 mo, and most women need treatment for 12 to 18 mo. Patients with a relatively short history of hirsutism may respond better to oral contraceptives than patients with long-standing hyperandrogenism and its resultant coarse, dark, terminal hair. Therefore, electrolysis should not be recommended until the patient has received 4 to 6 mo of treatment. Upon discontinuation of oral contraceptives, abnormal hair growth usually recurs.

A number of other medications have also been used to treat the hirsutism associated with PCO. Those include medroxyprogesterone acetate (a progestin that decreases GnRH release and suppresses gonadotropins), spironolactone[92] (a competitive inhibitor of intracellular DHT receptor within the hair follicle), cimetidine (Smith, Kline & French) (a histamine H_2 receptor antagonist that is weakly antiandrogenic), and cyproterone acetate[84] (a synthetic progestin derived from 17-hydroxyprogesterone with potent antiandrogenic properties). The nonsteroidal pure antiandrogenic flutamide has proven itself an excellent treatment option for hirsutism. Unfortunately, because it is not a contraceptive and therefore must be used in conjunction with birth control, and because it carries a small risk of severe hepatic disease, its role must be viewed with caution.[93] In recent years the most popular and potentially beneficial treatment of the hyperandrogenism associated with PCO has been the use of GnRH agonists. Both GnRHa and cyproterone acetate have been shown capable of suppressing ovarian steroids with no effect on DHEAS levels. The result is a marked clinical improvement with decreased seborrhea and acne and normalization of ovarian size. Although GnRH agonists cause a "medical castration" with a resultant hypoestrogenic state, estrogen may be provided concurrently in the form of either Premarin (Wyeth/Ayerst) or ethinyl estradiol as the estrogen per se is not contributing to the hirsutism. In this fashion, ovarian androgen biosynthesis can be potently suppressed without the patient's experiencing the side effects of a hypoestrogenic state (see Chap 20).

SUMMARY

PCO represents a complex state of hormonal imbalance involving the hypothalamus, pituitary, ovaries, adrenal, and peripheral tissues. The end result is a self-perpetuating state of chronic hormonal imbalance. The most common symptoms leading patients with PCO to seek medical care are menstrual disturbances, infertility, and hirsutism. As advances in the understanding of the pathophysiology of PCO occur, greater insights can be gained into the treatment of this complex endocrine condition.

REFERENCES

1. Jacobs HS. Polycystic ovary syndrome. In: *Infertility: A Comprehensive Text*, 2nd ed. Norwalk, Conn., Appleton & Lange, 1997: 121–133
2. Jacobs HS. Prevalence and significance of polycystic ovaries. *Ultrasound Obstet Gynecol.* 4:3, 1994
3. Bridges NA, Cooke A, Healy MJ, et al. Standards for ovarian volume in childhood and puberty. *Fertil Steril.* 60:456, 1993
4. Rebar R, Judd HL, Yen SSC, et al. Characterization of the inappropriate gonadotropin secretion in polycystic ovary syndrome. *J Clin Invest.* 57:1320, 1976
5. Kazer RR, Kessel B, Yen SSC. Circulating luteinizing hormone pulse frequency in women with polycystic ovary syndrome. *J Clin Endocrinol Metab.* 65:233, 1987
6. Knobil E. The neuroendocrine control of the menstrual cycle. *Rec Prog Horm Res.* 36:53, 1980
7. Seibel MM, Claman P, Oskowitz SP, et al. Events surrounding the initiation of puberty with long-term subcutaneous pulsatile gonadotropin-releasing hormone in a female patient with Kallmann's syndrome. *J Clin Endocrinol Metab.* 61:575, 1985
8. Zumoff B, Freeman R, Coupey S, et al. A chronobiologic abnormality in luteinizing hormone secretion in teenage girls with polycystic ovary syndrome. *N Engl J Med.* 309:1206, 1983
9. Soule SG. Neuroendocrinology of the polycystic ovary syndrome. *Baillieres Clin Endocrinol Metab.* 10:205, 1996
10. Chehab FF, Lim ME, Ronghua L. Correction of sterility defect in homozygous obese female mice by treatment with the human recombinant leptin. *Nat Genet.* 12: 318, 1996
11. Stephens TW, Basinski M, Bristow PK, et al. The role of neuropeptide Y in the antiobesity action of the obese gene product. *Nature.* 377:530, 1995
12. Seifer DB, Collins RL. Current concepts of β-endorphin physiology in female reproductive dysfunction. *Fertil Steril.* 54:757, 1990

13. Cummings DC, Reid RL, Quigley ME, et al. Evidence for decreased endogenous dopamine and opioid inhibitory influences on LH secretion in polycystic ovary syndrome. *Clin Endocrinol.* 20:643, 1984

14. Barnes RB, Lobo RA. Central opioid activity in polycystic ovary syndrome (PCO) with and without dopaminergic modulation. *J Clin Endocrinol Metab.* 61:779, 1985

15. Reid RL, Hoff JD, Yen SSC, et al. Effects of exogenous β-endorphin on pituitary hormone secretion and its disappearance rate in normal human subjects. *J Clin Endocrinol Metab.* 52:1179, 1981

16. Van Loon GR. Brain opioid peptide regulations of autonomic function. In: Givens, ed. *The Hypothalamus.* Chicago, Ill., Year Book Publishers, 1984: 39

17. Rotsztejn WH, Drouva SV, Pattou E, Kordon C. Metenkephalin inhibits dopamine-induced LH-RH release from mediobasal hypothalamus of male rats. *Nature.* 274:281, 1978

18. Aleem FA, McIntosh T. Elevated plasma levels of β-endorphin in a group of women with polycystic ovary disease. *Fertil Steril.* 42:686, 1984

19. Petraglia F, D'Ambrogio G, Comitini G, et al. Impairment of opioid control of luteinizing hormone secretion in menstrual disorders. *Fertil Steril.* 43:534, 1985

20. Chang RJ, Mandel FP, Wolfsen AR, et al. Circulating levels of plasma adrenocorticotropin in polycystic ovary disease. *J Clin Endocrinol Metab.* 54:1265, 1982

21. Lobo RA, Granger LR, Paul WL, et al. Psychological stress and increases in urinary norepinephrine metabolites, platelet serotonin, and adrenal androgens in women with polycystic ovary syndrome. *Am J Obstet Gynecol.* 145:496, 1983

22. Kimball CD. Do opioid peptides mediate appetites and love bonds? *Am J Obstet Gynecol.* 156:1463, 1987

23. Herzog AG. Neurologic considerations. In: Seibel MM, ed. *Infertility: A Comprehensive Text.* Norwalk, Conn., Appleton & Lange, 1977

24. Herzog AG, Seibel MM, Schomer DL, et al. Reproductive endocrine disorders in women with partial seizures of temporal lobe origin. *Arch Neurol.* 43:347, 1986

25. Renaud LP. Influence of amygdala stimulation on the activity of identified tuberoinfundibular neurons in the rat hypothalamus. *J Physiol.* 260:237, 1976

26. Erickson LB, Wada JA. Effects of lesions in the temporal lobe and rhinencephalon on reproductive function in adult female rhesus monkeys. *Fertil Steril.* 21:434, 1970

27. Krieger DT, Martin JB. Brain peptides. *N Engl J Med.* 304:876, 1981

28. Zolovnik AJ. Effects of lesions and electrical stimulation of the amygdala on hypothalamic–hypophyseal regulation. In: Eleftheriou, ed. *The Neurobiology of the Amygdala.* New York, N.Y., Plenum, 1972: 745–762

29. Herzog AG. A relationship between particular reproductive endocrine disorders and the laterality of epileptiform discharges in women with epilepsy. *Neurology.* 43:1907, 1993

30. Bilo L, Meo R, Valentino R, et al. Abnormal patterns of luteinizing hormone pulsatility in women with epilepsy. *Fertil Steril.* 55:705, 1991

31. Drislane FW, Coleman AE, Schomer DL, et al. Altered pulsatile secretion of luteinizing hormone in women with epilepsy. *Neurology.* 44:306, 1994

32. Sata M, Nakashima T. Kindling: Secondary epileptogenesis, sleep and catecholamines. *Cam J Neurol Sci.* 2:349, 1975

33. Sommers SC, Wadman PJ. Pathogenesis of polycystic ovaries. *Am J Obstet Gynecol.* 72:160, 1956

34. Futterweit W, Krieger DT. Pituitary tumors associated with hyperprolactinemia and polycystic ovary disease. *Fertil Steril.* 31:608, 1979

35. Espinosa de las Monteros A, Cornejo J, Parra A. Differential prolactin response to oral metoclopramide in nulliparous versus parous women throughout the menstrual cycle. *Fertil Steril.* 55:885, 1991

36. Quigley ME, Rakoff JS, Yen SSC. Increased luteinizing sensitivity to dopamine inhibition in polycystic ovary syndrome. *J Clin Endocrinol Metab.* 52:231, 1981

37. Falaschi P, Rocco A, Del Pozo E. Inhibitory effect of bromocriptine treatment of luteinizing hormone secretion in polycystic ovary syndrome. *J Clin Endocrinol Metab.* 62:348, 1986

38. Erickson GF, Hsueh AJW, Quigley ME, et al. Functional studies of aromatase activity activity in human granulosa cells from normal and polycystic ovaries. *J Clin Endocrinol Metab.* 49:514, 1979

39. Tanabe K, Gagliano P, Channing CP, et al. Levels of inhibin-F activity and steroids from human follicular fluid from normal women and women with polycystic ovary disease. *J Clin Endocrinol Metab.* 57:24, 1983

40. Poretsky L, Kalin MF. The gonadotropic function of insulin. *Endocrine Rev.* 8:132, 1987

41. Dunai FA. Hyperadrenogenic anovulation (PCOS): A unique disorder of insulin action associated with an increased risk of non-insulin dependent diabetes mellitus. *Am J Med.* 98:33S, 1995

42. Stuart CA, Peters EJ, Prince MJ, et al. Insulin resistance with acanthosis nigricans: The role of obesity and androgen excess. *Metabolism.* 35:197, 1986

43. Chang RJ, Nakamura RM, Judd HL, Kaplan SA. Insulin resistance with acanthosis nigricans: The role of obesity and androgen excess. *Metabolism.* 35:197, 1987

44. Jialal I, Naiker P, Reddi K, et al. Evidence for insulin resistance in nonobese patients with polycystic ovarian disease. *J Clin Endocrinol Metab.* 64:1066, 1987

45. Conway GS: Polycystic ovary syndrome: Clinical aspects. *Baillieres Clin Endocrinol Metab.* 10:263, 1996

46. Conway GS, Agrawal R, Betteridge DJ, Jacobs HS. Risk factors for coronary artery disease in lean and obese women with the polycystic ovary syndrome. *Clin Endocrinol.* 37:119, 1992

47. Geffner ME, Kaplan SA, Bersch N, et al. Persistence of insulin resistance in polycystic ovarian disease after inhibition of ovarian steroid secretion. *Fertil Steril.* 45:327, 1986

48. Stuart CA, Prince MJ, Meyer WJ. Hyperinsulinemia and hyperandrogenemia: In vivo androgen response to insulin infusion. *Obstet Gynecol.* 69:921, 1987

49. Elkind-Hirsch KE, Valdes CT, McConnell TG, Malinak LR. Androgen responses to acutely increased endogenous

insulin levels in hyperandrogenic and normal cycling women. *Fertil Steril.* 55:486, 1991

50. Stuart CA, Nagamani M. Insulin infusion acutely augments ovarian androgen production in normal women. *Fertil Steril.* 54:788, 1990

51. Barbieri RL, Makris A, Randall RW, et al. Insulin stimulates androgen accumulation in incubations of ovarian stroma obtained from women with hyperandrogenism. *J Clin Endocrinol Metab.* 62:904, 1986

52. Savion N, Lui GM, Laherty R, et al. Factors controlling proliferation and progesterone production by bovine granulosa cells in serum-free medium. *Endocrinology.* 109:409, 1981

53. Poretsky L, Smith D, Seibel M, et al. Specific insulin-binding sites in human ovary. *J Clin Endocrinol Metab.* 59:809, 1984

54. Poretsky L, Grigorescu F, Seibel M, et al. Distribution and characterization of insulin and insulin-like growth factor I receptors in normal human ovary. *J Clin Endocrinol Metab.* 61:728, 1985

55. Jarrett JC, Ballijo G, Tsibris JCM, Spellacy WN. Insulin binding to human ovaries. *J Clin Endocrinol Metab.* 60:460, 1985

56. Gates GS, Bayer S, Seibel MM, et al. Characterization of insulin-like growth factor binding to human granulosa cells obtained during in vitro fertilization. *J Recept Res.* 7:885, 1987

57. Lessman CA, Schuetz AW. Role of follicle wall in meiosis reinitiation induced by insulin in Rana pipiens oocytes. *Am J Physiol.* 241:E51, 1981

58. Diamond MP, Webster BW, Carr RK, et al. Human follicular fluid insulin concentrations. *J Clin Endocrinol Metab.* 61:990, 1985

59. Adashi EY, Hsueh AJW, Yen SSC. Insulin enhancement of luteinizing hormone and follicle-stimulating hormone release by cultured pituitary cells. *Endocrinology.* 108:1441, 1981

60. Van Houten M, Posner BI, Kopriwa BM, et al. Insulin enhancement of luteinizing hormone and follicle-stimulating hormone release by cultured pituitary cells. *Endocrinology.* 108:1441, 1981

61. Van Houten M, Posner BI, Kopriwa BM, et al. Insulin binding sites localized to nerve terminals in rat median eminence and arcuate nucleus. *Science.* 207:1081, 1980

62. Brodie BL, Wentz AC. Late-onset congenital adrenal hyperplasia. *N Engl J Med.* 316:1519, 1987

63. White PC, New MI, Dupont B. Congenital adrenal hyperplasia. *N Engl J Med.* 316:1519, 1987

64. Wells G, Azziz R. Late onset adrenal hyperplasia: Mutation at codon 282 of the functional 21 hydroxylase gene is not ubiquitous. *Fertil Steril.* 54:819, 1990

65. Rivier C, Rivier J, Vale W. Stress induced inhibition of reproductive functions: Role of endogenous corticotropin-releasing factor. *Science.* 231:607, 1986

66. Lobo RA, Kletzky OA, Kaptein EM, Goebelsman U. Prolactin modulation of dehydroepiandrosterone sulfate secretion. *Am J Obstet Gynecol.* 138:632, 1980

67. Knudsen JF, Costoff A, Mahesh VB. Dehydroepiandrosterone-induced polycystic ovaries and acyclicity in the rat. *Fertil Steril.* 26:807, 1975

68. Sperling MR, Pritchard PB, Engel J Jr, et al. Prolactin in partial epilepsy: An indicator of limbic seizures. *Ann Neurol.* 20:716, 1986

69. Parra A, Velasco M, Cervantes C, et al. Plasma prolactin increase following electric stimulation of the amygdala in humans. *Neuroendocrinology.* 31:60, 1980

70. Levesque LA, Herzog AG, Seibel MM. The effect of phenytoin and carbamazepine on serum dehydroepiandrosterone sulfate in men and women who have partial seizures with temporal lobe involvement. *J Clin Endocrinol Metab.* 63:243, 1986

71. Siiteri PK, MacDonald PC. Role of extraglandular estrogen in human endocrinology. In: Greep RO, Astwood EB, eds. *Handbook of Physiology,* vol 2. Washington, D.C., American Physiology Society, 1973: 615–629

72. Anderson DC. Sex-hormone binding globulin. *Clin Endocrinol.* 104:419, 1979

73. Cramer DM, Parker CR, Porter JC. Estrogen inhibition of dopamine release into hypophyseal portal blood. *Endocrinology.* 104:419, 1979

74. Chang RJ, Mandel FP, Lu JKH, Judd HL. Enhanced disparity of gonadotropin secretion by estrone in women with polycystic ovarian disease. *J Clin Endocrinol Metab.* 54:490, 1982

75. Seibel MM. Polycycstic ovary disease. In: *Infertility: A Comprehensive Text.* Norwalk, Conn., Appleton & Lange, 1990: 61–82

76. Hatch R, Rosenfield RL, Kim MH, et al. Hirsutism: Implications, etiology, and management. *Am J Obstet Gynecol.* 140:815, 1981

77. Yen SSC. The polycystic ovary syndrome. *Clin Endocrinol.* 12:177, 1980

78. Kim HM, Rosenfield RL, Dupon C. The effects of dexamethasone on plasma free androgens during the normal menstrual cycle. *Am J Obstet Gynecol.* 126:982, 1976

79. Hann LE, Hall DA, McArdle CR, Seibel MM. Polycystic ovarian disease: Sonographic spectrum. *Radiology.* 150:531, 1984

80. Bates GW. Body weight and reproduction. In: Seibel MM, ed. *Infertility: A Comprehensive Text,* Norwalk, Conn., Appleton & Lange, 1997

81. Givens JR, Andersen RN, Wiser WL, et al. The effectiveness of two oral contraceptives in suppressing plasma androstenedione, testosterone, LH, and FSH, and in stimulating plasma testosterone binding capacity in hirsute women. *Am J Obstet Gynecol.* 124:333, 1976

82. Suikkari AM, Tiitinen A, Stenman UH, et al. Oral contraceptives increase insulin-like growth factor binding protein-1 concentration in women with polycystic ovary disease. *Fertil Steril.* 55:895, 1991

83. Armar NA, McGarrigle HHG, Honour J, et al. Laparoscopic ovarian diathermy in the management of anovulatory infertility in women with polycystic ovaries: Endocrine changes and clinical outcome. *Fertil Steril.* 53:45, 1990

84. Miller JA, Jacobs HS. Treatment of hirsutism and acne with cyproterone acetate. *Clin Endocrinol Metabol.* 15:373, 1986

85. Chamoun D, McClamrock HD, Adashi EY. Ovulation initiation. In: Seibel MM, ed. *Infertility: A Comprehensive Text,* 2nd ed. Norwalk, Conn., Appleton & Lange, 1997: 495–506

86. Seibel MM. Ovulation induction with follicle stimulating hormone. In: Seibel MM, ed. *Infertility: A Comprehensive Text,* 2nd ed. Norwalk, Conn., Appleton & Lange, 1997: 525–536

87. Dodson WC, Haney AF. Controlled ovarian hyperstimulation and intrauterine insemination for treatment of infertility. *Fertil Steril.* 55:457, 1991

88. Stein IF, Cohen MR. Surgical treatment of bilateral polycystic ovaries, amenorrhea and sterility. *Am J Obstet Gynecol.* 38:465, 1939

89. Bernstein J, Seibel MM. New reproductive technologies and polycystic ovary syndrome. In: Pittaway D, ed. *Infertility and Reproductive Medicine Clinics of North America.* Philadelphia, Pa., W. B. Saunders

90. Bar-Ami S, Seibel MM. Oocyte development and meiosis in humans. In: Seibel MM, ed. *Infertility: A Comprehensive Text.* Norwalk, Conn., Appleton & Lange, 1997: 81–110

91. Adashi E. The use of GnRH agonists in reproduction. In: Seibel M, Kiessling A, Bernstein J, Levin S, eds. *Technology and Infertility: Psychosocial, Legal and Ethical Implications.* New York, N.Y., Springer-Verlag, 1992

92. Shaw JC. Spironolactone in dermatologic therapy. *J Am Acad Dermatol.* 24:236, 1991

93. Gomez JL, Dupont A, Cusan L, et al. Incidence of liver toxicity associated with the use of flutamide in prostate cancer patients. *Am J Med.* 92:465, 1992

Chapter 20

HIRSUTISM AND VIRILISM

Rogerio A. Lobo

While it is not uncommon for women to present with the complaint of hirsutism, virilism is rarely encountered. This chapter will begin with a general discussion of androgen secretion and metabolism contributing to these disorders. This will be followed by the clinical presentations of hirsutism and virilism and the differential diagnosis and diagnostic approach. Finally, treatment will be discussed from the vantage point of suppressing the abnormality in androgen secretion and/or action.

ANDROGEN SECRETION AND ACTION IN WOMEN

Androgen production in women can be discussed according to three separate sources of production: the ovaries, the adrenal glands, which are glandular sources, and the peripheral compartment, which comprises all extrasplanchnic and nonglandular areas of androgen production. The peripheral compartment includes many tissues, the largest of which is the skin. Furthermore, the peripheral compartment modulates androgens produced by both the ovaries and the adrenals.

The ovary directly secretes testosterone and Δ^4-androstenedione (Adione) and, to a lesser degree, dehydroeipandrosterone (DHEA). The adrenal gland normally does not secrete testosterone but does secrete Adione in amounts equal to that produced by the ovary in the follicular phase.[1] Also, it is the adrenal that almost exclusively secretes dehydroeipandrosterone sulfate (DHEAS). DHEAS is secreted systemically in larger quantities than any other androgen and its serum concentration correlates significantly with urinary 17-ketosteroid excretion, but it appears to be a more specific marker of adrenal androgen production.[2] DHEA and Δ^5-androstenediol (Δ^5-diol) are also secreted by the adrenal and in quantities greater than by the ovary.[3]

Recently, 11β-hydroxyandrostenedione (11β-A) has been evaluated as an adrenal marker because 11β-hydroxylation normally occurs only in the adrenal. This measurement has proved to be extremely useful in that

it accurately reflects adrenal androgen secretion. It, however, does not correlate well with serum DHEAS, suggesting that 11β-A and DHEAS are produced from separate pools.[4] Although the measurement of 11β-A may have a slightly greater sensitivity and specificity than DHEAS for diagnosing adrenal androgen excess, it is subject to diurnal changes and therefore requires early morning (8:00 to 10:00 AM) sampling.

Distinguishing Ovarian from Adrenal Androgen Secretion

Investigators have used various stimulation and suppression protocols to determine the sources of androgen production in normal and hyperandrogenic women. Selective catheterization of adrenal and ovarian veins also has been attempted. However, none of these techniques adequately reflects the contribution of these glands to the total androgen pool. Recently, selective venous catheterization data confirmed that almost all exogenously administered agents (dexamethasone, human chorionic gonadotropin [hCG], corticotropin [ACTH], etc) affect both the ovary and adrenal.[5] Although these catheterization techniques may be useful in the detection of androgen-producing neoplasms, they have no place in the evaluation of other hyperandrogenic conditions.

The only probe that currently has the potential ability to distinguish ovarian from adrenal androgen secretion is the gonadotropin-releasing hormone (GnRH) agonist.[6] By downregulating the gonadotrope and ovary, ovarian androgens (testosterone and Adione) can be clearly distinguished from adrenal androgens (DHEA, DHEAS, 11β-A) in both normal women and those with polycystic ovary syndrome (PCOS) (Fig 20–1). Because Adione is secreted in equal quantities by both the ovary and adrenal, serum testosterone is the better ovarian marker. Although only one third of testosterone production (0.25 to 0.35 mg/day) is secreted directly by the ovary, the remaining two thirds is derived in nearly equal proportions from both ovarian and adrenal precursors. Therefore, normally two thirds of circulating testosterone

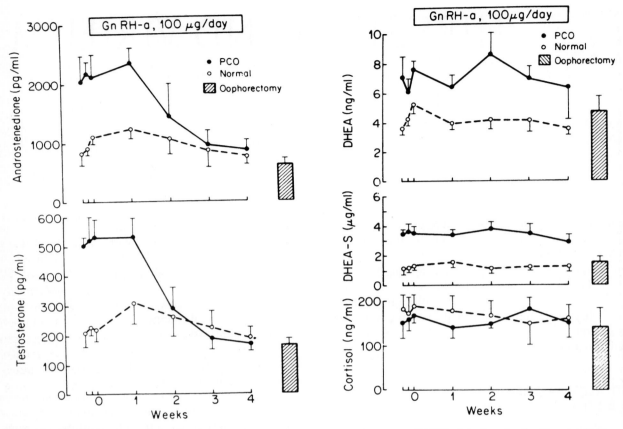

Figure 20–1. Mean serum androstenedione, testosterone, dehydroepiandrosterone (DHEA), dehydroepiandrosterone sulfate (DHEAS), and cortisol concentrations in polycystic ovary syndrome (PCOS) and normal ovulatory subjects before and during gonadotropin-releasing hormone agonist (GnRH-A) treatment and in oophorectomized women. *(Reproduced, with permission, from Chang RJ, Laufer LR, Meldrum DR, et al. Steroid secretion in polycystic ovarian disease after ovarian supression by long-acting gonadotropin-releasing hormone agonist. J. Clin Endocrinol Metab. 56:897, 1983[6])*

may originate from the ovary. These concepts, supported by data using the GnRH agonist, allow the conclusion that serum testosterone is the primary marker of ovarian androgen production, while DHEAS is the best serum marker of adrenal androgen production.

It has been noted that some women with PCOS who have elevated levels of DHEAS, have reductions in these levels with GnRH-A therapy.[7] When this occurs it has been assumed that ovarian DHEA production is increased in these women and is reduced by the agonist. The conversion of DHEA to DHEAS does not appear to be affected. Alternatively, it is possible that the GnRH-A can inhibit adrenal DHEAS production in these individuals.

SERUM MARKERS FOR ANDROGENICITY IN WOMEN

Although testosterone exerts significant androgenic activity, DHEAS is relatively inert as an androgen. As much as 20 mg/day DHEAS is produced, compared to only 3 mg/day Adione and 8 mg/day DHEA. These weak adrenal androgens exert their effects largely after conversion to more potent androgens such as testosterone, although this conversion rate is low. Testosterone, Δ^5-diol, dihydrotestosterone (DHT), and 3α-androstenediol (3α-diol) are classified as 17β-hydroxyandrogens and are the most potent circulating androgens, being largely formed from other precursor androgens.[8]

To exert effects in the periphery (skin and external genitalia), even the more potent androgens such as testosterone must be converted to DHT. Androgen action in peripheral tissues requires receptor occupancy by DHT, which in turn requires significant 5α-reductase activity within the cell. A more distal metabolite of DHT, 3α-diol, is also produced exclusively in peripheral tissues and is one of the 17β-hydroxyandrogens known to exert a biologic effect. However, most of the activity of 3α-diol is linked to DHT production. In the peripheral compartment, other enzymatic activities, such as 17-ketoreductase and aromatase activities, are largely responsible for producing less potent androgens (like Adione from testosterone) as well as estrogens. Thus, there appears to be a balance between the "step-up" of androgen action when DHT is formed and the "step-down" when less potent androgens and estrogens are formed. An understanding of the relative control of these enzymatic processes is key to an appreciation of the effects of androgen on skin.

Logically, DHT should serve as the primary marker of peripheral androgen production. However, because of rapid cellular turnover of DHT and its great affinity for sex hormone-binding globulin (SHBG), serum DHT does not reflect the step-up phenomenon in peripheral tissues in terms of androgenicity. Investigators have therefore focused on more distal metabolites of DHT. Of these, the most studied to date are 3α-diol and its glucuronide (3α-diol G).[9] While both 3α-diol and 3α-diol G are exclusively produced in peripheral tissues, 3α-diol G serves as a better marker of androgen action because, once formed, there is no back-conversion to DHT. There is an excellent correlation between serum 3α-diol G and the manifestation of androgenicity.[10,11] There also is a good correlation between androgenicity and the level of skin 5α-reductase activity[11] (Fig 20–2).

Another excellent marker of peripheral androgen action is androsterone glucuronide (AoG). This is primarily formed from the peripheral metabolism (5α-reductase activity) of Adione (Fig 20–3). Serum AoG may be more valuable in states such as acne,[12] but in hirsutism its measurement complements and is at times more useful than measurements of serum 3α-diol G.

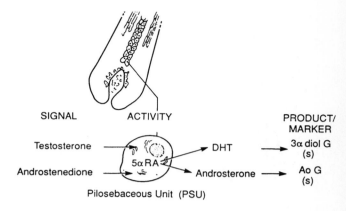

Figure 20–3. Peripheral androgen metabolism and markers of this activity.

Thus, each of the three principal compartments of androgen production has a serum marker that may be helpful clinically. Serum testosterone primarily signifies ovarian production, DHEAS is an adrenal marker, and serum 3α-diol G reflects androgen action in the peripheral compartment. As more clinical information becomes available, 11β-A may also be used to signify adrenal androgen production and AoG may also be used as a peripheral marker.

MODULATORS OF ANDROGEN ACTION

The principal modulator of androgen action in the periphery is determined by the inherent state of 5α-reductase activity and the androgen receptor. It appears, however, that the androgen receptor is less important than 5α-reductase activity. Receptor concentrations alone do not explain differences in clinical androgenicity.[13] Any factor that specifically modulates 5α-reductase activity can affect the expression of androgenicity. Several antiandrogens with these properties have been used successfully for the treatment of androgen excess. Moreover, it appears that estrogen may exert some antiandrogen activity, primarily by interfering with receptor function.

In blood, the primary modulator of the androgen signal is the transport protein, SHBG (also known as testosterone–estradiol-binding globulin). Conditions that decrease SHBG binding (androgen, obesity, acromegaly, hypothyroidism, liver disease) also increase unbound concentrations of the active 17β-hydroxyandrogens, thus augmenting their effect. Hence, unbound estradiol (normally, 35 percent is SHBG bound) would also increase. Total circulating testosterone includes three moieties. The first is that which is specifically bound to SHBG; the second includes that portion not bound to SHBG but associated with albumin ("loosely bound testosterone");

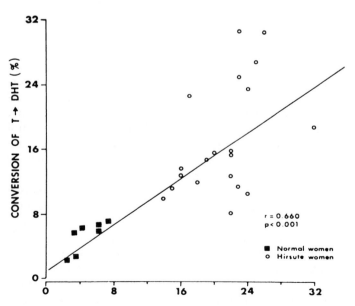

Figure 20–2. In vivo percentage conversion of testosterone (T) to dihydrotestosterone (DHT) by 5α-reductase in a genital skin preparation and the correlation with the clinical evaluation of hirsutism (Ferriman–Gallwey score). *(Reproduced, with permission, from Serafini P, Lobo RA. Increased 5 α-reductase activity in pubic skin fibroblasts from hirsute patients. Fertil Steril. 43:74, 1985[11])*

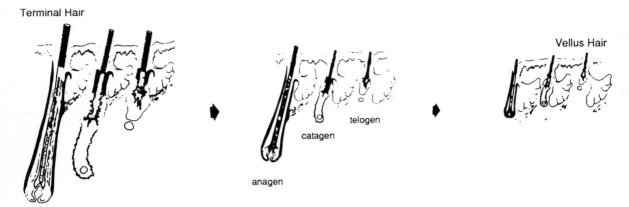

Figure 20–4. Changes occurring after several generations of hair cycles that result in the transition from terminal to vellus hair. (Under the influence of androgens, some of the hair changes from vellus to terminal. However, in postpuberty, for uncertain reasons, an increase in the normally low level of 5α-reductase activity in the scalp may induce a transition from terminal to vellus hair, leading eventually to alopecia.) *(Modified, with permission, from Montagna W, Parakkal PF. The Structure and Function of Skin, 3rd ed. New York, N.Y., Academic Press, 1974: 250.)*

and the third is that fraction not bound by either SHBG or albumin ("dialyzable free testosterone"). The measurement of those non-SHBG-bound moieties has been advocated in states of androgen excess to more accurately detect subtle forms of hyperandrogenism.[14] Although the diagnostic yield of this measurement is clearly superior to that of total serum testosterone, the correlation between total and non-SHBG-bound testosterone is excellent and frequently can be predicted.[15] Therefore, while dialyzable free or non-SHBG-bound testosterone is the preferred measurement for research purposes and detection of subtle androgenicity, this more expensive test may not be necessary clinically and treatment is rarely altered by its measurement. The purpose of measuring serum testosterone should be to determine the source of androgen production and to detect excessively high values that might suggest the presence of a neoplasm.

The normal serum levels for these sex steroids in women are as follows: testosterone, 20 to 70 ng/dl (some laboratories report values up to 100 ng/dl); dialyzable free testosterone, 1 to 8 pg/ml (free, by dialysis); non-SHBG-bound testosterone, 1 to 10 ng/dl (dialyzable free + loosely bound); androstenedione, 20 to 250 ng/dl; DHEA, 130 to 980 ng/dl, DHEAS, 0.5 to 2.8 μg/ml (some laboratories report values to 3.3 μg/ml); Δ^5-diol, 20 to 80 ng/dl; DHT, 5 to 30 ng/dl; 3α-diol, 0.5 to 6.5 ng/dl; and 3α-diol G, 60 to 300 ng/dl (range has been extended with refinements in the assay).

CLINICAL PRESENTATION

An understanding of the clinical conditions associated with hyperandrogenism requires some background information about the pilosebaceous unit (PSU), the common structure in skin that gives rise to hair and sebaceous glands. PSUs are present over virtually the entire body except the palms and soles. Thus, hair is distributed bodywide. If the sebaceous component of the PSU is prominent, the hair is merely vellus—soft, fine, and unpigmented—and may remain unrecognized (Fig 20–4). If the pillary component is prominent, a "terminal" hair is noted that differs from vellus hair by its darker color, greater length, and coarseness.

Before puberty, the predominant body hair is vellus. During puberty, some of the vellus hair normally is transformed into terminal hair, particularly in the pubic and axillary regions. After puberty, terminal hair in turn undergoes normal cyclic changes, the control of which is only partly understood.

The characteristics and distribution of body hair differ greatly among women and are strongly influenced by ethnic and racial factors (American Indians, Asians, light-skinned whites, and some blacks have less hair). Body hair is also influenced by immediate genetic factors; family members frequently have similar hair characteristics. Elderly women often have increased facial hair, which may be associated with a diminution in pubic and axillary hair. Body hair is more noticeable in women with dark hair.

The attitude toward body hair varies among different societies and individuals. In some societies, a relatively large amount of body hair in women is admired; in others, it is considered unattractive. Similarly, the psychology and immediate environment of a woman may markedly alter her attitude toward a degree of body hair that most women would not consider excessive but that she finds alarming or intolerable.

Hirsutism should not be confused with hypertrichosis, which simply implies any generalized increase in

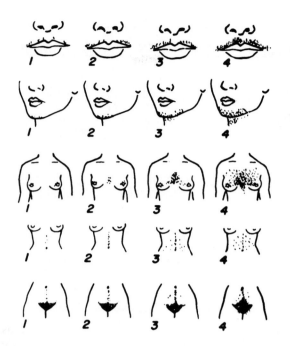
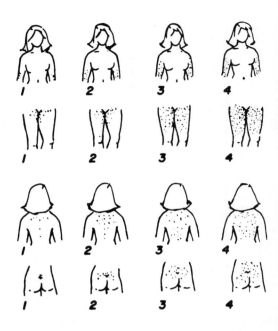

Figure 20–5. Hirsutism scoring from 1 to 14 from nine body sites. *(Reproduced, with permission, from Hatch R, Rosenfield RL, Kim MH, Tredway D. Hirsutism: Implications, etiology, and management. Am J Obstet Gynecol.140:815, 1981[16])*

body hair. Hirsutism is defined as the presence of hair in locations where hair is not commonly found in women. It refers particularly to "midline" hair (Fig 20–5). This includes facial hair on the cheeks (sideburns), above the upper lip (mustache), and on the chin (beard). Chest hair is significant if it is intermammary. In addition, a male escutcheon, hair on the inner aspects of the thighs, and midline lower back hair entering the intergluteal area are hair growth patterns compatible with the hirsute state. A moderate amount of hair on the forearms and lower legs by itself may not be abnormal, although it may be viewed by the patient as undesirable and may be mistaken for hirsutism. Figure 20–5 illustrates the midline distribution of hair and represents a modified scoring system for hirsutism that has been useful and has been adapted from the work of Ferriman, Gallwey, and Lorenzo.[16]

Virilization results from excessive amounts of androgen, with its defeminizing (antiestrogenic) and masculinizing actions. Any or all of the following signs constitute virilization: temporal balding, deepening of voice, decreased breast size, increased muscle mass, loss of female body contours, clitoral enlargement, and amenorrhea.

While virilism usually denotes an abnormal secretion of androgen from ovary or adrenal, it may also result occasionally in a more isolated form due to end-organ sensitivity. Progressive clitoral enlargement and temporal balding may occur with androgen levels that are not extremely high but that remain elevated for some time. Usually, however, a marked increase in androgen secretion, as occurs from neoplastic production, leads to a more full-blown picture of virilism over a short duration of time.

Virilism has been difficult to quantify, unlike the Ferriman–Gallwey and other scores used for hirsutism. Because clitoromegaly is often thought to be a cardinal finding in virilism, the use of the clitoral index may be useful.[17] This measurement determines the width and height of the glans clitoris. Any value >35 mm^2 is abnormal. Indeed, an important point to be stressed is that total clitoral length is relatively unimportant, but clitoral diameter at the glans (usually <7 mm) is what is important.

ANDROGEN AND HIRSUTISM

Three major concepts link androgen with hirsutism:

1. Androgen is necessary to recruit terminal hair development.
2. Androgen prolongs the time spent in anagen.
3. 5α-Reductase activity within the PSU modulates the androgenic signal.

On the scalp, a generally androgen-unresponsive area, anagen lasts 3 yr, whereas on the face it lasts approximately 4 mo if not abnormally stimulated by androgen. Telogen phases average 3 mo for both scalp and facial hair. The prolonged anagen of scalp hair explains the greater length of the hair in this area. Anagen on the thighs of men averages 54 days but is only 22 days in women. Moreover, axillary hair growth in men is 10

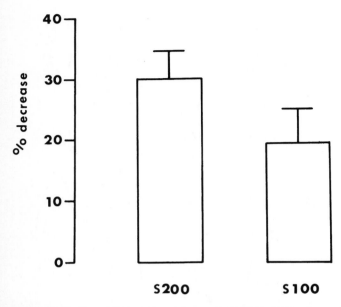

Figure 20–6. Percentage decrease in anagen hair shaft diameters with spironolactone (S) 200 and 100 mg. *(Reproduced, with permission, from Lobo RA, Shoupe D, Serafini P, et al. The effects of two doses of spironolactone on serum androgens and anagen hair in hirsute women. Fertil Steril. 43:200, 1985[42])*

percent faster than in women. Thus, with stimulation by androgen in androgen-responsive areas, the length of anagen is longer, terminal rather than vellus hairs appear, and the hair is thicker.

The latter findings, which explain hair density in hirsutism, have been inferred from antiandrogen therapy with both cyproterone acetate and spironolactone. A major effect of antiandrogen therapy is to convert terminal to vellus hairs. Figure 20–6 illustrates the dose–response effect of spironolactone in changing the thickness of anagen hair. This will be discussed in greater detail below.

Although the usual factors that control the shift between phases of hair growth remain elusive, androgen is known to be one factor that influences hair growth in responsive areas. It has long been assumed that androgen recruits the undifferentiated PSU with a dominant pillary component into a phase of growth or anagen.[18] However, although we do not adequately understand how hair in various phases of growth undergoes changes, the cyclicity of PSUs remains a major modulating factor in hirsutism.

The final and perhaps most important modulator of the biologic responses of androgens is 5α-reductase activity in PSUs. As discussed above, 5α-reductase is a pivotal enzyme that allows for an exaggeration or attenuation of the biologic signal (eg, levels of circulating unbound testosterone). If enzymatic activity is increased, hirsutism may result, whereas if there is a low level of activity, hirsutism may not occur even if circulating androgen levels are elevated. A schematic representation of this concept is illustrated in Figure 20–7. The level of 5α-reductase in

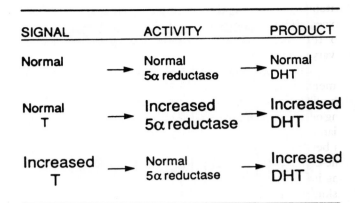

Figure 20–7. Influence of androgen substrate (signal, eg, testosterone or androstenedione) and 5α-reductase activity (in pilosebaceous units) on local production of biologically active androgens.

skin has been shown to correlate extremely well with the presence as well as severity of hirsutism in women.[11]

Androgens may accelerate and potentiate anagen. However, the balance between 5α-reductase activity and other enzymes influences hair growth. For example, in the scalp, which is not normally androgen responsive, 5α-reductase activity is low and hair cycles are more tightly controlled. However, in genital skin, where high 5α-reductase activity occurs, androgen and responsive hair growth are dominant. We used genital skin as a model to study 5α-reductase activity and the effects of androgen in women because the levels of the enzyme are highest in this site and representative of overall activity.

CAUSES OF ANDROGEN EXCESS

Only a limited number of disorders can cause hirsutism or virilization (Table 20–1). If one eliminates iatrogenic or drug-induced androgen excess, abnormal gonadal or sexual development (eg, androgen excess in conjunction with primary amenorrhea), and conditions unique to pregnancy (luteoma of pregnancy and hyperreactio

TABLE 20–1. DIFFERENTIAL DIAGNOSIS OF HIRSUTISM AND VIRILIZATION[a]

Source	Diagnosis
Nonspecific	Exogenous/iatrogenic; abnormal gonadal or sexual development
Peripheral	Idiopathic hirsutism
Ovarian	Polycystic ovary syndrome; stromal hyperthecosis; ovarian tumors
Adrenal	Adrenal tumors; Cushing syndrome; adult onset congenital adrenal hyperplasia

[a]Idiopathic hirsutism and polycystic ovary syndrome do not present with virilization.

luteinalis), there remain only seven causes of androgen excess. These have been listed in Table 20–1 according to the compartment or source of hyperandrogenism: ovary, adrenal, or peripheral.

When androgen excess is associated with primary amenorrhea, abnormal gonadal or sexual development should be strongly suspected. Furthermore, before embarking on a major workup for hirsutism or virilization, the physician is well advised to rule out exogenous androgen use. It is best to ask the patient to list all prescriptions and over-the-counter medications that she takes on her own, including injections. This is usually more rewarding than simply asking the patient whether she takes any androgens.

Medications that can cause hirsutism or virilization are related to testosterone. These include anabolic steroids, 19-norsteroids or synthetic progestins (eg, norethindrone, levo-norgestrel), and similar compounds (eg, danazol, an isoxazole derivative of 17α-ethinyl-testosterone).

A description of disorders associated with androgen excess and a simplified approach to the differential diagnosis of hirsutism and virilization follow.

"Idiopathic" Androgen Excess

Hirsutism labeled "idiopathic" (also referred to as constitutional or familial hirsutism) occurs more frequently in certain ethnic populations, particularly in women of Mediterranean ancestry. This common disorder associated with androgen excess, together with hyperandrogenic chronic anovulation (HCA) or PCOS, accounts for more than 90 percent of all patients presenting with hirsutism. It is defined as hirsutism in conjunction with regular menstrual cycles and normal levels of serum testosterone and DHEAS. Idiopathic hirsutism is never associated with any sign of virilization. Its cause has remained enigmatic for a long time. A relative increase in unbound or non-SHBG-bound testosterone has been thought responsible. However, unbound testosterone is not elevated in all women with clinical signs of the disorder and levels in normal and hirsute women overlap. Some investigators have suggested a subtle increase in either ovarian or adrenal production of androgens in this disorder. Even if this occurs, however, this elevation by itself is not of sufficient magnitude to explain the disorder.

A plausible hypothesis for the cause of idiopathic hirsutism is altered androgen action at the PSU due to increased 5α-reductase activity. As noted above, 3α-diol G has been found to be elevated in almost all hirsute patients. Recent work in our laboratory has also confirmed that there is increased 5α-reductase activity in the skin of patients with idiopathic hirsutism. However, in using our biochemical marker, 3α-diol G, not all patients will show an abnormality. In our original study, virtually all patients had elevated levels of 3α-diol G. With further experience and refinement in the assay, it was found that only 80 percent of patients will have elevated levels[19] (Fig 20–8).

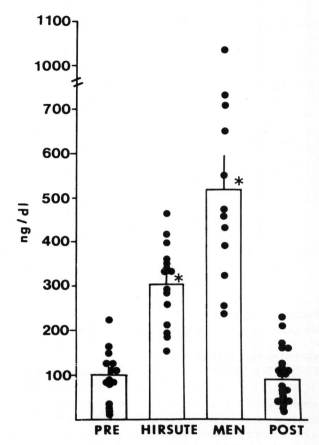

Figure 20–8. Serum 3α-androstenediol glucuronide (3α-diol G) in premenopausal nonhirsute women (PRE), hirsute women, normal men, and postmenopausal nonhirsute women (POST). The asterisks denote $P < .05$, as compared with PRE. *(Reproduced, with permission, from Paulson RJ, Serafini PC, Catalino JA, Lobo RA. Measurements of 3α-, 17β-androstenediol glucuronide in serum and urine and the correlation with skin 5α-reductase activity. Fertil Steril. 46:222, 1986[19])*

This suggests that idiopathic hirsutism is largely a misnomer and that, in fact, it is a disorder of peripheral androgen metabolism in the majority of patients. It also suggests that antiandrogen therapy, discussed below, which interferes with androgen action and 5α-reductase activity in the PSU, should be specific for this type of hirsutism.

A rare patient with idiopathic hirsutism may not have an androgen abnormality, even with measurements of skin 5α-reductase activity. In this situation, our contention has been that these rare patients have abnormalities in the cyclic process of hair growth and responsiveness of the hair follicle to trophic hormones and growth factors. Increased DNA content in the hair of some of these patients has been described.

HCA and PCOS

In brief, HCA is a combination of androgen excess and anovulation, usually manifested as hirsutism with oligomenorrhea, amenorrhea, or dysfunctional uterine bleeding.[20] PCOS is the "classic" form of HCA which includes the pathognomonic ovarian findings of polycystic changes. HCA or PCOS begins with menarche when both hirsutism and menstrual irregularities occur. Serum testosterone levels are usually mildly to moderately elevated but are generally below 1.5 ng/ml; levels of DHEAS may be normal or elevated, indicating an adrenal component of the disorder. Serum luteinizing hormone (LH) and the LH:follicle-stimulating hormone (FSH) ratio are typically, but not always, elevated.

HCA, in its broadest definition, which also includes adrenal androgen excess but not congenital adrenal hyperplasia (CAH), is probably the most common disorder associated with hirsutism.

Hirsutism is present in most (about 70 percent) but not all of these patients. Virilization, which requires higher serum testosterone levels, is virtually never encountered. The presence of virilization should raise the physician's suspicion of a more serious disorder.

Stromal Hyperthecosis

An occasional patient may give a history consistent with HCA or PCOS and present with slowly but persistently progressing signs of virilization, such as temporal balding, decreased breast size, and clitoral enlargement. Usually, such patients gain weight and muscle strength through the anabolic effect of their markedly increased ovarian testosterone production. Serum testosterone levels are markedly elevated above those seen in PCOS, whereas serum DHEAS levels are normal.

By the time this disorder has progressed to virilization, the serum testosterone level may be as high as in patients with androgen-producing tumors, often exceeding 2 ng/ml. However, stromal hyperthecosis is usually associated with a long history of anovulation and amenorrhea and of slowly but relentlessly progressing androgen excess, whereas androgen-producing tumors characteristically cause rapidly progressing signs of androgen excess.[21]

If retrograde ovarian vein catheterization is carried out and testosterone is measured in the ovarian venous effluent, it will be found that both ovaries produce large quantities of testosterone. Ovarian biopsy will reveal nests of luteinized theca cells within the stroma of bilaterally enlarged ovaries, which will have thickened capsules but lack the subcapsular cysts characteristic of PCOS.[22] The theca cells are thought to be the source of the excessive testosterone production.

Although LH levels are in the normal range, which also helps distinguish these patients from classic PCOS, there is evidence that the androgen levels are responsive to LH. The GnRH agonist has been used successfully to suppress androgen levels in hyperthecosis.[23]

Androgen-Producing Ovarian Tumors

This category includes Sertoli–Leydig cell tumors (formerly known as arrhenoblastomas), hilus cell tumors, lipoid cell (adrenal rest) tumors, and, infrequently, granulosa theca tumors. The androgen-producing ovarian stroma may also secrete excessive levels in association with other neoplasms such as epithelial cystadenomas, cystadenocarcinomas, Brenner tumors, or Krukenberg's tumors. Sertoli–Leydig cell tumors, which account for less than 1 percent of all solid ovarian tumors, tend to occur during the second to fourth decades of life, whereas hilus cell tumors occur more frequently in postmenopausal women.

By the time the signs and symptoms of androgen excess cause the patient to seek medical assistance, Sertoli–Leydig cell tumors are usually (in more than 85 percent of cases) so large that they are readily palpable on pelvic exam, while hilus cell tumors are still small. In women with either type of tumor, serum testosterone is much more elevated than serum DHEAS. Granulosa theca tumors primarily produce estradiol but may also produce testosterone.

Rapidly progressing symptoms of androgen excess should always suggest the presence of an androgen-producing tumor. This rapid progression is typical of both ovarian and adrenal androgen-producing tumors. The progression is usually from defeminizing signs (loss of female body contour, decrease in breast size) to the androgenic signs. As the tumor continues to grow, more and more testosterone is produced, resulting in rapidly worsening hirsutism and progressive virilization. With all ovarian tumors, except the lipoid cell tumors, serum testosterone is characteristically elevated in conjunction with normal or mildly elevated serum DHEAS levels. The lack of a significant increase in DHEAS distinguishes ovarian from adrenal androgen-producing tumors. The testosterone levels produced by certain ovarian tumors (eg, the Sertoli–Leydig cell tumor) may be suppressed with GnRH-A.[24] Therefore, use of GnRH-A cannot be relied upon to distinguish a neoplasm from another functional state.

In interpreting testosterone levels, the clinician should first be familiar with the normal ranges of the clinical laboratory used. A value of $2^{1}/_{2}$ times the upper normal range is suggestive of a neoplasm, particularly if the clinical history supports the possible diagnosis.

Once an elevated level is found and confirmed by clinical history, ovarian ultrasound should be able to detect the abnormality. It is important to remember that these tumors are unilateral in location.

Androgen-Producing Adrenal Tumors

These can be classified as adenomas and carcinomas (non-testosterone-producing) and testosterone-producing adenomas. Testosterone-producing adrenal adenomas are much more rare. Their cells resemble ovarian hilus cells, which are analogous to Leydig cells. These tumor cells produce testosterone and are stimulated by both LH and hCG. Thus, in patients with testosterone-producing adrenal adenomas, testosterone secretion usually decreases after LH suppression and increases after hCG stimulation.

Most commonly, androgen-producing adrenal adenomas and carcinomas secrete large quantities of DHEAS, DHEA, and androstenedione; testosterone is produced by extraglandular conversion of these prehormones and may also be secreted directly by the tumor. Levels of serum DHEAS are highly elevated. When DHEAS levels exceed 8 µg/ml, a scan either by computed axial tomography (CAT) or magnetic resonance imaging (MRI) should be ordered unless the history is more suggestive of PCOS (long onset and no virilization). In this case, a functional abnormality of the adrenal is likely to be present: either an enzymatic defect, such as CAH, or an unexplained hyperfunctional state. Under these circumstances, the scan can be deferred until further investigation has been carried out (eg, ACTH, dexamethasone).

Adrenal adenomas and carcinomas may produce various corticosteroids and sex hormones in various combinations. It is therefore impossible to establish a definite hormonal pattern that is pathognomonic of all tumors of this type. In general, high levels of serum DHEAS (>8 µg/ml) suggest an adrenal adenoma or carcinoma. Although the adrenal normally does not produce testosterone, an adrenal adenoma may be testosterone producing. If a patient has a history compatible with a tumor and the ovaries are normal on palpation and ultrasonography, the adrenal should be evaluated next.

Small Neoplasms of the Ovary or Adrenal

The diagnosis of small neoplasms of the ovary or adrenal may be challenging. In general, testosterone levels $2^{1}/_{2}$ times the upper normal range and DHEAS levels >8 µg/ml have been used to help with the diagnosis. However, there are several exceptions to this general principle:

1. Because tumors secrete androgens episodically, more than one value may be required.[25]
2. Different precursor steroids are often elevated as well (particularly androstenedione) and their measurement should be considered.
3. Androgen levels in postmenopausal women may be considerably lower (testosterone levels of 100 ng/dl and DHEAS levels of 4 µg/ml are abnormal and suspicious for a tumor).[26]
4. Any virilized patient warrants further investigation.

Because androgen-secreting tumors are usually virilizing, the presence of severe symptoms and signs, even if testosterone and/or DHEAS are not sufficiently high, warrants further investigation. With improvements in scanning techniques—vaginal ultrasound (which is most useful for

the ovary, particularly with color flow Doppler), CAT, and MRI—the diagnosis of even a small tumor may be easily made. However, if no neoplasm can be localized then selective venous catheterization is necessary (this technique is valuable only if carried out by an experienced angiographer). Imaging of the ovary or adrenal after administration of labeled iodomethylnorcholesterol (NP-59) (which should "light up" active steroid-producing tumors) has also proved useful.[27] If available, this procedure may preclude the need for catheterization studies, especially in cases that are difficult to manage. Figure 20–9 illustrates a proposed scheme for the management of cases of elevated testosterone, particularly if the history is suggestive of a tumor.

Cushing Syndrome

Cushing syndrome is caused by excessive production of glucocorticoid hormones. This may be due to increased hypothalamic–pituitary ACTH secretion, adrenal adenomas or carcinomas, or ectopic ACTH secretion such as with bronchogenic carcinoma. The well-known clinical findings of Cushing syndrome are centripetal obesity; abdominal striae; supraclavicular and dorsal neck fat pads; muscle wasting and weakness; thin skin with easy

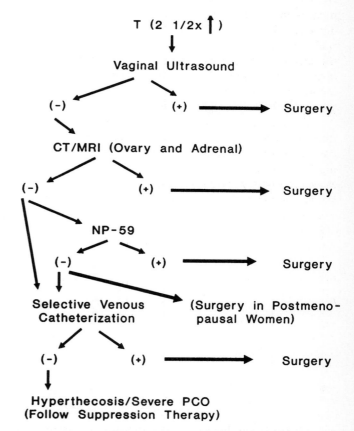

Figure 20–9. Proposed evaluation of a patient with elevated serum testosterone, a history compatible with an androgen-producing neoplasm and/or virilization.

bruising; fine hair (lanugo hair) on face, back, and extremities; hypertension, potassium loss, and alkalosis; overt or latent diabetes mellitus; osteoporosis; amenorrhea; and psychosis. Serum cortisol levels are increased and lack the typical diurnal cyclicity.

It is extremely unusual for a patient to present with Cushing syndrome with the chief complaint of hirsutism. However, on the basis of the clinical findings, if Cushing syndrome cannot be ruled out an overnight dexamethasone suppression test and/or measurements of urinary free cortisol are indicated. Dexamethasone (1.0 mg) is given orally at 11:00 PM and plasma cortisol is measured at 8:00 AM the next morning. If plasma cortisol is suppressed to less than 5 µg/100 ml, Cushing syndrome is ruled out. If cortisol is not suppressed, a further evaluation for Cushing syndrome is indicated. Urinary free cortisol levels above 250 µg/24 hr are suspicious.

Adult-Onset CAH

Although some controversy exists, it is clear that adult-onset (attenuated or incomplete) CAH does exist. This form of CAH is caused by a partial deficiency in 21hydroxylase ac-

tivity. The clinical presentation is identical to that of patients with HCA/PCOS.[28] The prevalence of this disorder varies according to ethnic background (frequency of genetic disequilibrium); the prevalence reported by different investigators has varied widely. Patients of northern European ancestry have a low frequency of this disorder, whereas Ashkenazi Jews, Hispanics, and patients of central European ancestry have a much higher prevalence.[29] Therefore, it is recommended that high-risk ethnic groups be screened. Screening may first be carried out by obtaining an early morning (8:00 AM) serum 17-hydroxyprogesterone (17-OHP) level. Because 17-OHP levels normally rise in the luteal phase due to ovarian production, values have to exceed 3 ng/ml to be elevated. However, baseline 17-OHP levels may be less than 3 ng/ml in cases involving only a mild 21-hydroxylase defect, which requires an ACTH stimulation test to diagnose. Patients with ovarian hyperandrogenism (eg, PCOS) may also have basal 17-OHP levels up to 5 ng/ml. The only way to distinguish CAH from PCOS under these circumstances would be with an ACTH test[30] (Fig 20–l0).

Besides the attenuated form of CAH, which presents like PCOS, 21-hydroxylase deficiency may also be

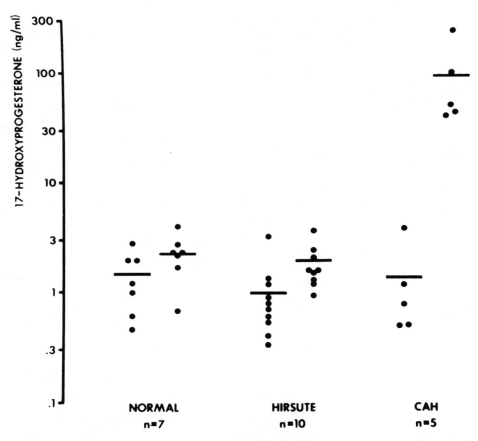

Figure 20–10. Serum 17-hydroxyprogesterone before and 60 min after intravenous administration of a single bolus of 0.25 mg ACTH in 7 normal female control and 10 hirsute oligomenorrheic women and in 5 patients with congenital adrenal hyperplasia. *(Reproduced, with permission, from Lobo RA, Goebelsmann U. Adult manifestation of congenital adrenal hyperplasia due to incomplete 21-hydroxylase deficiency mimicking polycystic ovarian disease. Am J Obstet Gynecol. 138:720, 1980[28])*

"cryptic" and may occur in the absence of hirsutism. The diagnosis can be made only by ACTH stimulation. Random ACTH testing in asymptomatic patients may be indicated only in families in whom there is a high prevalence of the disorder. In general, it is not an approach to be advocated. Other details of this disorder may be found in other chapters.

We do not routinely administer ACTH to all hirsute patients. In a patient with androgen excess who belongs to an ethnic group of high CAH prevalence, early morning (8:00 AM) 17-OHP should be measured. Also, the following patients should have a screening baseline 17-OHP level obtained: symptomatic patients who are young, women with a significant degree of androgen excess or virilization, patients with strong family histories of androgen excess, women with high levels of androgens, and patients with hypertension and androgen excess.

If basal 17-OHP levels are >8 ng/ml, the diagnosis of CAH is clear. (ACTH stimulation may still be done to confirm the diagnosis and determine whether 11-deoxycortisol is also elevated. Elevation of this steroid would suggest a case of the much more rare disorder, 11-hydroxylase deficiency. This uncommon disorder is sometimes associated with hypertension, while 21-hydroxylase is not. Whereas 11-hydroxylase is an autosomal recessive trait, it is not associated with human leukocyte antigen haplotypes nor is it known to be clustered in particular ethnic groups.) If basal levels of 17-OHP are between 3 and 8 ng/ml, an ACTH stimulation test is needed to distinguish CAH from other causes of hyperandrogenemia. Many methods have been used to diagnose CAH according to the 17-OHP response after ACTH (with and without dexamethasone pretreatment). We pretreat with 1 mg dexamethasone given at 11:00 PM prior to the day of the test. After 0.25 mg intravenous ACTH 1-14 (Cosyntropin), we diagnose CAH if the 60-min 17-OHP value is >20 ng/ml. However, other approaches can also be used, and recent evidence suggests that dexamethasone pretreatment is not necessary. A rise of 17-OHP as low as 10 ng/ml 60 min after ACTH has been considered diagnostic. A useful nomogram has been developed by New et al for the diagnosis utilizing basal and ACTH-stimulated values of 17-OHP[31] (Fig 20–11). Recent data have also concurred with our view of using early morning basal values as a primary screening procedure. Values as low as 2 ng/ml in the absence of ovulatory function have been considered diagnostic.

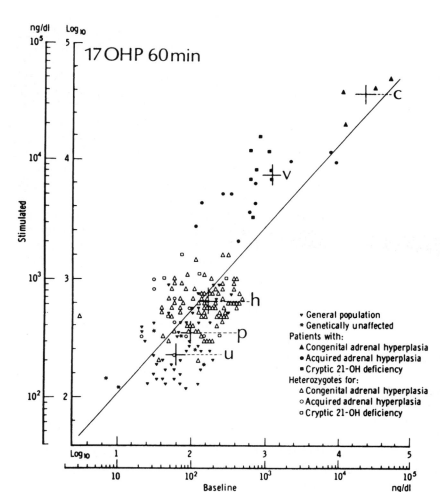

Figure 20–11. Nomogram relating baseline and 60-min ACTH-stimulated serum 17-hydroxyprogesterone concentrations. The mean values for each group are as follows: (c), congenital adrenal hyperplasia (CAH); (v), patients with nonclassic symptomatic or asymptomatic (cryptic, acquired, or late-onset) 21-hydroxylase (21-OH) deficiency; (h), heterozygotes for classic CAH, nonclassic symptomatic CAH (acquired or late-onset adrenal hyperplasia), and nonclassic asymptomatic CAH (cryptic 21-OH deficiency); (u), family members predicted by human lymphocytes antigen genotyping to be unaffected; and (p), general population (not human lymphocytes antigen genotyped). *(Reproduced, with permission, from New MI, Lorenzen F, Lerner AJ, et al. Genotyping steroid 21-hydroxylase deficiency: Hormonal reference data.* J Clin Endocrinol Metab. *57:320, 1983[31])*

Other enzymatic deficiencies may also result in hirsutism. The most common of these is 3β-hydroxysteroid-dehydrogenase isomerase deficiency.[32] A defect in 17-ketoreductase has also been postulated. The latter defect usually results in ambiguous genitalia and hirsutism in a 46,XY individual, but a milder form has been thought to give rise to patients diagnosed to have PCOS.[33]

THERAPY

Therapy for hirsutism and virilization should be directed toward its specific cause and at suppression of abnormal androgen secretion. Treatment of specific causes will be discussed first.

Specific treatments for hirsutism and virilization would be indicated for the following conditions: ovarian and adrenal tumors, stromal hyperthecosis, and the adrenal causes (Cushing syndrome and CAH).

Neoplasms warrant surgical intervention and will not be discussed in greater detail at this time. The ovarian hyperandrogenism of stromal hyperthecosis may be suppressed with a GnRH agonist or the older patients with this disease may prefer surgery with oophorectomy being performed. Patients with adrenal disease are treated specifically. For Cushing syndrome, this is according to the source of hypercortisolism and corticosteroid suppression used for patients with CAH. Greater details on such therapy may be found elsewhere.

Suppression According to the Abnormality

The approach advocated here is the specific suppression of the abnormal compartment, be it ovary, adrenal, or periphery. In some circumstances, there is more than one source contributing to the hyperandrogenism.

Ovarian Suppression. Listed in Table 20–2 are agents that have an inhibitory effect on ovarian androgen production. Some of these (eg, oral contraceptives) have a principal role in ovarian suppression while others, such as corticosteroids, do not exhibit major effects but can influence steroidogenesis to some degree because of gonadotropin suppression.

Oral Contraceptives. If testosterone is elevated, ovarian hyperandrogenism is best suppressed with oral contraceptives. The combination of progestin and synthetic estrogen decreases LH-dependent ovarian androgen production. Also, the estrogen increases the production of SHBG such that the lowered androgen (testosterone) is more avidly bound, yielding much lower serum unbound testosterone levels. Therefore, progestins alone are less effective than combination oral contraceptives. Certain oral contraceptives will decrease adrenal androgen production by at least 30 percent and will be helpful with

TABLE 20–2. AGENTS AVAILABLE TO INHIBIT VARIOUS SOURCES OF ANDROGEN PRODUCTION

Ovarian
  Oral contraceptives
  Progestins, including depo-medroxyprogesterone acetate
  Gonadotropin-releasing hormone agonist
  Antiandrogens (cyproterone acetate, spironolactone)
  Ketoconazole
  Corticosteroids

Adrenal
  Corticosteroids
  Oral contraceptives
  Spironolactone
  Ketoconazole

Peripheral
  Cyproterone acetate
  Spironolactone
  Cimetidine
  Flutamide
  Progesterone (topical)
  Oral contraceptives
  5α-Reductase inhibitors

mild adrenal function (DHEAS levels <4 µg/ml).[34] Oral contraceptives may also have an inhibitory effect on 5α-reductase activity and in inhibiting androgen receptor action. However, these latter effects are relatively mild.

In choosing an oral contraceptive, 35 µg ethinylestradiol is sufficient to increase SHBG significantly; therefore, treatment with higher-dose estrogen pills should not be routine. However, there is much more latitude with the progestin component. The most androgenic 19-norgestogen is levo-norgestrel. Thus, it is best to avoid formulations such as Ovral and Lo/Ovral. Ethynodiol diacetate (Demulen 1/35) is least androgenic and somewhat estrogenic. Norethindrone and its acetate are only mildly androgenic. Least androgenic are the oral contraceptive formulations containing norgestimate and desogestrel. These low-dose pills (eg, Orthocyclen, Orthocept, Desogen) offer a theoretical advantage in being potent oral contraceptives yet more estrogen dominant and only very weakly androgenic.

Progestins. Medroxyprogesterone acetate in doses of 20 to 40 mg daily suppresses LH and ovarian and androgen production by 50 to 70 percent. Medroxyprogesterone acetate may also increase the hepatic clearance of testosterone, resulting in a 23 percent increase in its metabolic clearance. However, because SHBG is unaffected, unbound testosterone is not decreased to a major extent. Intramuscular depo-medroxyprogesterone acetate has been used effectively, but because of the persistence of serum levels for up to 9 mo after a single injection we have not recommended its routine use in women of reproductive age.

GnRH Agonist. The GnRH agonist is a useful agent for suppressing ovarian androgen production. However, GnRH agonists have not yet been approved for this indication. Daily treatment of patients with PCOS using the GnRH agonist subcutaneously reduced ovarian androgen levels into the oophorectomized range over 4 wk[6] (Fig 20–1). Although immunoreactive LH is not dramatically reduced, LH bioactivity decreases significantly. GnRH agonists have been shown to be effective in treating hirsutism in combination with either estrogen replacement or an oral contraceptive. While added estrogen alleviates many of the side effects of GnRH agonist therapy, it does not detract from the efficacy of this treatment and may even enhance it.[35–37] Figure 20–12 suggests the added benefits of estrogen on suppressing androgen and clinical parameters. We have shown that GnRH-A therapy with added estrogen is as effective as high-dose cyproterone acetate therapy. Cyproterone acetate (an antiandrogen with gonadotropin-suppressing effects) has been used worldwide (except in the United States) for patients with significant complaints of hirsutism.

Antiandrogens. Among antiandrogens, two in particular are known for their inhibition of ovarian androgen production: cyproterone acetate and spironolactone. These properties have to be viewed as secondary to the major role of antiandrogens, that of blocking androgen effects in peripheral tissue.

Cyproterone acetate is most studied in this regard. It is available in Europe, Canada, and other countries but not in the United States. Cyproterone acetate was developed as a progestin and is a C21 steroid with a progestational potency similar to that of medroxyprogesterone acetate. As a progestin, it inhibits LH and androgen production. Cyproterone acetate is usually prescribed with ethinylestradiol, as described in greater detail below. In doses of 50 mg, cyproterone acetate is responsible for a variable reduction of androstenedione and testosterone that may be up to 50 percent of baseline values.[38]

Spironolactone is an aldosterone antagonist with a major inhibitory effect on peripheral androgen metabolism. However, it inhibits cytochrome P_{450}-linked enzymes involved in ovarian, testicular, and adrenal steroidogenesis.[39,40] In addition to the decrease in testosterone production, an increase in the metabolic clearance of testosterone has been reported.[41] In most patients studied, LH has not been noted to decrease and may be higher in earlier stages of treatment. This suggests that the inhibition of androgen production is primarily due to enzymatic inhibition. The inhibition is dose related. Unbound testosterone levels are usually not affected and SHBG is not suppressed.[42] Adrenal androstenedione production is decreased, but serum DHEAS levels are not affected.

The principal effects of the antiandrogens are in inhibiting the peripheral compartment. However, these inhibiting effects on ovarian and adrenal steroidogenesis are an important adjunct to therapy, particularly in the patients with PCO. In the hirsute, hyperandrogenic patient with idiopathic hypertension, spironolactone may

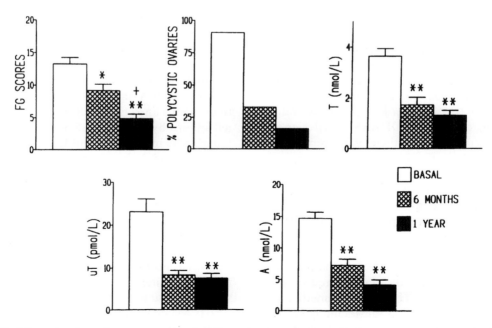

Figure 20–12. Effect of prolonged treatment with a GnRH agonist plus low doses of estrogens and progestin. *(Reproduced with permission from Carmina E, Janni A, Lobo RA. Physiological estrogen replacement may enhance the effectiveness of the gonadotropin-releasing hormone agonist in the treatment of hirsutism.* J Clin Endocrinol Metab. *78:126, 1994.)*

be useful, whereas oral contraceptives may be relatively contraindicated.

Ketoconazole. Ketoconazole, an imidazole derivative, inhibits ergosterol synthesis in fungi. However, in larger doses it interferes with glandular cytochrome P_{450}-linked steroidogenesis.[43] Its principal inhibitory role involves inhibition of the 17,20-desmolase step in steroidogenesis, which explains why androgen suppression is greater than with cortisol, although both adrenal and ovary are affected. In addition, ketoconazole inhibits cholesterol side-chain cleavage as well as 17-, 11-, and 18-hydroxylase activities.

Some clinical experience has been gained with ketoconazole in the treatment of Cushing syndrome and prostatic cancer. However, because of its significant ovarian suppressive effects, its use has been suggested for ovarian androgen suppression in hirsutism. Improvement has been noted with 400 mg/day in PCO,[44] as well as with 1000 mg/day in stromal hyperthecosis.

There is some concern about side effects, which include gastrointestinal complaints, pruritus, and alterations in hepatic function. Although some 10 percent of patients may have some transient hepatic dysfunction, true hepatotoxicity is rare (<1 percent) and apparently is not increased by the use of larger doses (up to 1200 mg/day).

Adrenal Suppression. Several agents may be used to suppress adrenal androgen production (Table 20–2). The principal agents are glucocorticoids and oral contraceptives.

Corticosteroids. Dexamethasone and prednisone are the two corticosteroids that have been most studied and adrenal androgens are extremely sensitive to corticosteroid suppression. There is some evidence that dexamethasone sensitivity may not be reflected solely by elevated levels of DHEAS. Nevertheless, we have relied heavily upon elevated levels of DHEAS or 11β-A as criteria for choosing corticosteroid therapy. Extremely low doses of dexamethasone effectively suppress adrenal androgen production and this suppression is greater than that of cortisol.[45] This provides for a certain margin of safety in that the ACTH–cortisol axis is not overwhelmingly suppressed. Moreover, after cessation of corticosteroid suppression, adrenal androgens remain suppressed for a longer period.[46]

For these reasons, low doses of dexamethasone have been advocated (0.25 mg), usually administered at night to suppress the nocturnal ACTH surge. Dexamethasone, being more potent and having less salt-retaining properties than prednisone, offers some advantages. However, for the same reasons, the margin of safety in terms of oversuppression and cushingoid changes favors the use

of prednisone, which is recommended for long-term use. Equivalent doses of prednisone (2.5 to 5 mg) may be used. At this small dose, salt-retaining properties of dexamethasone and prednisone are negligible. It has been suggested that, for adrenal androgen suppression, alternate-day prednisone therapy may be safer and as effective. However, there is no evidence for such an advantage.

There is, however, considerable variability in adrenal responses (DHEAS and cortisol) to suppression. This, in part, is due to the diverse etiologies of hyperandrogenism, but occurs also because of individual differences in the metabolism of corticosteroids. It is imperative, therefore, to measure DHEAS as a marker of suppression. Significant suppression usually occurs by 2 wk and doses should be adjusted to maintain DHEAS levels below 1 µg/ml. Although monitoring weight, blood pressure, and symptoms is important, it has been suggested that the measurement of 8:00 AM cortisol levels aids therapy in preventing excessive suppression.[47] Doses may be titrated to keep cortisol levels detectable, at least around 2 µg/dl. In most patients who need to have adrenal androgens suppressed, low doses are sufficient. However, in patients with a significant ACTH drive, such as those with CAH, doses near or equal to full adrenal replacement may be required (eg, 0.5 to 0.75 mg dexamethasone or 5 to 7.5 mg prednisone).

When larger doses of corticosteroids are used, it is imperative to increase coverage during times of stress and/or infection. Because of such concerns, long-term corticosteroid therapy should be prescribed only with clear-cut indications. Minor elevations in levels of DHEAS may not be significant and may allow for suppression with alternative regimens such as oral contraceptives.

In dexamethasone-sensitive patients, in spite of complete normalization of androgen levels, hirsutism is only modestly suppressed.[48] Indeed, even in those patients with a known adrenal abnormality, such as congenital adrenal hyperplasia, use of an antiandrogen has been found to be more efficacious than dexamethasone.[49] Our preference, therefore, is not to use dexamethasone as a primary agent for hirsutism and to use it selectively for adjunctive therapy in certain individuals.

Oral Contraceptives. Whether it is the progestin component alone that might interfere with steroidogenesis or the combination of progestin with ethinylestradiol, it is clear that most oral contraceptives suppress adrenal androgens significantly. The magnitude of this decrement varies from 30 to 60 percent in terms of DHEAS levels.

It has been postulated that oral contraceptives may exert a direct inhibitory role on cytochrome P_{450} or decrease the ACTH drive. Lower doses of oral contraceptives (30 to 35 µg of ethinylestradiol) appear to be equally effective in suppressing DHEAS. This effect does not appear to be related to the progestin dose (1 or 0.4 mg norethindrone having similar effects), but may be related to the type of progestin.[50] In our study, levo-norgestrel did not appear to be as effective. Because of the simplicity of this approach and the overall safety of oral contraceptives, this agent should be the drug of choice for patients with only mild to moderate elevations in DHEAS (<5 μg/ml). Testosterone, both total and unbound, should also be lowered even if they are initially in the normal range. In addition, there is the potential for a direct peripheral inhibitory effect of oral contraceptives that will be discussed below.

Our data[48] suggest that in hirsute patients with a proven dexamethasone sensitivity, corticosteroid suppression does not provide ideal therapeutic efficacy despite euandrogenemia. Thus, although androgen levels are well suppressed by dexamethasone or prednisone, hirsutism scores are only seen to decrease substantially if a peripheral blocking agent such as spironolactone is used. These data also provide evidence that peripheral events, specifically, 5α-reductase activity, are the most important determinants of hirsutism.

Suppression of the Peripheral Compartment.

The goal of this therapy is to block androgen action at peripheral sites such as the PSU. This is directed at competitive inhibition of the androgen receptor and inhibition of 5α-reductase activity. The principal agents having these properties are listed in Table 20–2.

Cyproterone acetate is mostly administered in doses of 50 to 100 mg from days 5 through 15 of the cycle. Because of its slow metabolism, it is administered early in the cycle whereas ethinylestradiol, when added, is usually ingested at 50-μg doses between days 5 and 26. This regimen is needed for menstrual control and is usually referred to as the reverse sequential regimen. In smaller doses (2 mg), cyproterone acetate has been administered as an oral contraceptive in daily combination with 50 or 35 μg ethinylestradiol (Diane). This regimen is primarily suited for individuals with a milder form of hyperandrogenism.

Apart from inhibition of the androgen receptor, there is some evidence that cyproterone acetate and ethinylestradiol in combination can inhibit 5α-reductase activity in skin.[51] This competitive inhibition is probably related to cyproterone acetate itself but is poorly documented. Clinical improvement of hyperandrogenism with cyproterone acetate is considered excellent. Metabolic changes, which may be subtle, do occur with the reverse sequential regimen. There is a tendency toward hyperinsulinemia and glucose intolerance in patients ingesting cyproterone acetate. Also, there are small decrements in high-density lipoprotein cholesterol, although the ratio of total high-density lipoprotein/low-density lipoprotein rises.

Cimetidine. This H_2 receptor antagonist is included here for its known androgen receptor-inhibiting properties. However, it appears to be relatively weak and, in clinical terms, is ineffective for the treatment of hirsutism.

Flutamide. Flutamide is a nonsteroidal compound that inhibits the androgen receptor and is considered a pure antiandrogen.[52] At high doses, it may reduce the synthesis of androgens or increase their metabolism.[53,54]

Several studies, using different doses of the product (ranging from 250 to 750 mg/day), have shown that flutamide is an effective therapy of hirsutism.[55–57] Concerns have been expressed about side effects—mostly hepatotoxicity[58]—that can appear with high doses (500 to 750 mg/day) but have been reported with doses of 375 mg/day as well.[6]

Although prolonged experience with flutamide is lacking, current protocols call for use of this agent at low doses (250 to 500 mg/day) accompanied by monitoring of liver enzymes. With these precautions, flutamide is probably safe and can be considered an alternative to other antiandrogen products.

In terms of efficacy, 100 mg of spironolactone has a therapeutic effect similar to that seen with 250 to 500 mg of flutamide.

Spironolactone. Spironolactone is an excellent inhibitor of the androgen receptor. In this regard, it appears far superior to the action of cyproterone acetate. It is postulated that spironolactone couples with the receptor to create a biologically inactive spironolactone–receptor complex.

Apart from the inhibition of steroidogenesis referred to previously and the inhibition of the androgen receptor, spironolactone has a significant effect in inhibiting 5α-reductase activity. This has been shown in vitro as well as in vivo[42] (Fig 20–6). These and several clinical studies clearly point to the efficacy of spironolactone for hyperandrogenism and suggest that the principal effect is in its peripheral blocking ability.

Doses of spironolactone have varied in clinical studies from 50 to 200 mg daily. We have found a dose–response difference in patients treated and suggested that most patients require at least 100 mg if not 200 mg.[42] In Europe, doses up to 400 mg have been used safely.

In patients with normal renal function, hyperkalemia is almost never seen. Hypotension is rare except in older women. Monitoring, however, is imperative for electrolytes and blood pressure within the first 2 wk at each dose level. Adjustments in dose should only be made after 3 to 6 mo, as with other antiandrogens, to account for changes in the hair cycle. Patients usually note an initial transient diuretic effect, but many women with normal cycles will complain of menstrual irregularity on spironolactone. The latter complaint is remedied by either a downward dose adjustment or the addition of a low-dose oral contraceptive. The mechanism for abnormal bleeding is unclear. In women with oligomenorrhea, such as those with PCOS, resumption of normal menses may occur. In part, this may be due to an alteration in levels of circulating androgens,[59] although LH levels have only occasionally been noted to decrease.

Both spironolactone and canrenone, its major metabolite, have been used topically with some success.[60] There is evidence that with a 5 percent cream mixture delivering 25 mg canrenone daily to the skin peripheral levels are not affected. However, for practical reasons, this therapy is useful only for fairly localized types of hirsutism.

Progesterone (Topical). Topical therapy in general will not be covered in detail here. However, this is an area of emerging interest. Cyproterone acetate, spironolactone (or canrenone), progesterone, and other specific 5α-reductase inhibitors have been studied topically. None of these has been marketed for use.

Progesterone, being the classical 5α-reductase inhibitor, has been used with some success.[61] Liposomal formulations are most useful in this regard. The major drawback of the use of progesterone in general is its rapid dissipation, creating the need for frequent doses.

Oral contraceptives appear to have some peripheral blocking effect, although this effect is of secondary importance. The inhibitory effect of oral contraceptives is due, in part, to the inhibitory effect of the progestin on 5α-reductase activity and the effect of estrogen in inhibiting androgen action at a postreceptor site.[62]

5α-Reductase Inhibitors

Specific 5α-reductase inhibitors are available and have been studied in animal models. Inhibition of rat, human, and dog prostatic tissue of 5α-reductase activities has been demonstrated. The 4-azasteroids are considered pure inhibitors because they are devoid of specific effects on the androgen receptor.[63]

Finasteride. Finasteride, a drug that inhibits 5α-reductase activity, has been mostly used for the treatment of prostatic hyperplasia.[63] It can also be used in the treatment of hirsutism.[64-66] At a dose of 5 mg/day, a significant improvement of hirsutism is observed after 6 mo of therapy, without significant side effects. In hirsute women, the decline in DHT levels is small and cannot be used to monitor therapy. Although this treatment regimen increases testosterone levels, SHBG levels remain unaffected (Fig 20–13).[64]

Finasteride primarily inhibits type II 5α-reductase activity. As hirsutism is a combination of type I and type II effects, this agent was expected to be only partially effective. Our own data suggest an overall efficacy similar to that seen with 100 mg of spironolactone.[64]

Although prolonged experience with finasteride is lacking, one of the potential advantages of this agent appears to be its benign side-effect profile. A recent study showed efficacy with 1 yr of treatment.[67] More studies, however, are needed to establish the role of this product in the therapy of hirsutism.

Treatment Choices and Follow-Up

Although treatment has been presented based on an approach of suppressing the compartment which is abnormal, in reality and for practical reasons, patients will be

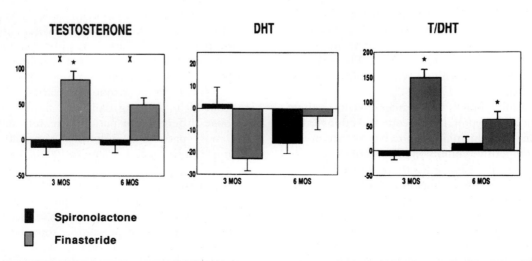

Figure 20–13. Serum testosterone and DHT changes after treatment with spironolactone or finasteride. *(Reproduced with permission from Wong IL, Morris RS, Chang L, et al. A prospective randomized trial comparing finasteride to spironolactone in the treatment of hirsute women. J Clin Endocrinol Metab. 80:233, 1995.)*

treated with an agent to suppress only the ovary and/or the peripheral compartment. Even in those women with a "pure" peripheral abnormality (idiopathic hirsutism), the addition of an oral contraceptive can improve efficacy and prevent abnormal bleeding. For women with only minor complaints of hirsutism, the use of an oral contraceptive alone may be an appropriate first approach.

In general, no responses should be expected for hirsutism before 3 mo. Objective means should be used to assess changes in hair growth. Whereas scoring systems and evaluation of anagen hair shafts are difficult, photographs may be used. Pictures of selected midline body areas before and during therapy have been useful. Patients are often unaware that change is indeed taking place unless there is some objective measurement; this is often essential in dealing with the psychological needs of the patient.

Once androgen levels are suppressed and some change is occurring, existent hair should be removed; this is best accomplished by electrolysis. Tweezing, in particular, is not a good method, as the irritant to PSUs may induce growth in surrounding areas.

The overall expected successful response rate is approximately 70 percent by 9 mo to 1 yr. Patients should be encouraged to continue treatment for at least 1 yr if not 2. After this, depending upon the wishes and clinical responses of patients, therapy can be stopped and the patient re-evaluated. Although in some patients hirsutism does not recur, in many treatment may need to be reinitiated.

Regression of virilism due to a tumor or stromal hyperthecosis occurs gradually, and while body contour and muscle mass change fairly rapidly temporal balding and clitoromegaly may not completely resolve. In those rare women who develop clitoral hypertrophy due to an increased end-organ sensitivity to androgens and do not have a neoplasm, clitoral reductive surgery may be indicated.

SUMMARY

Androgen excess in women exhibits a variety of manifestations but may be cryptic where hyperandrogenemia does not result in the typical skin manifestations. While hirsutism is fairly common, virilization is rare in women and denotes a more serious underlying disorder. The expression of hirsutism is largely explained by "peripheral" or skin 5α-reductase activity. An approach to the differential diagnosis of hirsutism is discussed where "peripheral," ovarian, and adrenal causes are distinguished. Overlap does exist between these "compartments" of androgen production. High levels of ovarian and adrenal androgen often signify tumors and warrant further evaluation by sensitive imaging techniques. This is of particu-

lar importance in the case of virilism. Treatment should be directed toward the offending cause. While the treatment of tumors is surgical, in other often mixed causes, suppression of androgen production and peripheral blockade are the mainstay of therapy. The most successful treatments for hirsutism involve peripheral blockade.

REFERENCES

1. Bardin CW, Lipsett MB. Testosterone and androstenedione blood production rates in normal women and women with idiopathic hirsutism or polycystic ovaries. *J Clin Invest.* 46:891, 1967
2. Lobo RA, Paul WL, Goebelsmann U. Dehydroepiandrosterone sulfate as an indicator of adrenal androgen function. *Obstet Gynecol.* 57:69, 1981
3. Bird CE, Morrow L, Fukumoto Y, et al. Δ^5-Androstenediol: Kinetics of metabolism and binding to plasma proteins in normal men and women. *J Clin Endocrinol Metab.* 43:1317, 1976
4. Stanczyk FZ, Chang L, Carmina E, et al. Is 11β-hydroxyandrostenedione a better marker of adrenal androgen excess than dehydroepiandrosterone sulfate? *Am J Obstet Gynecol.* 165:1837, 1991
5. Moltz L, Schwartz UD. Gonadal and adrenal androgen secretion in hirsute females. In: Horton R, Lobo RA, eds. *Androgen Metabolism in Hirsute and Normal Females. Clinics in Endocrinology and Metabolism*, vol 15. Philadelphia, Pa., W. B. Saunders, 1986: 229–245
6. Chang RJ, Laufer LR, Meldrum DR, et al. Steroid secretion in polycystic ovarian disease after ovarian suppression by a long-acting gonadotropin-releasing hormone agonist. *J Clin Endocrinol Metab.* 56:897, 1983
7. Carmina E, Gonazalez F, Chang L, Lobo RA. Reassessment of adrenal androgen secretion in women with polycystic ovary syndrome. *Obstet Gynecol.* 85:971, 1995
8. Rosenfield RL. Relationship of androgens to female hirsutism and infertility. *J Reprod Med.* 11:87, 1973
9. Morimoto I, Edmiston A, Hawks D, Horton R. Studies on the origin of androstenediol and androstenediol glucuronide in young and elderly men. *J Clin Endocrinol Metab.* 52:772, 1981
10. Lobo RA, Goebelsmann U, Horton R. Evidence for the importance of peripheral tissue events in the development of hirsutism in polycystic ovary syndrome. *J Clin Endocrinol Metab.* 57:393, 1983
11. Serafini P, Lobo RA. Increased 5α-reductase activity in idiopathic hirsutism. *Fertil Steril.* 43:74, 1985
12. Carmina E, Stanczyk FZ, Matteri RK, Lobo RA. Serum androsterone conjugates differentiate between acne and hirsutism in hyperandrogenic women. *Fertil Steril.* 55:872, 1991
13. Mowszowicz I, Melanitou E, Doukani A, et al. Androgen binding capacity and 5α-reductase activity in pubic skin fibroblasts from hirsute patients. *J Clin Endocrinol Metab.* 56:1209, 1983
14. Cumming DC, Wall SR. Non-sex hormone binding globulin-bound testosterone as a marker for hyperandrogenism. *J Clin Endocrinol Metab.* 61:873, 1985

15. Schwartz U, Moltz L, Brotherton J, Hammerstein J. The diagnostic value of plasma free testosterone in non-tumorous and tumorous hyperandrogenism. *Fertil Steril.* 40:66, 1983

16. Hatch R, Rosenfield RL, Kim MH, Tredway D. Hirsutism: Implications, etiology, and management. *Am J Obstet Gynecol.* 140:815, 1981

17. Tagatz GE, Kopher RA, Nagel TC, Okagaki T. The clitoral index: A bioassay of androgenic stimulation. *Obstet Gynecol.* 54:562, 1979

18. Ebling FJ. Hair. *J Invest Dermatol.* 67:98, 1976

19. Paulson RJ, Serafini PC, Catalino JA, Lobo RA. Measurements of 3α-, 17β-androstenediol glucuronide in serum and urine and the correlation with skin 5α-reductase activity. *Fertil Steril.* 46:222, 1986

20. Lobo RA. The syndrome of hyperandrogenic chronic anovulation. In: Mishell DR Jr, Davajan V, Lobo RA, eds. *Infertility, Contraception and Reproductive Endocrinology*, 3rd ed. Cambridge, Mass., Blackwell Scientific Publications, 1991: 447–487

21. Judd HL, Scully RE, Herbst AL, et al. Familial hyperthecosis: Comparison of endocrinologic and histologic findings with polycystic ovarian disease. *Am J Obstet Gynecol.* 117:976, 1973

22. Behrman SJ, Scully RE. Case records of the Massachusetts General Hospital: Infertility and irregular menses in a 27-year-old woman. *N Engl J Med.* 287:1192, 1972

23. Steingold KA, Judd HL, Nieberg RK, et al. Treatment of severe androgen excess due to ovarian hyperthecosis with a long-acting gonadotropin-releasing hormone agonist. *Am J Obstet Gynecol.* 154:1241, 1986

24. Kennedy L, Traub AI, Atkinson AB, et al. Short-term administration of gonadotropin-releasing hormone analog to a patient with testosterone-secreting tumor. *J Clin Endocrinol Metab.* 64:1320, 1987

25. Friedman CI, Schmidt GE, Kim MH, Powel J. Serum testosterone concentrations in the evaluation of androgen-producing tumors. *Am J Obstet Gynecol.* 153:44, 1985

26. Surrey ES, de Ziegler D, Gambone JC, Judd HL. Preoperative localization of androgen-secreting tumors: Clinical, endocrinologic, and radiologic evaluation of ten patients. *Am J Obstet Gynecol.* 158:1313, 1988

27. Taylor L, Ayers JWT, Gross MD, et al. Diagnostic considerations in virilization: Iodomethyl-norcholesterol scanning in the localization of androgen secreting tumors. *Fertil Steril.* 46:1005, 1986

28. Lobo RA, Goebelsmann U. Adult manifestation of congenital adrenal hyperplasia due to incomplete 21-hydroxylase deficiency mimicking polycystic ovarian disease. *Am J Obstet Gynecol.* 138:720, 1980

29. Speiser PW, Dupont B, Rubinstein P, et al. High frequency of nonclassical steroid 21-hydroxylase deficiency. *Am J Hum Genet.* 37:650, 1985

30. Lobo RA. Adult onset 21-hydroxylase deficiency: A significant problem in gynecology? *Gynecol Rep.* 2:266, 1990

31. New MI, Lorenzen F, Lerner AJ, et al. Genotyping steroid 21-hydroxylase deficiency: Hormonal reference data. *J Clin Endocrinol Metab.* 57:320, 1983

32. Lobo RA, Goebelsmann U. Evidence for reduced 3β-ol-hydroxysteroid dehydrogenase activity in some hirsute

33. Pang S, Softness B, Sweeney WJ III, New MI. Hirsutism, polycystic ovarian disease, and ovarian 17-ketosteroid reductase deficiency. *N Engl J Med.* 316:1295, 1987

34. Wild RA, Umstot ES, Andersen RN, Givens JR. Adrenal function in hirsutism. II. Effect of an oral contraceptive. *J Clin Endocrinol Metab.* 54:676, 1982

35. Carmina E, Janni A, Lobo RA. Physiological estrogen replacement may enhance the effectiveness of the gonadotropin-releasing hormone agonist in the treatment of hirsutism. *J Clin Endocrinol Metab.* 78:126, 1994

36. Carr BR, Breslau NA, Givens C, et al. Oral contraceptive pills, gonadotropin-releasing hormone agonists, or use in combination for treatment of hirsutism: A clinical research center study. *J Clin Endocrinol Metab.* 80:1169, 1996

37. Heiner JS, Greendale JA, Kawakami AK, et al. Comparison of a gonadotropin-releasing hormone agonist and a low dose oral contraceptive given alone or together in the treatment of hirsutism. *J Clin Endocrinol Metab.* 80:3412, 1995

38. Kuttenn F, Rigaud C, Wright F, Mauvais-Jarvis P. Treatment of hirsutism by oral cyproterone acetate and percutaneous oestradiol. *J Clin Endocrinol Metab.* 51:1107, 1980

39. Menard RH, Guenthner TM, Kon H, Gillette JR. Studies on the destruction of adrenal and testicular cytochrome P-450 by spironolactone. Requirement for the 7α-thio group and evidence for the loss of the heme and apoproteins of cytochrome P-450. *J Biol Chem.* 254:1726, 1979

40. Corvol P, Michaud A, Menard J, et al. Antiandrogenic effect of spironolactone: Mechanism of action. *Endocrinology.* 97:51, 1975

41. Boisselle A, Tremblay RR. New therapeutic approach to the hirsute patient. *Fertil Steril.* 32:276, 1979

42. Lobo RA, Shoupe D, Serafini P, et al. The effects of two doses of spironolactone on serum androgens and anagen hair in hirsute women. *Fertil Steril.* 43:200, 1985

43. Sonino N. The use of ketoconazole as an inhibitor of steroid production. *N Engl J Med.* 317:812, 1987

44. Pepper G, Brenner SH, Gabrilove JL. Ketoconazole use in the treatment of ovarian hyperandrogenism. *Fertil Steril.* 54:438, 1990

45. Cutler GB Jr, Davis SE, Johnsonbaugh RF, Loriaux DL. Dissociation of cortisol and adrenal androgen secretion in patients with secondary adrenal insufficiency. *J Clin Endocrinol Metab.* 49:604, 1979

46. Rittmaster RS, Loriaux DL, Cutler GB Jr. Sensitivity of cortisol and adrenal androgens to dexamethasone suppression in hirsute women. *J Clin Endocrinol Metab.* 61:462, 1985

47. Boyers SP, Buster JE, Marshall JR. Hypothalamic–pituitary–adrenocortical function during long-term low-dose dexamethasone therapy in hyperandrogenized women. *Am J Obstet Gynecol.* 142:330, 1982

48. Carmina E, Lobo RA. Peripheral androgen blockade versus glandular androgen suppression in the treatment of hirsutism. *Obstet Gynecol.* 18:845, 1991

49. Carmina E, Lobo RA. Ovarian suppression reduces clinical and endocrine expression of late-onset congenital

adrenal hyperplasia due to 21-hydroxylase deficiency. *Fertil Steril.* 62:738, 1994

50. Klove KL, Roy S, Lobo RA. The effect of different contraceptive treatments on the serum concentration of dehydroepiandrosterone sulfate. *Contraception.* 29:319, 1984

51. Mowszowicz I, Wright F, Vincens M, et al. Androgen metabolism in hirsute patients treated with cyproterone acetate. *J Steroid Biochem.* 20:757, 1984

52. Simard J, Luthy I, Guay J, et al. Characteristics of interaction of the antiandrogen flutamide with the androgen receptor in various target tissues. *Mol Cell Endocrinol.* 44:261, 1986

53. Ayub M, Levell MJ. Inhibition of rat testicular 17α-hydroxylase and 17,20-lyase activities by antiandrogens (flutamide, hydroxyglutamide RU 23908, cyproterone acetate) in vitro. *J Steroid Biochem.* 28:43, 1987

54. Brochu M, Belanger A, Dupont A, et al. Effects of flutamide and aminoglutathimide on plasma 5α-reduced steroid glucuronide concentrations in castrated patients with cancer of the prostate. *J Steroid Biochem.* 28:619, 1987

55. Marconides JAM, Minnani SL, Luthold WW, et al. Treatment of hirsutism in women with flutamide. *Fertil Steril.* 57:543, 1992

56. Fruzzetti F, De Lorenzo D, Ricci C, Fioretti P. Clinical and endocrine effects of flutamide in hyperandrogenic women. *Fertil Steril.* 60:806, 1993

57. Moghetti P, Magnani CM, Castello R, et al. Flutamide in the treatment of hirsutism: Long-term clinical effects, endocrine changes and androgen receptor behavior. *Fertil Steril.* 64:511, 1995

58. Wysowski DK, Freiman JP, Tourtelot JB, Horton ML. Fatal and nonfatal hepatotoxicity associated with flutamide. *Ann Intern Med.* 118:860, 1993

59. Evron S, Shapiro G, Diamant YZ. Induction of ovulation with spironolactone (Aldactone) in anovulatory oligomenorrheic and hyperandrogenic women. *Fertil Steril.* 36:468, 1981

60. Gamborg Nielsen P. Treatment of moderate idiopathic hirsutism with a cream containing canrenone (an antiandrogen). *Dermatologica.* 165:636, 1982

61. Rowe TC, Mezei M, Hilchie J. Treatment of hirsutism with liposomal progesterone. *Prostate.* 5:346, 1984

62. Cassidenti DL, Paulson RJ, Serafini P, et al. Effects of sex steroids on skin 5α-reductase activity in vitro. *Obstet Gynecol.* 78:103, 1991

63. Brooks JR. Treatment of hirsutism with 5α-reductase inhibitors. In: Horton R, Lobo RA, eds. *Androgen Metabolism in Hirsute and Normal Females. Clinics in Endocrinology and Metabolism*, vol 15. Philadelphia, Pa., W. B. Saunders, 1986: 391–405

64. Rittmaster RS. Finasteride. *N Engl J Med.* 330:120, 1994

65. Wong LI, Morris RS, Chang L, et al. A prospective randomized trial comparing finasteride to spironolactone in the treatment of hirsute women. *J Clin Endocrinol Metab.* 80:233, 1995

66. Fruzzetti F, De Lorenzo D, Parrini D, Ricci C. Effects of finasteride, a 5α-reductase inhibitor, on circulating androgens and gonadotropin secretion in hirsute women. *J Clin Endocrinol Metab.* 79:831, 1994

67. Castello R, Tosi F, Perrone F, et al. Outcome of long-term treatment with the 5α-reductase inhibitor finasteride in idiopathic hirsutism: Clinical and hormonal effects during a 1-year course of therapy and 1-year follow-up. *Fertil Steril.* 66:734, 1996

Chapter 21

ENDOCRINE ALTERATIONS IN FEMALE OBESITY

Barbara A. Gower and Ricardo Azziz

Obesity is the most prevalent nutritional disorder of affluent nations, with a broad and significant impact on many endocrinologic parameters. While obesity is rarely the result of endocrinologic disorders, the presence of obesity is associated with a number of disturbances in androgen, estrogen, binding globulin, insulin/glucose, gonadotropin, prolactin, and growth hormone/growth factor metabolism. Additionally, the newly discovered hormone leptin, produced in and secreted by adipose tissue, affects the neuroendocrine–reproductive axis in animal models. It is possible that some or all of these physiologic alterations play a role in the genesis of obesity-related ovulatory dysfunction, or hormone-sensitive carcinomas.

DEFINITION AND MEASUREMENT OF OBESITY

Obesity is the presence of excess body fat, a definition that requires a measurement of adiposity. Alternatively, *overweightness* denotes a body weight above some reference weight. The deviation of body weight in relationship to an arbitrary standard is referred to as *relative weight*. Excess body fat and overweightness do not necessarily correlate, this relationship being determined by variations in body build and muscle mass.

Direct measurements of total body fat are extremely difficult, usually requiring autopsy analysis. Indirect measurements of adiposity include the following.[1]

1. *Simple rules for establishing overweightness or obesity.* For example, the Broca index, whereby height in cm − 100 = appropriate weight in kg; or the "magic 36"

rule, a whereby height in inches − waist circumference in inches denotes obesity if less than 36.

2. *Dilutional techniques.* The injection of a known quantity of an isotope or other substance can, after equilibration, allow an estimation of total body water, body potassium, or fat cell mass.

3. *Measures of body density.* The measurement of body density by submersion into a water tank utilizes an assumed average density for fat and nonfat tissues for calculating total body fat.

4. *Dual-energy x-ray absorptiometry (DEXA).* Developed for diagnosis of osteoporosis, DEXA scanning has become a useful tool for determining whole or regional body composition. DEXA relies on the principle that soft tissue versus bone, and fat versus fat-free soft tissue, will cause differential attenuation of two intensities of x-ray beams as they pass through the body.[2]

5. *Computed tomography (CT) scanning and magnetic resonance imaging (MRI).* Single or multiple-slice CT scanning or MRI, in conjunction with appropriate imaging software, can be used to quantify adipose or other tissue in two-dimensional images.[3]

6. *Anthropometric measurements.* Significantly less accurate than dilutional or scanning techniques, or measures of body density, anthropometric measurements have the highest clinical utility. Height, weight, skinfold thickness, and body or limb circumferences and diameters have been correlated with body fat content. It appears that the *body mass index* (BMI) or *weight/height*^{2} in kilograms and meters is relatively accurate, although in women the weight/height may be more appropriate.[1] The *ponderal index* (height in inches^3/weight in pounds) appears to be the least satisfactory assessment of body fat when compared to measurements of body density or skinfold thickness measurements.[1] Measurement of subcutaneous skinfold thickness are also clinically useful, although there are a number of problems with this technique including the selection

Supported in part by National Cancer Institute grant CA-28103 of the Clinical Nutrition Research Unit of the University of Alabama at Birmingham (RA), and National Institute of Aging grant K01AG00740 (BG).

of an appropriate instrument, the selection of sites for measurement, and observer reproducibility. There is no single skinfold measurement that is a reliable index of total body fat for both men and women, and usually a combination of sites must be assessed. Furthermore, the utility of skinfold thickness as a predictor of body fat decreases with age, since body fat deposition occurs in areas other than the subcutaneous tissue in older subjects.[1] The measurement of limb or body circumferences and diameters can also give a reliable estimate of body fat. Steinkamp and colleagues reported that in white females aged 25 to 44 years, the measurement of waist, iliac crest, arm, and thigh circumferences had a greater than 85 percent correlation coefficient with body fat as measured by ^{40}K and ^{137}Cs dilution techniques.[4] They also noted that weight alone had an 87 percent coefficient of correlation with estimated body fat.

Establishing the presence and degree of overweightness requires the use of standardized weight/height tables. These tables will be variously based on "average or mean" population weight (which is not very useful due to variations in the prevalence of obesity among the different populations studied), or "ideal" weight based on a reduced mortality risk (of which cardiovascular disease is the principal component). Various standards are available in the literature, the most popular being those of "ideal" weights of the Metropolitan Life Insurance Company, either from 1959[5] or 1983.[6] The body weights at which the least mortality occurs (ideal body weight or IBW) are slightly higher in the 1983 tables. Unfortunately, these IBWs are well below the average weight for United States residents. The use of these tables in clinical investigation has a number of drawbacks. First, they are based on individuals who are seeking life insurance, which may not represent a true cross-section of the population to be studied, or even of the United States population. In addition, each subject is measured wearing shoes and clothes. Notwithstanding the arbitrary nature of these standards, they provide a reasonable method for clinically screening and categorizing large populations.

Prevalence of Obesity

The prevalence of obesity in a population entirely depends on the criteria used, since the degree of adiposity represents a continuum. If a body weight above 20 percent IBW is considered the lower end of obesity (using the 1959 Metropolitan Life Insurance Company standards), 40, 46, and 45 percent of women aged 40 to 49, 50 to 59, and 60 to 69 yr are defined as obese, respectively.[7] Alternatively, using the 95th percentile for BMI, only 5 percent of men and 3.8 percent of women in the United States are obese,[8] due to the high *average* body weight. If

obesity is arbitrarily defined as a BMI over 30 kg/m^2, 12 percent of females in the United States are considered obese.[9] Unfortunately, the proportion of obese women in the United States is steadily increasing, regardless of race.[10]

Obesity can be further classified into mild, moderate, and severe. For example, mild obesity may denote individuals weighing between 20 and 40 percent above IBW, comprising about 90.5 percent of all obese persons.[11] Individuals who are between 41 percent and 100 percent overweight demonstrate moderate obesity and constitute 9 percent of obese subjects. Severe obesity (>100 percent IBW) is extremely rare and afflicts approximately 0.5 percent of obese subjects.

Obesity correlates with a number of demographic characteristics. Women have a greater percentage of body fat even in the same relative weight category as men. This difference is noticeable in early childhood, becoming more marked after puberty.[12] In a complex fashion, socioeconomic status is negatively correlated with obesity in the United States.[1] Obesity is consistently more common in white than in black males. Conversely, black women show a higher prevalence of obesity at all ages than do white women.[1]

Adipocyte Hyperplasia and Hypertrophy in Obesity

There appear to be two forms of excessive fat tissue. The first occurs through adipocyte hypertrophy or increased cell size. The second presents as a hyperplasia of adipose tissue or an increase in the number of adipocytes.[13] It was originally proposed that fat cells proliferate only in early life and that their number cannot be subsequently reduced, the propensity for obesity being determined in early life.[14] Subsequently, investigators have noted that the weight of each individual fat cell increases until the total body fat approximates 30 kg.[15] With increases in total body fat beyond 30 kg, very little increase in the size of individual adipocytes occurs, although the number of fat cells rises in a linear fashion. Thus, all obese individuals demonstrate adipocyte hypertrophy, unless ill or attempting to lose weight. Patients with more severe obesity will also have an increased fat cell number or adipocyte hyperplasia.[13] Unfortunately, it appears true that once the number of fat cells has increased it cannot be reduced by dieting alone.

Although there appears to be a closer association between metabolic disturbances and adipocyte size (particularly of abdominal fat cells) than with fat tissue hyperplasia, this may not hold true in all instances. For example, peripheral aromatase activity is correlated with the number of adipocytes and adipose tissue stromal cells, and not with cell size, particularly of the gluteofemoral area (discussed later).

Endocrinologic Consequences Related to Topographic Distribution of Fat

Vague suggested in 1956 that upper body obesity (the so-called "android" obesity) leads to a number of metabolic disturbances in both males and females, and was associated with premature arteriosclerosis and diabetes.[16] Metabolically, abdominal obesity and the size of the abdominal adipocytes have been associated with higher circulating triglyceride (TG), insulin, and total, low-density lipoprotein (LDL), and very low-density lipoprotein (VLDL) cholesterol levels; and with lower high-density lipoprotein (HDL) levels and reduced glucose tolerance in both men and women.[15,17–24]

The negative health effects of upper-body obesity are now thought to be due primarily to intra-abdominal or visceral adipose tissue, in contrast to simply the presence of subcutaneous abdominal fat.[25] Visceral fat is associated with insulin resistance, hyperinsulinemia, high TG, low HDL, high apolipoprotein-B, small LDL particle size, and high LDL particle density. Relative to other depots, visceral fat is more sensitive to lipolytic stimuli, and less sensitive to the antilipolytic effects of insulin. Because of this ability to readily mobilize free fatty acids, visceral fat may increase hepatic exposure to lipids, resulting in decreased insulin extraction, increased glucose production, and increased triglyceride production. So striking is the association between visceral fat and metabolism, that it has been proposed[26,27] that visceral obesity be included as a component of the "metabolic syndrome," a constellation of metabolic disorders comprised of hyperinsulinemia, insulin resistance, dyslipidemia (hypertriglyceridemia, low HDL), and hypertension.[28]

In premenopausal women, who may be protected to some extent from visceral obesity,[29,30] obesity is nonetheless associated with metabolic disturbances. But in this instance, it is unclear whether it is total obesity or subcutaneous abdominal obesity that confers disease risk. Subcutaneous upper-body fat, although less of a health risk than visceral fat, is more lipolytically sensitive than lower-body fat and also appears to be less sensitive to insulin-induced glucose utilization.[31] Total body obesity is associated with hyperinsulinemia and increased pancreatic insulin production. In a group of premenopausal women, obese individuals had greater basal and stimulated lipolysis in adipocytes from abdominal subcutaneous adipose tissue than lean individuals, a characteristic due primarily to greater adipocyte size.[21] In the group as a whole, subcutaneous abdominal adipocyte lipolysis was correlated both with total body obesity and with insulin and triglyceride concentrations. Thus, the negative metabolic profile associated with "simple" obesity in premenopausal women may occur secondary to enlarged adipocyte size and increased lipolysis/lipid mobilization, particularly from abdominal subcutaneous tissue.

Abdominal obesity appears to be associated with androgenicity. In premenopausal women a decrease in circulating sex hormone-binding globulin (SHBG) and/or an increase in free testosterone (T) was associated with an increase in waist to hip ratio (WHR), independent of obesity level (Fig 21–1).[18,32] Women with androgen excess have a higher mean WHR than euandrogenic controls.[33] Furthermore, free T was positively correlated, and SHBG negatively correlated, to the size of the abdominal, but not femoral, adipocytes.[18] Differential steroid metabolism in upper versus lower-body adipose tissue may partially account for the differences in hormone profile in abdominal versus gluteofemoral obesity.[32] Women with upper-body obesity had higher T and dihydro-testosterone (DHT) production rates, while women with lower-body obesity had increased estrone (E_1) levels due to a higher degree of peripheral aromatization.

The possibility that androgens stimulate upper-body, particularly visceral, fat deposition in women has been discussed,[33–35] and is supported by studies involving androgen administration.[36,37] However, the physiologic relevance of these observations is unclear; in men, testosterone administration decreases, rather than increases, visceral fat,[38] and the role of decreased female sex steroid hormones as a contributing factor in studies with women cannot be discounted. Estrogens, possibly in conjunction with progesterone, promote fat deposition in the gluteofemoral area, leading to the characteristic gynoid fat distribution in obese, cyclic, premenopausal women. Thus, low estrogens/progesterone may, by default, promote upper-body obesity. Additionally, progesterone competes for binding sites with glucocorticoids,[39] hormones associated with abdominal/visceral fat accumulation.[40–44] Upper-body obesity in women is observed in individuals with depressed ovarian estrogen production/action, such as smokers[45] and postmenopausal women (see "Obesity and the Menopause" near the end of the chapter). Not all studies support a strong association between androgens and abdominal adiposity.[34] And, in prospective analyses, *low* rather than high total testosterone predicted deposition of upper-body fat in postmenopausal women, whereas bioavailable testosterone was not related to change in WHR.[46] Taken together, data suggest that hyperandrogenicity occurs either secondary to, or in conjunction with, the development of upper-body obesity, but is unlikely to be a causal factor.

Greater relative androgenicity may partly explain the metabolic defects observed in women with abdominal fat distribution. In women, the decrease in hepatic insulin extraction and peripheral insulin sensitivity noted with upper body obesity was, in part, mediated by the increased androgenic activity.[47] Haffner and colleagues noted that after adjusting for overall obesity, the SHBG level still remained positively correlated to HDL cholesterol, but not to

TG, in premenopausal women.[23] Adipocyte size has been observed to correlate both with various measures of androgenicity, and with the insulin response to glucose loading.[18] However, the degree of androgenicity does not fully explain all the metabolic alterations observed in upper body obesity in men[20] and postmenopausal women,[19] especially that of lipoproteins.

The presence of abdominal obesity is often estimated using the waist to hip circumference ratio (WHR). However, this index correlates with metabolic parameters less well than waist circumference.[48] Furthermore, it is of limited usefulness for diagnosing visceral obesity, as it cannot discriminate between intra-abdominal and subcutaneous abdominal fat, particularly in some populations. The correlation of WHR with visceral fat is lower in 20- to 40-year-old Caucasian women (r = 0.28) than in same-aged Caucasian men (r = 0.84),[29] and is lower in African-American women (aged 35 ± 7, r = 0.35) than in Caucasian women (aged 39 ± 6, r = 0.71).[49] In women aged 40 and greater, waist circumference is the best anthropometric index of visceral obesity (r = 0.82).[29] Additionally, prediction equations have been developed for women that use simple anthropometric indices and age to estimate visceral fat.[50,51] Intra-abdominal fat increases with age, and

perhaps with menopause, and is higher in sedentary than active individuals.[29,30,52,53] In women, an increase in abdominal or truncal obesity is associated with an increase in the incidence of gallbladder disease,[54] menstrual irregularities,[54] diabetes mellitus,[54] hypertension,[54,55] cardiovascular disease,[56] and premature death.[56] Furthermore, the WHR is significantly higher in obese individuals who smoke cigarettes, and weight loss in smokers is associated with a further increase in WHR.[57]

ANDROGEN METABOLISM IN OBESITY

Circulating Androgen Concentrations in Obesity

In adults or adolescents with eumenorrheic obesity, total androgen circulating levels do not appear to be increased, and may actually be lower than in normal weight controls.[47,58–62] However, unbound T may be increased in otherwise euandrogenic obesity.[59] Evans et al[18] noted that BMI and WHR correlated inversely with SHBG levels and directly with the proportion of free T (Fig 21–1). In our laboratory we have observed higher free T levels in obese eumenorrheic non-hirsute women, in spite of a

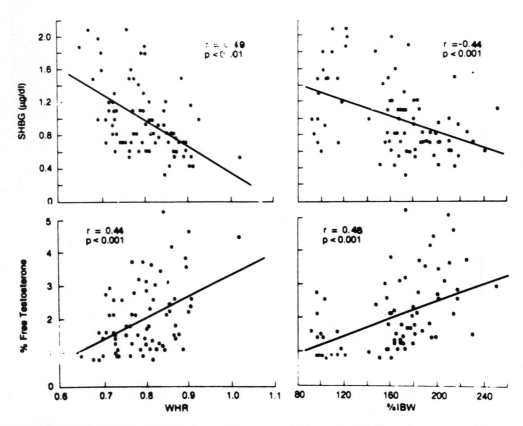

Figure 21–1. Relationship of body fat topography and obesity level to SHBG and percentage of free testosterone (n = 80). *(Reproduced, with permission, from Evans DJ Hoffman RG, Kalkhoff RK, Kissebah AH. Relationship of androgenic activity to body fat topography, fat cell morphology, amd metabolic aberrations in premenopausal women. J Clin Endocrinol Metab. 57:304, 1983.[18])*

similar WHR to non-obese controls, suggesting that the increase in free T is more closely associated with total, rather than abdominal, obesity.[63] Wajchenberg and colleagues observed higher total and free T levels in obese eumenorrheic non-hirsute women.[64] While some other studies have not confirmed the increase in free T levels in obese premenopausal[62] and postmenopausal[65] women, such a finding is consistent with the lower SHBG binding activity noted in obese subjects (discussed later).

In summary, it appears that circulating levels of plasma total androgens do not vary significantly with weight, and in fact may be slightly lower in overweight subjects. However, because of an obesity-related decrease in the circulating level of SHBG, the percentage of free T may be somewhat elevated, in particular in those women with upper body fat distribution.

Androgen Clearance in Obesity

Samojlik et al[58] reported a higher metabolic clearance rate (MCR), as well as production rate (PR), of T, DHT, and 3α-androstenediol (3α-diol) in obese eumenorrheic women when compared to normal-weight subjects. The MCR of T was 1256 ± 145 L/day and 740 ± 40 L/day, in obese and normal-weight women, respectively. Because serum androgen levels were the same or slightly lower, the calculated production rates of T, DHT, and 3α-diol were 1.5 to 3-fold higher in obese subjects. This obesity-related increase in MCR and PR was also reported for androstenedione (A) and dehydroepiandrosterone (DHEA) (Fig 21–2).[66] Both BMI and WHR correlated with the MCR of A and DHEA, and the PR of A. The PR of DHEA did not appear to be associated with the WHR. The etiology of the obesity-related increase in androgen MCR is not clear, but may relate to both decreased SHBG, and increased sequestration by adipose tissue. T and DHT are bound by SHBG in the circulation.[67] This carrier protein has a high affinity for these steroids, but a low carrying capacity. As will be discussed, the circulating levels of SHBG decrease with obesity, probably secondary to hyperinsulinemia. As SHBG levels decrease, the MCR of T increases, probably due to the increase in unbound T available for hepatic extraction and clearance.[68,69] Because A, DHEA, or dehydroepiandrosterone sulfate (DHEAS) are not bound significantly by SHBG, variations in the concentration of this carrier protein with obesity do not explain their increased MCR. The increased clearance of these and other androgens may reflect adipose tissue sequestration or metabolism.

Fat tissue is able to sequester various steroids including androgens, probably secondary to their lipid solubility. The observation that clearance of T, A, and estradiol correlated with body weight in women infused with radiolabeled hormones may support the importance of adipose tissue sequestration as a significant component of clearance.[70] Most sex hormones appear to be preferentially concentrated within human adipocytes

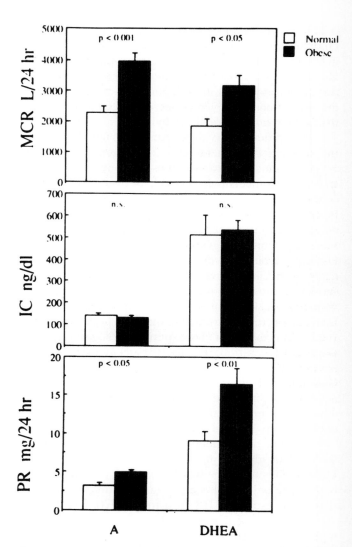

Figure 21–2. Mean (± SEM) metabolic clearance rate (MCR), 24-hr integrated plasma concentration (IC), and production rate (PR) of androstenedione (A) and dehydroepiandrosterone (DHEA) in normal and obese eumenorrheic women. *(Reproduced, with permission, from Kurtz BR, Givens JR, Komindr S, et al. Maintenance of normal circulating levels of delta-4 androstenedione and dehydroepiandrosterone in simple obesity despite increased metabolic clearance rates: Evidence for a servo-control mechanism.* J Clin Endocrinol Metab. *64:1261, 1987.[66])*

TABLE 21–1. STEROID CONCENTRATION RATIOS: HUMAN ADIPOSE TISSUE TO PERIPHERAL BLOOD

Steroid[a]	Tissue/Serum Ratio[b]
F	0.4 ± 0.7
DHEA	13.2 ± 4.4
A	7.7 ± 3.4
T	7.0 ± 3.0
$E_1 + E_2$	2.2 ± 1.5
Progesterone	6.3 ± 7.0
17-Hydroxyprogesterone	4.0 ± 2.5

[a]For abbreviations, see text.
[b]Mean ± standard error.
(Modified, with permission, from Feher T, Bodrogi L. A comparative study of steroid concentrations in human adipose tissue and peripheral circulation. Clin Chim Acta. *126:135, 1982.[71])*

rather than in plasma (Table 21–1).[71] Only cortisol and DHEAS are not significantly stored in fat tissue. Since the volume of fat in obese subjects is much larger than their intravascular space, and because tissue steroid concentrations are 2- to 13-fold higher than those in plasma, the steroid pool of severely obese subjects is far greater than that of normal-weight individuals.

In addition to serving as a reservoir, fat tissue can be the site of steroid metabolism. Androgens can be irreversibly aromatized to estrogens, or converted to other androgens, a reversible process.[72] Between 1 and 5 percent of circulating A is converted to E_1 in women.[69,72–74] Peripheral aromatization is responsible for a large fraction of androgen clearance and will be discussed further in the section on estrogen metabolism and obesity. 17β-Hydroxysteroid dehydrogenase, the activity of which leads to the interconversion of A and T, has been observed in vitro in adipose tissue by some,[75–77] but not all[78] investigators. Interconversion of T and A may occur in both adipocytes and stromal tissue, with preferential conversion of A to T.[75] In vivo experiments suggest that adipose tissue contributes 5 to 10 percent of the overall conversion of A to T, but less than 2 percent of T to A.[79] Conversion of T to A may be regulated by the circulating level of unbound T, with which it is correlated.[68] There does not appear to be a significant correlation between obesity and the conversion of T and A in vivo.[73]

Adipose tissue metabolism of estrogens may be influenced by the androgen environment. In vitro, both DHEA and DHEAS were observed to inhibit 17β-hydroxysteroid dehydrogenase (as measured by the conversion of estradiol $[E_2]$ to estrone $[E_1]$).[76] Aromatase activity in adipose tissue (A to E_1 conversion) was not inhibited by adrenal androgens.

5α-Reductase activity was not observed in adipose tissue in vitro,[78] and hepatic metabolism is estimated to be sufficient to explain observed in vivo conversion of DHEA to A or T (3β-dehydrogenase activity).[80] 3α-Hydroxysteroid-oxido-reduction, a process that encourages the formation of the less androgenic 3α-diol from DHT, has been noted in hamster adipose tissue.[78]

Obesity-related alterations in hepatic and urinary metabolism/excretion may also influence the clearance of androgens. Feher and Halmy[81] observed a deficient metabolism of DHEA to DHEAS, and a ten-fold higher urinary excretion of DHEA in overweight subjects. These data suggested an obesity-related decrease in the sulfoconjugation of DHEA or an increase in the desulfation of DHEAS. The increased urinary excretion of DHEA may be secondary to the higher glomerular filtration rate observed in obese women, or to the intrinsic natriuretic action of DHEA. In addition, Samojlik et al noted an increase in plasma and urinary levels of T and 3α-diol glucuronide, with normal plasma concentrations of unconjugated steroids.[58] These data suggest that obesity is associated with an accelerated rate of hepatic conjugation

and extraction, factors that may explain the observation of normal circulating androgen levels in obesity.

Androgen Production in Obesity

As mentioned, PR of A, T, DHT, 3α-diol, and DHEA are increased in obesity. It is possible that the obesity-related increase in androgen PR occurs in response to the increase in MCR observed, a type of servocontrol mechanism.[66] Alternatively, an increase in the ovarian or adrenal production of androgens may initially result in higher circulating levels, which then are cleared following suppression of SHBG production, resulting in an increased MCR of unbound steroids.

There is no evidence that ovarian enzymatic function is altered in euandrogenic obesity. However, the hyperinsulinemia that accompanies obesity may affect ovarian steroidogenesis in certain predisposed individuals, and could be partly responsible for the hyperandrogenism associated with some cases of obesity. High levels of insulin stimulate androgen production in vivo, and insulin augments responsiveness to LH in vitro, indirectly stimulating steroidogenesis and androgen production.[82–86] Reduction of insulin with metformin reduced ovarian cytochrome P450c17α activity in obese women with polycystic ovary syndrome (PCOS).[87] Treated women showed decreases in insulin area-under-the-curve during an oral glucose tolerance test (OGTT), basal serum 17α-hydroxyprogesterone, leuprolide-stimulated 17α-hydroxyprogesterone, and basal serum LH. Insulin may stimulate ovarian steroid production through either the insulin or IGF-I receptor, as both are present in the ovary.

Adrenocortical Function in Obesity

Adrenocortical Dynamics. Obese individuals display evidence of alterations in adrenocortical dynamics. Brody and associates reported a positive correlation between body weight and the change in DHEA and the ratio of the increment (>) in DHEA to >17-hydroxyprogesterone following adrenocorticotropic hormone (ACTH) administration, suggesting a hyper-responsiveness of adrenal androgens in obesity.[88] The relative sensitivity and responsiveness of serum F, A, and DHEA to exogenous ACTH stimulation was studied in 16 obese eumenorrheic premenopausal women.[89] Utilizing incremental doses of 1-24 ACTH, the relative responsiveness of the steroids to ACTH was the same in obese and normal weight women: F > DHEA > A (Fig 21–3). The slope of the DHEA response versus time was higher in obese women, indicating a greater "responsivity" to stimulation. Furthermore, in obese women, the ACTH dose at which A began to rise was significantly lower (greater sensitivity) than in normal-weight subjects. The sensitivity of the response of F or DHEA to incremental doses of ACTH was not different in obese subjects. These investigators postulated an enhancement of ACTH-stimulated adrenal androgen pro-

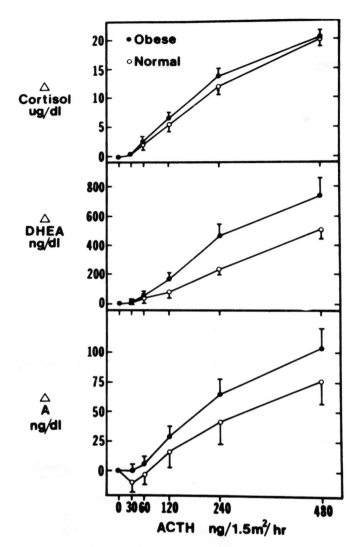

Figure 21–3. Mean (± SEM) incremental (>) responses of cortisol (F), dehydroepiandrosterone (DHEA), and androstenedione (A) to the continuous infusion of 1-24 ACTH in normal and obese non-hirsute eumenorrheic women. The ACTH dose was doubled every hr. *(Reproduced, with permission, from Komindr S, Kurtz BR, Stevens MD, et al. Relative sensitivity and responsivity of serum cortisol and adrenal androgens to adrenocorticotropin (1-24) in normal and obese, nonhirsute, eumenorrheic women. J Clin Endocrinol Metab. 63:860, 1986.[89])*

duction in asymptomatic obese women. Data from our laboratory have not demonstrated any significant difference in the adrenal response to acute ACTH stimulation between eumenorrheic obese and normal-weight premenopausal women, with the exception of a higher A.[63]

Plasma cortisol (F), its circadian secretion, and the response of F to ACTH are not altered in obesity.[89–93] Normal plasma F levels are maintained in spite of an accelerated PR and MCR.[92,94,95] A 30 to 50 percent increase in the urinary excretion of 17-hydroxy-corticosteroids is noted in obesity,[91,92,95] but this increase does not completely normalize when corrected for body surface area.[92]

It is felt that the increased MCR of F in obesity is secondary to a decrease in cortisol binding globulin plasma concentrations. Slavnov and associates have reported a slight increase in plasma ACTH levels in obese subjects, possibly explaining the increased F production.[96] This obesity-related acceleration in the overall adrenocortical function may also lead to an increase in adrenal androgen production.

Urinary 17-ketosteroids measure various androgen metabolites including etiocholanolone, androsterone, DHEA, and epiandrosterone, and have been reported to be elevated in obesity,[97,98] although not all investigators agree.[99,100] The causes of these alterations in adrenocortical function in obesity are not known, but may relate to the hyperinsulinism/insulin resistance associated with obesity.

Possible Role of Insulin. As previously noted, the circulating levels of DHEA, A, and DHEAS are normal or slightly decreased in obese subjects.[18,60,66] In spite of this, increased adrenal androgen PR and MCR have been reported.[66,81] In some cases, obesity-related increases in adrenal androgen production are associated with upper-body obesity, an observation that led to investigations into the possible cause of this relationship.

Associations between upper-body obesity and adrenal function may be related to perturbations in insulin action. Receptors for both insulin and IGF-I (which demonstrate some cross-reactivity with respect to ligands) are present on human adrenals,[101,102] and hyperinsulinemia, which occurs secondary to visceral obesity-induced insulin resistance, may affect steroidogenesis. Women infused with insulin, or in whom endogenous insulin was increased, showed decreased serum DHEA and DHEAS.[103–107] Likewise, a pharmacologic decrease in hyperinsulinemia resulted in an increase in serum levels of DHEAS.[108] Acute hyperinsulinemia in vivo inhibits adrenal 17,20-lyase activity.[109,110] Likewise, 17,20-lyase activity is inhibited by exposure of adrenal cells to insulin in vitro.[109] These studies suggest that hyperinsulinemia decreases synthesis of DHEA and DHEAS.

However, the effect of insulin on adrenal androgen production is not consistent. Reduction in the insulin responsiveness following pharmacologic improvement in insulin sensitivity resulted in a decrease in DHEAS (rather than an increase), as well as a decrease in A.[111] Women with PCOS, who demonstrate both insulin resistance and hyperinsulinemia, may have either increased or decreased levels of DHEA and DHEAS.[108] Among hyperandrogenic women, neither basal androgen levels nor the response of DHEAS or A to a 1-24 ACTH challenge differed between those who were hyperinsulinemic and those who were normoinsulinemic.[112] Thus, although insulin may affect adrenal androgen production, the precise effect may depend upon the experimental or physiologic circumstances, one of which is insulin resistance; in mild cases, adrenal androgens may be depressed due to hyperinsulinemia, whereas in severe cases, insulin resistance may extend to the adrenal, which may become insensitive to the inhibitory effects of insulin on androgen production.

Insulin also may have a role in clearance of adrenal androgens. Clearance (as well as production) of DHEA was strongly and positively correlated with insulin in healthy obese and non-obese women.[113] Increased clearance may be partly independent of insulin-induced suppression of SHBG, as it was observed during continuous infusion of DHEA and A.[66]

Weight Loss and Androgen Metabolism

If the alterations in androgen metabolism noted in obesity are due to the excess body fat, normalization of the metabolic aberration should be observed following weight loss. Kopelman et al[114] observed increased T and A, and decreased SHBG circulating concentrations in massively obese women compared to normal-weight individuals. Following jejuno-ileal bypass surgery and an average weight loss of 39.5 kg, a normalization of the T, A, and SHBG levels was observed. Neither serum DHT nor F values varied with weight loss.[114] Alternatively, most reports have not observed a difference in total T levels between normal and obese females, and consequently do not report any change with weight loss.[60,115,116] However, it should be noted that the average weight loss in these studies ranged from 6.5 to 18 kg, somewhat less than was observed in Kopelman's study. Kim et al[116] reported a decrease in free T levels following weight reduction, dependent on the degree of weight loss. In their study, only women with an increase in the ponderal index of greater than 0.5 demonstrated a significant decrease in free T and an increase in SHBG. Total T did not change.

Kopelman et al noted a decrease in the plasma concentration of A following weight reduction.[114] Alternatively, Grenman et al[60] observed an increase in A levels after an average weight loss of 13.2 kg, although these investigators had reported a lower initial A level in their obese subjects compared to normal-weight women. Other investigators have also observed an increase in A levels with weight reduction.[117] Pintor et al, investigating peripubertal girls, reported a decrease in DHEA levels after weight loss while the plasma concentration of A decreased only in older prepubertal children.[118] This report did not specify the degree of weight loss.

Starvation, independent of weight loss, may alter sex hormone levels. Acute fasting (7 to 10 days), with little weight loss, has a well-documented detrimental effect on adrenocortical function. Urinary and serum measurements of adrenal androgens and cortisol are noted to decrease acutely during the fasting period.[119–121] Nevertheless, O'Dea and colleagues studied obese postmenopausal women before and during a supplemented fast, and on a stable postreduction diet, and did not observe a change in the total T level during these periods.[115] The metabolic alterations due to acute starvation, independent of weight loss, must be considered when interpreting steroid changes during weight reduction. It appears that obesity-related aberrations in the plasma concentration of androgens normalize following weight reduction in a linear fashion.

Summary

In eumenorrheic obesity the PR and MCR of ovarian and adrenal androgens are increased while serum levels are usually maintained normally. The exception is the increase in free T and decrease in SHBG levels noted in obese eumenorrheic non-hirsute individuals. The increased MCR may be due to an obesity-related decrease in the plasma concentration of SHBG. Steroid sequestration by fat may also increase steroid clearance, but also leads to an extremely large pool of sex hormones in obese individuals. Increased metabolism of steroids by adipose tissue, including aromatization and 17β-hydroxysteroid dehydrogenation, and alterations in hepatic conjugation and extraction may also contribute to the increased MCR of androgens. The increased PR of androgens noted in obese individuals may occur to compensate for the increased MCR, or may be secondary to insulin action on ovarian or adrenal steroidogenic enzymes. In addition, changes in adrenocortical dynamics may favor adrenal androgen secretion in obese eumenorrheic women. The increased ovarian and adrenal androgen production noted in obesity may reflect accompanying hyperinsulinemia, or changes in the intraglandular and/or circulating concentration of androgens, estrogens, prolactin, or other unidentified factors. Weight reduction corrects any abnormality noted in steroid levels, although it is not known whether the elevated PR and MCR of androgens also normalize following weight reduction.

ESTROGEN METABOLISM IN OBESITY

Excess body fat leads to alterations in estrogen metabolism, which in turn may affect the hypothalamic–pituitary–ovarian axis leading to ovulatory dysfunction. Functional hyperestrogenism in obesity has also been associated with an increased risk of breast and endometrial carcinoma.

Estrogen Plasma Concentrations in Obesity

The production of estrogen and its precursors, including A and T, decreases with age and menopause.[122] In reviewing estrogen metabolism in eumenorrheic obesity, premenopausal and postmenopausal patients need to be considered separately. In premenopausal women, Trichopoulos et al did not observe a difference in spot urinary E_1 and E_2 concentrations in women of varying weights.[123] Other investigators have noted that the circulating levels of total E_1 and E_2 were not different between obese and normal weight premenopausal eumenorrheic women,[62,124] or were slightly lower.[60] In an attempt to eliminate the variability of single plasma measurements, the serum levels of E_1 and E_2 were assayed every 20 min for 24 hr, and no significant difference was observed between normal-weight and obese women.[59,125] Eumenorrheic obese women demonstrate lower circulating SHBG levels (Fig 21–1),[18] suggesting that the free fraction of circulating E_2 may be higher in obesity. Nonetheless, Dunaif et al were unable to confirm this.[62]

In contrast to premenopausal individuals, serum levels of E_1 and E_2 are mildly correlated with the degree of obesity and fat mass in postmenopausal obese women.[126–129] Sex-hormone binding globulin activity is also lower in these older obese women, suggesting elevated free E_2 concentrations. Investigating the role of free E_2 in postmenopausal women with and without endometrial cancer, Davidson et al noted that body size correlated positively with total and free E_2 plasma levels.[130] Estrone and E_2 circulating concentrations progressively decrease with age in postmenopausal females,[126,127] and this drop begins 4 to 5 yr earlier in obese women compared to normal-weight controls.[126]

These data suggest that the circulating levels of E_1, and total and/or free E_2 are slightly higher in obese postmenopausal women. These increments are overshadowed in premenopausal women by the ovarian estrogen production, although free E_2 may also be slightly elevated.

Peripheral Production of Estrogens in Obesity

West et al first reported the aromatization of T to estrogens in oophorectomized adrenalectomized women.[131] The aromatization of A to E_1 by human adipose tissue has been demonstrated in vitro,[132,133] and in vivo in premenopausal[72,74] and in postmenopausal[73,134] women. Aromatase activity is detected primarily in the stroma of adipose tissue and not in intact adipocytes.[135,136] Although adipose tissue is a significant source of aromatase activity in women, Longcope et al noted that muscle accounts for 25 to 30 percent of total peripheral aromatization and adipose tissue for only 10 to 15 percent in men.[137] The liver and other organs account for the remaining portion of extragonadal aromatization. Nevertheless, the rate of peripheral A to E_1 conversion is clearly correlated with body weight in premenopausal[74] and postmenopausal women (Fig 21–4).[73,134,138] Since the majority of adipose tissue aromatase resides within the stromal compartment and most overweight patients do not have hyperplastic obesity, it is surprising to observe such a consistent rise in A to E_1 conversion with excess body fat. Either the quantity of adipose

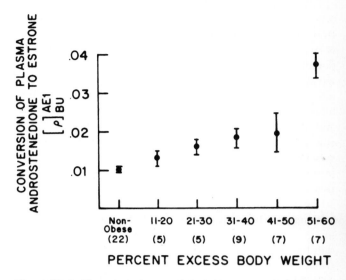

Figure 21–4. The extent of conversion of plasma androstenedione to estrone as a function of the percentage of excess body weight in ovulatory and anovulatory young women. The bars represent the standard error of the mean for each group. The numbers in parenthesis represent the number of patients in that group. *(Reproduced, with permission, from Edman CD, MacDonald TC. Effect of obesity on conversion of plasma androstenedione to estrone in ovulatory and anovulatory young women.* J Obstet Gynecol. *130:456, 1978.[74])*

tissue stroma increases regardless of obesity cell type, or the activity of other sources of extragonadal aromatization (eg, hepatic) increase as well. This latter possibility is suggested by the data of Takaki et al, who observed a *rise* in A to E_1 conversion following significant weight loss.[139] In addition, in vitro studies have suggested that the increase in A to E_1 conversion observed in obesity occurs because of an increase in fat cell numbers and not due to a change in the specific activity of the enzyme.[140,141]

Peripheral aromatization increases with age and is 2- to 4-fold higher in postmenopausal women.[142] This age-related increase in the efficiency of aromatization occurs secondary to a rise in the specific activity of the aromatase enzyme in the adipose stromal cells, which is independent of the higher gonadotropin levels associated with menopause but linearly correlated with chronologic age.[140,141] In two separate reports from the same laboratory, the average A to E_1 conversion rate for premenopausal women was 1.5[74] compared to 3.9 percent in postmenopausal women.[134]

Androstenedione is the major substrate for peripheral estrogen formation, 0.74 percent of which is aromatized. Only 0.15 percent of T is converted to E_2, although this may become clinically significant because this estrogen is much more potent than E_1. Longcope et al reported a significant association between body weight and the conversion of T to E_2.[73] Dehydroepiandrosterone contributes very little to circulating estrogens via A, with only 0.05 percent being converted.[143]

The interconversion of E_1 to E_2 has been demonstrated in vivo[144] and in vitro[76] in adipose tissue. The conversion of E_1 to E_2 is approximately 5 percent, while 15 percent of E_2 is converted back to E_1 in premenopausal women.[144] Adipose tissue 17β-hydroxysteroid dehydrogenase activity (measured by the conversion of E_1 to E_2) was higher in premenopausal than in postmenopausal women, and all females had a greater activity than males.[76] The conversion of E_1 to E_2 was also greater in omental than in subcutaneous abdominal fat, and was noncompetitively inhibited by DHEA and DHEAS. The significance of this finding is not clear, but it appears that circulating adrenal androgens may influence peripheral estrogen metabolism. Although estrogen interconversion is observed in adipose tissue in vitro, Longcope et al were not able to demonstrate an association between body fat and interconversion rates in vivo.[73]

The catabolism of estrogens may also be altered in obesity. Normal estrogen metabolism begins with E_2, which is subsequently oxidized to E_1. Estrone is metabolized to estriol (E_3) via the 16α-hydroxylation pathway, or to catechol-estrogens via C_2-hydroxylation. Schneider et al reported that obesity was associated with a decrease in C_2-hydroxylation, and little alteration in 16α-hydroxylation activity.[145] These metabolic alterations can result in a higher E_3 to catechol-estrogen ratio. Since E_3 has significantly more estrogenic activity than 2-hydroxyestrone (a catechol-estrogen), the altered estrogen metabolism may contribute to the functional hyperestrogenism noted in obesity. Notwithstanding these metabolic disturbances, E_3 probably contributes little to the overall estrogenic activity of normal premenopausal women regardless of weight.[146]

Estrogens are not a passive byproduct of obesity but can also help promote adipose tissue proliferation. 17β-estradiol, but not 17α-estradiol, induced the replication and proliferation of adipocyte precursors in vitro. This growth stimulation was noted at physiologic concentrations of 17β-estradiol.[147]

Weight Loss and Estrogen Metabolism

The effect of weight reduction on estrogen metabolism has not been clearly defined. DeWaard et al reported that following an average weight loss of 4.5 kg, urinary concentrations of E_2 and E_1 were slightly decreased in postmenopausal females.[148] Kopelman and associates observed a decrease in serum E_2 levels after a mean 13.2 kg weight reduction in premenopausal women, while E_1 levels remained unchanged.[114] Alternatively, other investigators have observed that following a 13- to 14-kg weight loss, serum E_1 levels increased while E_2 remained the same in postmenopausal[92] and premenopausal obese women.[60] The stromal cells of adipose tissue are the major source of peripheral aromatase activity,[136] and reduction in the size of the adipocytes should not signifi-

cantly alter the stromal component or the A to E_1 conversion rate. The effect of starvation, independent of weight reduction, was studied by O'Dea and associates,[115] who noted a significant decrease in serum E_2 levels with fasting. However, these values returned to normal when the thinned subjects began eating. Surprisingly, Takaki et al[139] demonstrated an increase in the conversion of A to E_1 in obese women losing an average of 45 kg. These authors suggested that starvation and weight loss may actually accentuate any obesity-related increase in hepatic aromatization.

Summary

There is an increased production of estrogens, in particular E_1, in obese women. The bulk of the increase in estrogen PR is due to aromatization of circulating androgens by adipose tissue stromal cells. The major substrate for peripheral estrogen production is A through conversion to the weak estrogen E_1. Testosterone contributes to a lesser degree via its conversion to E_2, although this activity may be clinically significant due to the greater estrogenic activity of E_2. Notwithstanding the increased peripheral aromatization noted in obesity, no consistent alteration in the plasma levels of E_1 and E_2 is observed in premenopausal women, due to the large quantity of ovarian estrogen secretion. Postmenopausal females demonstrate a slight increase in circulating E_1, E_2, and free E_2 concentrations. Weight reduction per se does not significantly change circulating levels of E_2, while E_1 levels and the conversion of A to E_1 may actually increase.

SEX HORMONE BINDING GLOBULIN IN OBESITY

Sex hormone-binding globulin (SHBG) is a circulating α-globulin produced by the liver that binds, in a high-affinity but low-capacity fashion, many of the circulating sex steroids.[149] Some of these same steroids are also bound by albumin and by other less well-described carrier proteins.[150]

Traditionally, only the free fraction of sex hormone has been considered available for tissue action. More recently, the albumin-bound fraction of sex steroids also appears to be available for tissue interaction. Using a rat-brain perfusion model, Partridge et al have demonstrated that albumin-bound steroid is readily transported into the brain substance, while antibody or SHBG-bound hormone is not.[67] Tissue utilization of albumin-bound steroid depends on how closely the tissue–capillary transit time approximates the half-time of the hormone–protein dissociation rate. Tissues with high capillary transit time (eg, liver, ±5 sec) will "strip" the steroid from albumin better than organs with short transit times (eg, brain, ±1 sec).

The percentage of E_2 not bound to SHBG or albumin is 2 to 3 percent in normal women, while unbound T constitutes 1.5 to 2 percent of the total, as determined by in vitro experiments.[151] Alterations in SHBG levels have a profound impact on the metabolism and action of bound steroids. A decrease in SHBG plasma concentration is associated with an increase in the MCR and free fraction of T[68] and E_2.[152,153] Furthermore, the blood conversion rates of T to A and T to DHT are positively correlated with the free T fraction but are independent of total plasma T.[68,154]

Circulating SHBG concentrations are influenced by a number of factors including estrogens, androgens, and insulin. It is known that the administration of exogenous estrogen, particularly oral, leads to the increased hepatic production of various carrier proteins including cortisol-binding globulin (CBG), thyroxine-binding globulin, ceruloplasmin, plasminogen, and transferrin. Alternatively, albumin, haptoglobins, and total protein are decreased.[155–157] The dosages of exogenous estrogens required to alter SHBG levels are usually large, achieving plasma levels similar to those observed during pregnancy.[158] Lesser elevations, such as the endogenous rise in E_2 during the normal menstrual cycle, do not cause any significant change in SHBG levels.[158,159] Androgens decrease the circulating levels of SHBG and CBG,[154,160,161] although they do not appear to alter the level of total proteins, albumin, haptoglobins, ceruloplasmins, or plasminogen. Thus, the effect of androgens on the hepatic production of carrier proteins is not exactly opposite to that of estrogens. In addition, glucocorticoids may inhibit, and thyroid hormones increase, SHBG levels in normal subjects.[151]

SHBG levels appear to be relatively sensitive to circulating androgens and estrogens throughout life, although other factors are clearly involved. Prior to puberty there are no sexual differences in the levels of SHBG. At puberty, plasma SHBG concentrations decrease slightly in females and markedly in males.[151] However, this decrease is likely due to the increase in insulin observed at this time,[162,163] with increased androgen production further decreasing SHBG production in males. Cunningham and associates studied men with untreated isolated gonadotropin deficiency and subjects with complete androgen insensitivity.[164] They observed a decrease in SHBG levels during the second decade of life irrespective of androgen activity. These data suggest that the decrease in SHBG levels during the second decade of life is in part independent of the increasing androgen levels. A fall in total T levels in men after age 50 yr is associated with a slight increase in SHBG plasma concentrations.[151] In the normal female population, SHBG is not correlated with androgen levels,[165] and there does not appear to be any consistent change in SHBG with age in postmenopausal women.[151]

Obesity is clearly associated with lower SHBG levels in otherwise normal women (Fig 21–1)[59,60,63,124,166] and prepubertal and pubertal children.[167] Women who weigh greater than 65 pounds above their IBW have an SHBG capacity one third that of individuals within 5 pounds of their IBW.[166] As noted above, various investigators have observed an inverse correlation between SHBG binding capacity and WHR.[46,168] Some investigators have not observed such an association.[60] Reduction in SHBG binding capacity and concentration in obese postmenopausal females is not due to impaired steroid binding but to a decrease in the number of circulating SHBG molecules.[169]

The mechanism by which obesity decreases the production of SHBG is likely hyperinsulinemia. In vitro[170] and in vivo,[171] insulin decreases SHBG production, and circulating SHBG concentrations are inversely related to insulin in healthy controls and hyperandrogenic women.[172,173] In obese hyperandrogenic women,[174] and in women with PCOS,[111] a reduction in insulin was associated with an increase in SHBG and a decrease in free T. In premenopausal women of various body weights, percent free T correlated directly with fasting insulin and the insulin response to an OGTT.[18] Furthermore, low SHBG was an independent risk factor for the development of non-insulin dependent diabetes mellitus (NIDDM) in a longitudinal study of 1462 women,[175] suggesting a link between SHBG concentration and derangement in insulin–glucose metabolism. Although many studies have documented the association between fasting insulin and SHBG levels,[18,173,176] fasting insulin may not be the only parameter with an impact on SHBG. In a study that examined multiple aspects of insulin secretion, the insulin secretory pulse frequency was more closely related to SHBG concentration than fasting insulin concentration.[177] In a cross-sectional study, insulin sensitivity emerged as independently related to SHBG after statistically controlling for fasting insulin, C-peptide, obesity, and abdominal fat.[178] These results support the role of insulin in influencing SHBG production, and suggest that multiple aspects of insulin secretion (fasting concentrations, postprandial serum profile, 24-hour circulating concentrations) may be important.

Reed et al presented data correlating dietary lipid intake with plasma levels of SHBG.[179] Six normal men consuming a high-fat diet for 2 wk demonstrated an increase in mean plasma cholesterol levels and a decrease in SHBG level. Changing to a low-fat diet resulted in a significant reduction in plasma cholesterol and an increase in mean SHBG levels.[179] Overweight women consume a greater amount of fat in their diet than do normal-weight individuals, and the decreased SHBG levels observed in obesity may be in part secondary to this dietary preference. The exact mechanism for the decrease in SHBG associated with the intake of greater quantities of lipids is not clear.

Most investigators report an increase in SHBG plasma concentrations following weight reduction,[114,117] and the extent of the rise in SHBG correlates linearly with the amount of weight loss.[116] This increase is independent of whether exercise is part of the dietary plan. It appears that starvation has a synergistic effect with weight reduction in increasing SHBG levels.[115] Women who were fasting and lost an average of 20 kg had higher SHBG levels than subjects who lost an average of 25 kg but were not fasting.

Summary

Obesity lowers the plasma concentration of SHBG by decreasing hepatic production, an effect that may be secondary to elevated insulin. The drop in circulating SHBG leads to greater levels in the unbound fraction of free E_2, T, and other sex steroids. As SHBG levels are reduced, the MCR for both E_2 and T subsequently increases, and the conversion of T to DHT and T to A increases. Weight reduction serves to normalize the SHBG plasma concentrations.

INSULIN/GLUCOSE HOMEOSTASIS IN SIMPLE OBESITY

Insulin Concentrations in Simple Obesity

It is generally agreed that most obese women have an increased insulin resistance demonstrated by an elevated fasting serum insulin–glucose ratio, increased insulin levels following a glucose tolerance test (GTT), and an increased requirement for insulin during euglycemic clamp testing.[180–183] Although fasting glucose plasma levels are similar in obese and non-obese women throughout the day, plasma insulin concentrations are significantly higher in obese individuals.[184,185] The insulin resistance noted in most obese subjects appears to be secondary to a decrease in receptor number in the various tissues involved.[182,186,187] In more severely obese individuals, postreceptor defects are also noted in vivo[186] and in vitro.[182] The abnormalities in insulin–glucose homeostasis resolve upon weight reduction.[188–191]

Although insulin is a potent anti-lipolytic hormone, free fatty acid levels are higher in obese hyperinsulinemic euglycemic individuals than normal.[184] This decreased ability of insulin to regulate free fatty acid levels in obesity appears to be independent of plasma glucagon or growth hormone concentrations. It appears that obese individuals have elevated levels of insulin and fatty acids in the face of normal circulating plasma glucose and glucagon concentrations.

Insulin and Regional Adiposity

Regional differences in insulin binding and action may explain gender differences in fat distribution.[31] Prior to menopause, women deposit fat primarily in the gluteofemoral region. In contrast, men exhibit abdominal obesity, particularly as they age. Insulin receptors appear to be more numerous in the femoral fat of obese women.[31] It is suggested that the higher number of insulin receptors of femoral fat leads to an increase in glucose metabolism and promotes the formation of α-glycerol phosphate, which enhances the ability of femoral adipocytes to synthesize and store acylglycerols.

Effects of Androgens on Insulin Action

Obesity, especially abdominal obesity, is a risk factor for development of NIDDM in women.[192] Although cause-and-effect relationships have not been fully established, disturbances in androgen production could play a role. Insulin resistance, a precursor to NIDDM, is present both in women with PCOS and in women with abdominal obesity. Furthermore, women with NIDDM were found to be hyperandrogenic, having high circulating free testosterone secondary to depressed SHBG.[193] Thus, in two disorders involving hyperandrogenism, insulin resistance is the common denominator.

Studies with rats have shown that testosterone administration causes a suite of responses similar to those observed in women with abdominal obesity. Testosterone-treated female rats became insulin resistant, and developed a type of muscle morphology characterized by a relatively higher proportion of insulin-insensitive type IIb (fast twitch) fibers, relatively low capillarization, reduced glycogen synthase activity, and a reduced proportion of insulin-sensitive glycogen synthase.[193,194] Although causal relationships cannot be inferred from these observations, such a muscle morphology would be compatible with a decrease in insulin sensitivity. Thus, both clinical and experimental observations support the hypothesis that obesity-related disturbances in androgen metabolism may be involved in the pathogenesis of NIDDM, a disease commonly observed in obese women.

The relationship of insulin and androgens has received considerable attention in the study of hyperandrogenic patients. Nevertheless, the insulin/androgen relationship in obese eumenorrheic subjects is not clear. Experimental administration of insulin is reported to increase A in obese and non-obese women,[195] decrease DHEAS in non-obese women,[103] and have no effect on T.[103,195] In normal-weight women, Schriock et al[196] observed a positive correlation between the insulin response curve levels following an oral GTT and the basal serum T. A negative correlation was noted between the basal DHEAS and the insulin response. Likewise in obese women, basal insulin and the insulin response to GTT correlated with A and T.[197] However, these results were not observed in a similar study,[62] nor in a study of 80 premenopausal women of varying weight.[18] The tentative conclusion that could be drawn from these observations is that DHEAS may enhance insulin action, whereas T and A may have the opposite effect.

Summary

Simple obesity is associated with hyperinsulinemia. When visceral obesity is present, hyperinsulinemia is accompanied by insulin resistance and postreceptor defects in insulin action. These abnormalities resolve with weight loss. There appears to be a positive correlation between insulin responsiveness and circulating levels of androgens, in particular free T and A, in eumenorrheic women. This correlation is nevertheless weak, and is independent of body weight. It is possible that a stronger correlation between androgens, insulin, and obesity would be present if body fat topography were considered. Whereas T and A may have a detrimental influence on insulin activity, DHEAS may have a favorable effect.

GROWTH HORMONE/INSULIN-LIKE GROWTH FACTOR AXIS IN OBESITY

Growth Hormone

Obesity is associated with decreased secretion[198] and increased clearance[199] of growth hormone (GH), resulting in depressed serum concentrations of GH. Low GH appears to be a consequence rather than a cause of obesity, as weight loss restores normal GH levels.[200] The precise mechanism through which obesity alters GH release is not known, but may be related to associated hyperinsulinemia. Insulin suppresses hepatic production of insulin-like growth factor (IGF) binding protein-1 (IGFBP-1),[201–205] thus increasing free IGF-I and IGF bioavailability. Negative feedback action of IGF-I on somatostatin-containing hypothalamic neurons may then depress pituitary GH release.

The clinical implications of depressed GH for reproductive function are not known. However, studies showing that the ovary is targeted by GH, and is a site of GH reception and action, have led some investigators to propose labeling GH a gonadotropin.[206] In the human ovary, GH stimulated E_2 synthesis both independently and in synergy with FSH.[207] Human GH both stimulated progesterone synthesis in human luteinized granulosa cells, and enhanced the ability of low, generally ineffective, concentrations of hCG to stimulate progesterone production.[208] Additionally, GH treatment facilitates gonadotropin-induced ovulation in vivo in patients with amenorrhea and anovulatory infertility.[209–211] It is probably more accurate to consider GH a facilitator of gonadotropin action (a "co-gonadotropin"), as most of its effects depend upon the concurrent presence of physiologic gonadotropin concentrations. If GH has a role in normal ovarian physiology, the possibility exists that obesity-related changes in GH status could affect reproductive function.

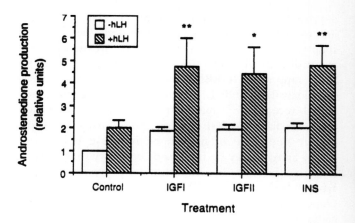

Figure 21–5. Effects of IGF-I (30 ng/ml), IGF-II (30 ng/ml), and insulin (30 ng/ml), in the presence and absence of LH, on A production in thecal cell monolayers established from euandrogenic women. *(Reproduced, with permission, from Nahum R, Thong KJ, Hillier SG. Metabolic regulation of androgen production by human thecal cells in vitro. Hum Reprod. 10:75, 1995.[216])*

Insulin-Like Growth Factors

Circulating insulin-like-growth factor-I (IGF-I; somatomedin-C) is derived largely from hepatic production, which is stimulated by GH. Serum IGF-I (of hepatic origin) has mitogenic effects on muscle and perhaps other tissues. In addition to its endocrine role, IGF-I has several postulated paracrine/autocrine functions. It is produced in adipose, bone, and muscle tissue, where it is hypothesized to act locally to stimulate cellular proliferation. IGF-I and IGF-II also are produced in the ovary, where they may affect steroidogenesis. In vitro studies have indicated that IGF-I stimulates aromatase activity[212] and estradiol secretion,[213] both independently and in response to FSH. It also increases the expression of LH receptors,[214] and stimulates LH-induced androgen synthesis in cultured thecal–interstitial cells from rats.[215] Both IGF-I and IGF-II stimulate LH-induced androgen synthesis in cultured thecal cells from euandrogenic women (Fig 21–5).[216] The importance of locally produced IGFs in ovarian function was demonstrated by inhibiting IGF action with binding proteins.[217] Addition of IGFBP-1 to granulosa cell culture decreased FSH-stimulated progesterone accumulation; this inhibition was prevented by concomitant administration of monoclonal antibodies to IGFBP-1. Regulation of ovarian IGF production is not entirely clear; although it may be affected by GH in the pig and rat, local IGF-I production in the human ovary probably is independent of circulating GH.[206]

The effect of obesity on serum IGF levels and on IGF action is not clear. Obese individuals are reported to have elevated,[218,219] depressed,[200,220,221] or unchanged[219,222] levels of IGF-I. Discrepant observations may derive from differences both in the type of obesity assessed (simple versus visceral) and from the method of assessing IGF-I (total versus free). Visceral fat, but not adiposity per se, was associated with depressed levels of total IGF-I.[221,223] Both types of obesity are associated to some degree with hyperinsulinemia. As mentioned, insulin suppresses IGFBP-1 production, thereby increasing bioavailable IGF-I. Additionally, insulin acting at the IGF-I receptor[86,224] may further augment events normally mediated by IGF-I. Thus, even if total IGF-I levels are depressed or unchanged in obese individuals, IGF-I activity may be increased secondary to associated hyperinsulinemia. In support of this hypothesis, high free IGF-I, high IGFBP-3, low IGFBP-1,[225] and unchanged total IGF-I have been observed in obese individuals.[226]

Although the clinical implications of these obesity-related alterations in the IGF axis are not known, several observations suggest that changes in IGF action could affect reproductive condition. PCOS is associated with decreased IGFBP-1.[227–229] IGFBP-2, IGFBP-4, and a 29K IGF binding protein were increased in the follicular fluid of women with PCOS when compared to that from unaffected individuals.[230] And, in hyperandrogenic adolescents, IGFBP-3 was inversely associated with the free androgen index.[231] This observation could imply that greater IGF bioavailability was causally related either to androgen production, via direct action on the ovary, or to concentrations of free androgens, via reduction in SHBG. IGF-I also has been found to increase steroid production in cultured human adrenocortical cells.[232]

Obesity-related alterations in IGF action have been implicated both in the etiology of PCOS, and in the heterogeneity of the syndrome. According to one hypothesis,[224,233] relatively thin women predisposed to PCOS may develop the syndrome secondary to increased circulating GH. High GH may increase ovarian IGF-I synthesis, and subsequently A production. In contrast, obese women may develop PCOS secondary to hyperinsulinemia and associated defects: decreased IGFBP-1 and increased activation of ovarian IGF-I receptors, either by the greater free IGF or the greater exposure to insulin. This hypothesis is based on the observation that lean PCOS patients had greater GH pulse amplitude than lean controls, and that insulin resistance, although present in all PCOS subjects and obese controls, was greatest in obese PCOS patients. However, compensatory hyperinsulinemia was less in the lean than obese PCOS patients. These data suggest that women who develop PCOS are inherently predisposed to do so (as evidenced by insulin resistance and LH hyperpulsatility), and that obesity serves only to exacerbate underlying defects leading to hyperandrogenic chronic anovulation and polycystic ovary morphology. The possible role of insulin and IGFs in the etiology of PCOS is illustrated in Figure 21–6.

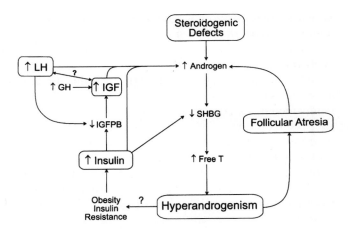

Figure 21–6. Hypothetical mechanism underlying functional ovarian hyperandrogenism. *(Reproduced, with permission, from Cara JF. Insulin-like growth factors, insulin-like growth factor binding proteins and ovarian androgen production.* Horm Res. *42:49, 1994.[338])*

Although much evidence suggests that the IGF system may affect both normal and abnormal aspects of human ovarian function, the role of systemic versus local factors remains unresolved. According to some investigators, it is local IGF-I, rather than that of hepatic origin, that is important in ovarian function.[206] However, intraovarian IGF action may be regulated in part by circulating IGFBPs, which can be derived from the circulation, at least in some species.[234] Production of hepatic IGFBP-1 in humans, and of local IGFBP-3 in porcine follicles,[235] is influenced by insulin (which is elevated in obesity). Furthermore, production of intraovarian IGF-I may be affected by circulating insulin.[235] Other authors do hypothesize a role for serum IGF-I in human ovarian function,[233] and speculate that serum IGF-I can gain entry into at least some ovarian compartments.[234]

Summary

Obesity decreases circulating GH, and is likely to affect IGF action at some level; secondary to obesity-related hyperinsulinemia, the ovary or adrenal may be exposed to increased circulating free IGFs or to increased insulin-binding of IGF-I receptors. Additionally, the ovary may be exposed to decreased IGFBPs, resulting in increased (local) free IGFs. Changes in GH or IGF action at the level of the ovary or adrenal could affect steroidogenesis, resulting in reproductive dysfunction or promoting the development of PCOS.

LEPTIN

The newly discovered hormone leptin is synthesized in, and secreted from, adipocytes of white adipose tissue.[236] In genetically altered obese (*ob/ob*) mice, leptin promotes satiety and increases resting energy expenditure,[237–239] thereby comprising part of a postulated feedback loop regulating energy balance. These actions presumably are mediated centrally, as specific leptin receptors have been identified in various regions of the brain.[240,241] *Ob/ob* mice do not synthesize leptin and therefore become obese. Normal mice synthesize and secrete leptin in direct proportion to the amount of adipose tissue stored; thus, fatter mice have higher levels of circulating leptin.

Both leptin and the gene that codes for it (*ob*) have been identified in human sera and adipose tissue, respectively.[242–244] Like in animal models, people with greater fat stores have higher circulating leptin concentrations. However, to date no physiologic action of leptin has been identified in humans, and defects in leptin production or receptors have not been implicated in the etiology of human obesity.[245]

A role for leptin in normal reproductive physiology is suggested by numerous observations indicating that energy balance affects reproductive function and the secretion of reproductive hormones. Food deprivation, calorie restriction, or negative energy balance induced by exercise or other means can result in delayed puberty, suppressed ovulatory cycles, altered reproductive behavior, and altered gonadotropin secretion in animals and humans.[246–250] Resumption of normal energy intake or energy balance allows normal reproductive function to resume. Because these changes can occur in the absence of, or prior to, appreciable changes in body or fat mass, it is assumed that the change in metabolic status per se is the driving factor.[250] Although the actual signaling molecule(s) has not been identified, its primary effect appears to be suppression of GnRH secretion.[250]

The possibility that leptin may serve as such a signal of metabolic status is suggested by its sensitivity to energy balance. Changes in energy balance are reflected in analogous changes in circulating leptin concentrations in humans,[244,251] and in *ob* gene expression in animals.[252–255] Experiments with *ob/ob* mice, which are infertile,[256] and with normal mice support a role for leptin as a signal of metabolic status to the hypothalamic/hypophyseal centers that regulate reproductive processes. Treatment of *ob/ob* mice with leptin increased circulating concentrations of LH, and increased uterine and ovarian weights in females[257]; increased serum follicle stimulating hormone (FSH), and testicular and seminal vesicle weights in males; promoted histologic changes in ovaries and seminal vesicles indicative of stimulation; and restored fertility.[258] Treatment of normal prepubertal mice with leptin accelerated maturation of the reproductive tract, concomitantly advancing age at first reproduction by 9 days,[259] and resulted in earlier onset of puberty, as indicated by vaginal opening, estrus, and cycling.[260] Although the reproductive effects of leptin are likely to be mediated centrally,[261] re-

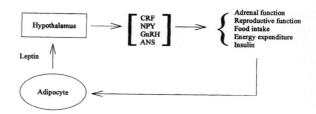

Figure 21–7. Hypothesized feedback loop between energy intake/storage and energy expenditure/reproductive function. Leptin administration (or increased adipocyte leptin production) decreases hypothalamic neuropeptide-Y (NPY), food intake, and insulin, and increases corticotropin-releasing factor (CRF), energy expenditure, and ovarian/uterine weight. See text, Barash et al,[257] and Rohner-Jeanrenaud and Jeanrenaud[261] for additional discussion. *(ANS = autonomic nervous system.)*

ceptors for the hormone also have been found in the ovary,[262] indicating the possibility of local effects. The hypothesized effects of leptin on reproductive and metabolic physiology are illustrated in Figure 21–7.

Few studies have examined the potential role of leptin in human reproductive physiology. Brzechffa et al[263] examined circulating leptin concentrations in women with PCOS, a type of ovulatory dysfunction common in obesity. Leptin was positively correlated with body mass index in both control, cyclic women, and in women with PCOS. However, 29 percent of the PCOS women had levels of leptin above the 99 percent prediction interval for BMI, and none had levels lower than predicted. In contrast, none of the body mass-matched control women had higher-than-expected leptin concentrations. These data suggest that leptin production may be abnormally regulated in women with PCOS. Leptin overproduction could suggest a lack of sensitivity to leptin action, and compensatory hypersecretion. Whether a regulatory defect actually exists in PCOS, or contributes to the etiology of the syndrome, remain to be determined, as does the importance of leptin for normal reproductive function in humans.

Butte et al[264] examined leptin concentrations in women sequentially during both late gestation (36 wk) and lactation (3 mo and 6 mo). The relationship between fat mass and serum leptin (slope of regression line) was the same during both gestation and lactation, but the intercept was greater during gestation. Furthermore, the amount of variance in serum leptin explained by fat mass was greater during lactation ($R^2 = 0.66$) than during gestation ($R^2 = 0.39$). These results imply that at any given fat mass, pregnant women have greater leptin levels, and that factors other than fat mass affect leptin secretion during pregnancy. Both of these observations may be explained by the positive energy balance (and individual differences in the degree of positive energy balance) associated with pregnancy. Leptin was inversely associated with serum prolactin in lactating women, suggesting that central leptin action may affect prolactin production or release. This observation agrees with those from animal studies; leptin-treated female *ob/ob* (sterile) mice were able to bear young, but not lactate.[258] Although the clinical implications of high leptin concentrations on lactation are not known, these limited observations suggest that women who remain in positive energy balance postpartum may produce less milk.

GONADOTROPIN SECRETION IN OBESITY

Comparing premenopausal obese women to normal-weight subjects of the same age, most investigators have noted no difference in the basal or 24-hr luteinizing hormone (LH) and FSH plasma concentrations,[59,62,94] while some have observed a decrease in basal[60] and 24-hr mean concentrations.[265] No significant difference in LH pulsatility has been observed between normal-weight and obese adolescent[88] or premenopausal women.[59] No abnormality in the LH and FSH response to the intravenous administration of gonadotropin-releasing hormone (GnRH)/thyrotropin-releasing hormone (TRH),[124] or to GnRH alone,[62] was observed in eumenorrheic obese women. Obese, ovulatory women have higher A levels than non-obese women, indicating that obesity may result in hyperandrogenism even when ovulation is not affected.[266] FSH and LH circulating levels are similar in obese and normal weight perimenopausal and postmenopausal women. Although the perimenopausal rise in FSH is reported to occur 3 to 4 yr earlier in overweight subjects,[117,126] menopause may be delayed.[267]

Weight reduction does not appear to have a great influence on premenopausal basal LH and FSH circulating levels.[60,114,268] The response of gonadotropins to GnRH was reported to be the same in obese subjects before and after weight reduction.[265] Weight loss in postmenopausal females appears to increase FSH,[115,117] with LH having a similar but less marked trend.[115] Short-term fasting led to the excretion of large quantities of urinary gonadotropins in obese postmenopausal women, although the serum concentrations of LH and FSH did not change.[269] The increased urinary concentration of gonadotropins was attributed to a starvation-related inability of the renal proximal tubular cells to reabsorb and metabolize small proteins, including gonadotropins.

In general, eumenorrheic obesity does not appear to be associated with gross alterations in gonadotropin levels or their hypothalamic–pituitary control. Weight reduction may slightly increase FSH levels in obese postmenopausal women, although it has little effect on premenopausal circulating levels.

PROLACTIN IN EUMENORRHEIC OBESITY

Most reports note that the basal or 24-hr concentration of prolactin (PRL) is normal in obese premenopausal and postmenopausal women,[59,97,270–272] although a slight increase in the basal level of PRL was noted for obese prepubertal girls aged 7 to 9 yr.[89] No such difference was observed in overweight girls aged 10 to 11 yr. Weight reduction appears to have a limited effect on circulating PRL levels,[60] although a slight decrease in the 24-hr concentration was observed after a 12-day fast.[269] In spite of normal serum PRL values in obese subjects the MCR, and consequently the PR, of PRL correlates with body surface area.[273]

It is known that PRL levels demonstrate a nocturnal sleep-entrained peak. Copinschi and associates reported that the PRL peak was significantly delayed in obese patients under basal conditions, occurring between 4:30 and 11:00 AM and after awakening in 4 of 5 subjects.[270] This abnormality was corrected by a 12-day fast (average weight loss of 8 kg). Alternatively, Kwa et al[274] noted that evening blood samples (5:30 to 8:30 PM) revealed higher PRL levels in nulliparous postmenopausal women weighing over 70 kg than in their normal-weight counterparts. This difference was not observed in parous postmenopausal women and was not confirmed by other studies of nocturnal hormonal profiles in obesity.[275] In addition, neither the study by Kwa and associates[274] nor Copinscki et al[270] specify the clinical characteristics of their patients. In eumenorrheic premenopausal women, Zhang and associates did not observe a difference in the 24-hour PRL pulse frequency or amplitude between obese and normal-weight subjects.[59]

Evidence has been presented supporting an abnormality of PRL hypothalamic–pituitary control in obesity. The intravenous administration of TRH has been associated with a deficient rise in PRL in obese women.[271,272] Impaired PRL release was also noted following insulin administration[271,276] and arginine.[277] Alternatively, Wilcox reported a normal PRL and thyroid-stimulating hormone (TSH) response to the administration of TRH in obese premenopausal women.[277] Although Cavagnini et al[276] also reported a normal PRL response to TRH in obese premenopausal subjects, the PRL rise following insulin and arginine infusion was impaired. Differences in PRL response to the administration of TRH could be attributed to the greater intravascular volume of obese subjects. Nevertheless, in obese women Donders et al[272] demonstrated a decreased PRL secretion following TRH infusion, but an increased TSH response. These authors hypothesize that a central deficiency in serotonin may account for the disparity in TSH and PRL responses to TRH in obesity.

Hyperprolactinemia has been associated with elevations in the serum levels and the PR of DHEAS.[278] Increasing WHR is related to greater androgenicity, and Grenman et al noted a significant correlation between the WHR and PRL levels.[60] These data suggest that obesity-related androgenicity, rather than obesity itself, is associated with subtle increases in serum PRL concentrations.

In summary, obese women do not appear to demonstrate any significant difference in baseline or 24-hr PRL concentrations. The circadian secretion of PRL and its hypothalamic control may be subtly impaired, although this remains to be confirmed. Obesity-related abnormalities in PRL metabolism may be more closely associated with androgenicity than with excess body fat.

CLINICAL IMPLICATIONS OF OBESITY

The various endocrinologic aberrations associated with obesity in females result in a number of clinical problems.

Obesity and Pubertal Development

Juvenile obesity is associated with an earlier age at menarche.[267,279,280] Furthermore, the peripubertal, and possibly the prepubertal, onset of obesity is associated with a higher risk of menstrual irregularities and oligo-ovulation.

Obese girls exhibit accelerated rates of linear growth and skeletal maturation, changes that may be due to higher circulating concentrations of insulin and IGF-I, and lower IGFBP-1 (despite lower levels of GH).[219] As discussed earlier, these hormones affect ovarian steroidogenesis in vitro and possibly in vivo, and therefore potentially could affect normal pubertal events.

The hyperinsulinemia associated with childhood obesity may play a role in peripubertal ovulatory disturbances. Hyperinsulinemia was more prevalent in postpubertal females who had experienced premature pubarche, or who were hyperandrogenic, than in control girls, and was positively correlated with the free androgen index.[231,281] Insulin sensitivity, often a cause of hyperinsulinemia, was inversely correlated with obesity. As discussed earlier, insulin may augment ovarian androgen production via specific receptors, or via IGF-I receptors. Whether insulin, and obesity-related hyperinsulinemia, are involved in the early phases of reproductive dysfunction remains to be determined. However, this possibility is support by the observation that ovarian volume and androgen production were associated with insulin concentration in adolescent girls with hyperandrogenism.[282]

Androgen status tracks from childhood to adulthood, and is related to fertility; higher serum androgen concentrations were associated with lower fertility.[283] Thus, aberrations in androgen production during puberty due to obesity or related metabolic complications may have long-lasting effects on reproductive function.

Oligo-Ovulation and Obesity

Bayer[284] reported in 1939 that increased body weight and decreased sugar tolerance was associated with menstrual disturbances. Rogers and Mitchell[285] noted that of 100 patients with menstrual disorders, 43 were more than 20 percent overweight. In a control group of eumenorrheic women the incidence of obesity was only 13 percent. The association of corpulence and ovulatory disturbances has been confirmed in subsequent reports.[286,287]

One of the principal causes of oligo-ovulation is the so-called PCOS,[288] or the hyperandrogenic chronic anovulatory syndrome. This syndrome is a heterogeneous disorder characterized by enlarged ovaries containing multiple small (<5 mm) atretic follicles, hyperandrogenemia, an LH/FSH ratio above 3, oligo-ovulation, and/or hirsutism. Goldzieher and Green[289] noted that the incidence of obesity among patients with PCOS ranged from 16 to 49 percent. These investigators nevertheless felt that there was a higher prevalence of obesity among women with this syndrome than normal. Hartz and associates[290] reported that oligo-ovulatory hirsute women were 30 or more pounds heavier than women with no menstrual abnormalities, after adjusting for height and age. In this study, the incidence of anovulatory cycles was 8.4 percent for women weighing more than 74 percent above IBW as compared to 2.6 percent for women within 20 percent of their ideal weight. In addition, a longer duration of obesity was associated with increased facial hair.

The relationship between excess body fat and ovulatory disturbances appears to be stronger for early-onset obesity. Hartz and associates noted that the incidence of teenage obesity was greater among nulligravid married women than for previously pregnant married females.[290] In this study, teenage obesity was also more frequent among women undergoing surgery for polycystic ovaries than those having ovarian surgery for other reasons. In another report, 96 percent of women with the onset of obesity after menarche reported normal menses as compared to 69 percent of women with a premenarcheal onset of excess weight.[291] Alternatively, Combes et al[286] reported that juvenile onset obesity was less likely to be associated with later menstrual disorders (31 percent) when compared with pubertal or adult onset obesity (53 and 51 percent, respectively). The relationship of peripubertal obesity and oligo-ovulation has been stressed by other investigators.[292]

It is clear that weight loss will re-establish normal menstrual cycles in some of these obese oligo-ovulatory women. In the study by Mitchell and Rogers,[293] there was no clear correlation between the amount of weight lost and the return of menses. In another study, 13 obese anovulatory women, experiencing a reduction in body weight of more than 15 percent, resumed regular menstrual function.[294] Ten of these women (77 percent) became pregnant without additional therapy. These observations have been confirmed by others.[295] It should be noted that dietary restriction and starvation, independent of weight loss, have a significant effect on many endocrinologic systems. Both negative energy balance and weight loss were associated with improved ovarian function in women with PCOS, perhaps due to a reduction in insulin and an increase in SHBG.[296] Nevertheless, weight loss clearly has a salutary effect on ovulatory function.

Women with PCOS exhibit multiple small (< 5 mm) immature follicles throughout the ovarian cortex. Although there appears to be an association between obesity and PCOS, the ovarian changes observed in women with morbid obesity did not appear to be similar to the pathologic findings in PCOS[297] or those seen following long-term androgen treatment.[298] Thus, the etiology and symptomology of PCOS may reflect complications not present in simple obesity-related oligo-ovulation; such complications may be related to insulin resistance and the effects of concomitant hyperinsulinemia on ovarian steroidogenesis.

Observation of elevated A in obese women with normal, ovulatory menstrual cycles suggests that hyperandrogenicity may be involved in the subsequent development of anovulatory cycles.[266] A may undergo peripheral conversion to E_1, which in turn may trigger an increase in LH, leading to increased ovarian androgen production and ovulatory dysfunction.

Obesity and the Development of Hormone-Sensitive Carcinoma

Wynder et al[299] reported that 48 percent of patients with endometrial carcinoma were overweight, compared to 18 percent of the control population. The association between obesity and endometrial cancer has been stressed by others.[300,301] The risk appears to increase linearly with the degree of excess weight and is 10-fold higher in subjects weighing 25 kg in excess of their IBW.[302]

The incidence of breast cancer also appears to be higher in obesity,[303,304] although results differ,[305] and some investigators have argued that body size or body mass are the critical parameters with respect to breast cancer development.[306] The mortality associated with a breast malignancy and the risk of recurrence are increased in overweight women.[307,308] Early menarche, common in obese girls, is a risk factor for breast cancer,[309] perhaps due to early exposure to estrogens or progesterone.

Several mechanisms have been postulated to account for the association between obesity and the development of hormone-sensitive carcinomas. Dietary fat has been implicated as a possible cause due to epidemiologic

and experimental observations of an association between fat intake and breast/mammary cancer.[310,311] Additionally, overweight women may ingest greater quantities of lipid-soluble pre-carcinogens due to their preference for high-fat foods.[312] However, not all studies have found a positive association between fat consumption and breast cancer risk.[313,314] Alternatively, exogenous carcinogens or pre-carcinogens may be lipid soluble, leading to a greater accumulation in the adipose tissue in obese subjects, regardless of their particular dietary preference.[315] A change in the enteric flora of obese women, with the production of endogenous carcinogens from biliary steroids, may also occur.[316] More prevalent is the hypothesis that stresses the association between the endocrinologic alterations of obesity, in particular estrogen metabolism, and cancer risk. Recent evidence suggests that fat distribution, rather than obesity per se, may affect breast cancer risk. Central adiposity is associated with greater risk of postmenopausal breast cancer[317–319] (reviewed in ref. 320), possibly due to the presence of greater visceral fat. Women with breast cancer had greater visceral fat, as assessed with CT scanning, than did control women matched for age, weight, and waist circumference.[321] The relative risk for breast cancer increased with increasing visceral-to-total fat ratio and decreasing subcutaneous abdominal-to-visceral fat ratio. Since visceral obesity is associate with insulin resistance and hyperinsulinemia, the association between visceral obesity and breast cancer may secondary to insulin action. Breast tissue growth may be stimulated either directly by insulin or by the increase in free IGF-I that may occur with insulin-mediated suppression of IGFBP-1. Alternatively, the insulin-induced suppression of SHBG may increase circulating bioavailable estrogens, which in turn could promote the growth of estrogen-sensitive tissue.[322]

The importance of obesity to breast cancer risk appears to be stronger in postmenopausal women[317,323,324] (reviewed in ref. 320). Prior to menopause, obesity actually may have a "protective" effect against the development of breast cancer[325,326] (reviewed in ref. 320). The different relationships between obesity and cancer risk with reproductive status may reflect different etiologies of the disease. In premenopausal women, peripheral production of relatively weak estrogens may interfere with the action of estradiol (or other agonists) at the level of the receptor. Alternatively, obese premenopausal women may produce less progesterone,[320] also a stimulator of breast tissue growth. In postmenopausal women, in whom endogenous estrogens are normally very low, peripheral production of estrogens may stimulate growth of estrogen-sensitive tissue.

Obesity and the Menopause

Obesity may affect menopause and postmenopausal symptomatology. Sherman and colleagues noted that obesity was associated with a later age at menopause.[267] Campagnoli and colleagues, studying women from a geriatric center, noted that overweight women seemed to suffer fewer "somatic" symptoms, such as hot flushes, than normal-weight individuals independent of their socioeconomic level.[327] In contrast, "psychic" (anxiety, depression, irritability, crying spells) problems seemed to be more frequent and incapacitating in severely obese women of all socioeconomic classes, and those minimally obese of the lower socioeconomic group. The authors postulated that while some of these differences may be due to cultural factors, the effect of endogenous estrogens in overweight women may account for the decrease in somatic symptomatology. While Bottiglioni and colleagues were not able to confirm these differences in climacteric symptoms between overweight and normal-weight women, it should be noted that they studied patients from a menopausal clinic, that is, a select population.[328]

It appears that the menopause aggravates the metabolic disturbances already present in overweight subjects, including lipid and glucose regulation.[328] Furthermore, with the onset of menopause the plasma level of testosterone fell in normal-weight women, while it increased in overweight subjects. While obesity in the menopause may be associated with an aggravation of the lipid and glucose tolerance profile, overweight women are at less risk for the development of osteoporosis in the postmenopause.[329] The differences in bone mineral density between obese and normal-weight women is observable in the premenopause, and may account for the lower incidence of osteoporosis and hip fractures in obese postmenopausal women.[330,331]

Menopause may affect both the amount and distribution of adipose tissue deposited. Poehlman et al[332] examined a group of women aged 44 to 48 both at baseline (premenopausal) and 6 yr later, when a portion of the group had become postmenopausal. The investigators observed that those women who became postmenopausal over the 6-yr period gained more fat, and showed a greater increase in waist-to-hip ratio, than did those who remained premenopausal (Fig 21–8). Likewise, cross-sectional analysis of body composition in pre- and postmenopausal women with DXA indicated that total and upper-body fat were greater, and lower-body fat lesser, in the postmenopausal group.[333] Data obtained with CT scanning suggest that the increase in upper-body fat seen in postmenopausal women is visceral.[30] The increase in visceral fat with menopause may be associated with the increased risk for insulin resistance, dyslipidemia, and associated diseases seen in older women.

Limited data suggest that hormone replacement therapy may prevent or reverse the effects of menopause on fat distribution. Haarbo et al,[334] using densitometric scanning, found that women on estrogen–progestin therapy showed less of an increase in abdominal fat over a 2-yr

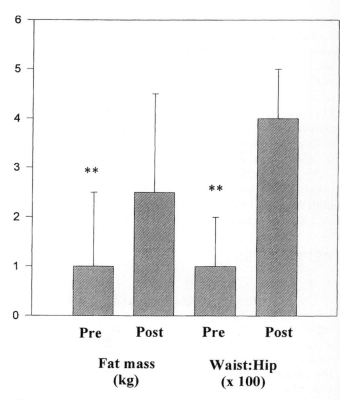

Figure 21–8. Change in total body fat and waist-to-hip ratio in same-aged women who did (Post) or did not (Pre) traverse the menopause during the 6-yr study period. *(Drawn, with permission, from Poehlman ET, Toth MJ, Gardner AW. Changes in energy balance and body composition at menopause: a controlled longitudinal study.* Ann Intern Med. *123:673, 1995.[332])*

study period than did women receiving placebo medication. More recently, Reubinoff et al[335] reported that estrogen/progestin-treated women failed to show an increase in waist-to-hip ratio over a 1-yr study period, whereas women receiving placebos showed a significant increase. Thus, in addition to having direct, beneficial effects on blood lipids,[336,337] hormone therapy also may indirectly benefit metabolic health by minimizing central fat deposition.

CHAPTER SUMMARY

Upper-body/visceral obesity is associated with greater metabolic perturbation than generalized obesity due, at least in part, to a greater degree of insulin resistance and hyperinsulinemia. Female obesity is associated with a suppression of SHBG, an increase in free testosterone, and increases in both the production and clearance rates of a number of androgens. Adipose tissue aromization of androgens may increase circulating estrogens in postmenopausal women.

Obesity is associated with lower circulating GH; nonetheless, effects on total and free IGF-I are variable.

Levels of the newly discovered hormone leptin, produced in human adipose tissue, are higher in obese women and may affect energy expenditure and intake, and possibly reproductive function. Simple obesity is not, however, associated with alterations in gonadotropin or prolactin concentrations.

Obesity is associated with earlier menarche, and increased risk for oligo-ovulation, PCOS, endometrial cancer, and following menopause, breast cancer. Menopause occurs later in obese women, with fewer somatic symptoms and less risk for osteoporosis. Both total and abdominal fat increase around the time of menopause, perhaps contributing to the hyperlipidemia/dyslipidemia and glucose intolerance of aging.

REFERENCES

1. Bray GA. The obese patient. In: Smith LH Jr, ed. *Major Problems in Internal Medicine.* Philadelphia, W. B. Saunders Co., 1976; 9: 1

2. Lohman TG. Dual energy X-ray absorptiometry. In: Roche AF, Heymsfield SB, Lohman TG, eds. *Human Body Composition.* Champaign, Ill., Human Kinetics, 1996: 63

3. Despres JP, Ross R, Limieux S. Imaging techniques applied to the measurement of human body composition. In: Roche AF, Heymsfield SB, Lohman TG, eds. *Human Body Composition.* Champaign, Ill., Human Kinetics, 1996: 149

4. Steinkamp RC, Cohen NL, Gaffey WR, et al. Measures of body fat and related factors in normal adults, II. *J Chronic Dis.* 18:1291, 1965

5. Metropolitan Life Insurance Company. New weight standards for men and women. *Stat Bull.* 40:1, 1959

6. Metropolitan Life Insurance Company. 1983 Metropolitan height and weight tables. *Stat Bull.* 64:3, 1988

7. Metropolitan Life Insurance Company. Frequency of overweight and underweight. *Stat Bull.* 41:4, 1960

8. Health implications of obesity. *Ann Intern Med.* 103:1073, 1985

9. Bray GA. Overweight is risking fate. In: Wurtman RJ, Wurtman JJ, eds. *Human Obesity.* New York, New York Academy of Sciences, 1987: 14

10. Harlan WR, Landis JR, Flegal KM, et al. Secular trends in body mass in the United States, 1960–1980. *Am J Epidemiol.* 128:1065, 1988

11. Stunkard AJ, Stinnett JL, Smoller JW. Psychological and social aspects of the surgical treatment of obesity. *Am J Psychiatry.* 143:417, 1986

12. Weil WBJ. The demographic characteristics of fatness and obesity. In: Hansen BC, ed. *Controversies in Obesity.* New York, Paeger, 1983: 274

13. Sjostrom L. Fat cells and body weight. In: Stunkard AJ, ed. *Obesity.* Philadelphia, W. B. Saunders Co., 1980: 72

14. Hirsch J, Knittle JL. Cellularity of obese and nonobese human adipose tissue. *Fed Proc.* 29:1516, 1970

15. Krotkiewski M, Bjorntorp P, Sjostrom L, Smith U. Impact of obesity on metabolism in men and women. Importance of regional adipose tissue distribution. *J Clin Invest.* 72:1150, 1983

16. Vague J. The degree of masculine differentiation of obesities: A factor determining predisposition to diabetes, atherosclerosis, gout, and uric calculous disease. *Am J Clin Nutr.* 4:20, 1956

17. Kissebah AH, Vydelingum N, Murray R, et al. Relation of body fat distribution to metabolic complications of obesity. *J Clin Endocrinol Metab.* 54:254, 1982

18. Evans DJ, Hoffmann RG, Kalkhoff RK, Kissebah AH. Relationship of androgenic activity to body fat topography, fat cell morphology, and metabolic aberrations in premenopausal women. *J Clin Endocrinol Metab.* 57:304, 1983

19. Soler JT, Folsom AR, Kaye SA, Prineas RJ. Associations of abdominal adiposity, fasting insulin, sex hormone binding globulin, and estrone with lipids and lipoproteins in postmenopausal women. *Atherosclerosis.* 79:21, 1989

20. Terry RB, Wood PD, Haskell WL, et al. Regional adiposity patterns in relation to lipids, lipoprotein cholesterol, and lipoprotein subfraction mass in men. *J Clin Endocrinol Metab.* 68:191, 1989

21. Mauriege P, Despres JP, Marcotte M, et al. Abdominal fat cell lipolysis, body fat distribution, and metabolic variables in premenopausal women. *J Clin Endocrinol Metab.* 71:1028, 1990

22. Ostlund REJ, Staten M, Kohrt WM, et al. The ratio of waist-to-hip circumference, plasma insulin level, and glucose intolerance as independent predictors of the HDL_2 cholesterol level in older adults. *N Engl J Med.* 322:229, 1990

23. Haffner SM, Katz MS, Stern MP, Dunn JF. Association of decreased sex hormone binding globulin and cardiovascular risk factors. *Arteriosclerosis.* 9:136, 1989

24. Despres JP, Allard C, Tremblay A, et al. Evidence for a regional component of body fatness in the association with serum lipids in men and women. *Metabolism.* 34:967, 1985

25. Despres JP. Dyslipidaemia and obesity. *Clin Endocrinol Metab.* 8:629, 1994

26. Despres JP. The insulin resistance-dyslipidemia syndrome: The most prevalent cause of coronary heart disease? *Can Med Assoc J.* 148:1339, 1993

27. Despres JP. Abdominal obesity as important component of insulin-resistance syndrome. *Nutrition.* 9:452, 1993

28. Reaven GM. Role of insulin resistance in human disease. *Diabetes.* 37:1595, 1988

29. Seidell JC, Oosterlee A, Deurenberg P, et al. Abdominal fat depots measured with computed tomography: Effects of degree of obesity, sex, and age. *Eur J Clin Nutr.* 42:805, 1988

30. Zamboni M, Armellini F, Milani MP, et al. Body fat distribution in pre- and post-menopausal women: Metabolic and anthropometric variables and their interrelationships. *Int J Obesity.* 16:495, 1992

31. Bolinder J, Engfeldt P, Ostman J, Arner P. Site differences in insulin receptor binding and insulin action in subcutaneous fat of obese females. *J Clin Endocrinol Metab.* 57:455, 1983

32. Kirschner MA, Samojlik E, Drejka M, et al. Androgen-estrogen metabolism in women with upper body versus lower body obesity. *J Clin Endocrinol Metab.* 70:473, 1990

33. Evans DJ, Barth JH, Burke CW. Body fat topography in women with androgen excess. *Int J Obesity.* 12:157, 1988

34. Pasquali R, Casimirri F, Cantobelli S, et al. Insulin and androgen relationships with abdominal body fat distribution in women with and without hyperandrogenism. *Horm Res.* 39:179, 1993

35. Kissebah AH, Peiris AN. Biology of regional body fat distribution: Relationship to non-insulin-dependent diabetes mellitus. *Diabetes Metab Rev.* 5:83, 1989

36. Lovejoy JC, Bray GA, Bourgeois MO, et al. Exogenous androgens influence body composition and regional body fat distribution in obese postmenopausal women—A clinical research center study. *J Clin Endocrinol Metab.* 81:2198, 1996

37. Elbers JMH, Asscheman H, Seidell JC, Gooren LJG. Increased accumulation of visceral fat after long-term androgen administration in women. *Int J Obesity.* 19(suppl 2):25, 1995. Abstract

38. Marin P, Holmang S, Gustafsson C, et al. Androgen treatment of abdominally obese men. *Obesity Res.* 1:245, 1993

39. Xu X, Hoebeke J, Bjorntorp P. Progestin binds to the glucocorticoid receptor and mediates antiglucocorticoid effect in rat adipose precursor cells. *J Steroid Biochem.* 36:465, 1990

40. Fried SK, Russell CD, Grauso NL, Brolin RE. Lipoprotein lipase regulation by insulin and glucocorticoid in subcutaneous and omental adipose tissues of obese women and men. *J Clin Invest.* 92:2191, 1993

41. Bjorntorp P. Visceral fat accumulation: The missing link between psychosocial factors and cardiovascular disease? *J Int Med.* 230:195, 1991

42. Marin P, Darin N, Amemiya T, et al. Cortisol secretion in relation to body fat distribution in obese premenopausal women. *Metabolism.* 41:882, 1992

43. Rebuffe-Scrive M, Krotkiewski M, Elfverson J, Bjorntorp P. Muscle and adipose tissue morphology and metabolism in Cushing's Syndrome. *J Clin Endocrinol Metab.* 67:1122, 1988

44. Rodin J. Determinants of body fat localization and its implications for health. *Ann Behav Med.* 14:275, 1992

45. Daniel M, Martin AD, Faiman C. Sex hormones and adipose tissue distribution in premenopausal cigarette smokers. *Int J Obesity.* 16:245, 1992

46. Goodman-Gruen D, Barrett-Connor E. Total but not bioavailable testosterone is a predictor of central adiposity in postmenopausal women. *Int J Obesity.* 19:293, 1995

47. Peiris AN, Mueller RA. Relationship of androgenic activity to splanchnic insulin metabolism and peripheral glucose utilization in premenopausal women. *J Clin Endocrinol Metab.* 64:162, 1987

48. Pouliot MC, Despres JP, Lemieux S, et al. Waist circumference and abdominal sagittal diameter: Best simple anthropometric indexes of abdominal visceral adipose tissue accumulation and related cardiovascular risk in men and women. *Am J Cardiol.* 73:460, 1994

49. Conway JM, Yanovski SZ, Avila NA, Hubbard VS. Visceral adipose tissue differences in black and white women. *Am J Clin Nutr.* 61:765, 1995

50. Ferland M, Despres JP, Tremblay A, et al. Assessment of adipose tissue distribution by computed axial tomography in obese women: Association with body density and anthropometric measurements. *Br J Clin Nutr.* 61:139, 1989

51. Kekes-Szabo T, Hunter GR, Nyikos I, et al. Anthropometric equations for estimating abdominal adipose tissue distribution in women. *Int J Obesity.* 20:753, 1996

52. Ryan AS, Nicklas BJ, Elahi D. A cross-sectional study on body composition and energy expenditure in women athletes during aging. *Am J Physiol.* 271:E916, 1996

53. Hunter GR, Kekes-Szabo T, Treuth MS, et al. Intra-abdominal adipose tissue, physical activity and cardiovascular risk in pre- and post-menopausal women. *Int J Obesity.* 20:860, 1996

54. Hartz AJ, Rupley DC, Rimm AA. The association of girth measurements with disease in 32,856 women. *Am J Epidemiol.* 119:71, 1984

55. Blair D, Habicht JP, Sims EAH, et al. Evidence for an increased risk of hypertension with centrally located body fat and the effect of race and sex on this risk. *Am J Epidemiol.* 119:526, 1984

56. Lapidus L, Bengtsson C, Larsson B, et al. Distribution of adipose tissue and risk of cardiovascular disease and death: A 12-year follow-up of participants in the population study of women in Gothenburg, Sweden. *Br Med J.* 289:1257, 1984

57. Shimokata H, Muller DC, Andres R. Studies and the distribution of body fat. III. Effects of cigarette smoking. *JAMA.* 261:1169, 1989

58. Samojlik E, Kirschner MA, Silber D, et al. Elevated production and metabolic clearance rates of androgens in morbidly obese women. *J Clin Endocrinol Metab.* 59:949, 1984

59. Zhang YW, Stern B, Rebar RW. Endocrine comparison of obese menstruating and amenorrheic women. *J Clin Endocrinol Metab.* 58:1077, 1984

60. Grenman S, Ronnemaa T, Irjala K, et al. Sex steroid, gonadotropin, cortisol, and prolactin levels in healthy, massively obese women: Correlation with abdominal fat cell size and effect of weight reduction. *J Clin Endocrinol Metab.* 63:1257, 1986

61. Kaufman ED, Mosman J, Sutton M, et al. Characterization of basal estrogen and androgen levels and gonadotropin release patterns in the obese adolescent female. *J Pediatr.* 98:990, 1981

62. Dunaif A, Mandeli J, Fluhr H, Dobrjanski A. The impact of obesity and chronic hyperinsulinemia on gonadotropin release and gonadal steroid secretion in the polycystic ovary syndrome. *J Clin Endocrinol Metab.* 66:131, 1988

63. Azziz R, Zacur HA, Parker CRJ, et al. Effect of obesity on the response to acute adrenocorticotropin stimulation in eumenorrheic women. *Fertil Steril.* 56:427, 1991

64. Wajchenberg BL, Marcondes JAM, Mathor MB, et al. Free testosterone levels during the menstrual cycle in obese versus normal women. *Fertil Steril.* 51:535, 1989

65. Brody S, Carlstrom K, Lagrelius A, et al. Serum sex hormone binding globulin (SHBG), testosterone/SHBG index, endometrial pathology and bone mineral density in postmenopausal women. *Acta Obstet Gynecol Scand.* 66:357, 1987

66. Kurtz BR, Givens JR, Komindr S, et al. Maintenance of normal circulating levels of delta-4-androstenedione and dehydroepiandrosterone in simple obesity despite increased metabolic clearance rates: Evidence for a servo-control mechanism. *J Clin Endocrinol Metab.* 64:1261, 1987

67. Pardridge WM. Transport of protein-bound hormones into tissues in vivo. *Endocr Rev.* 2:103, 1981

68. Vermulen A, Ando S. Metabolic clearance rate and inter-conversion of androgens and the influence of the free androgen fraction. *J Clin Endocrinol Metab.* 48:320, 1979

69. Rosenfield RL. Studies of the relation of plasma androgen levels to androgen action in women. *J Steroid Biochem.* 6:695, 1975

70. Longcope C, Baker S. Androgen and estrogen dynamics: Relationship with age, weight, and menopausal status. *J Clin Endocrinol Metab.* 76:601, 1993

71. Feher T, Bodrogi L. A comparative study of steroid concentrations in human adipose tissue and peripheral circulation. *Clin Chim Acta.* 126:135, 1982

72. Longcope C, Kato T, Horton R. Conversion of blood androgens to estrogens in normal adult men and women. *J Clin Invest.* 48:2191, 1969

73. Longcope C, Baker R, Johnston CCJ. Androgen and estrogen metabolism: Relationship to obesity. *Metabolism.* 35:235, 1986

74. Edman CD, MacDonald TC. Effect of obesity on conversion of plasma androstenedione to estrone in ovulatory and anovulatory young women. *J Obstet Gynecol.* 130:456, 1978

75. Perel E, Killinger DW. The interconversion and aromatization of androgens by human adipose tissue. *J Steroid Biochem.* 10:623, 1979

76. Deslypere JP, Verdonck L, Vermeulen A. Fat tissue: A steroid reservoir and site of steroid metabolism. *J Clin Endocrinol Metab.* 61:564, 1987

77. Bleau G, Roberts KD, Chapdelaine A. In vitro and in vivo uptake and metabolism of steroids in human adipose tissue. *J Clin Endocrinol Metab.* 39:236, 1974

78. Blohm TR, Laughlin ME. Androgen metabolism in adipose tissue: Conversion of 5-α-dihydrotestosterone to 3-α-androstenediol by hamster tissue. *J Steroid Biochem.* 9:603, 1978

79. Longcope C, Pratt JH, Schneider SH, Fineberg SE. The in vivo metabolism of androgens by muscle and adipose tissue of normal men. *Steroids.* 28:521, 1976

80. Horton R, Tait JF. In vivo conversion of dehydroisoandrosterone to plasma androstenedione and testosterone in man. *J Clin Endocrinol Metab.* 27:79, 1967

81. Feher T, Halmy L. Dehydroepiandrosterone and dehydroandrosterone sulfate dynamics in obesity. *J Biochem.* 53:215, 1975

82. Poretsky L. On the paradox of insulin-induced hyperandrogenism in insulin resistant states. *Endocr Rev.* 12:3, 1991

83. Bergh C, Carlsson B, Olssonn JH, et al. Regulation of androgen production in cultured human thecal cells by insulin-like growth factor I and insulin. *Fertil Steril.* 59:323, 1993

84. Poretsky L, Piper B. Insulin resistance, hypersecretion of LH, and a dual-defect hypothesis for the pathogenesis of polycystic ovary syndrome. *Obstet Gynecol.* 84:613, 1994

85. Kitabchi AE, Buffington CK. Body fat distribution, hyperandrogenicity, and health risks. *Semin Reprod Endocrinol.* 12:6, 1994

86. Ehrmann DA, Barnes RB, Rosenfield RL. Polycystic ovary syndrome as a form of functional ovarian hyperandrogenism due to dysregulation of androgen secretion. *Endocr Rev.* 16:322, 1995

87. Nestler JE, Jakubowicz DJ. Decreases in ovarian cytochrome P450c17-alpha activity and serum free testosterone after reduction of insulin secretion in polycystic ovary syndrome. *N Engl J Med.* 335:617, 1996

88. Brody S, Carlstrom K, Lagrelius A, et al. Adrenal steroids in post-menopausal women: relation to obesity and bone mineral content. *Maturitas.* 9:25, 1987

89. Komindr S, Kurtz BR, Stevens MD, et al. Relative sensitivity and responsivity of serum cortisol and adrenal androgens to adrenocorticotropin (1-24) in normal and obese, nonhirsute, eumenorrheic women. *J Clin Endocrinol Metab.* 63:860, 1986

90. Kobberling J, Von zur MA. The circadian rhythm of free cortisol determined by urine sampling at two-hour intervals in normal subjects and in patients with severe obesity or Cushing's syndrome. *J Clin Endocrinol Metab.* 38:313, 1974

91. Scheingart DE, Gregerman RI, Conn JW. A comparison of the characteristics of increased adrenocortical function in obesity and in Cushing's syndrome. *Metabolism.* 12:484, 1963

92. Migeon CJ, Green OC, Eckert JP. Study of adrenocortical function in obesity. *Metabolism.* 12:718, 1963

93. Genazzani AR, Pintor C, Corda R. Plasma levels of gonadotropins, prolactin, thyroxin, and adrenal and gonadal steroids in obese prepubertal girls. *J Clin Endocrinol Metab.* 47:974, 1978

94. Dunkelman SS, Fairhurst B, Plager J, Waterhouse C. Cortisol metabolism in obesity. *J Clin Endocrinol Metab.* 24:832, 1964

95. O'Connell M, Danforth EJ, Horton ES, et al. Experimental obesity in men. III. Adrenocortical function. *J Clin Endocrinol Metab.* 36:323, 1973

96. Slavnov VN, Epshtein EV. Somatotrophic,thyrotrophic, and adrenocorticotrophic functions of the anterior pituitary in obesity. *Endocrinologie.* 15:213, 1977

97. Simkin V. Urinary 17-ketosteroid and 17-ketogenic steroid excretion in obese patients. *N Engl J Med.* 264:974, 1961

98. Cigolini M, Micciolo R, Pelloso M, Vosello O. Urinary excretion of androgens in obese women. In: Mancini M, Lewis B, Contaldo F, eds. *Medical Complications of Obesity.* Serono Symposia, vol. 26. New York, Academic Press, 1979: 289

99. Lobo RA, Paul WL, Goebelsmann U. Dehydroepiandrosterone sulfate as an indicator of adrenal androgen function. *Obstet Gynecol.* 57:69, 1981

100. Hendrikx A, Meulepas E, Heyns W, De Moor P. A comparative study of the urinary excretion of glucocorticoids in 11-deoxy-17-ketosteroids in a group of obese women. *Ann Endocrinol* (Paris). 35:508, 1974

101. Kamio T, Shigematsu K, Kawai K, Tsuchiyama H. Immunoreactivity and receptor expression of insulin-like growth factor I and insulin in human adrenal tumors. An immunohistochemical study of 94 cases. *Am J Pathol.* 138:83, 1991

102. Pillion DJ, Arnold P, Yang M, et al. Receptors for insulin and insulin-like growth factor-I in the human adrenal gland. *Biochem Biophys Res Comm.* 165:204, 1989

103. Nestler JE, Clore JN, Strauss JF, Blackard WG. Effects of hyperinsulinemia on serum testosterone, progesterone, dehydroepiandrosterone sulfate, and cortisol levels in normal women and in a woman with hyperandrogenism, insulin resistance and acanthosis nigricans. *J Clin Endocrinol Metab.* 64:180, 1987

104. Smith S, Ravnikar VA, Barbieri RL. Androgen and insulin response to an oral glucose challenge in hyperandrogenic women. *Fertil Steril.* 48:72, 1987

105. Falcone T, Finegood DT, Fantus IG, Morris D. Androgen response to endogenous insulin secretion during the frequently sampled intravenous glucose tolerance test in normal and hyperandrogenic women. *J Clin Endocrinol Metab.* 71:1653, 1990

106. Diamond MP, Grainger DA, Laudano AJ, et al. Effect of acute physiological elevations of insulin on circulating androgen levels in nonobese women. *J Clin Endocrinol Metab.* 72:883, 1991

107. Hubert GD, Schriock ED, Givens JR, Buster JE. Suppression of circulating delta-4-androstenedione and dehydroepiandrosterone sulfate during oral glucose tolerance test in normal females. *J Clin Endocrinol Metab.* 73:781, 1991

108. Nestler JE. Insulin and adrenal androgens. *Semin Reprod Endocrinol.* 12:1, 1994

109. Nestler JE, McClanahan MA, Clore JN, Blackard WG. Insulin inhibits adrenal 17,20-lyase activity in man. *J Clin Endocrinol Metab.* 74:362, 1992

110. Moghetti P, Castello R, Negri C, et al. Insulin infusion amplifies 17alpha-hydroxycorticosteroid intermediates response to adrenocorticotropin in hyperandrogenic women: Apparent relative impairment of 17,20-lyase activity. *J Clin Endocrinol Metab.* 81:881, 1996

111. Dunaif A, Scott D, Finegood D, et al. The insulin-sensitizing agent troglitazone improves metabolic and reproductive abnormalities in the polycystic ovary syndrome. *J Clin Endocrinol Metab.* 81:3299, 1996

112. Azziz R, Bradley EL Jr, Potter HD, et al. Chronic hyperinsulinemia and the adrenal androgen response to acute corticotropin-(1-24) stimulation in hyperandrogenic women. *Am J Obstet Gynecol.* 172:1251, 1995

113. Sarah MJ, Givens JR, Kitabchi AE. Bimodal correlation between the circulating insulin level and the production rate of dehydroepiandrosterone: Positive correlation in controls and negative correlation in the polycystic ovary syndrome with acanthosis nigricans. *J Clin Endocrinol Metab.* 70:1075, 1990

114. Kopelman PG, White N, Pilkington TRE, Jeffcoate SL. The effect of weight loss on steroid secretion and binding in massively obese women. *Clin Endocrinol.* 14:113, 1981

115. O'Dea JPK, Wieland RG, Hallberg MC, et al. Effect of dietary weight loss on sex steroid binding, sex steroids and gonadotropins in obese postmenopausal women. *J Lab Clin Med.* 93:1004, 1979

116. Kim MH, Friedman CI, Barrows H, Rosenfield RL. Serum androgen concentrations in the massively obese reproductive woman: The response to weight loss. *Trans Am Gynecol Obstet Soc.* 1:26, 1982

117. Klinga K, von Holst TH, Runnebaum B. Serum concentrations of FSH, oestradiol, oestrone and androstenedione in normal and obese women. *Maturitas.* 4:9, 1982

118. Pintor C, Genazzani AR, Buggioni R, et al. Effect of weight loss on adrenal androgen plasma levels in obese prepubertal girls. In: Genazzani AR, Thijssen JHH, Siiteri PK, eds. *Adrenal Androgens.* New York, Raven Press, 1980: 259

119. Van Riet HG, Schwarz F, Der Kinderen PJ. Metabolic observations during the treatment of obese patients by periods of total starvation. *Metabolism.* 13:291, 1964

120. Schultz AL, Kerlow A, Ulstrom RA. Effect of starvation on adrenal cortical function in obese subjects. *J Clin Endocrinol Metab.* 24:1253, 1964

121. Hendrikx A, Heyns W, de Moor P. Influence of a low-calorie diet fasting on the metabolism of dehydroepiandrosterone sulfate in adult obese subjects. *J Clin Endocrinol Metab.* 28:1525, 1968

122. Judd HL. Hormonal dynamics associated with the menopause. *Clin Obstet Gynecol.* 19:775, 1976

123. Trichopoulos D, Polychronopoulou A, Brown J, MacMahon B. Obesity, serum cholesterol, and estrogens in premenopausal women. *Oncology.* 40:227, 1983

124. Kopelman PG, Pilkington TRE, White N, Jeffocate SL. Abnormal sex steroid secretion and binding in massively obese women. *Clin Endocrinol.* 12:363, 1980

125. Zumoff B, Strain GW, Kream J, et al. Obese young men have elevated plasma estrogen levels but obese premenopausal women do not. *Metabolism.* 30:1011, 1981

126. Klinga K, von Holst T, Runnebaum B. Influence of severe obesity on peripheral hormone concentrations in pre- and postmenopausal women. *Eur J Obstet Gynecol Reprod Biol.* 15:103, 1983

127. Vermeulen A. Sex hormone status of the postmenopausal woman. *Maturitas.* 1:81, 1980

128. Meldrum DR, Davidson BJ, Tataryn IV, Judd HL. Changes in circulating steroids with aging in postmenopausal women. *Obstet Gynecol.* 57:624, 1981

129. Vermeulen A, Verdonck L. Sex hormone concentrations in post-menopausal women. *Clin Endocrinol.* 9:59, 1978

130. Davidson BJ, Gambone JC, Lagasse LV. Free estradiol in postmenopausal women with and without endometrial cancer. *J Clin Endocrinol Metab.* 52:404, 1981

131. West CD, Damast BL, Sarro SD, Pearson OH. Conversion of testosterone to estrogens in castrated, adrenalectomized human females. *J Biol Chem.* 218:409, 1956

132. Schindler AE, Ebert A, Friedrich E. Conversion of androstenedione to estrone by human fat tissue. *J Clin Endocrinol Metab.* 35:627, 1972

133. Nimrod A, Ryan KJ. Aromatization of androgens by human abdominal and breast fat tissue. *J Clin Endocrinol Metab.* 40:367, 1975

134. MacDonald PC, Edman CD, Hemsell DL, et al. Effect of obesity on conversion of plasma androstenedione to estrone in postmenopausal women with and without endometrial cancer. *Am J Obstet Gynecol.* 130:448, 1978

135. Ackerman GE, Smith ME, Mendelson CR, et al. Aromatization of androstenedione by human adipose tissue stromal cells in monolayer culture. *J Clin Endocrinol Metab.* 53:412, 1981

136. Cleland WH, Mendelson CR, Simpson ER. Aromatase activity of membrane fractions of human adipose tissue, stromal cells and adipocytes. *Endocrinology.* 113:2155, 1983

137. Longcope C, Pratt JH, Schneider SH, Fineberg SE. Aromatization of androgens by muscle and adipose tissue in vivo. *J Clin Endocrinol Metab.* 46:146, 1978

138. Rizkallah TH, Tovell HMM, Kelly WG. Production of estrone and fractional conversion of circulating androstenedione to estrone in women with endometrial carcinoma. *J Clin Endocrinol Metab.* 40:1045, 1975

139. Takaki NK, Siiteri PK, Williams J, et al. The effect of weight loss on peripheral estrogen synthesis in obese women. *Int J Obesity.* 2:386, 1978

140. Forney JP, Milewich L, Chen GT, et al. Aromatization of androstenedione to estrone by human adipose tissue in vitro. Correlation with adipose tissue mass, age, and endometrial neoplasia. *J Clin Endocrinol Metab.* 53:192, 1981

141. Cleland WH, Mendelson CR, Simpson ER. Effects of aging and obesity on aromatase activity of human adipose cells. *J Clin Endocrinol Metab.* 60:174, 1985

142. MacDonald PC, Edman CD, Kerber IJ, Siiteri PK. Plasma precursors of estrogen. III. Conversion of plasma dehydroisoandrosterone to estrogen in young nonpregnant women. *Gynecol Invest.* 7:165, 1976

143. Hemsell DL, Grodin JM, Brenner PF, et al. Plasma precursors of estrogen. II. Correlation of the extent of conversion of plasma androstenedione to estrone with age. *J Clin Endocrinol Metab.* 38:476, 1974

144. Longcope C, Layne DS, Tait JF. Metabolic clearance rates and interconversions of estrone and 17-β-estradiol in normal males and females. *J Clin Invest.* 47:93, 1968

145. Schneider J, Bradlow HL, Strain G, et al. Effects of obesity on estradiol metabolism: Decreased formation of nonuterotropic metabolites. *J Clin Endocrinol Metab.* 56:973, 1983

146. Flood C, Pratt JH, Longcope C. The metabolic clearance and blood production rates of estriol in normal, non-pregnant women. *J Clin Endocrinol Metab.* 42:1, 1976

147. Roncari DAK, Van RLR. Promotion of human adipocyte precursor replication by 17-β-estradiol in culture. *J Clin Invest.* 62:503, 1977

148. De Waard F, Poortman J, de Pedro-Alvarez Ferrero M, Baanders-van Halewisn EA. Weight reduction and oestrogen excretion in obese post-menopausal women. *Maturitas.* 4:155, 1982

149. Kato T, Horton R. Studies of testosterone binding globulin. *J Clin Endocrinol Metab.* 28:1160, 1968

150. O'Brien TJ, Higashi M, Kanasugi H, et al. A plasma/serum estrogen-binding protein distinct from testosterone-estradiol-binding globulin. *J Clin Endocrinol Metab.* 54:793, 1982

151. Anderson DC. Sex-hormone-binding globulin. *Clin Endocrinol.* 3:69, 1974

152. Pardridge WM, Mietus LJ, Frumar AM, et al. Effects of human serum on transport of testosterone and estradiol into rat brain. *Am J Physiol.* 239:E103, 1980

153. Nisker JA, Hammond GL, Davidson JB, et al. Serum sex hormone-binding globulin capacity and the percentage of free estradiol in postmenopausal women with and without endometrial carcinoma. *Am J Obstet Gynecol.* 138:638, 1980

154. Vermeulen A, Verdonck L, Van Der Straeten M, Orie N. Capacity of the testosterone-binding globulin in human plasma and influence of specific binding of testosterone on its metabolic clearance rate. *J Clin Endocrinol Metab.* 28:1470, 1969

155. Doe RP, Mellinger GT, Swaim WR, Coseal US. Estrogen dosage effects on serum proteins: A longitudinal study. *J Clin Endocrinol Metab.* 27:1081, 1967

156. Musa BU, Doe RP, Coseal US. Serum protein alterations produced in women by synthetic estrogens. *J Clin Endocrinol Metab.* 27:1463, 1967

157. Laurell CB, Kullander S, Thorell J. Effect of administration of a combined estrogen-progesterone contraceptive on the level of individual plasma protein. *Scand J Clin Lab Invest.* 21:337, 1968

158. Pearlman WH, Crepy O, Murphy M. Testosterone-binding levels in the serum of women during the normal menstrual cycle, pregnancy, and the post-partum period. *J Endocrinol Metab.* 27:1012, 1976

159. Wu CH, Motohashi T, Abdel-Rahman HA, et al. Free and protein-bound plasma estradiol 17-β during the menstrual cycle. *J Clin Endocrinol Metab.* 43:436, 1967

160. Dickinson P, Zineman HH, Swaim WR, et al. Effects of testosterone treatment on plasma proteins and amino acids in men. *J Clin Endocrinol Metab.* 29:837, 1969

161. Azziz R, Gay F, Potter SR, et al. Effect of prolonged hypertestosteronemia on adrenocortical biosynthesis in oophorectomized women. *J Clin Endocrinol Metab.* 72:1025, 1991

162. Bloch CA, Clemons P, Sperling MA. Puberty decreases insulin sensitivity. *J Pediatr.* 110:481, 1987

163. Holly JMP, Smith CP, Dunger DB, et al. Relationship between the pubertal fall in sex hormone binding globulin and insulin-like growth factor binding protein-I. A synchronized approach to pubertal development. *Clin Endocrinol.* 31:277, 1989

164. Cunningham S, Loughlin T, Culliton M, McKenna TJ. Plasma sex hormone-binding globulin levels decrease during the second decade of life irrespective of pubertal status. *J Clin Endocrinol Metab.* 58:915, 1984

165. Pugeat M, Crave JC, Elmidani M, et al. Pathophysiology of sex hormone binding globulin (SHBG): Relation to insulin. *J Steroid Biochem Molec Biol.* 40:841, 1991

166. Siiteri PK, Hammond GL, Nisker JA, Tataki N. Adrenal androgen, metabolism and conversion in humans. In: Genazzani AR, Thijssen JHH, Siiteri PK, eds. *Adrenal Androgens.* New York, Raven Press, 1985: 109

167. Dunkel L, Sorva R, Voutilainen R. Low levels of sex hormone-binding globulin in obese children. *J Pediatr.* 107:95, 1985

168. Bernasconi D, Del Monte P, Meozzi M, et al. The impact of obesity on hormonal parameters in hirsute and nonhirsute women. *Metabolism.* 45:72, 1996

169. Lee IR, Greed LC, Hahnel R. Comparative measurements of plasma-binding capacity and concentration of human sex hormone binding globulin. *Clin Chim Acta.* 137:131, 1984

170. Plymate SR, Matej LA, Jones RE, Friedel KE. Inhibition of sex hormone binding globulin production in the human hepatoma (HepG2) cell line by insulin and prolactin. *J Clin Endocrinol Metab.* 66:460, 1988

171. Fendri S, Arlot S, Marcelli JM, et al. Relationship between insulin sensitivity and circulating sex hormone binding-globulin levels in hyperandrogenic obese women. *Int J Obesity.* 18:755, 1994

172. Robinson S, Kiddy D, Gelding SV, et al. The relationship of insulin insensitivity to menstrual pattern in women with hyperandrogenism and polycystic ovaries. *Clin Endocrinol.* 39:351, 1993

173. Preziosi P, Barrett-Connor E, Papoz L, et al. Interrelation between plasma sex hormone-binding globulin and plasma insulin in healthy adult women: The telecom study. *J Clin Endocrinol Metab.* 76:283, 1993

174. Nestler JE, Powers LP, Matt DW, et al. A direct effect of hyperinsulinemia on serum sex hormone-binding globulin levels in obese women with the polycystic ovary syndrome. *J Clin Endocrinol Metab.* 72:83, 1991

175. Lindstedt G, Lundberg PA, Lapidus L, et al. Low sex-hormone-binding globulin concentration as independent risk factor for development of NIDDM. *Diabetes.* 40:123, 1991

176. Haffner S, Katz M, Stern M, Dunn J. Relationship of sex hormones to hyperinsulinemia and hyperglycemia. *Metabolism.* 37:683, 1988

177. Peiris AN, Stagner JI, Plymate SR, et al. Relationship of insulin secretory pulses to sex hormone-binding globulin in normal men. *J Clin Endocrinol Metab.* 76:279, 1993

178. Birkeland KI, Hanssen KF, Torjesen PA, Vaaler S. Level of sex hormone-binding globulin is positively correlated with insulin sensitivity in men with type 2 diabetes. *J Clin Endocrinol Metab.* 76:275, 1993

179. Reed MJ, Cheng RW, Simmonds M, et al. Dietary lipids: An additional regulator of plasma levels of sex hormone binding globulin. *J Clin Endocrinol Metab.* 64:1083, 1987

180. Arendt EC, Pattee CJ. Studies on obesity. I. *Metabolism.* 16:367, 1956

181. Sims EAH, Danforth E Jr, Horton ES, et al. Endocrine and metabolic effects of experimental obesity in man. *Recent Prog Horm Res.* 29:457, 1973

182. Pagano G, Cassader M, Bozzo C, et al. Insulin resistance in human obesity: In vivo studies by "insulin clamping" and in vitro by insulin binding and biologic activity on isolated adipocytes. In: Enzi G, Grepaldi G, Pozza G, Renold AE, eds. *Obesity: Pathogenesis and Treatment.* Serono Symposia, vol. 28. New York, Academic Press, 1981: 175

183. Debry G, Martin JM, Pointel JP, et al. Comparative study of glucose tolerance and stimulated insulin secretion in obesity by oral and intravenous glucose tolerance and tolbutamide tests. In: Mancini M, Lewis B, Contaldo F, eds. *Medical Complications of Obesity.* Serono Symposia, vol. 26. New York, Academic Press, 1979: 59

184. Golay A, Swislocki ALM, Chen YDI, et al. Effect of obesity on ambient plasma glucose, free fatty acid, insulin, growth hormone, and glycogen concentrations. *J Clin Endocrinol Metab.* 63:481, 1986

185. Koivisto VA, Yki-Jarvinen H, Hartling SG, Pelkonen R. The effect of exogenous hyperinsulinemia on proinsulin secretion in normal man, obese subjects, and patients with insulinoma. *J Clin Endocrinol Metab.* 63:1117, 1986

186. Kolterman OG, Insel J, Saekow M, Olefsky JM. Mechanisms of insulin resistance in human obesity. *J Clin Invest.* 65:1272, 1980

187. Grunberer G, Taylor SI, Dons RF, Gorden P. Insulin receptors in normal and diseased states. *Clin Endocrinol Metab.* 12:191, 1983

188. Bagdade JD, Bierman EL, Porte D Jr. The significance of basal insulin levels in the evaluation of insulin response to glucose in diabetic and nondiabetic subjects. *J Clin Invest.* 46:1549, 1967

189. El-Khodary AZ, Ball MF, Oweiss IM, Canary JJ. Insulin secretion in body composition in obesity. *Metabolism.* 21:641, 1972

190. Olefsky J, Reaven JM, Farquhar JW. Effects of weight reduction on obesity. *J Clin Invest.* 53:64, 1974

191. Bar RS, Gorden P, Roth J, et al. Fluctuations in the affinity and concentration of insulin receptors on circulating monocytes of obese patients. *J Clin Invest.* 58:1123, 1976

192. Lungren H, Bengtsson C, Blohme G, Lapidus L. Adiposity and adipose tissue distribution in relation to incidence of diabetes in women: Results from a prospective population study in Goteborg, Sweden. *Int J Obesity.* 13:413, 1989

193. Bjorntorp P. Androgens, the metabolic syndrome, and non-insulin-dependent diabetes mellitus. *Ann NY Acad Sci.* 676:242, 1993

194. Holmang A, Svedberg J, Jennische E, Bjorntorp P. Effects of testosterone on muscle insulin sensitivity and morphology in female rats. *Am J Physiol.* 259:E555, 1990

195. Stuart CA, Prince MJ, Peters EJ, Meyer WJ III. Hyperinsulinemia and hyperandrogenemia: In vivo androgen response to insulin infusion. *Obstet Gynecol.* 69:921, 1987

196. Schriock ED, Buffington CK, Hubert GD, et al. Divergent correlations of circulating dehydroepiandrosterone sulfate and testosterone with insulin levels and insulin receptor binding. *J Clin Endocrinol Metab.* 66:1329, 1988

197. Burghen GA, Givens JR, Kitabchi AE. Correlation of hyperandrogenism with hyperinsulinism in polycystic ovarian disease. *J Clin Endocrinol Metab.* 50:113, 1980

198. Veldhuis JD, Liem AY, South S, et al. Differential impact of age, sex steroid hormones, and obesity on basal versus pulsatile growth hormone secretion in men as assessed in an ultrasensitive chemiluminescence assay. *J Clin Endocrinol Metab.* 80:3209, 1995

199. Dubey AK, Hanukoglu A, Hansen BC, Kowarski AA. Metabolic clearance rates of synthetic human growth

hormone in lean and obese male rhesus monkeys. *J Clin Endocrinol Metab.* 67:1064, 1988

200. Rasmussen MH, Hvidberg A, Juul A, et al. Massive weight loss restores 24-hour growth hormone release profiles and serum insulin-like growth factor-I levels in obese subjects. *J Clin Endocrinol Metab.* 80:1407, 1995

201. Conover CA, Lee PDK, Kanaley JA, et al. Insulin regulation of insulin-like growth factor binding protein-1 in obese and nonobese humans. *J Clin Endocrinol Metab.* 74:1355, 1992

202. Mogul HR, Marshall M, Frey M, et al. Insulin like growth factor-binding protein-1 as a marker for hyperinsulinemia in obese menopausal women. *J Clin Endocrinol Metab.* 81:4492, 1996

203. Orlowski CC, Ooi GT, Brown DR, et al. Insulin rapidly inhibits insulin-like growth factor binding protein-1 gene expression in H4-II-E rat hepatoma cells. *Molec Endocrinol.* 5:1180, 1991

204. Ooi GT, Tseng LYH, Tran MQ, Rechler MM. Insulin rapidly decreases insulin-like growth factor binding protein-1 gene transcription in streptozocin-diabetic rats. *Molec Endocrinol.* 6:2219, 1992

205. Lee PDK, Jensen MD, Divertie GD, et al. Insulin-like growth factor-binding protein-1 response to insulin during suppression of endogenous insulin secretion. *Metabolism.* 42:409, 1993

206. Katz E, Ricciarelli E, Adashi EY. The potential relevance of growth hormone to female reproductive physiology and pathophysiology. *Fertil Steril.* 59:8, 1993

207. Mason HD, Martkaninen H, Beard RW, et al. Direct gonadotrophic effect of growth hormone on oestradiol production by human granulosa cells. *J Endocrinol.* 126:R1, 1990

208. Lanzone A, Di Simone N, Castellani R, et al. Human growth hormone enhances progesterone production by human luteal cells in vitro: Evidence of a synergistic effect with human chorionic gonadotropin. *Fertil Steril.* 57:92, 1990

209. Homburg R, West C, Ostergaard H, Jacobs HS. Combined growth hormone and gonadotropin treatment for ovulation induction in patients with non-responsive ovaries. *Gynecol Endocrinol.* 5:33, 1991

210. Homburg R, West C, Torresani T, Jacobs HS. Cotreatment with human growth hormone and gonadotropin for induction of ovulation: A controlled clinical trial. *Fertil Steril.* 53:254, 1990

211. Homburg R, Eshel A, Abdalla HI, Jacobs HS. Growth hormone facilitates ovulation induction by gonadotropins. *Clin Endocrinol.* 29:113, 1988

212. Erickson G, Gabriel GV, Magoffin D. Insulin-like growth factor-I regulates aromatase activity in human granulosa cells and granulosa luteal cells of polycystic ovaries. *J Clin Endocrinol Metab.* 69:716, 1989

213. Mason HD, Margara R, Winston RML, et al. Insulin-like growth factor-I (IGF-I) inhibits production and IGF-binding protein-1 while stimulating estradiol secretion in granulosa cells from normal and polycystic human ovaries. *J Clin Endocrinol Metab.* 76:1275, 1993

214. Cara JF, Fan J, Azzarello J, Rosenfield RL. Insulin-like growth factor-I enhances luteinizing hormone binding to rat ovarian theca-interstitial cells. *J Clin Invest.* 86:560, 1990

215. Cara JF, Rosenfield RL. Insulin-like growth factor-I and insulin potentiate luteinizing hormone-induced androgen synthesis by rat ovarian theca-interstitial cells. *Endocrinology.* 123:733, 1988

216. Nahum R, Thong KJ, Hillier SG. Metabolic regulation of androgen production by human thecal cells in vitro. *Hum Reprod.* 10:75, 1995

217. Adashi EY, Resnick CE, Rosenfeld RG, et al. Insulin-like growth factor (IGF) binding protein-1 is an antigonadotropin: evidence that optimal follicle-stimulating hormone action in ovarian granulosa cells is contingent upon amplication by endogenously-derived IGFs. *Adv Exp Med Biol.* 343:377, 1993

218. Loche S, Cappa M, Borrelli P, et al. Reduced growth hormone response to growth hormone-releasing hormone in children with simple obesity: Evidence for somatomedin-C mediated inhibition. *Clin Endocrinol.* 27:145, 1987

219. Vanderschueren-Lodeweyckx M. The effect of simple obesity on growth and growth hormone. *Horm Res.* 40:23, 1993

220. Minuto F, Barreca A, Del Monte P, et al. Spontaneous growth hormone and somatomedin-C/insulin-like growth factor-I secretion in obese subjects during puberty. *J Endocrinol Invest.* 11:489, 1988

221. Rasmussen MH, Frystyk J, Andersen T, et al. The impact of obesity, fat distribution, and energy restriction on insulin-like growth factor-I (IGF-I), IGF-binding protein-3, insulin, and growth hormone. *Metabolism.* 43:315, 1994

222. Slowinska-Srzednicka J, Zgliczynski W, Makowska A, et al. An abnormality of the growth hormone/insulin-like growth factor-I axis in women with polycystic ovary syndrome due to coexistent obesity. *J Clin Endocrinol Metab.* 74:1432, 1992

223. Marin P, Kvist H, Lindstedt G, et al. Low concentrations of insulin-like growth factor-I in abdominal obesity. *Int J Obesity.* 17:83, 1993

224. Insler V, Shoham Z, Barash A, et al. Polycystic ovaries in non-obese and obese patients: Possible pathophysiological mechanism based on new interpretation of facts and findings. *Hum Reprod.* 8:379, 1993

225. Weaver JU, Holly JM, Kopelman PG, et al. Decreased sex hormone binding globulin (SHBG) and insulin-like growth factor binding protein (IGFBP-1) in extreme obesity. *Clin Endocrinol.* 33:415, 1990

226. Frystyk J, Vestbo E, Skjaerbaek C, et al. Free insulin-like growth factors in human obesity. *Metabolism.* 44:37, 1995

227. Laatikainen T. How IGF-I and IGF-I binding protein can be modulated in polycystic ovarian syndrome. *Ann NY Acad Sci.* 687:90, 1993

228. Suikkari AM, Ruutiainen K, Erkkola R, Seppala M. Low levels of low molecular weight insulin-like growth factor binding protein in patients with polycystic ovarian disease. *Hum Reprod.* 4:136, 1989

229. Pekonen F, Laatikainen T, Buyalos R, Rutanen EM. Decreased 34K insulin-like growth factor binding protein in polycystic disease. *Fertil Steril.* 51:972, 1989

230. San Roman GA, Magoffin DA. Insulin-like growth factor binding proteins in ovarian follicles from women with polycystic ovarian disease: Cellular source and levels in follicular fluid. *J Clin Endocrinol Metab*. 75:1010, 1992

231. Ibanez L, Potau N, Georgopoulos N, et al. Growth hormone, insulin-like growth factor-I axis, and insulin secretion in hyperandrogenic adolescents. *Fertil Steril*. 64:1113, 1995

232. Pham-Huu-Trung MT, Villette JM, Bogyo A, et al. Effects of insulin-like growth factor I (IGF-I) on enzymatic activity in human adrenocortical cells. Interactions with ACTH. *J Steroid Biochem Molec Biol*. 39:903, 1991

233. Morales AJ, Laughlin GA, Butzow T, et al. Insulin, somatotropic, and luteinizing hormone axes in lean and obese women with polycystic ovary syndrome: Common and distinct features. *J Clin Endocrinol Metab*. 81:2854, 1996

234. Armstrong DG, Hogg CO, Campbell BK, Webb R. Insulin-like growth factor (IGF)-binding protein production by primary cultures of ovine granulosa and theca cells. The effects of IGF-I, gonadotropin, and follicle size. *Biol Reprod*. 55:1163, 1996

235. Edwards JL, Hughey TC, Moore AB, Cox NM. Depletion of insulin in streptozocin-induced-diabetic pigs alters estradiol, insulin-like growth factor (IGF)-I, and IGF binding proteins in cultured ovarian follicles. *Biol Reprod*. 55:775, 1996

236. Zhang Y, Proenca R, Maffei M, et al. Positional cloning of the mouse obese gene and its human homologue. *Nature*. 372:425, 1994

237. Weigle DS, Bukowski TR, Foster DC, et al. Recombinant *ob* protein reduces feeding and body weight in the *ob/ob* mouse. *J Clin Invest*. 96:2065, 1995

238. Halaas JL, Gajiwala KS, Maffei M, et al. Weight-reducing effects of the plasma protein encoded by the obese gene. *Science*. 269:543, 1995

239. Pellymounter MA, Cullen MJ, Baker MB, et al. Effects of the obese gene product on body weight regulation in *ob/ob* mice. *Science*. 269:540, 1995

240. Lee G, Proenca R, Montez JM, et al. Abnormal splicing of the leptin receptor in diabetic mice. *Nature*. 379:632, 1996

241. Tartaglia LA, Dembski M, Weng X, et al. Identification and expression cloning of a leptin receptor, OB-R. *Cell*. 83:1263, 1995

242. Lonnqvist F, Arner P, Nordfors L, Schalling M. Overexpression of the obese (*ob*) gene in adipose tissue of human obese subjects. *Nature Med*. 1:950, 1995

243. Maffei M, Halaas J, Ravussin E, et al. Leptin levels in human and rodent: Measurement of plasma leptin and *ob* RNA in obese and weight-reduced subjects. *Nature Med*. 1:1155, 1995

244. Considine RV, Shinha MK, Heiman ML, et al. Serum immunoreactive leptin concentrations in normal weight and obese humans. *N Engl J Med*. 334:292, 1996

245. Maffei M, Stoffel M, Barone M, et al. Absence of mutations in the human OB gene in obese/diabetic subjects. *Diabetes*. 45:679, 1996

246. Wade GN, Schneider JE. Metabolic fuels and reproduction in female mammals. *Neurosci Biobehav Rev*. 16:235, 1992

247. Stewart D. Reproductive functions in eating disorders. *Ann Med*. 24:287, 1992

248. De Souza M, Metzger D. Reproductive dysfunction in amenorrheic athletes and anorexic patients: A review. *Med Sci Sports Exerc*. 23:995, 1991

249. Griffin M, South S, Yankov V, et al. Insulin-dependent diabetes mellitus and menstrual dysfunction. *Ann Med*. 26:331, 1994

250. Wade GN, Schneider JE, Li HY. Control of fertility by metabolic cues. *Am J Physiol*. 270:E1, 1996

251. Kolaczynski JW, Ohannesian JP, Considine RV, et al. Response of leptin to short-term and prolonged overfeeding in humans. *J Clin Endocrinol Metab*. 81:4162, 1996

252. Becker DJ, Ongemba LN, Brichard V, et al. Diet-induced and diabetes-induced changes of *ob* gene expression in rat adipose tissue. *FEBS Lett*. 371:324, 1995

253. Cusin I, Sainsbury A, Doyle P, Rohner-Jeanreanaud B. The ob gene and insulin. A relationship leading to clues to the understanding of obesity. *Diabetes*. 44:1467, 1995

254. Trayhurn P, Thomas MEA, Duncan JS, Rayner DV. Effects of fasting and refeeding on *ob* gene-expression in white adipose tissue of lean and obese (*ob/ob*) mice. *FEBS Lett*. 368:488, 1995

255. Saladin R, De Vos P, Guerre-Millo M, et al. Transient increase in obese gene expression after food intake or insulin administration. *Nature*. 377:527, 1995

256. Coleman DL. Obese and diabetes: Two mutant genes causing diabetes-obesity syndromes in mice. *Diabetologia*. 14:141, 1978

257. Barash IA, Cheung CC, Weigle DS, et al. Leptin is a metabolic signal to the reproductive system. *Endocrinology*. 137:3144, 1996

258. Chehab FF, Lim ME, Lu R. Correction of the sterility defect in homozygous obese female mice by treatment with the human recombinant leptin. *Nature Genet*. 12:318, 1996

259. Chehab FF, Mounzih K, Lu R, Lin ME. Early onset of reproductive function in normal female mice treated with leptin. *Science*. 275:88, 1997

260. Ahima RS, Dushay J, Flier SN, et al. Leptin accelerates the onset of puberty in normal female mice. *J Clin Invest*. 99:391, 1997

261. Rohner-Jeanrenaud F, Jeanrenaud B. Obesity, leptin, and the brain. *N Engl J Med*. 334:324, 1996

262. Cioffi JA, Shafer AW, Zupancic TJ, et al. Novel B219.OB receptor isoforms: Possible role of leptin in hemato-poiesis and reproduction. *Nature Med*. 2:585, 1996

263. Brzechffa PR, Jakimiuk AJ, Agarwal SK, et al. Serum immunoreactive leptin concentrations in women with polycystic ovary syndrome. *J Clin Endocrinol Metab*. 81:4166, 1996

264. Butte NF, Hopkinson JM, Nicholson MA. Leptin in human reproduction: Serum leptin levels in pregnant and lactating women. *J Clin Endocrinol Metab*. 82:585, 1997

265. Zumoff B, Strain GW, Kream J, et al. Subnormal 24-hour mean plasma LH concentration and elevated plasma FSH/LH ratio in obese premenopausal women. *J Reprod Med*. 28:843, 1983

266. Unzer SRM, dos Santos JE, Moreira AC, et al. Alterations in plasma gonadotropin and sex steroid levels in

obese ovulatory and chronically anovulatory women. *J Reprod Med.* 40:516, 1995

267. Sherman B, Wallace R, Bean J, Schlabaugh. Relationship of body weight to menarcheal and menopausal age: Implications for breast cancer risk. *J Clin Endocrinol Metab.* 52:488, 1981

268. Newmark SR, Rossini AA, Aftolin FI, et al. Gonadotropin profiles in fed and fasted obese women. *Am J Obstet Gynecol.* 133:75, 1979

269. Beitins IZ, Shah A, O'Loughlin K, et al. The effects of fasting on serum and urinary gonadotropins in obese postmenopausal women. *J Clin Endocrinol Metab.* 51:26, 1980

270. Copinscki G, De Laaet MH, Brion JP, et al. Simultaneous study of cortisol, growth hormone and prolactin nyctohemeral variations in normal and obese subjects: Influence of prolonged fasting in obesity. *Clin Endocrinol.* 9:15, 1978

271. Kopelman PG, Pilkington TRE, White N, Jeffocate SL. Impaired hypothalamic control of prolactin secretion in massive obesity. *Lancet.* 1:747, 1979

272. Donders SHJ, Peiters J, Heevel JG, et al. Disparity of thyrotropin (TSH) and prolactin response to TSH-releasing hormone in obesity. *J Clin Endocrinol Metab.* 61:56, 1985

273. Cooper DS, Ridgway EC, Kliman B, et al. Metabolic clearance and production rates of prolactin in man. *J Clin Invest.* 64:1669, 1979

274. Kwa HG, Bulbrook RD, Clenton F, et al. An abnormal early evening peak of plasma prolactin in nulliparous and obese postmenopausal women. *Int J Cancer.* 22:691, 1978

275. Kalucy RS, Crisp AH, Chard T, et al. Nocturnal hormonal profiles in massive obesity, anorexia nervosa in normal females. *J Psychosom Res.* 20:595, 1976

276. Cavagnini F, Maraschini C, Pinto M, et al. Impaired prolactin secretion in obese patients. *J Endocrinol Invest.* 4:149, 1981

277. Wilcox RG. Triiodothyronine, TSH, and prolactin in obese women. *Lancet.* 1:1027, 1977

278. Schiebinger RJ, Chrousos GP, Cutler GBJ, Loriaux DL. The effect of serum prolactin on plasma adrenal androgens and the production and metabolic clearance rate of dehydroepiandrosterone sulfate in normal and hyperprolactinemic subjects. *J Clin Endocrinol Metab.* 62:202, 1986

279. World Health Organization Task Force on Adolescent Reproductive Health. World Health Organization multicenter study on menstrual and ovulatory patterns in adolescent girls. *J Adolesc Health Care.* 7:229, 1986

280. Vignolo M, Naselli A, DiBattista E, et al. Growth and development in simple obesity. *Eur J Pediatr.* 147:242, 1988

281. Ibanez L, Potau N, Zampolli M, et al. Hyperinsulinemia in postpubertal girls with a history of premature pubarche and functional ovarian hyperandrogenism. *J Clin Endocrinol Metab.* 81:1237, 1996

282. Apter D, Butzow T, Laughlin GA, Yen SSC. Metabolic features of polycystic ovary syndrome are found in adolescent girls with hyperandrogenism. *J Clin Endocrinol Metab.* 80:2966, 1995

283. Apter D, Vihko R. Endocrine determinants of fertility: Serum androgen concentrations during follow-up of adolescents into the third decade of life. *J Clin Endocrinol Metab.* 71:970, 1990

284. Bayer LM. Build in relation to menstrual disorders and obesity. *Endocrinology.* 24:260, 1939

285. Rogers J, Mitchell GWJ. The relation of obesity to menstrual disturbances. *N Engl J Med.* 247:53, 1952

286. Combes R, Altomare E, Tramoni M, Vague J. Obesity in menstrual disorders. In: Mancini EM, Lewis B, Contaldo F, eds. *Medical Complications of Obesity.* Serono Symposia, vol. 26. New York, Academic Press, 1979: 285

287. Nagata I, Kato K, Seki K, Furuya K. Ovulatory disturbance. *J Adolesc Health Care.* 7:1, 1986

288. Adams J, Polsom DW, Franks S. Prevalence of polycystic ovaries in women with anovulation and its idiopathic hirsutism. *Br Med J.* 292:355, 1986

289. Goldzieher JW, Green JA. The polycystic ovary I. Clinical and histologic features. *J Clin Endocrinol Metab.* 22:325, 1962

290. Hartz AJ, Barboriak PN, Wong A, et al. The association of obesity with infertility and related menstrual abnormalities in women. *Int J Obesity.* 3:57, 1979

291. Friedman CI, Kim MH. Obesity and its effect on reproductive function. *Clin Obstet Gynecol.* 28:645, 1958

292. Yen SSC, Chaney C, Judd HL. Functional aberrations of the hypothalamic-pituitary system in polycystic ovary syndrome: A consideration of the pathogenesis. In: James VHT, Serio M, Guisti G, eds. *Endocrine Function of the Human Ovary.* New York, Academic Press, 1976: 373

293. Mitchell GWJ, Rogers J. The influence of weight reduction on amenorrhea in obese women. *N Engl J Med.* 249:835, 1953

294. Bates GW, Whitworth NS. Effect of body weight reduction on plasma androgens in obese, infertile women. *Fertil Steril.* 38:406, 1982

295. Harlass FE, Plymate SR, Farris BL, Belts RP. Weight loss is associated with correction of gonadotropin and sex steroid abnormalities in the obese anovulatory female. *Fertil Steril.* 42:649, 1984

296. Kiddy DS, Hamilton-Fairley D, Bush A, et al. Improvement in endocrine and ovarian function during dietary treatment of obese women with polycystic ovary syndrome. *Clin Endocrinol.* 36:105, 1992

297. Fisher ER, Gregorio R, Stephan T, et al. Ovarian changes in women with morbid obesity. *Obstet Gynecol.* 44:839, 1974

298. Amirikia H, Savoy-Moore RT, Sundareson AS, Moghissi KS. The effects of long-term androgen treatment on the ovary. *Fertil Steril.* 45:202, 1986

299. Wynder EL, Escher GC, Mantel N. Epidemiological investigation of cancer of the endometrium. *Cancer.* 19:489, 1966

300. Damon A. Host factors in cancer of the breast and uterine cervix and corpus. *J Natl Cancer Inst.* 24:483, 1960

301. MacMahon B. Risk factors for endometrial cancer. *Gynecol Oncol.* 2:122, 1974

302. Elwood JM, Cole P, Rothman KJ, Kaplin SD. Epidemiology of endometrial cancer. *J Natl Cancer Inst.* 59: 1055, 1977

303. Staszewski J. Breast cancer and body build. *Prev Med.* 6:410, 1977

304. Paffenbarger RSJ, Kampert JB, Chang HG. Characteristics that predict risk of breast cancer before and after the menopause. *Am J Epidemiol.* 112:258, 1980

305. London SJ, Colditz GA, Stampfer MJ, et al. Prospective study of relative weight, height, and risk of breast cancer. *JAMA.* 262:1853, 1989

306. DeWaard F. Breast cancer incidence and nutritional status with particular reference to body weight and height. *Cancer Res.* 35:3351, 1975

307. Donegan WL, Hartz AJ, Rimm AA. The association of body weight with recurring cancer of the breast. *Cancer.* 41:1590, 1978

308. Tartter PI, Papatestas AE, Iannovich J, et al. Cholesterol and obesity as prognostic factors in breast cancer. *Cancer.* 47:222, 1981

309. Lipworth L. Epidemiology of breast cancer. *Eur J Cancer Prev.* 4:7, 1990

310. Armstrong B, Doll R. Environmental factors and cancer incidence and mortality in different countries, with special reference to dietary practices. *Int J Cancer.* 15:617, 1975

311. Howe GR, Hirohata T, Hislop TG, et al. Dietary factors and risk of breast cancer: Combined analysis of 12 case-controlled studies. *J Natl Cancer Inst.* 82:561, 1990

312. Miller AV, Kelly A, Choi NW, et al. A study of diet and breast cancer. *Am J Epidemiol.* 107:499, 1978

313. Graham S, Marshall J, Mettlin C, et al. Diet in the epidemiology of breast cancer. *Am J Epidemiol.* 116:68, 1982

314. Hunter DJ, Spiegelman D, Adami HO, et al. Cohort studies of fat intake and the risk of breast cancer—a pooled analysis. *N Engl J Med.* 334:356, 1996

315. Beer AE, Billingham RW. Adipose tissue, a neglected factor in etiology of breast cancer? *Lancet.* 2:296, 1978

316. Hill MJ, Goddard P, Williams REO. Gut bacteria and etiology of cancer of the breast. *Lancet.* 2:472, 1971

317. Bruning PR, Bonfrer JMG, Hart AAM, et al. Body measurements, estrogen availability and the risk of human breast cancer: A case-control study. *Int J Cancer.* 51:14, 1992

318. Sellers TA, Kushi LH, Potter JD, et al. Effect of family history, body fat distribution, and reproductive factors on the risk of postmenopausal breast cancer. *N Engl J Med.* 326:1323, 1992

319. Folsom AR, Kaye SA, Prineas RJ, et al. Increased incidence of carcinoma of the breast associated with abdominal adiposity in postmenopausal women. *Am J Epidemiol.* 131:794, 1990

320. Ballard-Barbash R. Anthropometry and breast cancer. Body size—a moving target. *Cancer.* 74:1090, 1994

321. Schapira DV, Clark RA, Wolff PA, et al. Visceral obesity and breast cancer risk. *Cancer.* 74:632, 1994

322. Toniolo PG, Levitz M, Zeleniuch-Jacquotte A, et al. A prospective study of endogenous estrogens and breast cancer in postmenopausal women. *J Natl Cancer Inst.* 87:190, 1995

323. Hseih C, Trichopoulos D, Katsouyanni K, Yuasa S. Age at menarche, age at menopause, height and obesity as risk factors for breast cancer: Associations and interactions in an international case-control study. *Int J Cancer.* 46:796, 1990

324. Parazzini F, La Vecchia C, Negri E, et al. Anthropometric variables and risk of breast cancer. *Int J Cancer.* 45:397, 1990

325. Brinton LA, Swanson CA. Height and weight at various ages and risk of breast cancer. *Ann Epidemiol.* 2:597, 1992

326. Vatten LJ, Kvinnsland S. Prospective study of height, body mass index and risk of breast cancer. *Acta Oncol.* 31:195, 1992

327. Campagnoli C, Morra G, Belforte P et al. Climacteric symptoms according to body weight in women of different socio-economic groups. *Maturitas.* 3:279, 1981

328. Bottiglioni F, de Aloysio D, Nicolett G, et al. Physiopathological aspects of body overweight in the female climacteric. *Maturitas.* 5:153, 1984

329. Slemenda CW, Hui SL, Longcope C, et al. Predictors of bone mass in perimenopausal women. A prospective study of clinical data using photon absorptiometry. *Ann Int Med.* 112:96, 1990

330. Dequeker J, Goris P, Uytterhoeven R. Osteoporosis and osteoarthritis (osteoarthrosis). Anthropometric distinctions. *JAMA.* 249:1448, 1983

331. Liel Y, Edwards J, Shary J, et al. The effects of race and body habitus on bone mineral density of the radius, hip, and spine in premenopausal women. *J Clin Endocrinol Metab.* 66:1247, 1988

332. Poehlman ET, Toth MJ, Gardner AW. Changes in energy balance and body composition at menopause: a controlled longitudinal study. *Ann Intern Med.* 123:673, 1995

333. Ley CJ, Lees B, Stevenson JC. Sex- and menopause-associated changes in body-fat distribution. *Am J Clin Nutr.* 55:950, 1992

334. Haarbo J, Marslew U, Gotfredsen A, Christiansen C. Postmenopausal hormone replacement therapy prevents central distribution of body fat after menopause. *Metabolism.* 40:1323, 1991

335. Reubinoff BE, Wurtman J, Rojansky N, et al. Effects of hormone replacement therapy on weight, body composition, fat distribution, and food intake in early postmenopausal women: A prospective study. *Fertil Steril.* 64:963, 1995

336. Vaziri SM, Evans JC, Larson MG, Wilson PWF. The impact of female hormone usage on the lipid profile. *Arch Intern Med.* 153:2200, 1993

337. Sitruk-Ware R. Cardiovascular risk at the menopause—Role of sexual steroids. *Horm Res.* 43:58, 1995

338. Cara JF. Insulin-like growth factors, insulin-like growth factor binding proteins and ovarian androgen production. *Horm Res.* 42:49, 1994

Chapter 22

BREAST DISEASE

Richard E. Blackwell and Karen R. Hammond

The breast has assumed a prominent role in art and literature throughout history. It is identified as an object of beauty and sexuality, and as such its role goes far beyond its primary function of lactation. Because of the importance attached by society to the breast, any pathology of the organ is viewed by the patient with alarm. With the exception of carcinoma, disorders of the breast are not life threatening; however, any deviation from normal size and appearance must be thoroughly evaluated.

BENIGN PATHOLOGY OF THE BREAST

Developmental Anomalies

Nipple inversion, breast hypertrophy, hypoplasia of the breast, and breast asymmetry represent a family of congenital anomalies. These anomalies are uncommon and may consist of amastia (congenital absence of the breast), athelia (congenital absence of the nipple), polymastia (multiple breasts), and polythelia (multiple nipples). Polythelia, for instance, occurs in about 1 to 2 percent of the population and has a familial tendency.[1] Thelarche may occur in children under 8 yr old and present with either bilateral or unilateral breast development occurring independent of other events associated with puberty. Premature thelarche is self-limited and usually no therapy is required; these children have prepubertal serum gonadotropin and estrogen levels (see Chap 5).

Patients often present with breast asymmetry and are quite concerned about this condition. Presumably, this occurs secondary to a difference in end-organ sensitivity to estrogens and progestogens. The condition may be treated with oral contraceptive agents, which often may result in acquisition of full symmetry. Often, once the patient understands that the breasts are subject to the same asymmetry as other body parts, no therapy is requested. However, in extreme cases of breast asymmetry, augmentation and/or reduction mammoplasty can be carried out.

Breast hypoplasia is likewise a common complaint that presents to the reproductive endocrinologist (see Chap 6). The breasts may be small secondary to a transient delay in puberty, or there may be a genetic tendency toward hypoplasia (see Fig 6–9). Obviously, small breasts increase in size physiologically during pregnancy secondary to an altered hormonal milieu, and the affected person usually will lactate normally and can breast-feed without difficulty. Breast augmentation, however, is often sought by affected women because of social pressure to have "normal-sized breasts." It should be noted that augmentation mammoplasty does not interfere with lactation or breast-feeding, yet it complicates the self-examination process and radiographic surveillance for malignancies. Further, breast implants have been reported to leak or become displaced and concern has been raised in the lay press regarding the alleged role of silicone in the development of autoimmune dysfunction. Breast hypoplasia can be found in patients who have systemic diseases such as eating disorders or other variances of hypothalamic amenorrhea associated with a decreased body weight or extremes in exercise. These patients demonstrate hypogonadotropic hypoestrogenism, which results in breast atrophy.[2] Further, women taking medication such as GnRH analogs will experience a transient reduction in breast size. Finally, breast hypoplasia can occur in association with genetic disorders such as female pseudohermaphrodism or Turner syndrome variance.

Nipple inversion is common and the situation can be rectified with cosmetic surgery. Unfortunately, following these procedures, breast-feeding is difficult because of interruption of the lactiferous ducts. Nipple inversion can resolve during pregnancy, and it is rare for inversion to pose difficulty for the breast-feeding mother. However, it should also be recalled that unilateral nipple inversion may be a sign of breast malignancy.

Gigantomastia (macromastia or breast hypertrophy) is very commonly encountered in adults and adolescents (see Fig 6–7). Breast hypertrophy may be unilateral or bilateral, and patients often present seeking treatment for chest wall or shoulder pain secondary to the weight of the breast. Further, these women often have difficulty finding clothes to fit the upper body, have difficulty with their self-image, and are frequently under intense sexual pressure. Young women are often embarrassed by peers when appearing in gymnasium classes or in swimsuits.

Therefore, reduction mammoplasty is frequently a benefit for relief of both physical and emotional symptoms associated with that condition (Fig 22–1).

Functional Disorders of the Breast

Galactorrhea is a common problem encountered by the gynecologist, and is frequently seen in association with menstrual dysfunction or disorders of puberty. Milk secretion may be intermittent, continuous, unilateral, bilateral, expressible, or free flowing. On microscopy, fat globules are detected, which can be used to separate simple galactorrhea from discharge secondary to infection or benign or malignant tumors. If cells are present on microscopic exam, the discharge should be fixed as it is for a Papanicolaou smear and examined by a pathologist. The patient who presents with galactorrhea should have a measurement of serum prolactin level repeated (see Chap 15). Prolactin secretion is physiologically stimulated by stress, breast examination, and food intake, and follows a sleep-entrained pattern. In the past it was recommended that prolactin be measured an hour away from meals, preferably in the late morning or early afternoon. Recently these beliefs have been challenged in that prospective controlled studies evaluating the effect of amino acids such as tyrosine, tryptophan, and arginine

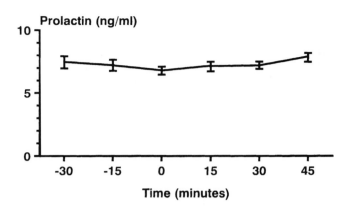

Figure 22–2. Failure of high-dose oral intake of amino acids (tryptophan, tyrosine, arginine) to elevate serum prolactin levels in normal cycling women.

in normal cycling reproductive age women failed to show significant elevation in prolactin with an hour's follow-up (Fig 22–2). Likewise, breast examination carried out in a similar group of women failed to result in the acute release of prolactin (Fig 22–3). Although breast examination or suckling will result in an elevated prolactin level in women who are pregnant or in postpartum women, and the infusion of pharmacologic doses of arginine or other amino acids may elevate prolactin levels in men, it appears that these events taken in the context of daily practice do not influence the measurement of this hormone. Further, it is advisable to repeat the measurement of prolactin because tabulations from the College of American Pathologists standards suggest that there is a great variation in laboratory stability to measure this hormone. For instance, in 1985 the data suggested that multiple assays carried out in nearly 400 laboratories resulted in a mean value of 95 ng/ml, with the range extending from 5 to 135 ng/ml. It should be recalled that most contemporary prolactin assays were developed from monoclonal antibodies and the measurement is carried out on a single serum sample, although analyzed by automated systems. However, room for error exists, and no data are available concerning the likelihood of obtaining a normal level after measurement of an elevated level.

Further, patients with hyperprolactinemia should be evaluated for compensated hypothyroidism with a high-sensitivity TSH assay. Large pituitary lesions have been demonstrated in patients with hypothyroidism, and these problems are corrected with the administration of Synthroid.[3] Finally, it should be mentioned that macroprolactinemia is present with considerable frequency in pregnant women; the formation of big big prolactin is due to different etiologies.[4,5]

Once the presence of a pituitary tumor and its size has been determined by MRI or CT scanning, therapy is often instituted with dopamine agonists (see Chap 15). In the Middle Ages it was noted that women who ate bread made from rye flour contaminated with the fungus

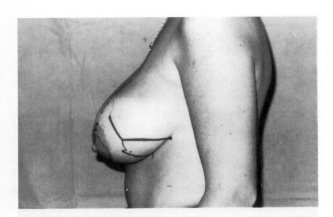

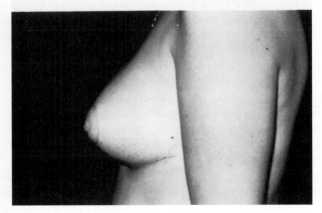

Figure 22–1 Lateral view of patient before and after classic reduction mammoplasty.

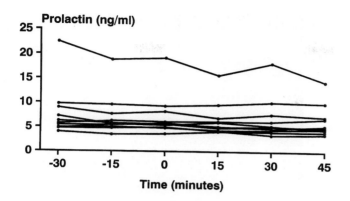

Figure 22–3. Failure of breast examination to elevate serum pro-lactin levels in normal cycling women.

Claviceps purpura, developed gangrenous ergotism and failure to lactate. A disease called St. Anthony's fire resulted from the ingestion of ergot alkaloids (ergopeptines). Later these compounds were extracted for obstetrical use, and in the mid-1970s the first dopamine agonist (Parlodel) was developed, which revolutionized the care of patients with hyperprolactinemia. This compound inhibits prolactin secretion and synthesis, both in vitro and in vivo, and normalizes the prolactin level in the vast majority of patients. Further, it can cause astounding shrinkage of large prolactinomas.[6] Bromocriptine is usually administered orally in doses ranging from 1.25 to 160 mg, the latter dose for patients with Parkinson's disease. However, the majority of patients with hyperprolactinemia respond to doses of 2.5 to 15 mg/day. Bromocriptine ingestion results in a number of side effects including nausea. Some patients are hypersensitive to the drug, and intractable vomiting will develop. Likewise, nasal stuffiness, dysphoria, and lethargy are common side effects, and at very high doses psychosis or fatal tachyarrhythmias can occur.[7] The drug is frequently administered at bedtime to maximize its effectiveness, and it has been suggested that vaginal delivery will attenuate some of the side effects.[8] It has been demonstrated that oral and vaginal administration may result in different kinetics; the vaginal route resulting in a slower rise in serum levels but a longer maintenance.[9] It is suggested that the drug be administered at 1.25 mg at bedtime and increased until prolactin levels are suppressed over the next 4 wk.

Other drugs are available for the treatment of hyperprolactinemia, although they are used in an off-label manner. Pergolide mesylate (Permax, Eli Lilly), is a nonergoline dopamine agonist that is three times more potent than bromocriptine and is taken once a day. Its active dose range is 50 to 100 μg and it is highly effective in suppressing hyperprolactinemia in patients with and without tumors.[10] The drug carries FDA approval for the treatment of Parkinson's disease; however, it is widely used in Europe and Canada for the treatment of hyperprolactinemic disorders.

CV205-052 is a new nonergoline dopamine agonist that suppresses hyperprolactinemia in the 60- to 80-μg range. It has a 30 percent better side-effect profile than bromocriptine[11] Like bromocriptine and pergolide mesylate, patients can experience dysphoria, lethargy, nasal stuffiness, and at times nausea. The drug is sold in Europe under the trade name Norprolac; it is unclear whether it will ever be approved for use in the United States.

Several new forms of bromocriptine have been introduced into the European market. Parlodel SRO is a long-acting oral bromocriptine.[12] The drug suppresses the prolactin level with a single dose for greater than 24 hr. After 1 mo therapy, 63 percent of patients have normal prolactin levels and 43 percent have a return of menstruation. Likewise, Parlodel LAR is a long-acting repeatable injectable form of bromocriptine.[13] The polymer matrix has a total mass degradation of less than 3 mo and is being used every 28 days for prolactin suppression. It should be noted that these drugs are not available on the current U.S. market.

Cabergoline is a new potent dopamine agonist that inhibits prolactin levels from 7 to 14 days. It can be administered by oral or vaginal routes and is thought to be better tolerated than bromocriptine, although gastrointestinal side effects are frequently reported.[14] Like bromocriptine, it has been demonstrated to improve menstrual cyclicity in certain categories of women with polycystic ovary syndrome.[15]

Mastodynia is a painful engorgement of the breast and is usually cyclic. It is generally worse before menstruation, and is frequently treated with cyclic analgesics or nonsteroidal anti-inflammatory drugs.[16] Mastodynia may be a component of the premenstrual tension syndrome, which is often treated by rendering the patient acyclic with either oral contraceptive agents or low-dose danazol.

Breast infections may present with unilateral or bilateral discharge and are often confused with galactorrhea. Fat globules are not demonstrated on microscopic examination, and Gram stain or culture will frequently demonstrate the presence of staphylococcus, streptococcus, *E coli*, or pseudomonas. If the discharge has a greenish tint to it, it is very likely that pseudomonas forms will be isolated. These infections are treated with systemic antibiotics; if an abscess forms, incision and drainage may be required.

Galactoceles or retention cysts occur frequently after the cessation of lactation and are probably secondary to mechanical duct obstruction. These cysts can masquerade as mastitis, and lesions will be palpated that lie below the areola and are tender. Pressure can often cause emptying of the cyst; however, incision and drainage frequently must be carried out. Untreated galactoceles may be a site of future sepsis; they can calcify and cause confusion with malignancy. When drained, the galactocele produces a milky to clear to green, yellow-green, purulent-appearing material, yet the lesions are sterile.

Fibrocystic Changes

Women frequently present to the gynecologist with a history of breast pain and lumpiness. Usually, these represent benign processes, but they are frequently referred to as fibrocystic disease. Other terms such as chronic lobular hyperplasia, cystic hyperplasia, and chronic cystic mastitis have been used. However, the appropriate terminology applied to this condition is benign breast disease of mammary dysplasia, and the term cystic mastitis should be discarded because inflammation is not present in the disorder. Mammary dysplasia is perhaps the most common lesion of the female breast; it can be bilateral or unilateral, and is frequently seen in the upper outer quadrant (Fig 22–4). The disorder tends to exacerbate during menstrual periods, and patients usually complain of pain or lumps in the breast. The breast may be tender in many locations, but axillary adenopathy is not found. Breast lumps are frequently cystic, and they tend to fluctuate with the menstrual cycle and shrink after menstruation. The natural history of the disease varies and it may resolve after menopause.[17,18] Nipple discharge can accompany mammary dysplasia and this is often confused with galactorrhea. The discharge may be clear or bloody in 15 percent of individuals, and this may be confused with carcinoma. A Papanicolaou smear of the discharge, mammography, and needle aspiration may be necessary to rule out a malignancy. Breast aspiration will usually yield a gray, dirty-green fluid. The cysts may vary in size from 1 mm to many cm, and they are usually unilocular. When examined histologically, the cysts are lined with cells that contain a large number of mitochondria, and secretory granules. They yield a pink color on eosin staining. The cells are columnar and may have a protuberance that appears to be bleb-like (snouts).

Treatment for mammary dysplasia is usually directed at suppressing breast lumpiness and pain. Pain at times can be relieved by avoiding methylxanthine. Some patients respond well to cyclic oral contraceptive use, and in more extreme cases danazol therapy at doses of 100 to 800 mg a day can be used. Likewise, GnRH analog therapy with leuprolide (Lupron) could be instituted; however, treatment beyond 6 mo will require add-back therapy with estrogens. The empiric use of bromocriptine while suppressing prolactin secretion has not been demonstrated in placebo-controlled trials to be effective in treating cyclic mastodynia.

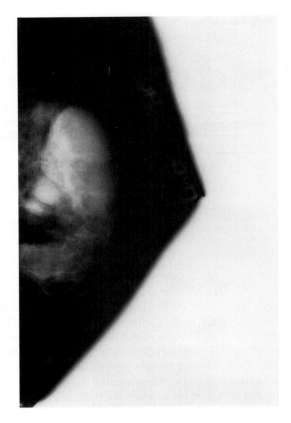

Figure 22–4. Mammogram of patient with fibrodysplasia.

Benign Breast Tumors

Apocrine metaplasia is often associated with ductal hyperplasia. When viewed histologically, metaplastic epithelial cells are characterized by dense eosinophilic cytoplasm, often with evident apical apocrine secretions. The cells exhibit hyperplastic features; capillary hyperplasia is particularly common in association with apocrine change. Although rare forms of mammary carcinoma show apocrine features, apocrine metaplasia is usually considered a benign phenomenon and is seldom associated with atypical hyperplasia.

Hyperplasia is defined as an increased number of cells relative to a specific basement membrane. The breast hyperplasias range from mild forms, which are characterized by the presence of three or more cells above the basement membrane and carry no increased risk of formation of carcinoma; to atypical ductal or lobular hyperplasia, which contains some features of well-differentiated carcinoma, and is associated with an increased risk of carcinoma in situ of 8- to 10-fold. A special feature of the lobular neoplasias is their tendency to undermine normal cell populations. To complete the transition of carcinoma in situ, one must find a uniform group of neoplastic cells populating the entire basement membrane space. Some investigators still advocate that this alteration must involve two or more spaces. It has also been suggested that an intercellular pattern of rigid arches and even placement of cells must be present along with the findings of hyperchromatic nuclei.[19]

Adenosis refers to increased numbers of acini within a lobular unit. Adenosis with or without mild sclerosis is not a marker of malignant potential. Florid sclerosing adenosis, on the other hand, has been recognized as an indicator of slightly increased cancer risk. Sclerosing adenosis mimics invasive carcinoma of the breast. These lesions are usually smooth and circumscribed, contain a double cell layer, and are confined to a lobular unit. The central spaces are most often flattened and there is rarely the finding of an atypical cytoplasmic snout. Elastic tissue mass is usually not present. These lesions are characterized by proliferation of ductal tissue that produce a palpable lesion. These lesions are commonly found in younger women, especially in the third and fourth decades of life, and they are rarely seen after menopause. Grossly, breast carcinoma is firm and gritty to palpation whereas adenosis is usually rubbery.

Fat necrosis may present as a hard lump and may be tender. It rarely enlarges and may be associated with a history of trauma. The histology of fat necrosis in the breast is no different from that appearing in other organs. One will find chronic inflammatory cells including lymphocytes and histiocytes. Clinically, the acute phase develops approximately 1 wk after an inciting event with the findings of white cells and oily lipid material. In the acute stage, swelling, redness, and warmth are found. In the later stage, caliginous scarring may be found and surround an oily cyst. Skin retraction may be seen along with irregularity of the edges, and fine stipple calcifications have been demonstrated on mammography. Over one half of the patients give a history of breast trauma, and excisional biopsy is the treatment of choice.[20,21]

The interductal papilloma is a benign lesion of the lactiferous duct wall that usually occurs below the areola (75 percent of cases). Such lesions present with pain or bloody discharge. They are generally soft, small masses. They are extremely difficult to locate. The presentation of a bloody nipple discharge in association with a small palpable mass is associated with a 75 percent chance of interductal papilloma. If no mass can be palpated, Paget's disease of the nipple or carcinoma should be considered. The interductal papilloma is not pre-malignant and is best managed by incision of the duct. Interductal papillomas are usually found in women of the late childbearing years, although they have been reported in adolescents. In younger patients the lesions are found in the periphery of the breast and multiple ducts may be involved. There may be cystic dilation of the lesions and

they have been called Swiss cheese or juvenile papillomatosis.[22,23]

Duct ectasias include a group of entities that involve duct dilation. These lesions present as lumps and are frequently found under the areola. Nipple discharge is commonly found, scarring occurs, and the majority of cases show nipple inversion. Periductal inflammation is the hallmark of the condition and it is most frequently found in the perimenopausal female.

Perhaps the most common benign neoplasm of the adolescent and adult breast is the fibroadenoma (Fig 22–5). These lesions are small, firm, nodular, or large, rapidly growing, and multiple up to 20 percent of the time. The lesions may be painful, and the fibroadenoma may be hormonally responsive and grow rapidly during pregnancy and/or lactation. The lesions are easily movable and are not fixed to surrounding tissue; they are usually sharply circumscribed and have very smooth boundaries.

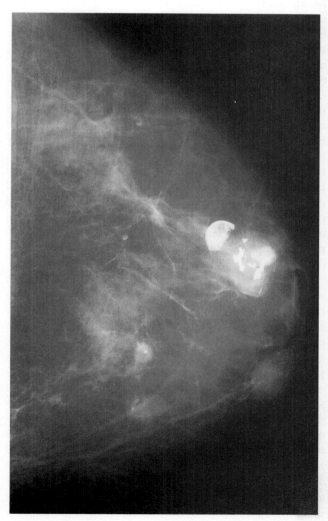

Figure 22–5. Mammogram of patient with fibroadenoma.

On gross specimen the cut surface is white with tissue whirls being present. These lesions are not associated with an increased risk of carcinoma; however, more than 100 cases of carcinoma have been reported arising in fibroadenomas. On microscopic examination the fibroadenoma is composed of fibrous tissue, and the stoma may be surrounded by round duct-like epithelial structures, or they may be arranged in a curvilinear manner. Fibroadenomas have a racial predilection, with the lesions being more common in blacks than in whites; likewise, the recurrence rate is greater in blacks than in whites. The lesions are usually treated by excisional biopsy or followed expectantly.[24,25]

BREAST SCREENING AND SELF-EXAMINATION

The subject of breast screening and self-examination has come under attack from both federal agencies and epidemiologic studies. Several factors should be considered before instituting screening for any disease. First, the disease must be important from a clinical prospective; that is, it should be common and be associated with significant mortality or morbidity. The prevalence may be influenced by sample size, race, sex, age, geography, or other parameters. Second, the screening test to be used must be available. It must be acceptable to the patient population, and it must not be too costly. It should be easy to perform, involve little or no patient discomfort, be sensitive and specific, and not yield false positive or false negative results. Third, the disease to be screened should have a defined natural history and a detectable presymptomatic stage. Fourth, the disease must have an available and efficacious treatment, and screening for untreatable disease at this juncture in history is not cost effective.

The breast examination is one of the most important methods for the diagnosis of breast disease, either benign or malignant. Studies conducted by the American Cancer Society found that physicians play a very important role in encouraging patients to practice breast self-examination. When a patient receives personal instruction from a physician, 92 percent continue to practice breast self-examination regularly.[26] Women should be taught breast self-examination by the age of 20, and the patient needs to be aware of what is normal in terms of the look and feel of the breast and be aware of the changes that may occur through the menstrual cycle. They should be encouraged to report any changes without delay and present for examination. Patients should be told that they need to look for any change in size or contour of the breast, puckering or dimpling of the skin, any discrete mass (particularly one that is not movable), asymmetric nodularity of the breast that persists (particularly after menstruation), and any pain or discomfort that deviates from the normal. Further, they should examine the nipples for any discharge, either serous or bloody, and look for nipple retraction or inversion. Examination should be carried out at least once per month, and it is generally recommended that the exam be done after menstruation when the breast is least tender. For women who are postmenopausal or who have undergone hysterectomy, examination on the first day of each month is suggested. The examination technique is standardized and consists of six steps: the first involves observation of the breasts for the changes described as well as visualization of the breasts during movement to accentuate contour. The woman should place her hands on her hips, flex the shoulders forward, and then raise the hands behind the head. Palpation of the breast should be carried out with the contralateral hand, and it is recommended that the breast be moistened with a soapy solution. Examination can be carried out systematically with the fingertips or in a circumferential fashion with the palm of the hand. Finally, the nipple should be inspected and the areola compressed to assess the presence of any discharge.

Despite the perceived benefit of self-examination, many women do not practice it.[27] Many false positive results occur and many women are examined for benign lesions. Examinations give rise to anxiety and worry about finding lumps that may or may not represent cancer. Some women feel guilty about not performing breast examinations or about not carrying out proper exams. The reward for carrying out thorough breast self-examination is the detection of a disease, and this is a negative reinforcement. The overall sensitivity of breast examination is poor and the percentage of false negative results is high.[28,29] The World Health Organization, Russian Federation, randomized self-breast examination study enrolled 60,000 women in each group. One hundred ninety cancers were detected in the examination group and 192 in the control group. The detection rate was 3.15 per thousand in the breast examination group, and 3.19 per thousand in the control group. The investigators concluded that there was no difference in cancer detection rate or in the tumor characteristics; and that patients had a significantly higher rate of visits to specialists, a significantly higher rate of referrals for their investigations, and significantly more incisional biopsies in the breast self-examination group. Further, the positive predictive value of self-examination in younger women is very poor, 4 percent to 6 percent. The large majority of women who have positive results do not have significant breast disease. This is in contrast to older women, which shows that 48 percent of lumps detected in women over 55 yr of age were malignant, compared with 3 percent in women under 44 yr of age. Therefore, at present there appears to be no compelling evidence that breast self-examination is effective in reducing the morbidity or mortality of breast cancer. However, because over 90 percent of breast cancers are found by women themselves, it seems that the teaching of efficient breast examination techniques should continue. Despite this controversy with self-examinations, the breast examination should be part of the annual examination rendered to women by all primary care specialists. Patients should be questioned about a family history of breast cancer, particularly in a first-order female relative. Attention should be paid to their ethnic origin, history of breast radiation, alcohol consumption, diet consisting of high fat intake, menstrual irregularity, parity, and age at birth of their first child.[30–39] Physical examination should be carried out both in the sitting and lying positions. The breasts should be inspected for symmetry at rest and symmetry during motion, thickening of the skin, any dimpling of the breast surface, areola or nipple inversion, discharge from the nipple, and any discoloration of the skin. The breasts should be examined bilaterally using the fingertips; the axilla should be palpated and an attempt made by both physician and patient to express discharge from the nipples.

It is recommended that a baseline mammographic examination be obtained by 40 years of age or earlier if a patient is at risk. Mammography should be performed every 1 to 2 yr from age 40 to 50, and yearly in women 50 years and older. There is considerable controversy about the need for baseline mammograms before 40 yr of age in asymptomatic women and about the frequency with which mammography should be performed in women age 40 to 50.[40,41] However, the effect of mammography cannot be overemphasized as a means for reducing mortality from breast cancer. For instance, the health insurance plan program in New York showed a 30 percent decrease in mortality in women older than 50 yr who were screened.[42] Studies from the Netherlands suggest a reduction in breast cancer rates by 50 percent in patients undergoing annual mammography.[43] It has been argued that if screening has saved the lives of women in the 50-yr and older age group, it should detect similar disease in the 40-yr-old group. It has been pointed out that the current studies do not have significant power to show benefit for screening women age 40 to 49; however, the studies do not disprove the benefit. The Canadian breast screening trial is the only prospective attempt to evaluate women in the fourth decade of life. It failed to show any advantage of screening women on the basis of a power calculation of 40 percent. In a 7-yr follow-up of women aged 40 to 49, it was found that 25,214 received annual mammography and clinical examination, and that they displaced a statistically insignificant excess of death resulting from breast cancer compared with 25,216 women

who received a single clinical examination of the breast and returned to normal community care. Unfortunately, normal community care might mean that patients receive mammography as well as physician examination, and apparently some 26 percent of these women received mammograms, which could have easily eschewed or obliterated the statistical difference.

Analysis conducted by Elwood on all screening studies published before 1992 indicates the total number of observed person-years at 7-yr follow-up. In women 40 to 49 yr of age, 601,380 person-years have been observed for screened women and 528,848 person-years for controlled subjects, for a total of 1.13 million person-years in the age group. Despite these numbers, the efficacy of screening could not be demonstrated, at least with the population-based technique. As a result of these types of reports, the National Cancer Institute no longer recommends that women age 40 to 49 have routine mammographic screening. Proponents of the guidelines claim that screening mammography does not work for these women because of their high breast density and the fact that the lumps that are detected are usually benign and resolve without surgery. Although it has been demonstrated that five times as many cancers per thousand first-screening mammographic examinations are diagnosed in women age 50 yr and older compared with younger women, women aged 40 to 49 yr with a positive family history of breast cancer had a higher positive predictive value compared with women without such a history; 0.3 versus 0.04 with a peak value of 1.00.

In view of this controversy, it seems reasonable to recommend (1) frequent breast self-examinations to all women older than 20 yr, (2) annual examinations beginning at least by age 35 yr, (3) baseline mammography at approximately 40 yr, (4) mammography every other yr after age 50 yr, and (5) mammography used liberally in women 40 yr and older with a positive family history of breast cancer or increased risk factors.

CARCINOMA OF THE BREAST

The National Cancer Database, which is a joint project of the commission on cancer for the American College of Surgeons and the American Cancer Society, drives data from cancer diagnosed and treated in more than 1000 hospitals throughout the United States.[44] In 1991, reports were submitted from 937 hospitals, including 507,203 cases. More than 50 percent of overall cancers were reported in individuals age 60 to 79; 85 percent were non-Hispanic whites, and the majority were derived from the South Atlantic, East, North Central, and Pacific regions; 52 percent of the individuals had incomes between $32,000 and $50,000, and the majority lived in urban regions. These highlights from the database suggest a marked increase in the percentage of patients being staged by the American Joint Committee on Cancer/International Union Against Cancer criteria, and that the percentage of patients diagnosed with stage II and III disease decreased; however, the percentage of patients with stage IV disease remained constant. The stage of presentation was found to be related to income; a large percentage of high-income patients presented with lower stages, as expected. The database also suggested a relationship to ethnicity in that a larger percentage of white women presented with a lower stage of disease. These findings are further amplified by racial difference in survival from breast cancer. Seventy-five percent of the difference may be accounted for by sociodemographic variables rather than by race.[45] This is further reflected by the finding that when one compares the stage of disease by census region, there are some minor variations; patients living in the South Central regions, both east and west, show less early stage disease than patients in other regions. The youngest and oldest cohorts present with the higher stages, that is, stage III or IV.

Marked regional variations in the use of partial mastectomy was the highest in New England and the lowest in the East and South Central regions. This is confirmed by reports suggesting that breast-conserving surgery with radiation therapy is not performed on the majority of women with stage I or II disease as recommended by the National Institutes of Health. Against this background, when one evaluates cohorts from 1973 to 1987, cardiovascular disease was found to decrease among the populations in both the United States and Sweden, whereas cancer among whites increased, and this increase could not be linked to either age or smoking.[46]

Unfortunately, breast cancer strikes 180,000 women in the United States and kills 46,000 annually, leaving in its wake a survivor group of 1.5 million.[47] The National Breast Disease Cancer Coalition is a political force, and through lobbying efforts has persuaded Congress to double the amount of money spent on breast cancer research. The National Cancer Institute (NCI) budget for breast cancer research has increased from $133 to $197 million; and $210 million more went to the Department of Defense to be administered by the Department of the Army. For NCI alone, this represents a 177 percent increase in commitment to breast cancer research over the recent years, whereas the overall NCI budget has grown by 35 percent. As a result of the increased funding, the NCI has established special programs for research excellence (SPORES), which is aimed at the transfer of basic science into clinical treatment trials as rapidly as possible.

Despite this enormous investment, little headway has been made in explaining the relentless increase in the disease. Women living in the United States have a risk of 1 in 8 by age 85, which is twice that seen in 1940. At age 25 a woman has a 1 in 19,608 risk of developing breast cancer, yet by age 40 this increases to 1 in 217. By age 50 it is 1 in 50, by age 70 it is 1 in 14, and by age 85 it is 1 in 8 to 1 in 9. A number of established risk factors have been determined for breast cancer. These include family history, diet, obesity, smoking, ethyl alcohol consumption, nulliparity, age at parity, age at menarche, and menopause. Possible risk factors include exposure to diethylstilbestrol, a history of mammary dysplasias, and caffeine consumption.[48–50] Epidemiologic risk factors are beginning to suggest that hormones, particularly estrogen, may play an important role in allowing the expression of breast cancer. The origin of estrogen may be exogenous or endogenous, as demonstrated by the following observations. Breast cancer occurs more frequently in older than in younger women, and more frequently in Northern Europe and North America than in Asia or Africa. Upper socioeconomic women are at greater risk than in women in lower classes. Women who have never been married are at higher risk than those who have been married, and women who delay childbearing past the age of 30 have a much higher incidence than women who conceive at age 20 or younger. Obese women have a higher incidence of breast cancer than thin women, women who undergo early menarche are at higher risk than those whose menstrual periods begin later, and women who have delayed menopause are at higher risk than those who have early menopause. Further, a family history of premenopausal breast cancer increases a woman's risk for this disorder, as does having cancer in one breast. Further, having a first-degree relative with breast cancer increases a woman's risk, as does a history of primary cancer of either the ovary or endometrium.

Review of Risk Factors

Family History. There appears to be a 2- to 3-fold increased risk in the incidence of breast cancer in women who have a female relative with the disease. For the patient with an affected mother or sister there is a 2.3 relative risk, and with an affected aunt or grandmother a 1.5 relative risk. Fortunately, hereditary forms of breast cancer make up 8 percent of the disease; unfortunately, women with a strong family history develop the disease at a younger age.

One of the most exciting events to occur in breast cancer research is the identification of genes that predispose to breast cancer.[51–54] These findings appeared in three papers published in the September 30 and October 7, 1994, issues of *Science*. The two genes are called BRAC1 and BRAC2, and together account for about two thirds of familial breast cancer, or roughly 5 percent of all cases. BRAC1 is also associated with a predisposition for ovarian cancer, and it is located on a locus on chromosome 17Q. BRAC2 is mapped by the International Breast Cancer Linkage Consortium. The predisposing gene lies within six centimorgan intervals on chromosome 13Q12.13, centered on D13S260. The loss of this gene appears to result in elimination of suppressor function.

Cigarettes, Coffee, Alcohol, and Diet.

Tobacco accounts for approximately 400,000 deaths in the United States. It is responsible for 17 percent of all deaths, yet more than 50 million Americans continue to smoke. The incidence of smoking in women has risen at an alarming rate, and it is of interest that the rate nearly parallels the increased occurrence of lung cancer in women. The impact on breast cancer is not clear, but this question deserves careful attention.

The consumption of methylxanthine-containing compounds has been implicated as a causative factor in the development of fibrocystic disease of the breast and cancer. The Boston Collaborative Drug Surveillance Program evaluated 16,000 patients and found 210 women with fibrocystic disease and 204 women with breast cancer. An increased risk was detected in women who drank between 1 and 3 cups of coffee or tea per day.[55]

Women who consume more than three drinks per day are reported to have a 40 percent increased risk of breast cancer. Consumption of one alcoholic drink a day is associated with the relative risk of 1.6. The National Health and Nutrition Examination Survey Cohort Study revealed a 40 to 50 percent increased risk in breast cancer in women who drank fewer than three alcoholic drinks per week; however, the risk increased in women who drank more than 5 grains of alcohol per day. The mechanism by which alcohol increased the risk of breast cancer is unclear; however, given its hepatotoxic effects one could postulate that this may be secondary to altered estrogen metabolism.[56]

Diet, particularly the intake of fat, is associated with an increased risk of breast cancer. It is noted that postmenopausal women in the United States have a much higher risk of breast cancer than women in Asia. This does not appear to be geographic, because the movement of Asian women to the Hawaiian Islands or the Pacific Coast of the United States seems to eradicate the difference in incidence. The assumed alteration is thought to be secondary to an increased consumption of fats; however, populations with a low risk of breast cancer, such as those found in Greece or Spain, have been shown to use monounsaturated fats composed primarily of oleic acid.

Hormonal Replacement Therapy.

At least 30 epidemiologic studies designed to identify an association between hormone replacement therapy in the postmenopausal woman and breast cancer have been published since 1974. Four large meta-analyses have been published since 1988. Two concluded that estrogen replacement therapy does not increase the risk of breast cancer, and two concluded that it does. It is unclear whether estrogen replacement therapy increases the risk of breast cancer; however, it appears that progesterone therapy neither increases nor decreases the risk.[57-59] Concerning the use of hormonal replacement therapy in women with a past history of breast cancer, the American College of Obstetricians and Gynecologists in April 1994 rendered a committee opinion that said "There are no data to indicate an increased risk of recurrent breast cancer in postmenopausal women receiving replacement estrogen therapy." (See also Chap 38.)

Treatment of Breast Cancer

A number of factors influence the treatment and prognosis of breast cancer, including the presence or absence of estrogen receptors in the tumor, lymph node and vascular metastasis, the histologic grade of the tumor, and the size and histologic type of the primary cancer and differentiation. Those lesions that are estrogen receptor-negative frequently occur in the premenopausal age group. Patients who are receptor positive tend to survive longer and have longer disease-free intervals. Patients who have estrogen receptor-positive tumors generally have slower growth of the lesion. The best prognosis is seen in patients whose tumors are positive for both estrogen and progesterone.

Stage I or II cancers can be treated with either modified radical mastectomy or wide local excision and axillary resection followed by radiation therapy. Survival and recurrence figures are as good as those with radical mastectomy.[60,61] The current guidelines from the National Cancer Institute regarding adjunct therapy depends on whether the woman is pre- or postmenopausal, and with or without nodes. The premenopausal woman with positive nodes is treated with chemotherapy regardless of receptor status; those with negative nodes are only treated if they are at high risk. Postmenopausal women with positive nodes are treated with estrogen antagonists such as tamoxifen if they are receptor positive; if they are receptor negative, other chemotherapy is considered. Considering the high rate of recurrence (30 percent), more aggressive forms of therapy have been advocated in the postmenopausal woman.

Special mention needs to be made of the use of tamoxifen in the premenopausal woman with a functional uterus and ovaries. Most of the patients seen in our practice have developed ovarian cysts and an endometrium whose thickness exceeds 1.5 to 1.7 cm. The vast majority have experienced irregular bleeding and pain, and these side effects are probably secondary to the fact that tamoxifen is similar to clomiphene citrate, stimulates gonadotropin production while antagonizing the biological effect of 17-β-estradiol and has an estrogen agonist effect of its own. Further, it should be noted that women who are treated with tamoxifen can rapidly develop well-differentiated carcinomas of the uterus. In an attempt to manage these patients, we have utilized the administration of 3.75 mg of leuprolide acetate, which in all cases has resulted in the suppression of ovarian cysts and resolution of the hypertrophic endometrium. Treatment generally lasts for 1 to 2 mo. Leuprolide therapy does not necessitate discontinuation of tamoxifen, and does not interfere with this form of therapy. In fact, leuprolide therapy has been used for the treatment of certain types of breast cancers. Unfortunately, these side effects do not seem to be of great concern to the medical oncologists, who often leave these problems to the gynecologist or reproductive endocrinologist for management. Nevertheless, these side effects could be a challenging clinical dilemma for those treating the problems.

SUMMARY

Diseases of the breast are commonly seen in gynecologic practices. These physicians are to a great deal responsible for training women in breast self-examination and tumor detection. Fortunately, a significant amount of breast disease is benign and involves developmental anomalies or functional disorders that are not life threatening. These include nipple inversion, breast hypertrophy, hypoplasia of the breast, galactorrhea, mastalgia, galactocele, breast infections, and fibrocystic change. In fact, the most common factors—such as fat necrosis, interductal papilloma, and fibroadenoma—are benign disorders.

Carcinoma of the breast is one of the most feared and common malignancies encountered in women. It rises relentlessly with age, and by age 85 afflicts 1 in 8 women. It affects 180,000 women in the United States per year and kills 46,000 annually. Risk factors that seem to influence the occurrence of breast cancer include family history, diet, obesity, smoking, ethyl alcohol consumption, nulliparity, age at parity, age at menarche, menarche, and menopause. Despite these dim statistics, breast cancers are detected early in many cases and treated with local excision and radiation therapy. Those women who experience recurrences with certain receptor profiles respond favorably to therapy with drugs such as tamoxifen.

REFERENCES

1. Pellegrini J, Wanger R. Polythelia and associated conditions. *Am Fam Physician*. 28:129, 1983
2. Aksu MF, Tzingounis VA, Greenblatt RB. Treatment of benign breast disease with danazol: A follow-up report. *J Reprod Med*. 31:181, 1978
3. Atchison JA, Lee PA, Albright AL. Reversible suprasellar pituitary mass secondary to hypothyroidism. *JAMA*. 262:3175, 1989
4. Sinhu YN. Prolactin variants. *Trends Endocrinol Metab*. 3:100, 1992
5. Larrea F, Escorza A, Valero A, et al. Heterogeneity of serum prolactin throughout the menstrual cycle and pregnancy in hyperprolactinemic women with normal ovarian function. *J Clin Endocrinol Metab*. 68:982,1989
6. Molitch M, Elton R, Blackwell RE, et al, and the Bromocriptine Study Group. Bromocriptine as primary therapy for prolactin secreting macroadenomas: Results of a prospective, multicenter study. *J Clin Endocrinol Metab*. 60:698-705, 1985
7. Barbieri RL, Ryan KJ. Bromocriptine: Endocrine pharmacology and therapeutic applications. *Fertil Steril*. 39:72, 1982
8. Vermesh M, Fosum GT, Kletzky OA. Vaginal bromocriptine: Pharmacology and effect on serum prolactin in normal women. *Obstet Gynecol*. 72:693, 1988
9. Katz E, Weiss BE, Hassell A, et al. Increased circulating levels of bromocriptine after vaginal compared with oral administration. *Fertil Steril*. 55:882, 1991
10. Blackwell RE, Bradley EL Jr, Kline LB, et al. Comparison of dopamine agonists in the treatment of hyperprolactinemic syndromes: A multicenter study. *Fertil Steril*. 39:744, 1983
11. Vance ML, Cragun JR, Reimnitz C, et al. CV205-502 treatment of hyperprolactinemia. *J Clin Endocrinol Metab*. 68:336, 1989
12. Chenette PE, Siegel MS, Vermesh M, Kletzky OA. Effect of bromocriptine on sperm function in vitro and in vivo. *Obstet Gynecol*. 77:935, 1991
13. Ciccarelli E, Miola C, Avataneo T, et al. Long-term treatment with a new repeatable injectable form of bromocriptine, Parlodel LAR, in patients with tumorous hyperprolactinemia. *Fertil Steril*. 52:930, 1989
14. Motta T, de Vincentis S, Marchini M, et al. Vaginal cabergoline in the treatment of hyperprolactinemic patients intolerant to oral dopaminergics. *Fertil Steril*. 65:440, 1996
15. Paoletti AM, Cagnacci A, Depau GF, et al. The chronic administration of cabergoline normalizes androgen secretion and improves menstrual cyclicity in women with polycystic ovary syndrome. *Fertil Steril*. 66:527, 1996
16. Pilnik S. Clinical diagnosis of benign breast disease. *J Reprod Med*. 22:277, 1979
17. Love S, Gelman R, Silen W. Fibrocystic "disease" of the breast: A nondisease? *N Engl J Med*. 307:1010, 1982
18. Hutter RVP. Goodbye to "fibrocystic disease." *N Engl J Med*. 312:179, 1985
19. Page DL, Dupont WD, Rogers LW, Rados MS. Atypical hyperplastic lesions of the female breast: a long-term follow-up study. *Cancer* 55:2698, 1985
20. Pilnik S. Clinical diagnosis of breast disease. *J Reprod Med*. 22:277, 1979
21. Oberman HA. Benign breast lesions confused with carcinoma. In: McDiutt RW, Oberman HA, Ozello L, Kaufman N, eds. International Academy of Pathology monograph: *The Breast*. Baltimore, Williams & Wilkins, 1984

22. Colman M, Mattheiem W. Imaging techniques in breast cancer: Workshop report. *Eur J Cancer Clin Oncol.* 24:69, 1988

23. Carter D. Intraductal papillary tumors of the breast: A study of 78 cases. *Cancer.* 30:1689,1977

24. Hertel B, Zaloudek C, Kemson R. Breast adenomas. *Cancer.* 37:2891, 1976

25. Fechner RE. Fibroadenomas and related lesions. In: Page DL, Anderson TF, eds. *Diagnostic Histopathology of the Breast.* New York, Churchill Livingstone, 1987, 72

26. Dodd GD. 1988 American Cancer Society guidelines for breast cancer screening. *Cancer.* 69:1885, 1992

27. Austoker J. Cancer prevention in primary care. *Br Med J.* 309:168, 1994

28. Kopans DB, Halpern E, Hulka CA. Statistical power in breast cancer screening trials and mortality reduction among breast cancer screening trials and mortality reduction among women 40–49 years of age with particular emphasis on the National Breast Screening Study of Canada. *Cancer.* 74:1196, 1994

29. Baines CJ. A different view on what is known about breast screening and the Canadian National Breast Screening Study. *Cancer.* 74:1207, 1974

30. Stoll BA. Diet and exercise regimens to improve breast carcinoma prognosis. *Cancer.* 78:2465, 1996

31. Tremollieres FA, Pouilles JM, Ribot CA. Relative influence of age and menopause on total and regional body composition changes in postmenopausal women. *Am J Obstet Gynecol.* 175:1594, 1996

32. Anderson KE, Sellers TA, Chen PL, et al. Association of Stein–Leventhal syndrome with the incidence of postmenopausal breast carcinoma in a large prospective study of women in Iowa. *Cancer.* 79:494, 1997

33. Kumar NB, Lyman GH, Allen K, et al. Timing of weight gain and breast cancer risk. *Cancer.* 76:243, 1995

34. Manson JE, Willett WC, Stamper MJ, et al. Body weight and mortality among women. *N Engl J Med.* 333:677, 1995

35. Melbye M, Wohlfahrt J, Olsen JH, et al. Induced abortion and the risk of breast cancer. *N Engl J Med.* 336:81, 1997

36. Zhang S, Folsom AR, Sellers TA, et al. Better breast cancer survival for postmenopausal women who are less overweight and eat less fat. *Cancer.* 76:275, 1995

37. Bagga D, Ashley JM, Geffrey SP, et al. Effects of a very low fat, high fiber diet on serum hormones and menstrual function. *Cancer.* 76:2491, 1995

38. Newcomb PA, Storer BE, Longnecker MP, et al. Pregnancy termination in relation to risk of breast cancer. *JAMA.* 275:283, 1996

39. Hunter DJ, Spiegelman D, Adami HO, et al. Cohort studies of fat intake and the risk of breast cancer—a pooled analysis. *N Engl J Med.* 334:356, 1996

40. Dupont WD. Evidence of efficacy of mammographic screening for women in their forties. *Cancer.* 74:1204, 1994

41. Kerkikowske K, Grady D, Barclay J, et al. Positive predictive value of screening mammography by age and family history of breast cancer. *JAMA.* 270:2444, 1993

42. Shapiro S, Venet W, Strax P, et al. Ten to fourteen year effect of screening on breast cancer mortality. *J Natl Cancer Inst.* 69:349, 1982

43. Verbeck ALM, Holland R, Sturmans F, et al. Reduction of breast cancer mortality through mass screening with modern mammography. *Lancet.* 1:222, 1984

44. Steele GD, Osteen RT, Winchester DP, et al. Clinical highlights from the National Cancer Data Base, 1994. *Cancer.* 44:71, 1994

45. Eley JW, Hill HA, Chen VW, et al. Racial differences in survival from breast cancer. *JAMA.* 272:947, 1994

46. David DL, Dinse GE, Hoel DG. Decreasing cardiovascular disease and increasing cancer among whites in the United States from 1973 through 1987. *JAMA.* 271:431, 1994

47. Marshall E. The politics of breast cancer. *Science.* 259:616, 1993

48. Marshall E. Search for a killer: Focus shifts from fat to hormones. *Science.* 259:618, 1993

49. Colton T, Greenberg ER, Noller K, et al. Breast cancer in months prescribed diethylstilbestrol in pregnancy. *JAMA.* 269:1096, 1993

50. Brenner H, Engelsmann B, Stegmaier C, Ziegler H. Clinical epidemiology of bilateral breast cancer. *Cancer.* 72:3629, 1993

51. Futreal PA, Liu Q, Shattuck-Eldens D, et al. BRAC1 mutations in primary breast and ovarian carcinomas. *Science.* 266:120, 1994

52. Miki Y, Swensen J, Shattuck-Eldens D, et al. A strong candidate for the breast and ovarian cancer susceptibility gene BRAC1. *Science.* 266:66, 1994

53. Nowak R. Breast cancer gene offers surprises. *Science.* 265:1796, 1994

54. Wooster R, Neuhausen SL, Mangion J, et al. Localization of a breast cancer gene. BRAC2 to chromosome 13q12-13. *Science.* 265:2088, 1994

55. Welsch CW. Caffeine and the development of the normal and neoplastic mammary gland. *Proc Soc Exp Biol.* 207:1, 1994

56. Willett WC, Colditz G, Stampfer MJ, et al. A prospective study of alcohol intake and risk of breast cancer. *Am J Epidemiol.* 124:540, 1986

57. Harding C, Knox WF, Faragher EB, et al. Hormone replacement therapy and tumour grade in breast cancer: Prospective study in screening unit. *Br Med J.* 312:1646, 1996

58. Dhodapkar MV, Ingle JN, Ahmann DL. Estrogen replacement therapy withdrawal and regression of metastatic breast cancer. *Cancer.* 75:43, 1995

59. Pritchard KI, Sawka CA. Menopausal estrogen replacement therapy in women with breast cancer. *Cancer.* 75:1, 1995

60. Schover LR, Yetman RJ, Tuason LJ, et al. Partial mastectomy and breast reconstruction. *Cancer.* 75:54, 1995

61. Early Breast Cancer Trialists' Collaborative Group. Effects of radiotherapy and surgery in early breast cancer. *N Engl J Med.* 333:1444, 1995

Chapter 23

PSYCHOLOGICAL ASPECTS OF MENSTRUATION

Premenstrual Syndrome

Robert L. Reid

The many conflicting theories about the pathophysiology of premenstrual syndrome (PMS) and a host of unproved remedies have both confused and frustrated practitioners in their attempts to answer questions and provide efficacious treatment for women with this disorder.[1] Critical review of the published literature on PMS reveals a multitude of methodologically flawed epidemiological studies and poorly controlled therapeutic trials.[2,3] Although definitive answers to many questions relating to the epidemiology and pathophysiology of PMS are not yet available, this does not preclude the development of rational guidelines for evaluation and therapy based upon present knowledge. This chapter will summarize available evidence on the prevalence and epidemiology, pathophysiology, and treatment options while, at the same time, considering the social ramifications of this diagnosis.

DIAGNOSIS

PMS has been defined as "the cyclic recurrence in the luteal phase of the menstrual cycle of a combination of distressing physical, psychological, and/or behavioral changes of sufficient severity to result in deterioration of interpersonal relationships and/or interference with normal activities.[1]

Originally called "premenstrual tension" to highlight the tension and anxiety that eclipsed other symptoms in some women,[4] this condition has now been renamed "premenstrual syndrome" or "premenstrual syndromes" to take into account the varied clinical presentations that may exist. Until recently, these terms referred to any woman with troublesome symptomatology prior to menstruation. It has become clear, however, that it is inappropriate to extrapolate information from a small subgroup of women with premenstrual functional impairment to the larger group of women experiencing only minor premenstrual symptoms.[5,6] The term "premenstrual molimina" is now used to describe symptoms of lesser severity that affect most women to some degree in the late luteal phase.

The facts that PMS represents the severe end of the spectrum of physiological premenstrual changes, and that there exists no simple biochemical test for PMS, inevitably results in some imprecision in diagnosis.

Four critical parameters must be evaluated in establishing a diagnosis of PMS: (1) the nature of symptoms; (2) the severity of symptoms (degree of functional impairment); (3) the timing of symptoms in relation to menstruation; and (4) the baseline (follicular phase) level of symptoms upon which premenstrual symptoms are superimposed. Although the actual symptoms occurring in the premenstrual phase of the cycle may be myriad, there are certain common symptoms (Table 23–1). To meet the severity criteria for PMS, one or more of these symptoms should be rated by the patient as severe or temporarily disabling in repeated menstrual cycles. Four temporal patterns have been defined according to onset and duration of symptoms (Fig 23–1) with the majority experiencing patterns A and B.[1] Approximately 5 to 10 percent of patients will experience midcycle symptoms (pattern C) during the transient period of estrogen withdrawal that follows ovulation (Fig 23–2).[1,7,8] In each case, however, symptoms onset at or after ovulation and resolve within 6 to 7 days following onset of menstruation. During the second half of the follicular phase, the patient should have at least 1 wk during which she is asymptomatic to differentiate this condition from other, more chronic mood or behavioral disorders.

This information is best confirmed with a prospective symptom record maintained for a minimum of two complete cycles.[2,9–11] One such calendar record, the PRISM

TABLE 23–1. COMMON COMPLAINTS OF WOMEN SUFFERING FROM PMS

Psychological
 Irritability
 Fatigue
 Anger
 Labile mood
 Depression
 Restlessness
 Anxiety
 Lack of control
 Low self-esteem
 Guilt
 Suicidal thoughts

Life-style Impact
 Physically or verbally aggressive toward others
 Unreasonable behavior
 Wish to be alone
 Neglect of housework or time off work
 Disorganized, distractible
 Uneasy about driving the car
 Avoid social activities
 Increased use of alcohol

Physical
 Breast tenderness
 Abdominal bloating
 Edema of extremities
 Headaches
 Constipation or diarrhea

Other
 Increased thirst
 Cravings for sweets or salty foods
 Alteration in sexual drive
 Menopausal-like hot sweats or chills
 Palpitations
 Insomnia
 Sensitivity to noise

calendar, allows rapid visual confirmation of the nature, timing, and severity of menstrual cycle-related symptomatology (Fig 23–3).[1] The American Psychiatric Association recently outlined research diagnostic criteria for what they termed "Premenstrual Dysphoric Disorder" (PMDD) in an effort to ensure standardization in ongoing research.[12] Premenstrual changes may be sufficiently distressing to warrant counseling or treatment even though they do not meet severity criteria for a diagnosis of PMS. Research diagnostic criteria for PMS were developed to standardize future research investigations and not to determine who should and should not receive therapeutic interventions.

PREVALENCE

Up to 80 to 90 percent of women will experience symptoms that forewarn them about impending menstruation, so-called premenstrual molimina. Available data suggest that 30 percent of women of reproductive age range will experience some temporary distress each month related to premenstrual symptomatology; however, the number of women in whom one or more symptoms are severe or temporarily disabling falls between 3 and 5 percent.[13–15]

EPIDEMIOLOGY

Some authors have suggested that PMS is a Western culture-specific disorder.[16] Recent studies have documented typical premenstrual syndrome in a variety of races, cultures, and socioeconomic strata[17–19] and, in-

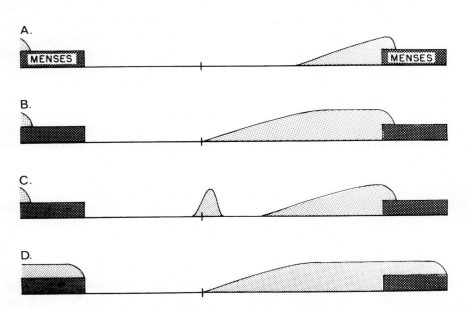

Figure 23–1. Variations in the onset and duration of PMS symptoms. *(Reproduced, with permission, from Reid RL, Yen SSC. Premenstrual syndrome. Clin Obstet Gynecol. 27:710. 1983.)*

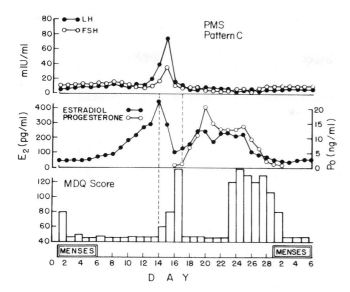

Figure 23–2. Correlation of hormonal data and mood ratings (Moos Menstrual Distress Questionnaire) for a subject with severe midcycle and premenstrual depression and irritability. *(Reproduced, with permission, from Reid RL. Endogenous opioid activity in premenstrual syndrome. Lancet. 2:786. 1983.)*

deed, PMS-like behavior has been observed in the subhuman primate who, like the human female, has a 28-day menstrual cycle.[20–22] In cultures where women experience few menstrual cycles because of repeated episodes of pregnancy and breast-feeding, PMS is uncommon.[19]

Premenstrual syndrome may begin at any phase of reproductive life but is more commonly reported by women in the later reproductive years and in those with more years of "natural" menstrual cycles.[23,24] It is uncommon for PMS to onset suddenly. Most women with severe PMS will report that symptoms became gradually worse over a number of years. Typically, at the outset, symptoms will vary in severity from month to month and according to concurrent life stresses. Later, symptoms may become very consistent and predictable from cycle to cycle. It is unusual for PMS to disappear suddenly without major life-style modifications or some form of medical intervention. No good data exist on the natural history of PMS during the menopausal transition, although menopause does bring relief.

There is no convincing evidence to support the notion that premenstrual symptomatology begins or worsens after pregnancy,[1] and recent data indicate that the incidence of PMS is not increased following tubal ligation.[25] It is likely that feelings of well-being during the antecedent pregnancy make PMS symptomatology seem worse postpartum (especially with the additional stresses of a newborn). Cohabitation and parenting are reported to exacerbate PMS.[26] Little is known about hereditary

influences on PMS, although limited data suggest genetic factors may be operant.[23,26,27]

Although PMS and dysmenorrhea may coexist, the variable nature of this association suggests that different pathophysiological mechanisms are involved. The prevalence and severity of dysmenorrhea fall with increasing parity, which may explain why PMS and dysmenorrhea coexist more frequently in adolescents than they do in women in their later reproductive years.[1,24]

Whether or not PMS is more common in women with a lifetime diagnosis of psychiatric illness remains controversial.[28–30] Depression and its associated symptoms, such as alteration in sleep, appetite, energy level, and concentration, are common in women with PMS.[31] Unlike typical endogenous depression, PMS is characterized by features of labile mood, hypersomnia, anxiety, agitation, irritability, and feelings of inability to cope.[32] Suicidal thoughts may be recorded on prospective symptom records and several authors have noted the increased risk of suicide in this group.[32–34] It is hardly surprising that women with a history of psychiatric disease might be more vulnerable to premenstrual depression and that such a population would be more likely to return to psychiatrists who had formerly been their caregivers.

Spitzer reported that 57 percent of women with major depressive disorder had a history of premenstrual depression compared to 14 percent in a control group who were not depressed.[35] Endicott et al[32] found that 84 percent of women with premenstrual depression had already met research diagnostic criteria for major depressive disorder at some time in the past while only 9 percent had no history of this condition. Both sleep deprivation and exposure to bright light (photoperiod extension) have been shown to alleviate premenstrual depression.[31,36] One interpretation of such data is that PMS merely represents an entrainment or synchronization of a chronic mood disorder to the menstrual cycle.

Several lines of evidence, however, argue against this. Detailed psychological studies comparing women with precisely defined PMS to unaffected controls revealed no differences between the two groups in the follicular phase yet significantly higher levels of depression in PMS subjects during the luteal phase.[37] Further, comparison of psychological profiles and cortisol secretory dynamics in women with PMS, women with endogenous depression, and control women showed the depressive episodes in PMS were distinct from those of endogenous depression as measured both by cortisol secretory parameters and psychological indices.[38] The findings from both of these studies suggest that PMS in many women is specific luteal phase disorder superimposed on a background free of psychiatric or physiologic illness.[37,38]

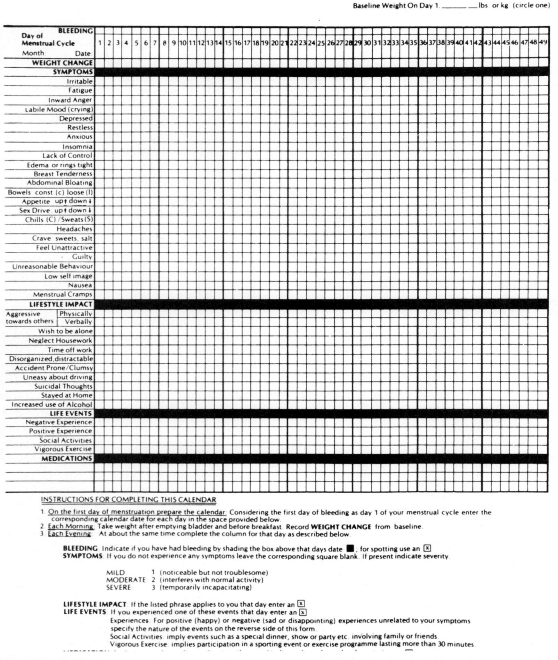

Figure 23–3. Prospective record of the impact and severity of menstrual symptomatology (PRISM calendar). *(Developed by R. L. Reid and S. Maddocks.)*

SOCIAL IMPACT

Although the precise impact of PMS on afflicted women, their families, and society is impossible to quantitate accurately, published reports[39] lend credence to commonly expressed concerns of PMS sufferers about premenstrual marital discord,[40] irritability leading to more harsh disciplining of children,[41] alcohol or drug abuse,[42–45] uneasi-

ness about driving the car,[46] and depression that may, at times, reach suicidal proportions.[47,48] A recent Swedish survey reported that 10 percent of women missed 1 or more days of work during the premenstrual wk in the preceding 6 mo.[13]

Caution is required in interpretation of such studies, however, as investigator bias and methodological shortcomings are common. Despite frequent claims about premenstrual cognitive impairment by PMS sufferers, no such abnormality has been demonstrated. More carefully constructed epidemiologic studies are needed to gain insight into the true familial and societal impact of PMS. The legal implications of the PMS diagnosis are unfolding in a complex way (mitigating responsibility in some criminal acts, yet undermining women's competence in civil matters) such that even legal experts are hesitant to introduce PMS into the courts until there is further scientific clarification about this condition.[41,47]

CLINICAL MANIFESTATIONS

The earliest changes reported generally include sensations of breast swelling and tenderness together with lower abdominal bloating and constipation. These changes, which may contribute to a distorted perception of bloating and weight gain,[49] occur after ovulation and generally persist until the onset of menstruation. Many women note a change to loose stool or diarrhea in the 24 hr prior to menstruation and the first 1 to 2 days of menstruation.[50] At times, these changes may be severe enough to suggest a diagnosis of irritable bowel syndrome. Indeed, a recent publication reported treatment of "irritable bowel syndrome" employing medical ovarian suppression with a gonadotropin-releasing hormone (GnRH) agonist.[51] Some women report that bloating is severe enough to necessitate a change to looser clothing as the menses approach. Although frequently attributed to a generalized fluid retention, these symptoms often exist in the absence of weight gain or edema, suggesting that they may result either from local fluid shifts within the body or from progesterone-induced alteration in other hormones, such as motilin, which influence gastrointestinal motility.[52] Premenstrual mastalgia bears no relationship to total body water,[53] making it likely that breast swelling and tenderness are, in part, the result of intralobular edema and ductal–acinar growth.

A dramatic increase in appetite and unusual cravings for chocolate and salty foods are common.[54,55] The premenstrual increase in appetite has been shown to correlate with the degree of premenstrual depression[56] and to be suppressed by the antidepressant, d-fenfluramine.[57] Alcohol use is often also increased premenstrually.

Coincident with these annoying but generally well-tolerated physical changes, many women experience marked fatigue, emotional lability, and depression. Sexual drive is frequently reduced, and affected women may choose to withdraw from family and friends, physically isolating themselves or relinquishing parental responsibilities to the spouse. Not uncommonly, the severely afflicted woman may defer important decisions or cancel social commitments in the premenstrual week. In other women, anxiety and inward tension may lead to physical unrest, irritability, and combativeness. Insomnia may be marked and nightmares are more frequently reported. Typical menopausal-like hot flushes are frequently seen in PMS sufferers during the symptomatic period[58] and night sweats may coincide with waking episodes. Migraine-like headaches may occur both in the periovulatory and menstrual phases of the cycle and may be debilitating in some women.

Positive changes such as increased energy and creativity are reported by some women premenstrually. In addition, many women with PMS report a period of abundant energy and a sense of well-being bordering on euphoria in the postmenstrual week.[59]

A variety of other medical conditions such as asthma, epilepsy, and arthritis may show cyclic changes with deterioration in the late luteal or menstrual phases of the cycle.[60–62] Menstrual cycle phase may have important effects on the immune system with the potential to have a significant impact not only on disease but also on its treatment.[63]

THEORIES OF PATHOPHYSIOLOGY

Psychosocial Theory

Menstrual and premenstrual attitudes and behavior are undoubtedly influenced by a complex interplay of cultural beliefs, socialization factors, actual experiences, and concomitant life stresses.[64] Less certain, however, is the respective influence of endocrine events and psychosocial variables on the expression of premenstrual symptomatology. Ruble's study,[65] in which university women recorded higher symptom scores when they were misled to believe that they were premenstrual than if they were led to believe they were in other phases of their cycle, appears to lend support to the primary role of psychological factors. However, it must be remembered that subjects in this investigation represent a nonclinical sample of students in whom shifts in physical symptoms and mood would normally be minimal and perhaps more susceptible to suggestion than the extreme symptoms of PMS clinic attenders. Physicians confronted by patients with severe menstrual cycle-related mood and behavioral disturbances often find it difficult to accept that these changes could simply be the result of learned attitudes and expectations. The sudden onset and rapid recovery from severe symptoms at midcycle in women with pattern C PMS,[66] the elimination of symptoms by medical ovarian suppression[67–70] or oophorectomy,[71,72] and the persistence of cyclic symptoms in women following hysterectomy in whom ovarian function remains intact[73] all suggest a primary role for hormonal shifts in the genesis of distressing premenstrual symptoms.

Others have advanced an attributional theory to explain PMS,[74] emphasizing that it is human nature to seek a biologic event (menstruation) on which to blame negative outcomes (adverse mood or physical symptoms). This theory argues that when negative behavioral patterns are internally attributed (blamed on an uncontrollable biologic cycle) and situational factors (such as life events and stresses) are discounted as an explanation, a vicious cycle of condemnation, anxiety, and lowered self-esteem ensues. Although attribution may be a well-established phenomenon, it is common for those treating PMS to see women with recurrent episodes of severe depression for whom the association with menstruation goes unnoticed until they begin prospective charting. At times, such women are managed by psychiatrists for "so-called" manic depressive disorders because a satisfactory menstrual history has never been obtained. These findings seem to argue against attribution as the sole cause of premenstrual symptomatology.

Recent detailed psychological comparisons between women with well-characterized PMS and carefully screened controls turned up no evidence to indicate that women with PMS were more likely than control women to attribute negative feelings or behavior to specific biologic events, thus casting doubt on a simple explanation of "learned helplessness."[37]

Thyroid Dysfunction

In 1986, a letter to the editor in the *New England Journal of Medicine* claimed that 94 percent of a group of PMS sufferers showed subclinical hypothyroidism and that prompt symptomatic relief followed thyroid supplementation.[75] Although it is likely that occasional patients with hypothyroidism will present to PMS clinics, the claim that hypothyroidism was the cause of PMS has been refuted by several groups.[76–78]

Chronic Infection

Bacterial. Doxycycline has been reported to relieve PMS in a double-blind clinical trial.[79] To date, the rationale for such a therapeutic trial is obscure and no etiologic agent has been identified. Replication of these findings is essential prior to acceptance of a bacterial causation.

Candidal. Claims have been made that chronic candidal infection may cause a host of illnesses including PMS.[80] To date, there has been no convincing documentation of any such association or of any effect of treatment.[81]

Evolutionary Theory

The finding by zoologists that primates show a variety of premenstrual changes in behavior and appetite similar to those reported in women with PMS[20-22] led to a search for an evolutionary explanation. Morriss and Keverne[82]

suggested that continued bouts of hostility in the premenstrual period would tend to break down the pair bond for a given primate couple. This, they argued, would continue only as long as the couple remained infertile and would resolve either with pregnancy or with dissolution of the pair bond and the formation of a new coupling with renewed chance for successful mating. While such a theory contributes little to our understanding of PMS, it may be of interest to those who seek a teleological explanation.

Nutritional Abnormalities

Vitamins and Trace Element Deficiency. The vitamin B_6 deficiency hypothesis, although primarily a nutritional theory about the causation of PMS, invokes an interrelationship between vitamin levels and endocrine function. To date, however, there has been no objective evidence to support the existence of either an absolute or relative vitamin B_6 deficiency occurring in women with PMS[83,84] nor is there any established link between ovarian function and levels of activity of vitamin B_6 that would explain the cyclic nature of symptoms in PMS. In controlled trials, vitamin B_6 has been shown to improve mood in depressed oral contraceptive users[85]; however, studies in women with PMS have produced contradictory results with reports both of improvement and no change.[86–93] Long-term use of vitamin B_6 has been associated with peripheral neuropathy; hence, if patients are treated with B_6 they must be cautioned about the risk of overdosage.[94,95]

Negative findings have been reported for a variety of other vitamins (vitamin A, vitamin E) and trace elements (magnesium and zinc) in PMS.[83,91,96,97]

Prostaglandin E_1 Deficiency. Horrobin has postulated that a defect in the conversion of essential free fatty acids to prostaglandin E_1 may result from a competitive enzyme block at the conversion of γ-linoleic acid to dihomo-γ-linoleic acid, a precursor of prostaglandin E_1.[98] Treatment with 9 percent γ-linoleic acid in the form of evening primrose oil (EPO) has been postulated to overcome this competitive block. Despite widespread promotion of this therapy for PMS, there has been no convincing documentation of its efficacy. The studies[99,100] widely cited by proponents of this approach either fail to show superiority of EPO to placebo or contain serious methodologic flaws that cast doubt on the conclusions. Recent double-blind placebo-controlled trials have failed to show the superiority of γ-linoleic acid supplements to placebo in the treatment of PMS.[101–104] Based upon these findings, and insufficient evidence about product safety, the U.S. Food and Drug Administration, in 1988, issued an "Import Alert" on EPO, seizing all products at point of entry into the United States.[105]

Hypoglycemia. Similarities between the symptoms of hypoglycemia and certain manifestations of PMS (fatigue, hunger, nervousness, sweating, and vague gastrointestinal complaints) led investigators to study hypoglycemia as a possible causative factor in PMS as early as the 1950s. A number of studies of glucose, insulin, and glucagon levels in response to either oral or intravenous glucose tolerance tests at different phases of the menstrual cycle, in both PMS patients and controls, have failed to show significant differences, thus casting doubt on this theory.[106–109] However, more recent studies employing sensitive analytic methods have shown declining insulin sensitivity in the luteal phase of the menstrual cycle.[110] In addition, the euglycemic insulin clamp technique has demonstrated premenstrual abnormalities of cellular glucose uptake in women with PMS[111] although not in normal controls.[112] Whether or not these changes can account for some of the varied clinical manifestations of PMS is uncertain. The role of "hypoglycemic" diets in the treatment of PMS is likewise unresolved.

Fluid Retention

The popular notion that fluid retention explains symptoms of PMS has received little support from scientific studies.[113] Some women with PMS do experience minor peripheral edema premenstrually but this most likely results from fluid shifts within the body. When weight is followed prospectively, changes appear random, and weight gain, when it does occur, seldom correlates with the severity of other premenstrual manifestations. Studies of a variety of fluid-retaining hormones failed to demonstrate any clear abnormalities in women with PMS. Diuretic therapy may transiently improve self-esteem by allowing the woman to fit into her tight clothing; however, it may provoke further fluid retention by activation of the renin–angiotensin–aldosterone system.

Progesterone Deficiency

The concept that progesterone deficiency was the etiologic trigger for PMS was popularized in the mid-1950s by Katharina Dalton.[114] Since that time, treatment with progesterone vaginal suppositories has been promoted in PMS clinics throughout Europe and North America. Critical evaluation of publications purporting to demonstrate the efficacy of progesterone therapy reveals only uncontrolled studies and anecdotal observation. Other investigators have attempted to replicate Dalton's findings in properly controlled studies and have not been able to confirm the efficacy of progesterone vaginal suppositories for the treatment of PMS.[115–118]

Initial enthusiasm for oral micronized progesterone[119] has been tempered by the result of a controlled trial showing no benefit for PMS.[120] Schmidt et al[120A] recently presented the results of a unique experimental model in which they were able to determine the results of truncation of luteal phase steroidogenesis. Their findings demonstrated that whether or not progesterone secretion was abolished in the midluteal phase there was no change in the timing or severity of subsequent premenstrual symptoms.[5] Other investigators have shown that severe PMS may occur in a high progesterone environment during the luteal phase.[121] Both of these observations argue against progesterone deficiency as an inciting factor in the genesis of PMS.

Neuroendocrine Hypotheses

Endogenous Opiate Peptides. Endogenous opiate peptides (EOPs) are widely distributed throughout the body and are known to have a variety of diverse actions such as modulation of hormone secretion, mood, behavior, appetite, sleep, temperature regulation, and bowel function. Their activity is known to be modulated in primates by changes in ovarian steroid secretion, suggesting the possibility of a unique interaction between the hypothalamic–pituitary–ovarian system and these central neurotransmitters, which might explain some of the diverse physical, psychological, and behavioral manifestations of PMS.[1] Studies in the rhesus monkey, which has a 28-day menstrual cycle with endocrine changes similar to those of the human, have shown that EOP activity is increased in the luteal phase of the menstrual cycle with a return to normal levels during the luteal–follicular transition.[122] It has been hypothesized that exposure to high levels of EOPs may induce a form of transient opiate addiction with secondary effects on a variety of other neurotransmitter systems with which EOPs interact.[1] This, in turn, may cause changes in mood, appetite, temperature regulation, etc. It is presently impossible to achieve access to sites of synthesis and secretion of EOPs in the human to directly address levels of EOPs in women with PMS at different times of the cycle or in comparison to unaffected controls.

It is doubtful whether the reported changes in peripheral endorphin levels truly reflect central EOP activity in view of the fact that secretion from these two sites is dissociated in many circumstances.[123] A clinical trial indicating a possible therapeutic effect of the opiate antagonist, naltrexone, in women with PMS requires verification before such an approach can be advocated.[124]

Serotonin Deficiency. Evidence from a variety of different sources suggests that serotonin metabolism may be disturbed in depression.[125] In subjects with PMS, the concentration of 5-hydroxytryptamine (5-HT) in whole blood[126] as well as platelet uptake of 5-HT[127,128] are diminished during the luteal phase. Competition between L-tryptophan and other large neutral amino acids for the same saturable carrier protein for transport across the blood–brain barrier has been advanced as a possible mechanism resulting in reduced 5-HT levels in the central nervous system.[129] This theory has recently been called into question by the finding that no abnormalities exist in the ratio of circulating tryptophan to other amino acids in subjects with PMS when compared to controls.[130] This is in contrast to evidence that patients with major depressive disorders do have an alteration in the ratio of these amino acids.[131]

The precise mechanism by which a deficiency of serotonin production could contribute to the development of premenstrual symptomatology remains speculative. Studies employing serotonergic agonists[57] and serotonin reuptake inhibitors[132] have shown beneficial effects in some women with PMS. Acceptance of a serotonin deficiency hypothesis, however, must await further evidence demonstrating a true serotonin deficiency.

Summation

Any etiologic theory for PMS must take into account the need to link symptoms to hormonal fluctuations of the menstrual cycle. In support of such an obligatory role of ovarian hormone secretion are the observations that: (1) PMS does not appear prior to activation of the hypothalamic–pituitary–ovarian axis at puberty; (2) midcycle (pattern C) PMS symptoms are intimately related to periovulatory hormonal shifts[66]; (3) PMS disappears both during brief anovulatory periods[133] and during more prolonged intervals of hyper- or hypogonadotropin amenorrhea or pregnancy; (4) PMS persists following hysterectomy if ovarian function remains intact[73,134]; and (5) medical[69,70,135] or surgical[71,72] therapy to suppress ovarian function will eliminate PMS.

Why some women develop PMS and others do not is unknown although such differences may result from hereditary and life-style variables affecting regulation of central neurotransmitter systems. There is now ample anecdotal evidence to indicate that PMS symptoms are accentuated at times of increasing life stress. The paradigm shown in Figure 23–4 expresses this dual input of ovarian steroidogenesis and psychological stress into the genesis of premenstrual syndrome.

ASSESSMENT AND MANAGEMENT

Selection of appropriate interventions for PMS will rely greatly on the adequacy of the initial diagnostic assessment. A wide spectrum of problems may present under the guise of PMS and misdirected therapeutic efforts have been the cause of frustration for many physicians. Clinical history alone, although suggestive, is insufficient to confirm the diagnosis.

Investigation of PMS begins with a complete history and physical examination. The nature, severity, and

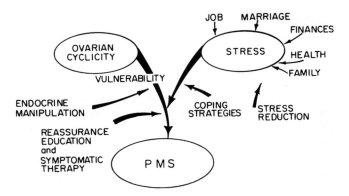

Figure 23–4. Schematic diagram showing the respective contributions of cyclic ovarian hormone secretion and life stress on the expression of menstrual cycle-related physical and psychological symptoms (so-called premenstrual syndrome [PMS]). Therapeutic interventions may be directed at stress reduction, improved coping, symptomatic therapy, or manipulation of the ovarian cycle. (*Reproduced, with permission, from Reid RL. Premenstrual syndrome: Social phenomenon or real medical entity? In: Soules MR, ed.* Controversies in Reproductive Endocrinology and Infertility. *New York, N.Y., Elsevier, 1989: 79–93.*)

chronologic appearance of symptoms in the course of the menstrual cycle should be determined. Information should be sought about stresses related to the woman's occupation and family life as these may tend to exacerbate PMS. Past medical and psychiatric diagnoses may be relevant in that a variety of medical and psychiatric disorders may show premenstrual exacerbation. Medical conditions such as arthritis, asthma, epilepsy, and irritable bowel syndrome have all been chronologically linked to the menstrual cycle.

Organic causes of PMS-like symptoms must be ruled out.[136] Marked fatigue may result from anemia, leukemia, hypothyroidism, or diuretic-induced potassium deficiency. Headaches may be due to intracranial lesions. Gynecologic assessment should be part of the initial evaluation of all women with PMS. Pelvic pain, dysmenorrhea, dyspareunia, and menorrhagia are not unusual features in patients presenting with PMS and may be indicative of coexisting gynecologic disorders. Pelvic examination may reveal pathology such as endometriosis or pelvic inflammatory disease to account for sensations of lower abdominal pain or bloating.

There are no specific diagnostic laboratory tests for PMS although a complete blood count and thyroid function tests may occasionally reveal an unsuspected cause for symptoms.

Charting

Retrospective recall by a patient correlates poorly with prospective symptom records. Daily prospective symptom records, such as the PRISM calendar,[1] will provide at a glance an indication of the nature, timing, and severity of symptoms, as well as the baseline level of symptoms in

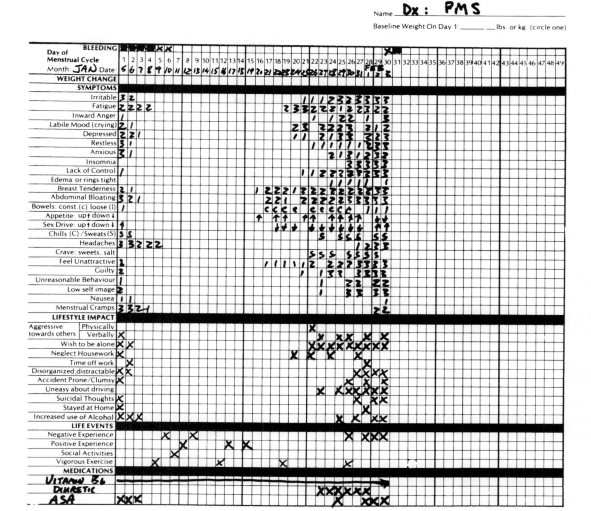

Figure 23–5. Typical prospective record of the impact and severity of menstrual symptoms (PRISM calendar) from a patient with severe PMS. Resolution of symptoms coincides with menstrual flow shown in shaded boxes at top. Symptoms resume shortly after ovulation and persist for remainder of the cycle. *(Reproduced, with permission, from Reid RL. Premenstrual syndrome: Social phenomenon or real medical entity? In: Soules MR, ed.* Controversies in Reproductive Endocrinology and Infertility. *New York, N.Y., Elsevier, 1989: 79–93.)*

the late follicular phase upon which these are superimposed.[137,138] Such a record allows the patient to record her perception of the life-style impact of her symptoms, as well as other positive or negative life events that may influence the perception of symptom severity (Fig 23–5). A record of medication used is also valuable in assessing response to therapy and the patient's perception of her requirement for treatment.

In addition, the PMTS Self-Rating Scale[139] can be completed twice each month, on days 9 and 24. This concise 36-point self-rating scale (Fig 23–6) has been shown to reliably identify women with PMS if symptom scores are low on day 9 and high on day 24. Patients with chronic mood or behavioral disorders will

show little change in symptom levels between these 2 days whereas patients with PMS will show a marked increase in symptoms on day 24. To identify depression, which may be a major component for some women, the Beck Depression Inventory[140] may be applied in the same fashion with comparison of scores between days 9 and 24.

Psychiatric consultation should be sought if there is evidence of risk for suicide, concern about possible violence directed toward children or others, or psychotic behavior. Additional medical consultations may be warranted for unusual premenstrual complaints such as asthma, epilepsy, migraine, arthritis, tinnitus, or vertigo.

Name: Date:

Instructions: The following questions are concerned with the way you feel or act today.

Please answer *all* questions by circling YES or NO as indicated.

1. Do you find yourself avoiding some of your social commitments?	YES	NO
2. Have you gained 5 or more pounds during the past week?	YES	NO
3. Is your coordination so poor that your are unable to use kitchen utensils, garden tools or unable to drive?	YES	NO
4. Do you feel more angry than usual ?	YES	NO
5. Do you avoid family activities and prefer to be left alone?	YES	NO
6. Do you doubt your judgement or feel that you are prone to hasty decisions?	YES	NO
7. Do you feel more irritable than usual?	YES	NO
8. Is your efficiency diminished?	YES	NO
9. Do you feel tense and restless?	YES	NO
10. Do you feel a marked change in your sexual drive or desire during the last week?	YES	NO
If YES, is it *increased* or *decreased*? ⬆ ⬇		
11. Are your present physical symptoms causing so much pain and discomfort that you are unable to function?	YES	NO
12. Have you recently cancelled previously scheduled social activities?	YES	NO
13. Do you feel as if you were unable to relax at all?	YES	NO
14. Do you feel confused?	YES	NO
15. Do you suffer from painful or tender breasts?	YES	NO
16. Do you have an increased desire for specific kinds of food (e.g. cravings for candy, chocolate, etc.)?	YES	NO
17. Do you scream/yell at family members (friends, colleagues) more than usual? Are you "short-fused"?	YES	NO
18. Do you feel sad, gloomy, and hopeless most of the time?	YES	NO
19. Do you feel like crying?	YES	NO
20. Do you have difficulty completing your daily household/job routine?	YES	NO
21. Was there a marked change in your sexual drive with definite change in your sexual behavior during the last week? If YES, is it *increased* or *decreased*? ⬆ ⬇		
22. Do you find yourself being more forgetful than usual or unable to concentrate?	YES	NO
23. Do you happen to have more "accidents" with your daily housework/job (cut fingers, break dishes, etc.)?	YES	NO
24. Have you noticed significant swelling of your breasts and/or ankles and/or bloating of your abdomen?	YES	NO
25. Does your mood change suddenly without obvious reason?	YES	NO
26. Are you easily distracted?	YES	NO
27. Do you think that your restless behavior is noticeable by others?	YES	NO
28. Are you clumsier than usual?	YES	NO
29. Are you obviously negative and hostile towards other people?	YES	NO
30. Are you so fatigued that it interferes with your usual level of functioning?	YES	NO
31. Do you tend to eat more than usual or at odd irregular hours (sweet, snacks, etc.)?	YES	NO
32. Do you become more easily fatigued than usual?	YES	NO
33. Is your handwriting different (less neat than usual)?	YES	NO
34. Do you feel jittery or upset?	YES	NO
35. Do you feel sad or blue?	YES	NO
36. Have you stopped calling or visiting some of your best friends?	YES	NO

Figure 23–6. Self-rating scale for PMS. *(Adapted, with permission, from Steiner M, Haskett RF, Carrol BJ, Premenstrual tension syndrome: The development of research diagnostic criteria and new rating scales. Acta Psychiatr Scand. 62:177, 1980.[139])*

Therapy

Charting and Counseling. Common concerns expressed by women with severe PMS include feelings of fear (that they are "losing their minds") and guilt (over the negative impact of their behavior on relationships with colleagues and family members). Embarrassment and frustration at the skepticism of the medical profession result if their concerns are not taken seriously or they are told to simply "put mind over matter."[6] Counseling and reassurance about the nature of premenstrual mood and behavioral changes are the first important step in allowing such patients to cope with their symptoms.

The chart itself may provide much needed reassurance that other women experience similar symptoms in order that such a symptom record could have been developed. The completed chart may demonstrate to the patient for the first time that there is cyclicity to her symptoms suggesting a link to hormonal swings of the menstrual cycle.

While it is useful for PMS sufferers to learn to anticipate times in the month when vulnerability to emotional upset and confrontation may be greatest, the strategy of making important decisions "only on the good days," as espoused in some clinics, falls apart if premenstrual symptoms last for more than just a few days per month. For some women, premenstrual symptoms may last for a full 3 wk and advising them to restrict their important activities to the remaining days of the month is neither helpful nor warranted. Interventions aimed at reducing symptoms are more appropriate in this circumstance.

Life-style Modification. When an individual is suffering to a degree that requires more than simple counseling and reassurance, measures aimed at life-style modification should be explored first.[25,141] The woman and her family must develop strategies for coping and stress reduction.[142] Communication skills and assertiveness may be improved with counseling. Group counseling in a program supervised by a clinical psychologist may be invaluable.[143] Participation in a "support group" of heterogeneous self-diagnosed PMS sufferers may do more harm than good and patients should be cautioned about the need for qualified group supervision.[144,145]

While there have been many books written that describe specific "PMS diets," few of the recommendations contained therein are founded on scientific fact. Several simple dietary measures may afford relief for women with PMS. Reduction of the intake of salt and refined carbohydrates may help prevent edema and swelling in some women.[146] Although a link between methylxanthine intake and premenstrual breast pain has been suggested, available data are not convincing.[147] Nevertheless, a reduction in the intake of caffeine may prove useful in women where tension, anxiety, and insomnia predominate.[148] Anecdotal evidence suggests that small, more frequent meals may occasionally alleviate mood swings. Based upon recent evidence that cellular uptake of glucose may be impaired premenstrually,[111] there is, at least, some theoretical basis for this dietary recommendation. Several lines of evidence indicate that there is a tendency toward increased consumption of alcohol premenstrually,[42–45] and women should be cautioned that excessive use of alcohol is frequently an antecedent factor in family discord.

Exercise is reported to reduce premenstrual molimina in women running in excess of 50 km/cycle.[149] Even lesser amounts of regular exercise may benefit PMS sufferers.[150] As part of an overall program of life-style modification, exercise may reduce stress by providing a quiet period of time alone and by diverting any pent-up tension or anxiety in a constructive direction.

Medication. As a general rule, the degree of medical intervention for treatment of PMS should be tailored to the severity of symptoms. For women in whom symptoms are transient or where a specific symptom (such as in-

somnia or headache) predominates, symptomatic therapy during affected days of the month may be most appropriate. Conversely, if symptoms are myriad and long lasting, then intervention aimed at modifying the underlying process may be necessary. Accordingly, the treatment options outlined below will be divided into first and second-level interventions.

First-level Interventions. Attention should always initially be directed to symptoms for which established treatments exist. For example, dysmenorrhea or menorrhagia may be satisfactorily relieved with prostaglandin synthetase inhibitors or oral contraceptives. Persisting heavy menstrual flow, despite these interventions, may be an indication for alternate therapies such as tranexamic acid or evaluation of the intrauterine cavity employing ultrasound or hysteroscopy. Although oral contraceptives by no means guarantee relief from PMS, they may afford sufficient relief from associated symptoms that, for some women, remaining premenstrual manifestations become more tolerable.

Two relatively safe, inexpensive, and simple interventions, which may be tried for the initial management of mild premenstrual symptomatology, include pyridoxine 100 to 200 mg daily throughout the menstrual cycle[85,86] and mefenamic acid 250 to 500 mg po qid in the premenstrual and menstrual week.[151–153] There have been some contradictory data published in regard to the efficacy of pyridoxine; however, this medication in proper dosages is, at worst, a safe placebo that becomes one part of an overall management plan including life-style modification and changes in diet.[152] Patients should be cautioned that these medications do not work for all women and that increasing the dose of pyridoxine in an effort to achieve complete relief of symptoms may lead to peripheral neuropathy. Pyridoxine should be discontinued if there is evidence of tingling or numbness of the extremities.

Mefenamic acid has outperformed placebo for the treatment of PMS in some[151,153] but not all[154] clinical trials. It is a valuable intervention for any woman with co-existing dysmenorrhea and menorrhagia; however, its effectiveness for premenstrual symptomatology seems quite variable. Mefenamic acid is contraindicated in women with known sensitivity to aspirin or those at risk for peptic ulcers.

Premenstrual mastalgia has been shown to respond to tamoxifen (10 mg daily),[155] bromocriptine (2.5 mg tid),[11] and danazol (100 to 400 mg OD),[156,157] but not to pyridoxine.[158]

The routine use of diuretics in the treatment of PMS should be abandoned. Only if a reduction of salt and refined carbohydrates in the diet fails to relieve premenstrual fluid accumulation (documented by evidence of pitting edema or consistent weight gain) should consideration be given to the use of a potassium-sparing diuretic such as spironolactone.[159]

Some women report overriding symptoms of anxiety and tension or insomnia in the premenstrual week. New short-acting anxiolytics or hypnotics such as alprazolam (0.25 mg po bid) or triazolam (0.25 mg po qhs), respectively, may be prescribed sparingly for such individuals.[160]

Estrogen withdrawal has been implicated in menstrually related migraines,[161] and recent evidence indicates that estrogen supplementation commencing in the late luteal phase and continued through menstruation may alleviate headaches in some women.[162,163] As discussed below, if headaches are severe and unrelieved by short-term estrogen supplementation, they can often be nicely controlled by overriding the normal menstrual cycle.[164–166]

Oral contraceptives fail to relieve PMS symptoms in most circumstances[167,168] and may actually result in earlier onset of symptoms.[169] A switch to an alternate means of contraception is often attended by a substantial reduction in symptoms.

Second-level Interventions. Two classes of medications have been used in an attempt to afford relief to the severely affected woman when life-style modification and symptomatic therapies are unrewarding.

MEASURES AIMED AT OVARIAN SUPPRESSION

MEDICAL OVARIAN SUPPRESSION. Suppression of cyclic ovarian function may afford dramatic relief for the woman with severe and long-lasting symptoms. In each case, therapy should be directed toward suppression of cyclic ovarian activity while ensuring a constant low level of estrogen sufficient to prevent menopausal symptomatology and side effects. As a rule, oral contraceptives do not work, perhaps because ovarian steroidogenesis is replaced by exogenous synthetic steroids.[167] Danazol 200 mg bid will effect ovarian suppression in approximately 80 percent of women with prompt relief from symptoms.[67] Higher doses up to 200 mg qid may be required in the remaining women to achieve complete menstrual suppression. Danazol, at a dosage of 200 mg bid, has relatively few side effects; these may include hot flushes, muscle cramps, and occasional cases of epigastric pain, fine tremor, or insomnia. In the woman without pre-existing hair growth, hirsutism is rarely a problem at these dosages when treatment is limited to 1 yr or less. In the individual with pre-existing acne or increased body hair, alternative interventions should be considered. The use of danazol causes a shift to a more unfavorable lipid profile, likely to have little impact when danazol is used on a short-term basis. In the patient who tolerates danazol well and in whom symptomatic relief is dramatic, this effect is the primary concern that will influence decision making about long-term treatment.

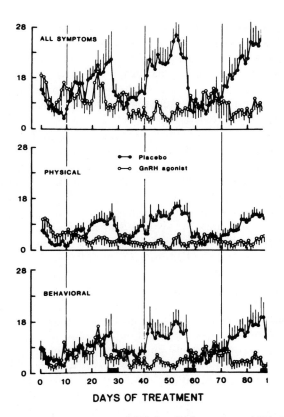

Figure 23–7. Mean scores (±SE) for all 15 symptoms (10 behavioral and 5 physical) during GnRH agonist treatment and placebo administration. *(Reproduced, with permission, from Muse KN, Cetel NS, Futterman LA, Yen SC, The premenstrual syndrome. Effects of "medical ovariectomy." N Engl J Med. 311:1345, 1984.)*

Luteinizing hormone-releasing hormone (LHRH) agonists effect rapid medical ovarian suppression, thereby inducing a pseudomenopause and affording relief from PMS (Fig 23–7).[69,70] This approach is unsatisfactory in the long term not only because of the troublesome menopausal symptoms it evokes but also because it creates an increased risk for osteoporosis and ischemic heart disease. When combined with replacement doses of estrogen and Provera (as one would do in menopausal hormone replacement therapy), LHRH agonists afford excellent relief from premenstrual symptomatology without the attendant risks and symptoms resulting from premature menopause.[135,170] The major drawback to this therapeutic approach is the expense of medication and the need for the patient to take multiple medications. Regrettably, the cyclic addition of progestin induces a recrudescence of symptoms in many PMS sufferers.

A simpler and less expensive approach involves the use of continuous oral medroxyprogesterone (15 mg daily) or depo-medroxyprogesterone acetate (150 mg IM q 2–3 mo). Both routes of administration result in rapid suppression of cyclic ovarian function without attendant menopausal symptomatology. The major drawback to this approach is that a substantial percentage of women will get irregular bleeding or nuisance spotting.[171] The ideal situation, in which depo-medroxyprogesterone acetate induces amenorrhea, may be problematic for the woman who wishes future fertility. Patients should always be counseled about the potential for protracted amenorrhea following use of this medication.

Another method for overriding the spontaneous cycle is to use exogenous estrogen in the form of a subcutaneous implant or a transdermal patch (Estraderm two 100-µg patches changed every 3 days) combined with cyclic or continuous Provera to prevent endometrial hyperplasia.[164,172] This intervention can afford quite dramatic relief not only for menstrual migraines but also for other premenstrual symptoms.

SURGICAL THERAPY. For the woman in whom premenstrual symptoms have been severe and unresponsive to conservative approaches, but dramatically improved with medical ovarian suppression, a surgical option may be discussed.[71,72] In the circumstance where family is complete and permanent contraception is a desire, the pros and cons of oophorectomy for lasting relief from premenstrual symptomatology should be discussed with the patient. If a decision is made to proceed to oophorectomy, this can be relatively innocuously performed by laparoscopy. Continuous estrogen replacement therapy would be necessary thereafter, combined with either cyclic or continuous progestin therapy to prevent endometrial hyperplasia. To avoid progestin-associated return of PMS-like symptoms the patient may choose to have concomitant hysterectomy, allowing subsequent treatment with estrogen replacement alone (Fig 23–8).

Initial treatment for PMS should involve conservative measures such as life-style modification and symptomatic therapies. If these are ineffective and symptoms are severe and disruptive to life-style, a course of medical ovarian suppression may be tried. If practical, this treatment should be maintained for 6 to 12 mo to ensure a lasting symptomatic improvement. Subsequent treatment options include discontinuation of therapy, continuing medical ovarian suppression, or surgery.[72] Should the patient opt for a surgical approach, she should be advised to discontinue medication for at least 3 to 4 mo prior to surgery to ensure that surgery is still warranted based upon the reappearance of severe symptoms.

ANTIDEPRESSANT THERAPY. A range of newer antidepressant medications that augment central serotonin activity have been shown to alleviate severe premenstrual syndrome.[132,173–175] Since these agents will also relieve endogenous depression, a pretreatment diagnosis, achieved by prospective charting, is very important. Practically speaking, many women who attend a gynecology clinic to seek relief from premenstrual symptoms express reservations about taking an antidepressant, particularly if a

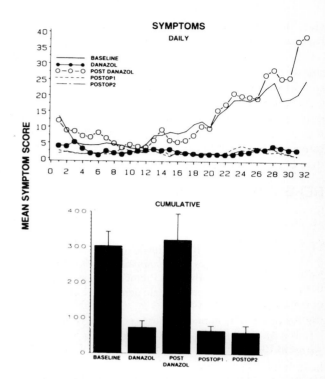

Figure 23–8. Mean daily (upper panel) and monthly cumulative (lower panel) symptom scores for 14 women with severe PMS. Baseline (solid), danazol treatment (closed circles), postdanazol (open circles), and two postoperative months (dotted lines) approximately 4 and 8 mo following hysterectomy and oophorectomy are represented. Day 0 is first day of menses for spontaneous cycles or start of calendar month for danazol and postoperative cycles. *(Reproduced, with permission, from Casson P, Hahn PM, Van Vugt DA, Reid RL, Lasting response to ovariectomy in severe intractable premenstrual syndrome. Am J Obstet Gynecol. 162:99, 1990.)*

short-term end point (3 to 6 mo away) is not likely. Long-term therapy may be required to control symptoms of PMS from the late 30s until menopause, and data on safety and the consequences of discontinuation of long-term antidepressant treatment in this population are unknown. Studies to evaluate long-term outcomes for the thousands of PMS sufferers started on antidepressant medications in the mid-1990s are urgently required.

For patients in whom PMS symptoms are severe and menstrual cycle suppression is not a desired option, antidepressant therapy may provide excellent results. Selective serotonin reuptake inhibitors (SSRIs), such as fluoxetine, sertraline, paroxetine, fluvoxamine, and velafaxine (a serotonin and norepinephrine reuptake inhibitor), have all been successfully employed.[132,173–174]

Symptom profiles may help in selecting the most appropriate agent (eg, fluoxetine in patients where fatigue and depression predominate; sertraline if insomnia, irritability, and anxiety are paramount). SSRIs have been associated with loss of libido and anorgasmia, which are particularly distressing to patients, and appropriate pretreatment counseling is essential.

Tricyclic antidepressants (TCAs) have not generally been effective with the exception of clomipramine, a TCA with strong serotoninergic activity.[175] Intolerance to the side effects of TCAs is common.

Most PMS sufferers would prefer to medicate themselves only during the symptomatic phase of the menstrual cycle. Efforts are presently underway to evaluate the efficacy of an antidepressant administered in the luteal phase only.[176]

REFERENCES

1. Reid RL. Premenstrual syndrome. *Curr Probl Obstet Gynecol Fertil.* 2:1, 1985
2. Halbreich U, Endicott J. Methodological issues in studies of premenstrual changes. *Psychoneuroendocrinology.* 10:15, 1985
3. Rubinow DR, Roy-Byrne P. Premenstrual syndromes: Overview from a methodologic perspective. *Am J Psychiatry.* 141:163, 1984
4. Frank FT. The hormonal causes of premenstrual tension. *Arch Neurol Psychiatry.* 26:1053, 1931
5. Reid RL. Premenstrual syndrome. *N Engl J Med.* 324: 1208, 1991
6. Reid RL. Premenstrual syndrome: A time for introspection. *Am J Obstet Gynecol.* 155:921, 1986
7. Geringer E, Mittelwahn L. A reconsideration of premenstrual phenomena. *J Obstet Gynaecol Br Commonw.* 58:1010, 1951
8. Altmann M, Knowles E, Bull HD. A psychosomatic study of the sex cycle in women. *Psychosom Med.* 111:199, 1941
9. Mortola JF, Girton L, Beck L, Yen SS. Diagnosis of premenstrual syndrome by a simple, prospective, and reliable instrument: The calendar of premenstrual experiences. *Obstet Gynecol.* 76:302, 1990
10. Casper RF, Powell AM. Premenstrual syndrome: Documentation by a linear analog scale compared with two descriptive scales. *Am J Obstet Gynecol.* 155:862, 1986
11. Rubinow DR, Roy-Byrne P, Hoban MC, et al. Prospective assessment of menstrually related mood disorders. *Am J Psychiatry.* 141:684, 1984
12. American Psychiatric Association. *Diagnostic and Statistical Manual of Mental Disorders,* 4th ed (DSM-IV), Washington, D.C., APA, 1994
13. Andersch B, Wendestam C, Hahn H, Ohman R. Premenstrual complaints: I Prevalence of premenstrual symptoms in a Swedish urban population. *J Psychosom Obstet Gynaecol.* 5:39, 1986
14. Woods NF, Most A, Dery GK. Prevalence of perimenstrual symptoms. *Am J Public Health.* 72:1257, 1982
15. Rivera-Tovar AD, Frank E. Late luteal phase dysphoric disorder in young women. *Am J Psychiatry.* 147:1634, 1990
16. Johnson TM. Premenstrual syndrome as a western culture-specific disorder. *Cult Med Psychiatry.* 11:337, 1987
17. Janiger O, Riffenburgh R, Kersh R. Cross cultural study of premenstrual symptoms. *Psychosomatics.* 13:226, 1972
18. Adenaike OC, Abidoye RO. A study of the incidence of the premenstrual syndrome in a group of Nigerian women. *Public Health.* 101:49, 1987
19. Cenac A, Maikibi DK, Develoux M. Premenstrual syndrome in Sahelian Africa. A comparative study of 400 literate and illiterate women in Niger. *Trans R Soc Trop Med Hyg.* 81:544, 1987
20. Gilbert C, Gillman J. The changing pattern of food intake and appetite during the menstrual cycle of the baboon (papio ursinus) with a consideration of some of the controlling endocrine factors. *S Afr J Med Sci.* 21:75, 1956
21. Sassenrath EN, Rowell TE, Hendrickx AG. Perimenstrual aggression in groups of female rhesus monkeys. *J Reprod Fert.* 34:509, 1973
22. Hausfater G, Skoblick B. Perimenstrual behavior changes among female yellow baboons: Some similarities to premenstrual syndrome (PMS) in women. *Am J Primatology.* 9:165, 1985
23. Wilson CA, Turner CW, Keye WR. Firstborn adolescent daughters and mothers with and without premenstrual syndrome: A comparison. *J Adolescent Health.* 12:130, 1991
24. Warner P, Bancroft J. Factors related to self-reporting of the pre-menstrual syndrome. *Br J Psychiatry.* 157:249, 1990
25. DeStefano F, Perlman JA, Peterson HB, Diamond EL. Long-term risk of menstrual disturbances after tubal sterilization. *Am J Obstet Gynecol.* 152:835, 1985
26. Coppen A, Kessel N. Menstruation and personality. *Br J Psychiatry.* 109:711, 1963
27. Dalton K, Dalton ME, Guthrie K. Incidence of the premenstrual syndrome in twins. *Br Med J.* 295:1027, 1987
28. Hamilton JA, Parry BL, Blumenthal SJ. The menstrual cycle in context I: Affective syndromes associated with reproductive hormonal changes. *J Clin Psychiatry.* 49:474, 1988
29. Stout AL, Steege JF, Blazer DG, George LK. Comparison of lifetime psychiatric diagnoses in premenstrual syndrome clinic and community sample. *J Nerv Ment Dis.* 174:517, 1986
30. Diamond SB, Rubinstein AA, Dunner DL, Fieve RR. Menstrual problems in women with primary affective illness. *Compr Psychiatry.* 17:541, 1976
31. Parry BL, Wehr TA. Therapeutic effect of sleep deprivation in patients with premenstrual syndrome. *Am J Psychiatry.* 144:808, 1987
32. Endicott J, Halbreich U, Schacht S, Nee J. Affective disorder and premenstrual depression. In: Osofsky HJ, Blumenthal SJ, eds. *Progress in Psychiatry,* American Psychiatric Press, Washington, D.C., 1985: 3–11
33. Tonks CM, Rack PH, Rose MJ. Attempted suicide and the menstrual cycle. *J Psychosom Res.* 11:319, 1968
34. Pallis DJ, Holding TA. The menstrual cycle and suicidal intent. *J Biosoc Sci.* 8:27, 1976
35. Spitzer RL, Endicott J, Robins R. Research diagnostic criteria: Rationale and reliability. *Arch Gen Psychiatry.* 35:773, 1978
36. Parry BL, Rosenthal NE, Tamarkin L, Wehr TA. Treatment of a patient with seasonal premenstrual syndrome. *Am J Psychiatry.* 144:762, 1987
37. Trunnell EP, Turner CW, Keye WR. A comparison of the psychological and hormonal factors in women with and without premenstrual syndrome. *J Abnorm Psychol.* 97:429, 1988
38. Mortola JF, Girton L, Yen SS. Depressive episodes in premenstrual syndrome. *Am J Obstet Gynecol.* 161:1682, 1989

39. Brown MA, Zimmer PA. Personal and family impact of premenstrual symptoms. *J Obstet Gynecol Neonatal Nurs.* 15:31, 1986

40. Clare AW. Psychiatric and social aspects of premenstrual complaint. *Psychol Med Monogr Suppl.* 4:1, 1983

41. Meehan E, MacRae K. Legal implications of premenstrual syndrome: A Canadian perspective. *Can Med Assoc J.* 135:601, 1986

42. Halliday A, Bush B, Cleary P, et al. Alcohol abuse in women seeking gynecologic care. *Obstet Gynecol.* 68:322, 1986

43. Mello NK, Mendelson JH, Lex BW. Alcohol use and premenstrual symptoms in social drinkers. *Psychopharmacology.* 101:448, 1990

44. Mello NK. Drug use patterns and premenstrual dysphoria. *NIDA Res Monogr.* 65:31, 1986

45. Sutter PB, Libet JM, Allain AN, Randall CL. Alcohol use, negative mood states and menstrual cycle phases. *Alcoholism.* 7:327, 1983

46. Stewart NL. Premenstrual tension in automobile accidents. *Cleveland-Marshall Law Rev.* 6:17, 1957

47. Mandell AH, Mandell MP. Suicide and the menstrual cycle. *JAMA.* 200:792, 1967

48. Patel S, Cliff KS, Machin D. The premenstrual syndrome and its relationship to accidents. *Public Health.* 99:45, 1985

49. Faratian B, Gapar A, O'Brien PM, et al. Premenstrual syndrome: weight, abdominal swelling, and perceived body image. *Am J Obstet Gynecol.* 150:200, 1984

50. Wald A, Van Thiel DH, Hoechsteller L, et al. Gastrointestinal transit: The effect of the menstrual cycle. *Gastroenterology.* 80:1497, 1981

51. Mathias JR, Ferguson KL, Clench MH. Debilitating "functional" bowel disease controlled by leuprolide acetate, gonadotropin-releasing hormone analog. *Dig Dis Sci.* 34:761, 1989

52. Host N, Jenssen TG, Burhol PG, et al. Plasma gastrointestinal hormones during spontaneous and induced menstrual cycles. *J Clin Endocrinol Metab.* 68:1160, 1989

53. Preece PE, Richards AR, Owen GM, Hughes LE. Mastalgia and total body water. *Br Med J.* 4:498, 1975

54. Davit SP. The effect of the menstrual cycle on patterns of food intake. *Am J Clin Nutr.* 34:1811, 1981

55. Tomelleri R, Grunewald KK. Menstrual cycle and food cravings in young college women. *J Am Diet Assoc.* 87:311, 1987

56. Both-Orthman B, Rubinow DR, Hoban MC, et al. Menstrual cycle phase-related changes in appetite in patients with premenstrual syndrome and in control subjects. *Am J Psychiatry.* 145:628, 1988

57. Brzezinski AA, Wurtman JJ, Wurtman RJ, et al. D-fenfluramine suppresses the increased calorie and carbohydrate intakes and improves the mood of women with premenstrual depression. *Obstet Gynecol.* 76:296, 1990

58. Casper RF, Graves GR, Reid RL. Objective measurement of hot flushes associated with the premenstrual syndrome. *Fertil Steril.* 47:341, 1987

59. Halbreich U, Endicott J, Schacht S, Nee J. The diversity of premenstrual changes as reflected in the Premenstrual Assessment Form. *Acta Psychiatr Scand.* 65:46, 1982

60. Pauli BD, Reid RL, Munt PW, et al. Influence of the menstrual cycle on airway function in asthmatic and normal subjects. *Am Rev Respir Dis.* 140:358, 1989

61. Magos A, Studd J. Effects of the menstrual cycle on medical disorders. *Br J Hosp Med.* 33:68, 1985

62. Case AM, Reid RL. Effects of the menstrual cycle on medical disorders. *Arch Intern Med.* 158, 1998. In press.

63. Badwe RA, Gregory WM, Chandry MA, et al. Timing of surgery during menstrual cycle and survival of premenopausal women with operable breast cancer. *Lancet.* 337:1261, 1991

64. Brooks-Gunn J. The experience of menarche. *Child Dev.* 53:1557, 1982

65. Ruble DN. Premenstrual symptoms: A reinterpretation. *Science.* 197:291, 1977

66. Reid RL. Endogenous opioid activity and the premenstrual syndrome. *Lancet.* 2:786, 1983

67. Watts JF, Butt WR, Logan Edwards R. A clinical trial using danazol for the treatment of premenstrual tension. *Br J Obstet Gynaecol.* 94:30, 1987

68. Bancroft J, Boyle H, Warner P, Fraser HM. The use of an LHRH agonist, buserelin, in the long-term management of premenstrual syndromes. *Clin Endocrinol.* 27:171, 1987

69. Hammarback S, Backstrom T. Induced anovulation as treatment of premenstrual tension syndrome. A double-blind cross-over study with GnRH-agonist versus placebo. *Acta Obstet Gynecol Scand.* 67:159, 1988

70. Mortola JF, Girton L, Fischer U. Successful treatment of severe premenstrual syndrome by combined use of gonadotropin-releasing hormone agonist and estrogen/progestin. *J Clin Endocrinol Metab.* 72:252A, 1991

71. Casper RF, Hearn MT. The effect of hysterectomy and bilateral oophorectomy in women with severe premenstrual syndrome. *Am J Obstet Gynecol.* 162:105, 1990

72. Casson P, Hahn PM, Van Vugt DA, Reid RL. Lasting response to ovariectomy in severe intractable premenstrual syndrome. *Am J Obstet Gynecol.* 162:99, 1990

73. Backstrom CT, Boyle H, Baird DT. Persistence of symptoms of premenstrual tension in hysterectomized women. *Br J Obstet Gynaecol.* 88:530, 1981

74. Koeske RW, Koeske GF. An attributional approach to moods and the menstrual cycle. *J Pers Soc Psychol.* 31:473, 1975

75. Brayshaw ND, Brayshaw DD. Thyroid hypofunction in premenstrual syndrome. *N Engl J Med.* 315:1486, 1986

76. Casper RF, Patel-Christopher A, Powell AM. Thyrotropin and prolactin responses to thyrotropin-releasing hormone in premenstrual syndrome. *J Clin Endocrinol Metab.* 68:608, 1989

77. Nikolai TF, Mulligan GM, Gribble RK, et al. Thyroid function and treatment in premenstrual syndrome. *J Clin Endocrinol Metab.* 70:1108, 1990

78. Roy-Byrne PP, Rubinow DR, Hogan MC, et al. TSH and prolactin responses to TRH in patients with premenstrual syndrome. *Am J Psychiatry.* 144:480, 1987

79. Toth A, Lesser ML, Naus G, et al. Effect of doxycycline on premenstrual syndrome: A double-blind randomized clinical trial. *J Int Med Res.* 16:270, 1988

80. Crook WG. *The Yeast Connection*, 3rd ed. Jackson, Tenn, Professional Books, 1989

81. Dismukes WE, Wade JS, Lee JY, et al. A randomized double blind trial of nystatin therapy for the candidiasis hypersensitivity syndrome. *N Engl J Med.* 323:1717, 1990

82. Morriss GM, Keverne EB. Premenstrual tension. *Lancet.* 2:1317, 1974. Letter

83. Mira M, Stewart PM, Abraham SF. Vitamin and trace element status in premenstrual syndrome. *Am J Clin Nutr.* 47:636, 1988

84. Van den Berg H, Louwerse ES, Bruinse HW, et al. Vitamin B$_6$ status of women suffering from premenstrual syndrome. *Hum Nutr Clin Nutr.* 40:441, 1986

85. Adams PW, Wynn V, Seed M. Vitamin B$_6$, depression and oral contraception. *Lancet.* 2:516, 1974

86. Hallman J. The premenstrual syndrome: Epidemiological, biochemical and pharmacological studies (dissertations from the Faculty of Medicine). Uppsala, Sweden, Acta Universitatis Upsaliensis, 1987: 1

87. Doll H, Brown S, Thurston A, Vessey M. Pyridoxine (vitamin B$_6$) and the premenstrual syndrome: A randomized crossover trial. *J R Coll Gen Pract.* 39:364, 1989

88. Kleijnen J, Ter Riet G, Knipschild P. Vitamin B$_6$ in the treatment of the premenstrual syndrome—a review. *Br J Obstet Gynaecol.* 97:847, 1990

89. Mattes JA, Martin D. Pyridoxine in premenstrual depression. *Hum Nutr Appl Nutr.* 36:131, 1982

90. Williams MJ, Harris RI, Dean BC. Controlled trial of pyridoxine in the premenstrual syndrome. *J Int Med Res.* 13:174, 1985

91. Hagen I, Nesheim BI, Tuntland T. No effect of vitamin B$_6$ against premenstrual tension. A controlled clinical study. *Acta Obstet Gynecol Scand.* 64:667, 1985

92. Kendall KE, Schnurr PP. The effects of vitamin B$_6$ supplementation on premenstrual symptoms. *Obstet Gynecol.* 70:145, 1987

93. Abraham GE, Hargrove JT. Effect of vitamin B$_6$ on premenstrual symptomatology in women with premenstrual tension syndromes: A double blind crossover trial. *Infertility.* 3:155, 1980

94. Schaumburg H, Kaplan J, Windebank A, et al. Sensory neuropathy from pyridoxine abuse. *N Engl J Med.* 309: 445, 1983

95. Parry GJ. Sensory neuropathy with low dose pyridoxine. *Neurolog.* 35: 1466, 1985

96. Chuong CJ, Dawson EB, Smith ER. Vitamin E levels in premenstrual syndrome. *Am J Obstet Gynecol.* 163:1591, 1990

97. Chuong CJ, Dawson EB, Smith ER. Vitamin A levels in premenstrual syndrome. *Fertil Steril.* 54:643, 1990

98. Horrobin DF. The role of essential fatty acids and prostaglandins in the premenstrual syndrome. *J Reprod Med.* 28:465, 1983

99. Puolakka J, Makarainen L, Viinikka L, Ylikorkala O. Biochemical and clinical effects of treating the premenstrual syndrome with prostaglandin synthesis precursors. *J Reprod Med.* 30:149, 1985

100. Ockerman PA, Backrack I, Glasu S, Rassner S. Evening primrose oil as a treatment of the premenstrual syndrome. *Recent Adv Clin Nutrition.* 2:404, 1986

101. Khoo SK, Munro C, Battistutta D. Evening primrose oil and treatment of premenstrual syndrome. *Med J Aust.* 153:189, 1990

102. Callender K, McGregor M, Kirk P, Thomas CS. A double-blind trial of evening primrose oil in the premenstrual syndrome: nervous symptom subgroup. *Hum Psychopharmacol.* 3:57, 1988

103. Collins A, Cerin A, Coleman G, Landgren BM. Essential fatty acids in the treatment of premenstrual syndrome. *Obstet Gynecol.* 81:93, 1993

104. Budeiri D, Li Wan Po A, Dorman J. Is evening primrose oil of value in the treatment of premenstrual syndrome? *Control Clin Trials.* 17:60, 1996

105. McCollum JR. FDA alert on evening primrose oil. *J Am Diet Assoc.* 89:622, 1989

106. Reid RL, Greenaway-Coates A, Hahn PM. Oral glucose tolerance during the menstrual cycle in normal women and women with alleged premenstrual "hypoglycemic: attacks: Effects of naloxone. *J Clin Endocrinol Metab.* 62:1167, 1986

107. Spellacy WN, Ellingson AB, Keith G, et al. Plasma glucose and insulin levels during the menstrual cycles of normal women and premenstrual syndrome patients. *J Reprod Med.* 35:508, 1990

108. Bonora E, Zavaroni I, Alpi O, et al. Influence of the menstrual cycle on glucose tolerance and insulin secretion. *Am J Obstet Gynecol.* 157:140, 1987

109. Toth EL, Suthijumroon A, Crockford PM, Ryan EA. Insulin action does not change during the menstrual cycle in normal women. *J Clin Endocrinol Metab.* 64:74, 1987

110. Valdes CT, Elkind-Hirsch KE. Intravenous glucose tolerance test-derived insulin sensitivity changes during the menstrual cycle. *J Clin Endocrinol Metab.* 72:642, 1991

111. Diamond M, Simonson DC, DeFronzo RA. Menstrual cyclicity has a profound effect on glucose homeostatis. *Fertil Steril.* 52:204, 1989

112. Yki-Jarvinen H. Insulin sensitivity during the menstrual cycle. *J Clin Endocrinol Metab.* 59:350, 1984

113. Reid RL, Yen SS. Premenstrual syndrome. *Am J Obstet Gynecol.* 139:85, 1981

114. Greene R, Dalton K. The premenstrual syndrome. *Br Med J.* 1:1007, 1953

115. Sampson GA. Premenstrual syndrome: A double-blind controlled trial of progesterone and placebo. *Br J Psychiatry.* 135:209, 1979

116. Andersch B, Hahn L. Progesterone treatment of premenstrual tension—a double blind study. *J Psychosom Res.* 29:489, 1985

117. Van der Meer YG, Benedek-Jaszaan LJ, Van Loenan AC. Effects of high dose progesterone on premenstrual syndrome: A double blind crossover trial. *J Psychosom Obstet Gynecol.* 2:220, 1983

118. Maddocks S, Hahn P, Moller F, Reid RL. A double-blind placebo-controlled trial of progesterone vaginal suppositories in the treatment of premenstrual syndrome. *Am J Obstet Gynecol.* 154:573, 1986

119. Dennerstein L, Spencer-Gardner C, Gotts G, et al. Progesterone and the premenstrual syndrome: a double blind crossover trial. *Br Med J.* 290:1617, 1985

120. Magos A, Studd J. Progesterone and the premenstrual syndrome: A double blind crossover trial. *Br Med J.* 291:213, 1985. Letter

120A. Schmidt PJ, Nieman LK, Grover GN, et al. Lack of effect of induced menses on symptoms in women with premenstrual syndrome. *N Engl J Med.* 324:1174, 1991

121. Backstrom T, Sanders D, Leask R, et al. Mood, sexuality, hormones, and the menstrual cycle. II. Hormone levels and their relationship to the premenstrual syndrome. *Psychosom Med.* 45:503, 1983

122. Wardlaw SL, Wehrenberg WB, Ferin M. Effect of sex steroids on B-endorphin in hypophyseal portal blood. *J Clin Endocrinol Metab.* 55:877, 1982

123. Reid RL. Neuropeptides and PMS. *Fertil Steril.* 46:738, 1986. Letter

124. Chuong CJ, Coulam CB, Bergstralh EJ, et al. Clinical trial of naltrexone in premenstrual syndrome. *Obstet Gynecol.* 72:332, 1988

125. Asberg M, Thoren P, Traskman I. Serotonin depression: A biochemical subgroup within the affective disorders. *Science.* 191:478, 1976

126. Rapkin AJ, Edelmuth E, Chang LC, et al. Whole-blood serotonin in premenstrual syndrome. *Obstet Gynecol.* 70: 533, 1987

127. Ashby CR Jr, Carr LA, Cook CL, et al. Alteration of platelet serotonergic mechanisms and monoamine oxidase activity in premenstrual syndrome. *Biol Psychiatry.* 24:225, 1988

128. Taylor DL, Mathew RJ, Ho BT, Weinman ML. Serotonin levels and platelet uptake during premenstrual tension. *Neuropsychobiology.* 12:16, 1984

129. Fernstrom JD. Role of precursor availability in control of monoamine biosynthesis in brain. *Physiol Rev.* 63:484, 1983

130. Rapkin AJ, Reading AE, Woo S, Goldman LM. Trytophan and neutral amino acids in premenstrual syndrome. *Am J Obstet Gynecol.* 165:1830, 1991

131. Joseph MS, Brewerton TD, Reus VI. Plasma L tryptophan/neutral amino acid ratio and dexamethesone suppression in depression. *Psychiatry Res.* 11:185, 1984

132. Stone AB, Pearlstein TB, Brown WA. Fluoxetine in the treatment of premenstrual syndrome. *Psychopharmacol Bull.* 26:331, 1990

133. Hammarback S, Johansson UB, Backstrom T. Spontaneous anovulation causing disappearance of cyclical symptoms in women with the premenstrual syndrome. *Acta Endocrinol* 125:132, 1991

134. Silber M, Carlstrom K, Larsson B. Premenstrual syndrome in a group of hysterectomized women of reproductive age with intact ovaries. *Adv Contracept.* 5:163, 1989

135. Muse KN, Cetel NS, Futterman LA, Yen SC. The premenstrual syndrome. Effects of "medical ovariectomy." *N Engl J Med.* 311:1345, 1984

136. Keye WR Jr, Hammond DC, Strong T. Medical and psychologic characteristics of women presenting with premenstrual symptoms. *Obstet Gynecol.* 68:634, 1986

137. Chisholm G, Jung SO, Cumming CE, et al. Premenstrual anxiety and depression: Comparison of objective psychological tests with a retrospective questionnaire. *Acta Psychiatr Scand.* 81:52, 1990

138. West CP. The characteristics of 100 women presenting to a gynecological clinic with premenstrual complaints. *Acta Obstet Gynecol Scand.* 68:743, 1989

139. Steiner M, Haskett RF, Carroll BJ. Premenstrual tension syndrome: The development of research diagnostic criteria and new rating scales. *Acta Psychiatr Scand.* 62:177, 1980

140. Beck AT, Ward CH, Mendelson M, et al. An inventory for assessing different kinds of hostility. *J Consult Clin Psychol.* 21:343, 1957

141. Heinz SA. Premenstrual syndrome: An assessment, education, and treatment model. *Health Care Women Int.* 7:153, 1986

142. Ensign JE, Rowe J, Kowalski K. Premenstrual syndrome. Etiology and treatment possibilities. *AORN J.* 47: 962, 1988

143. Hicks RA, Olsen C, Smith-Robison D. Type A-B behavior and the premenstrual syndrome. *Psychol Rep.* 59:353, 1986

144. Keye WR Jr, Trunnell EP. A biopsychological model of premenstrual syndrome. *Int J Fertil.* 31:259, 1986

145. Walton J, Youngkin E. The effect of a support group on self-esteem of women with premenstrual syndrome. *J Obstet Gynecol Neonatal Nurs.* 16:174, 1987

146. Taylor D, Bledsoe L. Peer support, PMS, and stress: A pilot study. *Health Care Women Int.* 7:159, 1986

147. MacGregor GA, Roulston JE, Markander ND. Is idiopathic edema idopathic? *Lancet.* 1:397, 1979

148. Minton JP, Foecking MK, Webster DJT. Caffeine cyclic nucleotides and breast disease. *Surgery.* 86:105, 1979

149. Rossignol AM, Bonnlander H. Caffeine-containing beverages, total fluid consumption, and premenstrual syndrome. *Am J Pub Health.* 80:1106, 1990

150. Prior JC, Vigna Y, Alojada N. Conditioning exercise decreases premenstrual symptoms. A prospective controlled three month trial. *Eur J Appl Physiol.* 55:349, 1986

151. Mira M, McNeil D, Fraser IS, et al. Mefenamic acid in the treatment of premenstrual syndrome. *Obstet Gynecol.* 68:395, 1986

152. Mitwalli A, Blair G, Oreopoulos DG. Safety of intermediate doses of pyridoxine. *Can Med Assoc J.* 131:14, 1984

153. Wood C, Jakubowicz D. The treatment of premenstrual symptoms with mefenamic acid. *Br J Obstet Gynaecol.* 87:627, 1980

154. Gunston KD. Premenstrual syndrome in Cape Town. Part II. A double-blind placebo-controlled study of the efficacy of mefenamic acid. *S Afr Med J.* 70:159, 1986

155. Messinis IE, Lolis D. Treatment of premenstrual mastalgia with tamoxifen. *Acta Obstet Gynecol Scand.* 67:307, 1988

156. Gorins A, Perret F, Tourant B, et al. A French double-blind crossover study (danazol vs placebo) in treatment of severe fibrocystic breast disease. *Eur J Gynaecol Oncol.* 5:85, 1984

157. Mansel RE, Wisbey JR, Hughes LE. Controlled trial of the antigonadotropin danazol in painful nodular benign breast disease. *Lancet.* 1:928, 1982

158. Smallwood J, Ah-Kye D, Taylor I. Vitamin B_6 in the treatment of pre-menstrual mastalgia. *Br J Clin Pract.* 40:532, 1986

159. O'Brien PM, Craven D, Selby C, Symonds EM. Treatment of premenstrual syndrome by spironolactone. *Br J Obstet Gynaecol.* 86:142, 1979

160. Harrison WM, Endicott J, Nee J. Treatment of premenstrual dysphoria with alprazolam. A controlled study. *Arch Gen Psychiatry.* 47:270, 1990

161. Somerville BW. Estrogen-withdrawal migraine. *Neurology.* 25:239, 1975

162. Magos AL, Zilkha KJ, Studd JW. Treatment of menstrual migraine by oestradiol implants. *J Neurol Neurosurg Psychiatry.* 46:1044, 1983

163. De Lignieres B, Vincens M, Mauvais-Jarvis P, et al. Prevention of premenstrual migraine by percutaneous oestradiol. *Br Med J.* 293:1540, 1986

164. Watson NR, Studd JW, Savvas M, et al. Treatment of severe premenstrual syndrome with oestradiol patches and cyclical oral norethisterone. *Lancet.* 2:730, 1989

165. Calton GJ, Burnett JW. Danazol and migraine. *N Engl J Med.* 310:721, 1984

166. Murray S, Muse KN. Effective treatment of severe menstrual migraine headaches with gonadotropin-releasing agonist and "add-back" therapy. *Fertil Steril.* 67:390, 1997

167. Cullberg J. Mood changes and menstrual syndromes with different gestagen/estrogen combinations. A double blind comparison with a placebo. *Acta Psychiatr Scand Suppl.* 236:1, 1972

168. Graham CA, Sherwin BB. A prospective treatment study of premenstrual symptoms using a triphasic oral contraceptive. *J Psychosom Res.* 36:257, 1992

169. Forrest ARW. Cyclical variations in mood in normal women taking oral contraceptives. *Br Med J.* 1:1403, 1979

170. Mezrow G, Shoupe D, Spicer D, et al. Depot leuprolide acetate with estrogen and progestin add-back for long term treatment of premenstrual syndrome. *Fertil Steril.* 62:932, 1994

171. West CP. Inhibition of ovulation with oral progestins—effectiveness in premenstrual syndrome. *Eur J Obstet Gynecol Reprod Biol.* 34:119, 1990

172. Watson NR, Studd JW, Savvas M, Baber RJ. The long-term effects of estradiol implant therapy for the treatment of premenstrual syndrome. *Gynecol Endocrinol.* 4:99, 1990

173. Freeman EW, Rickels K, Sondheimer SJ, et al. Sertraline versus desipramine in the treatment of premenstrual syndrome: An open-label trial. *J Clin Psychiatry.* 57:7, 1996

174. Eriksson E, Hedberg MA, Andersch B, et al. The serotonin reuptake inhibitor paroxetin is superior to the noradrenaline reuptake inhibitor maprotline in the treatment of premenstrual syndrome: A placebo-controlled study. *Neuropsychopharmacology.* 12:167, 1995

175. Sunblad C, Modigh K, Andersch B, Eriksson E. Clomipramine effectively reduces premenstrual irritability and dysphoria: A placebo-controlled trial. *Acta Psychiatr Scand.* 85:39, 1992

176. Sunblad C, Hedberg MA, Eriksson E. Clomipramine administered during the luteal phase reduces the symptoms of premenstrual syndrome: A placebo-controlled trial. *Neuropsychopharmacology.* 9:133, 1993

Chapter 24

CHRONIC PELVIC PAIN: ORIGIN, PHYSIOLOGY, EVALUATION, AND TREATMENT

Richard E. Blackwell

Reproductive endocrinologists deal with pain on a daily basis. The pain may be psychological, physiologic, or a mixture of the two. We are quite aware of the psychic pain associated with infertility and pregnancy loss as well as physiologic pain associated with ovarian cyst formation and ovarian hyperstimulation syndrome associated with ovulation induction protocols. We subject patients to surgical and diagnostic procedures that generate pain from an obvious cause. Yet frequently our therapies induce much more subtle pain, such as migratory arthralgia that may be associated with GnRH analog therapy. Many of the conditions that we treat are not only associated with infertility but pain—for instance, pelvic adhesive disease, endometriosis, fibroids, or abnormal uterine bleeding. Therefore, it is the purpose of this chapter to give the reproductive endocrinologist an overview of the state of pain.

The sensation of pain varies among individuals, with one person's nuisance being another person's agony. Pain presents to the gynecologist that may be distributed anywhere from the diaphragm to the knees. Pain is often complicated by the fact that it can be associated with other symptoms such as nausea, diarrhea, vomiting, dizziness, palpitations, syncope, and migraine headaches. Many of these symptoms are associated with aberrant prostanoid or sex hormone production. Pelvic pain can also come from bone, the neuromuscular system, nerve compression or irritation, bowel, bladder, connective tissue, the reproductive system, or the psyche. Pain may be point specific or very diffuse; it may be intermittent or continuous; cyclic or noncyclic; and related to activity and exercise as well as diet. Our patients often present with chronic abdominopelvic pain and have a history of pelvic inflammatory disease or endometriosis, may have undergone multiple surgical procedures, and often are taking multiple drugs. Unfortunately, in the later stages a great deal of abdominal pain has an iatrogenic underlying component that has been introduced into the situation as a result of appropriate or inappropriate surgery.[1]

PHYSIOLOGY OF PAIN

The acquisition of pain avoidance is a major step in evolutionary biology. Most likely, organisms were randomly selected that could evolve systems to detect pain and institute appropriate avoidance. This did not occur in a teleologic sense, as organisms cannot "will" structural changes that benefit their survival, but evolve in terms of the laws of general adaptation.[2] Pain is generally divided into distinct entities consisting of acute pain (somatic and visceral), neuropathic pain, terminal pain, postoperative pain, chronic (behavioral) pain, and psychogenic pain.[3]

Both visceral organs and skin have *nociceptors*, which are free nerve endings that respond to various noxious stimuli. These may be of high intensity, thermal, chemical, or mechanical types. The signaling is mediated by A-Δ and C-afferent fibers. Receptors are *modality specific* in that they respond to distinct stimuli, such as heat. A fibers are divided into types 1 and 2 based on their response threshold, and these nociceptors function as transducers and convert various energy forms to electrical signals that can then be processed centrally.[4] Receptor activation involves changes in membrane structure, depolarization, and in some cases mechanical deformation, which result in the release of chemical mediators such as substance P, serotonin, potassium, and bradykinin.[5] Receptors function in a *proportional* manner in that the magnitude of stimulus is directly related to the response. Further, when a receptor is activated a state of *hyperalgesia* is induced, which results in a decrease in the pain threshold.

Nociceptors have been identified in all visceral tissues, yet are different from cutaneous receptors. There are fewer receptors in the viscera than in the skin, and they respond to different types of activation. For instance, cutting or burning of mesentery, uterine cervix, or other organs may not necessarily produce pain; however, ischemia, distention, and traction will result in the induction of pain signals. These types of pain are diffuse, generally have an autonomic component, and are poorly localized. Afferent transmission occurs in the spinal cord and is associated with autonomic fibers usually of the sympathetic type, and projects to the same area in the dorsal horn as a corresponding somatic efference. This reception is widely distributed over the cord, makes localization of visceral pain quite difficult, and accounts for the phenomenon of referred pain. This type of pain information is transmitted centrally in unmyelinated A-Δ fibers and C fibers. Transmission in the A-Δ fibers occurs at a velocity of 2 to 30 m/sec, and in C fibers at less than 2 m/sec.[6,7]

The signals transmitted from A and C fibers are integrated in the dorsal horn.[8] This structure is divided into six lamina, which to some degree segregates pain into certain categories. The cells of the dorsal horn are involved in the processing of pain. They do so when the nerve fibers enter the spinal cord and separate in the dorsal root, so that large fibers are located medially and small fibers are located laterally. Also, neurotransmitters are restricted to specific lamina including substance P, somatostatin, vasoactive intestinal peptide, serotonin, dopamine, glycine, norepinephrine, the enkephalins, neurotensin, acid phosphatase, and gamma-aminobutyric acid.[9–11] For instance, substance P may be the primary afferent neurotransmitter; likewise, the enkephalins inhibit primary afferent transmission, and this seems to involve multiple opioid receptor mechanisms. Serotonin and norepinephrine play prominent roles in descending inhibitory mechanisms, yet the picture is far from complete. There are at least 20 neuropeptides, 4 amino acids, and 3 monoamines that are involved in spinal cord physiology.

Painful stimuli result in the release of a neurotransmitter from a nociceptive neuron. Activation of a second neuron occurs, which ultimately results in the transmission of a higher center. Neurons in the substantia gelatinosa can release enkephalins, which serve as prejunctional inhibitory neurotransmitters. Serotonin and norepinephrine also act within the substantia gelatinosa by activating descending inhibitory pathways. Suppression of response to noxious stimuli into substantia gelatinosa can be mediated via large alpha/beta fibers, which results in so-called gate closure. This process is mediated by gamma-aminobutyric acid, and this represents the classic *gate theory* proposed by Melzack and Wall in 1968.[12] While the gate theory has received extensive evaluation it does not apply well to mechanisms other than those involved in nociceptor systems.

The ascending pathways consist of the spinothalamic tract, spinoreticular tract, spinomesocephalic tract, and spinocervical tract. These tracts project signals to a variety of structures including the reticular formation, hypothalamus, thalamus, limbic forebrain structure, pons, periaqueductal gray matter, mesencephalon, medial interlamina thalamic nuclei, limbic forebrain bundle, caudal medulla, nucleus gracilis, nucleus cuneatus, nucleus lemniscus, and posterior thalamic nuclei.[13–16]

EVALUATION OF THE PATIENT WITH PELVIC PAIN

The objectives of the investigation of pelvic pain are to (1) identify the likely cause of pain if possible; (2) determine whether the cause of pain is treatable, and if so by what means; (3) educate the patient and her family about the nature of the pain; and (4) prevent the development or interrupt the process of the chronic pain syndrome. It is best to frame questions about pain in terms of the menstrual cycle, as folliculogenesis induces stretching of the follicles. Pain could be present prior to, during, or after ovulation. The presence of both follicular fluid and blood on the pelvic lining could produce pain for 30 min to multiple days. Further, corpus luteum formation can be associated with pain. Both folliculogenesis and corpus luteum formation generate pain if the adnexa are bound by adhesions to the pelvic sidewall. Finally, menstruation can give rise to pain secondary to ischemia brought about by the action of prostanoids on the vascular system.[17]

First, attention should be turned to the patient's affect, response to pain, and relationship to her spouse or family members. At times, social dysfunction such as the adolescent adjustment reaction, marital discord, or midlife transition may be somatized and present as pain.[18–20] Sociopathic behavior should be suspected if there is a chronic history of discord with employers, family members, or previous treating physicians. The time course of the onset and progression of pain can be defined in terms of limitation of life functions, alterations, and interpersonal relationships, as well as effect on work. Daily variation may give a clue as to the pain's origin, and changes in pain during the work week versus weekends may suggest either family discord or work stress. If family members are present, it is advisable to obtain a separate history from them, as the presentation or the effect of pain may be remarkably different from that given by the patient. At times, when other family members are questioned regarding the history, substance abuse and addictive behavior may be uncovered, which predicts a poor prognosis. Finally, when parents, spouse, or family members are present, pathologic family dynamics are often observed.

One should also explore the possibility that the patient with chronic pelvic pain has been sexually abused as a child. This will frequently not be revealed on the initial consultation, but should be pursued once a trusting physician/patient relationship has been established. One should discuss sexual practices, both date and marital; past history of IUD use; abortion, legal or criminal; known or suspected pelvic infections; and history of a partner with various forms of venereal disease.

One should ask about bowel function with emphasis on both constipation and diarrhea. If diarrhea is found, then information should be gathered about the source of water consumed by the individual such as wells, foreign travel, and hobbies such as hiking, as these individuals are very likely to contract *Giardia lamblia* infections in the southern Appalachian regions. Further, competitive athletes and dancers may be affected with bulimia or anorexia, and may abuse laxatives or diuretics. It should be remembered that factitious diarrhea has been reported that represents a variation of Münchhausen syndrome.[21] A careful history should be taken, since alcohol, lactulose, magnesium-containing antacids, nonsteroidal anti-inflammatory drugs, antibiotics, digitalis, colchicine, quinidine, theophylline, bile salts, and prostaglandins can cause diarrhea. Further, consumption of large quantities of diet colas can induce diarrhea secondary to lack of absorption of the sugar substitute. Drugs such as opiates, heavy metals, calcium-channel blockers, barium sulfate, antacids, various agents used to treat Parkinson's disease, antihypertensives, anticonvulsants, anticholinergics, and antidepressants can cause constipation.[22,23] Further, systemic disorders such as irritable bowel syndrome, Crohn's disease, and postgastrectomy syndrome can result in diarrhea.[24,25] Malabsorption can result in bacterial overgrowth, from radiation enteritis, enteric fistulas, ileal resection, short bowel syndrome, pancreatic dysfunction, diabetic neuropathies, hyper- and hypothyroidism, and the Zollinger–Ellison syndrome. Further, carcinoid can present with both pain and diarrhea. It should be recalled that diabetes and hypothyroidism are very frequently associated with constipation. Eighty percent of diabetics have either anatomic or peripheral neuropathy. Hypothyroidism has also been associated with the formation of toxic megacolon. Pain and bowel dysfunction may be associated with 10 percent of patients with Parkinson's dis-

ease and 40 percent of those with multiple sclerosis. Fifty percent of patients over age 65 who present with both pain and constipation have diverticular disease, and irritable bowel syndrome has a marked predilection for women over age 35.

There is a frequent association between vague abdominal pain, bloating, and bowel dysfunction. These types of disorders have psychological overtones, and frequently occur in younger women who are practicing weight control. It has been estimated that 4 to 50 percent of acute abdominal pain is nonspecific. One might suspect that stool passing through the intestine rapidly might be the etiology of this type of pain. Irritable bowel syndrome is a common cause of chronic abdominal pain. It is generally located in the hypogastric and periumbilical area and may be associated with constipation, change in consistency of stool, bloating, or intermittent constipation. Depression can be associated with irritable bowel syndrome.

The association of endometriosis and bowel symptoms deserves special comment, as this condition is often unrecognized and goes undiagnosed. A patient with endometriosis involving the small or large bowel, uterosacral ligaments, or cul-de-sac, will frequently present with constipation or diarrhea that is cyclic in nature (Fig 24–1). In fact, it follows the typical presentation of endometriosis with the onset occurring just prior to menses and ending as flow decreases (see Chap 32). At times implants on the colon may cause chronic constipation as well. Further, the patient who presents with bowel complaints and endometriosis may have associated interior thigh pain accompanying menstruation or cyclic dysuria that cannot be attributed to urinary tract infections or other causes (Fig 24–2). In all of these cases, endometriosis should be suspected and ruled out by laparoscopy. Frequently, these patients have been approached either with sigmoidoscopy or cystoscopy and invariably have negative results. At times, sigmoidoscopy has been carried out following the detection of blood in the stool with heme occult positive examination. However, it is suggested that care be taken in interpreting heme occult results, and that the test be repeated after the patient has been cautioned not to eat red meat or take iron supplements for several days. In addition, when carrying out rectovaginal examination after a bimanual examination, gloves should be changed to avoid transfer of menses to the heme occult card.

PHYSICAL AND LABORATORY EVALUATION OF THE PATIENT WITH PELVIC PAIN

The most powerful tool in the armamentarium for the management of pelvic pain is the use of a careful history

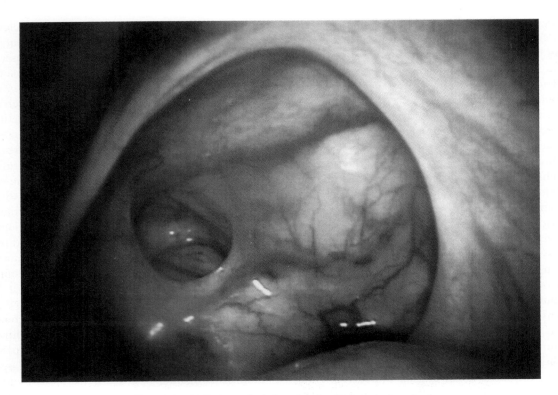

Figure 24–1. Endometriosis invading the rectovaginal septum.

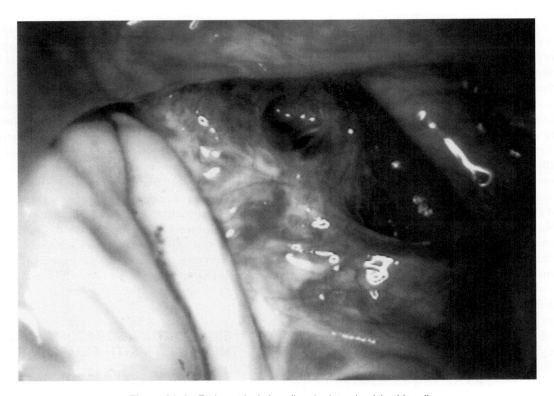

Figure 24–2. Endometriosis invading the lateral pelvic sidewall.

and clinical acumen. Physical examination should be directed to the diagnosis of systemic diseases including malignancies. Attention should be paid to height and body weight, and information should be obtained about weight loss or gain. A pelvic examination should be carried out including transvaginal sonography if needed, a rectal examination, and examination of the stool for blood. One also may wish to submit a stool sample for the identification of ova and parasites. Urine should be examined for the presence of white or red blood cells, bacteria, and glucose. If these are negative, one might wish to proceed with evaluation of the GI tract with a barium enema or flexible sigmoidoscopy; evaluation of the urinary tract with IVP, sonography, or cystoscopy; and evaluation of the gynecologic system with either laparoscopy or hysteroscopy. Occasionally, abdominopelvic CT scanning may be useful in diagnosing retroperitoneal disease. If this type work-up is negative, one must redouble the effort to evaluate the social and emotional picture with consultation with psychiatric or pain service as needed.

PAIN ASSOCIATED WITH THE URINARY TRACT

Acute pelvic pain associated with a urologic cause can usually be pinpointed to a specific etiology and treated appropriately. The patient with chronic pelvic pain may present with a much wider spectrum of disease.[26] If symptoms are mild, reassurance and behavioral modification may be useful. More trying problems may result in radical surgery. In the absence of an obvious pathology, one must consider a diagnosis such as interstitial cystitis, urethral syndrome, irritable bladder syndrome, and sensory neuropathic urgency. The etiology is not well understood, and oftentimes therapy is empiric. An example would be interstitial cystitis, which is thought to occur with an incidence of about 1.2 per 100,000 women. It is associated with urinary frequency, urgency, urethral or bladder pain, and often abdominal, genital, or pelvic pain. The patients disabled by this disorder have major depression, and suicidal ideation is often present in this group. Interstitial cystitis affects ten times as many women as men and is more prevalent in Caucasians. The etiology is unclear and may be multifactorial, including infection, inflammatory reactions, autoimmune reactions, mass cell infiltrates, glycosaminoglycan deficiency, urinary toxins, and reflux sympathetic dystrophy. Evaluation includes a thorough history and physical examination and cystoscopy under anesthesia with bladder hydrodistention and biopsy. Urodynamic evaluation is controversial. The treatment of this disorder includes hydrodistention, oral and intravesical drug therapy, behavior modification, and surgery. Bladder distention, for instance, pro-

duces mechanical pain relief due to local ischemic changes and damage to the submucosal nerve plexus and stretch receptors. The goal of this therapy is to increase bladder capacity, relieve pain, and reduce urinary frequency. In fact, 20 percent of patients actually benefit from this form of therapy. Medications that have been instilled into the bladder include dimethyl sulfoxide (DMSO), heparin, silver nitrate, oxychlorosene sodium, corticosteroids, and bupivacaine. At times, a "cocktail" is administered. Oral agents have proven useful, including amitriptyline with its anticholinergic antihistaminic, analgesic, and antidepressive effects, and nifedipine, a calcium-channel blocker that inhibits bladder contractions.[27–30]

PAIN ASSOCIATED WITH BOWEL DISEASE

Gastrointestinal causes of chronic pelvic pain include functional bowel disorders such as the irritable bowel syndrome, spastic colon, and constipation; primary colon and rectal diseases including inflammatory bowel disease, diverticulitis, colorectal cancer, radiation enteritis, ischemic colitis, infectious colitis, appendicitis, and intestinal endometriosis; pelvic floor dysfunctional disorders including rectal prolapse, solitary rectal ulcers, proctalgia fugax, coccyodynia, and descending perineum syndrome; and retrorectal tumors such as congenital cysts, teratomas, teratocarcinomas, chordoma, and neural defects.[31] The GI tract evaluation includes a careful history and physical with particular emphasis placed on familial history of colon cancer, evaluation of GI symptoms, and symptoms with bowel movements. A rectal examination should be carried out with an evaluation for occult blood. Barium enema or colonoscopy, CT scanning, flexible sigmoidoscopy, or endoscopy may be used to evaluate the problem. The most common gastrointestinal causes of pelvic pain in women include irritable bowel syndrome, chronic idiopathic constipation, and a number of pelvic floor disorders.[32,33] Further discussion will be restricted to these conditions. The irritable bowel syndrome is a common gastrointestinal cause of abdominal pain and is generally characterized by a complex of symptoms including spastic colon associated with chronic abdominal pain and constipation, intermittent painless diarrhea, and alternating diarrhea and constipation with abdominal pain. Further, as mentioned earlier, patients may present with abdominal distention, bloating, fatigue, headaches, and irritability. Symptoms are exacerbated at certain points during the menstrual cycle, and they are affected by diet, stress, menses, and underlying psychic disorders such as bipolar depression or hysteria. There is no good diagnostic test for the syndrome, and one must strive to eliminate other etiologies such as inflammatory bowel disease, colorectal carcinoma, or diverticulitis. The barium enema is helpful in ruling out an organic etiology. The treatment of irritable bowel syndrome is supportive; one strives for dietary changes including the addition of bran and other bulking agents. Drug therapy is directed toward resistant symptoms and consists of antispasmodics, tranquilizers, antidepressants, and calcium-channel blockers. Patients benefit from a stress-relief program, and underlying depression should be treated.

Inflammatory bowel disease of the colon or rectum may be due to either ulcerative colitis or Crohn's disease.[34] A problem may result from an inflammation of the bowel, obstruction, perforation, fissure, or abscess formation. Symptoms include bloating, abdominal distention, constipation, and incomplete evacuation. Ulcerative colitis is confined to the colonic mucosa and most commonly involves the rectum. Patients may also present with weight loss and mucous discharge as well as other symptoms associated with the disease. Diagnosis is made by sigmoidoscopy even of the unprepared bowel, which will show a friable surface and the presence of pseudopolyps. The risk of colon and rectal cancer is significant in these patients over time; ulcerative colitis is usually treated with a combination of steroids, oral or rectal, and nonsteroidal preparations—5-amino salicylic acid. Crohn's disease, in contrast, involves the full thickness of the bowel and may appear anywhere along the gastrointestinal tract from the mouth of the anus. Symptoms include intermittent or cramping pain and fever. Crohn's disease commonly involves the terminal ileum (41 percent) and small bowel or colon (29 and 27 percent, respectively). The condition is diagnosed by barium enema, upper GI series, and CT scanning. The treatment of Crohn's disease includes the use of anti-inflammatory and immunosuppressive agents as well as azathioprine. Immunosuppressive agents such as methotrexate, cyclosporine, and metronidazole have been used with success.

MYOFASCIAL PAIN AND THE CONCEPT OF TRIGGER POINTS

Fibromyalgia, or myofascial pain syndrome, is usually associated with widespread muscle or joint pain, and affects multiple sites in the body. It may present as a steady, aching discomfort often associated with fatigue, insomnia, or symptoms of chronic pain syndrome. There are no specific diagnostic or laboratory tests that make the diagnosis; however, on clinical examination one finds tender areas in the muscles and their supporting structures that have been defined as "trigger points." It is suspected that the mechanism involved in the trigger point may be caused by stress-induced ischemia causing either muscular or vascular spasm. At times, a trigger point can

develop after trauma or may develop as the result of pain in a distant site. The lower back is the most common source of myofascial pain, and is frequently encountered by the gynecologist. This is best treated by counseling, stress reduction, improved physical fitness, and local therapy such as the application of hot or cold packs, massage, or a TENS unit. Some patients improve following dry needling of the trigger point site or injection with local anesthetics, corticoids, or saline. Likewise, treatment of insomnia with drugs such as Elavil or Restoril may improve the management of the overall syndrome.[35]

ATYPICAL ENDOMETRIOSIS

Endometriosis may present with infertility, sacral pain during menstruation, progressive dysmenorrhea, or progressive deep dyspareunia. Atypical disease can present with the same symptoms or may present with vague interior thigh pain that may or may not be related to menstruation. It should be recalled that the interior thigh lies in dermatomes L2 and L3, and sensory nerves of the interior thigh pass under the peritoneum on the sidewalls lateral to the uterosacral ligaments. Compression of these nerve roots by fixation of the ovaries or implants to the pelvic sidewall induce pain. Often, the interior thigh pain is unilateral and frequently involves the left leg, which should increase one's suspicion of endometriosis. Obviously, one must rule out inguinal hernia or, more commonly, femoral hernia in women. The second most common presentation of atypical endometriosis is cyclic dysuria either with or without hematuria. These patients will have had a history of vague suprapubic pain, and they have been treated multiple times with antibiotics for supposed urinary infections; however, on careful questioning, neither a urinalysis nor microscopic examination was performed prior to treatment and no bacteria were noted when examination was carried out. At times, white or red blood cells may be present, and these patients may have a negative cystoscopic examination. Virtually always when these patients undergo diagnostic laparoscopy, endometriosis will be found on the bladder flap, and at times accumulation of endometriosis seen several cm in diameter involving the uterine fundus and the bladder reflection.

Another common presentation of endometriosis involves cyclic pain with defecation with or without melena. These dyschezias can be associated with diarrhea, constipation, or both, as endometriosis implants are not representative of classic endometrium but mixed as of glandular-like and stromal tissue, and thus produce different mixtures of F2 and E2 prostanoids. These types of lesions may be atypical or classic, and care should be taken to look between the rectum and the most posterior aspect of the uterosacral ligament to identify them. Further, when carrying out laparoscopy, care should be taken to aspirate all of the peritoneal fluid that is present so that a very clear image can be obtained of the entire cul-de-sac. It should be recalled that atypical endometriosis does not present with white stellate scarring, powder burn lesions, or blue dome cysts. Atypical disease will be distributed primarily in the cul-de-sac, on the ovaries, with lesions found on the bladder, appendix, or small or large bowel. Further, atypical endometriosis may be found on the anterior abdominal wall, above the pelvic brim, on round ligaments, in the inguinal canal, in abdominal incisions, in vaginal incisions including episiotomy, posterior colpotomy, and on the diaphragm. Atypical endometriosis presents with a variety of subtle patterns, and biopsy is always advisable. Disorders such as psammoma bodies, cancers, or endosalpingitis may masquerade as atypical endometriosis (Fig 24–3). The endometriosis may present as a hypervascular pattern, a small bleb that is either red, white, clear, yellow, or orange in color. These lesions may be interspersed over hypervascular areas, and there may be subtle enfoldings of the peritoneum accompanied by yellow discoloration or hypervascularity. There may be pockets in the peritoneum in which the ovary may rest or be entirely engulfed. It should also be recalled that minimal disease may be seen

at the peritoneal surface; however, the studies of Donnez and Koninckx have demonstrated extensive invasion of tracks of endometriosis that can result in nerve entrapment or compression. Endometriosis, as described elsewhere in this text, can be treated medically with a drug such as norethindrone acetate or GnRH analogs, or with endoscopic or open abdominal surgery. Therefore, care should be taken in exercising a surgical option, particularly in the younger patient, as this may exacerbate the chronic pelvic pain syndrome secondary to scarring.[36–40]

CHRONIC PELVIC PAIN SYNDROME

Failure to adequately diagnose and treat the patient with pelvic pain frequently leads to the development of chronic pain syndrome. These individuals present taking multiple medications; they have undergone multiple surgical procedures; they show signs of drug dependence, depression, inappropriate affect, and inappropriate limitation of activity; and they will invariably have been seen by a large number of physicians. These patients may have a history of eating disorders, stringent appetite control, or gorging, and generally problems with insomnia. These patients have a marginal pain tolerance and have adopted the sick role. At times, this is reinforced by

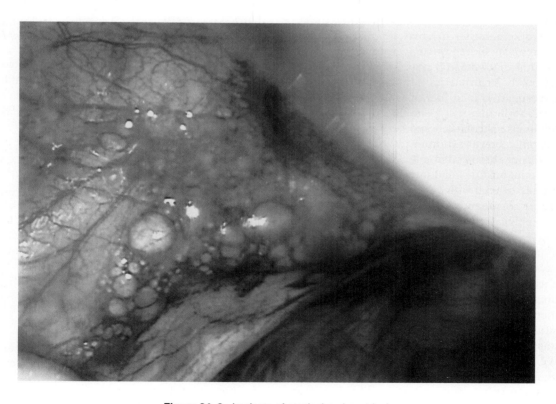

Figure 24–3. Implants of atypical endometriosis.

friends and family as well as the medical system, and patients derive positive reinforcement and sometimes secondary gain from these experiences. The best approach with these patients is a careful history and physical examination and meticulous review of previous tests. If the evaluation is appropriate and no evidence of serious disease is indicated, little is to be gained by further diagnostics. However, it should be emphasized that the work-up of these patients, however difficult, should be thorough and if need be, extensive. Once a diagnosis is established, sedative, hypnotic, and narcotic treatment should be withdrawn, even if inpatient detoxification is necessary. The patients may be treated with tricyclic antidepressants such as amitriptyline to facilitate sleep. Both the patient and her family should be involved in psychological counseling, and she should be enrolled in a pain management program. An exercise program and adequate diet should be prescribed as well. Physical therapy and transdermal electrical stimulation may also be used as an adjunct therapy. The ultimate goal of this form of therapy is to eliminate the sick role and restore the patient to both psychological and physical function. This may or may not involve resolution of the pain, but assists the patient in placing it in proper perspective.[41,42]

SUMMARY

Chronic pelvic pain is frequently encountered by the reproductive endocrinologist, and may be emitted from a variety of systems including urinary, gastrointestinal, gynecologic, and musculoskeletal systems. Visceral pain by its nature is poorly localized and often referred, and the object of investigation is to identify the likely cause of pain, determine whether it is treatable and if so by what means, and educate the patient and her family about the problem. Irritable bowel syndrome is one of the most common causes of chronic abdominal pain, and presents with constipation, bloating, and intermittent pain. It may or may not be associated with endometriosis involving either the large or small bowel. Interstitial cystitis is a common cause of pelvic pain involving the urinary system; it is associated with frequency, urgency, and abdominal, genital, or pelvic pain. Likewise, pain of the musculoskeletal system often presents as fibromyalgia with its respective trigger points. These patients suffer from fatigue, insomnia, and chronic pain. Individuals with atypical endometriosis may present with interior thigh pain, cyclic painful defecation or urination, and painful intercourse. Almost all of the patients afflicted with these disorders will experience either major or minor depression, and it is not uncommon for these individuals to enter the state of a chronic pelvic pain syndrome. This results in individuals' taking multiple medications, being subjected

to multiple surgical procedures, often developing drug dependence and an inappropriate affect, inappropriately limiting activity, and becoming chronically debilitated. It is the goal in treating all of these disorders to return patients to reasonably normal life functions and avoid introducing iatrogenic components to their pain.

REFERENCES

1. Bonica JJ. General considerations of chronic pain. In Bonica JJ, ed. *The Management of Pain*. Philadelphia, Lea & Febiger, 1990: 180
2. Kavaliers M. Evolutionary and comparative aspects of nociception. *Brain Res Bull*. 21:923, 1988
3. Merskey DM, Bond MR, Bonica JJ, et al. Classification of chronic pain for the Study of Pain Subcommittee. *Pain Suppl*. 12:S1, 1986
4. Willis WD Jr. The pain system: The neural basis of nociceptive transmission in the mammalian nervous system. In: Edenberg P, ed. *Pain and Headache*. Basel, Karger, 1985: 8
5. Yaksh TL, Bailey J, Roddy DR, et al. Peripheral release of substance P from primary afferents. In: Dubner R, Gebhart GF, Bond MR, eds. Proceedings of the Fifth World Congress on Pain. Amsterdam, Elsevier, 1988: 3
6. Foreman RD. Spinal substrates of visceral pain. In: Yaksh TL, ed. *Spinal Afferent Processing*. New York, Plenum Press, 1986: 217-242
7. Dubner R, Bennett GJ. Spinal and trigeminal mechanisms of nociception. *Annu Rev Neurosci*. 6:381, 1983
8. LaMotte CC. Organization of dorsal horn neurotransmitter systems. In: Yaksh TL, ed. *Spinal Afferent Processing*. New York, Plenum Press, 1986: 97-116
9. LaMotte CC, Pert CB, Snyder SH. Opiate receptor binding in primate spinal cord: Distribution and changes after dorsal root section. *Brain Res*. 112:407, 1976
10. Yaksh TL, Hammond DL. Peripheral and central substrates involved in the rostrad transmission of nociceptive information. *Pain*. 13:1, 1982
11. Ruda MA, Bennett GJ, Dubner R. Neurochemistry and neural circuitry in the dorsal horn. *Prog Brain Res*. 66:219, 1986
12. Melzack R, Wall PD. Pain mechanisms: A new theory. *Science*. 150:971, 1978
13. Willis WD, Kenshalo DR Jr., Leonard RD. The cells of origin of the primate spinothalamic tract. *J Comp Neurol*. 188:543, 1979
14. Kevetter GA, Haber LH, Yesierski RP, et al. Cells of origin of the spinoreticular tract in the monkey. *J Comp Neurol*. 207:61, 1982
15. Hylden JL, Hayashi H, Bennett GJ. Lamina I spinomesencephalic neurons in the cat ascend via the dorsolateral funiculi. *Somatosens Res*. 4:31, 1986
16. Truex RC, Taylor JM, Smyth MQ, Goldenberg PL. The lateral cervical nucleus of the cat, dog, and man. *J Comp Neurol*. 139:93, 1970
17. Leffler CW. Prostanoids: Intrinsic modulators of cerebral circulation. *News Physiol Sci*. 12:71, 1997

18. Kaplan C, Lipkin M Jr., Gordon GH. Somatization in primary care: Patients with unexplained and vexing medical complaints. *J Gen Int Med.* 3:177, 1988

19. Katon W, Lin E, Von Korff M, et al. Somatization: A spectrum of severity. *Am J Psychiatry.* 148:34, 1991

20. Quill TE. Somatization: One of medicine's blind spots. *JAMA.* 254:3075, 1985

21. Brownlee HJ (ed). Symposium on management of acute nonspecific diarrhea. *Am J Med.* 88:1S, 1990

22. Johnason JF, Sonnenberg A, Kioch TR. Clinical epidemiology of chronic constipation. *J Clin Gastroenterol.* 11:525, 1989

23. Wald A, Hinds JPJ, Caruana BJ. Psychological and physiological characteristics of patients with severe idiopathic constipation. *Gastroenterology.* 97:932, 1989

24. Freidman G. Treatment of the irritable syndrome. *Gastroenterol Clin North Am.* 20:325, 1991

25. Klein KB. Controlled treatment trials in the irritable bowel syndrome. A critique. *Gastroenterology.* 94:232, 1988

26. Summitt L. *The Developing Human: Clinically Oriented Embryology,* 3rd ed. Philadelphia, W. B. Saunders, 1982: 280

27. Krishnan R, Khoury J, Marson L. Interstitial cystitis. *Mediguide to Urology.* 9: 3, 1996

28. Domingue GJ, Ghoniem GM, Bost KL, et al. Dormant microbes in interstitial cystitis. *J Urol.* 153:1321, 1995

29. Koziol JA, Clark DC, Gittes RF, et al. The natural history of interstitial cystitis: A survey of 374 patients. *J Urol.* 149:465, 1993

30. Hanno PM, Levin RM, Monson FC, et al. Diagnosis of interstitial cystitis. *J Urol.* 143:278, 1990

31. Rapkin AJ, Mayer EA. Gastroenterologic causes of chronic pelvic pain. *Obstet Gynecol Clin North Am.* 20:663, 1993

32. Moriarty KJ. ABC of colorectal diseases. The irritable bowel syndrome. *Br Med J.* 304:1166, 1992

33. Thompson WG. Irritable bowel syndrome. Pathogenesis and management. *Lancet.* 341:1569, 1993

34. Hanauer SB. Inflammatory bowel disease. *N Engl J Med.* 334:841, 1996

35. Goldenberg DL. Fibromyalgia syndrome: An emerging but controversial condition. *JAMA.* 257:2782, 1987

36. Konnickx PR, Meuleman C, Oosterlynck D, Cornillie FJ. Diagnosis of deep endometriosis by clinical examination during menstruation and plasma CA-125 concentration. *Fertil Steril.* 65:280, 1996

37. Spuijroek MDEH, Dunselman GAJ, Menheere PPCA, Evers JLH. Early endometriosis invades the extracellular matrix. *Fertil Steril.* 58:929, 1992

38. Koninckx PR, Martin DC. Deep endometriosis: A consequence of infiltration or retraction or possibly adenomyosis externa? *Fertil Steril.* 48:924, 1992

39. Donnez J, Nisolle M, Somes P, et al. Peritoneal endometriosis and "endometriotic" nodules of the rectovaginal septum are two different entities. *Fertil Steril.* 66:361, 1996

40. Murphy AA, Green WR, Bobbie D, et al. Unexpected endometriosis documented by scanning electron microscopy in visually normal peritoneum. *Fertil Steril.* 46:522, 1986

41. Merskey DM, Bond MR, Bonica JJ, et al. Classification of chronic pain for the Study of Pain Subcommittee. *Pain Suppl.* 13:51, 1986

42. Turk DC, Rudy TE. A cognitive-behavioral perspective on chronic pain: Beyond the scalpel and syringe. In: Tollison CD, ed. *Handbook of Chronic Pain Management.* Baltimore, Williams & Wilkins, 1989

Chapter 25

CLINICAL TRIALS FOR THE REPRODUCTIVE ENDOCRINOLOGIST: DESIGN, POWER ANALYSIS, AND BIOSTATISTICS

Dale W. Stovall and David S. Guzick

In order to practice evidence-based medicine, clinicians must have access to data that provide sufficient information about the efficacy of clinical interventions. With regard to evidence on medical and surgical therapies, a hierarchy of the quality of data has been established. The poorest quality comes from case reports. Better evidence comes from well-designed observational and retrospective analyses, while properly designed randomized clinical trials yield the best quality of evidence of efficacy.

A randomized clinical trial is a prospective comparative study with an intervention group and a control group that utilizes a method of assignment of participants such that all participants are equally likely to be assigned to either the intervention or control group. Randomized clinical trials are accepted as the standard by which investigators can best evaluate the efficacy, efficiency, and effectiveness of clinical therapies. Although a properly planned and executed clinical trial is a powerful experimental tool, the development and completion of a clinical trial often requires significant time, effort, and monies as well as collaboration and cooperation from a mixture of statisticians, epidemiologists, and clinical scientists.

The evolution of the clinical trial dates back beyond the 18th century.[1] During the twentieth century, substantial advancements in the design of clinical trials were introduced by several investigators. Most of the early foundations for the design of controlled experiments were established in the agricultural field. R.A. Fisher is credited with introducing the principle of randomization to clinical trials,[2] and J.B. Amberson's manuscript, published in 1931, regarding the use of sanocrysin in pulmonary tuberculosis was the first to introduce the concept of blindness in clinical trials.[3] In that same decade, H.S. Diehl was the first to use the term placebo in reference to a saline solution given to participants of a trial evaluating the efficacy of a cold vaccine.[4] It was not until the early 1950s that the need for a control group in clinical trials was widely accepted.[5] In 1964, clinical trials received unequivocal federal support in the form of legislation requiring the Food and Drug Administration (FDA) to obtain proof of efficacy before approving any new drug for the U.S. market. This decision came on the heels of the reports that thalidomide was responsible for producing phocomelia in infants of exposed mothers in Europe.[6] The irony of this turn of events is that the FDA does not currently require clinical trials of new drugs to include pregnant women, and therefore, if thalidomide were developed today, it could very well gain FDA approval without any knowledge of its teratogenic effects.

Recently, there has been some concern that women have been underrepresented in clinical trials. One example is in the evaluation of the effects of aspirin on the risk of myocardial infarction.[7] Some progress has been made in this specific area with an ongoing trial in women.[8] Furthermore, there are now requirements stating that minority populations be included in appropriate numbers in clinical trials.[9]

Few randomized clinical trials were reported in the infertility literature until the 1980s. Of those reported, many lacked sufficient statistical power because of small samples. Although multicenter trials would address this problem, funding for multicenter trials remains limited. The need for clinical trials in reproductive medicine is urgent and long overdue. The purpose of this chapter is to review the phases of the clinical trial including its uses, development, design, execution, close-out, data analysis, and interpretation, and to discuss some of the ethical concerns surrounding the implementation of a clinical trial.

USES

Clinical trials have three primary uses. First, they can be used to evaluate the efficacy, efficiency, and effectiveness of pharmaceutical agents. For example, clinical trials may be used to assess the effectiveness of a new contraceptive agent or the efficacy of a new drug in the treatment of obesity. The FDA requirements for approval of new drug applications into the U.S. market has had a significant impact on the number of trials being conducted by pharmaceutical companies. Assisting in the conduct of these pharmaceutical trials are investigators in both the academic and private practice sector.

In addition to testing the efficacy of pharmacologic agents, clinical trials can be used to evaluate the therapeutic value of new technologies. Such trials might evaluate procedures performed in the laboratory, such as intracytoplasmic sperm injection (ICSI) or assisted hatching of embryos, or procedures performed in the operating room, such as endometrial ablation or metroplasty.

Finally, clinical trials can be used to evaluate the effectiveness of screening tests. In this regard, the clinical trial is designed to evaluate the sensitivity, specificity, and predictive value of a test at given cut points and to determine if the beneficial information provided by the test offsets its costs. These trials might be used to evaluate the use of serum androstenedione or Dehydroepiandrosterone sulfate levels in the evaluation of hirsutism, ultrasound in the evaluation of polycystic ovarian syndrome, and laparoscopy or the postcoital test in the evaluation of the infertile female.

Clinical trials do not seem appropriate or cost effective to evaluate small variations in a clinical procedure or to assess the impact of therapeutic agents on rare events. For example, if a previously approved drug is made available as a depot form, and the depot form has been shown to have acceptable bioavailability, a new clinical trial evaluating the depot formulation is not warranted. Likewise, the effects of pharmaceutical agents on rare events such as the effect of human menopausal gonadotropins on the incidence of ovarian cancer should be evaluated by case-control studies instead of clinical trials. Once an unproven pharmaceutical agent or procedure

has become part of accepted clinical practice, carrying out a clinical trial is made more difficult.

DESIGN

The ideal clinical trial is one that is randomized, double-blinded, and placebo controlled. The design is the key to the clinical trial. The basic components of a clinical trial are outlined in Table 25–1.

Developing a Hypothesis

The planning of a clinical trial depends on the development of a testable hypothesis. The hypothesis should be clearly defined and stated as specifically as possible before the trial is designed. The hypothesis should contain the primary question the investigator(s) is interested in answering. The investigator may wish to evaluate changes in severity of a disease or functional changes in various biologic parameters. Usually, the study hypothesis states that no difference in outcome exists between two given therapies (ie, the null hypothesis). For example, in patients with chronic anovulation, treatment with compound A at daily dose X is no better at reducing hirsutism over a 6-mo period than treatment with compound B at daily dose Y. The clinical trial is designed to determine whether or not the null hypothesis can be rejected. When selecting a hypothesis, the investigator must take several issues into account: Has the question been sufficiently addressed by other investigators? Does the question have significant clinical importance and interest, and are the results of the trial likely to change clinical management? Can the response to therapy be precisely and reliably measured? Given the resources available, can the trial be completed in a reasonable time at a finite cost? And finally, is the trial ethical?

Besides the primary question(s) to be addressed by the trial there may also be several secondary hypotheses to be addressed. For example, in a trial evaluating ablation of endometriosis, one primary question might be whether a subject's morbidity is altered after therapy. A secondary question might address the incidence of

---

TABLE 25–1. COMPONENTS OF A CLINICAL TRIAL

Central research hypothesis
Concurrent comparison of interventions
Placebo control
Blinding
Randomized allocation of interventions
Homogeneous study population
Power analysis
Clearly defined and measurable outcome events
Analysis method(s) defined before data collection

cause-specific morbidity from anesthesia, abdominal incisions, and injury to intra-abdominal organs. Secondary hypothesis may address the analysis of certain subgroups. In the endometriosis example, the investigator may want to determine if the stage of the disease alters outcome. Whenever subgroup analyses are to be performed they should be specified before the trial is begun. The same is not the case in regards to the assessment of adverse events.

Choosing a Baseline State

During the development of the hypothesis, the investigator takes the first step in selecting a study population, which is to identify a group of patients with an important therapeutic need. The subjects that will actually be included in the clinical trial are further defined by a set of eligibility and exclusion criteria that constitute the admission criteria. A set of clearly defined admission criteria needs to be established to avoid the enrollment of ineligible participants. The eligibility criteria are used to define the disease state to be studied. The eligibility criteria as well as the reason for the selection of each criterion should be precisely defined. For example, when studying a new therapy for the treatment of unexplained infertility, it is important to define what history and diagnostic tests will be used to identify patients with unexplained infertility. Furthermore, it should be specified when, with what instruments, how often, and by whom the tests are to be performed. With tests such as semen analyses that have more than one parameter, it should be determined whether a single abnormal parameter on one occasion is evidence of abnormality. It should be made clear whether or not inclusion is based upon previously measured parameters, measurements obtained during screening of participants, or on investigator judgment. An example of the latter might occur in a trial evaluating a new treatment for endometriosis-associated infertility. With regard to the diagnosis of endometriosis, one needs to specify whether or not all participants have biopsy-proven disease or if the diagnosis is based upon the surgeon's judgment that a participant has endometriosis. This approach is advantageous because of its simplicity and cost savings, yet not all of the scientific community may agree with this definition.

The eligibility criteria not only defines the disease to be studied; it also attempts to select participants who will benefit from the study and who have a high probability of having the hypothesized result. For example, in a trial of postmenopausal estrogen replacement for the prevention of heart disease, choosing a high-rate group, such as women with previous myocardial infarction, will reduce the number of subjects needed to detect an effect. Commonly, an investigator uses what is known about the mechanism of action of a new intervention to select which participants have the greatest potential to benefit from therapy. For example, women with a history of thromboembolic disease with menopausal symptoms are appropriate to enroll in a study of a new selective estrogen receptor modulator that has been demonstrated to act as an agonist in the brain and bone but as an antagonist in the liver and uterus. If the mechanism of action of a new drug is unknown, or if it has more than one potential mechanism of action, it may be difficult to select a specific group of participants that is most likely to respond to the new therapy.

Once the eligibility criteria have been selected, the exclusion criteria are defined. The exclusion criteria contain those criteria but for which a participant would have been eligible. One common example is an age restriction. When age restrictions are used, it should be made clear when the age limit applies. For example, in a trial on assisted reproduction therapy in which 41 is used as an exclusionary age, it should be made clear whether a patient is eligible who is 40 on the day of screening but will be 41 before the day of oocyte retrieval. Exclusionary criteria are often used to eliminate participants at high risk for a particular adverse event. In a trial involving a new oral contraceptive or hormone replacement therapy, a history of a deep venous thrombosis might be used as an exclusion criteria. In this case, the investigator should define how the thrombosis is to be diagnosed. Is the participant's history sufficient or is documentation from one or more diagnostic tests required. Often, these decisions are based on the severity of the adverse event. Exclusion criteria are also used to exclude subjects that have medical conditions that might obscure the assessment of the outcome of interest. For example, in a trial on a new therapy in the treatment of endometriosis-associated pelvic pain, women with a history of gastrointestinal diseases that may cause pelvic pain, such as Crohn's disease, might be excluded from enrollment, as their intestinal disease might preclude the assessment of their response to the therapy being investigated. Pregnancy is often used as an exclusion criteria. Whether or not pregnant women should be excluded from drug trials in which pregnancy is not the focus of the intervention is controversial.[10]

In the development of the ideal admission criteria, one must maintain an appropriate balance between practicality and fastidiousness. On the one hand, it is desirable for the criteria to allow enrollment of a *heterogeneous* population of patients. This has three major advantages. First, recruitment will benefit. By including a heterogeneous population of patients one will increase the percentage of subjects screened that are eligible for the study, making the performance of the study more feasible. Second, if a heterogeneous population is studied, the results of the study will be more likely to be generalizable to a broader population of patients with the disease.

Furthermore, studying a diverse population provides a greater opportunity to evaluate the effectiveness of the intervention in several subgroups or stages of a disease. On the other hand, however, enrollment of a *homogeneous* study group has its advantages. Strict admission criteria simplify the conduct of the study and sharpen the statistical precision of the results. Moreover, if the study population is too diverse, a less susceptible study group may be selected, diluting the effect and decreasing the probability of finding a significant benefit. Clearly, there are instances when selecting a homogeneous study population is not feasible because the technology to do so is not available. Examples would include clinical trials evaluating the treatment of a new therapy for premenstrual syndrome or pelvic pain. In this case, the mechanism(s) that cause premenstrual syndrome and pelvic pain are often unclear, making it difficult to identify a homogeneous population based on the etiology of the disease.

Issues regarding homogeneity and heterogeneity of study populations extend beyond the influences of the admission criteria. There is some evidence to suggest that subjects who agree to sign an informed consent to participate in a study are different from those who do not volunteer.[11,12] Volunteers tend to be healthier and are more likely to be compliant with the study protocol. The influence of these observations on those who participate in clinical trials and how to account for these influences is still unclear. By no means should this undermine the importance of selecting the baseline state, as one cannot claim that a therapy is or is not effective unless one can clearly define the population in which the intervention was tested. This level of detail not only allows the reader to identify which patients in his or her practice are appropriate for therapy, but also allows other investigators to analyze the appropriateness of the study and to perform confirmatory trials if necessary. In general, the admission criteria should exclude those individuals who are not likely to benefit from the therapy, might be harmed by the therapy, and/or are not likely to comply with the study protocol. A qualification period should be considered before the treatment(s) are imposed to demonstrate that the admission criteria have been fulfilled. Exclusion criteria only apply to subjects who have not been enrolled in the trial. If a participant that has been enrolled in a trial develops a condition that would have excluded him or her from enrollment, the participant may be removed from the trial but should be included in the final analysis of the trial. Table 25–2 includes a brief checklist of the important components of the admission criteria.

Selection of Interventions and Comparisons

As the natural history of most diseases is still unclear and because a broad variability of individual responses to medical intervention is common, the need for a defined control or comparison group can rarely be disputed. The choice of the comparative treatment depends on whether the comparison is intended to show the treatment's efficacy, efficiency, or effectiveness.[13] If a clinical trial is to evaluate a new therapy's efficacy (ie, whether it is better than nothing), the appropriate comparison is against a placebo.

There has been considerable debate regarding the ethics of using placebos in clinical trials.[14] Placebo-controlled trials can best be supported under two specific conditions.[15] First, there should be no standard intervention that is clearly superior to placebo. If such a standard therapy does exist, it could be used in combination with the new intervention and placebo. Second, the informed consent for participation in the clinical trial should clearly state that the participant may receive a placebo and what the chances are of receiving either the placebo or alternative.

If a trial is to determine a new treatment's efficiency, the decision that the treatment works better than a previously proven standard therapy, the comparison is against the standard therapy. In this case the new therapy would be used as an alternative to the previously proven therapy.

Finally, a trial may be developed to determine a new therapy's effectiveness. Effectiveness refers to the impact of a therapeutic agent on a population and is not necessarily the result of a comparison. Although a new therapy may be proven to be efficacious or efficient, it may be ineffective if it is so expensive, uncomfortable to administer, or inconvenient to take that patients refuse to use it. A new therapy may also be ineffective if participants are simply not motivated to sustain its use. If a new therapy is to be used as a supplement, then the combination of the new and existing treatment should be compared to the existing treatment alone.

When selecting an intervention for investigation, the investigator must consider several issues. First, the intervention's potential for benefit should be maximized while keeping adverse events to a minimum. In the case of a new hormone replacement regimen, this would mean determining the best dose, route, and frequency of

---

TABLE 25–2. CHECKLIST FOR ADMISSION CRITERIA

Eligibility Criteria
Define the basic disease process
Select the most susceptible participants
Select participants with a high event rate
Select participants most likely to adhere to the protocol

Exclusion Criteria Address
Subjects with competing disease processes
Subjects with insufficient prognostic susceptibility
Subjects with a high risk of therapeutic vulnerability
The presence of confounding therapies
Referral bias

administration. Second, the intervention should be standardized and made stable over the course of the trial so that variations in the intervention will not affect the outcome(s). This is especially true when new procedures are being tested and when multicenter trials are being performed. Furthermore, the duration of intervention needs to be determined. This may be impacted by potential side effects of the therapy, such as the problems with loss of bone density found with gonadotropin-releasing hormone agonist therapy or with the length of time needed to obtain the outcome of interest such as in infertility therapies. The investigator must also determine if multiple drug doses are to be evaluated. If a procedure or new device is being evaluated, the investigator must determine who will perform the procedure or will operate the device. The total number and types of treatments to be evaluated should be kept to a minimum, as increasing the number of treatment arms will decrease the feasibility of the study.

Allocation of Treatments

Randomization. Historical control studies compare a group of participants on a new therapy or intervention with a previous group of participants on standard or control therapy. Clinical trials compare a group of participants being administered a new therapy to a group of participants who are concurrently being administered a standard or control therapy. Although there is little debate that concurrent controls are the most appropriate with regard to drug evaluation, there is still some controversy and debate regarding the evaluation of new procedures and devices.[16]

The preferred method of assigning participants to intervention and control groups is by randomization. Randomization is a process of assignment that gives each participant the same chance of being assigned to either the intervention or control group. Normally, study participants are not chosen for participation in a study in a random manner. However, once an individual has decided to participate in a clinical trial, placement into the control or treatment group should be a random event. Although sometimes used as a randomization surrogate, an alternating assignment of participants to the intervention and control groups is not a form of randomization. The two most common mechanisms from which randomized assignments are obtained are from a random digit table and a computer-generated random-number algorithm. Randomized treatment allocations have several advantages.[17] First, randomization tends to create comparable study groups. If participants are assigned to two study groups by chance, the distribution of both known and unknown prognostic variables will tend to be evenly balanced between the two groups. This is probably more important for unknown prognostic variables as the distribution of known prognostic variables can be evaluated and con-

trolled for when the data is analyzed. In large studies involving several hundred or more participants, the chance that randomization will fail to achieve a balance of prognostic factors is negligible; however, small clinical trials involving less than 100 subjects are much more likely to contain an unbalanced distribution of prognostic factors.[18] Another advantage of a randomized allocation schedule is the potential for the removal of allocation bias. If participants are randomly assigned, neither the participant nor the investigator can influence the choice of intervention. For example, in a trial evaluating the efficacy of preoperative therapy with a gonadotropin-releasing hormone agonist in the treatment of leiomyoma-associated anemia, if referring physicians would only refer their patients with large leiomyomas to the study if they would be guaranteed allocation of the agonist, the allocation would be biased. Again, neither the participant nor the investigator should know what the intervention assignment will be before the participant's decision to enter the study. Otherwise, the potential for bias will not be affected by the randomization procedure. The third, and probably most often overlooked advantage of a randomized allocation schedule is for the validation of statistical tests.[19] The validity of statistical tests (eg, chi-square test and Student's *t*-test) can be justified on the basis of randomization alone. Otherwise, further assumptions regarding the comparability of the study groups must be established to validate these statistical comparisons. If this is not done, the P values obtained may not be valid.

Randomization protocols can be either equal or proportional. In an equal randomization schedule, the allocations are constrained so that the same numbers of subjects are assigned to each of the maneuvers under investigation. Proportional assignments are used to create an unbalanced, yet proportional, assignment of the comparative agents. For example, a randomization schedule may be arranged so that two thirds of subjects receive a new hormone therapy for oligospermia, and one third of the subjects receive a placebo. There are two potential advantages to this 2:1 intervention-to-control allocation schedule. First, more information regarding participant responses to the new intervention, such as adverse events, will be gained. Second, if the therapy was found to be beneficial, more subjects will have benefited from the new therapy. Of course, the therapy may be found to be nonefficacious. Allocations proportionally can be tilted toward the control group. If a new intervention is expensive or believed to have a significant chance for one or more toxic side effects, a 1:2 or 1:3 intervention to control allocation could be selected. The disadvantages of any proportional allocation schedule are substantial. Most importantly, proportional allocations are less sensitive and have less statistical power as compared to equal allocation methods,[20] and a proportional allocation schedule may suggest a bias for or against a new intervention, especially in the eyes of the referring physician.

Besides simply randomizing participants into different study groups, participants can be randomized by blocks or strata.[21–23] One disadvantage to a simple stratification procedure is that at any one time during the study, and potentially at the end of the study, a significant imbalance in the number of participants in each group may exist. For example, in a trial of 20 participants, with a simple stratification method, there is a 50 percent chance that at the end of the study there will be a 12:8 unbalanced distribution of participants or worse. The advantage of a blocked randomization is that balance between the number of participants in each group is assured during the course of the study. An example of a blocked randomization would be in the assignment of 100 participants to a new therapy (T) for premenstrual syndrome and to a placebo (P). A schedule could be devised so that participants are randomized in 25 blocks each with 4 assignments. In this example there are 6 different combinations of group assignments (eg, TTPP, TPTP, etc). In this example, one of the 6 assignments is selected at random for the purpose of group assignment and this is repeated 25 times until all participants have been randomized.

In contrast, a stratified randomization schedule is used to randomized participants not over time but with regard to one or more prognostic characteristics. Stratification will help to evenly distribute prognostic variables that are strongly associated. If only one prognostic factor is used, it is divided into several subgroups or strata. Otherwise, more than one prognostic factor can be used. For example, in a study comparing two different ovarian stimulation protocols, one might want to stratify subjects based upon their cycle day 3 FSH level (eg, 0 to 10 mIU/ml, 11 to 20 mIU/ml, $\geq$ 21 mIU/ml) and smoking history (never smoker, ever smoker, current smoker). When two or more variables are used the total number of strata is the product of the number of subgroups in each factor; therefore, the number of prognostic factors should be kept to a minimum. In this example, the total number of strata is 9. Once a subject has been placed in one of the nine strata, she can then be randomized to receive one of the two stimulation protocols using either a simple or blocked stratification method. Using a blocked randomization method as opposed to a simple randomization method does have important statistical implications.[24] If the appropriate analysis is performed, a blocked randomization scheme will increase the power of the study. Stratified randomizations are usually reserved for smaller studies (eg, <100 participants). An alternative to stratifying participants at the time of randomization is to stratify participants during analysis. Evaluation by subgroups may help to elucidate the mechanism(s) of action of the intervention.

Crossover Designs. The crossover study design is a variation of the randomized clinical trial. In the beginning of a crossover study, each participant is randomly assigned to either the intervention or control group. After a defined period, the control group is "crossed over" and begins receiving treatment and vice versa with the treatment group. Both single and double crossover periods have been described, known as two-period and three-period cross-over studies, respectively. Crossover study designs have several advantages. First, because the measured effect of the intervention is the difference in an individual's response to intervention and control, the statistical variance is reduced. Therefore, fewer participants are required to detect a specific difference in response. Some evidence suggests that parallel study designs require as many as 2.5 to 3 times as many participants as three-period crossover designs.[25] This could result in significant cost savings especially in regards to recruitment. However, crossover designs have one significant disadvantage. To use a crossover design a very important assumption must be made; that is, the effects of the therapy in the first or second period must not carry-over to the second or third period. This carry-over effect can be avoided if a sufficiently long washout or no treatment period is used before crossing over. Washout periods lengthen the trial and therefore increase costs and reduce participant retention. Furthermore, outcome events may occur during the washout period, such as pregnancies in an infertility therapy trial, making the results difficult to interpret. A statistical test to assess period–treatment interaction has been described but it has limited power.[26] The most appropriate use for crossover study designs is in conditions that are not cured by therapy such as hyperprolactinemia, chronic anovulation and osteoporosis; otherwise, the participant cannot return to the initial state. Finally, crossover designs are only recommended if there is clear evidence that no carry-over effect exists.

Blinding the Study. Blinding refers to the process of concealing the identity of the assigned intervention. The principal function of blinding is to avoid problems of bias during data collection and analysis that might lead to false conclusions. A study is particularly susceptible if the response variables are subjective. There are three separate groups that can be blinded: the participants, the investigators and staff, and committees that monitor response variables or adverse events. In a double-blind study, both the participants and the investigators and staff are kept unaware of the identity of the intervention assignment. If participants are blinded, their reporting of symptoms and side effects are less likely to be biased. Participants' preconceived notions regarding a particular therapy or placebo might yield biased reporting of subjective outcome variables. Blinding participants can help prevent study withdrawal that occurs when participants learn they have been placed on what they think is an undesirable treatment arm. Blinding the investigators and staff can help prevent bias in both data collection and analysis and the unequal administration of concomitant non-study treatment that is likely to influence the outcome variables. For example, in a trial of hormone replacement therapy versus placebo in which quality-of-life parameters were being evaluated, if an investigator is not blinded to the intervention assignment he or she might tend to unequally prescribe concomitant hormonal therapy to the treatment group in cases of vaginal bleeding or other known side effects of hormone replacement therapy. Furthermore, if the investigator's bias is that hormone replacement therapy does improve the quality of life, he or she may subconsciously counsel the placebo group regarding lifestyle changes to improve their quality of life or vice versa if he or she wants the study results to be positive. To bias the outcome of a trial, concomitant therapy must be effective and it must be prescribed to a significant proportion of the participants.

In a single-blind study, only the participants are unaware of the identity of the intervention. These studies are easier to carry out. However, the preconceived ideas of the investigator may lead to bias in data collection and concomitant therapy. If a trial is not double-blind, the outcome of response variables should be assessed by investigators who are not involved in follow-up of the participants and are blinded to the treatment group. Some investigators prefer single-blind study designs as this design allows investigators to use their judgment to do what is best for a participant's health and safety should an adverse event occur. Some trials are very difficult to single or double blind. Unblinded or open studies are most commonly used when a medical therapy is compared against a surgical therapy or laparotomy is compared against laparoscopy. It is possible to design a blinded study comparing two surgical procedures if only the surgeon and not the investigator know the type of surgery being performed. Clearly, initiating and maintaining a blinded study design can be very difficult.[27] In pharmaceutical trials, if a drug has one or more identifying characteristics such as its shape, color, or taste, the blind can be broken.[28] In a study involving hormone replacement therapy, certain side effects, including telltale changes on mammography, may tip off the staff to the participants who are on study drug. Included in the protocol of any blinded trial should be the reason(s) why and the mechanisms for breaking the blind.

Choosing Outcome Events

Anything that happens after the initiation of therapy can be regarded as an outcome event, also called a response variable. Certain outcomes will be carefully chosen and will represent the specific focus of the study, such as the

primary and secondary outcome events, and these events should be clearly stated as such before the trial begins. Other outcomes may be unanticipated, yet may also be of critical importance to the conclusions or completion of the study. These outcomes are known as adverse events and are discussed in the next section. Because decisions regarding sample size will depend in large part on the primary outcome event, careful consideration should be made when choosing the outcome(s) that relate to the principal hypothesis of the study. It is important to have only objective, unambiguous response variables that are not too costly to measure and can be accurately measured. Ascertainment of all outcomes must be complete and honest. The investigator must be capable of measuring the primary response variable(s) in all study participants. By the same accord, all response variables must be measured by the same mechanism in all participants, and if possible, by the same investigator. In a study evaluating a new therapy in the treatment of luteal phase deficiency in a group of women with infertility, pregnancy rates would be a preferred outcome over correction of an abnormal endometrial biopsy, and delivery rates would be a preferred outcome over pregnancy rates.

In general, a single response variable should be chosen to answer the primary question. In some situations, combining response variables may be considered. For example, in a hormone replacement study involving women with cardiovascular disease, combined events might include death from coronary heart disease and nonfatal myocardial infarction. Here, both events measure a similar outcome, a cardiac event, so it may be acceptable to use this combined response variable if it is defined as such before the trial begins. When combined responses are used, only one response event is counted per participant. If a single or combined response variable cannot be chosen, the feasibility of conducting the trial should be reconsidered. Response variables are categorized as either continuous or noncontinuous, and may change from one noncontinuous variable (not pregnant) to another (pregnant) or from one noncontinuous variable (stage I endometriosis) to any one of a number of others (stage II or III endometriosis). Response variables may also change from one level of a continuous variable (eg, a serum estradiol level) to another. Both the type and quantity of the response variable has implications on the sample size. For example, if the primary response is continuous (eg, serum estradiol levels), change is easier to detect when the initial level is extreme.

Adverse Events

Any event or outcome that occurs after the beginning of the study can be categorized as desirable, undesirable, or neutral. Adverse events are the undesirable signs, symptoms, and clinical events that occur during the clinical trial. Unlike the events that define the primary and secondary outcome variables, adverse events are not always well defined or anticipated. The assessment and reporting of adverse events is important for development of the risk: benefit ratio that is considered when a new treatment is appraised. For example, if a new treatment is being compared against a known efficacious therapy and no difference in the primary outcome variable(s) is found between the two groups, the therapy of choice might be decided upon based on the frequency of adverse events. Before beginning a clinical trial, the investigator(s) should make a list of the adverse events that have been associated with the intervention and are clinically important. A clear definition of each event, based on history, physical examination, and laboratory criteria, should be denoted in the procedure manual. This allows the investigators to record important adverse events in a consistent manner. There is some controversy as to whether or not the investigator or staff should elicit specific adverse events from participants or if adverse events should be volunteered by participants.[29–31] We prefer a combination of these two approaches. A limited checklist of what are considered the most important adverse events should be reviewed with the participant, followed by a general question regarding any health-related problems encountered by the participant. This allows for accurate and consistent assessment of what are considered to be the most important adverse events. Another alternative is to use an event diary. The advantage of this technique is a potential reduction in recall bias. One clear disadvantage is the exorbitant amount of time required to review the diaries. No matter which technique is used, the frequency of each event in each participant during the duration of the trial should be recorded. Clear step-by-step instructions should be developed that define what evaluation, therapy, and follow-up will be performed for certain adverse events. An example would be in a clinical trial assessing hormone replacement therapy in which clear guidelines for vaginal bleeding would need to be developed. Several points should be considered when reporting adverse events. Besides reporting the frequency of specific events, it should be clear whether or not a particular adverse event was defined before the study, how the event was diagnosed, and whether or not its presence was elicited by the investigator or volunteered by the participant. The impact of the event should be reported: for example, whether it required hospitalization, surgery, additional medical therapy, discontinuation of the study drug, or a reduced drug dosage.

The Operations Manual

All large or complex clinical trials, especially multicenter trials, require the development of an operations manual.

TABLE 25–3. THE STUDY PROTOCOL

1. Title of the study
2. Specific aims
   a. Primary aim
   b. Secondary aims
3. Background and significance
4. Investigators
5. Experimental design and methods
   a. Study population
   b. Recruitment plan
   c. Schedule and description of visits
   d. Treatment regimen
   e. Randomization
   f. Blinding
   g. Compliance
   h. Adverse events
   i. Sample size calculations
6. Statistical analysis
7. Appendices
   a. Admission criteria
   b. Definition of outcome variables
   c. Definition of adverse events

Contained within the operations manual is a definitive description of all aspects of the trial including the study protocol. An example of the contents of a study protocol is given in Table 25–3. Besides the study protocol, the operations manual will contain the standard operating procedures, including protocol amendments, a timetable for initiation and completion of the trial, recruitment information, a description of clinical and laboratory procedures, protocols on early termination, protocols on how and when to inform participants about the identity of their study intervention, quality control procedures, algorithms for the evaluation and treatment of specific adverse events, and all clinical research forms. Research forms are developed to record the data that will be collected during the study. Forms need to be developed to record the results of the preliminary screening procedures, information from follow-up visits, concomitant therapies, and adverse events. The list of standard operating procedures will most likely grow as the study progresses and new clinical issues arise. Completion dates are especially helpful to inform both participants and co-investigators as to when the results of the study will become available.

The Budget

Making a budget for the clinical trial may be one of the most difficult duties for the investigator. It is helpful to use the resources available from the hospital or university, including personnel, when compiling a budget. A clinical trial contains numerous direct and indirect costs. Table 25–4 lists the potential costs of a clinical trial. As clinical trials involve screening procedures, there are

TABLE 25–4. THE STUDY BUDGET (COSTS)

1. Personnel
    a. Investigator(s)
    b. Study coordinator
    c. Recruitment staff
    d. Data entry staff
    e. Secretary or clerk
2. Equipment
    a. Mammography, ECG machine
    b. Centrifuge, autoclave, freezer
    c. Computer hardware/software
3. Supplies
    a. Clinical supplies for Pap smear, blood draws, endometrial biopsies
    b. Medications/placebos
    c. Postage/shipping of materials
4. Travel for investigators and staff for off-site training and national meeting
5. Other expenses
    a. Travel reimbursement for study participants
    b. Participant parking
    c. Recruitment mailings
    d. Recruitment advertising (newspaper, radio, television)
    e. Long distance phone calls
    f. Rent
6. Indirect costs

likely to be positive tests that require further follow-up or therapy. It should be clear in the consent form whether or not tests or procedures not included in the initial screening will be covered by the investigators or trial; this is usually not the case. An example would be a positive pap smear or mammogram that requires more than an annual follow-up.

Calculating the Sample Size (Power Analysis)

Analysis of the sample size needed for a trial is one of the most important and commonly overlooked components of the clinical trial. Several good reviews of the basic concepts used in sample size calculations are available.[32,33] Sample size calculations should be performed before any study is begun to address the feasibility of testing the null hypothesis. In other words, sample size calculations are important to assure that a clinical trial will have sufficient statistical power to detect differences between treatment and control groups that would be considered clinically important. Sample size calculations are based on the primary outcome defined in the null hypothesis. The admission criteria are also important in sample size calculations because these criteria define a specific baseline state with a specific, although not always known, therapeutic susceptibility. Regarding sample size calculations, it is desirable to study participants with a high probability of an anticipated outcome event. Of course, sample size calculations are only estimates of the true sample size required for a study, and therefore the inves-

tigator should considering being conservative and error on overestimating the sample size.

The components of a power analysis are listed in Table 25–5. A sample size is chosen that will adequately test the null hypothesis. When stating a null hypothesis, investigators generally state that no difference exists regarding the primary outcome between the two study groups. The study is then conducted to determine whether this hypothesis is true and should be accepted or is false and should be rejected. Because differences in outcomes can occur by chance alone, the investigator may falsely reject the null hypothesis when in fact it is true. When an investigator falsely rejects the null hypothesis he or she is said to have made a type I error. The probability that a type I error will occur is denoted by α and is called the significance level. On the other hand, if the investigator fails to find a difference between the outcome variable of interest when in fact a difference does exist, this is called a type II error. The probability of a type II error is denoted by β. The power of a study is a quantification of its ability to correctly reject the null hypothesis and is denoted by $1-\beta$. Traditionally, investigators have set α at 0.01 or 0.05, making the probability of a type I error low (1 to 5 percent). Investigators have accepted a greater probability for a type II error. For example, β is often set at 0.20, making the power of the study 80 percent.

The total sample size (control plus treatment group) is a function of α, β, and the effect size. The effect size is the difference in the primary outcome variable that the investigator would consider clinically important. With a fixed sample size, the power of a study is dependent on the size of the difference of the primary outcome, as shown in the power curve in Figure 25–1. As α and β are generally fixed at 0.05 and 0.20, the only variable needed to calculate the sample size is the effect size. Therefore, the investigator is forced to define what difference in outcomes he or she thinks would be considered successful treatment. For example, in a study of a fertility-enhancing procedure, does the intervention need to increase the chance for conception by 10 percent, 25 percent, 50 percent, or greater before it can be recommended for general use? As the magnitude of the difference in response is decreased, the sample size must increase at a given α and β. If the calculated sample size is larger than can be realistically obtained, then one of

TABLE 25–5. COMPONENTS OF A POWER ANALYSIS

Significance level or probability of a type I error (α)
Probability of a type II error (β)
Power ($1-\beta$)
Effect size
Sample size
One-sided versus two-sided hypothesis
Variable type (categorical versus continuous)

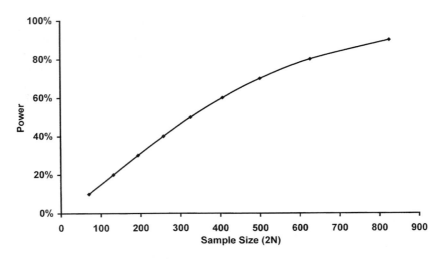

Figure 25–1. Power curve for increasing sample size with baseline pregnancy rate 20 percent, effect size 50 percent, and α = 0.05.

the parameters could be modified. For example, one may relax α if a therapy is being tested that has no side effects and is inexpensive but may provide benefit for an illness with significant morbidity and cost. In this scenario, it would be unfortunate to discard such a therapy without further consideration because a type II error was made. However, if no compromise in α, β, or the effect size can be agreed upon, and the sample size is still unattainable, serious consideration should be given to abandoning the trial.

Once an α, β, and effect size have been chosen, power can be calculated from standard tables once three additional pieces of information are known.[34,35] First, the investigator must categorize the outcome variables as categorical (dichotomous), such as pregnant or not pregnant; or continuous, such as mean serum androgen levels, as power calculations are different for different types of variables. Second, it must be determined if the treatment allocation method will result in an equal or unequal proportion of participants in each group. If the variability in the responses for the two groups is approximately the same, equal allocation of interventions will provide a more powerful design. If the variability in the treatment groups is significantly different, an uneven allocation may be more powerful. Third, the investigator must decide if he or she is interested in differences that are in one direction only—a one-sided test—or if differences in either direction are important—a two-sided test. In general, a two-sided test is recommended, unless it is clear that the only changes to be expected are in one direction. In other words, it is clear that a given therapy can only be better and not worse than another. If a one-sided test is used, in most circumstances the significance level should be reduced by one half of what would have been used for a two-sided test. Both methods require the same documentation to declare a treatment effec-

tive. This methodology in effect provides two one-sided (eg, 0.025) hypothesis tests, for an overall 0.05 significance level.

UNIQUE CLINICAL TRIAL DESIGNS

Pharmaceutical Trials

The first step in the development of a new drug comes in preclinical studies performed in an animal model, in vitro, or both. After basic safety and bioavailability information are obtained, clinical trials are initiated. Pharmaceutical clinical trials are divided into three or four phases. Phase I studies are designed to determine the metabolic and pharmacologic actions of a new drug and to determine how well the drug is tolerated.[36] Phase I studies are not true clinical trials in that the proposed intervention is not compared against a control. In contrast, during phase I trials a relatively small group of participants, often in groups of three, are administered a drug in a step-up manner to determine the pharmacologic actions and maximally tolerated dose (MTD) of the drug. Usually, the MTD is the dosage at which approximately one third of the participants experience significant toxicity.

If the phase I study reveals that a new drug is sufficiently well tolerated, a phase II study can be initiated. Phase II studies involve small numbers of participants and are designed to evaluate the adverse events of a new drug and to provide preliminary evidence of efficacy.[37] Phase II studies often involve less than 50 participants, and therefore are usually not sufficient to obtain a precise estimate of the true percentage of patients who would respond to therapy (ie, the response rate). Furthermore, the eligibility criteria of phase II trials are often more restrictive than phase III trials and the primary outcome(s) of a phase II trial may be more short-term oriented as compared to those used in phase III trials.

Phase III studies are true clinical trials performed to evaluate the effectiveness and safety of a new pharmacologic agent and thus determine its role in clinical practice. Phase III studies usually include several hundred to several thousand subjects and can precisely estimate the true response rate to a given therapy. There are some shortcomings of the phase III trial. Their size makes both cost and quality control significant problems, especially since they are almost always multicenter trials and may involve as many as 80 different centers. In addition to the problems associated with their size, phase III studies are often designed with short follow-up intervals. This is particularly problematic when evaluating treatments in chronic disease states such as endometriosis. For this reason, trials with long-term follow-up, known as phase IV studies, are sometimes performed in subjects with chronic illnesses. Phase IV studies do not include a control group.

Surgical Trials

The reproductive endocrinology literature contains few appropriately conducted clinical trials evaluating new surgical procedures or instruments. The difficulty in the timing of the performance of a clinical trial that evaluates a new surgical procedure may be one reason why. When deciding when to initiate a trial evaluating a new surgical procedure, one must consider the evolution of the procedure. Enough time must have passed since the introduction of the new technique to allow for its optimization before it is appropriate to conduct a trial. On the other hand, if one waits too long, a new procedure may become an integrated part of general medical practice, and the opportunity to conduct a new study may no longer exist because of a loss of clinical equipoise. The medical community may be unwilling to refer patients for randomization once a bias towards the benefit(s) of a procedure has been established. If this occurs, a clinical trial with sufficient power might never be conducted to determine if a given procedure is better than any other therapy or if only a selected group of patients will benefit from the procedure. Furthermore, if various methods of performing a procedure exist, the best method may never be established.

Surgical trials have specific outcomes of interest. Which outcomes are the most important depends on one's perspective. Outcomes that are most important to the surgeon might not be as important to the patient, third party payor, or an employer. Because of the expense of surgical procedures and new surgical instruments, cost is commonly one of the primary outcomes of interest. There are many costs associated with any surgical procedure and calculating these costs can be laborious. Surgical procedures

harbor both direct and indirect costs. The direct costs include the surgeon's fee, the anesthesiologist's fee, operating room costs, the cost of a hospital room, laboratory fees, the cost of postoperative pain control, and the cost of the surgical instruments. The cost of surgical instruments can be calculated from two perspectives, the cost to the hospital and the cost (price) to the consumer. Thus, when performing a cost analysis, one must differentiate between the cost of acquisition of materials and the cost to the patient. The indirect costs of surgical procedures include the cost of time off work, which may be difficult to measure; and the cost of diagnosing and treating complications from the procedure. Besides costs, another outcome of particular interest in surgical trials is patient satisfaction and the effects on a surgical procedure on the patient's quality of life. One recent article utilized a patient satisfaction scale to evaluate the differences in satisfaction between patients undergoing either endometrial ablation or hysterectomy.[38] A patient's satisfaction with a procedure may include the procedure's impact on the patient's physical, psychological, and social functioning.[39] Additionally, the procedure may influence the patient's personal productivity, pain perception, sexual functioning, and sleep habits.

There are several potential risks for bias in surgical trials. Like other clinical trials, the study population may be affected by the selective referral of the most difficult surgical cases and the participants may be self-selected based upon their beliefs. Unlike some pharmaceutical trials, it is especially difficult to blind surgical trials. It is possible to design a study in which the surgeon performing the procedure is the only one that knows the type of surgical procedure, but neither the participant nor the study investigators do. However, this is not possible when a laparoscopic procedure is being compared to a laparotomy procedure, or when either of these two procedures is being compared to a hysteroscopic or other transvaginal procedure. Therefore, it is especially important to use objective outcomes, such as delivery rates, whenever possible. Still, the selection of objective outcomes will not alleviate the bias that occurs with regard to the level of skill of the surgeon. For example, if several surgeons are performing the procedures in a trial comparing laparoscopic fimbrioplasty to fimbrioplasty via laparotomy, if the laparoscopic skills of one of the surgeons is particularly good or poor, the results of the trial may be positively or negatively biased toward laparoscopy. Further, if there are only a small number of surgeons participating in a trial, the skill of one surgeon will have an even greater impact on the outcome. One way to overcome this problem is to randomize patients to a few selected surgeons who only perform one of the two procedures being evaluated and who do not assess the outcome variables. Failing to blind a surgical trial will tend to decrease the effect seen, not unlike failing to randomize participants tends to increase the effect seen.[40]

Multicenter Trials

As discussed in the section on sample size, studies evaluating infrequent events and those attempting to detect small differences between study groups require large sample sizes. Recruitment of the necessary number of participants (eg, hundreds to several thousand) within an acceptable length of time by a single center would not be possible; therefore, multicenter trials were developed. A multicenter trial is a collaborative trial in which several university and/or non-university based investigators contribute subjects to a common protocol.[41] Besides making a large trial feasible, multicenter trials have several other advantages. First, multicenter trials enable numerous investigators with similar interests to work together to answer a particularly difficult or important clinical question. Second, recruitment of participants from several geographic areas allows for evaluation of a study population that may be more representative of the general population, making the results of the trial more generalizable. The multicenter study design has been used in several recently completed and ongoing studies in women's health, including the PEPI study, the HERS study, and the WHI.

Developing a multicenter trial requires the establishment of an organizing group. Members of the organizing group may be primarily investigators from academic institutions but may also be from governmental agencies or private industry. The organizing group has the task to organize and oversee all phases of the trial including whether or not a particular trial is worth pursuing, the timeliness of the trial, the feasibility of the study, planning of the study, sample size analysis, cost of the trial, participant follow-up, and data analysis. Occasionally, a pilot study is needed to answer some of these questions. The organizing group will select at least some of the clinical centers that will participate in the trial. Out of these centers, a coordinating center will be selected. The coordinating center will help with the design, management, and analysis of the trial, including implementation of the randomization process, evaluation of data quality from the various clinical centers, and the day-to-day running of the trial. Therefore, the coordinating center must have particular expertise in clinical, epidemiologic, and biostatistical issues, and must be readily accessible and free of any overriding interest in the outcome of the trial. Once the coordinating center and some of the clinical centers have been selected, the final work on the organizational structure, including establishing lines of authority and the final protocol, may begin.

A steering committee, made up of a subset of investigators in the trial, is developed to oversee development of the protocol and study forms, approve all scientific publications, select members of subcommittees, and make final decisions regarding safety issues. Some multicenter trials will elect an executive committee from the members of the steering committee. The executive committee may help set the agenda for the steering committee by setting the priorities of the trial and make quick operational decisions when necessary. A data-monitoring committee, independent of the investigators and the study sponsor, is charged with periodic monitoring of response-variable data, and assessment of intervention toxicity and center performance.[42] Subcommittees are often developed to carry out numerous important functions including patient recruitment, quality control, publication functions, and protocol adherence. Furthermore, specialized centers may need to be selected to prepare medications and perform specialized laboratory assays. During the initial meeting of the investigators, the final and usually most difficult protocol decisions are made. All investigators must agree to follow a common protocol. To expedite some of these decisions, a small group of investigators may be assembled with particular expertise in a given area. Continued communication between the coordinating center and the clinical centers is important through all stages of the trial. Because of the complexity of a multicenter trial, successful monitoring of the trial can be difficult.[43,44] Periodic meetings of the steering committee and the investigators are necessary to maintain the quality of the data and address problems that arise. Training workshops are useful for the investigators and clinical coordinators of multicenter studies and can significantly improve the quality of a clinical trial. Finally, issues regarding publications, presentations, and authorship should be addressed before the trial is begun. A diagram of the structure of a hypothetical, two-site trial is presented in Figure 25–2.

CONDUCTING THE CLINICAL TRIAL

Recruitment

A common mistake in clinical trials is the underestimation of the time and effort needed to recruit participants. The investigator must ensure that an adequate amount of time, funds, and energy will be appropriated to the recruitment of participants. A well thought-out plan for recruitment is essential. Obtaining the institutional review board's approval of the study is part of the planning process. Several recruitment strategies should be devised,[45] and the necessary staff, facilities, and equipment for recruitment and screening of participants needs to be secured. An experienced and organized coordinator in charge of recruitment is helpful.

There are several recruitment strategies available. No one strategy will work in all geographic locations, and some strategies may not work in any geographic lo-

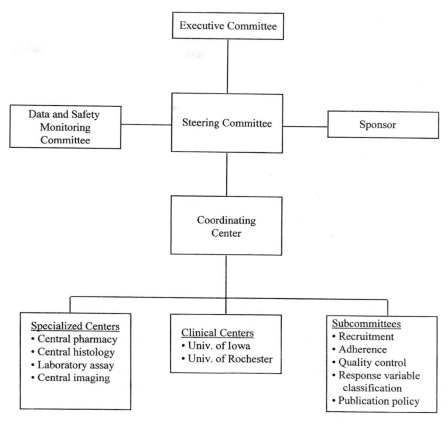

Figure 25–2. Example of the administrative structure in a multicenter trial.

cation. The success of recruitment will depend on the recruitment strategies used, the prevalence of the disease being studied, the study design, the admission criteria, and the population base of the clinical center. No matter what recruitment strategy is used, potential participants should undergo a screening evaluation, in person or by phone, before the baseline assessment is initiated to eliminate participants who do not meet the admission criteria. Most clinical trials in reproductive endocrinology require a community-based screening program. One way to identify eligible study participants is by reviewing office records. Once eligible participants are identified, the appropriate channels should be followed before subjects are contacted. Another recruitment strategy is to advertise the study through various media including mass mailings, various newspapers, and radio and television stations. All advertisements must be approved through the institutional review board. A combination of approaches will tend to yield the best results. Records should be kept of recruiting activities, including which activities yield the most participants for a given cost. Regular meetings should be held to keep the investigators and staff up to date on how recruitment is progressing. A timetable for recruitment of all partici-

pants should be set, as well as short-term (monthly) recruitment goals.

Problems that may occur in recruitment include inadequate funding for the screening process, unwillingness of physicians to refer patients,[46,47] overestimation of the prevalence of the disease, and strenuous requirements of the admission criteria.[48] When recruitment lags there are several possible solutions. First, if the trial is a multicenter study, investigators can solicit solutions from centers that have had success with their recruitment strategies. Second, depending on costs, the length of recruitment can be extended. This might be particularly attractive if recruitment was initiated during a holiday season, when recruitment might be expected to lag. Another idea is to determine if there were potential participants who failed their screening process because of self-limiting problems, such as a washout period that was not completed or lack of transportation for a given period of time. These participants could be given a second opportunity to be screened. Attention to detail is important during the recruitment phase in order to avoid enrolling ineligible patients. When recruitment lags, the investigator and staff should avoid any temptation to begin to loosely interpret or alter the inclusion criteria. Changes in the admission criteria are appropriate only after a thorough analysis has determined that the design of the study will not suffer. Recently, the U.S. Congress has directed the National Institutes of Health to establish guidelines for the recruitment and inclusion of women and minorities in clinical research.[49]

Executing the Study

Once participants pass the initial screening evaluation, a baseline assessment is performed. Depending on the admission criteria, the baseline assessment may measure variables by history, physical examination, blood tests, tissue samples, and imaging studies. Because of cost concerns, only factors that are pertinent to the study and admission criteria should be evaluated. One prerequisite for inclusion into a study is the participant's willingness to comply with the study protocol. For example, in a study that requires an endometrial biopsy be performed at the baseline visit and at additional follow-up visits, a participant who does not tolerate the baseline endometrial biopsy may not be a good candidate for the study. Occasionally, when evaluating continuous variables such as prolactin levels, the serum level obtained in an office setting may have met the inclusion criteria but the evaluation at the baseline visit, with no interim therapy, may not meet the inclusion criteria. This is particularly problematic when the inclusion criteria include an extreme cut-point, such as >150 ng/ml in this example. One possible reason for this occurrence is that successive samples of continuous variables tend to yield values that are closer to the mean of the population. This is known as regression toward the mean.[50] This problem can be decreased by using a higher cut-point in the screening visit or using a mean of two or three samples during the screening visit. The later technique may not be cost effective or tolerable depending on the variable being evaluated. With either technique, to assure that the baseline data reflect the true condition of the participants, some time limit should be set for the interval between the baseline evaluation and the allocation of interventions.

Monitoring and maintaining participant compliance to the study protocol is critical to the success of the study. Usually, minimal compliance guidelines are established. For example, in studies involving pharmaceutical agents a 90 percent minimum compliance rate per individual may be reasonable. If the compliance rate is as low as 80 percent, a significant increase in the sample size (≥50 percent) may be necessary to maintain the power of the study.[51] Study protocols that are short and contain simple (eg, single-dose) interventions yield higher compliance rates.[52,53] Better-informed participants and those with a higher level of education are more likely to comply with the study protocol.[54,55] Further, participant compliance is improved if participants think their health will be improved by the intervention.[56] Therefore, it is important

for the staff to stay in close contact with study participants, especially after randomization, and to spend time answering participants' questions and reminding them of upcoming visits, and making each clinic visit a pleasant experience by decreasing waiting times and increasing the accessibility of the clinic. In trials that include elderly participants, involving family and friends can help improve compliance. Pill dispensers help keep track of medications taken.[57] Monitoring compliance can be difficult. Frequent follow-up visits can ease the task of compliance monitoring. In pharmaceutical trials, pill counts and diaries can be useful in monitoring compliance. In a study of insulin administration for the treatment of diabetes mellitus, assessment of hemoglobin A1c levels could be useful to assess compliance. Both noncompliance and losses to follow-up need to be monitored. Noncompliance is the better of these two evils, as one still has the data and may be able to adjust one's analysis appropriately. Usually with losses to follow-up, information bias is lost to the treatment arm at a greater rate than the control arm.

Proper execution of the study is required to maintain data quality and therefore reduce bias. Special attention should be given to controlling the quality of the assessment and recording of important information such as baseline characteristics and outcome measures. To help maintain high-quality data, all investigators and staff should be well versed in the study protocol and have a clear understanding of how all variables are defined and assessed. The operations manual should be constantly updated, made available to all staff, and consulted anytime their is a question regarding the definition or assessment of any variable. Maintaining the quality of data includes assessing all variables in a similar manner in all participants, consistently and completely filling out all data forms, properly labeling tissue specimens, asking questions in a consistent manner, calibrating instruments on a regularly scheduled basis, and using technology instead of technicians to assess variables whenever possible. Histology slides should be evaluated by a single pathologist if possible. Imaging procedures should be assessed by a single radiologist. Whenever possible, repetitive measures should be performed. For example, in a study using ultrasonography to evaluate the endometrial effects of a new hormone replacement regimen, the mean of three endometrial stripe measurements should be used for analysis instead of the results from a single measurement. Data forms should be easy to follow and complete and be devoid of any essay-type questions.[58,59] During the study, data forms should be reviewed for completeness. Extreme values, such as an FSH of 0.5 mIU/ml or an estradiol of 3000 pg/ml, should be checked. Finally, computers and data-entry programs should be used to assess data quality when available.

During the execution phase of the trial, an ongoing statistical evaluation of the differences in response variables between the intervention groups is important to determine if early termination of the trial is necessary in cases of unanticipated toxicity, greater-than-expected benefit, or high likelihood of indifferent results. If any of these suspicions are confirmed, the trial may be terminated before its scheduled completion. It is preferred that this analysis be performed by a person or group who has no formal involvement with the participants or the investigators,[60] but who has experience in clinical trials, epidemiology, and statistical analysis.[61,62] There is no best formula to determine how often the data should be reevaluated. One possibility is to use discrete intervals of time (eg, every other month); another possibility is to re-analyze the data when a given percentage of the total number of participants has received therapy (eg, 20 percent, 40 percent, 60 percent).[63] Repetitive testing is not without its problems. For example, if one reevaluates the data 100 times, 5 of these evaluations, on average, will show a significant difference based on chance alone if a 0.05 level of significance is used. More specifically, if a hypothesis is tested twice, first when half of the data is known and again at the end of the trial, the probability of a type I error increases from 5 percent to 8 percent.[64]

The solution to this problem is to adjust the critical value used in each analysis so that the overall probability of a type I error remains at the level desired. One method that is commonly used to monitor the accumulating data in a clinical trial is known as the group sequential method.[65,66] In this procedure, the number of repeat analyses that will be performed is specified before the trial is begun, and the analysis is performed only with equal numbers of participants or after an equal number of events have occurred between analyses. In a multi-center trial, monitoring committees may not be able to meet at prespecified intervals, making this method less useful for multicenter trials. Another method known as a flexible group sequential procedure does not require an equal number of participants or events to have occurred between analyses or a pre-specified number of analyses.[67] Comparisons of life-table analysis curves, means, proportions, and linear regression slopes, as well as linear and nonlinear random effects models for continuous data and repeated measure methods for discrete data; can be monitored using the group sequential approach.[68–72] Computer programs are available for statistical calculations using these various procedures.[73] Confidence intervals can also be used to monitor data using the group sequential approach.[74] Before deciding to terminate a trial early, several factors must be evaluated, including the distribution of prognostic factors, data quality of all intervention groups, consistency of results across subgroups, presence of concomitant therapy, and whether or not randomization errors have occurred. A trial should not be terminated without definitively resolving whether or not the intervention effects are harmful. Otherwise, an intervention may continue to be used in practice although its harmful effects were deemed significant enough to terminate a clinical trial.

Closing Out the Study

The close-out of a clinical trial begins with the last follow-up visit of the first participant randomized, and ends with the archiving of study material. During the close-out phase of the trial, every effort is made to assure that the final data regarding the outcome variables are as complete as possible. This process involves both verification of incomplete data and assessment of missing data when possible. All efforts should focus on obtaining data in regards to the primary outcome(s) of interest. To minimize the delay in the final data analysis, a reasonable time is allotted for data clean-up before the data are locked. Most clinical trials close out participants after a defined period of follow-up per participant. Other trials follow all participants to a preselected month or year, during which the close-out process is completed in all participants. Depending on the size of the study and the close-out interval the latter method may not be feasible. After the data is finalized, it should be stored in an easily retrievable form. The investigator may have to choose if all biologic specimens and seemingly less important data not directly related to the outcomes of interest should be stored. Archiving of data will allow investigators and other interested groups to audit the results of the trial and may be important for future meta-analysis.

Several additional points are important to consider at the conclusion of a clinical trial. First, when should the participants be told which intervention they received? Second, how does the investigator advise the participant regarding future therapy? Third, should a participant wish to continue therapy, how will treatment and follow-up be performed? Fourth, how will the results of the study be disseminated to referring physicians and other health care providers? And finally, is a poststudy follow-up warranted for ascertainment of additional data?

The investigator has several obligations during the close-out phase of the study. One of these obligations is to inform each participant which intervention she received. As soon as all of the data from an individual have been collected, the participant can be unblinded. In some studies, to determine if the study was truly blinded, participants and study coordinators may be asked, before being unblinded, if they can guess which intervention they had received. Participants should be advised regarding future therapy at close-out. This may be difficult, as the final results of the study may not be known for many months or longer. In any case, the participant needs to be referred to a local physician for continued medical care. Both participants and referring physicians may have to be contacted at a later date when the results of the study are known. It is best if participants and referring physicians can be informed of the study results before the data are made public.[75] The NIH has issued guidelines for informing the public and physicians regarding the benefit or harm of therapies of significant importance to public health.[76] In the case of a trial that is investigating a new drug or device, specific regulatory agencies may need to be informed of the study conclusions.

Because the actions and mechanisms of action of a new therapy are rarely understood and because the beneficial or adverse effects of an intervention may last long after the intervention has been discontinued, some investigators have designed follow-up visits to evaluate poststudy events. The optimal interval of the poststudy follow-up depends on the intervention under investigation and the outcomes of interest. In a trial involving hormone replacement therapy, if a positive cardiovascular effect was obtained, an investigator may want to determine if the cardiovascular benefit continues for a period of 5 or 10 yr after therapy has been discontinued. In the same trial, women with vaginal bleeding or other adverse events could be followed to determine how long these events persist or if other adverse events, such as breast disease, occur 1 or 2 yr after discontinuation of therapy. Poststudy follow-up has been used to determine whether participants changed their lifestyles based on results from a clinical trial or if participants comply with the therapeutic recommendations given to them by the study coordinator or investigator.[77,78] Clearly, it may be very difficult to maintain contact with participants over an extended period, making poststudy follow-up complex and expensive.

ANALYSIS

Analysis and interpretation of data collected during a clinical trial is affected by decisions made during the development of the protocol, the performance and modification of the protocol during the trial, the compliance of study participants, and the quality of the data.[79] In addition to the outcomes of interest, several other parameters must be evaluated. Included are the admission eligibility, evaluation for randomization, participant compliance, and placebo response. Follow-up of control groups allows investigators to learn about the natural history of a disease. Just as the hypotheses to be tested are stated a priori, so are the statistical tests that will be used to evaluate these hypotheses. Otherwise, numerous statistical tests may be performed on the data, increasing the probability of a type I error, and falsely concluding that a difference

in outcomes exists. Stated another way, data analysis should be used for formal hypothesis testing and not as a method to determine how one can manipulate the data so that a significant difference can be found.[80]

The first question to be answered in the data analysis is which participants and which events will be included in the analyses. An investigator may want to exclude participants who dropped out of the study, were noncompliant with their intervention, took competing interventions, or had incomplete data. A policy regarding withdrawal of participants should be stated in the study protocol before initiation of the study. Any withdrawals should be done early in the study, preferably before any outcome(s) have occurred. Participants should never be excluded from analysis based upon their outcome status, as this will tend to bias the study.[81] In general, an "intention to treat" analysis is recommended for all clinical trials. In other words, all participants who were randomized to an intervention should be included in the initial analysis. The reason for adopting this strategy is that the reason a participant may have dropped out of a study or been noncompliant with therapy may be related to the adverse effects or complexity of the intervention. This type of analysis will give the investigator a better understanding of the impact an intervention will have on the population—its effectiveness. Likewise, all events should be included in the initial analysis. One might argue that including noncompliant participants in the analysis will not allow the investigator to evaluate the true efficacy of an intervention. For this reason, it is also recommended that the data be analyzed without including participants who were determined to be noncompliant based on a pretrial definition of noncompliance.

No matter how good of an effort is made to have participants come in for all follow-up visits, subjects may be lost to follow-up, yielding missing data. The participants lost to follow-up in one group may be very different in terms of their prognosis or susceptibility to therapy as compared to the subjects lost to follow-up in the comparison group. Life-table analysis, which assumes that losses to follow-up are random, can be used to assess differences in dichotomous response variables, such as pregnant or not pregnant, in situations in which the length of follow-up is variable.[82–84] Many methods for imputation of missing values have been described. Included are the method of end-point analysis or carrying the last observation forward.[85] Others use the derivation of a regression equation that is used for the basis of the input of missing data.[86] One potential problem with these methods of imputation of missing data is that each model assumes that the reason for missing data is simply a random event.[87] In any case, if more than one method is used to assess outcomes in cases of missing data, the results of all analyses should be presented.

Even if randomization is used in a trial, all of the baseline prognostic factors may not be perfectly balanced. If this is the case and if the baseline variables are highly correlated with outcome, the analysis may require that the data are adjusted for this imbalance. If stratification was used in the randomization, the analysis should be stratified. The type of adjustment used depends on the type of baseline variable being adjusted and the type of outcome variables being analyzed. If the baseline variables are not discrete (see definition below), these variables can be redefined into strata and made discrete. If the outcome variable is discrete, then a Mantel–Haenszel statistic can be used.[88] If the outcome variable is continuous (see definition below) and there is a linear relationship between the two variables, then the stratified analysis is called an analysis of covariance.[89,90]

If the overall comparison between the intervention and the outcome(s) is significant for beneficial or harmful effects, then the investigator may want to determine which subgroup of participants is most susceptible to therapy.[91] Subgroup analysis is only appropriate if the subgroups were specified in the study protocol.[92] Only baseline variables are used to define subgroups; outcome variables should never be used to define subgroups. In a subgroup analysis, the investigator is only concerned about intervention and control comparisons within one or more subgroups. Because of reductions in sample size per group, the probability of finding a significant difference is reduced. Post hoc analysis of subgroups that are not predefined but are suggested by the data, have less credibility. This type of retrospective subgroup analysis should be used to generate new hypotheses for future study.

BIOSTATISTICAL METHODS

The decision as to which statistical test to use to assess differences between two or more groups of participants depends upon several factors. First, the type of variable being evaluated must be categorized. Variables are either discrete (ie, categorical) or continuous. Discrete variables are intrinsically "gappy," in the sense that between two potentially attainable values lies at least one unattainable value. The simplest example in reproductive endocrinology is in counting the number of pregnancies after a given therapy. One can have 1, 2, 3, or more pregnancies but 2.5 pregnancies is impossible. On the other hand, if a variable can take potentially any value within a range, it is called a continuous variable. Examples of continuous variables include mean serum blood levels, height, and body temperature. In addition to defining the type of variable under investigation, several assumptions must be accepted before the appropriate statistical test is selected. Certain assumptions involve how the data were

collected, while other assumptions involve the distribution of the data. Appropriate questions about a set of data would include, are the treatment groups a random sample of the population, are the study groups independent, were the interventions randomly assigned, are the variances of the study groups equal, and are the distributions of the variable of interest normal? If these assumptions are not considered, the wrong statistical test may be applied. Tests are available to evaluate most of these assumptions. Furthermore, data can be transformed so that one might work with a variable's logarithm instead of its original value.

In general terms, statistical tests can be categorized into parametric and nonparametric tests. Parametric tests are used when the distribution of the data is known, or can be assumed to be, normal. Nonparametric tests are distribution-free methods of hypothesis testing. Nonparametric tests are much easier to calculate but are often less sensitive and lack statistical power as compared to parametric tests. In general, when the appropriate assumptions are met, if the variables being evaluated are both discrete, a chi-square test should be performed. If one variable is discrete and one is continuous, either a Student's t-test or analysis of variance is appropriate. If both variables are continuous, either a correlation or regression analysis is appropriate. An annotated list follows of some of the most commonly used statistical tests in reproductive endocrinology.

Statistical Tests

The **chi-square (χ^2) test** is used to evaluate associations between two variables. It is particularly useful for noncontinuous co-variates such as proportions. A χ^2 test is not appropriate if any expected frequency is less than one or if over 20 percent of the expected frequencies are less than five. The χ^2 test is not normally distributed and therefore is a nonparametric test. The exact distribution of χ^2 depends on the number of degrees of freedom.

The **Fisher's exact test** is one form of "correction" of the χ^2 test, and can be used with small sample sizes when expected frequencies are less than one. Another example of a correction of the χ^2 test is **Yates-corrected χ^2 statistic.**

The **Mantel–Haenszel statistic** has a χ^2 distribution with one degree of freedom.[93] This test is used for co-variates that are noncontinuous or for continuous co-variates that have been classified into intervals, such as age. Any value for the Mantel–Haenszel statistic greater than 3.84 is significant at the 0.05 level.

The **Student's t-test,** discovered by W. S. Gosset, is used to evaluate group mean differences in continuous variables (eg, the differences in mean androgen levels before and after treatment with an oral contraceptive). As described earlier, this design has the advantage of controlling for many extraneous sources of variation in the data. The T distribution is normal.

Both the **Wilcoxon signed rank test** and the **Spearman's rank correlation** are examples of nonparametric tests. The Wilcoxon signed rank test is used to compare mean differences for paired data while the Spearman's test is used when the assumptions for a parametric test cannot be met; however, one wishes to investigate the correlation between two random variables.

An **analysis of variance (ANOVA)** is used when one is comparing differences between three or more means. If a difference is found between the means, the investigator can then make comparisons between specific pairs or combinations of groups. **Multivariate analysis of variance (MANOVA)** is used when both multiple dependent variables as well as multiple independent variables are being evaluated. Conceptually, MANOVA is an extension of ANOVA.

Receiver operating curves (ROC) are used to assess differences between screening tests. The sensitivity of a test is plotted on the x axis against 1 − specificity on the y axis. Receiver operating curves are advantageous because they do not require the investigator to split continuous variables into two categories, for example, by an arbitrary cut-point, which must otherwise be done to assess sensitivity and specificity. The area under the curve or the equation of the lines can be used to assess differences between two ROC curves.

Life-table analysis is used in trials in which participants are entered into intervention over an extended period of time and followed after therapy for various lengths of time. This type of analysis could be used to evaluate pregnancy rates after myomectomy or metroplasty in infertile women as compared with pregnancy rates in participants who do not undergo surgical intervention. In this situation, participants may have varying intervals between surgery and pregnancy and may be lost to follow-up at various lengths of time. With life-table analysis, every month of follow-up can be used to calculate a cumulative pregnancy rate. Life-table analysis curves are generated for each intervention and comparisons can be made between two survival curves to determine if the pregnancy rates are significantly different. There are both parametric and nonparametric tests available to assess the significance of differences between life-table analysis curves. Regression models for the analysis of life-table data that allow for the variation of covariates over time are also available.[94]

Meta-analysis. When data from several clinical trials performed at different research centers, often over a period of several years, are pooled and analyzed together to answer one or more preselected questions, the overview is known as a **meta-analysis.**[95,96] Meta-analyses are performed to obtain sufficient power to detect small, yet clinically significant and generalizable, intervention effects.[97] Ideally, a meta-analysis should only be performed on randomized clinical trials that study the same type of participant, use precisely the same intervention, measure the same outcome variables, have similar lengths of follow-up, and have similar quality of data. One problem with meta-analysis is that some of the data regarding the question to be answered may not be available. A MEDLINE search may find only 30 to 60 percent of published trials.[98] Furthermore, trials that demonstrated a negative effect may not be available because of publication bias.[99] The results of a meta-analysis are usually summarized by calculating a relative risk or odds ratio with a 95 percent confidence interval. Both the relative risk and odds ratios are a product of the intervention success rate divided by the control success rate. A relative risk is calculated from prospective data and is a better estimate of the true risk than an odds ratio, which is inherently retrospective. The method used for calculation of the relative risk depends on whether or not the effects of therapy are similar (homogeneous) among trials or heterogeneous. If the effects are homogeneous then a Mantel–Haenszel method is appropriate; if the effects are found to be heterogeneous, a random effects model is used.[100]

Often, data are combined from several observational studies and are reported as a "meta-analysis." Such combined analyses suffer from the lack of reliability that flows from aggregating data across studies with widely varying entry criteria, methods of intervention, definitions of outcome variables, and methods of data management and analysis.

PRESENTATION AND PUBLICATION

A policy for presentation and publication should be agreed upon before initiation of the clinical trial. This may seem trivial and premature, but it can be extremely beneficial in the long run to clarify responsibilities and expectations. Each investigator has an obligation to critically review his or her study and its findings and to present sufficient information so that readers can properly evaluate the trial. Ideally, the manuscript should be completely prepared before the data are presented in a scientific setting, to decrease the delay between the presentation and publication of the data.[101] In any presentation or publication the hypotheses should be clearly stated, a clear but brief description of the randomization procedure should be included,[102] the selection of the study population should be clearly defined, and the methods used to assess the outcome variables should be described. All presentation and publications should state how the sample size was determined (eg, a sample size of

200 was required to detect a 25 percent relative increase in pregnancy rates after intervention, with a two-sided significance level of 5 percent and a power of 90 percent). The method(s) of analysis should be stated and the results of all analyses should be reported. Finally, the investigator should report all major outcome categories, such as total mortality, cause-specific mortality, and morbid events. This information will help other investigators assess the appropriateness of the methods and conclusions of the study.

ETHICS OF CLINICAL TRIALS

Questions regarding the participant's best interest surround most clinical trials. Ethical issues regarding clinical trials commonly center around the process of randomizing participants to interventions[103,104] and whether investigators are fully truthful when seeking informed consent. All investigators would agree that patients should receive the best therapy available, and that it is unethical to treat a patient with a therapy that is known to be inferior. Presumably, the reason a clinical trial is being conducted is because there is uncertainty about which therapy is best in regards to health benefits, adverse effects, and costs. Investigators should only recruit participants for a clinical trial if they believe that there is insufficient evidence to suggest that the intervention should be favored over a control. One could argue that clinical trials are a much more ethical method of approach to clinical problems than routinely prescribing medications or performing procedures that have never been proven to be beneficial and that might be harmful.

CONCLUSIONS

Designing and completing a clinical trial is a challenging undertaking. But, when appropriately performed, clinical trials allow one to compare the outcome in a treatment group to the outcome in a control group that is comparable to the treatment group in every way except for the treatment being studied. Clinical trials can also assist in determining the incidence of adverse events, cost implications of an intervention, and if the benefits of therapy outweigh the risks. The influence of the results of a clinical trial depend on the direction of the findings, the means used to disseminate the results, and any confirmatory evidence regarding the efficacy of the therapy in question. While well-designed clinical trials can provide sound rationale for the use of a given intervention, clinical trials that are poorly designed or executed can yield misleading data.

Well-run clinical trials with sufficient statistical power are costly and should be performed only after a given treatment has completely evolved and after preliminary data regarding efficacy looks promising. On the other hand, the consequences of delaying clinical trials can have a serious impact on health care as new procedures of unproven clinical benefit are allowed to become part of general medical practice.

Clinical trials do have limitations. Occasionally, the prevalence of a disease is so rare that a large enough population cannot be readily obtained, making a case-control study, not a clinical trial, the most appropriate method of evaluating the disease. Although a randomized trial could be developed to determine if cessation of an allegedly noxious agent, such as cigarette smoke, would prevent disease, one cannot ethically assign participants to begin using noxious agents. In the final analysis, no single study is definitive. Instead, each trial should be interpreted in regard to its consistency with known biologic and epidemiologic information.

REFERENCES

1. Lilienfeld AM. Ceteris paribus: The evolution of the clinical trial. *Bull Hist Med*. 56:1, 1982
2. Box JF. RA Fisher and the design of experiments, 1922–1926. *Am Stat*. 34:1, 1980
3. Amberson JB Jr, McMahon BT, Pinner M. A clinical trial of sanocrysin in pulmonary tuberculosis. *Am Rev Tuberc*. 24:401, 1931
4. Diehl HS, Baker AB, Cowan DW. Cold vaccines: An evaluation based on a controlled study. *JAMA*. 111:1168, 1938
5. Hill AB. Observation and experiment. *N Engl J Med*. 248:995, 1953
6. McBride WG. Thalidomide and congenital abnormalities. *Lancet*. 2:1358, 1961. Letter
7. Peto R, Gray R, Collins R, et al. A randomized trial of the effects of prophylactic daily aspirin among male British doctors. *Br Med J*. 296:320, 1988
8. Buring JE, Hennekens CH, for the Women's Health Study Research Group: The Women's Health Study: Rationale and background. *J Myocardial Ischemia*. 4:30, 1992
9. NIH Revitalization Act of 1993. Public Law 103–43.
10. Committee on the Ethical Issues Relating to the Inclusion of Women in Clinical Studies, Institute of Medicine. Mastroianni AC, Faden R, Federman D, eds. *Women and Health Research: Ethical and Legal Issues of Including Women in Clinical Studies*. Washington, DC, National Academy Press, 1994
11. Wilhelmsen L, Ljungberg S, Wedel H, Werko L. A comparison between participants and nonparticipants in a primary preventive trial. *J Chron Dis*. 29:331, 1976
12. Smith P, Arnesen H. Mortality in non-consenters in a post-myocardial infarction trial. *J Intern Med*. 228:253, 1990
13. Cochrane AL. *Effectiveness and Efficiency: Random Reflections on Health Services*. London, Nuffield Provincial Hospitals Trust, 1972

14. Bok S. The ethics of giving placebos. *Sci Am.* 231:17, 1974

15. Rothman KJ, Michels KB. The continuing unethical use of placebo controls. *N Engl J Med.* 331:394, 1994

16. Sapirstein W, Alpert S, Callahan TJ. The role of clinical trials in the Food and Drug Administration approval process for cardiovascular devices. *Circulation.* 89:1900, 1994

17. Byar DP, Simon RM, Friedewald WT, et al. Randomized clinical trials: perspectives on some recent ideas. *N Engl J Med.* 295:74, 1976

18. Lachin JM. Statistical properties of randomization in clinical trials. *Control Clin Trials.* 9:289, 1988

19. Armitage P. The role of randomization in clinical trials. *Stat Med.* 1:345, 1982

20. Brittain E, Schlesselman JJ. Optimal allocation for the comparison of proportions. *Biometrics.* 38:1003, 1982

21. Kalish LA, Begg CB. Treatment allocation methods in clinical trials: A review. *Stat Med.* 4:129, 1985

22. Lachin JM. Properties of simple randomization in clinical trials. *Control Clin Trials.* 9:312, 1988

23. Zelen M. The randomization and stratification of patients to clinical trials. *J Chronic Dis.* 27:365, 1974

24. Matts JP, Lachin JM. Properties of permutated-blocked randomization in clinical trials. *Control Clin Trials.* 9:327, 1988

25. Carriere KC. Crossover designs for clinical trials. *Stat Med.* 13:1063, 1994

26. Grizzle JE. The two period change-over design and its use in clinical trials. *Biometrics.* 21:467, 1965

27. Moscucci M, Byrne L, Weintraub M, Cox C. Blinding, unblinding, and the placebo effect: An analysis of patients' guesses of treatment assignment in a double-blind clinical trial. *Clin Pharmacol Ther.* 41:256, 1987

28. Farr BM, Gwaltney JM Jr. The problems of taste in placebo matching: An evaluation of zinc gluconate for the common cold. *J Chronic Dis.* 40:875, 1987

29. Avery CW, Ibelle BP, Allison B, Mandell N. Systematic errors in the evaluation of side effects. *Am J Psychiatry.* 123:875, 1967

30. Huskisson EC, Wojtulewski JA. Measurement of side effects of drugs. *Br Med J.* 2:698, 1974

31. Simpson RJ, Tiplady B, Skegg DCG. Event recording in a clinical trial of a new medicine. *Br Med J.* 280:1133, 1988

32. Lachin JM. Introduction to sample size determination and power analysis for clinical trials. *Control Clin Trials.* 2:93, 1981

33. Donner A. Approaches to sample size estimation in the design of clinical trials—A review. *Stat Med.* 3:199, 1984

34. Kraemer HC, Thiemann S. *How Many Subjects? Statistical Power Analysis in Research.* Newburgh Park, CA, Sage Publications, 1987

35. Brittain E, Schlesselman JJ. Optimal allocation for the comparison of proportions. *Biometrics.* 38:1003, 1982

36. Storer BE. Design and analysis of phase I clinical trials. *Biometrics.* 45:925, 1989

37. Chang MN, Therneau TM, Wieand HS, Cha SS. Designs for group sequential phase II clinical trials. *Biometrics.* 43:865, 1987

38. Sculpher MJ, Dwyer N, Byford S, Stirrat GM. Randomized trial comparing hysterectomy and transcervical endometrial resection: Effects on health related quality of life and costs two years after surgery. *Br J Obstet Gynecol.* 103:142, 1996

39. Berzon R, Hays RD, Shumaker SA. International use, application and performance of health-related quality of life instruments. *Qual Life Res.* 2:367, 1993

40. Miller JN, Colditz GA, Mosteller F. How study design affects outcomes in comparison of therapy. II. Surgical. *Stat Med.* 8:455, 1989

41. Meinert CL. *Clinical Trials: Design, Conduct and Analysis.* New York, Oxford University Press, 1986

42. Friedman L, DeMets DL. The data monitoring committee: How it operates and why. *IRB* 3:6, 1981

43. Fleming TR, DeMets DL. Monitoring of clinical trials: issues and recommendations. *Control Clin Trials.* 14:183, 1993

44. Cohen J. Clinical trial monitoring: Hit or miss? *Science.* 264:1534, 1994

45. Hunninghake DB. Summary conclusions. *Control Clin Trials.* 8:1S, 1987

46. Tognoni G, Alli C, Avanzini F, et al. Randomised clinical trials in general practice: Lessons from a failure. *Br Med J.* 303:969, 1991

47. Peto V, Coulter A, Bond A. Factors affecting general practitioners' recruitment of patients into a prospective study. *Fam Pract.* 10:207, 1993

48. Tilley BC, Shorck MA. Designing clinical trials of treatment for osteoporosis: Recruitment and follow-up. *Calcif Tissue Int.* 47:327, 1990

49. Freedman LS, Simon R, Foulkes MA, et al. Inclusion of women and minorities in clinical trials and the NIH Revitalization Act of 1993—The perspective of NIH clinical trial lists. *Control Clin Trials.* 16:277, 1995

50. James KE. Regression toward the mean in uncontrolled clinical studies. *Biometrics.* 29:121, 1973

51. Davis CE. Prerandomization compliance screening: A statistician's view. In: Shumaker SA, Schron EB, Ockene JK, eds. *Health Behavior Changes.* New York, Springer, 1990

52. Sackett DL, Snow JC. The magnitude of compliance and non-compliance. In: Hayes RB, Taylor DW, Sackett DL, eds. *Compliance in Health Care.* Baltimore, Johns Hopkins University Press, 1979

53. Pullar T, Kumar S, Feely M. Compliance in clinical trials. *Ann Rheum Dis.* 48:871, 1989

54. Shulman N, Cutter G, Daugherty R, et al. Correlates of attendance and compliance in the Hypertension Detection and Follow-up Program. *Control Clin Trials.* 3:13, 1982

55. Green LW. Educational strategies to improve compliance with therapeutic and preventive regimens: The recent evidence. In: Haynes RB, Taylor DW, Sackett DL, eds. *Compliance in Health Care.* Baltimore, Johns Hopkins University Press, 1979

56. Dunbar J. Predictors of patient adherence: Patient characteristics. In: Schumaker SA, Schron EB, Ockene JK, eds. *Health Behavior Changes.* New York, Springer, 1990

57. Moulding TS. The unrealized potential of the medication monitor. *Clin Pharmacol Ther.* 25:131, 1979

58. Knatterud GL, Forman SA, Canner PL. Design of data forms. *Control Clin Trials.* 4:429, 1983

59. Wright P, Haybittle J. Design of forms for clinical trials. *Br Med J.* 2:529, 1979

60. Fleming T, DeMets DL. Monitoring of clinical trials: Issues and recommendations. *Control Clin Trials.* 14:183, 1993

61. Fleming TR. Data monitoring committees and capturing relevant information of high quality. *Stat Med.* 12:565, 1993

62. Walters L. Data monitoring committees: The moral case for maximum feasible independence. *Stat Med.* 12:575, 1993

63. Li Z, Geller NL. On the choice of times for data analysis in group sequential trials. *Biometrics.* 47:745, 1991

64. Armitage P, McPherson CK, Rowe BC. Repeated significance tests on accumulating data. *J R Stat Soc.* 132 A:235, 1969

65. Popock SJ. Interim analyses for randomized clinical trials: The group sequential approach. *Biometrics.* 38:153, 1982

66. O'Brien PC, Fleming TR. A multiple testing procedure for clinical trials. *Biometrics.* 35:549, 1979

67. DeMets DL, Lan KKG. Interim analyses: The alpha spending function approach. *Stat Med.* 13:1341, 1994

68. Lan KKG, Lachin J. Implementation of group sequential log rank tests in a maximum duration trial. *Biometrics.* 46:759, 1990

69. Kim K, DeMets DL. Sample size determination for group sequential clinical trials with immediate response. *Stat Med.* 11:1391, 1992

70. Lee JW. Group sequential testing in clinical trials with multivariate observations: A review. *Stat Med.* 13:101, 1994

71. Su JQ, Lachin JU. Group sequential distribution-free methods for the analysis of multivariate observations. *Biometrics.* 48:1033, 1992

72. Gange SJ, DeMets DL. *Sequential Monitoring of Clinical Trials with Correlated Categorical Responses.* University of Wisconsin Department of Biostatistics, technical report no. 86, July 1994

73. Reboussin DM, DeMets DL, Kim K, Lan KKG. *Programs for Computing Group Sequential Bounds Using the Lan-Demets Method.* University of Wisconsin Department of Biostatistics, technical report no. 60, June 1992

74. Tsiatis AA, Rosnar GL, Mehta CR. Exact confidence intervals following a group sequential test. *Biometrics.* 40:797, 1984

75. Klimt CR, Canner PL. Terminating a long-term clinical trial. *Clin Pharmacol Ther.* 25:641, 1979

76. Healy B. From the National Institutes of Health. *JAMA.* 269:3069, 1993

77. Cutler JA, Grandits GA, Grimm RH, et al. Risk factor changes after cessation of intervention in the Multiple Risk Factor Intervention Trial. *Prev Med.* 20:183, 1991

78. Hypertension Detection and Follow-up Program Cooperative Group: Persistence of reduction in blood pressure and mortality of participants in the Hypertension Detection and Follow-up Program. *JAMA.* 259:2113, 1988

79. Sackett DL, Gent M. Controversy in counting and attributing of ends in clinical trials. *N Engl J Med.* 301:1410, 1979

80. Byars DB. Assessing apparent treatment—Covariant interactions in randomized clinical trials. *Stat Med.* 4:255, 1985

81. May GS, DeMets DL, Friedman LM, et al. The randomized clinical trial: Bias in analysis. *Circulation.* 64:669, 1981

82. Crowly J, Breslow N. Statistical analysis of survival data. *Annu Rev Public Health.* 5:385, 1984

83. Cox DR, Oakes D. *The Analysis of Survival Data.* New York, Chapman & Hall, 1984

84. Fleming T, Harrington D. *Counting Processes and Survival Analysis.* New York, John Wiley & Sons, 1991

85. Pledger GW. Basic statistics: Importance of adherence. *J Clin Res Pharmacoepidemiol.* 6:77, 1992

86. Espeland MA, Byington RP, Hire D, et al. Analysis strategies for serial multivariate ultrasonographic data that are incomplete. *Stat Med.* 11:1041, 1992

87. Laird NM. Missing data in longitudinal studies. *Stat Med.* 7:305, 1988

88. Bishop YM, Fienberg SE, Holland PW. *Discrete Multivariate Analysis: Theory and Practice.* Cambridge, MIT Press, 1975

89. Egger MJ, Coleman ML, Ward JR, et al. Uses and abuses of analysis of covariance in clinical trials. *Control Clin Trials.* 6:12, 1985

90. Thall PF, Lachin JM. Assessment of stratum-covariate interaction in Cox's proportional hazards regression model. *Stat Med.* 5:73, 1986

91. Simon R. Patient subsets and variation in therapeutic efficacy. *Br J Clin Pharmacol.* 14:473, 1982

92. Ingelfinger JA, Mosteller F, Thibodeau LA, Ware JH. *Biostatistics in Clinical Medicine.* New York, Macmillan, 1983

93. Mantel N, Haenszel W. Statistical aspects of the analysis of data from retrospective studies of disease. *J Natl Cancer Inst.* 22:719, 1959

94. Cox DR. Regression models and lifetables. *J R Stat Soc.* 34B:187, 1972

95. Meinert CL. Meta-analysis: Science or religion? *Control Clin Trials.* 10:257S, 1989

96. Sacks HS, Berrier J, Reitman D, et al. Meta-analyses of randomized controlled trials. *N Engl J Med.* 316:450, 1987

97. Peto R. Why do we need systematic overviews of randomized trials? *Stat Med.* 6:233, 1987

98. Chalmers TC, Frank CS, Reitman D. Minimizing the three stages of publication bias. *JAMA.* 263:1392, 1990

99. Berlin JA, Begg CB, Louis TA. An assessment of publication bias using a sample of published clinical trials. *J Am Stat Assoc.* 84:381, 1989

100. DerSimonian R, Laird N. Meta-analysis in clinical trials. *Control Clin Trials.* 7:177, 1986

101. Editorial. Reporting clinical trials: Message and medium. *Lancet.* 344:347, 1994

102. Williams DS, Davis CE. Reporting of assignment methods in clinical trials. *Control Clin Trials.* 15:294, 1994

103. Byar DP, Simon RM, Friedewald WT, et al. Randomized clinical trials: Perspectives on some recent ideas. *N Engl J Med.* 295:74, 1976

104. Levine RJ, Lebacqz K. Some ethical considerations in clinical trials. *Clin Pharmacol Ther.* 25:728, 1979

Chapter 26

REPRODUCTIVE MEDICINE AND THE MANAGED CARE MARKET

Richard E. Blackwell

Reproductive medicine is a very broad-based discipline, which renders primary, secondary, and tertiary care to women of all age groups and to infertile couples. The reproductive medicine practitioner has been in the forefront of the movements of outpatient surgery and minimally invasive surgery, has refined endocrine laboratory services, was the first to practice abdominal and then transvaginal ultrasonography, and most recently has developed the assisted reproductive technology culminating with intracytoplasmic sperm injection and the cloning of animal embryos.[1] Despite this broad base of activities, reproductive endocrinologists are often viewed as "infertility subspecialists," and specifically, practitioners of in vitro fertilization. Unfortunately, infertility is often viewed as an elective service to be rendered to couples by insurance carriers, employers, and the federal government. This attitude is the result of lack of public education and the fact that the subject is often sensationalized by the media. Further, the arrival of most multiple births are at least mentioned in the local newspaper if not the national press, and scandals involving implied mishandling of embryos have reached an international level.[2-7]

CLINICAL PRACTICE AT THE TURN OF THE CENTURY: EDUCATION, ECONOMICS, AND THEIR CONTRIBUTION TO TODAY'S MANAGED CARE ENVIRONMENT

In 1910, Abraham Flexner released the Flexner report on medical education in the United States and Canada. He was commissioned by the Carnegie Foundation for the Advancement of Teaching, and the report was divided into two parts. The first dealt with the history of medical education, the proper basis of a medical education, and the actual basis of medical education at the time. It also dealt with the course of study in the first through fourth years and reviewed the financial aspects of all medical institutions, various medical sects, licensing boards, women's medical education, and the medical education of blacks. The second part dealt with medical schools in each of the states and Canada, and contained a compendium of faculty, students, and fees. As an example, in the state of Alabama, the Birmingham Medical College had a faculty of 18 volunteers, 185 students, and a total annual revenue of $14,550. The University of Alabama Department of Medicine had a volunteer faculty of 18 members, 204 students, and an income of $17,300. Harvard University fared better with 23 faculty members, 285 students, and an income of $72,037 per year.

Prior to the Flexner report, there were literally hundreds of small medical schools in the United States. The larger eastern cities literally had dozens of schools, which were often housed in private residences and staffed by one or two private practitioners, with a course that consisted of dissection, reading, and demonstration. There was little laboratory instruction and little or no clinical experience.

In 1854, Mr. Hopkins bought a large tract of land overlooking the harbor in Baltimore. The building was previously occupied by the Maryland Hospital for the Insane. The university rented dwellings near the center of the city and formally opened in 1876 under the presidency of Daniel Coit Gilman. The trustees secured the service of John Shaw Billings, an authority on hospital construction and management, and the plans went forward to create the finest medical facility in the country, which would have the laboratories, operating rooms, and wards for the hospital. In 1889, the hospital was completed. Five years earlier, William Henry Welch had been called from Bellevue in New York to take the Chair of Pathology, William Osler was brought from Philadelphia to head the Department of Medicine, William Halstead was appointed to the Chair of General Surgery, and Howard Atwood Kelly was named as Chairman of Gynecology. These men were perhaps the first to serve as full-time faculty members, and Dr. Kelly was appointed at a salary of $3,000 per annum with a $500 allowance made for an assistant. In the early days there were no x-ray machines, and the technique of blood transfusion had not been developed, but antiseptic technique was practiced and surgeons wore thick white duct trousers under their sterile gowns and white caps on their heads. It was Kelly's custom, for instance, to scrub his hands and nails for 10 min in water that was frequently changed. He then soaked his hands and forearms in a saturated solution of permanganate, a potash, that stained them a deep mahogany, and then plunged them into a saturated solution of oxalic acid until the color disappeared. Subsequently, he removed the acid with sterilized water. The thumb, index, and middle fingers of both hands were covered with rubber finger stalls taken from a carbolic solution. In that day, bichloride of mercury was universally accepted as a disinfectant but caused considerable skin irritation. It was known that Dr. Halstead, the Chief of Surgery, commissioned the Goodyear Rubber Company to make a thin pair of rubber gloves for his scrub nurse. It was not until 1894 that Hunter Robb recommended that surgeons wear gloves themselves. As was practiced in the day, the hospital gynecologic services had one charity ward for white women and one for black women, each with 24 beds, and another floor for private patients.

The economics of medicine were relatively straightforward in those days. Many physicians did not charge for services to the poor, but would not hesitate to ask "exorbitantly large fees" from patients who could well afford to pay. Professor Kelly, for example, was criticized for his obstetric fee, which was $500. It was thought that he no doubt accepted this figure for the express purpose of discouraging obstetric practice, which he did not welcome. He often said, "A great temptation and danger in a physician's life is that he may be tempted to wear spectacles with dollar marks on them."

The life of J. Marion Sims brings into focus another dimension of the evolution of American medicine. Sims, after early failures in obstetrics and gynecology, vowed not to be further involved in the health of women. When presented with a problem of "strictly" female origin, he always told her promptly, "This is out of my line entirely and I know practically nothing about it." Sims, while working in Alabama, carried out many operative proce-

dures such as resection of malignancies of the sinus, which were done by blind dissection with his finger. The only anesthesia was brandy and water. Ironically, less than 300 miles away in the neighboring state of Georgia, a country doctor named Crawford W. Long had discovered that by giving his patients sulfuric ether to inhale, he could perform operations without pain. Long disliked writing and carried out these successful procedures for many years before reporting it in the medical literature after W.T.G. Morton successfully demonstrated the use of ether at Massachusetts General Hospital. This illustrates the difficulty of communication at the time, in that most medical information was transferred by case discussions at local medical societies or at world congresses. This demonstration of anesthesia at Massachusetts General also points out the differences in complexity of carrying out research at that point in history. Morton had attended an ether frolic; during the performance a man fell from the stage, driving a piece of wood through his leg. The man felt no pain despite considerable injury. Morton contacted the owner of the frolic, and arranged to have a gas cylinder brought to his studio. At that juncture, one of Morton's party had a tooth removed under anesthesia and reported that he felt no pain. At the demonstration at Massachusetts General Hospital, a medical student was selected from the audience, brought to the stage, anesthetized, and one of his teeth was removed with great success. This, of course, was carried out without approval of an institutional review board or the FDA.

Sims' contact with three remarkable women, Anarcha, Bessy, and Lucy, propelled him into the role of the woman's surgeon in the United States. These three young slave women endured tedious labors and had sloughing of the anterior vagina and bladder base, yielding enormous vesicovaginal fistulas. Prevailed upon by Mr. Westcott, Anarcha's master, Sims attempted to cure the problem. However, after an encounter with Mrs. Merrill, who suffered an acute retrodisplacement of the uterus, he subsequently developed the Sims' position and the method for allowing atmospheric pressure to dilate the vagina, thus permitting visualization of the vagina and the fistula site. This led to numerous operations on these young women, followed by numerous failures due to breakdown of the suture line. Finally, after having a jeweler prepare a wire of silver alloy, drawn to the diameter of a horse hair, in May 1849 he operated on Anarcha for the thirteenth time. He brought the edges of the fistula together with four fine sutures of the silver wire and cured the young woman's affliction.

Despite Sims' success both professionally and financially in Alabama, his move to New York met with disaster. Not only did he lack local connections and a European education, but New York in the 1850s was divided into warring factions who supported various hospitals and vested interests. As a result of this, Sims was unable to attain a hospital appointment in any of the established institutions. As he perceived a need for his services, he simply founded his own hospital. He was aided in this endeavor by a New Yorker of no small social stature, Henry Luther Stewart. He and Sims mobilized the medical community in support of a women's hospital. The effort, of course, required no certificate of need (CON).

In 1849, on the Minnesota frontier, other events were occurring that would change the face of American medicine. Minnesota had just been organized into a territory with a population of less than 5000 people. Dr. and Mrs. W. W. Mayo made their home in Lasuer from 1859 to 1863. Subsequently, the Mayos moved to Rochester in 1868 with their sons Will and Charlie, just as the railroad built a line to the city. Like their father, they pursued a medical career, Charlie graduating from the Chicago Medical College and Will from the University of Michigan. They were joined in practice by Christopher Graham, Augustus Stinchfeld, Marvin Millet, Gertrude Booker Granger, Edward Starr Judd, and Henry S. Plummer. This group formed the forerunner of the Mayo Clinic. Simultaneously, the Catholic sisters under the leadership of Mother Alford and Sister Joseph developed St. Mary's Hospital, which became Charlie and Will's primary admitting hospital. In 1914, following reorganization and construction of a new building, the Mayo Clinic emerged as a distinct institution. The clinic's marvelous case record system was established by Dr. Plummer, and it became a model for research. Thus, in this remarkable time in history around the turn of the century, many institutions of modern medicine were founded by physicians of strong personality. These include the development of contemporary medical curriculum, establishment of full-time medical facilities, development of the modern case report system, creation of specialty hospitals for women, and development of the multispecialty clinic.

Once the basic structure for medical practice was established around the turn of the century, many events in reproductive biology took place rapidly thereafter. Obstetrics and gynecology, which had previously been practiced as two different disciplines, merged into one specialty, and the American Board of Obstetrics and Gynecology was established. Subsequently, the American Fertility Society (now called the American Society of Reproductive Medicine) was founded in Birmingham, Alabama, in 1944. Today, it has grown to over 10,000 members and contains three subspecialty societies: the Society for Reproductive Endocrinologists, the Society for Reproductive Surgeons, and the Society for Assisted Reproductive Technology. In the 1960s, the radioimmunoassay was developed and laparoscopy was introduced. The late 1960s and 1970s saw the development of agents for the induction of ovulation and the treatment of various endocrinopathies; the mid-1970s saw sonography begin to flourish in obstetrics and gynecology; and on June 25, 1978, a 5-pound 12-ounce baby girl fertilized in a petri dish was born in Oldham General District Hospital in Lancaster, England. Louise Brown was the result of an assisted scientific effort by gynecologist Patrick C. Steptoe and physiologist Robert G. Edwards.

The introduction of in vitro fertilization into reproductive medicine not only changed the specialty in the way it was perceived by reproductive endocrinologists and the public, but also the economics of infertility practice. The young reproductive endocrinologists flocked to in vitro fertilization and became its stars. Insurance carriers at first liberally covered in vitro fertilization procedures under the practice of charge fragmentation. However, once the economic impact of ART technology became apparent to the insurance industry, restrictions were applied in almost every state. This was followed by the appearance of mandated coverage in Massachusetts, Maryland, Illinois, and other states, yet in most of the country out-of-pocket payment became the rule (Table 26–1). Primarily because of the threat of federal regulations, the Society for Assisted Reproductive Technology created a registry that *supposedly* accurately records IVF and GIFT activities in the United States. Once this data began to be accumulated, it was distributed to the public and, in fact, the take-home baby rate has now become the "currency" of IVF and GIFT programs and serves as its principal means of advertisement. Along with this notoriety has obviously come unwanted news releases, sensational press, magazine articles featuring such topics as "High Tech Baby Making," "The Next Front Page Scandal," and the recent international scandal involving alleged mishandling of cryopreserved embryos at the University of California at Irvine. In fact, the expense and risks have dissuaded 43 percent of couples from ever seeking help, and only approximately 10 to 12 percent seeking care in a given year. This should convince us that infertility does not exist in a social, political, or economic vacuum.

THE CURRENT PROBLEMS IN HEALTH CARE

In 1945, many young men and women returned to the United States from World War II to undertake educational endeavors in medicine under the newly created GI Bill. The United States entered an era of unprecedented prosperity, funding flowed into the U.S. medical establishment, subspecialization became the rule of the day, and, with the enactment of Medicare and Medicaid legislation, medical schools began to be paid handsome incentives to train ever-increasing numbers of physicians.

TABLE 26–1. MANDATED COVERAGE OF INFERTILITY BENEFIT

State	Commentary
Arkansas	Mandates insurance carrier to cover IVF, allows insurers to impose a lifetime benefit cap of $15,000.
California	Mandates insurance carriers to offer group policy holder coverage of infertility treatment, excluding IVF but including GIFT.
Connecticut	Mandates insurance carriers to offer coverage of comprehensive infertility diagnosis and treatment, including assisted reproductive technology procedures.
Hawaii	Mandates insurance carriers to cover one cycle of IVF, only after several conditions have been met.
Illinois	Mandates insurance carriers to cover the diagnosis and treatment of infertility, including assisted reproductive technology procedures, but limits first-time attempt for complete oocyte retrieval and two complete oocyte retrievals for a second birth. Insurance carriers are not required to provide this benefit to businesses (group policies) of 25 or fewer employees.
Maryland	Mandates insurance carriers, excluding HMOs, to cover IVF, only after several conditions have been met. Insurance carriers are not required to provide this benefit to businesses (group policies) of 50 or fewer employees.
Massachusetts	Mandates insurance carriers to cover comprehensive infertility diagnosis and treatment, including assisted reproductive technology procedures.
Montana	Mandates HMOs to cover infertility treatment as a "preventive service" benefit.
New York	Mandates insurance carriers to cover the "diagnosis and treatment of correctable medical conditions." Thus, insurers may not deny coverage for treatment of a correctable medical condition solely because the condition results in infertility.
Ohio	Mandates HMOs to cover infertility treatment as a "preventable service" benefit.
Rhode Island	Mandates insurance carriers to cover comprehensive infertility diagnosis and treatment, including assisted reproductive technology procedure, but permits insurers to impose up to a 20 percent co-pay requirement.
Texas	Mandates insurance carriers to offer coverage of IVF to group policy holders.
West Virginia	Mandates HMOs to cover infertility treatment as a "preventable service" benefit.

(Courtesy of Foster Higgins.)

This has resulted in a presumed oversupply of physicians (17,000/year U.S. graduates) and certainly a maldistribution as specialists tended to settle in large cities. Aggravating this manpower situation was the flow of foreign medical practitioners into the United States educational system (8000/year), which was and is encouraged today, because of the royalties received by the training institutions and their need for low-cost manpower to service their charity populations. Further, using various visa pathways, many of the foreign graduates have remained in the United States as permanent residents, often having spent several years in an underserved area as payment. Recently, the sentiment has been expressed by many U.S. physicians and legislators that visa distribution needs to be revamped such that foreign physicians training in the United States would be required to return to their parent country. This has been strongly opposed by foreign medical graduate groups, which argue that no other occupation in the United States is so protected by legislation. Despite one's opinion regarding these issues, the American College of Obstetricians and Gynecologists predicts that there will be about 1000 active practitioners in reproductive endocrinology, at least over the next 10 years.

The massive availability of highly skilled health care providers coupled with an unrestrained fee-for-service insurance reimbursement system gave rise to a health care system that consumed ever-increasing portions of the gross national product. It is no accident that the American Fertility Society grew at an unprecedented rate over the last 20 years, and that this interest in infertility mirrored an almost exponential demand for consumer services despite the fact that the incidence of infertility has remained somewhere between 9 and 25 percent of married couples. This rise in interest in "infertility" directly correlates with the flight of obstetrician/gynecologists from obstetrics. Many of these physicians turn their interest to surgical infertility, and coupled with the rise of operative endoscopy, this has led to a gross over-utilization of services. As is interpreted from Romans 6:16, "When we make something our slave and use it too freely or too frequently, it will soon master us." The events that were occurring in obstetrics and gynecology represent only one small part in the overall drama that was occurring across the United States. One has seen similar utilization of gastric endoscopic procedures, radiographic imaging, open heart surgery, invasive radiologic procedures, and so forth. This insatiable consumption of health care obviously is at the breaking point with employers and payers, and these concerns reached a sympathetic ear with the coming of the Clinton administration. Although the federal health care initiative failed, it accomplished its primary purpose by setting into motion a market-driven resolution to the health care crisis. Unfortunately, as we will see in subsequent sections, managed care has not addressed the aging U.S. population, the ultimate increase in chronic disease states that will be reflected in that population, our propensity for violent crime, the utilization of illicit drugs and alcohol as well as cigarettes, or the AIDS epidemic.[8–13]

MANAGED CARE, ITS FORM AND STRUCTURE

In the 1980s, managed care began to arise in many forms. First, in the southern United States came the preferred provider organization (PPO) introduced by Blue Cross/ Blue Shield. This type of organization essentially has open participation by physicians, yet rate discounts of up to 50 cents on the dollar were imposed. To counter this, the Individual Practice Association (IPA) was formed, often with unsatisfactory results. Likewise, this was based on decreased utilization, discounting, and taxation under the guise of creation of reserves. Following this, or in parallel, was the creation of the HMO with open staffing, or the staff model such as the Kaiser– Permanente program.

The 1990s have seen the rise of physician practice management (PPM) groups. Some of these have been formed by physicians and called medical service organizations (MSOs); others have tried to function as an IPA. At least 30 PPM companies are traded in the stock market, and they share a $200 billion annual market of physician services. About 8 percent of the nation's 527,000 practicing doctors are affiliated. One of the largest is Phycor, which has revenues of $766 million, net income of $36 million, stock market capitalization of $2.3 billion, 12,540 affiliated physicians, and 34 percent of revenues from capitated contracts. Joseph Hutts, the CEO, was quoted in Business Week (1997) as saying, "At this point the only constraints on our growth are self-imposed." Another major PPM leader is MedPartners, based in Birmingham, Alabama. Larry House, CEO, was quoted as saying, "You have to be bold and aggressive to build what we want to build and that's not going to change." MedPartners recently paid $190 billion to purchase Care Mark International, and $490 million to acquire In Phynet Medical Management. MedPartners has revenues of $2.5 billion, a net income of $134 million, stock market capitalization of $3.7 billion, 10,688 affiliated physicians, and 55 percent of total revenues from managed care contracts. Another principal player in the managed care process is Principal Care, based in Nashville, Tennessee. Dr. G. William Bates is the president of the company, whose long-range strategy is the acquisition of specialty obstetrics/gynecology practices in medium-sized cities. Integramed, based in New York City, specializes in the acquisition of practices that deliver assisted reproductive technology services, and most recently they have diversified into other areas of women's health care. Gyncor, based in Chicago, whose president is Dr. Norbert Gleicher, has been active in the acquisition of IVF practices throughout the country. The MSO is also becoming a popular approach to managed care. An MSO is a privately held entity, with the ownership generally split 50/50 between physicians and hospitals. Recent relaxation of the antitrust laws have allowed these organiza-

tions to flourish. It has been predicted that the MSO could curtail the PPM industry growth where their greatest threats are. "Minus profit margins and a heavy reliance on acquisition coupled with the intricacies of medical practice and the stubbornly independent ways of doctors, make physicians' practice management one of the most unforgiving businesses in health care."

RESPONSE TO MANAGED CARE BY THE OBSTETRICIAN/GYNECOLOGIST AND REPRODUCTIVE ENDOCRINOLOGIST

While obstetrician/gynecologists and reproductive endocrinologists have been some of the most entrepreneurial and medical businessmen, the era of managed care has created a dangerous and treacherous venue in which to operate.[14] The response of many physicians has been to deny that there has been a revolution in health care payment, and to resist the utilization of any tools to counter these trends such as networking or algorithms. The reproductive endocrinologists, in particular, seem to be divided along two courses of action: the first group seeks to enhance insurance coverage for infertility services, while the other seeks to further isolate infertility services into a boutique niche similar to that occupied by cosmetic surgery. Other groups have attempted to encourage legislators to add mandates to various state laws; in general, this has been moderately successful. Those physicians who have elected to deal with managed care have done so with the mechanisms mentioned previously or by direct contracting. Nevertheless, when one deals with infertility services, one must first counter a great deal of the bad publicity that is associated with advanced reproductive technologies; realize that insurance carriers are interested in providing good to average health care, not necessarily the absolute best; come to understand that one's individual data are therefore not special; and further understand that providers seek to purchase good care at low prices. Each physician's response to managed care will be based on services provided, geographic location, and level of competition.

ACADEMIC HEALTH SCIENCE CENTER— ITS SPECIAL PROBLEMS AND SOLUTIONS

From the viewpoint of the reproductive endocrinologist, the current problems besetting the typical academic health science center are similar to those perceived by the plastic surgeon.[15,16] Most reproductive endocrinologists deal with patients who carry commercial insurance or pay for services out of pocket. We operate in private practice settings, and generate income not only from assisted reproductive technology but from surgery, laboratory services, and radiographic services. The vast majority of our surgical procedures are carried out in an outpatient setting, and many of us carry out a great deal of our practice in large community private hospitals or outpatient surgical facilities. Likewise, our teaching is carried out in these settings as well as our clinical research, whether funded by industry or the federal government. Because we are generally a high-profit center, however, we are vulnerable to ever-increasing university taxation to supplement loss leaders. This results in the diversion of funds from teaching, research, and other academic activities. Along with these financial inconsistencies has come an ever-increasing load of administrative responsibilities and an expanding bureaucracy that more often than not hinders individual efforts, although it may facilitate institutional goals. As a result of this, there has been an exodus from academic reproductive medicine of a huge number of senior, highly talented reproductive endocrinologists. Many of these individuals are world-class physicians and some have established reproductive centers of excellence that rival, if not surpass, those seen in the academic environment. Further, the private practice gynecologists have been the driving force behind outpatient surgery and the development of advanced endoscopy, and industry more often than not is just as inclined to lend its support to these private endeavors as to furnish traditional funding to academic divisions. This evolution and revolution creates a special dilemma for academic divisions of reproductive endocrinology. It is hoped that these divisions will maintain their philosophy of furnishing broad-based reproductive medicine services, draw patients from the pediatric to the menopausal population, continue their role in research, perhaps enhance their role in technology transfer, limit their output of fellows to a level that can be absorbed by the marketplace, and increase their interaction with their referring obstetrician/gynecologists as well as other reproductive endocrinologists to establish regional centers of excellence.

SOLUTIONS

"No human endeavor relies more heavily on information than modern medicine, yet all too often we have an inability to conveniently and effectively access the scientific literature. All too often decisions are made by anecdotal impressions and imperfect literature recall, rather than a systematic overview of the pertinent information." These thoughts expressed by David L. Olive, MD, at the annual meeting postgraduate course of the American Society for Reproductive Medicine on November 3, 1996, bring to light a new movement in evaluation of reproductive medicine. For the first time, a course on evidence-based medicine, Contemporary Mode of Practice, was offered by a major organization in our specialty. Evidence-based medicine "is the conscientious, explicit, and judicious use of current best evidence in making decisions about the care of individual patients."[17–23] This is not cookbook medicine, but it forms the basis for construction of all medical algorithms. It uses blinded, randomized prospective trials, nonblinded trials, case-controlled studies, retrospective analysis, single-physician retrospective analysis, clinical acumen, and opinion, and it applies the appropriate weighting to this information to give the most accurate result. Meta-analysis is simply one tool used by the physician utilizing evidence-based medicine, and these techniques have been utilized in forming the algorithms and guidelines that will be discussed later in this chapter.[24,25]

Another shift that is occurring in reproductive medicine, as well as other specialties, is the utilization of cost-effective analysis.[26,27] This is a systematic approach to evaluate the outcomes and cost of interventions designed to improve health. As pressures to control health care costs grow, it is increasingly used by policy analysts, clinicians, and health care organizations in determining the cost and consequences of alternative treatments.[28–33] While this technique is only loosely employed in the construction of algorithms today, it will undoubtedly play a major role in the future.

Essentially three types of proposals have been presented for dealing with infertility from a financial point of view: a capitated plan such as the one implemented by U.S. HealthCare, the infertility protocol presented by Bates Consulting, and the Lewin VHI algorithm.[34–36] Under the U.S. HealthCare model, the basic infertility work-up can be carried out by anyone designated as a primary provider. This consists of a semen analysis, hysterosalpingogram, some assessment of ovulation, and postcoital testing. The majority of patients who finish this segment of the work-up are referred directly to a limited number of reproductive endocrinologists, completely bypassing the obstetrician/gynecologist. The patient may visit two reproductive endocrine practices, and at that juncture choose a health care provider. A capitated arrangement is reached between the corporate entity and the provider that is in the mid-four-figure region. Any means may be used to achieve conception such as intrauterine insemination, gonadotropins, gamete intrafallopian transfer, in vitro fertilization, or infertility surgery. The provider has 2 yr to achieve a pregnancy and must maintain a low 20 percent pregnancy rate to remain eligible for the plan. If a conception occurs early in the workup, the provider receives the remainder of the capitated payment.

An algorithm presented by Bates Consulting Company involves an initial evaluation of history and physical, semen analysis, hormonal evaluation in 35 percent of patients, and hysterosalpingogram in 30 percent of patients. One third of patients are thought to have disorders of ovulation; this is treated with correction of body weight if less than 95 or greater than 100 percent of ideal, and therapy with clomiphene citrate, bromocriptine, or prednisone for six cycles. If no pregnancy occurs, 30 percent of patients undergo office hysteroscopy, and then three cycles of in vitro fertilization. Thirty percent of the patients have ovulatory disorders and 24 percent of them undergo operative laparoscopy. Half are thought to have a good prognosis, and they attempt pregnancy for 6 mo. If no pregnancy occurs, approximately 40 percent undergo three cycles of in vitro fertilization. If they are poor prognosis patients, 50 percent with extensive tubal disease, they undergo three cycles of IVF. Forty percent of the couples have male factor, 80 percent are oligospermic, and varicocelectomy is used sparingly in this protocol; if no pregnancy occurs following surgery, then three cycles of IVF are carried out. The oligospermic patient, found 20 percent of the time, will undergo six cycles of therapeutic donor insemination. If no pregnancy occurs, then two cycles of IVF are carried out. It should be noted that in this algorithm the patient pays the cost of laboratory evaluation, the cost of all medications including gonadotropins, an additional charge for IVF cycles, and the cost of donor insemination.

The algorithm originally designed by Lewin VHI was prepared by a panel of infertility experts using literature review and a modified Delphi approach. Infertility was treated as being the result of a variety of disease processes including pituitary tumors, central nervous system dysfunction, diabetes mellitus, other systemic disorders, endometriosis, fibroids, adhesions, eating disorders, and so forth. The algorithm further depended on a working relationship between the obstetrician/gynecologist and the reproductive endocrinologist functioning together as a network. It continuously evolves based on outcome analysis. It sets boundaries on therapy based on literature review and outcome analysis. This is entirely different from the protocol concept which is derived from an individual anecdotal practice experience and often leads to failure or increased cost, dissatisfied subscribers, and ultimately litigation. Algorithms can be used to improve care, control cost, use resources efficiently, and increase the availability of coverage, because they allow the payer to predict the underlying worst-case scenario, which generally falls in the range of 40 to 50 cents per payer per month. This is much lower than is generally thought by the insurance industry.

The algorithm also has as its basis a number of facts that influence reproduction. Women in the United States age 15 through 45 who are trying to conceive show subfertility rates in the range between 8.5 and 25 percent.[37,38] Infertility acts against a background of change

in age in both men and women, with the age of menopause normally ranging between 35 and 57 with a mean of 51.4 years in the U.S. population. By age 35 there is an exponential fall in fecundity rate with the fertility rate, per thousand people being approximately 100 at age 40. Further, the number of clinically recognized trisomies rises exponentially at age 35, and by the age of 40 it represents 25 percent of pregnancies.[39] Likewise, the spontaneous miscarriage rate rises exponentially after the age of 35, and by the age of 40 it is approximately 30 percent. Ectopic pregnancies rise from 15 percent per thousand pregnancies at age 25 to 34, to nearly 20 percent between age 35 and 44.[40] In fact, every complication of pregnancy including abortion, ectopic pregnancy, congenital malformations, prematurity, intrauterine growth retardation, perinatal mortality, fetal death, macrosomia, neonatal death, placenta previa, infant mortality, abruptio placentae, pregnancy-induced hypertension, labor dysfunction, chronic hypertension, diabetes, cesarean section, maternal mortality, and maternal morbidity increase markedly beyond age 35.

In addition, the likelihood of conception is associated with age-related male sexual dysfunction. The conception rate with partners under the age of 25 with 6 mo of unprotected intercourse is 48.5 percent; at age 40 and over it is 22.7 percent. Frequency of intercourse falls with age, and with intercourse less than once per week the conception rate is 16.7 percent over 6 mo; greater than four times a week the conception rate is 83.3 percent. Finally, there is an exponential decrease in the number of orgasms per week, and an exponential rise in the number of episodes of impotency that begins around the age of 35. All of these factors result in decreased cost, decreased productivity of the couple, depression, marital discord, family discord, and isolation of the couple. These factors make a powerful argument to present to the infertility benefit providers. Further, as a way of reducing cost, the algorithm repeatedly stresses the use of underlying accurate diagnosis, the maximization of pregnancy using low-technology therapy, the appropriate use of laparoscopic surgery, and the appropriate use of ART technology early in the work-up if need be, all of which is cost effective. Such an algorithm helps codify the standard of practice, it controls cost, it limits other costs such as surgeries and ectopic pregnancies, it predicts outcome, and it makes therapy *finite*. As an example, clomiphene citrate ovulation induction is used for five ovulatory cycles, gonadotropin ovulation induction is used for six cycles, in vitro fertilization is used for four to six cycles. An infertility algorithm also sets the referral pattern; that is, it moves patients to the reproductive endocrinologist earlier in the work-up, which again is cost effective.[41-44]

The second revision of the VHI algorithm has been prepared in collaboration with Drs. Merrill Berger, Paul

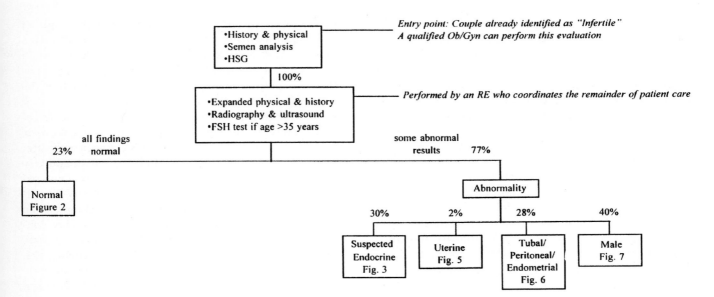

Figure 26–1. Basic work-up of the infertile couple, showing the type of abnormality and indicating referral points. *(Figure courtesy of the Lewin Group, Inc.)*

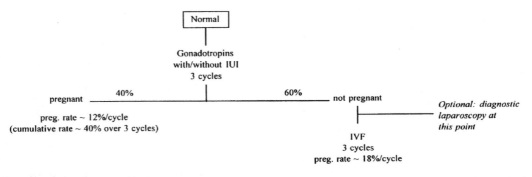

Figure 26–2. Treatment of the couple with a normal basic work-up. *(Figure courtesy of the Lewin Group, Inc.)*

Zarutskie, and Richard Blackwell. This represents a streamlined algorithm that reduces the initial number of tests used in the infertility evaluation, involves the reproductive endocrinologist at least as a consultant earlier in the work-up and treatment plan, moves to superovulation with gonadotropins and IVF in a more expedited manner, further decreases the utilization of surgery in the treatment of infertility, and increases the utilization of ICSI in the treatment of male infertility (Figs 26–1 to 26–7). (See also Chap 27 for additional algorithms.)

PAYMENT FOR SERVICES

Payment for infertility services usually falls into three general categories: capitation, discounted fee for service, and self-pay. Most reproductive endocrine practices op-erate with some form of all of these payments. There is little experience with capitated plans in the infertility arena, and to my knowledge no prospective data have been presented. Our own prospective payment plan designed for the VIVA University of Alabama at Birmingham (UAB) program uses the Lewin VHI algorithm to form the basis of the proposal. A figure of 47 cents per member per month was used to project our expenses in revenue. Eleven months into the first year, this figure appears to be correct. The plan covers a semen analysis, postcoital test, hysterosalpingogram or sono-hysterogram, hormone assay, and follicle monitoring by ultrasound. It also covers surgical procedures to diagnose or treat infertility, ovulation induction including clomiphene and gonadotropin therapy, artificial insemination by donor or husband, assisted reproductive technology including in vitro fertilization, and gamete intrafallopian transfer. There are exclusions and limitations,

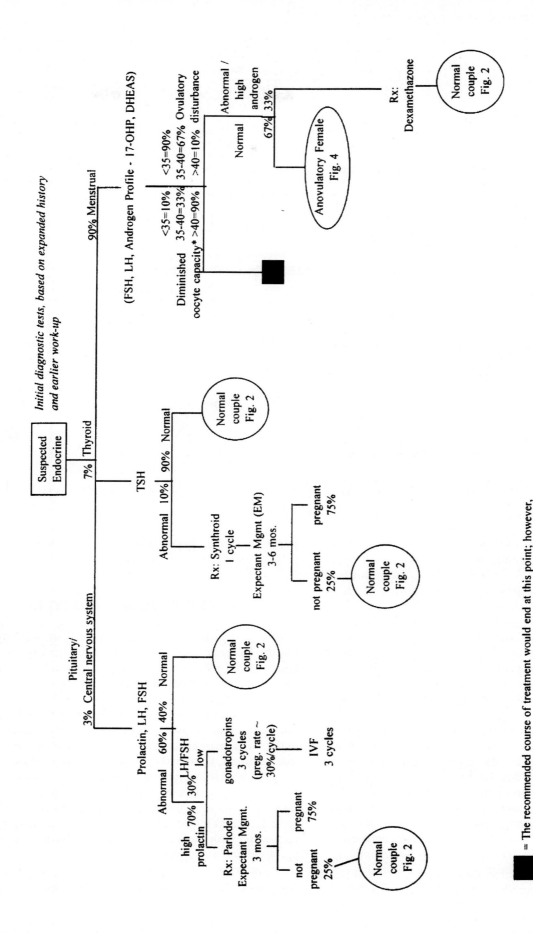

Figure 26–3. Evaluation of the woman who has a suspected endocrine abnormality as suggested by some dysfunction in ovulation. *(Figure courtesy of the Lewin Group, Inc.)*

525

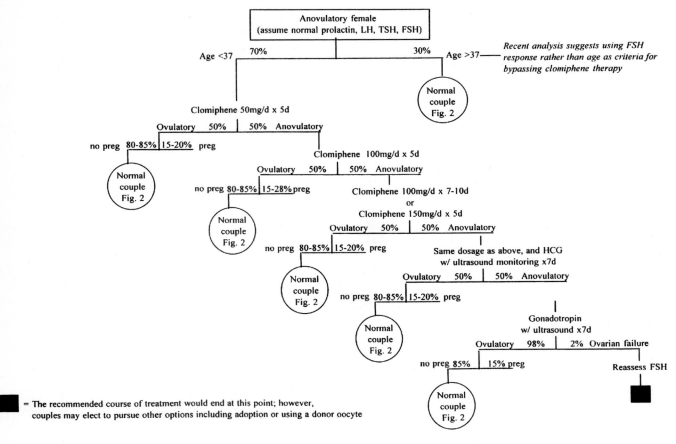

Figure 26–4. Treatment of the ovulatory female assuming normal LH, FSH, and TSH levels. *(Figure courtesy of the Lewin Group, Inc.)*

including a maximum lifetime coverage of nine ovulation induction cycles with clomiphene, six gonadotropin cycles, three artificial insemination cycles, and four assisted reproductive technology cycles. Further, in addition to a standard co-pay, any service related to hospitalization or outpatient surgical procedures has a 40 percent co-pay, and any drugs such as clomiphene citrate, gonadotropins, and GnRH analogs used for infertility treatment has a 40 percent co-pay. Sterilization reversal is excluded under this plan. Our experience over less than 1 yr suggests that there is not an unfavorable selection bias.

All of us are familiar with discounted fee for service. Currently, many practitioners receive between 30 and 50 cents on the dollar for services rendered. Other than those states having mandated coverage for ART technology, many commercial carriers discontinue therapy either at the level of gonadotropin plus or minus intrauterine insemination or following a limited number of treatment cycles with this mode of therapy. Many reproductive endocrinologists, as stated previously, favor out-of-pocket payment. However, caution should be used in isolating infertility services. While it may be convenient for calculating outcome

analysis and cost, this segregation makes it all too easy to exclude these services from any future health care plans.

DATABASE AND OUTCOME ANALYSIS

Following the publication of the article, "Are we exploiting the infertile couple?,"[45] Congress began to focus a great deal of effort on standardizing not only infertility but laboratory services. The outcome database was established by the Society for Assisted Reproductive Technology, and the CLIA regulations were modified. At the same time, following the failed Clinton health care initiative, a marketplace-driven revolution in managed care occurred. Carriers began to insist on accurate databases as an outcome analysis. The concept of underlying *disease management* was simultaneously introduced by both the insurance and pharmaceutical industries. This concept insists that diseases are treated in an incremental manner with the most cost-effective therapy based on literature and outcome analysis.[46]

These concepts appeal to some, are rejected by others, and raise many difficult issues. We have all seen databases

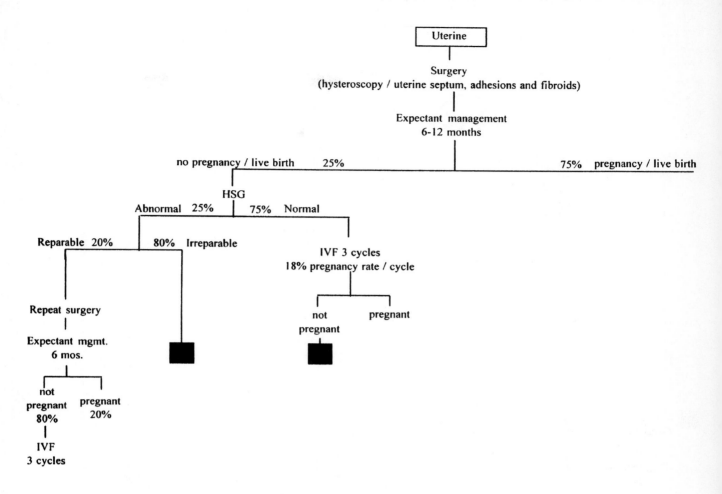

= The recommended course of treatment would end at this point; however,
couples may elect to pursue other options including adoption or using a gestational host

Figure 26–5. Evaluation and treatment of the woman with a uterine abnormality. *(Figure courtesy of the Lewin Group, Inc.)*

manipulated and outcomes skewed by patient selection and exclusion. Pregnancy rates are diagnosis and age dependent, and advanced therapies often yield impressive results when applied to those who don't need them. Further, disease management raises licensure issues, as with the recent criminal indictment by the state of Florida of a physician benefits manager who was charged with practicing medicine in the state without a license. While this particular physician was licensed to practice in another state, his direction of patient care in the state of Florida was viewed by the courts as a licensure violation. In this particular case, the Florida appellate court issued a summary judgment and dismissed the case. The same issues have been raised with regard to satellite offices, various satellite affiliations, and telemedicine. Likewise, recent advertisements appearing on the World Wide Web may fall under the same constraints.

CREDENTIALING

Another area that will come under intense focus involves licensing and credentialing. Those individuals who practice medicine in any state regardless of form will most likely be required to apply for a license in that state, be networked with physicians who are physically in that location, and be appropriately certified, particularly as we enter the area of virtual reality surgery. Certification in reproductive endocrinology will most likely be a requisite for a payment by insurance companies, and failure to be certified will probably result in de-selection, as has already been seen in some communities. Payment for sonography will probably be dependent on being certified by the American Registry of Diagnostic and Medical Sonographers (ARDMS) (600 Jefferson Plaza, Suite 360, Rockville, Md 20852). Laboratories will have to be

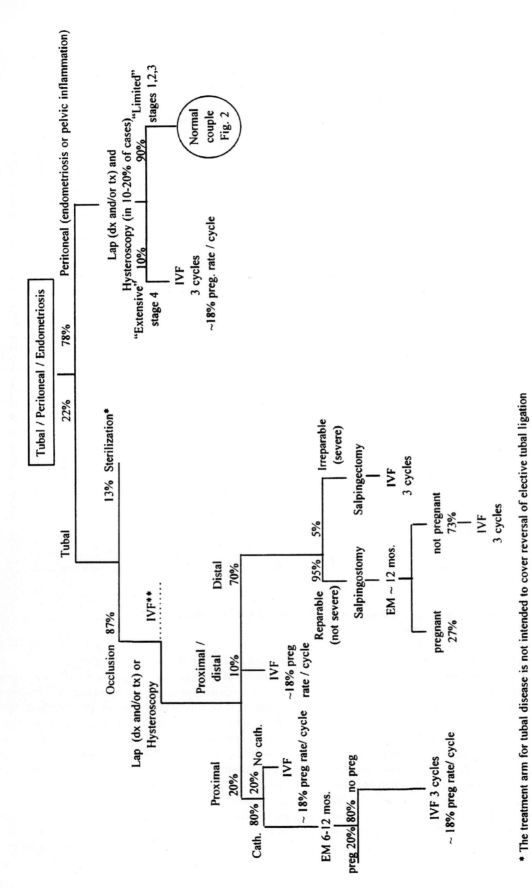

Figure 26–6. Evaluation and treatment of the woman with tubal/peritoneal disease, with or without the presence of endometriosis. *(Figure courtesy of the Lewin Group, Inc.)*

* The treatment arm for tubal disease is not intended to cover reversal of elective tubal ligation

* * Alternative treatment pathway, in some practice settings, may bypass surgery and proceed with IVF for 3 cycles

EM = Expectant Management

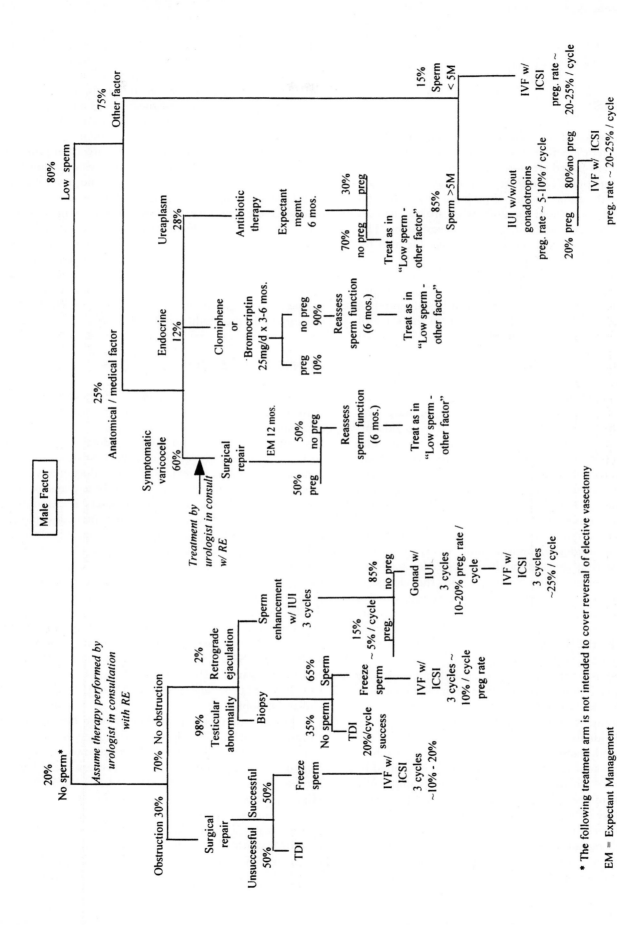

Figure 26–7. Evaluation and treatment of the male with an abnormal semen analysis. (*Figure courtesy of the Lewin Group, Inc.*)

* The following treatment arm is not intended to cover reversal of elective vasectomy

EM = Expectant Management

certified by CLIA and/or the College of Pathology to be competitive for contract bids.

NETWORKS

Networking is one of the most difficult social and legal issues facing reproductive endocrinologists. Many of us practice broad-based reproductive medicine, which means we function as a primary, secondary, and tertiary provider for the same patient. The issue of self-referral from one role to another is perilous as we are watched intensely by the insurance industry and government. The whole area of networking creates a special dilemma for those of us in academic medicine, for plans such as that presented by U.S. HealthCare seem to strike at the very purpose of a residency training program, since better programs prepare residents to manage broad-based reproductive medical and infertility problems up to the stage of assisted reproductive technology utilization. To bypass the skills of so many of our colleagues was seen to be an inefficient use of resources. The most efficient treatment of a patient with complex reproductive medical problems would seem to be an initial referral of this patient directly to the obstetrician/gynecologist by the primary care provider who works up the patient guided by algorithms and disease management concepts, frequent consultation with the reproductive endocrinologist during the work-up as part of a working team, and referral of the patient who fails to conceive to the reproductive endocrinologist in a timely manner, all of which would seem to limit cost and maximize the outcome. However, in this intense era of competition the formation of working networks between reproductive endocrinologists and the obstetrician/gynecologist is at times difficult since problems of ego, training, and practice often interfere with the successful function of such networks. The future of reproductive medicine will be dictated by the use of algorithms that are no more than a codification of the guidelines of practice advocated by the Subspecialty Division of the American Board of Obstetrics and Gynecology.

Another issue that one must deal with in networking is antitrust violation and percentage of market control in formal networks, which seem to attract the least attention from government antitrust forces. Under such arrangements, individuals could be members of a number of different networks, and admission to one would not exclude admission to another. Networks have been described by Nancy Foy[46,47] in these terms, "The effectiveness of a network is inversely proportional to its goal. A network needs to have a focus, not a goal. A network needs a spider at the center, not a chairman. A network needs a note or a newsletter, not a journal. A network needs a good list of members more than a set of by-laws. A network needs groups, not committees. A network needs a phone number, not a building."[47,48] In other words, one needs an informal network of providers who are willing to come together under a common philosophy and agree to treat patients accordingly. Such an organization, made up of a strong group of obstetrician/gynecologists and reproductive endocrinologists, would have great appeal to insurance carriers looking for providers or their subscribers, and many physician management firms are attempting to construct such networks. Such a network would allow the accumulation of enough data to furnish the payer meaningful outcome analysis. There will always be a dynamic process as the pendulum of managed care swings to and from, whether we are dealing with the extremes of capitation or the medical savings account. Those groups who will do well in such an environment will continue to strive to hone their clinical skills, to question their every practice, and to discard those that will not stand close analysis. These groups and only these groups will be able to compete in the medicine of the future.

CONTRACTS AND RESOURCES

Reproductive practitioners today are besieged by solicitations to become a part of various health care plans, often as a subspecialist, specialist, or primary care provider. Even those physicians who have considerable experience with these plans have often entered into unsatisfactory contracts and upon re-review of these documents have elected to discontinue participation in these plans for economic reasons. While obtaining contracts is certainly a physician-driven initiative, the contract process is probably best handled by our colleagues in the legal profession. It has been suggested that there are at least ten pitfalls in contracting, which include such things as retroactive payment denial, changes without consent, access to data, definition of terms, indemnification clauses, extracontractual liability, representations of high quality, appeals processes, post-termination care, and termination at will. Most large law firms now have divisions of medical contracting. One such group is Smith, Anderson, Blount, Dorsett, Mitchell, and Journeygan (LLP), 2500 First Union Capital Center, P.O. Box 2611, Raleigh, NC 27602-2611, 919-821-6612 (Julian D. Bobbitt, Jr.).

Further, there are a number of large benefits consulting firms who will help physicians prepare presentations for managed care plans. The best known is Foster Higgins, Survey and Research Services, 125 Broad Street, New York, NY 10004, 212-574-9025. Foster Higgins is best known for preparation of a national survey of employer-sponsored health care plans, and annually prepares a stratified random sample of all U.S. employers with 10 or more employees. Their reports are priced at $500 and tables at $1,000 each. The reports are usually broken out by West, Midwest, Northeast, and

TABLE 26–2. PERCENTAGE OF PLANS THAT INCLUDE COVERAGE FOR INFERTILITY TREATMENT

	West (%)	Midwest (%)	Northeast (%)	South (%)	All Employers (%)
Traditional medical indemnity	15	26	36	18	20
Preferred provider organizations	31	39	37	23	23
Point-of-service plans	31	38	63	34	25
Health maintenance organizations	40	45	38	25	28

(Reproduced, with permission, from Foster Higgins' National Survey of Employer-Sponsored Health Plans, *1995.)*

South regions. They plot changes in a variety of parameters, usually over a 3- to 4-yr period (Table 26–2).

Larger practices and institutions may need the services of a health care policy firm to develop algorithms and computer software to support them. Such a firm is the Lewin Group, 9302 Lee Highway, Suite 500, Fairfax, VA 22031, 703-218-5500. Legal advice on health law and health policy can be obtained from James F. Blumstein, Professor of Law, Vanderbilt Law School, Nashville, Tennessee 37240, 615-322-2613. At times, reproductive endocrinologists will need marketing analysts to evaluate regional or local demographics, prepare presentations, and support the practice in the field. Such a company is Medical Market Analysts, 4915 Foxbrier Trail, Charlotte, NC 28269.

FUTURE TRENDS

As stated previously in the chapter, I predict that evidence-based medicine and algorithms will define the way we practice. We will work in networks with economy of scale being in our favor. I believe that reproductive endocrinologists will regain control of managed care, because we are in the unique position of furnishing a service that can only be *gained* by *great personal sacrifice* and effort. Therefore, that means a loss of control of managed care by nonphysicians.[49] Further, there will be an elimination of risk sharing, patients will assume more of the responsibility for managing payment of their own health care, and thanks to our colleagues in the legal profession, an end of gatekeepers and restriction of health care benefits by corporate entities. As it must, the portion of our gross national product spent on health care will increase, but that increase will not be proportional as our aging population will require a greater proportion of our attention.

SUMMARY

The concept of managed care is a product of the 20th century, perhaps started with the emergence of the multispecialty clinic around 1914. Its creation is in part due to aging of the population, continuous rising demand for health services, the creation of new technology, and the expanded medical work force of both U.S. and international consistency. Managed care has taken many forms including the early preferred provider organization, followed by the individual practice association. Recently, the emergence of the physician practice management groups and medical service organizations has further complicated the field. In general, managed care has been translated into restriction of services; however, most parties agree that this is not an acceptable permanent solution. One suspects that the use of evidence-based medicine, cost-effective analysis, treatment algorithms, and disease management programs will be the wave of the future.

REFERENCES

1. Wilmut AE, Schnieke AE, McWhir J, et al. Viable offspring derived from fetal and adult mammalian cells. Nature. 385:810, 1997
2. Callahan TL, Hall JE, Ettner SL, et al. The economic impact of multiple-gestation pregnancies and the contribution of assisted-reproduction techniques to their incidence. N Engl J Med. 331:244, 1994
3. Collins JA, Bustillo M, Visscher RD, et al. An estimate of the cost of in vitro fertilization services in the United States in 1995. Fertil Steril. 64:1, 1995
4. Hecht BR. Iatrogenic multifetal pregnancy. Asst Reprod Rev. 3:75, 1993
5. Wilcox LS, Kiely JL, Melvin CL, et al. Assisted reproductive technologies estimates of their contribution to multiple births and newborn hospital days in the United States. Fertil Steril. 65:361, 1996
6. Neumann PJ, Gharib SD, Weinstein MC. The cost of a successful delivery with in vitro fertilization. N Engl J Med. 331:239, 1994
7. Goldfarb JM, Austin C, Lisbona H, et al. Cost-effectiveness of in vitro fertilization. Obstet Gynecol. 87:18, 1996
8. Drake DF. Managed care: A product of market dynamics. *JAMA.* 277:560, 1997
9. Lilford RJ. Hysterectomy: Will it pay the bills in 2007? *Br Med J.* 314:160, 1997
10. Fowles JB, Weiner JP, Knutson D, et al. Taking health status into account when setting capitation rates. *JAMA.* 276:1316, 1996

11. Donelan K, Blendon RJ, Hill CA, et al. Whatever happened to the health insurance crisis in the United States? Voices from a national survey. *JAMA*. 276:1346, 1996

12. Judge K. Income distribution and life expectancy: A critical appraisal. *Br Med J*. 311:1282, 1995

13. Hoffman C, Rice D, Sung HY. Persons with chronic conditions: Their prevalence and costs. *JAMA*. 276:1473, 1996

14. Soules MR. Now that we have painted ourselves in a corner. *Fertil Steril*. 66:693, 1996

15. Frye RL, Wood DL. The business of medicine. *Circulation*. 95:546, 1997

16. Feldman AM, Greenhouse PK, Reis SE, Sevco MS. Academic cardiology division in the era of managed care: A paradigm for survival. *Circulation*. 95:740, 1997

17. Evidence-Based Medicine Working Group. Evidence-based medicine. A new approach to teaching the practice of medicine. *JAMA*. 268:2420, 1992

18. Grimes DA. Introducing evidence-based medicine into a department of obstetrics and gynecology. *Obstet Gynecol*. 86:451, 1995

19. MacPherson DW. Evidence-based medicine. *Can Med Assoc J*. 152:201, 1995

20. Moher D, Jadad AR, Nichol G, et al. Assessing the quality of randomized controlled trials: An annotated bibliography of scales and checklists. *Controlled Clin Trials*. 16:62, 1995

21. Oxman AD, Scakett DL, Guyatt GH. Users' guides to the medical literature. I. How to get started. *JAMA*. 270:2093, 1995

22. Rosenberg W, Donald A. Evidence-based medicine: An approach to clinical problem solving. *Br Med J*. 310:1122, 1995

23. Schultz KF, Chalmers I, Hayes RJ, Altman DG. Empirical evidence of bias. Dimensions of methodological quality associated with estimates of treatment effects in controlled trials. *JAMA*. 273:408, 1995

24. Cappelleri JC, Ioannidis JPA, Schmid CH, et al. Large trials vs Meta-analysis of smaller trials. How do their results compare? *JAMA*. 276:1332, 1996

25. Begg C, Cho M, Eastwood S, et al. Improving the quality of reporting of randomized controlled trials. *JAMA*. 276:637, 1996

26. Russell LB, Gold MR, Siegel JE, et al. The role of cost-effectiveness analysis in health and medicine. *JAMA*. 276:1172, 1996

27. Siegel JE, Weinstein MC, Russell LB, et al. Recommendations for reporting cost-effectiveness analyses. *JAMA*. 276:1339, 1996

28. Alexander DA, Naji AA, Pinion SB, et al. Randomized trial comparing hysterectomy with endometrial ablation for dysfunctional uterine bleeding: Psychiatric and psychosocial aspects. *Br Med J*. 312:280, 1996

29. Unger JB, Meeks GR. Hysterectomy after endometrial ablation. *Am J Obstet Gynecol*. 175:1432, 1996

30. Stovall TG, Summitt RL Jr. Laparoscopic hysterectomy—Is there a benefit? *N Engl J Med*. 335:512, 1996

31. Weber AM, Lee JC. Use of alternative techniques of hysterectomy in Ohio, 1988–1994. *N Engl J Med*. 335:483, 1996

32. Dorsey JH, Holtz PM, Griffiths RI, et al. Costs and charges associated with three alternative techniques of hysterectomy. *N Engl J Med*. 335:476, 1996

33. Psaty BM, Smith NL, Siscovick DS, et al. Health outcomes associated with antihypertensive therapies used as first-line agents. *JAMA*. 277:739, 1997

34. Bates GW, Bates SR. The economics of infertility: Developing an infertility managed-care plan. *Am J Obstet Gynecol*. 174:1200, 1996

35. Blackwell RE. A proposed algorithm for evaluation and treatment of infertility: Update. *Infert Reprod Med*. 7:1, 1995

36. Blackwell RE. Clinical treatment of infertility: A practical algorithm. *Drug Benefit Trends*. 8:17, 1996

37. Page H. Estimation of the prevalence and incidence of infertility in a population: A pilot study. *Fertil Steril*. 51:571, 1989

38. Stein ZA. Reviews and commentary: A woman's age, childbearing and child rearing. *Am J Epidemiol*. 121:327, 1985

39. Hassold T, Chiu D. Maternal age-specific rates of numerical chromosome abnormalities with special reference to trisomy. *Hum Genet*. 70:11, 1985

40. Chow W-H, Daling VR, Cates WJ, et al. Epidemiology of ectopic pregnancy. *Epidemiol Rev*. 9:70, 1987

41. Gleicher N, Vanderlaan B, Karande V, et al. Infertility: Treatment dropout and insurance coverage. *Obstet Gynecol*. 88:289, 1996

42. Glatstein IZ, Harlow BL, Hornstein MD. Practice patterns among reproductive endocrinologists: The infertility evaluation. *Fertil Steril*. 67:443, 1997

43. Little P, Smith L, Carntrell T, et al. General practitioners' management of acute back pain: A survey of reported practice compared with clinical guidelines. *Br Med J*. 312:485, 1996

44. Tucker MH, Howie PW, et al. Should obstetricians see women with normal pregnancies? A multicentre randomized controlled trial of routine antenatal care by general practitioners and midwives compared with shared care led by obstetricians. *Br Med J*. 312:554, 1996

45. Blackwell RE, Carr BR, Change JR, et al. Are we exploiting the infertile couple? *Fertil Steril*. 48:25, 1987

46. Marwick C. Another health care idea: Disease management. *JAMA*. 274:1416, 1995

47. Foy N. *The Yin and Yang of Organizations*. London, Grant McIntyre, 1981

48. Handy C. *Gods of Management. The Changing Work of Organizations*. New York, Oxford University Press, 1995

49. McArthur JH, Moore FD. The two cultures and the health care revolution: Commerce and professionalism in medical care. *JAMA*. 277:985, 1997

Chapter 27

DIAGNOSTIC EVALUATION AND TREATMENT ALGORITHMS FOR THE INFERTILE COUPLE

Karen D. Bradshaw, Samuel J. Chantilis, and Bruce R. Carr

Involuntary infertility affects about 15 to 20 percent of couples or approximately 11 million reproductive age people in the United States.[1] Primary infertility occurs in couples with no previous history of conception; secondary infertility exists when a prior conception has been at a minimum documented by a positive β-human chorionic gonadotropin (β-hCG), histology, or ultrasound. The causes of infertility are equally distributed between the male and female and often the physician encounters multiple etiologies during the investigation. Most infertile couples have one or more of three major causes—a male factor, ovulatory dysfunction, or tubal–peritoneal disease.

With the tendency of more couples practicing contraception and delaying childbearing until the last two decades of a woman's reproductive life, the number of women aware of infertility and seeking care for this disorder is increasing. Several factors account for this. Because of the epidemic of sexually transmitted diseases such as chlamydia and gonorrhea, pelvic infection may lead to tubal occlusion, pelvic adhesions, and distortion of tubal–ovarian anatomy. As women enter the last decade of reproductive capacity, anovulation is more common, as are spontaneous abortions.[2–4] In addition, there may be an increased incidence of endometriosis and uterine pathology such as leiomyoma, intrauterine adhesions, and adenomyosis with advancing age. Also, due to increased use of and availability of contraception and abortion fewer infants are available for adoption. These factors place more demands on physicians who treat infertile couples to provide more accurate, thorough, and rapid evaluation and treatment.

Infertility evaluation and treatment is often expensive. Each year, an estimated 1 billion dollars is spent by infertile couples in pursuit of pregnancy.[5] Unfortunately, many major insurance carriers exclude infertility as a reimbursable diagnosis. Therefore, the financial burden is often left with the infertile couple. One must take these issues into consideration when counseling patients about treatment options available to them. Evaluation of fertility issues may be extremely stressful to some married couples. Loss of privacy, disruption of spontaneous sexual habits, and a feeling of reproductive failure or inadequacy are frequent causes of depression, anxiety, and grief in these patients. The practitioner must be aware of the psychological impact of infertility and be sensitive and understanding to the patient's needs. Referral for counseling or to local infertility support groups may be helpful.

The infertility evaluation serves to: (1) determine the etiology(ies) of infertility as expediently as possible; (2) provide the couple with recommended treatment protocols; (3) determine expected success rates for recommended therapy; (4) educate the couple about their specific disorder and available alternatives. A certain percentage of patients are merely seeking diagnosis and do not intend to pursue therapy or cannot afford recommended diagnostic tests or treatment. Some couples proceed with adoption, while others comply with specific medical and surgical therapy.

GENERAL PRINCIPLES

Definitions

Infertility is usually defined as the inability of a couple practicing frequent intercourse and not using contraception to conceive a child within 1 yr. This definition is based upon investigations by Tietze et al in 1950, who reported that 90 percent of 1727 couples followed for 1 yr became pregnant.[6] The chance of conception depends upon the length of exposure, coital frequency, and the age of the couple. In normal couples, the chances of conception after 1 mo of unprotected intercourse is 25 percent, 70 percent by 6 mo, and 90 percent by 1 yr.[7] Only an additional 5 percent will conceive after waiting an additional 6 to 12 mo. Once fertility therapy is initiated, couples must be counseled that at least 6 mo of therapy are required to test the adequacy for most given treatment regimens.

A thorough evaluation of the infertile couple often reveals one or more causes for failure to conceive. Motivated couples who comply with therapeutic guidelines can expect a 50 to 60 percent chance of conception. A spontaneous, treatment-independent cumulative pregnancy rate of about 30 to 40 percent exists in couples in whom no identifiable cause for the infertility can be determined.[8]

Age Factors

The peak rate of conception occurs in both men and women at age 24 and begins to decline significantly after age 35 so that for every 5 yr the length of time for conception doubles. Thus, in the couple over 30 who meets the definition of either primary or secondary infertility the workup should be initiated and completed as soon as possible. The rate of conception declines in advancing age in women (Table 27–1),[9] as well as the age of the husband.[10]

Causes of Infertility

The exact incidence of the various etiologic factors for infertility appears to vary with the population studied. Fifteen to 20 percent of causes of infertility are due to ovulatory dysfunction; 30 to 40 percent are due to pelvic factors such as endometriosis, adhesions, or tubal disease; 30 to 40 percent are due to male factors such as oligospermia, increased semen viscosity, decreased sperm motility, or decreased semen volume; and less

TABLE 27–1. EXPECTED PERCENTAGE OF NONSTERILE, CURRENTLY MARRIED WOMEN WHO WILL CONCEIVE WITHIN 12 MO OF UNPROTECTED INTERCOURSE

Age Group (yr)	Conceiving in 12 Mo (%)
20–24	86
25–29	78
30–34	63
35–39	52

(Data adapted, with permission, from Hendershot GE, et al, Infertility and Age: An unresolved issue. Family Plan Perspect. 14:287, 1982.[9])

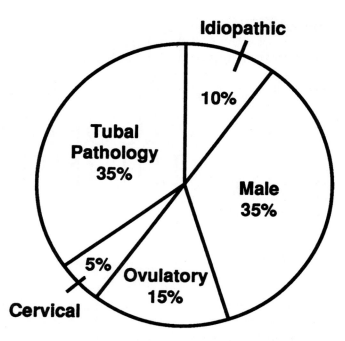

Figure 27–1. Cause and incidence of infertility in couples. In addition, 20 to 40 percent of couples may have multiple factors for infertility.

than 5 percent are due to abnormal sperm–cervical mucus penetration or antisperm antibodies. In about 10 to 15 percent of couples, no cause of their infertility can be found (Fig 27–1). The basic infertility evaluation is aimed at evaluating couples for these disorders. The initial workup of the infertile couple consists of a semen analysis, detection of ovulatory function by various methods, and evaluation of tubal patency by hysterosalpingogram (HSG) with concomitant fluoroscopy. Further evaluation of pelvic anatomy, either by laparoscopy and/or hysteroscopy, is considered a part of the initial workup if there is an abnormality on HSG or later if no cause for infertility can be found. Other procedures such as postcoital testing, antisperm antibodies, sperm penetration assay, or other tests of sperm function may be employed in certain cases.

Evaluation of the Couple as a Unit

It is extremely important to regard infertility as a "two-patient disorder." Male and female partners must be thoroughly evaluated, counseled, and included in the therapeutic decision-making processes. Exclusion of the male partner, for example, leads to feelings of isolation in the female and disinterest and lack of cooperation of the male partner. A questionnaire is often helpful prior to the first visit and should include questions regarding prior conceptions, contraception, coital frequency, and techniques. This document serves as a basis for review and in-depth questioning, not to replace the history. Both partners should be screened for the use of drugs or alcohol that may affect fertility. Studies in males with heavy marijuana use show reduced testosterone levels, decreased sperm counts, and impotency.[11] Alcohol is well known to affect libido and potency as well. Decreases in gonadotropin levels and ovulation are noted in females with frequent drug or alcohol ingestion. Cigarette smoking has also been implicated in subfertility. Early menopause, reduced spermatogenesis, and decreased steroid production have been noted in individuals who use cigarettes.[12] Life table analysis studies demonstrate a longer period of time to conception for smokers as compared to nonsmokers.[13]

INITIAL CONSULTATION

Complete Medical and Gynecologic History

The basic evaluation of an infertile couple is generally agreed upon (see Fig 27–2). The evaluation consists of a detailed history, physical examination, an assessment of ovulation, semen evaluation, and utero-tubal assessment. In addition, estradiol and FSH levels obtained on the third day of the menstrual cycle may be useful in women older than 35.[14]

Female. A thorough workup is based upon an extensive history and physical examination. The woman should be asked about the timing of her pubertal development and menarche. Menstrual history should include cycle length, duration and amount of bleeding, associated dysmenorrhea, and premenstrual symptoms. A history of spontaneous, regular, cyclic predictable menses is, in almost all women, consistent with ovulation, while a history of amenorrhea or abnormal or unpredictable bleeding suggests anovulation or uterine pathology. Previous pregnancies, abortions, and birth control history is also documented. The patient should be asked about dyspareunia and dysmenorrhea that may be linked to endometriosis. A history of pelvic inflammatory disease, sexually transmitted disease, ruptured appendix or other abdominal surgery, and past use of an intrauterine device may be associated with tubal disease. A history of galactorrhea may be an indication of elevated prolactin levels, while a history of pubertal onset of progressive hirsutism associated with oligomenorrhea may indicate polycystic ovarian disease or other disorders of androgen excess. Excessive weight loss or gain, stress, and exercise are often associated with ovulatory disorders. Sexual, social, and psychological issues should be explored. Any prior infertility evaluation, surgery, or medical therapy is essential

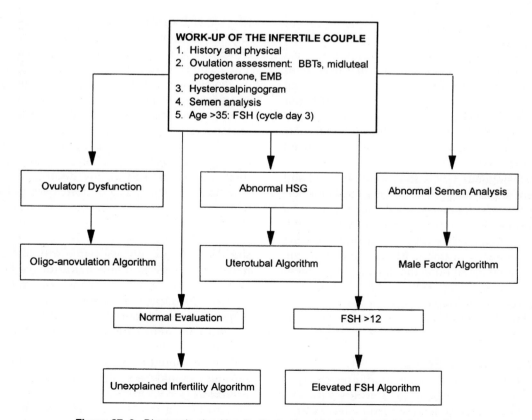

Figure 27–2. Diagnostic algorithm for the basic evaluation of an infertile couple.

information and therefore records, films, or photos should be sought and carefully re-evaluated.

Male. The husband should be questioned about prior fertility, general health, medications, genital surgery, trauma, infection, and impotence. A history of drug or alcohol abuse, frequent hot tub baths, constricting underwear, excess stress, fatigue, and excessive or infrequent coitus should be elicited. Medical conditions that may result in infertility include diabetes (retrograde ejaculation), any serious debilitating disease, mumps orchitis, and pituitary hypofunction, which all may lead to hypogonadism. Herniorrhaphy, varicocele, and bladder neck suspensions are surgical procedures that may potentially be associated with infertility.

Careful Review of Records

Most infertile couples have had some prior evaluation for causes of their infertility, and this information is extremely important and should be reviewed. Couples may not understand the complexity of a thorough infertility evaluation. Many times, the proper infertility evaluation might have been satisfactory by standards set 20 or 30 yr ago, but is far from adequate by today's standards. In addition, review of the couples' records and reports may suggest a different interpretation: For instance, the woman who is proven to be ovulatory may have a cycle length of 25 days with a biphasic rise of basal body temperature but the temperature elevation only lasts 7 to 11 days, which indicates a short luteal phase. An HSG that was reported as normal may be of such poor quality to adequately rule out uterine filling defects or evaluate tubal patency. In addition, it is not uncommon to see couples who have experienced an extensive female evaluation and treatment for 5 or 6 years who have not had a semen analysis or one re-evaluated during that time.

Therefore, previous HSGs should be obtained and films reviewed. If previous pelvic surgery has been performed, operative notes, photos, or videotapes should be obtained and reviewed. Hormonal studies including follicle-stimulating hormone (FSH), luteinizing hormone (LH), progesterone, thyrotropin (TSH), and prolactin should be evaluated based upon the day within the menstrual cycle the sample was collected. Prior treatment regimens should be evaluated as to efficacy and length of treatment. All medications used by the couple should be reviewed.

Physical Examination: Female

A thorough general physical examination is necessary to help define factors that may lead to infertility with special attention to signs of endocrine disturbance such as abnormal size or consistency of the thyroid gland, skin pigmentation, or the presence of abdominal stria. The presence of acne, oily skin, and hirsutism indicates androgen excess. Acanthosis nigricans, the presence of galactorrhea, surgical scars, or significant variation from normal body weight or percent body fat should be noted. The degree of estrogenization of the vagina and the quality and quantity of cervical mucus should be observed in the context of the current phase of the menstrual cycle. The presence of vaginal or cervical infection should be evaluated by microscopic exam of a wet prep of a vaginal smear. The cervix is also carefully examined for anatomic abnormalities due to intrauterine exposure to diethylstilbestrol or prior cervical surgery, including cryotherapy, cautery, or laser. Cervical cultures for gonococcus, chlamydia, and Pap smears may be obtained. A thorough pelvic examination should detect the presence of cervical, uterine, adnexal tenderness, and pelvic masses. The size and contour of the uterus and adnexa should also be described. A careful rectovaginal exam should be performed to palpate uterosacral nodularity found in endometriosis. The length and direction of uterine cavity should be gently measured with a sterile plastic catheter to check for cervical stenosis, as well as depth and direction of the uterine cavity. This information may aid in future intrauterine inseminations or embryo transfers.

Physical Examination: Male

Physical examination of the male can be performed by either the gynecologist, urologist, or family physician. The exam should focus on the degree of secondary sexual development, general body habitus, height, arm span, and presence of gynecomastia. A general physical exam is performed and should include evaluation of perineal sensation and rectal sphincter tone.

Examination of the male genitals begins with careful inspection of the penis. Size and location of the urethral meatus, as well as any discharge or evidence of stricture, is evaluated. The testes are individually palpated, and the relative weights, sizes, and consistency should be evaluated. The average volume for an adult testis is 25 ml or approximately 5×3 cm. Very small or soft testes are usually associated with a decrease in germinal tissue mass due to either testicular failure or some abnormality in the hypothalamic–pituitary axis leading to hypogonadotropic hypogonadism. The epididymis is palpated along its course to evaluate for swelling or tenderness consistent with epididymitis. The vas deferens should be evaluated by palpation. The presence of a varicocele should be looked for following valsalva. The prostrate should be evaluated for size and evidence of prostatitis (see Chap 28).

Following the history and physical examination of both partners, an initial diagnosis should be made. The history and physical examination may clearly point to one or more etiologies. During the first evaluation, initial laboratory and diagnostic tests should be ordered.

INITIAL LABORATORY AND DIAGNOSTIC TESTS

Basic Laboratory Testing

While routine preobstetrical screening of infertile women is not mandatory, it is extremely helpful to screen patients for anemia; blood type, including RH; and antibody status. Women may need RhoGAM following early spontaneous abortions or ectopic pregnancies. Women with a negative titer for rubella will require immunization prior to therapy for infertility. Acquired immunodeficiency syndrome (AIDS) testing and hepatitis screening are essential in high-risk populations, those undergoing assisted reproductive techniques, and those receiving cryopreserved gametes. Some physicians screen all patients, with appropriate patient consent, yet the widespread screening for AIDS in low-risk women has not been shown to be cost effective.

Hormonal Testing

Ovulation Documentation

EVALUATION OF OVULATION. Ovulatory factors account for up to 25 percent of infertility and may be due to a multitude of factors that may be elicited in the initial history. This includes a history compatible with polycystic ovarian disease, oligomenorrhea, or amenorrhea associated with weight loss or excessive obesity, exercise, eating disorders, and galactorrhea. If the woman is experiencing cyclic menses, adequate ovulation and follicle development should be assessed by a number of methods in multiple cycles. Basal body temperature charting, sonographic follicle monitoring, urinary LH testing, midluteal progesterone levels, and endometrial biopsy are important tests to evaluate ovulation and subsequent corpus luteum function.

BASAL BODY TEMPERATURE. The basal body temperature chart, although much maligned, is still a useful and cost-effective index of evaluating ovulation. A biphasic temperature chart characterized by a sustained increased temperature of at least 0.4 °F for 12 to 15 days is consistent with ovulation and an adequate luteal phase length (Fig 27–3). The day of ovulation is usually suggested by day of the lowest temperature (nadir) and is followed by a sustained rise in temperature of 0.4 °F. However, significant variation in temperature may occur and it may be difficult to predict the time or presence of ovulation in some cycles. Luteal phase length less than 11 days as measured by basal body temperature chart recording correlates well with luteal phase defects diagnosed by endometrial biopsy. Finally, the temperature chart serves as a visual reminder for the couple and physician as to the frequency and timing of intercourse and the timing of medications and studies in the infertility evaluation. It is our practice to write the various steps of the workup in

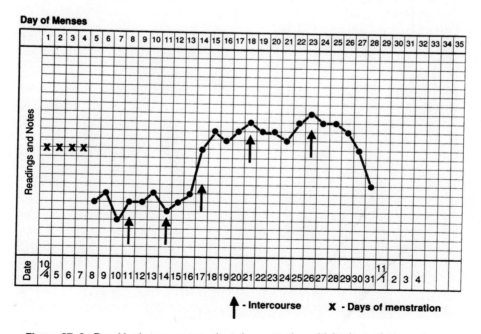

Figure 27–3. Basal body temperature chart demonstrating a biphasic, ovulatory pattern.

the margins of a temperature chart and on the first consultation give the patient a written outline as to the steps that will be involved in their infertility workup. This reassures the couple that a plan has been established and will be carried out within a reasonable period of time.

SERUM PROGESTERONE. The use of serum progesterone levels obtained at midluteal phase evaluates the occurrence and adequacy of ovulation and corpus luteum function. Most clinicians agree that a level of 10 ng/ml or greater is indicative of adequate ovulation (luteinization). Other investigators have suggested that three samples obtained in the luteal phase totaling 15 ng/ml constitutes normal ovulation. However, it should be remembered that progesterone is secreted in a pulsatile manner and a single low level may not indicate a defect of luteal function. Therefore, one might suggest that if progesterone is to be used as an index for ovulation, it should be used in multiple cycles or that multiple levels should be drawn every other day during the luteal phase and averaged to yield a single result.

ENDOMETRIAL BIOPSY. The endometrial biopsy may also be used to confirm ovulation and diagnose a luteal phase defect. It is usually performed late in the cycle,

1 to 2 days before expected menstruation. It is recommended that the couple refrain from intercourse or use barrier contraception during the cycle that the endometrial biopsy is obtained. The sample of endometrium is obtained with a curette from the anterior or lateral walls of the uterus fundus. The dating of the endometrium is best correlated with the timing of the ovulation as detected by sonography or LH timing rather than backdating from the onset of the subsequent menstrual cycle. It should also be noted that a delay in maturation of a single endometrial biopsy is a common finding and therefore must be repeated in another cycle before it may be interpreted as indicative of the presence of a luteal phase defect. Further, as stated previously, the use of sonography or urinary LH monitoring may enhance the predictive value of both midluteal progesterone measurement and endometrial biopsy.

Preovulatory transvaginal sector sonography is a highly useful tool for evaluating adequate follicle development, endometrial assessment, and oocyte release (Fig 27–4). A triple-line endometrial pattern seen on sonography before ovulation is predictive of subsequent pregnancy.[15] Sonography is best used in combination with home LH urinary testing kits. It has been proposed that a considerable amount of previously unexplained

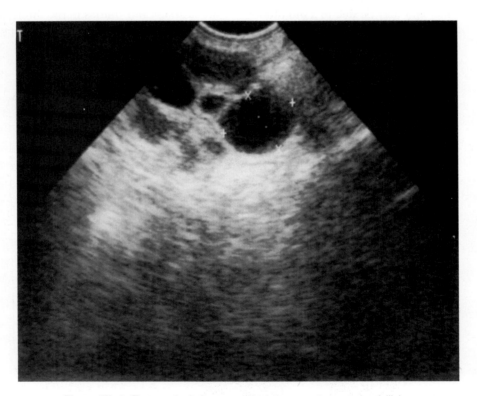

Figure 27–4. Transvaginal ultrasound depicting a mature ovarian follicle.

infertility may be due to dysfolliculogenesis (ie, development of multiple small follicles that bring about premature or inadequate luteinization). Regardless of the method chosen to assess adequate ovulation, we suggest that luteal abnormalities be detected by various methods in multiple cycles before instituting therapy. We usually will obtain a serum thyroid-stimulating hormone (TSH) and prolactin in most women with infertility but in all women with amenorrhea and/or galactorrhea. Serum androgens are only obtained in hirsute women and gonadotropins are obtained only in women with amenorrhea. However, we suggest that a day 3 FSH level be obtained in women over the age of 35 to detect rises in FSH consistent with early ovarian failure.

In women with ovulatory dysfunction with normal TSH, prolactin, and FSH (if indicated), ovulation induction can be initiated with clomiphene citrate in appropriate doses to effect ovulation (see also Chap 29). Figure 27–5 outlines a treatment algorithm for infertile couples with oligo-anovulation. In women who have not conceived after 6 ovulatory cycles, a diagnostic laparoscopy may be considered to evaluate for the presence of asymptomatic endometriosis or pelvic adhesions. Three cycles of menotropin therapy should then be initiated with estradiol and sonographic monitoring followed by intrauterine insemination with washed husband's sperm (IUH; see Chap 29). If pregnancy has still not been achieved, up to 3 cycles of in vitro fertilization (IVF)

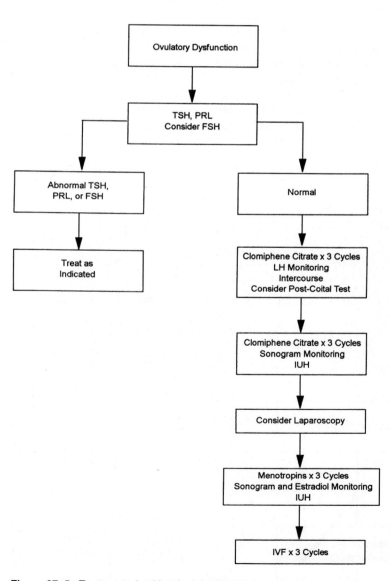

Figure 27–5. Treatment algorithm for infertile couples with oligo-anovulation.

should be offered to the infertile couple (see Chap 33). Patients with a day 3 FSH >12 mIU/ml should have a repeat FSH and estradiol. With persistent elevation of these values, oocyte donation may be considered (Fig 27–6).

Semen Analysis

A semen specimen should be examined in all couples presenting with infertility. The specimen is obtained by masturbation into a sterile collection cup. Forty-eight to 72 hr of abstinence is recommended prior to analysis. The sample should be delivered to the laboratory within 1 hr of collection. The test should be *insisted* upon despite a history of past paternity, as paternity may in fact be in doubt in a troubled relationship. Frequently, one encounters the infertile couple who have had a normal postcoital test in the past and this has been interpreted as adequate evaluation of the male. However, the postcoital test does not substitute for a formal semen analysis. Often, reluctance to obtain a semen analysis may be due to embarrassment or hesitation about masturbation. This can be overcome by the use of silicon condoms, which allow the man to produce a semen sample by intercourse. It should be noted, however, that most condoms are made with latex and should not be used for collection

purposes because latex may be toxic and most of these condoms are also coated with nonoxynol-9, a detergent that will disrupt cell membranes and is therefore a potent spermicide.

The semen analysis should have a volume of 2 to 5 cc, 20 to 200 million sperm/cc with 50 percent directional motility, 0 to 40 percent abnormal forms, liquefication at room temperature in 1 to 20 min, and a pH of 7.5 with a range of 7.0 to 8.0. There is a great variation from sample to sample in terms of volume, number, and motility, and in addition there may be seasonal variation in these values. Therefore, it is recommended that if an abnormality is found, a repeat analysis should be carried out 2 to 3 mo later to determine the presence of a male factor. It is *inappropriate* to designate a male as infertile based upon a single semen analysis.

The use of IUI for the primary treatment of male factor infertility associated with severe oligospermia or oligoasthenospermia remains controversial because of extremely low pregnancy rates.[16,17] For couples with severe oligospermia or those with sperm-directed antibodies, IVF may be a better choice. Couples with mild-moderate oligospermia, on the other hand, may be treated with IUI in conjunction with menotropins for

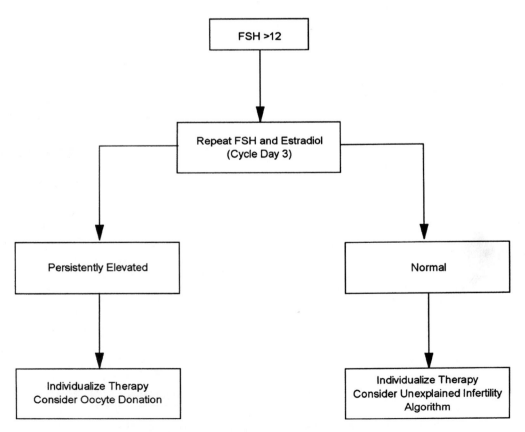

Figure 27–6. Treatment algorithm for elevated cycle day 3 FSH.

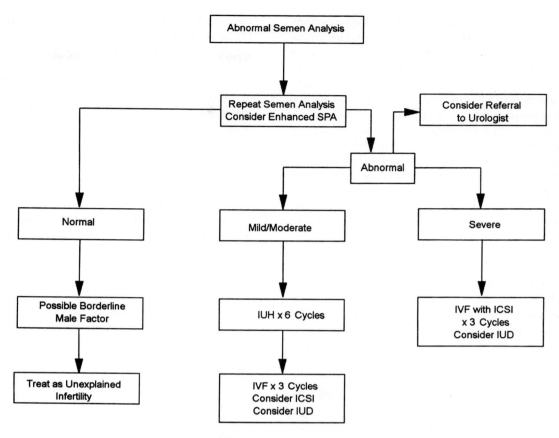

Figure 27–7. Treatment algorithm for male factor infertility.

controlled ovarian hyperstimulation prior to IVF. A treatment algorithm for male factor infertility is outlined in Figure 27–7 (see also Chap 28). In men with repeat abnormal semen analysis, an enhanced sperm penetration assay (SPA) as well as referral to a urologist specializing in male infertility may be considered. Persistent infertility can be treated with IVF with consideration of intracytoplasmic sperm injection (ICSI) or the use of donor sperm.

TUBAL–UTERINE EVALUATION

HSG

The HSG is an important tool in infertility evaluation.[18] The HSG provides information regarding the shape of the uterine cavity and patency of the fallopian tubes. It should be performed in the early follicular phase of the cycle, as soon as menstrual bleeding has ceased. This eliminates the risk of reflux of blood or performing the procedure during early conception. It is our practice to reduce the small chance of infection (1 to 3 percent)[19] following this procedure by: (1) avoiding performing the procedure in a woman with significant pelvic tenderness

or adnexal mass suspected to be a tubo-ovarian complex; (2) chlamydia and/or gonococcal screening; (3) prophylactic antibiotics (usually doxycycline 100 mg bid beginning the day before procedure and continuing until the day after; and (4) Betadine application to the cervix before this procedure. There has been some evidence that an HSG itself is therapeutic, and pregnancies have been reported following the procedure.[20]

For best results, it is recommended that not only the radiologist but also the physician be present during the hysterosalpingography. In this way, the actual procedure can be adapted to specific needs as determined by the appearance on the monitor. The dye may be oil or water based: There are as yet limited data to resolve which dye is preferred although there are some indications that the pregnancy rates are somewhat higher when an oil-based medium is used.[21] Hysterosalpingography can, in rare instances, result in allergic reactions or infections. Women who are allergic to iodine or are suspected of having occult infections should not undergo this procedure.

Following an initial film, 3 to 5 ml dye should be injected slowly to allow adequate visualization of the uterine cavity. A second film is then taken. Cervical traction is often necessary to completely evaluate the uterine cavity.

A small acorn tip is preferred over balloon-type catheters, as the latter obstructs the visualization of the cavity (Fig 27–8). Following this, another 5 ml is injected to evaluate tubal patency, followed by a third film. A follow-up film is taken to evaluate peritubal adhesions and usually is performed in 10 min (using water-soluble media) or 24 hr (oil-based media).

El-Yahia recently described the results of laparoscopic investigation in 130 women following a normal HSG.[22] Diagnostic laparoscopy was performed following an evaluation including normal semen analysis, pelvic examination, historical screening for pelvic inflammatory disease, prolactin and thyroxine assays, postcoital test, and confirmation of ovulation. All of the women reported at least 1 yr of unprotected intercourse without conception. In this retrospective review, only 42.3 percent of the women were noted to have normal pelvic anatomy at laparoscopy. Pelvic adhesive disease was observed in 20 percent (27 patients). The remainder of abnormalities included pelvic endometriosis, pelvic inflammatory disease, and uterine leiomyoma. Cundiff et al suggest the following for infertile couples who have a normal HSG: (1) Laparoscopy should not be performed until 3 months after a normal HSG because of the potential therapeutic effect of HSG; (2) however, laparoscopy should be performed after a normal HSG if pregnancy has not occurred by 6 mo to 1 yr because of the high incidence of pelvic pathology; and (3) HSG using water-soluble contrast media has a therapeutic effect comparable to that described for oil-soluble contrast media.[23]

Mild distal tubal disease may be amenable to laparoscopic tuboplasty, while moderate to severe tubal occlusion (Fig 27–9) is most effectively managed with IVF (see Chap 31). When a proximal tubal occlusion is evident on HSG, a laparoscopy and hysteroscopy with tubal cannulation should be performed (Fig 27–10). Uterine filling defects are evaluated with office hysteroscopy and treated appropriately. Patients with a normal HSG and laparoscopy evaluation are treated according to the unexplained infertility algorithm (Fig 27–11).

Timing of Testing. In the first month of evaluation, the use of condoms or barrier contraceptives is suggested. On day 1, the woman begins the basal body temperature (BBT). An HSG is scheduled for days 7 to 11 of the cycle to avoid menstruation and the possibility of radiation exposure to a potential embryo. Home urine LH testing is begun on days 10 through 18. A serum progesterone level is obtained on day 21 or more accurately 7 days after the LH surge. An endometrial biopsy is taken on days 25 to 28, again most accurately dated to LH surge. During this time, a semen analysis is also obtained.

In the second month, a follow-up visit is scheduled. This may be done on days 12 to 14 or following the LH surge, at which time a PCT is performed if indicated. At this time, test results, HSG films, and other data are reviewed with the couple (Table 27–2).

Following these tests, further evaluation may be indicated. If all tests are normal, or if the HSG suggests tubal pathology (Fig 27–9), a laparoscopy (hysteroscopy is optional unless uterine pathology is suggested from an abnormal HSG) is indicated.

FURTHER DIAGNOSTIC TESTING

Laparoscopy

The next test frequently done in an infertility evaluation is a laparoscopy and/or hysteroscopy. A laparoscopy is performed when all other tests have been normal or when there is reason to suspect intra-abdominal pathology (such as endometriosis, pelvic adhesions, or uterine leiomyoma) (Fig 27–10). Laparoscopy is scheduled in the early to mid-follicular phase of the cycle to avoid disrupting a pregnancy or a well-vascularized corpus luteum. At this stage of the

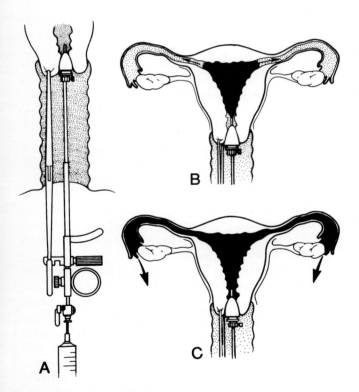

Figure 27–8. Technique of hysterosalpingography. **A.** A tenaculum is placed on the anterior cervical lip and a Jarco cannula is placed in the external cervical os. **B.** With gentle traction on the cervix, a small amount of radio-opaque dye is instilled in the uterine cavity under fluoroscopic control. **C.** Additional dye is instilled to check for patency of fallopian tubes. (Note: the tenaculum is placed on the side of the cervix for diagrammatic purposes only; it is usually placed on the anterior lip of the cervix.)

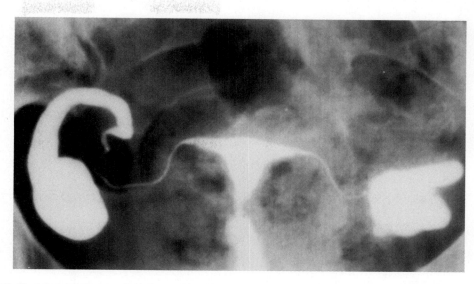

Figure 27–9. Hysterosalpingogram depicting a normal endocervical canal, uterine cavity, and large bilateral hydrosalpinx.

cycle, the thickness of the endometrium is low, allowing for accurate evaluation of the uterine cavity. If hysteroscopic surgery is planned due to a suggestive abnormality of the HSG (and adhesions, septums, or leiomyomas), it may be useful to pretreat the patient with gonadotropin-releasing hormone (GnRH) analogs or Danazol to reduce the height of the endometrium, thereby increasing visualization.

Most infertility procedures (lysis of adhesions, removal or ablation of endometriosis lesions, or tubal surgery) can be performed via the laparoscope using video monitoring. Thus, the infertility surgeon should be able to perform these procedures if indicated. An inex-

perienced gynecologist or one who only rarely performs laparoscopic (operative laparoscopy, pelviscopic surgery) or hysteroscopic surgery should refer the patient to a reproductive endocrinologist or reproductive surgeon. Hysteroscopy usually requires dilation of the cervix and use of distending medium such as Hyscon, sorbitol, or glycine. Following this procedure, a cannula or catheter should be inserted into the cervix so that methylene blue or indigo carmine dye can be injected during laparoscopy to evaluate tubal patency.

The laparoscopic procedure should be performed under general anesthesia in steep Trendelenburg position.

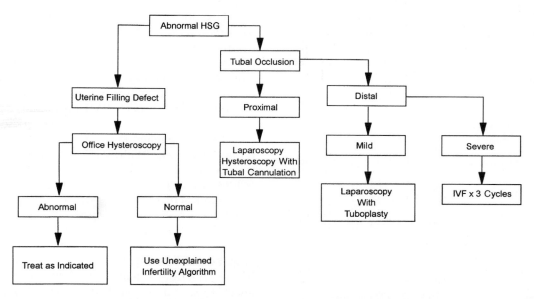

Figure 27–10. Treatment algorithm for utero-tubal infertility diagnosed by an abnormal HSG.

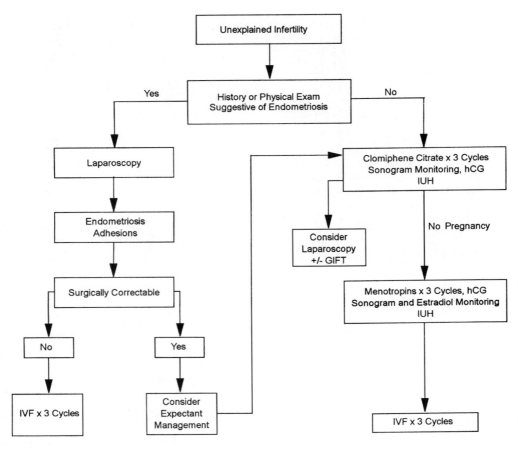

Figure 27–11. Treatment algorithm for unexplained infertility.

The laparoscope is usually inserted following CO_2 insufflation with a verris needle through the umbilicus, although recent studies suggest that similar results and safety can be obtained with direct trocar insertion, followed by CO_2 instillation.[24] After the peritoneal cavity is visualized, one or two secondary punctures are required to adequately visualize pelvic structures. A thorough evaluation in a planned, clockwise, organized manner is required to rule out pelvic pathology including the undersurface of the ovaries. Proper staging by the American Society for Reproductive Medicine for pelvic adhesions, tubal disease, and endometriosis is performed.[25] Photos or videotaping is often helpful to document disease. In women who have a normal laparoscopy or who have undergone surgical correction of either endometriosis or adhesions, expectant management or a more aggressive treatment for "unexplained infertility" may be pursued (Fig 27–11). Utilizing this algorithm, patients undergo 3 cycles of clomiphene citrate stimulation with sonogram monitoring, hCG, and IUI. If no pregnancy results, laparoscopy with GIFT or 3 cycles of menotropin therapy and IUI should be offered prior to proceeding to IVF (see also Chaps 26, 29, 31, and 32).

ADDITIONAL OPTIONAL TESTS

Postcoital Testing

A postcoital test has been advocated to evaluate the presence of cervical factors. Unfortunately, most poor postcoital tests are the result of inadequate timing. Most often, the test is performed on day 12 of the cycle, but if

TABLE 27–2. TIMING AND COORDINATION OF INFERTILITY TESTING

Month 1 following first visit (barrier contraceptives recommended)

Day 1	Initiate BBT
Days 7–11	HSG
Days 10–18	LH urine testing
Day 21 (or 1 week after LH surge)	Progesterone level
Days 25–28	Endometrial biopsy (dated to LH surge)
Days 1–28	Semen analysis

Month 2

Days 12–14	PCT (or at LH surge)
	Review test results, confirm diagnosis, and plan treatment or schedule other tests if indicated

ovulation occurs earlier or later, the test will often result in immobile sperm. It has been our observation that many so-called cervical factors have as their origin poor timing or inadequate follicle development with poor estrogen production.

There is considerable lack of standardization in postcoital testing. We advocate that the test be done 24 to 36 hr prior to ovulation determined by urinary LH testing and that 0 to 4 hr elapse between intercourse and the examination. At that time, one should find an open cervix and clear cervical mucus with spinbarkeit 8 to 10 cm and 5 to 15 directionally motile sperm per high-power field. Despite the manner in which the postcoital test is carried out, some investigators have suggested that it provides little information regarding potential fertility.[26] Support for this contention comes from the finding of sperm in the peritoneal fluid at laparoscopy in patients having poor postcoital tests and the finding that 27 percent of fertile couples show either no sperm or less than one sperm per high-power field in their postcoital test.[27] Nevertheless, at a minimum, information is gained about the adequacy of coital technique if a normal postcoital test is obtained.

Sperm Antibodies

The incidence of antisperm antibodies is less than 2 percent in serum, sperm, and cervical mucus in fertile men and women. However, the levels range from 5 to 25 percent in serum, sperm, and cervical mucus of infertile couples.[28,29]

Some considerations are helpful in choosing which couples should be tested for antisperm antibodies. Clinical conditions in which the blood–testis or excurrent ductal system is breached, such as a history of testicular biopsy, vasectomy reversal, or obstructive lesion of the male ductal system, should be tested. Sperm agglutination is frequently a result of genital tract infection due to prostatitis, urethritis, or epididymitis. These disorders should be treated with antibiotics before testing for sperm antibodies. The absence of motile sperm in midcycle cervical mucus after intercourse has been correlated with sperm-associated antisperm antibodies in approximately 50 percent of men.[30] As many as 17 percent of women in couples with unexplained infertility are found to have serum antisperm antibodies. Women with a history of frequent receptive anal or oral intercourse should be considered for antisperm antibody testing.[29]

Clumping found on the standard semen analysis may also be consistent with antibodies. Specific tests for antisperm antibodies in cervical mucus, serum, and seminal plasma are available, and at present the immunobead test is recommended. The significance of these tests in regard to infertility workup, however, is not always clear because some couples have been known to conceive in the presence of high levels of antisperm antibodies.

However, physicians believe that decreased or impaired movement of sperm through genital tract secretions and failure of fertilization may be due to sperm antibodies. Patients with high levels of antibodies and prolonged infertility should be offered IVF with possible ICSI.

Hamster Egg Penetration Test

This test is aimed at assessing the ability of spermatozoa to undergo capacitation and achieve fertilization. Egg penetration equal to or greater than 10 percent is considered normal in most centers. In the absence of any other abnormal findings, a test that reveals less than 10 percent penetration may suggest the existence of subtle factors that affect the ability of sperm to penetrate and fertilize the egg. However, the clinical relevance of such results remains to be established, especially because pregnancy can still occur under these circumstances.

PSYCHOLOGICAL EVALUATION

Every aspect of the infertility evaluation evokes some emotional and psychological stresses for the couples involved. Many times, in a large, busy medical practice, it may be difficult for physicians to spend the time necessary to allow frustrated couples to ventilate their feelings and give feedback on management and outcomes. Investigators have found a higher incidence of emotional disturbance in infertile women than among matched controls.[31] Infertile couples have described themselves as being "damaged," "defective," "hollow," and "empty."[32,33]

The physical and mental consequences of the infertility workup, subsequent treatment, and lack of success may either cause or greatly exacerbate a psychological problem. Physicians who treat infertile couples should be aware of the enormous stress infertility places on both partners and able to understand the psychological interventions that are effective in alleviating some of the stress.[34] Probably all couples experiencing infertility could greatly benefit from counseling and in our practice all new patients are offered follow-up with a professional psychologist who is trained with associated infertility problems. There are three times in the evaluation and therapy that intervention is encouraged: (1) with the beginning of the infertility evaluation; (2) when psychiatric indications are obvious; and (3) at the termination of unsuccessful treatment or with a pregnancy loss. Couples participating in artificial insemination with donor (AID) or donor oocyte are all strongly encouraged to seek counseling.

Anxiety often occurs during the infertility evaluation. However, depression seems to be the most common reaction to failed fertility treatment. Because many couples believe this is their last hope for a biologic child and because their expectations are great, this reaction is consistent. In fact, failed outcome may translate into loss of a loved one, which is commonly associated with depression. The percentage of patients who develop an episode of depression after failed IVF ranges from approximately 25 to 40 percent.[35-37] There is also a suggestion that the severity of the response varies over time. One group found that women with 2 to 3 yr of infertility had higher depression scores than women who had either longer or shorter durations of infertility.[36]

Therapy of infertility rarely offers a clear end point for cessation after repeated failures. Paulson[34] suggests that all couples establish an ongoing relationship with a qualified counselor, be given the option of stopping treatment from the start, and be encouraged to seek second opinions throughout treatment. Some couples require time off from treatment to regroup, decrease their level of stress, and re-evaluate their decision to continue treatment. Arbitrary time limits, based upon known success rates and life table analysis, should be set at the beginning of treatment regimens so that if conception does not occur, prognosis and options can be re-assessed. For some couples, this may be the time to stop or interrupt treatment for a period of time or begin adoption proceedings (see also Chap 35).

REFERENCES

1. Menning BE. The psychology of infertility. In: Aimen J, ed. *Infertility: Diagnosis and Management*. New York, N.Y., Springer-Verlag, 1984: 17–29
2. Federation CECOS, Schwartz D, Mayaux MJ. Female fecundity as a function of age: Results of artificial insemination in 2193 nulliparous women with azoospermic husbands. *N Engl J Med*. 306:404, 1982
3. Gindoff PR, Jewelewicz R. Reproductive potential in the older woman. *Fertil Steril*. 46:989, 1986
4. James W. The causes of the decline in fecundability with age. *Soc Biol*. 26:330, 1979
5. U.S. Congress, Office of Technology Assessment. *Infertility: Medical and Social Choices*. OTA-BA 358. Washington, D.C., U.S. Government Printing Office, 1988, pp 1–402
6. Tietze C, Guttmacher AF, Rusin S. Time required for conception in 1727 planned pregnancies. *Fertil Steril*. 1:338, 1950
7. Fundamental considerations. In: Keller DW, Strickler RC, Warren JC, eds. *Clinical Infertility*. Norwalk, Conn., Appleton-Century-Crofts, 1984: 1–9
8. Collins JA, Wrixon W, Janes LB, Wilson EH. Treatment-independent pregnancy among infertile couples. *N Engl J Med*. 309:1201, 1983
9. Hendershot GE, Mosher WD, Pratt WF. Infertility and age: An unresolved issue. *Family Plan Perspect*. 14:287, 1982
10. Guzick D, Bradshaw KD, Grun B, et al. Factors affecting the probability of pregnancy in a cycle of donor insemination. *Proc Am Fert Soc*. 35, abstr 170, 1986
11. Hembree WC, Zeidenberg P, Nahas GG. Marijuana's effect on human gonadal function. In: Nahas GG, ed. *Marijuana, Chemistry, Biochemistry and Cellular Effects*. New York, N.Y., Springer-Verlag, 1976: 521–532
12. Hammond EC. Smoking in relation to physical complaints. *Arch Environ Health*. 3:146, 1961
13. Baird DD, Wilcox AJ. Cigarette smoking associated with delayed conception. *JAMA*. 253:2679, 1985
14. Scott RT Jr, Hofmann GE. Prognostic assessment of ovarian reserve. *Fertil Steril*. 63:1, 1995
15. Serafini P, Batzofin J, Nelson J, Olive D. Sonographic uterine predictors of pregnancy in women undergoing ovulation induction for assisted reproductive treatments. *Fertil Steril*. 62:815, 1994
16. Dodson WC, Haney AF. Controlled ovarian hyperstimulation and intrauterine insemination for treatment of infertility. *Fertil Steril*. 55:457, 1991
17. Arici A, Byrd W, Bradshaw KD, et al. Evaluation of clomiphene citrate and human chorionic gonadotropin treatment: A prospective, randomized, crossover study during intrauterine insemination cycles. *Fertil Steril*. 61:314, 1994
18. Marshak RH, Roole CS, Goldberger MA. Hysterography and hysterosalpingography. *Surg Gynecol Obstet*. 91:182, 1950
19. Measday B. An analysis of the complications of hysterosalpingography. *J Obstet Gynecol Br Emp*. 67:663, 1960
20. Alper MM, Garner PR, Spence JEH, et al. Pregnancy rates after hysterosalpingography with oil- and water-soluble contrast media. *Obstet Gynecol*. 68:6, 1986
21. Mackey RA, Glass RH, Olson LE, Vaidya R. Pregnancy following hysterosalpingography with oil- and water-soluble dye. *Fertil Steril*. 22:504, 1971
22. El-Yahia AW. Laparoscopic evaluation of apparently normal infertile women. *Aust NZ J Obstet Gynaecol*. 34:440, 1994
23. Cundiff G, Carr BR, Marshburn PB. Infertile couples with a normal hysterosalpingogram: Reproductive outcome and its relationship to clinical and laparoscopic findings. *J Reprod Med*. 40:19, 1995
24. Byron JW, Fujiyoshi CA, Miyazawa K. Evaluation of the direct trocar insertion technique at laparoscopy. *Obstet Gynecol*. 74:423, 1989
25. Buttram VC. Evolution of the revised American Fertility Society classification of endometriosis. *Fertil Steril*. 43:347, 1985
26. Griffith CS, Grimes DA. The validity of the post-coital test. *Am J Obstet Gynecol*. 162:615, 1990
27. Asch RH. Sperm recovery in peritoneal aspirate after negative Sims–Huhner test. *Int J Fertil*. 23:57, 1978
28. Kutteh WH, McAllister D, Byrd W, Mestecky J. Antisperm antibodies: Current knowledge and new horizons. *Mol Androl*. 4:183, 1992
29. Marshburn PB, Kutteh WH. The role of antisperm antibodies in infertility. Fertil Steril. 61:799, 1994
30. Mathur S, Williamson HO, Baker ME, et al. Sperm motility on postcoital testing correlates with male autoimmunity to sperm. *Fertil Steril*. 41:81, 1984
31. Eisner B. Some psychological differences between fertile and infertile women. *J Clin Psychol*. 19:391, 1963
32. Seibel M, Taymor M. Emotional aspects of infertility. *Fertil Steril*. 37:137, 1982
33. Sandelowski M. Sophie's choice: A metaphor for infertility. *Health Care Women Int*. 7:439, 1986

34. Paulson RJ, Sauer MV. Counseling the infertile couple: When enough is enough. *Obstet Gynecol.* 78:462, 1991

35. Beaurepaire J, Jones M, Thiering P, et al. Psychosocial adjustment to infertility and its treatment: Male and female response at different stages of IVF/ET treatment. *J Psychosom Res.* 38:229, 1994

36. Boivin J, Takefman JE, Tulandi T, Brender W. Reactions to infertility based on extent of treatment failure. *Fertil Steril.* 63:801, 1995

37. Domar AD, Broome A, Zuttermeister PC, et al. The prevalence and predictability of depression in infertile women. *Fertil Steril.* 58:1158, 1992

Chapter 28

DIAGNOSIS AND TREATMENT OF MALE INFERTILITY

John D. McConnell

In approximately one half of infertile couples, the male is at least partially responsible for the inability to conceive. In one third of cases, significant male-factor abnormalities are found in the man alone, while in an additional 20 percent of cases concomitant factors are found in both the man and woman.[1,2] This high incidence of concomitant disease mandates a basic evaluation of both partners (see also Chap 27). Often, when a male factor is identified, completion of the female workup is inappropriately halted. Even when the male is found to have azoospermia, it is usually prudent to complete a basic female factor workup.

The evaluation of male infertility should proceed in the same logical fashion followed in the assessment of other disease states. Although it is certainly appropriate for the semen analysis to be the first step in evaluation of the male, a detailed history and physical examination should precede more sophisticated laboratory tests. The trend to proceed with complex andrology testing before a history and physical examination is not cost effective and often leads to inappropriate therapy. Even in the era of intracytoplasmic sperm injection (ICSI), a thorough male factor evaluation is prudent and cost effective.[3]

DIAGNOSIS

History

After initial semen analyses demonstrate the possibility of male subfertility, a careful history should be taken to determine whether the patient has any potential risk factors. It is critical to determine whether the patient has had prior pregnancies with current or past partners, since this effectively rules out most genetic spermatogenic defects. A general review of the couple's sexual habits—including coital frequency and pattern, as well as the use of vaginal lubricants—often identifies easily reversible problems. Since frequent ejaculation will deplete epididymal sperm reserves, especially in oligospermic men, the couple should be advised to have intercourse every 48 hr around the ovulatory peak. The frequency of masturbation should be determined in a private consultation with the patient.

Past Medical History. A variety of developmental abnormalities, even when recognized and treated successfully, often result in male subfertility. Of particular importance is a history of cryptorchidism. Men born with undescended testes, repaired by appropriate surgical or hormonal intervention, are known to have decreased semen quality.[4,5] Approximately one half of men with bilateral cryptorchidism and one third of men with unilateral cryptorchidism will have sperm densities below 20 million/ml.[6] Whether the observed decrease in sperm production is due to the effects of increased temperature or other factors on an intrinsically normal testis, or to intrinsic developmental defects in the testis itself, is unclear. Both the timing and extent of pubertal development should be determined. Severe degrees of hypospadias or marked delays in pubertal development suggest endocrinopathy.

Systemic illness may affect reproduction function in a variety of ways. Diabetes mellitus and multiple sclerosis can lead to impotency as well as ejaculatory dysfunction. Cystic fibrosis may be associated with epididymal or vasal abnormalities.

Chemotherapy for prior malignancy, especially Hodgkin's and non-Hodgkin's lymphoma, leukemias, sarcomas, and testicular cancer, can cause both acute and chronic defects in sperm production. Chemotherapeutic protocols that result in significant spermatogonial stem-cell destruction usually lead to azoospermia or severe oligospermia. The alkylating agents and procarbazine, both commonly used for the treatment of lymphomas, often result in azoospermia.[7] Other medications such as sulfasalazine, cimetidine, and nitrofurantoin have been implicated as gonadotoxic agents. Anabolic steroids, commonly abused by athletes, may act as a male contraceptive by depressing gonadotropin secretion and suppressing normal spermatogenesis.

Febrile illnesses within the preceding sperm production cycle (70 to 90 days) may result in transient abnormalities in sperm production, which are invariably reversible. In contrast, infectious diseases affecting the testis or epididymis may significantly impair fertility. Viral orchitis is the most common cause of acquired testicular failure in the subfertile male.[8] Although mumps virus is responsible for the majority of cases, echovirus, group B arboviruses, and others can produce similar effects.[9] Orchitis occurs in as many as one fourth of postpubertal males who develop mumps parotitis.[10] Approximately one third of men who develop orchitis will develop unilateral testicular atrophy within 1 to 6 mo, while in 10 percent the atrophy may be bilateral. Histologically, the atrophic testis will show progressive tubular sclerosis and hyalinization. Even in cases of unilateral clinical involvement, degenerative changes may be seen in the contralateral testis. Plasma luteinizing hormone (LH) and follicle-stimulating hormone (FSH) are elevated, and plasma testosterone (T) is decreased during acute orchitis.[10] Chronically, low T production with resultant gynecomastia may occur in association with bilateral atrophy. Although the incidence of subfertility in men with a prior history of mumps orchitis is unknown, fewer than one third of men with bilateral orchitis have a return of semen parameters to normal and one third have azoospermia.[11] In unilateral cases, however, 75 percent of men have normal semen analyses within 1 to 2 yr despite the presence of decreased sperm density on the majority of analyses obtained within 3 mo of the infection.[11] A history of testicular pain and swelling, especially associated with urethral discharge, may suggest a prior episode of epididymitis. Both gonococcal and chlamydia epididymitis can result in epididymal obstruction.

Chronic sinopulmonary disease may be associated with two specific types of male infertility. Men with congenital absence of the vas may have gene abnormalities at the cystic fibrosis gene locus. Patients with Young syndrome have epididymal obstruction and resultant azoospermia secondary to inspissated epididymal secretions, as well as sinopulmonary disease.[12] The immotile-cilia syndrome, a spectrum of disorders characterized by genetic defects in the axonemal structure of both the cilia and sperm flagella, leads to the classic triad of chronic sinopulmonary disease, situs inversus, and nonmotile sperm (Kartagener syndrome).[13]

Modern molecular techniques will undoubtedly identify other genetic causes of male infertility. Deletions of the Y chromosome involving the DAZ (deleted in azoospermia) gene have been described in approximately 3 percent of men with azoospermia.[14]

Past Surgical History. Prior retroperitoneal or pelvic surgery may lead to genital duct obstruction or ejaculatory dysfunction. Retroperitoneal lymph node dissection, commonly performed for treatment of non-seminomatous testicular cancer, may result in either a loss of ejaculation (anejaculation) or retrograde ejaculation.[15] In addition, patients with a history of testicular malignancy may have altered sperm production in the contralateral testis as a sequela of chemotherapy, radiation therapy, or inherent abnormality. Y-V plasty of the bladder neck, commonly performed in the 1960s for treatment of assumed bladder neck obstruction in boys, usually leads to retrograde ejaculation. Herniorrhaphy or other types of inguinal or pelvic surgery may result in iatrogenic vasal occlusion.

Social History. A social and environmental history should be taken to determine whether the patient has had significant exposure to gonadotoxins. Environmental exposure to pesticides,[16] radiation, and hyperthermia should be noted. Chronic marijuana use may lead to subfertility by depressing plasma T levels, and by direct spermatogenic effects.[17] Sperm abnormalities have also been associated with cigarette smoking.[18,19] In addition, ethanol in significant doses may impair spermatogenesis directly, or indirectly through nepotic disease. Unfortunately, data establishing the critical usage level of these three forms of substance abuse are lacking. However, if other causes of subfertility cannot be elucidated, it is reasonable to recommend that the patient curtail the usage of these substances, at least for a trial period.

There is clear evidence in experimental animals that elevations of testicular temperature impair spermatogenesis. It is reasonable (although unproven) to assume that the routine use of hot tubs or saunas may impair spermatogenesis. In contrast, there are no data to suggest that scrotal temperature alterations induced by "brief" underwear or exercise lead to male subfertility.

PHYSICAL EXAMINATION

In addition to a comprehensive physical examination, the infertile male should have a careful assessment of virilization, secondary sexual characteristics, and the scrotal contents. Specifically, the presence or absence of gynecomastia, pubic and axillary hair, and normal penile development should be noted. The urethral meatus should be carefully examined, since a hypospadic urethra may lead to impaired sperm transport into the cervical mucus. Measurement of testicular size is the most important aspect of the examination. Testis size can be estimated by measuring the length of the testis (normal >4 cm) or by determining the volume with an orchidometer (>20 ml). The paratesticular area should be palpated to rule out epididymal induration or cystic abnormality, to note the presence or absence of the vas deferens, and to determine whether there is a clinical varicocele. Ninety percent of clinical varicoceles occur on the left side. Examination for a varicocele can be difficult depending upon the scrotal anatomy. The patient should be examined in a warm room after standing in the upright position for several minutes. Although the size of the palpable varicocele does not correlate with the severity of the spermatogenic defect, identification of a "subclinical" varicocele using a Doppler stethoscope, radioisotope scanning, scrotal thermography, or venography has not been proven to improve pregnancy rates.

Rectal examination to palpate the prostate and analyze expressed prostatic secretion is indicated if there is true pyospermia.

LABORATORY TESTING

Semen Analysis

Because of the variability in sperm density from ejaculate to ejaculate (largely dependent upon the abstinence interval), it is critical that multiple semen analyses be obtained. An assessment of semen quality should not be made until 2 or 3 analyses have been performed over a 1- to 2-mo period of time. A standard abstinence period of 2 to 3 days should be utilized. Upon arrival in the laboratory, motility should be promptly assessed and viscosity of the specimen analyzed. Sperm concentration should be determined by counting in a standard Neubauer blood cell counting chamber after an appropriate dilution. Normally, a 1:20 dilution with distilled water is utilized to immobilize the sperm. For severely oligospermic specimens, however, a lower dilution should be used to obtain an accurate count. Motility is assessed by determining the percentage of motile sperm in a sample size of at least 200 cells. The quality of the movement (linearity and velocity) is then assessed qualitatively (scale 1 to 4) or specific measurements of linearity and velocity are made by computer-assisted motion analysis. The presence of agglutination or pyospermia should be noted. Seminal fructose should be measured in men with azoospermia or semen volumes below 1 ml. Absence of fructose in the semen demonstrates ejaculatory duct obstruction, hypoplasia/aplasia of the seminal vesicles, or (since fructose production in the seminal vesicle is androgen dependent) hypoandrogenemia. In these conditions, the seminal volume should also be decreased. Assessment of sperm morphology is the most difficult part

TABLE 28–1. SEMEN ANALYSIS: MINIMUM STANDARDS

Ejaculate volume	1.15–5.0 cc
Sperm density	>20 MIL/cc
Motility	>60%
Forward progression	>2 (scale 1–4)
Morphology	>60% normal (or >15% "strict")
Absence of significant:	
Agglutination	
Pyospermia	
Hyperviscosity	

of the examination. After air drying, the spermatozoa should be stained with a Papanicolaou stain and 100 cells analyzed. Generally, sperm morphology is categorized by one of five categories: normal (oval), amorphous (including large and small sperm), tapered, duplicated, and immature.[20] Sperm morphology is one of the more sensitive indicators for fertility.[21,22] Many andrology laboratories now utilize "strict" morphology criteria, although the predictive value of this approach is debated.[23–27]

The average sperm density in fertile men ranges between 60 and 80 million/ml. However, the probability of conception does not decrease until the sperm density is under 20 million/ml, assuming normal motility and morphology.[20] Therefore, it is more appropriate to talk about "minimal standards of seminal adequacy," rather than "normal" semen parameters (Table 28–1). With the exception of azoospermia, the semen analysis is a poor "fertility" test. The "stress pattern" consisting of combined decreases in sperm density, motility, and normal oval forms is often said to be specific for varicocele. In fact, this is the semen pattern in most subfertile men, with or without varicocele. There is a suggestion, but no clear evidence, that mean sperm density is decreasing in developed countries.[28–30]

Endocrine Evaluation

The hormonal regulation of spermatogenesis has been reviewed elsewhere in detail.[31] Evaluation of the reproductive hormonal axis (hypothalamus, pituitary, and testes) is essential in the evaluation of men with azoospermia and severe oligospermia. Additional indications for endocrine evaluation (FSH, LH, T) are listed in Table 28–2. Semen volume is a sensitive indicator of androgen status in men.

TABLE 28–2. INDICATIONS FOR ENDOCRINE EVALUATION

Azoospermia
Significant oligospermia (<10 million/cc)
Oligospermia associated with:
   Low semen volume
   Testicular atrophy
   Gynecomastia
   Decreased libido or impotence
   History of cryptorchidism or hypospadias

Suggested tests: FSH, LH, and T.

Therefore, LH and testosterone should always be measured in men with semen volumes below 1 ml. The probability of finding a hormonal abnormality in men with mild oligospermia, or borderline sperm quality, is small.

Serum LH, FSH, and testosterone are all secreted in a pulsatile fashion, leading to short-term variations in serum concentration (see Chap 13). In theory, measurements of serum values at a single time point could lead to an incorrect interpretation of hormonal status. If this is a concern, three samples can be collected 20 min apart followed by pooling of the serum, and measurement of the concentrations of hormone in the pooled sample. Practically speaking, however, this is seldom necessary in the evaluation in the subfertile male. Bain et al have demonstrated that a single serum measurement is as accurate as the mean of three.[32] Analysis of pooled samples should be used when the results of an initial single sample are confusing, incompatible with the clinical picture, or when hypothalamic–pituitary disease is suspected.

Other endocrine tests are indicated in certain circumstances. Serum prolactin should be measured in patients with evidence of a pituitary tumor and in patients with a low serum T without an associated increase in LH. Estradiol (E_2) should be measured in patients with gynecomastia and in patients with suspected androgen resistance syndromes. Measure of serum inhibin levels may eventually prove useful in the evaluation of azoospermic men.[33] Assessment of adrenal, thyroid, parathyroid, and pancreatic hormones is recommended in patients suspected of having multiple end-organ failure; however, they should not be performed routinely. Measurement of adrenocorticotropic hormone, thyroid-stimulating hormone, and growth hormone is recommended in patients with documented LH and FSH deficiencies (hypogonadotropic hypogonadism). Gonadotropin-releasing hormone (GnRH) and clomiphene stimulation tests have been used for the assessment of male infertility.[34] In theory, a GnRH stimulation test may assist in distinguishing hypothalamic from pituitary disease, and in detecting subtle degrees of Sertoli and/or Leydig cell dysfunction. In practice, however, stimulation tests seldom provide information that affects patient management. The interpretation of endocrine tests is discussed next.

OPTIONAL DIAGNOSTIC TESTS

Correlation between the "bulk" semen parameters (density, motility, and morphology) and fertilization potential is limited at best.[35–37] Although the total number of motile sperm, especially after sperm processing, as well as sperm morphology may give indirect insight into the functional capacity of the patient's spermatozoa, traditional semen analysis usually fails to provide the specific etiology of the subfertility or an accurate assessment of the chances for pregnancy. For these reasons, a variety of supplemental diagnostic tests have evolved in recent years. Most of the tests accurately assess the given functional parameter for which they are designed; however, they suffer from either a lack of positive predictive value or low specificity.

Antisperm Antibody Tests

The plasma membrane of the spermatozoa contains antigens that are recognized as foreign by both the male and female immune systems.[38] The identity of the specific antigens has been elusive, but it is known that the major histocompatibility complex (MHC) and blood group antigens are not expressed on the mature sperm.[39] Sperm antigens first appear at puberty, after the fetal process of self-recognition has led to loss of those clones of immunoreactive cells capable of responding against the individual's own antigens.[40] Normally, tight junctions between adjacent Sertoli cells provide a barrier to prevent communication between the immune system and the developing spermatozoa. Outside of the testis, for example in the efferent ductal systems, sperm may gain access to immunoreactive cells. Witkin[41] has theorized that sperm antibody formation in subfertile males may be due to (1) a decrease in the quantity of genital tract T-suppressor cells, (2) a decline or depletion of factors in the male genital tract that recruit suppressor cells, and (3) an alteration in sperm antigenicity.

Antisperm antibodies are known to be present in some men following vasectomy,[42,43] testicular trauma, genital duct obstruction, testicular biopsy, and infection. Autoimmunity following torsion is uncertain.[38,44] In addition to these conditions, antisperm antibodies should be measured in subfertile men with isolated asthenospermia (decreased motility), and in both men and women with unexplained infertility.

There is little evidence to suggest that cellular or humoral immunity adversely affects spermatogenesis. Rather, antisperm antibodies bind to the sperm plasma membrane. Depending upon the location and nature of binding, antibodies may decrease motility in semen and cervical mucus[45] and inhibit normal sperm–egg interaction.[46–48]

The most sensitive and specific assays for antisperm antibodies are those that measure the presence of immunoglobulin directly on the surface of the patient's sperm (direct test) or in his blood (indirect test). These assays all employ an anti-antibody conjugated to a "reporter" that can be quantitated. Assuming appropriate precautions are taken to avoid exposure of internal sperm antigens during processing of the sample, the sensitivity and specificity of these assays are reasonable.[49,50] The immunobead assay utilizes conjugated polyacrylamide beads that permit localization of antibody binding (eg, head versus tail), as well as identification of immunoglobulin class.[51] Similar accuracy can be obtained using antibodies tagged with red blood cells (MAR-mixed agglutination reaction) or radioactive labels. Enzyme-linked immunosorbent assays (ELISAs) are widely used because of their ease of use[52]; however, false positives may be common.[50]

Hypo-osmotic Swelling

Sperm with functionally intact plasma membranes will swell when exposed to hypo-osmotic conditions. Initial studies showed a high degree of correlation between the results of the swelling test and fertilization capacity as measured by the sperm penetration assay. Subsequent studies, however, demonstrated poor correlation.[53] This assay may be helpful in establishing the effectiveness of individual sperm cryopreservation techniques.

Leukocytes in the Semen

Round cells are commonly seen in the semen of subfertile men. Phase contrast microscopy cannot easily distinguish immature sperm from leukocytes. Thus, a significant number of men reported to have pyospermia on routine semen analyses in fact have immature sperm forms. Cell staining with either Pap or peroxidase techniques can be helpful assessing the identity of a given round cell. Recently, leukocyte monoclonal antibodies have been used for this purpose as well.[20]

Cervical Mucus–Sperm Interaction

The postcoital test has been used for over 50 yr to assess sperm–cervical mucus interaction. If an appropriately timed postcoital test demonstrates motile sperm, then significant motility defects and antisperm antibodies are unlikely. A negative test, however, is difficult to interpret; improper timing, cervical mucus abnormalities, as well as sperm function defects can all lead to a negative postcoital test. To circumvent these difficulties a variety of in vitro assays have evolved that utilize bovine cervical mucus in prepackaged capillary tubes or similar containers. The distance and speed of sperm penetration into the mucus can be quantitated by microscopy. At present, there are conflicting reports about the predictive value of the test.[54,55]

Sperm Penetration Assay

Yanagimachi et al first reported the use of zona-free animal eggs (hamster) as a test system for the assessment of human sperm fertilization capacity in 1976.[56] Since that time, numerous studies have analyzed the predictive value of the sperm penetration test (SPA), as well as its limitations.[57–59] In general, the results of the SPA parallel the routine semen analysis: Men with severe oligoas-

thenospermia do poorly in the SPA. If a male is able to penetrate zona-free eggs the probability of impaired fertilization capacity is very low (ie, the false-positive rate is low). Unfortunately, in some studies as many as 20 percent of fertile men will test negatively on the SPA. Therefore, an abnormal SPA should not be used as evidence that a given male is "sterile." Because of its cost and significant false-negative rate, the SPA is not indicated as part of the initial evaluation of the subfertile male. The test may be of value in predicting the outcome of in vitro fertilization (IVF) and in the evaluation of the couple with unexplained infertility. Recent modifications have significantly enhanced the performance and availability of the SPA.[60]

The Hemizona Assay

The SPA assesses the sperm's ability to undergo capacitation and the acrosome reaction and to bind to the egg plasma membrane. Early steps in sperm–egg interaction are not assessed. Burkman et al developed the hemizona assay to assess the ability of sperm to bind to the zona pellucida.[61] Zonae from oophorectomy specimens are isolated, divided by microsurgery, and tested with sperm from the patient as well as a fertile control. Preliminary studies suggest a very high correlation with IVF outcome. Moreover, men who appear to have specific zona-binding defects have been identified.[61,62]

Assessment of Acrosomal Status

Several functional and ultrastructural acrosomal defects that lead to male infertility have been reported.[20] Special staining techniques have been developed that permit assessment of acrosomal status.[20,63] At present, these assays are limited to research environments.

Evaluation of Pyospermia

With the exception of viral orchitis and bacterial epididymitis, infection is an uncommon cause of male infertility in developed countries.[64] Many patients thought to have pyospermia in fact have immature sperm forms in the ejaculate as part of their spermatogenic defect. Moreover, the significance of true pyospermia is uncertain: seminal leukocyte counts in fertile men may be as high as 2 million/ml.[20] In vitro, leukocytes and bacteria inhibit sperm motility and impair sperm–egg interaction.[64] However, the etiology and importance of seminal leukocytes in the male presenting with subfertility is unknown. Certainly, genitourinary tract infection in symptomatic men should be excluded by appropriate urine and prostatic fluid cultures. Semen cultures are notoriously inaccurate because of normal urethral colonization. Mycoplasma and *Uurealyticum* are unproven as causes of male infertility.[64] Therefore, routine testing for these organisms is not justified. Likewise, the empirical use of antibiotics in subfertile men is not indicated.

Computer-assisted Motion Analysis

Isolated asthenospermia is the most common single parameter defect encountered in subfertile males.[20,65] In theory, precise assessment of sperm motion may be of greater predictive value than the standard motility evaluation performed as part of the routine semen analysis. Time-lapsed photography, video micrography, and computer-assisted motion analysis can accurately determine sperm velocity and linearity. The computer-based methods also allow for the measurement of more sophisticated parameters, like lateral head displacement and flagellar beat frequency. At present, it is unclear whether these measurements can be used to clarify the management of a given patient with infertility.[65]

Testis Biopsy and Vasography

In general, testicular biopsy is indicated only in the azoospermic patient with a normal serum FSH.[66,67] Biopsy is performed in this situation to rule out maturation arrest and those cases of germinal aplasia not associated with an FSH elevation.[67,68] Although testicular biopsy in patients with oligospermia can provide a quantitative assessment of spermatogenesis,[69] it neither demonstrates the specific etiology of the patient's defect nor provides insight into management strategy.[70] In addition to open surgical biopsy under local or general anesthesia, aspiration biopsy of the testis, with or without flow cytometry, can provide the needed information on presence of mature sperm.[71,72] The Biopty gun has also been utilized for minimally invasive testicular biopsy.[73] Recently, a touch-prep technique introduced by Lipshultz has been found to provide a more accurate assessment of mature sperm production than routine histology.[67] Late maturation arrest may be missed on frozen section and even formalin-fixed testicular tissue. Although multiple biopsies have been recommended to adequately sample the testis,[74] usually a single biopsy is sufficient. The presence of mature sperm on touch preparation assures complete spermatogenesis. Although the risk of testicular biopsy is minimal, the procedure should not be undertaken without good indication. In situations where the FSH is significantly elevated, testicular biopsy is not indicated, since the results of the biopsy can be predicted from the hormonal testing.[75]

Vasography is indicated in azoospermic men with biopsy-proven spermatogenesis. Vasography is best performed at the time of exploration for attempted microsurgical repair or resection of the ejaculatory ducts.

DIAGNOSTIC ALGORITHMS

After routine history, physical examination, and semen analyses, further workup can be determined after simple classification of the semen picture into one of three cate-

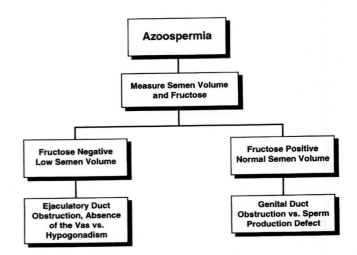

Figure 28–1. Flow diagram for evaluation of azoospermia.

gories: azoospermia (no sperm in the semen), aspermia (no semen), and oligospermia.

Azoospermia

Azoospermia should be confirmed on two semen analyses subjected to centrifugation (Fig 28–1). The presence of even a few spermatozoa in the centrifuged semen pellet suggests a sperm production defect rather than obstruction. Hormonal evaluation (FSH, LH, and T) is indicated in all patients with azoospermia. Once azoospermia is confirmed, subsequent workup will be determined by the presence or absence of fructose in the ejaculate. Although the absence of fructose and low semen volumes generally point to ejaculatory duct abnormalities, both of these parameters are androgen dependent; therefore, hypogonadism must be ruled out.

In cases of fructose-negative azoospermia, after hypogonadism has been ruled out, a careful assessment of the vas deferens should be performed by a physical examination (Fig 28–2). Careful examination of the scrotum will often demonstrate a nonpalpable vas (congenital aplasia of the vas deferens). Transrectal sonography may be helpful in confirming this diagnosis. However, it should be remembered that many patients with agenesis of the vas will have rudimentary seminal vesicles on imaging studies. Transrectal sonography may also demonstrate cystic abnormalities in the ejaculatory ducts or prostate producing obstruction. If the vas deferens is palpable, post-ejaculatory urine should be checked for sperm to rule out retrograde ejaculation. Although most patients with retrograde ejaculation will have aspermia, some will have small-volume fructose-negative ejaculates. If the post-ejaculatory urine test is negative, then ejaculatory duct obstruction is the most likely diagnosis. Vasography is required to confirm this diagnosis, but it is best done in conjunction with a

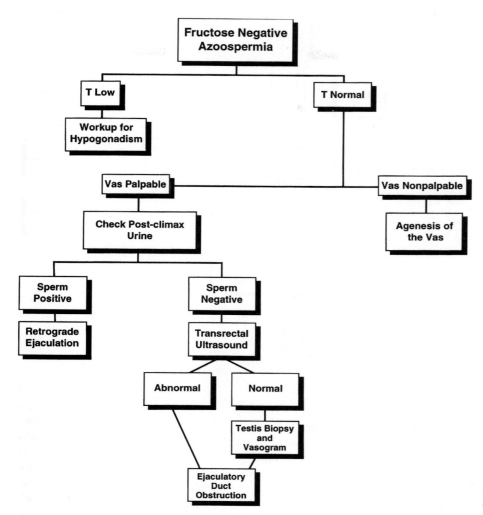

Figure 28–2. Flow diagram for evaluation of fructose-negative azoospermia.

planned surgical procedure to relieve the ductal obstruction (transurethral incision/resection).

In general, patients with fructose-positive azoospermia will have either a failure of sperm production or obstruction in the more proximal portions of the genital duct system (epididymis and vas). Assessment of the gonadotropin levels is crucial to determining the precise etiology of azoospermia (Fig 28–3). The azoospermic patient with significant elevation of the FSH and LH has testicular failure. This may be due to either acquired (eg, mumps orchitis) or genetic (eg, Klinefelter syndrome) causes. The hypogonadism associated with testicular failure can be successfully treated by testosterone placement, but fertility is not possible.

Isolated elevation of the FSH is indicative of germinal (spermatogenic) failure. Sertoli cell-only syndrome (germinal aplasia) is associated with FSH elevation in 90 percent of cases. The LH and T are normal since the pituitary–Leydig cell axis is unperturbed. This condition is not treatable.

Low to nondetectable levels of FSH and LH, associated with a significant reduction in the serum T, is indicative of hypogonadotropic hypogonadism. Usually, this is secondary to congenital disease (eg, Kallmann syndrome) or to acquired hypothalamic disease (eg, craniopharyngioma). Pituitary imaging and further endocrine workup is necessary to establish the cause of hypogonadotropic hypogonadism. However, the presence of anosmia confirms the presence of Kallmann syndrome. Fertility can often be achieved with gonadotropin or releasing hormone replacement therapy.

Mutations of the androgen receptor have been described that lead to infertility without other evidence of abnormal virilization. Although this is a rare cause of infertility, the hormonal findings are classic. Both the LH and T are elevated secondary to end-organ unresponsiveness. FSH levels are usually normal. The diagnosis can be confirmed by quantitative and qualitative analysis of the androgen receptor in cultured genital skin fibroblasts from the affected patient.

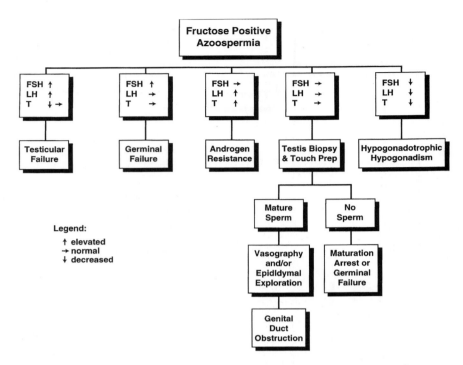

Figure 28–3. Flow diagram for evaluation of fructose-positive azoospermia.

If the azoospermic patient is found to have normal serum gonadotropin, then testis biopsy with touch preparation is indicated. If no sperm are identified on the touch preparation, then the etiology of the patient's azoospermia is clearly a production defect. Production failure may be secondary to maturation arrest, or uncommonly to germinal aplasia not associated with an elevated FSH. Maturation arrest is not a single disease entity. There are several known causes of maturation arrest, and probably many more that are not known. None of these conditions are currently treatable. If the touch preparation fails to show normal spermatogenesis, then vasography is not indicated.

If the testis biopsy shows normal spermatogenesis and the touch preparation demonstrates mature sperm, then formal scrotal exploration is indicated to determine the site of genital duct obstruction. In the absence of a history of inguinal or scrotal surgery to suggest iatrogenic vas obstruction, the most likely site of obstruction is the epididymis. Epididymal obstructions may be secondary to congenital malformation, prior epididymitis (inflammatory), or to obstructions more distal in the ductal system that produce epididymal "blow-out" (ie, vasectomy). Vasography will not demonstrate the level of obstruction in the epididymis. Rather, formal surgical exploration of the epididymis is required, using microscopic technique to analyze fluid in single epididymal tubules until spermatozoa are found.

Aspermia

The absence of an ejaculate can be due to a failure of the genital ducts to contract at the time of climax (anejaculation), or to flow of semen into the bladder at the time of climax (retrograde ejaculation). These two conditions can be distinguished by simple analysis of the urine after climax (Fig 28–4). If no sperm are seen in the urine of an aspermic patient, then anejaculation is clearly present. In contrast, the presence of sperm in

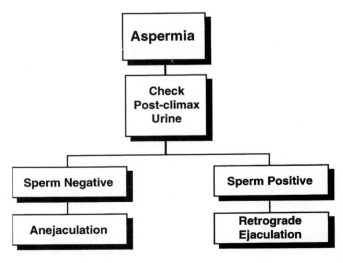

Figure 28–4. Flow diagram for evaluation of aspermia.

the bladder urine indicates retrograde ejaculation. Both conditions may be secondary to neurologic disease that disrupts either genital duct contraction or closure of the bladder neck at the time of climax (diabetic neuropathy, multiple sclerosis, spinal cord injury, retroperitoneal node dissection). In addition, retrograde ejaculation can occur following surgery at the bladder neck or prostate (Y-V plasty of the bladder neck, transurethral resection). In some cases, anejaculation/retrograde ejaculation may be idiopathic.

Oligoasthenospermia

The most common seminal pattern in men with subfertility is oligoasthenospermia. Isolated abnormalities in sperm density are uncommon. Most subfertile men have a "pan-defect," with decreased sperm density, decreased motility, and an increase in abnormal sperm forms. Hormonal evaluation should be performed in men with significant decreases in sperm density. Usually, however, the pituitary–gonadal axis will be normal in men with only marginal decreases in sperm number or quality. In men with more significant oligospermia (sperm concentrations <10 million/cc), measurement of gonadotropin may be of value (Fig 28–5). For example, if the patient with oligospermia already has elevation of FSH, it is unlikely that medical therapy designed to further increase gonadotropin (eg, clomiphene citrate) would result in improved sperm production. Although most patients with

hypothalamic–pituitary insufficiency will have azoospermia, severe oligospermia may be due to gonadotropin deficiency. If low gonadotropin is found in the patient with significant oligospermia, the hypothalamic–pituitary axis should be evaluated for evidence of other endocrine disease, and pituitary tumor ruled out by appropriate imaging studies. Replacement therapy may then begin with either specific gonadotropin therapy, or in cases of a partial deficiency, stimulation with clomiphene citrate. If a varicocele is present in the patient with evidence of hypogonadotropic hypogonadism, the endocrinopathy should be addressed first, and the varicocele repaired only if sperm density and quality do not normalize (Fig 28–5).

In the patient with normal gonadotropin, or in those patients with slight decreases in sperm concentration who do not need hormonal evaluation, a careful scrotal examination should be performed to rule out a clinical varicocele (Fig 28–5). If a varicocele is present and there are no other underlying causes for male subfertility, it is appropriate to consider varicocele repair. If a varicocele is not present in physical examination, then empirical therapy is indicated either by assisted reproductive techniques or by medical therapy. As previously mentioned, imaging techniques designed to identify the "subclinical/nonpalpable varicocele" have not been shown to improve pregnancy rates; therefore, they cannot be considered as the standard of care.

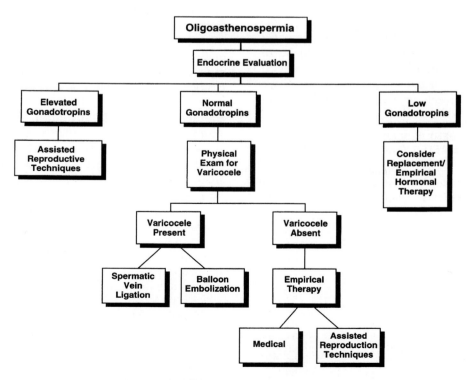

Figure 28–5. Flow diagram for evaluation of oligoasthenospermia.

In the workup of the oligoasthenospermic male, the other diagnostic tests outlined, such as the sperm penetration assay and antisperm antibody test, may be indicated in selected cases. However, they should be utilized only when the management plan will be altered by the results. Men with isolated asthenospermia should have antisperm antibody testing. In cases in which the sperm motility is below 10 percent, despite normal sperm density, ultrastructural study of the sperm tail by electron microscopy will usually demonstrate axonemal defects.[65] In men with severe oligospermia associated with decreased semen volume and low to absent fructose, consideration may be given to transrectal sonography to rule out cystic abnormalities in the prostate or ejaculatory duct, producing partial obstruction.

TREATMENT

Specific Therapy

Varicocele Repair. Varicocele ligation and balloon embolization have both been reported to improve semen quality and increase the chance of pregnancy (Table 28–3). The average pregnancy occurs at 6 mo following intervention. The significant incidence of varicocele in men without subfertility, as well as the 50 to 70 percent rate of treatment failure, mandates a thorough search for other causes of subfertility before recommending ligation or embolization. In a recent randomized, controlled trial, 44 percent of couples achieved a pregnancy following varicocele ligation compared to 10 percent in the control group.[89] Clinical varicoceles should be repaired in men with impaired sperm quality prior to ICSI.

There is little evidence to suggest the superiority of a given surgical approach or technique. Balloon em-

TABLE 28–3. IMPROVEMENT IN SEMEN QUALITY AND PREGNANCY RATE AFTER VARICOCELECTOMY

Selected Studies	No. Patients	Probability of Semen Improvement	Probability of Pregnancy
Tulloch[76]	30	66	30
Scott & Young[77]	166	70	31
Charney & Baum[78]	104	61	24
MacLeod[79]	108	74	41
Brown[80]	251	58	41
Glezerman et al[81]	51	53	26
Dubin & Amelar[82]	986	70	53
Lome & Ross[63]	80	78	51
Cockett et al[84]	56	NR	25
Newton et al[85]	149	66	34
Greenberg et al[86]	68	65	NR
Aafjes & van der Vijver[87]	157	NR	36
Marks et al[88]	130	51	39

NR = not reported.

bolization has the advantage of minimal recovery time. In addition, it is the procedure of choice for varicocele recurrence after surgery. However, balloon embolization is technically demanding, requiring a highly skilled interventional radiologist. Clearly, both options should be presented to the patient. Recurrence rates after surgery and balloon embolization are between 5 and 10 percent. Varicocele ligation has the additional complication of hydrocele formation in a small number of cases.

Vasoepididymostomy. Vasoepididymostomy is indicated in cases of proven epididymal obstruction. The etiology of epididymal obstruction includes congenital, inflammatory, and post-vasectomy defects. Older macroscopic techniques resulted in a very low patency rate and an even more dismal pregnancy rate. Modern two-layered microscopic techniques should yield patency rates greater than 60 to 70 percent, with a probability of pregnancy above 30 percent.[90–96]

Vasovasostomy. If vasography has demonstrated obstruction of the vas deferens secondary to prior inguinal or scrotal surgery, then microscopic vasovasostomy is indicated. Injury to the inguinal vas from prior herniorrhaphy may lead to loss of an extensive length of vas, making surgical reconstruction difficult. Moreover, obstruction in the distal portions of the genital duct system may be associated with secondary epididymal obstruction requiring vasoepididymostomy. Because of these technical difficulties, as well as the formation of antisperm antibodies in many men with obstruction, the overall pregnancy rates following vasovasostomy are generally in the 50 to 60 percent range. Epididymal sperm aspiration and ICSI are far less successful and more costly than microscopic vasectomy reversal.[97]

Ejaculatory Duct Obstruction. Ejaculatory duct obstruction can occur from inflammatory or developmental abnormality. Often the obstruction is present in only the distal portion of the ejaculatory duct, making the lesion amenable to transurethral incision or resection. At the time of vasography, methylene blue can be injected into the vas deferens proximal to the level of obstruction. Instruments can then be passed through the urethra to allow endoscopic incision of the floor of the prostate. This approach has a high initial success rate in terms of achieving sperm in the ejaculate. However, in some cases scarring will result in repeat obstruction.

Ejaculatory Disorders. Both retrograde ejaculation and anejaculation should be approached initially with medical therapy. Alpha-sympathomimetic drugs (eg, pseudoephedrine and ephedrine) increase smooth muscle tone at the bladder neck, as well as providing direct stimulation to the genital duct structures themselves.

Although data are lacking concerning the efficacy of medical therapy for these two conditions, at least 20 to 30 percent of patients will respond. In patients with retrograde ejaculation who are refractory to medical therapy, recovery of sperm from the bladder with subsequent insemination is highly effective. The urine pH and osmolarity are toxic to sperm, but there are several measures to circumvent this. First, oral alkalinization with bicarbonate or citrate may be attempted to bring the urine pH to 8 prior to ejaculation and sperm recovery. A more effective technique is to directly instill appropriately buffered sperm-processing media directly into the bladder, either by retrograde instillation or by catheterization. The patient subsequently climaxes and voids out sperm already present in appropriate media. Patients with anejaculation not responding to medical therapy may be treated by electroejaculation therapy or by harvest of sperm directly from the vas deferens using the microsurgical technique.[98–100]

Treatment of Antisperm Antibodies.

A variety of immunosuppressive drugs have been utilized for the treatment of immunologic infertility in the male, including steroids and cyclosporine. There is little question that high-dose immunosuppressive therapy will lower both the circulating level of antisperm antibody as well as the level of antibody on the sperm surface. Whether or not decreases in antibody titer lead to improved pregnancy rates is less certain. Randomized clinical trials have failed to provide convincing evidence of improved fertility. Since immunosuppressive drugs have significant side effects, the risk versus the benefit of therapy must be carefully discussed with the patient before embarking on treatment.

Empirical Therapy

When the specific etiology of a patient's decreased sperm density or quality cannot be determined, therapy by definition is empiric. The intent of empirical medical therapy is to improve sperm production so that a larger population of functional sperm is available for fertilization. In contrast, the intent of assisted reproductive techniques, which are also empiric by design, is to increase the probability of fertilization by decreasing natural barriers to fertilization. The low overall success rate of empirical therapy for the treatment of male factor infertility should not be surprising, since none of the empiric approaches specifically address the underlying pathophysiology.

The principle underlying empiric medical therapy is not always biologically correct: "If a little is good, more is better." Specifically, since gonadotropin is known to be necessary for normal spermatogenesis, it has been assumed that elevation of gonadotropin above normal levels would stimulate sperm production in men with oligospermia. Although elevation of gonadotropin levels with drugs such as clomiphene citrate will commonly increase production rates, sperm quality seldom improves. The use of medications that rely on the underlying principles of reproductive physiology, such as gonadotropin stimulation, is a *rational* approach. In contrast, some forms of empirical therapy are *irrational*, since the therapy has no underlying physiologic basis of action. It should be remembered that many commonly used *rational* therapies are unproven in terms of improvement in pregnancy rate.

Irrational Medical Therapy.

Testosterone has been used as a treatment for male-factor subfertility in two forms. First, low-dose testosterone has been used in an attempt to improve both sperm production and sperm quality. Second, high-dose testosterone has been used to suppress spermatogenesis, hoping for subsequent rebound of sperm production when gonadotropin rebounds. Low-dose testosterone does not increase the level of intratesticular or intraepididymal androgens. Rather, testosterone, even at low doses, suppresses pituitary LH release, thus *lowering* intratesticular androgen levels. This form of therapy is not only irrational, but recent clinical trials demonstrate a lack of efficacy. Testosterone rebound therapy should not be utilized since gonadotropin stimulation can be obtained by other approaches. Moreover, some patients suppressed to azoospermia with testosterone will not recover spermatogenesis.

Thyroid hormone as well as steroids in men without antisperm antibodies should not be utilized since there is no evidence that either of these hormonal approaches improve sperm production or fertility rates.

The use of zinc to improve sperm motility is controversial because of conflicting data in the fertility literature. However, it has been known for some time that the oral administration of zinc does not increase the level of zinc in the seminal plasma. Even though zinc may be an important co-factor for many spermatogenic processes, supplemental therapy does not appear to influence the level of zinc in the reproductive tissues. Its empirical use is therefore not justified.

Rational Medical Therapy.

The use of hormonal therapy to stimulate sperm production is a rational, albeit unproven, approach. Although there are more than 200 studies in the literature addressing the issue of empirical hormonal therapy in the subfertile male, there are only a small number of controlled trials (Table 28–4). Clomiphene citrate as well as cis-clomiphene citrate increase LH and FSH indirectly by inhibiting negative feedback. The available evidence suggests that improvements in sperm density are common. However, improvement in the sperm quality and function occurs uncommonly. Wang et al demonstrated in a well-controlled study that clomiphene does not improve sperm motility,

TABLE 28–4. EMPIRICAL THERAPY: RESULTS OF CONTROLLED TRIALS

Study	Dosage	No. Subjects	Probability of Semen Improvement (%)	Probability of Pregnancy (%)
Clomiphene Citrate				
Wieland et al, 1972[101]	5 mg/day	6	17	17
	10 mg/day	5	40	0
	Placebo	11	27	18
Foss et al, 1973[102]	100 mg × 10 day/mo	114	NR	NR
	Placebo	114		
Paulson, 1979[103]	25 mg × 25 day/mo	20	70	35
	Cortisone 10 mg/day	20	40	10
Rönnberg, 1980[104]	50 mg/day	27	78	10
	Placebo	29	21	3
Abel et al, 1982[105]	50 mg × 25 day/mo	98	0	17
	Vit. C 200 mg/day	89	0	13
Wang et al, 1983[106]	25 mg/day	11	NR	36
	50 mg/day	18	NR	22
	Placebo	7	NR	0
Mićić et al, 1985[107]	50 mg/day	56	32	13
	No Rx	45	7	0
Sokol et al, 1988[108]	25 mg/day	23	NR	9
	Placebo	23	NR	44
Tamoxifen Citrate				
Willis et al, 1977[109]	10 mg/day	9	11	11
	Placebo	9	0	0
Török, 1985[110]	20 mg/day	27	NR	33
	Placebo	27	NR	25
AinMelk et al, 1987[111]	20 mg/day	16	NR	13
	Placebo	16	NR	0
Testolactone				
Clark & Sherins, 1983[112]	2 g/day	20	NR	0
	Placebo	20	NR	0

NR = not reported.

morphology, or fertilization capacity as measured by the sperm penetration assay.[106] Randomized, placebo-controlled studies with clomiphene are largely negative.[102–108] Although there was initial enthusiasm for the use of the anti-estrogen tamoxifen in the treatment of male subfertility, subsequent controlled studies have demonstrated minimal effectiveness.[109–111] Likewise, aromatase inhibition with testolactone has been shown in a randomized, clinical trial to be ineffective in the treatment of male subfertility.[112]

More direct gonadotropin stimulation with the use of LH and FSH replacement therapy, and with the use of GnRH agonists, has been utilized in small series for the treatment of male subfertility. At the present time, efficacy has not been proven and cost is often prohibitive.

If empirical hormonal therapies are utilized, it should be done with the understanding that the benefits of therapy are marginal. If empirical therapy is utilized, the patient must be closely monitored to ensure that sperm production does not decrease, which can be a side effect of hormonal therapies that secondarily increase estrogen levels (eg, clomiphene). Moreover, if the serum FSH is already elevated, even slightly, the benefit of additional gonadotropin stimulation must be questioned. If a given empirical agent fails to significantly improve sperm density and quality within a 6-mo period, it is unlikely that further therapy will achieve the desired goal.

Assisted Reproductive Technologies. Several specific comments should be made related to the use of assisted reproductive technologies (ARTs) in male factor cases (see also Chap 33). Sperm-processing techniques underlie all ART approaches. It is still unclear whether sperm-processing techniques actually improve sperm function, or whether (more likely) a population of functioning cells is enriched in the final specimen. Despite much discussion in the literature concerning optimization of sperm-processing techniques, there is no clear evidence that one technique offers superior clinical outcome to another.

Intrauterine insemination (IUI) therapy has been extensively used in the treatment of male factor subfertility with variable results. IUI is a rational therapy for couples with moderate oligoasthenospermia.[113,114] However, motile sperm concentrations under 2 million are unlikely to result in pregnancy. IUI is feasible in men with a variety of ejaculatory disorders where sperm can be obtained by a variety of techniques.[115] (See Chaps 26 and 27.)

Gamete intrafallopian tube transfer (GIFT) and in vitro fertilization (IVF) have been used extensively for the treatment of male factor subfertility. Recent data from the United States IVF registry suggests that the overall live birth rate for male factor cases treated by GIFT and IVF approaches the overall success rates for the two techniques (Table 28–5).[116] GIFT is a less than ideal form of therapy for couples with severe male factor infertility, since no information is obtained concerning the ability of the male's sperm to achieve fertilization. Despite encouraging success rates with assisted reproductive techniques, overall they have made a negligible impact on the treatment of male infertility. This is primarily because men with severe oligoasthenospermia usually do not have a sufficient number of functional sperm to achieve fertilization. Moreover, the costs of the assisted reproductive techniques are simply prohibitive to many couples. It remains to be seen whether more recent advances, such as zona-drilling and micropuncture, will really achieve pregnancies when men have severe sperm production defects.

ICSI represents a significant advance in the management of couples with male factor infertility (see Chap 33). Fertilization rates with ICSI are considerably better than with IVF in cases of severe oligospermia. Acceptable fertilization and pregnancy rates have been reported in men with counts less than 5 million, severe asthenospermia, and antisperm antibodies.[117–120] In brief, ICSI in male factor cases has delivery rates roughly equivalent to the overall IVF success rates (25 to 30 percent). However, with further bypass of normal "biologic barriers," genetic issues have been raised[121]: Will the male offspring of ICSI couples have normal sperm production?

TABLE 28–5. UNITED STATES IVF REGISTRY DATA FROM 1994

Patient Category	Deliveries per Retrieval (%)	
	IVF-ET	*GIFT*
Women <40 yr with no male factor	24.5	33.5
Women ≥40 yr with no male factor	9.0	12.3
Women <40 yr with male factor	20.2	26.8
Women ≥40 yr with male factor	8.5	9.9

(Reproduced, with permission, from Society for Assisted Reproductive Technology and the American Society for Reproductive Medicine. Assisted reproductive technology in the United States and Canada: 1994 results generated from the American Society for Reproductive Medicine/Society for Assisted Reproductive Technology Registry. Fertil Steril. 66:697, 1996.)

SUMMARY

The diagnosis and treatment of male factor infertility is problematic, largely owing to insufficient insight into the pathophysiology of sperm production defects. As much as possible, however, the approach to the patient should be a rational one, with the selection of both diagnostic and treatment modalities firmly based upon the principles of male reproductive function. The physician's role in evaluating the male patient should be to (1) exclude specific, reversible causes of infertility; and (2) give an honest assessment to the couple concerning the probability of a given therapeutic intervention achieving a clinical pregnancy.

REFERENCES

1. MacLeod J. Human male infertility. *Obstet Gynecol Surv.* 26:325, 1971

2. Simmons FA. Human infertility. *N Engl J Med.* 225:1140, 1956

3. Oehninger S, Franken D, Kruger T. Approaching the next millennium: How should we manage andrology diagnosis in the intracytoplasmic sperm injection era? *Fertil Steril.* 67:434, 1997

4. Lipshultz LI. Cryptorchidism in the subfertile male. *Fertil Steril.* 27:609, 1976

5. Lipshultz LI, Caminos-Torres R, Greenspan CS, et al. Testicular function after orchiopexy for unilaterally undescended testes. *N Engl J Med.* 2925:15, 1976

6. Kogan SJ. Cryptorchidism. In: Kelalis PP, King LR, Belman AB, eds. *Clinical Pediatric Urology.* Philadelphia, W. B. Saunders, 1985: 876–930

7. Oates RD, Lipshultz LI. Fertility and testicular function in patients after chemotherapy and radiotherapy. In: Lytton B, ed. *Advances in Urology.* Chicago, Year Book Medical Publishers; 1989: 2–55

8. Werner CA. Mumps orchitis and testicular atrophy. 1. Occurrence. *Ann Intern Med.* 32:1066, 1950

9. Riggs S, Sanford JP. Viral orchitis. *N Engl J Med.* 266:990, 1962

10. Adamopoulos DA, Lawrence DM, Vassilopoulos P, et al. Pituitary testicular relationships in mumps orchitis and other viral infections. *Br Med J.* 1:1177, 1978

11. Bartak V, Skalova E, Nevarilova A. Spermiogram changes in adults and youngsters after parotitic orchitis. *Int J Fertil.* 13:2226, 1968

12. Handelsman DJ, Conway AJ, Boylan LM, et al. Young's syndrome: Obstructive azoospermia and chronic sinopulmonary infections. *N Engl J Med.* 310:3, 1984

13. Eilasson R, Mossberg B, Camner P, et al. The immotile-cilia syndrome. *N Engl J Med.* 297:1, 1988

14. Simoni M, Carani C, Gromoll J, et al. Screening for delection of the Y chromosome involving the DAZ (deleted in azoospermia) gene in azoospermia and severe oligozoospermia. *Fertil Steril.* 67:542, 1997

15. Kedia KR, Markland C, Fraley EE. Sexual function following high retroperitoneal lymphadenectomy. *J Urol.* 114:237, 1975

16. Lantz GD, Cunningham GR, Huckins C, et al. Recovery of severe oligospermia after exposure to dibromochloropropane (BCP). *Fertil Steril.* 35:46, 1981

17. Kolodny RC, Masters WH, Kolodny MR, et al. Depression of plasma testosterone levels after chronic intensive marihuana use. *N Engl J Med.* 290:872, 1974

18. Evans HF, Fletcher J, Torrance M. Sperm abnormalities and cigarette smoking. *Lancet.* 1:627, 1981

19. Vine MF, Tse CJ, Hu P, Truong KY. Cigarette smoking and semen quality. *Fertil Steril.* 65:835, 1996

20. Sigman M, Lipshultz LI, Howards SS. Evaluation of the subfertile male. In: Lipshultz LI and Howards SS, eds. *Infertility in the Male*, 3rd ed. St. Louis, Mosby-Year Book, 1997: 173–193

21. MacLeod J. Semen quality in one thousand men of known fertility and eight hundred cases of infertile marriages. *Fertil Steril.* 2:115, 1951

22. MacLeod J, Gold RZ. The male factor in fertility and infertility. II. Spermatozoan counts in 1000 men of known fertility and in 1,000 cases of infertile marriages. *J Urol.* 66:436, 1951

23. Karabinus DS, Gelety TJ. The impact of sperm morphology evaluated by strict criteria on intrauterine insemination success. *Fertil Steril.* 67:536, 1997

24. Hofmann GE, Scott RT, Santilli BA, et al. Intra observer, inter-observer variation of sperm critical morphology: Comparison of examiner and computer-assisted analysis. *Fertil Steril.* 65:1021, 1996

25. Matorras R, Mandiola M, Corcóstegui B, et al. Sperm morphology analysis (strict criteria) in male infertility is not a prognostic factor in intrauterine insemination with husband's sperm. *Fertil Steril.* 63:608, 1995

26. Davis RO, Gravance CG, Overstreet JW. A standardized test for visual analysis of human sperm morphology. *Fertil Steril.* 63:1058, 1995

27. Morgentaler A, Powers RD, Fung MY, et al. Sperm morphology and in vitro fertilization outcome: A direct comparison of World Health Organization and strict criteria methodologies. *Fertil Steril.* 64:1177, 1995

28. Lipshultz LI. "The debate continues"—The continuing debate over the possible decline in semen quality. *Fertil Steril.* 65:909, 1996

29. Fisch H, Feldshuh J, Goluboff ET, et al. Semen analyses in 1,283 men from the United States over a 25-year period: No decline in quality. *Fertil Steril.* 65:1009, 1996

30. Becker S, Berhane K. A meta-analysis of 61 sperm count studies revisited. *Fertil Steril.* 67:1103, 1997

31. Swerdloff RS, Wang C, Sokol RZ. In: Marshall DK, ed. *Infertility in the Male.* St. Louis, Mosby-Year Book, 1985: 211–222

32. Bain J, Langevin R, D'Costa M, et al. Serum pituitary and steroid hormone levels in the adult male: one value is as good as the mean of three. *Fertil Steril.* 49:123, 1988

33. Halvorson LM, DeCherney AH. Inhibin, activin, and follistatin in reproductive medicine. *Fertil Steril.* 65:459, 1996

34. Handelsman DJ, Swerdloff RS. Male gonadal dysfunction. *Clin Endocrin Metab.* 14:89, 1985

35. Aitken JR, Best FSM, Richardson DW, et al. An analysis of semen quality and sperm function in cases of oligozoospermia. *Fertil Steril.* 38:705, 1982

36. Amann R. A critical review of methods for evaluation of spermatogenesis from seminal characteristics. *J Androl.* 2:37, 1981

37. Battin D, Vargyas JM, Sato F, et al. The correlation between in vitro fertilization of human oocytes and semen profile. *Fertil Steril.* 44:835, 1985

38. Haas GG Jr. Male fertility and immunity. In: Marshall DK, ed. *Infertility in the Male.* St. Louis, Mosby-Year Book, 1985: 277–296

39. Anderson DJ, Bach DL, Unis EJ, et al. Major histocompatibility antigens are not expressed on human epididymal sperm. *J Immunol.* 129:452, 1982

40. Anderson DJ, Hill JA. Cell-mediated immunity in infertility. *Am J Reprod Immunol Microbiol.* 17:22, 1988

41. Witkin SS. Mechanisms of active suppression of the immune response to spermatozoa. *Am J Reprod Immunol Microbiol.* 17:61, 1988

42. Alexander NJ, Anderson DJ. Vasectomy: Consequences of autoimmunity to sperm antigens. *Fertil Steril.* 32:253, 1979

43. Ansbacher R, Hodge P, Williams A, et al. Vas ligation: Humoral sperm antibodies. *Int J Fertil.* 21:258, 1976

44. Fraser I, Slater N, Tate C, et al. Testicular torsion does not cause autoimmunization in man. *Br J Surg.* 72:237, 1985

45. Haas GG Jr. The inhibitory effect of sperm-associated immunoglobulins on cervical mucus penetration. *Fertil Steril.* 46:334, 1986

46. Haas GG Jr, Ausmanus M, Culp L, et al. The effect of immunoglobulin occurring on human sperm in vivo on the human sperm/hamster ova penetration assay. *Am J Reprod Immunol Microbiol.* 7:109, 1985

47. Clarke GN, Lopata A, McBain JC, et al. Effect of sperm antibodies in males on human in vitro fertilization (IVF). *Am J Reprod Immunol Microbiol.* 8:62, 1985

48. Bronson R, Cooper G, Rosenfield D. Ability of antibody-bound human sperm to penetrate zona-free hamster ova in vitro. *Fertil Steril.* 36:778, 1981

49. Haas GG Jr. Evaluation of sperm antibodies and autoimmunity in the infertile male. In: Santen RJ, Swerdloff Rs, eds. *Male Reproductive Dysfunction, Diagnosis and Management of Hypogonadism, Infertility, and Impotence.* New York, Marcel Dekker, 46:439, 1986

50. Haas GG Jr, DeBault LE, D'Cruz O, et al. The effect of fixatives and/or air-drying on the plasma and acrosomal membranes of human sperm. *Fertil Steril.* 50:487, 1988

51. Clarke GN, Elliott PJ, Smaila C. Detection of sperm antibodies in semen using the immunobead test: A survey of 813 consecutive patients. *Am J Reprod Immunol Microbiol.* 7:118, 1985

52. Golomb J, Vardinon N, Hommonnai ZT, et al. Demonstration of anti-spermatozoal antibodies in varicocele-related infertility with an enzyme-linked immunosorbent assay (ELISA). *Fertil Steril.* 45:397, 1986

53. Chan SYW, Fox EJ, Chan MMC, et al. The relationship between the human sperm hypoostmotic, routine semen analysis, and the human sperm zona-free hamster ovum penetration assay. *Fertil Steril.* 44:668, 1985

54. Moghissi KS, Darich D, Lebine J, et al. In vitro sperm–cervical mucus penetration: Studies in human and bovine cervical mucus. *Fertil Steril.* 37:823, 1982

55. Takemoto FS, Rogers BJ, Wiltbank MC, et al. Comparison of the penetration ability of human spermatozoa into bovine cervical mucus and zona-free hamster eggs. *J Androl.* 6:162, 1985

56. Yanagimachi R, Yanagimachi H, Rogers BJ. The use of zona-free animal ova as a test system for the assessment of the fertilizing capacity of human spermatozoa. *Biol Reprod.* 15:471, 1976

57. Mardin RRH, Taylor PJ. Reliability and accuracy of the zona-free hamster ova assay in the assessment of male infertility. *Br J Obstet Gynecol.* 89:951, 1982

58. Auzmanas M, Tureck RW, Blasco L, et al. The zona-free hamster egg penetration assay as a prognostic indicator in a human in vitro fertilization program. *Fertil Steril.* 43:433, 1985

59. Aitken JR. Diagnostic value of the zona-free hamster oocyte penetration test and sperm movement characteristics in oligospermia. *Int J Androl.* 8:348, 1985

60. Johnson A, Bassham B, Lipshultz LI, Lamb DJ. A quality control system for the optimized sperm penetration assay. *Fertil Steril.* 64:832, 1995

61. Burkman LJ, Coddington CC, Fraken DR, et al. The hemizona assay (HZA): Development of a diagnostic test for the binding of human spermatozoa to the human hemizona pellucida to predict fertilization potential. *Fertil Steril.* 49:688, 1988

62. Oehninger S, Kolm P, Mahony M, et al. Clinical significance of human sperm–zona pellucida binding. *Fertil Steril.* 67:1121, 1997

63. Byrd W, Wolf DP. Acrosomal status in fresh and capacitated human ejaculated sperm. *Biol Reprod.* 34:859, 1986

64. McConnell JD. The role of infection in male infertility. In: DeVere White, R, ed. *Problems in Urology.* Philadelphia, J. B Lippincott, 1987; 1: 467

65. McConnell JD. Abnormalities in sperm motility: Techniques of evaluation and treatment. In: Lipshultz LI, Howards SS, eds. *Infertility in the Male*, 3rd ed. St. Louis, Mosby, 1997: 249–267

66. Coburn M, Wheeler TM. Testicular Biopsy in Male Infertility Evaluation. In: Marshall DK, ed. *Infertility in the Male.* St. Louis, Mosby-Year Book, 1985;223–253

67. Turek PJ, Kim M, Gilbraugh JH, Lipshultz LI. The clinical characteristics of 82 patients with Sertoli cell-only testis histology. *Fertil Steril.* 64:1197, 1995

68. Aumuller G, Fuhrmann W, Krause W. Spermatogenetic arrest with inhibition of acrosome and sperm tail development. *Andrologia.* 19:9, 1987

69. Aafjes JH, van der Vijver JCM, Schenck PE. Value of a testicular biopsy rating for prognosis in oligozoospermia. *Br Med J.* 1:289, 1978

70. Coburn M, Wheeler T, Lipshultz LI. Testicular biopsy: Its use and limitations. *Urol Clin North Am.* 14:551, 1987

71. Linsk JA, Franzen S. Aspiration biopsy of the testis. In: *Clinical Aspiration Cytology.* Philadelphia, J. B. Lippincott, 1983: 267

72. Abyholm T, Clausen OF. Clinical evaluation of DNA flow cytometry of fine needle aspirates from testes of infertile men. *Int J Androl.* 4:505, 1981

73. Raifer J, Binder S. Use of Biopty gun for transcutaneous testicular biopsies. *J Urol.* 142:1021, 1989

74. Gottschalk-Subag S, Weiss DB, Folb-Zacharow N, Zukerman Z. Is one testicular specimen sufficient for quantitative evaluation of spermatogenesis? *Fertil Steril.* 64:399, 1995

75. Hargreave TB, Jequier AM. Can follicle stimulating hormone estimation replace testicular biopsy in the diagnosis of obstructive azoospermia? *Br J Urol.* 50:415, 1978

76. Tulloch WL. Varicocele in subfertility, results of treatment. *Br Med J.* 2:356, 1955

77. Scott LS, Young D. Varicocele: A study of its effects on human spermatogenesis and of the results produced by spermatic vein ligation. *Fertil Steril.* 13:335, 1962

78. Charney CW, Baum S. Varicocele and infertility. *JAMA.* 41:1, 1968

79. MacCleod J. Seminal cytology in the presence of varicoceles. *Fertil Steril.* 16:735, 1965

80. Brown JS. Varicocelectomy in the subfertile male: A ten-year experience with 295 cases. *Fertil Steril.* 27:1046, 1976

81. Glezerman M, Rakowszczyk M, Lunenfeld B, et al. Varicocele in oligospermic patients; Pathophysiology and results after ligation and division of the internal spermatic vein. *J Urol.* 115:562, 1976

82. Dubin L, Amelar RD. Varicocelectomy: 986 cases in a 12-year study. *Urology.* 10:446, 1977

83. Lome LG, Ross L. Varicocelectomy and infertility. *Urology.* 9:416, 1977

84. Cockett ATK, Urry RL, Dougherty KA. The varicocele. *Fertil Steril.* 26:1242, 1975

85. Newton R, Schinfeld JS, Schiff I. The effect of varicocelectomy on sperm count, motility, and conception rate. *Fertil Steril.* 34:250, 1980

86. Greenberg SH, Lipshultz LI, Morganroth J, et al. The use of the Doppler stethoscope in the evaluation of varicoceles. *J Urol.* 117:296, 1977

87. Aafjes JH, van der Vijver JCM. Fertility of men with and without a varicocele. *Fertil Steril.* 43:901, 1985

88. Marks JL, McMahon R, Lipshultz LI. Predictive parameters of successful varicocele repair. *J Urol.* 136:609, 1986

89. Madgar I, Karasik A, Weissenberg R, et al. Controlled trial of high spermatic vein ligation for varicocele in infertile men. *Fertil Steril.* 63:120, 1995

90. Dubin L, Amelar RD. Magnified surgery for epididymovasostomy. *Urology.* 23:525, 1984

91. Fogdestam I, Fall M, Nilsson S. Microsurgical epididymovasotomy in the treatment of occlusive azoospermia. *Fertil Steril.* 46:925, 1986

92. Lee HY. Corrective surgery of obstructive azoospermia. *Arch Androl.* 1:115, 1978

93. McLoughlin MG. Vasoepididymostomy: The role of the microscope. *Can J Sur.* 25:41, 1982

94. Schoysman RJ, Beford JM. The role of human epididymis in sperm maturation and sperm storage as reflected in the consequences of epididymovasostomy. *Fertil Steril.* 46:293, 1986

95. Silber SJ. Microscopic vasoepididymostomy: Specific microanastomosis to the epididymal tubule. *Fertil Steril.* 30:565, 1978

96. Thomas AJ. Vasoepididymostomy. *Urol Clin North Am.* 14:527, 1987

97. Pavlovich CP, Schlegel PN. Fertility options after vasectomy: a cost-effectiveness analysis. *Fertil Steril.* 67:133, 1997

98. Chung PH, Skinner L, Verkauf BS, et al. Correlation between semen parameters of electroejaculates and achieving pregnancy by intrauterine insemination. *Fertil Steril.* 67:129, 1997

99. Chung PH, Sanford EJ, Yeko TR, et al. Assisted fertility using electro-ejaculation in men with spinal cord injury—A review of literature. *Fertil Steril.* 64:1, 1995

100. Hakim LS, Lobel SM, Oates RD. The achievement of pregnancies using assisted reproductive technologies for male factor infertility after retroperitoneal lymph node dissection for testicular carcinoma. *Fertil Steril.* 64:1141, 1995

101. Wieland RG, Ansari AH, Klein DE, et al. Idiopathic oligospermia: Control observations and response to clomiphene. *Fertil Steril.* 23:471, 1972

102. Foss GL, Tindall VR, Birkett JP. The treatment of subfertile men with clomiphene citrate. *J Reprod Fertil.* 32:167, 1973

103. Paulson DF. Cortisone acetate versus clomiphene citrate in pre-germinal idiopathic oligospermia. *J Urol.* 121:432, 1979

104. Rönnberg L. The effect of clomiphene citrate on different sperm parameters and serum hormone levels in preselected infertile men: A controlled double-blind crossover study. *Int J Androl.* 3:479, 1980

105. Abel BJ, Carswell G, Elton R, et al. Randomized trial of clomiphene citrate treatment and vitamin C for male infertility. *Br J Urol.* 54:780, 1982

106. Wang C, Chan CW, Wong KK, et al. Comparison of the effectiveness of placebo, clomiphene citrate, mesterolone, pentoxifylline, and testosterone rebound therapy for the treatment of idiopathic oligospermia. *Fertil Steril.* 40:358, 1983

107. Mičić S, Dotlić R. Evaluation of sperm parameters in clinical trial with clomiphene citrate of oligospermic men. *J Urol.* 133:221, 1985

108. Sokol RZ, Petersen G, Steiner BS, et al. A controlled comparison of the efficacy of clomiphene citrate in male infertility. *Fertil Steril.* 49:865, 1988

109. Willis KJ, London DR, Bevis MA, et al. Hormonal effects of tamoxifen in oligospermic men. *J Endocrinol.* 73:171, 1977

110. Török L. Treatment of oligospermia with tamoxifen (open and controlled studies). *Andrologia.* 17:497, 1985

111. AinMelk Y, Belisle S, Carmel M, et al. Tamoxifen citrate therapy in male infertility. *Fertil Steril.* 48:113, 1987

112. Clark RV, Sherins RJ. Clinical trial of testolactone for treatment of idiopathic male infertility *J Androl.* 4:31, 1983. Abstract

113. Berg U, Brucker C, Berg FD: Effect of motile sperm count after swim-up on outcome of intrauterine insemination. *Fertil Steril.* 67:747, 1997

114. Nuojua-Huttunen S, Thomás C, Tuomivaara L, et al. Comparison of fallopian tube sperm perfusion with intrauterine insemination in the treatment of infertility. *Fertil Steril.* 67:939, 1997

115. Cha K, Oum K, Kim H. Approaches for obtaining sperm in patients with male factor infertility. *Fertil Steril.* 67:985, 1997

116. Society for Assisted Reproductive Technology and the American Society for Reproductive Medicine: Assisted reproductive technology in the United States and Canada: 1994 results generated from the American Society for Reproductive Medicine/Society for Assisted Reproductive Technology Registry. *Fertil Steril.* 66:697, 1996

117. Harari O, Speirs AL, Bourne H, et al. Intracytoplasmic sperm injection: A major advance in the management of severe male infertility. *Fertil Steril.* 64:360, 1995

118. Sherins RJ, Calvo LP, Thorsell LP, et al. Intracytoplasmic sperm injection facilitates fertilization even in the most severe forms of male infertility: Pregnancy outcome correlates with maternal age and number of eggs available. *Fertil Steril.* 64:369, 1995

119. Coulam CB, Dorfmann A, Opsahl MS, et al. Comparisons of pregnancy loss patterns after intracytoplasmic sperm injection and other assisted reproductive technologies. *Fertil Steril.* 65:1157, 1996

120. Palermo GD, Cohen J, Rosenwaks Z. Intracytoplasmic sperm injection: A powerful tool to overcome fertilization failure. *Fertil Steril.* 65:899, 1996

121. Wilkins-Haug LE, Rein MS, Hornstein MD. Oligospermic men: The role of karyotype analysis prior to intracytoplasmic sperm injection. *Fertil Steril.* 67:612, 1997

Chapter 29

OVULATION INDUCTION

Michael P. Steinkampf, Karen R. Hammond, and Richard E. Blackwell

Ovarian dysfunction is identified in as many as 20 percent of infertile women.[1] Managing the anovulatory infertility patient can be one of the most satisfying aspects of an infertility practice. The pretreatment evaluation is straightforward and easy to interpret, therapy is often inexpensive and relatively free of side effects, and success rates are generally high, with pregnancy rates approaching 90 percent in select patient groups. However, perhaps because ovulation induction can yield such dramatic results, this technique is too often abused by clinicians. A clear understanding of when and how (and how long) to treat patients for ovulatory disorders is important for any physician who deals with the infertile couple.

CLASSIFICATION OF OVULATORY DYSFUNCTION

A commonly used classification system for ovarian dysfunction is that proposed by the World Health Organization (WHO), in which ovulatory disorders are grouped into three broad categories based upon evidence of estrogen production and serum gonadotropin levels.[2] Patients who have amenorrhea associated with hypoestrogenic hypogonadism comprise WHO group I. These patients may not demonstrate withdrawal bleeding after progestin administration, estradiol levels are in the postmenopausal range, serum gonadotropin levels are low or normal, and prolactin levels are within the normal range. Group I includes patients with Kallmann syndrome, isolated gonadotropin deficiency, and functional causes of hypothalamic amenorrhea such as anorexia nervosa or exercise-related amenorrhea. Women with WHO group II amenorrhea are characterized by significant endogenous estrogen production with normal follicle-stimulating hormone (FSH) levels.[2] These patients usually have menstrual bleeding in response to discontinuation of a short course of progestins. Polycystic ovarian syndrome and hyperthecosis account for the majority of patients with group II amenorrhea. Women of reproductive age who have amenorrhea associated with elevated gonadotropins (particularly FSH) are classified in group III. This group, which includes patients with premature menopause or resistant ovary syndrome, represents those patients with primary gonadal failure.

OVULATION MONITORING IN INFERTILITY MANAGEMENT

The Medical History
If a patient gives a history of infrequent, irregular menses, she should be considered anovulatory. Only if the physical exam suggests some other cause for menstrual abnormality (such as severe cervical stenosis) should ovulation induction be postponed. Sending the amenorrheic patient home with basal body temperature charts is pointless and frustrating unless some treatment of her problem has been initiated at the same time. On the other hand, a history of regular, cyclic, predictable, painful menses usually indicates normal ovulatory function. Be cautious about starting such a patient on ovulation induction medications—there is usually another cause for her infertility.

Another worrisome sign is a past history of regular menses followed by the abrupt onset of amenorrhea. Unless this occurs along with a significant change in weight, such a history suggest some organic disorder (such as a hormone-producing tumor) as a cause for anovulation.

The patient interview should also attempt to elicit any history of pituitary, thyroid, or adrenal disease, any family history of similar problems, or whether the patient has noted any galactorrhea or symptoms of androgen excess such as hair growth, changes in body habitus, or deepening of the voice.

The Physical Exam
Clinical signs of disorders of the thyroid or adrenals (such as Cushing or Addison syndrome) should be elicited. The breasts should be examined for galactorrhea, although

in our experience the patient herself is better than the physician at finding this. Evidence of unopposed estrogen (pink, rugated vaginal mucosa and copious, clear, watery cervical mucus) should suggest WHO group II amenorrhea, while a patient in her late 30s with an atrophic vagina and scant cervical mucus will more often than not have primary ovarian failure. These women may give a history of previously regular menses followed by oligomenorrhea over the past few months. Although menstruation after progestin administration was once thought to rule out premature menopause, Rebar and Connelly documented progestin withdrawal bleeding in almost half of such patients.[3]

Laboratory Assessment

There are two steps to the laboratory assessment of ovulation: (1) determining whether the woman ovulates and (2) searching for specific, correctable causes of anovulation. As noted above, if the patient gives a menstrual history consistent with ovulation, proceed directly to step 2 rather than wasting time on temperature charts, progesterone assays, etc (see Chap 27).

Step 1: Documenting Ovulation.
There is a wide variety of choices for assessing ovulatory capacity. Our approach to documenting ovulation is to start with tests that are inexpensive, convenient, and noninvasive.

Basal Body Temperature Charting.
Basal body temperature (BBT) charting makes use of the thermogenic response to progesterone, which is produced by the ovary in significant quantities beginning at about the time of ovulation. There should be 11 to 16 days of elevated temperature[4]; a gradual temperature rise may indicate some dysfunction of ovulation, but in general the BBT is not considered a sensitive test for subtle defects in ovulatory capacity.[5] A BBT will be monophasic in 12 to 20 percent of cycles considered ovulatory by other hormonal criteria,[6,7] although Newill and Katz observed that the BBT was biphasic in all of 110 conception cycles.[5] A widely varying BBT usually indicates some technical problem (women who work rotating shifts may have unintelligible BBT charts). Although a temperature drop is occasionally observed on the day of ovulation, it is generally agreed that BBTs cannot *predict* the time of oocyte release except by referring to a previous cycle.[8] BBTs are inexpensive and reasonably convenient, although some patients find the procedure tedious.

Cervical Mucus Assessment.
Cervical mucus that is clear and watery with abundant spinnbarkeit and ferning is indicative of the immediate preovulatory period in normal cycling women, with mucus production most prominent on the day prior to ovulation in about 45 percent of patients.[9]

However, many patients with polycystic ovary syndrome have abundant cervical mucus production in the absence of ovulation. Cervical mucus may be adversely affected by antihistamines, clomiphene, or pelvic infections, but this probably has been overstated.

Mittelschmerz.
Cyclic pelvic pain is another clinical marker of ovulation. Although previously thought to be due to peritoneal irritation from blood released with ovulation, this symptom often occurs at a time that the preovulatory follicle is still visible by pelvic sonography.[10] The variability among patients of this ovulatory symptom limits its utility for insemination timing.

Luteinizing Hormone Surge.
Of the laboratory tests available to detect ovulation, identification of the luteinizing hormone (LH) surge is the most useful. Ovulation occurs about 32 hr (23.6 to 38.2) after the onset of the LH surge[11]; the midcycle rise of FSH tends to occur after that of LH and is more difficult to identify. Younger and colleagues[12] found serum LH measurements helpful for insemination timing. More recently, the development of commercial urinary LH assay kits has overcome the inconvenience and cost associated with serum assays. There is a lag of approximately 4 to 6 hr between serum and urinary LH surges. Because most LH surges begin between 5:00 and 9:00 AM,[13] more than 90 percent of LH surges can be detected by a single urinary test performed midafternoon to early evening.[14] The use of clomiphene does not interfere with urinary LH testing, but an occasional patient with elevated LH levels may test positive throughout the menstrual cycle. LH surges can occasionally be detected during cycles in which follicular collapse fails to occur; conversely, normal ovulation is not always preceded by the detection of an LH surge in urine.[15,16] The sensitivity and readability of these test kits vary considerably with the manufacturer; it is strongly recommended that clinicians become familiar with one or two widely available brands and limit their patients to these kits.

Progesterone Assay.
Because oocyte release is followed by the production of progesterone by the corpus luteum, it would seem logical to assess ovarian function simply by measuring progesterone levels directly. Early studies indicated that progesterone levels ≥3 ng/ml in the latter half of menstrual cycles were associated with the presence of secretory endometrium.[17] Cycles in which pregnancy is achieved are associated with considerably higher midluteal progesterone levels. Hull et al found that midluteal progesterone levels were ≥8.8 ng/ml in 95 percent of spontaneous conception cycles.[18] Similar findings have been reported by several other groups.[19,20] Hamilton et al found that follicular rupture is important for efficient progesterone release by the corpus luteum. In their study, pa-

tients in whom the dominant follicle failed to collapse had significantly lower midluteal progesterone levels.[21] Thus, luteal progesterone assays may be useful for the detection of subtle ovulatory disorders. We currently obtain a single sample 8 days after a urinary LH surge, with a progesterone level ≥10 ng/ml in spontaneous cycles confirming normal ovulatory function. Progesterone levels are higher in cycles stimulated with clomiphene or gonadotropins due to the presence of multiple corpora lutea; some clinicians feel that 15 ng/ml is the lower limit of normal for monitoring clomiphene cycles.[19] Progesterone or its metabolites can also be measured in urine or saliva, but the inconvenience and uncertain clinical utility of such assays have limited their acceptance except perhaps to ensure that the patient is not in the luteal phase when drawing blood samples or initiating therapy that must be done prior to ovulation.

Endometrial Biopsy. In the past, many clinicians felt that the gold standard for the confirmation of normal ovulatory function was the histological assessment of the endometrium. The characteristic changes on endometrial glands and stroma represent a biologic integration of both estrogen and progesterone secretion, and the test is widely available to gynecologists. Obviously, proliferative endometrium on a biopsy taken more than 3 wk after the last menses indicates an ovulation. In addition, a biopsy out of phase with the expected cycle dates on two occasions has been considered diagnostic of ovulatory dysfunction. However, there is disagreement about the degree of delay required for a biopsy to be regarded as abnormal, with either a 2- or 3-day discrepancy considered necessary.[22–24] It should be remembered that the menstrual day should be obtained using either the day of LH surge, BBT rise, or onset of the *next* menses. The optimal time for endometrial biopsy is thought to be 2 to 3 days prior to the expected menses. A biopsy performed with a disposable plastic catheter such as the Pipelle (Unimar, Wilton, Conn.) is considerably less painful than with a Novak curette. Although the risk of pregnancy interruption is small with endometrial biopsy, patients should be advised of this possibility prior to the procedure. Disadvantages of endometrial biopsy include expense, patient discomfort, and the requirement for two biopsies to ascertain subtle ovulatory disorders. In addition, some investigators have observed a decreased conception rate in cycles in which an endometrial biopsy is performed.[25] Recently, the validity of the endometrial biopsy as a test of ovulatory function has been called into question. Davis et al found that the incidence of abnormal endometrial biopsies in women of proven fertility was comparable to that observed in infertile populations.[26] Moreover, Balasch et al noted that even when an endometrial biopsy was inadvertently performed in a cycle in which conception occurred the endometrial histology was read as abnormal in over 20 percent of the

samples.[27] Interestingly, the midluteal phase progesterone levels were normal in these patients.

Sonography. The development of high-frequency transducers and transvaginal scanning techniques has resulted in a dramatic increase in the use of pelvic sonography in the diagnosis and treatment of the infertile couple. The normal mean diameter of a mature preovulatory follicle has been reported to range from 17 to 25 mm[28–31](Fig 29–1). These variations may be due in part to differences in sonographic technique or equipment design, but even within a given study there is considerable variation in the size of the dominant follicle before rupture among patients. Thus, the ability to predict the time of ovulation using sonography is limited. However, sonographic imaging is widely recognized as a reliable technique for monitoring follicular development in both spontaneous and stimulated cycles. In a review of over 600 menopausal gonadotropin ovulation induction cycles, March reported a significant increase in pregnancy rates when sonography was employed to monitor the response to treatment.[32] Sonography also may be useful in identifying patients in whom luteinization occurs without follicular rupture and ovum release. In one report, a sonographic abnormality of follicular development was observed in 58 percent of cycles among regularly menstruating infertile women in whom other causes for infertility had been ruled out.[33] However, other investigators have found the prevalence of recurrent dysfolliculogenesis in such patients to be about 5 percent or less, and such cycles are generally accompanied by low luteal progesterone levels.[34–36] Thus, the routine sonographic examination of all

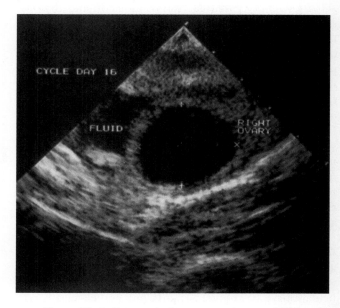

Figure 29–1. Transvaginal sonogram of mature follicle.

infertile women for subtle ovulatory dysfunction does not appear to be cost effective. In our own practice, sonography is used during gonadotropin treatment or when the response to other ovulatory stimulants is uncertain. When scanning is to be performed, a transvaginal approach should be used when possible because this eliminates the need for a full bladder and places the sonographic probe close to the structures of interest.

Other Methods. Serum estradiol monitoring is an integral part of the management of patients receiving menopausal gonadotropins. Haning et al demonstrated that the serum estradiol level was a more reliable predictor of ovarian hyperstimulation than sonography or urinary estrogen measurement in these patients.[37] However, the repeated testing necessary to assess follicular development renders this approach impractical for routine use in the infertile patient, and identification of the preovulatory estradiol peak is not a useful method for ovulation prediction.[11]

Measurement of electrical resistance in vaginal or oral secretions has been proposed as a reliable method of ovulation prediction; changes in cervical mucus production prior to ovulation could account for changes in vaginal resistance, but the mechanism for these effects is otherwise obscure. Little data exist on the reliability of this technique, and we found that patients generally prefer other methods of ovulation prediction.[38]

Step 2: Identifying Specific Causes of Ovulatory Dysfunction. Once a diagnosis of anovulation has been made, the initial tests ordered should in part depend upon the clinical appearance of the patient.

All Anovulatory Patients. Serum prolactin and thyroid-stimulating hormone (TSH) should be assessed in all patients in whom the cause of anovulation is uncertain because the treatments for hyperprolactinemia or hypothyroidism are specific for those disorders, and these illnesses have important health consequences for the patients. Semen analysis also should be preformed prior to ovulation induction. Obtaining a hysterosalpingogram (HSG) before ovulation induction is optional. In the absence of risk factors for tubal disease, we defer this exam until three ovulatory cycles have passed without pregnancy or if gonadotropin therapy is planned. Postcoital testing is often difficult to perform in the anovulatory patient due to abnormality of the cervical mucus and is usually deferred until after ovulation has been achieved.

Clinical Signs of Estrogen Deficiency. The most reliable test for ovarian failure is an FSH level. An FSH level >40 mIU/ml is diagnostic of ovarian failure. An early follicular phase FSH level >15 mIU/ml, and especially >25 mIU/ml, has been reported to predict lack of success

with IVF,[39] and we have found this to be a poor prognostic sign for other treatments involving ovulation induction as well. We usually assess gonadotropin levels in any patient in whom the cause for anovulation is not apparent clinically, especially in the woman over 30 yr of age.

Clinical Signs of Androgen Excess. Testosterone, dehydroepiandrosterone sulfate (DHEAS), and 17-hydroxy-progesterone levels should be obtained on these patients. Elevations of either testosterone or DHEAS to levels twice the upper limits of normal suggest the presence of an androgen-secreting tumor of either the ovary or adrenal. A 17-hydroxyprogesterone level >2 ng/ml (in the follicular phase of the menstrual cycle) indicates the possibility of late-onset congenital adrenal hyperplasia. These patients should be referred for corticotropin (ACTH) stimulation testing. Some investigators argue that androgens should be checked in *all* patients with anovulation because some clinically euandrogenic patients will have elevated serum androgens. However, we feel the chance of finding an androgen-secreting tumor in such patients is too small to make this approach cost effective.

CHOICE OF OVULATION-INDUCING AGENTS

The first step in ovulation induction is to encourage the patient to achieve her ideal body weight. Ovulatory disturbances increase significantly when body weight is less than 95 percent or greater than 120 percent of ideal. A well-planned diet supervised by a professional experienced in the management of obesity may result in spontaneous ovulation and pregnancy. Pharmacologic approaches to ovulation induction should vary with the nature of the underlying disorder. Induction of ovulation in patients with WHO group II amenorrhea can be accomplished with a variety of therapeutic agents; because of its low cost and well-documented efficacy, clomiphene citrate usually is the initial choice. Attempts to induce ovulation in patients with WHO group III amenorrhea have generally focused on administration of high-dose human menopausal gonadotropin (hMG), sometimes along with hormonal pretreatment to reduce endogenous gonadotropin levels. The rationale for this approach is to "sensitize" the ovary by upregulation of FSH receptors. Check and Chase[40] reported successful ovulation in three of five patients with hypergonadotropic amenorrhea using hMG after administration of oral conjugated estrogens to achieve a premenopausal FSH level. In contrast, Surrey and Cedars[41] were unable to consistently induce ovulation in any of 14 patients with premature ovarian failure who were suppressed with either high-dose estrogen or a gonadotropin-releasing hormone (GnRH) analog, and no pregnancies were obtained. At present, these regimens

hyperplasia) is usually best treated with a corticoid replacement therapy. Dexamethasone 0.5 mg administered at bedtime will normalize androgen levels in patients regardless of body weight. If the medication is discontinued, adrenal function will return to a baseline status within 8 to 11 hr. Alternately, patients with elevated testosterone levels indicating ovarian hyperfunction are usually best treated with clomiphene citrate as described above. Failure to produce ovulation with clomiphene doses in the 150- to 200-mg/day range may be augmented by the addition of dexamethasone therapy 0.5 mg every evening if DHEAS levels are found to be elevated. For those patients who fail to ovulate with such a protocol, gonadotropin therapy may be instituted using Metrodin (purified FSH).[55] Metrodin, like Pergonal, is administered via an IM route and is available at 75 and 150 IU units. Metrodin may be administered in two fashions; the short protocol, in which Metrodin is administered in a manner very similar to Pergonal beginning on cycle days 3 or 4 at 1 to 2 amp/day. The patient is stimulated with increasing doses of Metrodin until ovulation occurs between days 12 and 16. Many times, this protocol results in the induction of a large number of preovulatory follicles that predisposes to both hyperstimulation and multiple birth. Alternately, Metrodin can be used in an extended protocol with low doses (75 IU) being administered over as long as 26 days. Adequate follicle induction has been induced using the long protocol with successful pregnancy. Although it would appear advantageous to avoid LH administration in patients with elevated LH levels, the superiority of purified FSH (Metrodin) over a mixture of FSH and LH (Pergonal) has not yet been demonstrated.

Alternately, the patient with an androgen excess has been treated with GnRH and its analogs. Unfortunately, as opposed to the patient with hypothalamic amenorrhea, highly unpredictable patterns are obtained when GnRH is administered to patients with polycystic ovary syndrome.[56] Often, one will find a rapid rise in estrogen levels without appropriate folliculogenesis. In addition, both multiple births and hyperstimulation have been reported with native GnRH being administered to patients with PCOS.

Once the structure of GnRH is determined, many analogs were developed to this compound. These are the agonists (those agents that stimulate the GnRH receptor) or the antagonists (those that occupy the GnRH receptor and render it unavailable for occupancy by native GnRH). A number of analogs such as leuprolide, nafarelin, buserelin, and D-Tap[6]-LH-RH-Pamoate have been used worldwide to induce or facilitate ovulation. All these analogs have been modified to decrease their metabolic clearance rates and increase receptor occupancy. Administration of GnRH analogs continuously results in an initial increase in gonadotropin secretion

followed by down regulation of the receptor.[57] This results in hypogonadotropism and has been called a medical hypophysectomy or oophorectomy. This is a reversible phenomenon, and it has been used in patients with PCOS to render them "hormonally similar to patients with hypothalamic amenorrhea." Unfortunately, limited success is achieved in the concomitant use of GnRH analogs plus Pergonal.[58] Studies that have sought to evaluate this question have been uncontrolled and nonrandomized. Studies using the GnRH analog Lupron together with Metrodin have shown no advantage in the ovulation induction of patients with PCOS when compared to Metrodin alone (Serono collaborative study, unpublished data).

Recently, pretreatment of patients with GnRH analog followed by pulsatile native GnRH therapy has been proposed by Filicori et al.[59] Successful ovulation has been achieved in this group of patients, although reports by others have failed to substantiate this.

Surgical treatment of anovulation has long been known to induce ovulation in some patients with PCOS.[60] Bilateral wedge resection of the ovaries has been known to result in temporary normalization of ovarian function, with pregnancy resulting in 60 to 70 percent of infertile women.[61,62] The mechanism for this effect is unclear but may involve reduction in ovarian androgen production through a decrease in stromal mass or disruption of parenchymal blood flow. A number of alternatives to wedge resection at laparotomy have recently been proposed to decrease the morbidity and postoperative adhesion formation associated with laparotomy (Fig 29–3). Campo and co-workers[63] performed multiple ovarian biopsies at laparoscopy in 12 patients with PCOS in whom clomiphene was unable to induce pregnancy, with an increase in ovulatory cycles of 30 percent; pregnancy subsequently occurred in 5 patients. Gjonnaess described laparoscopic cauterization of the ovaries, with pregnancy occurring in 69 percent of patients after surgery.[64] More recently, Daniell and Miller noted comparable results with laser fulguration.[65] About half of their patients who were refractory to clomiphene ovulated spontaneously after surgery, and 85 percent of patients previously dependent upon clomiphene for cyclic ovarian function subsequently ovulated without medication. Pregnancy was achieved in 56 percent of patients.

Endocrine changes associated with laparoscopic ovarian fulguration in PCOS patients seem to correspond with those found after conventional ovarian wedge resection: a profound, temporary reduction in ovarian androgens (androstenedione and testosterone), reaching a nadir on the third or fourth postoperative day.[66,67] Some investigators have also noted a normalization of the LH:FSH ratio after surgery.[67–69] That comparable endocrine changes are associated with a variety of surgical

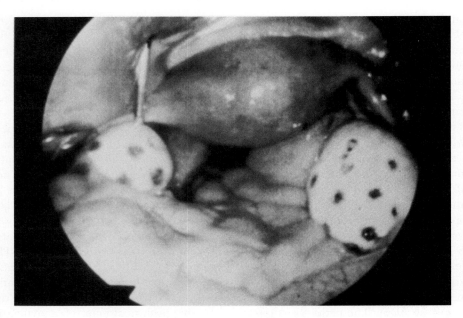

Figure 29–3. Laparoscopic cautery of polycystic ovaries.

procedures involving little or no reduction in ovarian mass suggests that the removal of stromal or cortical tissue is not the primary mechanism for the effects observed. Even the minor trauma of laparoscopic ovarian biopsy has been reported to result in spontaneous ovulation and pregnancy in women with PCOS unresponsive to clomiphene.[70,71] Interestingly, Cohen reported on a series of 149 PCOS patients who underwent laparoscopic puncture, with resumption of menses in 95 percent and pregnancy in 75 percent, compared to menstruation and pregnancy rates of only 75 and 56 percent, respectively, with classical wedge resection.[71] Thus, it is conceivable that less destructive surgical manipulation of the ovary than has been reported may be effective for the temporary normalization of ovarian function in women with PCOS. This would be a highly significant finding because a continuing concern of the surgical management of PCOS is postoperative adhesion formation that might itself result in infertility. Extensive intrapelvic adhesions after conventional ovarian wedge resection have been observed in virtually all patients who ovulate but fail to conceive after surgery, and the overall incidence of pelvic adhesions after wedge resection has been estimated to exceed 34 percent.[62,72,73] Little is known about the effect of ovarian cauterization on postoperative adhesion formation, although preliminary reports in animals[74] and humans[75] indicate a significant risk of this complication.

Hyperprolactinemia

The patient with hyperprolactinemia responds readily to dopamine agonist therapy. The treatment of choice of these individuals is bromocriptine mesylate (Parlodel, Sandoz Pharmaceuticals), which has been shown to induce ovulation in the 1.25-mg q.h.s. to 10-mg range[76] (Fig 29–4). Bromocriptine is available in 2.5- and 5-mg tablets and is administered orally. Although intermittent hyperprolactinemia has often been evoked as a cause of unexplained infertility, randomization of such patients to placebo or bromocriptine therapy has shown no significant difference in pregnancy outcome,[77] and induction of hyperprolactinemia with drugs such as metaclopramide 4 to 5 days prior to ovulation does not significantly affect folliculogenesis or ovulation. Therefore, bromocriptine should be reserved for the euthyroid patient with multiple elevated prolactin levels. Those patients who note side effects such as nausea and vomiting with bromocriptine may be treated with

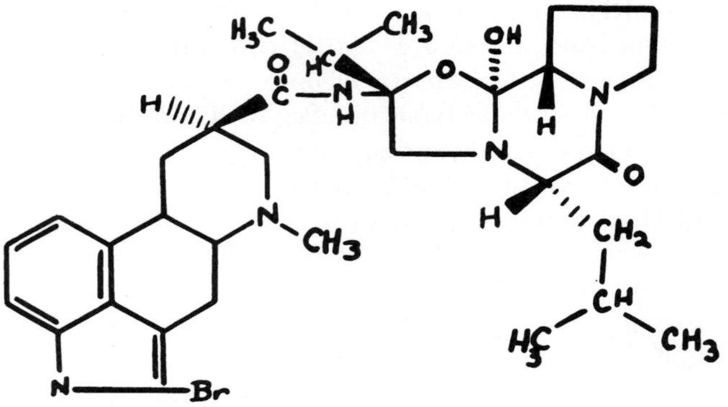

Figure 29–4. Structure of Parlodel (bromocriptine).

vaginal administration of bromocriptine.[78] Bromocriptine is readily absorbed in the vagina; although slower than by an oral route, it maintains blood levels for a longer period of time.[79] Further, incubation of sperm at different pHs with different concentrations of bromocriptine has shown this dopamine agonist not to be spermicidal.[80] Once patients are rendered euprolactinemic with bromocriptine, they often begin ovulation in the first cycle and conceive within 2 to 4 mo. Patients who conceive on bromocriptine should have their medication discontinued once conception occurs. However, it should be noted that exposure of pregnancies to dopamine agonists is not known to be associated with either an increased malformation or multiple birth rate. In fact, patients with pituitary adenomas (principally macroadenomas) have been treated throughout pregnancy with normal outcome. Further, at least four studies have demonstrated long-term follow-up of children exposed to bromocriptine.[81] No deficiency in either motor or learning skills has been demonstrated in an 8-yr follow-up. Although not approved for ovulation induction, pergolide mesylate (Permax, Eli Lilly) will induce euprolactinemia and ovulation at doses of 50 to 100 mg[82] (Fig 29–5). In addition, the nonergoline dopamine agonist CV205-502 (Sandoz) has been shown to render patients hypoprolactinemic with and without pituitary tumors and induce pregnancy.[83] The limited number of infants who were conceived on pergolide or CV205-502 and have been evaluated with long-term follow-up have not been shown to have developmental difficulties.

Dostinex (cabergoline) has been approved by the FDA for the treatment of hyperprolactinemic disorders of either idiopathic or pituitary adenoma cause. Cabergoline

is a dopamine receptor agonist with an empiric formula of $C_{26}H_{37}N_5O_2$, and a molecular weight of 451.62. The drug is long acting and has a high affinity for the D_2 receptor and very low affinity for the D_1, α_1- α_2- adrenergic 5-HT$_1$ and 5-HT$_2$ serotonin receptors. The agent is active orally and tablets contain 0.5 mg of active ingredient. The recommended dose is 0.25 mg twice a week, which may be increased to 1 mg twice a week. The dosage is associated with nasal congestion, syncope, and hallucinations. Side effects seem to be similar to those reported with bromocriptine (publication 816 989 000, N 808010530, Pharmacia & Upjohn Company, Kalamazoo, Michigan). Further, cabergoline has been shown to normalize androgen levels and to improve menstrual cyclicity in women affected with polycystic ovary syndrome.[84] As nausea has been demonstrated with all dopamine agonists, vaginal cabergoline has been reported to improve tolerance to the drug in a 35-year-old patient and a 22-year-old patient.[85]

Manipulation of the Immune System in Ovulation Induction

Independent therapy with glucocorticoids or in combination with clomiphene citrate has been used to induce ovulation in women with elevated levels of DHEAS. However, Trott et al have reported the use of clomiphene/dexamethasone in patients with normal DHEAS levels who demonstrate poor ovulatory response. Eleven of 13 women ovulated with five clinical pregnancies occurring with this form of therapy.[86] Further, Kim et al have reported an improvement in pregnancy rates in patients undergoing superovulation with intrauterine insemination who were treated with glucocorticoids. They demonstrated a pregnancy rate of 45.3 percent in treated groups compared with 29.3 percent in the controls.[87] These types of studies would suggest that further evaluation of the immune and endocrine interaction with regard to ovulation induction is warranted.[88]

Use of Metformin in Ovulation Induction

Metformin (binethylbiguanide) is an orally administrated drug used to lower blood glucose concentrations in noninsulin-dependent diabetics. It improves insulin sensitivity and decreases insulin resistance.[89] This agent is being investigated for use as an ovulation inducing agent in patients who have hyperandrogenemia, as is found in the polycystic ovary syndrome. Further, other androgen-affecting drugs such as Finasteride, a 5-α reductase inhibitor, have been shown to reduce androgens in men and women without altering gonadotropin secretion.[90,91] Likewise, European investigators have used subcutaneous pulsatile GnRH alone or in combination with clomiphene citrate or gonadotropins to induce ovulation in the clomiphene-resistant PCOS patient.[92]

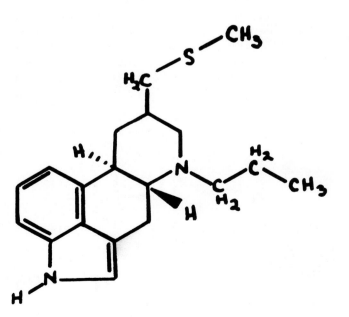

Figure 29–5. Structure of pergolide.

Use of Growth Hormone and Growth Hormone-Releasing Factor in Ovulation Induction

The use of concomitant or sequential growth hormone therapy to enhance ovulation has been used in Europe for a number of years. This hormone is thought to act either directly or indirectly through the production of insulin-like growth factor-1. Recently, growth hormone-releasing factor has been administered with FSH after pituitary down-regulation of the GnRH analog. The number of ampules of FSH needed to attain follicle growth was significantly reduced, and the number of follicles obtained was higher with this co-treatment.[93]

Future Trends in Ovulation Induction

Leptin, the weight-regulating hormone secreted from white adipose tissue, has recently been shown to rescue the sterility of genetically obese ob/ob male mice. Therapy restored testicular weight and normalized histology, indicating that as in the ob/ob female leptins play a significant role in reproduction.[94] Therefore, appetite-regulating agents may play an extremely important role in ovulation induction in the near future.

Perhaps the most exciting trend in ovulation induction to occur in the last decade was the introduction of Fertinex, an ultra-purified form of urinary FSH by the Aries-Serono group. This compound is 1000-fold purer than commercially available Metrodin, and can therefore be administered subcutaneously (Fig 29–6). This is extremely important to patients as a recent poll by Louis,

Harris & Associates (report 954011) showed that patients and their partners were more fearful of intramuscular injections involving gonadotropin therapy than most medical professionals perceive. Patients are very fearful of intramuscular self-injection and partners were also fearful of patient self-injecting. Further, patients and their partners indicated that their work schedules made it difficult to comply with the injection protocol, 30 percent of the patients interviewed believed they did not correctly follow the injection protocol, and unfortunately 13 percent of those patients did not notify the medical staff of the errors (Fig 29–7).

In addition to the availability of purified urinary products, a recombinant DNA technology is producing a generation of new gonadotropins. Gonal-F, manufactured by the Aries-Serono group, should be introduced into the market within the year, and although greater than 99 percent of protein has been removed from the ultrapurified urinary products, the possibility of allergic reactions, however small, still exists. The availability of recombinant FSH products should eliminate this event.[95]

FSH has been shown to have many isohormones[96]; therefore, purification of urinary products to ultrachemical grade or manufacture of gonadotropins by recombinant technology might be thought to alter clinical response and outcome. Thus far, Fertinex and Gonal-F have been shown to yield equivalent ovulation and pregnancy rates in conventional ovulatory disorders and in the in vitro fertilization setting and all randomized comparative trials (information derived from multiple stud-

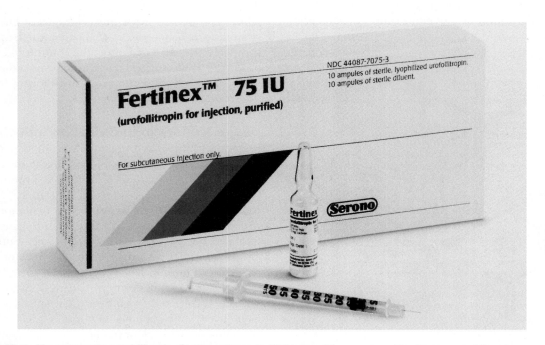

Figure 29–6. New generation urofollitropin, Fertinex, shown in 75 IU dose. The compound is ultrapure, and therefore may be administered by an insulin syringe. *(Reprinted, with permission from Serono Laboratories, Inc.)*

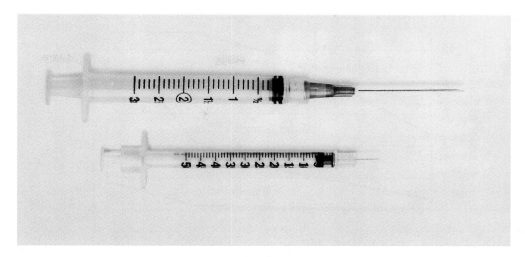

Figure 29–7. Comparison of insulin syringe to 1½-inch, 22-gauge needle used for intramuscular injection of less purified gonadotropins.

ies, Serono Laboratories, Norwell, Mass.) (Figs 29–8, 29–9). A second issue that has been raised is the necessity of LH for normal folliculogenesis. In fact, Regan's group considered LH levels above 10 to be associated with pregnancy loss. Recent studies from the group indicate that suppressing LH levels does not reduce the miscarriage rate.[97] Further, folliculogenesis has been induced in gonadotropin-deficient women with purified FSH preparations, suggesting that the two-cell hypothesis proposed by Short bears some modification.

Advances in Ovulation Induction

Two factors, the use of concomitant intrauterine insemination and endometrial sonographic monitoring, bear discussion. In 1995, the very important paper of Wilcox demonstrated that the probability of conception on the day of ovulation is approximately .35. Yet conceptions occurred at the .1 level 5 days prior to ovulation. An important feature of Wilcox's study was to demonstrate that no conceptions occurred following ovulation. This implies that the timing of sexual intercourse in relationship to ovulation is not under as strenuous constraints as previously thought. Further, a number of studies have demonstrated that in controlled hyperstimulation, the use of intrauterine insemination markedly enhances pregnancy rates when compared to gonadotropins alone.[98,99] Many investigators feel that this maneuver adds 7 to 10 percent additional pregnancy points to the treatment.

While the use of intrauterine insemination appears to have enhanced pregnancy rates, sonographic evaluation of

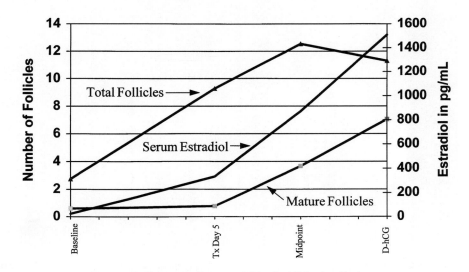

Figure 29–8. Mean efficacy variables in ART using Fertinex.

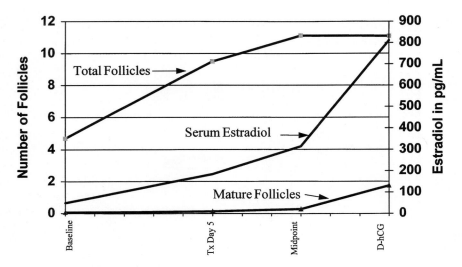

Figure 29–9. Mean efficacy variables in ovulation induction using Fertinex.

the endometrium seems to facilitate prediction of success or failure in ovulation induction (Fig 29–10). For instance, endometrial stripe thickness appears to have some predictive value in that intrauterine pregnancies have been reported to be 13.42 ± 0.68 mm. Patients who underwent spontaneous abortion exhibited endometrial thickness of 9.28 ± 0.88 mm, and ectopic pregnancy 5.95 ± 0.35 mm. Ninety-eight percent of pregnancies found to have an endometrial stripe less than 8 mm were abnormal.[100] Further,

in patients receiving menotropins, a homogeneous pattern detected on sonography was viewed as a bad prognostic sign regardless of endometrial thickness,[101] and in ovulation induction a preovulatory endometrial thickness of ≥10 mm defined 91 percent of conception cycles, and no pregnancies occurred in the series of Isaacs et al with an endometrium less than 7 mm.[102]

Although not currently in routine clinical use, the evaluation of endometrial integrins may be used to pre-

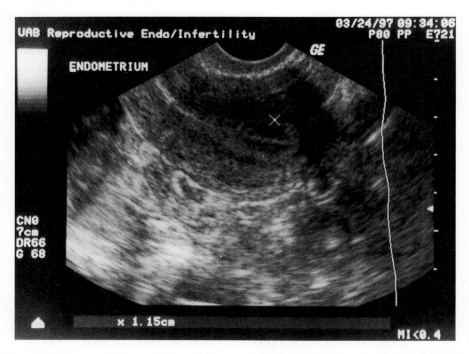

Figure 29–10. Transvaginal sonar of patient receiving gonadotropins immediately prior to induction of ovulation. The caliber marked the endometrial thickness.

dict success. The integrins are ubiquitous cell adhesion molecules that undergo dynamic alterations during the normal menstrual cycle. The αV-β3 vitronectin receptor integrin is expressed in the endometrium at the time of implantation, and its presence is delayed in situations of ovulatory dysfunction. This receptor appears to be present only after cycle day 19 in normal menstruating women, and the onset of its expression corresponds with the opening of the implantation window. Lessey et al have demonstrated that the β3-subunit expression is absent during this window in infertile women with maturation delay of the endometrium.[103]

COMPLICATIONS OF OVULATION INDUCTION

Some of the complications of ovulation induction include multiple gestation and hyperstimulation. Drugs utilized for ovulation induction are associated with multiple gestation. These include clomiphene citrate (8 to 10 percent incidence), Pergonal and Metrodin (17 to 35 percent incidence), and GnRH (sporadic cases reported). The incidence of multiple pregnancies is highest with gonadotropin treatment (about 5 percent of pregnancies); higher multiples have also been reported with clomiphene or GnRH therapy. Classically, estrogen levels were used to predict the risk of multiple births. Estrogen levels less than 1000 pg/ml were rarely associated with twins, whereas levels greater than 1700 pg/ml were frequently associated with multiple births greater than twins (Fig 29–11). With the

introduction of transvaginal sonography, much more precise evaluation of follicle progression can be carried out. Despite this precision, it is still impossible to absolutely predict the risk of high multiples in patients on either gonadotropin or GnRH therapy. The patient who conceives a multiple gestation has several options available. As the incidence of vanishing gestation is probably considerably higher than that reported in the literature, the patient may spontaneously reduce her pregnancy to a singleton or a set of twins. Alternately, the entire pregnancy could be terminated or the patient could elect to undergo selective embryo reduction to a more manageable gestation number.

Hyperstimulation of the ovaries, like multiple gestations, is associated with multiple folliculogenesis. Ovarian hyperstimulation syndrome is classified by Rabau et al into mild, moderate, and severe forms.[104] Those individuals with mild hyperstimulation have ovarian enlargement less than 5 cm, no ascites, and abdominal pain. Those with moderate hyperstimulation have ovaries less than 10 cm and may have ascites, nausea, and vomiting. Those with severe hyperstimulation have ovaries greater than 10 cm, ascites, and may have hydrothorax, dehydration, nausea, vomiting, and weight gain (Fig 29–12). Hyperstimulation syndrome occurs 7 to 8 days after ovulation and is most frequently associated with administration of hCG. Patients usually will begin to complain of abdominal fullness, weight gain, and pain followed by nausea and vomiting. Laboratory findings in patients who are hyperstimulated include an increased hematocrit, increased clotting factors, decreased serum sodium, and a compensatory increase in

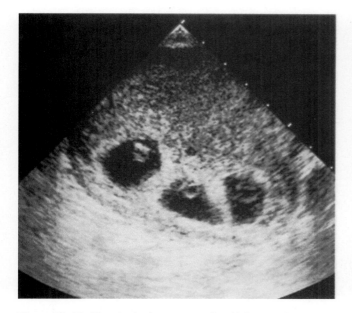

Figure 29–11. Transvaginal sonogram of multiple gestations secondary to Pergonal therapy.

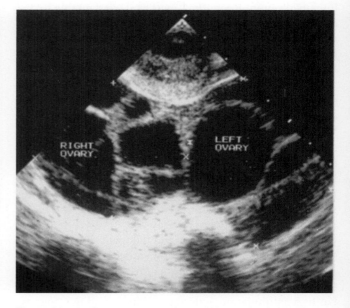

Figure 29–12. Transvaginal sonogram of hyperstimulation of the ovaries.

renin, aldosterone, and antidiuretic hormone. The cause of hyperstimulation is unknown, although it has been suggested to be due to increased prostaglandin production from hyperstimulated ovaries, resulting in peripheral vasodilation.[105] This, in association with the hyperestrogenism achieved with hyperstimulation, gives rise to "leaky blood vessels," resulting in intravascular dehydration and third spacing of fluid. The loss of fluid does not occur from the ovarian surface as exteriorization of ovaries in the rabbit model has failed to block hyperstimulation syndrome.

As hyperstimulation of the ovaries may result in dehydration, development of the hypocoagulable state, embolism, and death, it must be treated aggressively. Once the patient has been determined to be hyperstimulated, she should be hospitalized and hydrated until urinary output reaches 20 to 30 ml/hr. Then, fluid and salt restriction should be reinstituted and the patient maintained in hydration compatible with normal clotting and electrolyte balance. Hyperstimulation syndrome usually will resolve within 2 wk if not associated with pregnancy. However, pregnancy may extend the course of the disorder for 3 to 4 wk. Weight gain as great as 50 to 60 lb has been reported with hyperstimulation syndrome, and it has been suggested that transvaginal or transabdominal drainage of ascitic fluid may shorten hospitalization. Some of these patients have been treated with heparin and antihistamines in an attempt to alter the course of the disease, generally without consistent results.

It had been proposed by the groups of Ash and Shoham that ovarian hyperstimulation syndrome could be prevented by the intravenous administration of human albumin. Recently, Lewit et al were unable to duplicate these results and failed to prevent ovarian hyperstimulation with intravenous albumin infusion at the time of oocyte retrieval. They also administered doses at 12 and 24 hr after retrieval.[106]

Vascular endothelial growth factor (VEGF) is a potent mitogen for micro- and macrovascular endothelial cells derived from arteries, veins, and lymphatics.[107] VEGF promotes angiogenesis, inducing confluent microvascular endothelial cells to invade collagen gels and form capillary-like structures. There is a proven synergy between VEGF and BFGF in the induction of this effect.[107] VEGF mitogenic effect is mediated by binding the tyrosine kinase receptors and activation of the intercellular signaling induction pathways.[108] VEGF has been localized in the human ovary and fallopian tubes and may contribute to fluid formation in ovarian cysts.[109] Vascular endothelial growth factor plasma levels have been shown to correlate with the clinical picture seen in severe ovarian hyperstimulation syndrome. These findings suggest the involvement of this factor in the pathogenesis of cap-

illary leakage in ovarian hyperstimulation syndrome.[110] Further, increased levels of monocyte tissue factor expression is seen in patients with severe ovarian hyperstimulation syndrome. This may contribute to the adverse thrombotic events that are associated with the syndrome.[111]

While ovarian hyperstimulation syndrome is a rare complication of ovulation induction, ovarian cyst formation is commonly found with the use of all types of ovulation inducing agents. It was previously thought that the use of birth control pills hastened the resolution of these cysts. Recently, Steinkampf et al have demonstrated that Ortho-Novum 150 is no more efficacious in the resolution of cysts than expectant management,[112] and that the use of birth control pills markedly increased gonadotropin requirements in subsequent cycles.[113] Finally, Zanetta et al have demonstrated in a randomized study that surgical drainage of cysts proves to be no better than simple observation.[114]

Ovulation Induction, Infertility, and Ovarian Cancer Risk

The risk of ovarian cancer is closely associated with genetics, and particularly expression of BRCA1 and nulliparity.[115,116] In a review of the literature, Bistrow and Karlan found four case control studies and three retrospective cohort studies as well as a large meta-analysis of three additional case control studies that dealt with the subject of ovarian cancer risk and ovulation induction.[117] The three studies that are most frequently cited are those of Whittemore, Rossing, and Ron. Rossing's study showed that women who take clomiphene citrate longer than 1 yr have a slightly increased incidence of ovarian cancer. Those women taking the drug less than 1 yr had no increased risk; not enough data were present in their study to comment on gonadotropins.[118] The Collaborative Ovarian Cancer Group (Whittemore et al), evaluated 12 U.S. case control studies that suggested increased risks of ovarian cancer associated with advanced ovulation induction. These articles have been severely criticized for methodologic variances.[119,120] Finally, Ron et al evaluated the cancer incidence in a cohort of women over 10 yr and found no increased incidence of any cancer.[121] It should be pointed out that from 1982 to 1985, 12 investigators reported 15 individuals with in general serous low-grade malignancies of the ovary. It should be noted that in our own practice, since the advent of modern transvaginal sonography, we have diagnosed three 1A ovarian malignancies in women as part of their basic infertility workup who might have undergone ovulation induction. Obviously, if these patients had been treated with an ovulation induction agent, either clomiphene or gonadotropins, their pathology could easily have been falsely attributed to the ovulation-inducing agent. Therefore, caution should be taken in assigning a cause and effect relationship to ovarian cancer in the use of ovulation-inducing agents of any type.

REFERENCES

1. Hull MGR, Glazener CMA, Kelly NJ, et al. Population study of causes, treatment, and outcome of infertility. *Br Med J.* 291:1693, 1985

2. Breckwoldt M, Peters F, Geisthovel F, et al, eds. Classification and diagnosis of ovarian insufficiency. In: *Infertility: Male and Female.* Edinburgh, U.K., Churchill Livingston, 1986: 191

3. Rebar RW, Connolly HV. Clinical features of young women with hypergonadotropic amenorrhea. *Fertil Steril.* 53:804, 1990

4. Downs KA, Gibson M. Basal body temperature graph and the luteal phase defect. *Fertil Steril.* 40:466, 1983

5. Newill RGD, Katz M. The basal body temperature chart in artificial insemination by donor pregnancy cycles. *Fertil Steril.* 38:431, 1982

6. Johanssen EDB, Larsson-Cohn U, Gemzell CA. Monophasic basal body temperature in ovulatory menstrual cycles. *Am J Obstet Gynecol.* 113:933, 1972

7. Moghissi KS. Accuracy of basal body temperature for ovulation detection. *Fertil Steril.* 27:1415, 1976

8. Luciano AA, Peluso J, Edward I, et al. Temporal relationship and reliability of the clinical, hormonal, and ultrasonographic indices of ovulation in infertile women. *Obstet Gynecol.* 75:412, 1990

9. Templeton AA, Penney GC, Lees MM. Relation between the luteinizing hormone peak, the nadir of the basal body temperature and the cervical mucus. *Br J Obstet Gynaecol.* 89:985, 1980

10. O'Herlihy C, Robinson HP. Mittelschmerz is a preovulatory symptom. *Br Med J.* 280:986, 1980

11. World Health Organization. Temporal relationships between ovulation and defined changes in the concentration of plasma estradiol, luteinizing hormone, follicle-stimulating hormone, and progesterone. *Am J Obstet Gynecol.* 138:383, 1980

12. Younger JB, Boots LR, Coleman C. The use of a one-day luteinizing hormone assay for timing of artificial insemination in infertility patients. *Fertil Steril.* 30:648, 1978

13. Seibel MM, Shine W, Smith DM, Taynor ML. Biological rhythm of the luteinizing hormone surge in women. *Fertil Steril.* 37:709, 1982

14. Batzer FR, Corson SL. Indications, techniques, success rates, and pregnancy outcome: New directions with donor insemination. *Sem Reprod Endocrinol.* 5:45, 1987

15. Elkind-Hirsch K, Goldzieher JW, Gibbons WE, Besch PK. Evaluation of the Ovustick urinary luteinizing hormone kit in normal and stimulated menstrual cycles. *Obstet Gynecol.* 67:450, 1986

16. Ponto KL, Barnes RB, Holt JA. Quantitative and qualitative tests for urinary luteinizing hormone: Comparison in spontaneous and clomiphene-citrate-treated cycles. *J Reprod Med.* 35:1051, 1990

17. Israel R, Mishell DR, Stone SC, et al. Single luteal phase serum progesterone assay as an indicator of ovulation. *Am J Obstet Gynecol.* 112:1043, 1972

18. Hull MGR, Savage PE, Bromham DR, et al. The value of a single serum progesterone measurement in the mid-luteal phase as a criterion of a potentially fertile cycle ("ovulation") derived from treated and untreated conception cycles. *Fertil Steril.* 37:355, 1982

19. Hammond MG, Talbert L. Clomiphene citrate therapy of infertile women with low luteal phase progesterone levels. *Obstet Gynecol.* 59:275, 1982

20. Radwanska E, Swyer GIM. Plasma progesterone estimation in infertile women and in women under treatment with clomiphene and chorionic gonadotropin. *Obstet Gynecol Surv.* 30:205, 1978

21. Hamilton MPR, Fleming R, Coutts JRT, et al. Luteal cysts and unexplained infertility: Biochemical and ultrasonic evaluation. *Fertil Steril.* 54:32, 1990

22. Annos T, Thompson IE, Taymor ML. Luteal phase deficiency and infertility: Difficulties encountered in diagnosis and treatment. *Obstet Gynecol.* 55:705, 1980

23. March CM. Luteal phase defects. In: Mishell DR, Brenner PE, eds. *Management of Common Problems in Obstetrics and Gynecology.* Oradell, N.J., Medical Economics Books, 1983: 440

24. Jones GS. The clinical evaluation of ovulation and the luteal phase. *J Reprod Med.* 18:139, 1977

25. Jacobson A, Marshall JR. Detrimental effect of endometrial biopsies on pregnancy rate following human menopausal gonadotropin/human chorionic gonadotropin induced ovulation. *Fertil Steril.* 33:602, 1980

26. Davis OK, Berkeley AS, Naus GF, et al. The incidence of luteal phase defect in normal, fertile women, determined by serial endometrial biopsies. *Fertil Steril.* 51:582, 1989

27. Balasch J, Vanrell JA, Marquez M, Gonzalez-Merlo J. Endometrial biopsy inadvertently taken in the cycle of conception. *Int J Gynaecol Obstet.* 22:95, 1984

28. DeCherney AH, Romero R, Polan ML. Ultrasound in reproductive endocrinology. *Fertil Steril.* 37:323, 1982

29. Daly DC, Reuter K, Cohen S, Mastroianni J. Follicle size by ultrasound versus cervical mucus quality: Normal and abnormal patterns in spontaneous cycles. *Fertil Steril.* 51:598, 1989

30. Luciano AA, Peluso J, Koch EI, et al. Temporal relationship and reliability of the clinical, hormonal, and ultrasonographic indices of ovulation in infertile women. *Obstet Gynecol.* 75:412, 1990

31. Fossum GT, Vermesh M, Kletzky OA. Biochemical and biophysical indices of follicular development in spontaneous and stimulated ovulatory cycles. *Obstet Gynecol.* 75:407, 1990

32. March CM. Improved pregnancy rate with monitoring of gonadotropin therapy by three modalities. *Am J Obstet Gynecol.* 156:1473, 1987

33. Eissa MK, Sawers RS, Docker MF, et al. Characteristics and incidence of dysfunctional ovulation patterns detected by ultrasound. *Fertil Steril.* 47:603, 1987

34. Kerin JF, Kibry C, Morris D, et al. Incidence of the luteinized unruptured follicle phenomenon in cycling women. *Fertil Steril.* 40:620, 1983

35. Daly DC, Soto-Albors C, Walters C, et al. Ultrasonographic assessment of luteinized unruptured follicle syndrome in unexplained infertility. *Fertil Steril.* 43:62, 1985

36. Hamilton CJCM, Wetzels LGC, Evers JLH, et al. Follicle growth curves and hormonal patterns in patients with the luteinized unruptured follicle syndrome. *Fertil Steril.* 43:541, 1985

37. Haning RV Jr, Austin CW, Carlson IH, et al. Plasma estradiol is superior to ultrasound and urinary estriol glucuronide as a predictor of ovarian hyperstimulation during induction of ovulation with menotropins. *Fertil Steril.* 40:31, 1983

38. Hammond KR, Blackwell RE, Younger JB, et al. Monitoring techniques to predict ovulation: Evaluation of patient acceptance. *Am J Gynecol Health.* 5:88, 1991

39. Scott RT, Toner JP, Muasher SJ, et al. Follicle-stimulating hormone levels on cycle day 3 are predictive of in vitro fertilization outcome. *Fertil Steril.* 51:561, 1989

40. Check JG, Chase JS. Ovulation induction in hypergonadotropic amenorrhea with estrogen and human menopausal gonadotropin therapy. *Fertil Steril.* 42:919, 1984

41. Surrey ES, Cedars MI. The effect of gonadotropin suppression on the induction of ovulation in premature ovarian failure patients. *Fertil Steril.* 52:36, 1989

42. Reid RL, Fretts R, Van Vugt DA. The theory and practice of ovulation induction with gonadotropin-releasing hormone. *Am J Obstet Gynecol.* 158:176, 1988

43. Diamond MP, Wentz AC. Ovulation induction with human menopausal gonadotropins. *Obstet Gynecol Surv.* 41:480, 1986

44. Handelsman DJ, Jansen RPS, Boyland LM, et al. Pharmacokinetics of gonadotropin-releasing hormone: Comparison of subcutaneous and intravenous route. *J Clin Endocrinol Metab.* 59:739, 1985

45. Reid RL, Sauerbrei E. Evaluation of techniques for induction of ovulation in outpatients employing pulsatile gonadotropin-releasing hormone. *Am J Obstet Gynecol.* 148:648, 1984

46. Erickson GF, Magoffin DA, Dyer CA, Hofeditz C. The ovarian androgen-producing cells: A review of structure function relationships. *Endocrine Rev.* 6:371, 1985

47. Dor J, Itzkowic DJ, Mashiach S, et al. Cumulative conception rates following gonadotropin therapy. *Am J Obstet Gynecol.* 136:102, 1980

48. Lam SL, Baker G, Pepperell R, et al. Treatment-independent pregnancies after cessation of gonadotropin ovulation induction in women with oligomenorrhea and anovulatory menses. *Fertil Steril.* 50:26, 1988

49. Lunenfeld B, Blankenstein J, Ron E, et al. Short and long term survey of patients treated with HMB/HCG and follow-up of offspring. In: Gazziani AR, Volpe A, Faechinettle WW, ed. *Proceedings of the First International Congress on Gynecological Endocrinology.* Lancashire, U.K., Parthenon, 1987: 459

50. Wu CH, Winkel CA. The effect of therapy initiation day on clomiphene citrate therapy. *Fertil Steril.* 52:564, 1989

51. Hammond MG. Monitoring techniques for improved pregnancy rates during clomiphene ovulation induction. *Fertil Steril.* 42:499, 1984

52. Hammond MG, Halme JK, Talbert LM. Factors affecting the pregnancy rate in clomiphene citrate induction of ovulation. *Obstet Gynecol* 62:196, 1983

53. Lobo RA, Gysler M, Marcy CM, et al. Clinical and laboratory predictors of clomiphene response. *Fertil Steril.* 37:168, 1982

54. Hoffman DI, Lobo RA, Campeau JD, et al. Ovulation induction in clomiphene-resistant anovulatory women: Differential follicular response to purified urinary follicle-stimulating hormone (FSH) versus purified FSH in luteinizing hormone. *J Clin Endocrinol Metab.* 60:922, 1985

55. Seibel M. Ovulation induction: FSH. In: Seibel M, ed. *Infertility, A Comprehensive Text.* Norwalk, Conn., Appleton & Lange, 1990: 323–332

56. Saffan D, Seibel MM. Ovulation induction with subcutaneous pulsatile gonadotropin-releasing hormone in various ovulatory disorders. *Fertil Steril.* 45:475, 1986

57. Belchetz PE, Plant TM, Nakai Y, et al. Hypophyseal responses to continuous and intermittent delivery of hypothalamic gonadotropin-releasing hormone. *Science.* 202:631, 1978

58. Dodson WC, Hughs CL, Whitesides DB. The effect of leuprolide acetate on ovulation induction with human menopausal gonadotropins in polycystic ovary syndrome. *J Clin Endocrinol Metab.* 65:75, 1987

59. Filicori M, Campaniello E, Michelacci L, et al. Gonadotropin-releasing hormone (GnRH) analog suppression among polycystic ovarian disease patients more susceptible to ovulation induction with pulsatile GnRH. *J Clin Endocrinol Metab.* 66:327, 1988

60. Stein IF, Leventhal ML. Amenorrhea associated with bilateral polycystic ovaries. *Am J Obstet Gynecol.* 29:181, 1935

61. Adashi EY, Rock JA, Guzick D, et al. Fertility following bilateral ovarian wedge resection: A critical analysis of 90 consecutive cases of the polycystic ovary syndrome. *Fertil Steril.* 36:320, 1981

62. McLaughlin DS. Evaluation of adhesion reformation by early second-look laparoscopy following microlaser ovarian wedge resection. *Fertil Steril.* 42:531, 1984

63. Campo S, Garcea N, Caruso A, Siccardi P. Effect of celioscopic ovarian resection in patients with polycystic ovaries. *Gynecol Obstet Invest.* 15:213, 1983

64. Gjonnaess H. Polycystic ovarian syndrome treated by ovarian electrocautery through the laparoscope. *Fertil Steril.* 41:20, 1984

65. Daniell JF, Miller W. Polycystic ovaries treated by laparoscopic laser vaporization. *Fertil Steril.* 51:232, 1989

66. Judd HL, Rigg LA, Anderson DC, Yen SSC. The effects of ovarian wedge resection on circulating gonadotropin and ovarian steroid levels in patients with polycystic ovary syndrome. *J Clin Endocrinol Metab.* 43:347, 1976

67. Greenblatt E, Casper RF. Endocrine changes after laparoscopic ovarian cautery in polycystic ovarian syndrome. *Am J Obstet Gynecol.* 156:279, 1987

68. Katz M, Carr PJ, Cohen BM, Millow RP. Hormonal effects of wedge resection in polycystic ovaries. *Obstet Gynecol.* 51:437, 1978

69. Sakata M, Tasaka K, Kurachi H, et al. Changes of bioactive luteinizing hormone after laparoscopic ovarian cautery in patients with polycystic ovarian syndrome. *Fertil Steril.* 53:610, 1990

70. Yuzpe AA, Rioux JE. The value of laparoscopic ovarian biopsy. *J Reprod Med.* 15:57, 1975

71. Cohen MB. Surgical management of infertility in the polycystic ovary syndrome. In: Givens JR, ed. *The Infertile Female.* Chicago, Ill., Yearbook Medical Publishers, 1979: 273

72. Toaff R, Toaff ME, Peyser MR. Infertility following wedge resection of the ovaries. *Am J Obstet Gynecol.* 124:91, 1976

73. Buttran VC, Vaquero C. Post-ovarian wedge resection adhesive disease. *Fertil Steril.* 26:874, 1975

74. Awadalla SG, Mattox JH, Slichenmyer WJ. The effect of cauterization of the rabbit ovary on adhesion formation. *Fertil Steril.* 46:696, 1986

75. Lyles R, Goldzieher JW, Betts JW, et al. Early second look laparoscopy after the treatment of polycystic ovarian disease with laparoscopic ovarian electrocautery and/or ND:4.YAG laser photocoagulation American Fertility Society 45th annual meeting, 1989, abstract 0-061

76. Soto-Albors CE, Walters CA, Riddick DH, Daly DC. Titrating the dose of bromocriptine when treating hyperprolactinemic women. *Fertil Steril.* 41:58, 1984

77. McBain JC, Pepperell RJ. Use of bromocriptine in unexplained infertility. *Clin Reprod Fertil.* 1:145, 1982

78. Vermesh M, Fossum GT, Kletzky OA. Vaginal bromocriptine: Pharmacology and effect on serum prolactin in normal women. *Obstet Gynecol.* 72:693, 1988

79. Katz E, Weiss BE, Hassell A, et al. Increasing circulating levels of bromocriptine after vaginal compared with oral administration. *Fertil Steril.* 55:882, 1991

80. Rojas FJ, Djannati E, Rogas IM. The effect of bromocriptine on the motility of human spermatozoa and its capacity to penetrate the cervical mucus. *Fertil Steril.* 55:48, 1991

81. Trukalj I, Braun P, Krupp P. Surveillance of bromocriptine in pregnancy. *JAMA.* 247:1589, 1982

82. Blackwell RE, Bradley EL Jr, Kline LB, et al. Comparison of dopamine agonists in the treatment of hyperprolactinemic syndrome: A multicenter study. *Fertil Steril.* 39:744, 1983

83. Vance ML, Cragun JR, Reimnitz C, et al. CV205-502 treatment of hyperprolactinemia. *J Clin Endocrinol Metab.* 68:336, 1989

84. Paoletti AM, Cagnacci A, Depau GF, et al. The chronic administration of cabergoline normalizes androgen secretion and improves menstrual cyclicity in women with polycystic ovary syndrome. *Fertil Steril.* 66:527, 1996

85. Motta T, de Vincentis S, Marchini M, et al. Vaginal cabergoline in the treatment of hyperprolactinemic patients intolerant to oral dopaminergics. *Fertil Steril.* 65:440, 1996

86. Trott EA, Plouffe L Jr., Hansen K, et al. Ovulation induction in clomiphene-resistant anovulatory women with normal dehydroepiandrosterone sulfate levels: Beneficial effects of the addition of dexamethasone during the follicular phase. *Fertil Steril.* 66:484, 1996

87. Kim CH, Cho YK, Mok JE. The efficacy of immunotherapy in patients who underwent superovulation with intrauterine insemination. *Fertil Steril.* 65:133, 1996

88. Hoek A, Schoemaker J, Drexhage HA. Premature ovarian failure and ovarian autoimmunity. *Endocr Rev.* 18:107, 1997

89. Bailey CJ, Path MRC, Turner RC. Metformin. *N Engl J Med.* 29:574, 1996

90. Fruzzetti F, de Lorenzo D, Parrini D, Ricci C. Effects of finasteride, a 5α-reductase inhibitor, on circulating androgens and gonadotropin secretion in hirsute women. *J Clin Endocrinol Metab.* 79:831, 1994

91. Dallob AL, Sadick NS, Unger W, et al. The effect of finasteride, a 5α-reductase inhibitor, on scalp skin testosterone and dihydrotestosterone concentrations in patients with male pattern baldness. *J Clin Endocrinol Metab.* 79:703, 1994

92. Tan SL, Farhi J, Homburg R, Jacobs HS. Induction of ovulation in clomiphene-resistant polycystic ovary syndrome with pulsatile GnRH. *Obstet Gynecol.* 88:221, 1996

93. Busacca M, Fusi FM, Brigante C, et al. Use of growth hormone-releasing factor in ovulation induction in poor responders. *J Reprod Med.* 41:699, 1996

94. Mounzih K, Lu R, Chenhab F. Leptin treatment rescues the sterility of genetically obese ob/ob males. *Endocrinology.* 138:1190, 1997

95. Shoham Z, Insler V. Recombinant technique and gonadotropins production: New era in reproductive medicine. *Fertil Steril.* 66:187, 1996

96. Ulloa-Aquire A, Midgley AR Jr., Beitins IZ, Padmanabhan V. Follicle-stimulating isohormones: Characterization and physiological relevance. *Endocr Rev.* 16:765, 1995

97. Clifford K, Rai R, Watson H, et al. Does suppressing luteinizing hormone secretion reduce the miscarriage rate? Results of a randomized controlled trial. *Brit J Med* 312:1508, 1996

98. Wilcox AJ, Weinberg CR, Baird DD. Timing of sexual intercourse in relation to ovulation. *N Engl J Med.* 333:1517, 1995

99. Vollenhoven B, Selub M, Davidson O, et al. Treating infertility: Controlled ovarian hyperstimulation using human menopausal gonadotropin in combination with intrauterine insemination. *J Reprod Med.* 41:658, 1996

100. Spandorfer SD, Barnhart KT. Endometrial stripe thickness as a predictor of ectopic pregnancy. *Fertil Steril.* 66:474, 1996

101. Bohrer MK, Hick DL, Rhoads GG, Kemmann E. Sonographic assessment of endometrial pattern and thickness in patients treated with human menopausal gonadotropins. *Fertil Steril.* 66:244, 1996

102. Isaacs JD, Wells CS, Williams DB, et al. Endometrial thickness is a valid monitoring parameter in cycles of ovulation induction with menotropins alone. *Fertil Steril.* 65:262, 1996

103. Lessey BA, Castelbaum AJ, Sawin SW, et al. Aberrant integrin expression in the endometrium of women with endometriosis. *J Clin Endocrinol Metab.* 79:643, 1994

104. Rabau E, David A, Serr DM, et al. Human menopausal gonadotropins for anovulation and sterility. *Am J Obstet Gynecol.* 98:92, 1967

105. Navot D, Rebou A, Birkenfeld A, et al. Risk factors and prognostic variables in the ovarian hyperstimulation syndrome. *Am J Obstet Gynecol.* 159:210, 1988

106. Lewit N, Kol S, Romen S, Itskovitz-Eldor J. Does intravenous administration of human albumin prevent severe ovarian hyperstimulation syndrome? *Fertil Steril.* 66:654, 1996

107. Ferrara N, Davis-Smyth T. The biology of vascular endothelial growth factor. *Endocr Rev.* 118:4, 1996

108. Xia P, Alello LP, Isbil H, et al. Characterization of vascular endothelial growth factor's effect on the activation of protein kinase C, its isoforms, and endothelial cell growth. *J Clin Invest.* 98:2018, 1996

109. Gordon JD, Mesiano S, Zaloudek CJ, Jaffe RB. Vascular endothelial growth factor localization in human ovary and fallopian tubes: Possible role on reproductive function and ovarian cyst formation. *J Clin Endocrinol Metab.* 81:353, 1996

110. Abramov Y, Barak V, Nisman B, Schenker JG. Vascular endothelial growth factor plasma levels correlate to the clinical picture in severe ovarian hyperstimulation syndrome. *Fertil Steril.* 67:261, 1997

111. Balasch J, Reverter JC, Fabregues F, et al. Increased induced monocyte tissue factor expression by plasma from patients with severe ovarian hyperstimulation syndrome. *Fertil Steril.* 66:608, 1996

112. Steinkampf MP, Hammond KR, Blackwell RE. Hormonal treatment of functional ovarian cysts: A randomized, prospective study. *Fertil Steril.* 54:775, 1990

113. Steinkampf MP, Hammond KR, Blackwell RE. Effect of estrogen/progestogen administration on the ovarian response to gonadotropins: A randomized prospective study. *Fertil Steril.* 55:642, 1991

114. Zanetta G, Lissoni A, Torri V, et al. Role of puncture and aspiration in expectant management of simple ovarian cysts: A randomized study. *Brit J Med* 313:1110, 1996

115. Modan B, Gak E, Sade-Bruchim RB, et al. High frequency of BRCA1 185delAG mutation in ovarian cancer in Israel. *JAMA.* 276:1823, 1996

116. Rubin SC, Benjamin I, Behbakht K, et al. Clinical and pathological features of ovarian cancer in women with germ-line mutations of BRCA1. *N Engl J Med.* 335:1413, 1996

117. Bristow RE, Karlan BY. Ovulation induction, infertility, and ovarian cancer risk. *Fertil Steril.* 66:499, 1996

118. Rossing MA, Daling JR, Weiss NS, et al. Ovarian tumors in a cohort of infertile women. *N Engl J Med.* 331:771, 1994

119. Whittemore AS, Harris R, Itnyre J. The Collaborative Ovarian Cancer Group. Characterization relating to ovarian cancer risk: Collaborative analysis of 12 U.S. case-control studies. II. Invasive epithelial ovarian cancers in white women. *Am J Epidemiol.* 136:1184, 1992

120. Whittemore AS, Harris R, Itnyre J, Halpren J. The Collaborative Ovarian Cancer Group. Characteristics relating to ovarian cancer risk: Collaborative analysis of 12 U.S. case-control studies. III. Epithelial tumors of low malignant potential in white women. *Am J Epidemiol.* 136:1204, 1992

121. Ron E, Lunenfeld B, Menczer J, et al. Cancer incidence in a cohort of infertile women. *Am J Epidemiol.* 125:782, 1987

Chapter 30

DIAGNOSIS AND TREATMENT OF UTERINE PATHOLOGY

Craig A. Winkel

It is accepted generally that the uterus probably serves a limited role outside of reproduction, and yet this relatively small, muscular organ that the ancient Babylonians and Egyptians endowed with powers of controlling whim, mood, and compassion remains the source of a myriad of problems that bring women to their gynecologists. For many pathologic conditions of the uterus, when reproductive potential is no longer desired, extirpation of the offending organ has become standard therapy. Thus, some 600,000 hysterectomies are performed each year. On the other hand, for women of reproductive age, therapy must be directed at restoration or preservation of fertility, which in many cases might be altered by uterine pathology.

Most of the abnormalities of the uterus that result in reproductive failure, infertility and pregnancy wastage, or disordered cyclic function are the result of defective uterine development during fetal life, neoplastic or inflammatory conditions acquired during the reproductive years, iatrogenically induced conditions, or primary or secondary endocrine disorders. The purpose of this chapter is to provide the student of reproductive endocrinology with a practical approach to the clinical problems that result from any of the pathologic conditions of the uterus that might effect fertility potential. For this reason, the material presented is organized in a manner to enable the clinician to understand the normal physiology and the pathophysiology of the condition involved, the methods of diagnosis, alternatives of therapy, and the outcome results that can be expected when confronted by a woman with a uterine abnormality. Hysterectomy and the conditions for which hysterectomy may be the most appropriate therapy (cervical or endometrial malignancy, uterine prolapse, and pelvic inflammatory disease) are beyond the scope of this chapter. Furthermore, disorders of the en-

docrine system, such as polycystic ovarian disease, which may affect uterine function, are not discussed since they are covered elsewhere in this text.

DEVELOPMENTAL ABNORMALITIES

Embryology of the Müllerian Ducts

Since defective formation of the uterus during fetal life is the result of either arrested or deviant development of the Müllerian ducts, a brief review of the embryology of these structures has obvious practical value for the clinician (Fig 30–1). Between the 5th and 6th wk of embryonic life, the Müllerian ducts are formed.[1] Running longitudinally, cephalad to caudad, they lie in close proximity to the more well-developed Wolffian ducts. An important anatomic landmark is the insertion of the ligamentum inguinale, destined to become the round ligament, into the urogenital cord, thus dividing the Müllerian ducts into two segments: the segments above this insertion remain separate and become the fallopian tubes; the segments below this insertion move medially, will fuse eventually, and will form the uterus and upper portion of the vagina. During the 12th to 14th wk of embryonic life, the medial walls between the adjacent and parallel lower segments of the two fused Müllerian ducts begin to disintegrate from below upward. What remains is a lumen that begins to form at the cervical region and gradually migrates upward until the uterus is formed fully. At the same time that this sequence of events is occurring, the urinary system is developing in close anatomic proximity (Table 30–1).

By keeping a clear picture of these developmental processes in mind, the clinician should have little difficulty in understanding the resultant uterine anomalies

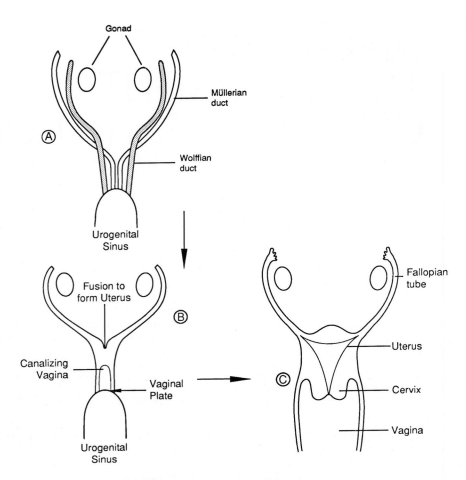

Figure 30–1. Embryology of the Müllerian system.

based upon the time at which an aberration occurs.[2] Unilateral or bilateral failure of the formation of the Müllerian duct(s) may occur anytime during the first 4 wk of development (Fig 30–2), while uterus didelphys or duplicated uterus and vagina may occur between 8 and 10 wk as a result of failure of the Müllerian ducts to fuse (Fig 30–3).

The formation of a bicornuate uterus, septated uterus, subseptated uterus, or arcuate uterus may occur between the 12th and 16th wk of gestational age as a result of failure of the mechanism of canalization to continue cephalad from the cervix to the fundus. Finally, it is possible also to observe asymmetric alterations in Müllerian duct development and the uterine defects that might ensue. For instance, complete or incomplete arrest of the development of a unilateral Müllerian duct might result in the formation of a bicornuate uterus or a unicornuate uterus with an accessory, rudimentary horn (Figs 30–4 and 30–5). Anomalies have also been reported that do not seem to follow any one specific area of dysfunction during the developmental processes. For exam-

ple, recently there was a report of a woman with a bicervical uterus and septate vagina.[3] In this case, the authors have proposed that a minor mesonephric defect might induce an isolated Müllerian defect, much in the same way that Gruenwald suggested that mesonephric defects might induce Wolffian abnormalities.[4] Other authors have recently described Müllerian abnormalities that appear to be supportive of this process as an additional mechanism to explain unusual Müllerian defects (see also Chap 6).[5–7]

Congenital Anomalies of the Uterus

Congenital anomalies of the Müllerian system are relatively common. The prevalence of these phenomena, based on the findings of postnatal examination of female infants, has been reported to be between 2 and 3 percent.[4] Anomalies of the uterus are the most common form of Müllerian system defects. Indeed, it has been suggested that congenital uterine anomalies may be demonstrated in 1 in 200 to 600 women of childbearing age.[5] However, because of the relatively low incidence of

TABLE 30–1. TIMING OF DEVELOPMENT OF GENITAL AND URINARY SYSTEMS

Wk	Crown–Rump Length (mm)	Genital	Urinary
4	5	—	Wolffian ducts reach cloaca, urethral buds form
5	8	—	Ureters, pelvis forming, kidneys move to lumbar region
6	12	Müllerian ducts form	Nephrogenesis, urorectal septum forming
7	17	—	Collecting tubules form, urorectal septum complete
8	23	Müllerian ducts cross medially to Wolffian ducts	—
	28	Müllerian ducts meet in midline below insertion ligamentum inguinale	—
	35	Müllerian ducts join urogenital sinus	—
10	40	Wolffian ducts degenerate	Kidney secretes
12	56	Uterine horns fused, canalization at cervix	—
	66	Canalization continues upward, vaginal wall forming	Urethral orifices appear
16	112	Uterus and vagina complete	—

symptoms attributable to developmental defects of the uterus outside of reproduction, the true incidence of these abnormalities is unknown. Since it has been reported that up to 57 percent of women with uterine defects have successful fertility and pregnancy, however, it is reasonable to conclude that the true incidence of congenital Müllerian defects that affect uterine function may be significantly understated. Nonetheless, a relatively large percentage of women with reproductive difficulty are found to have a uterine anomaly.

It is known that congenital uterine malformations may be responsible for reproductive failure but the magnitude is difficult to define. Consensus seems to exist with regard to the concept that more severe uterine developmental defects are associated with a high incidence of reproductive failures. It is generally agreed that uterine anomalies infrequently result in infertility but are more frequently associated with obstetrical difficulties. Indeed, up to 25 percent of women with uterine anomalies are reported to experience obstetric problems[6] such

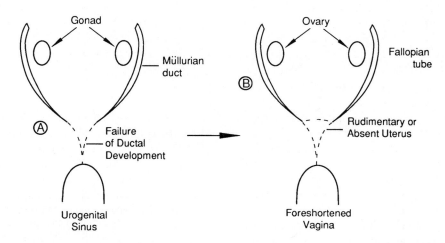

Figure 30–2. Müllerian anomalies that result from failure of development during the first 4 wk of embryonic life.

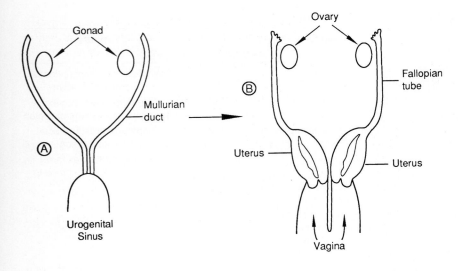

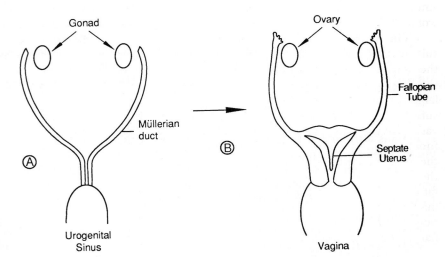

Figure 30–3. Müllerian anomalies that result from failure of fusion of the Müllerian ducts.

Figure 30–4. Failure to canalize during the final stages of Müllerian development may result in the formation of a uterine septum.

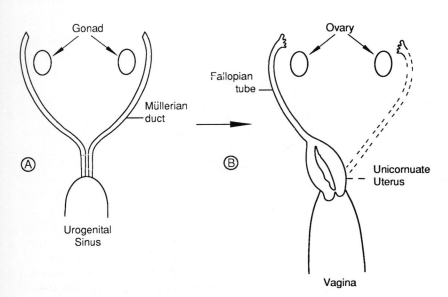

Figure 30–5. Incomplete arrest of development of one Müllerian duct may result in the formation of a unicornuate uterus with or without a remnant of the contralateral uterine horn.

as spontaneous abortion, fetal malpresentation, preterm labor, and ectopic cyesis.

Thus, there is relatively little reproductive impairment associated with true uterus didelphys or bicornuate uterus, although some authors have suggested some elevations in the incidences of infertility, miscarriage, and preterm labor over those expected in the normal population.[7] On the other hand, septate and subseptate uteri are associated with relatively high incidences of reproductive loss. Among women with these defects, there appears to be little difficulty conceiving, although very early miscarriage may be misconstrued as infertility. In fact, the incidence of infertility in one series of women with these disorders was 9.1 percent,[8] a value little different from the 10 percent incidence of infertility estimated for the general population. The incidence of spontaneous abortion is very high, however, approaching 90 percent among women with a complete septum and 70 percent in women with an incomplete septum.[9]

The mechanism(s) by which uterine anomalies result in reproductive failure are not clear. Distortion of the uterine cavity, disorganization of the uterine stroma that fails to allow for adequate compensation for the enlarging fetus and results in increased intrauterine pressure and relative cervical incompetence, and poor vascularization may be involved.[10–12] Luteal phase dysfunction has been suggested to occur more frequently in the malformed uterus because of altered blood supply to the endometrium.[13] It even has been suggested that the faulty Müllerian development that results in uterine malformation may be associated with defective formation of estrogen and progesterone receptors within internal reproductive tissues.[14]

A discussion of congenital anomalies of the Müllerian system would be incomplete without some mention of the female exposed as a fetus to diethylstilbestrol (DES) or other synthetic estrogens. In 1980, Kaufman et al reported the association between intrauterine exposure to DES and upper genital tract lesions that include constrictions within the uterine body, hypoplasia of the uterus, and the formation of a T-shaped uterus.[15] Subsequently, numerous authors have sought to define the relationship between in utero DES exposure, infertility, and reproductive failure. The results, however, are not very clear. Included in the role of the National Cooperative Diethylstilbesterol Adenosis (DESAD) project was an attempt to compare fertility rates among DES-exposed women to non-exposed controls. There were no differences in pregnancy rates observed between these two groups of women[16] or among women in a similar study undertaken in Southern California.[17] Other authors, however, have reported infertility rates up to 30 percent among women exposed to DES.[18,19]

While there is considerable disagreement whether or not DES exposure is linked closely with infertility, there is also disagreement as to whether women exposed in utero to DES are at significant risk for poor pregnancy outcome. Again, the etiologic factors remain to be elucidated, but alterations in uterine blood supply, diminished uterine volume and capacitance, and defective uterine or cervical connective tissues have been suggested as possible causative factors, similar to what has been suggested for the woman with Müllerian duct maldevelopments. Importantly, the presence of a hypoplastic or T-shaped uterus seems to predispose a particularly poor reproductive outcome, and there is little evidence to support any particular therapy for improving these results.

Diagnosis. Since the uterus is a relatively small organ within the female pelvis, evaluation without invasive examination or imaging techniques is difficult. Evaluation by bimanual vaginal examination is of limited value in detecting uterine malformation. On occasion, examination immediately following parturition may be suggestive of complete or partial uterine duplication. Detection of a cervical or vaginal malformation, however, at the time of routine pelvic examination should always induce suspicion of an associated uterine abnormality. Nonetheless, such examinations should be considered insufficient alone and further investigations should be undertaken to confirm or refute the diagnosis of a uterine anomaly.

The diagnostic tools available to the clinician for the purpose of demonstrating a uterine anomaly include hysterosalpingography, sonography, sonohysterography, magnetic resonance imaging, laparoscopy, and hysteroscopy. In most cases the clinician will find that the application of a combination of techniques is best suited to making an accurate diagnosis.

Hysterosalpingography. Since infertility alone is associated infrequently with uterine anomalies, the incidence of discovery of a uterine malformation during the performance of hysterosalpingogram (HSG) for evaluation of infertility is rather low. The HSG, however, is an excellent diagnostic technique to identify the presence of anomalies of the reproductive system and to evaluate the uterine cavity (Figs 30–6 and 30–7).

One cannot distinguish, however, between a bicornuate and a septate uterus on the basis of an HSG alone. Since the latter may be associated with a relatively high incidence of spontaneous abortion that may be overcome by surgical correction, certainty with regard to this diagnosis is mandatory. While hysterosalpingography may be suggestive of a septum or uterine duplication, and sonography and MRI may offer additional diagnostic accuracy, laparoscopy allows certainty in distinguishing the two. If

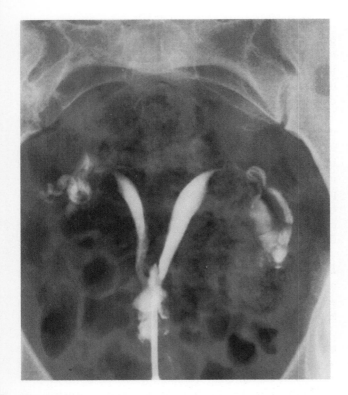

Figure 30–6. Hysterosalpingogram of a woman with a bicornuate uterus. *(Photograph courtesy of S. Karasick, MD.)*

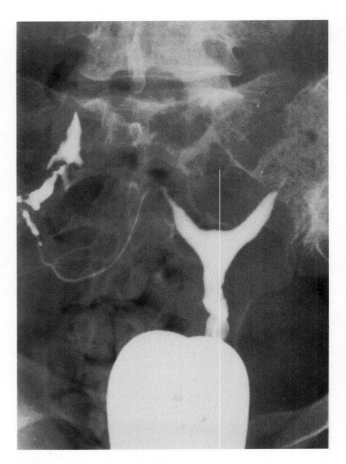

Figure 30–7. Hysterosalpingogram of a woman with a septate uterus. *(Photograph courtesy of S. Karasick, MD.)*

the uterus is septated, the fundal surface during direct visualization will be suggestive of a single myometrial mass, whereas the fundus will be bilobular in the presence of uterine duplication.

Sonography. In recent years there has been considerable interest in the use of ultrasonographic imaging as a means of detecting congenital uterine anomalies. The value of ultrasound for this use is limited in the nongravid state, and then dependent entirely upon the sonographer's or referring physician's index of suspicion. Furthermore, the major role for sonography under these circumstances is in the identification of defects in fusion that result in duplication (Fig 30–8). Early in pregnancy, when a gestation sac is visible as a landmark, the presence of a bicornuate or septate uterus may be identified readily if such an anomaly is considered. The more advanced the pregnancy, the more difficult it becomes to distinguish the uterine anomaly from an ectopic pregnancy, uterine leiomyomata, or premature separation of the placenta. For these reasons, it has been recommended that sonographic examination during pregnancy to rule out a congenital uterine abnormality should be performed no later than the end of the first trimester.[20]

The sonographic features most indicative of a midline uterine anomaly are best demonstrated on a high transverse image through the uterine fundus (Fig 30–8). In pregnancy, the combined findings of bilobed contour of the uterine fundus and a gestational sac in an eccentric location may be diagnostic of such an anomaly.[20] As pregnancy progresses, the bilobed contour and the eccentricity of the gestational sac become difficult if not impossible to delineate. Importantly, as with hysterosalpingography, sonography may not completely distinguish between the septate and the bicornuate or didelphic uterus, and additional evaluation must be undertaken prior to considering therapeutic intervention.

Sonohysterography. It has been suggested that fluid can be the "friend" of the sonographer. Experienced sonographers recognize that the accuracy of sonographic evaluation of virtually any organ is enhanced when that organ is immersed in or surrounded by fluid. The differences in density and the sharp delineation of those differences often allow for better measurement, evaluation of consistency, and definition of anatomy.

As a result, instillation of a small amount of fluid (usually saline) into the endometrial cavity has led to im-

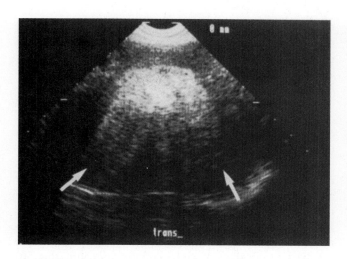

Figure 30–8. Pelvic sonogram of a woman with a bicornuate uterus. The arrows point to the two uterine horns.

proved techniques for evaluation of the endometrium sonographically.[16] Use of sonohysterography techniques have proven to be highly accurate in the diagnosis of Müllerian anomalies[17] and enable the clinician to overcome many of the pitfalls previously associated with difficulties in delineating septate from bicornuate defects.[17,18]

Magnetic Resonance Imaging. While sonography and hysterosalpingography may be used with some success in the identification of uterine anomalies, neither technique reliably distinguishes between the septate and the bicornuate uterus. Since each anomaly may be associated with different prognosis and treatment, such distinction is critical. Additionally, HSG involves ionizing irradiation, risks of infection and uterine perforation, and the potential for allergic response to contrast material. Magnetic resonance imaging techniques appear to offer an alternative, apparently accurate diagnostic tool.[16–18] Two basic patterns on MRI are demonstrated in patients with uterine

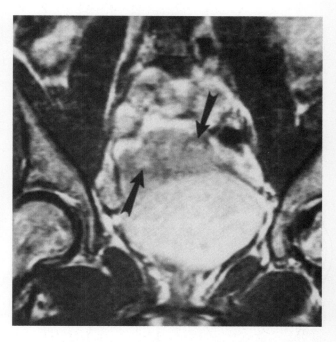

Figure 30–10. Magnetic resonance image of the uterus of a woman with a uterus didelphys. This image is through the fundus of the uterus. The two arrows point to the two uterine horns.

anomalies (Figs 30–9 and 30–10). In cases of bicornuate uterus, two high-signal areas (endometrium) are surrounded by a low-signal junctional zone, and the separation increases as the fundus is approached. With the septate uterus, only a low-intensity zone separates the cavities, and this is lost moving away from the fundus.

Hysteroscopy and Laparoscopy. The hysteroscope serves as a useful diagnostic tool as well as an excellent therapeutic tool. It may be difficult to determine the difference between a septate defect and a bicornuate uterus at the time of hysteroscopic examination (Fig 30–11). With the combination of hysteroscopy and laparoscopy, however, most uterine anomalies can be diagnosed accurately. In addition, hysteroscopy can allow the surgeon to evaluate the uterus for pathologic conditions that might appear on HSG to be congenital defects, such as intrauterine synechiae and uterine leiomyomata. Perhaps the greatest advantage of the hysteroscopic approach to diagnosis is the simultaneous ability to surgically correct the uterine defect.

Treatment. There is little disagreement that surgical correction is the only effective means of therapy of the patient with a congenital uterine anomaly. Before undertaking a surgical procedure to correct such a defect, however, there are a number of prerequisites. First, the surgeon must have a thorough understanding of the embryologic defect that resulted in the anomaly to ensure the selection

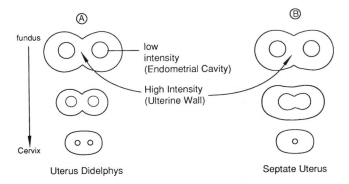

Figure 30–9. Patterns observed upon magnetic resonance imaging of the uterus of women with a bicornuate versus a septate uterus.

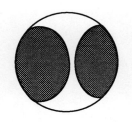

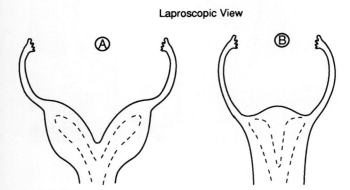

Figure 30–11. Artist's rendition of the view through the hysteroscope of a bicornuate or septate uterus.

resulting single cavity fully restores the normal intrauterine volume, and (4) converting the transverse incision into an anterior–posterior suture line ensures that the raw surfaces of the endometrium are not approximated during healing, thus avoiding formation of intrauterine adhesions. Thereafter, the partition between the two uterine cavities is incised creating a single space. The incision is closed in an anterior–posterior direction (Fig 30–12).

While Strassman originally suggested that this technique was useful in the treatment of women with either a didelphic, bicornuate, or septate uterus, if an abdominal approach is chosen, most surgeons employ either the Jones technique or the Thompkins technique for the removal of an intrauterine septum. The Jones technique involves removal of a wedge of myometrium that includes the septum.[22] Briefly, a wedge incision in the anterior–posterior direction is made in the fundus of the uterus incorporating the septum. The wedge of tissue is removed and the incision is closed in layers in the same anterior–posterior direction. The first layer incorporates the endometrium and is an interrupted layer. The second layer in the closure is an interrupted layer approximating

of the appropriate surgical technique. Second, it is essential that all other potential causes of either infertility or recurrent pregnancy loss have been excluded, since, for example, only 20 percent of patients with duplication of the uterus are likely to have difficulty with reproduction.[5,7,12] For this reason, assessment of male factors, endocrine function, luteal phase function, and other anatomic factors such as the condition of the fallopian tubes must be accurate and complete. Third, evaluation of the urinary tract should be accomplished; because of the close proximity of the Müllerian ducts and the primordial urinary tract structures, conditions that result in anomalous development of one often affect the other. A concomitant urinary tract malformation is observed in 9 to 20 percent of women with a Müllerian anomaly.[3,12] Fourth, before attempting any surgical procedure, the surgeon should discuss the potential outcome of surgical therapy compared to the results likely to occur without surgery.

The surgical approach to the correction of uterine anomalies must be chosen based upon an understanding of the embryology involved. The Strassman procedure is employed generally for the unification of the didelphic or bicornuate uterus.[21] In brief, an incision is made in the fundus of the uterus between the round ligaments. The reasons for a transverse incision from corner to corner are (1) reduced blood loss, (2) minimal loss of tissue, (3) the

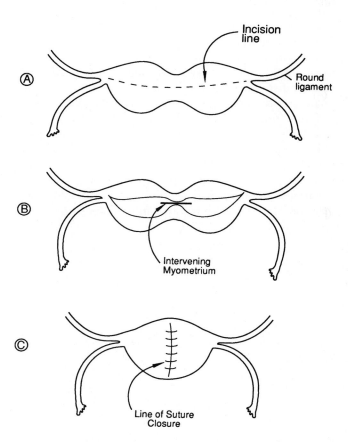

Figure 30–12. Technique for the performance of the Strassmann metroplasty.

the myometrium. The last layer is an inverted running stitch to approximate the serosa (Fig 30–13).

The Tompkins technique, on the other hand, avoids the removal of any myometrium, thus theoretically retaining maximal size of the uterine cavity following surgical correction.[23] This technique is commenced by making a single anterior–posterior incision in the fundus of the uterus directly over the midline septum and extending this incision through the lower extent of the septum. The septum is sharply incised on either side without the removal of any tissue. The single incision is then closed in layers in a manner similar to that described for the Jones technique. It should be noted that the first layer of suture that incorporates the endometrium includes also the edges of the respective septae (Fig 30–14).

The difficulties encountered in virtually all of the techniques for uterine correction that are performed at the time of laparotomy are similar: bleeding from myometrium (the septum, because of its recognizably diminished blood supply, bleeds very little) and postoperative adhesion formation. The use of a tourniquet around the lower uterine segment may temporarily reduce blood flow through the uterine fundus. In addition, injection of the site of the anticipated uterine incision with a dilute solution of Pitressin (usually 20 IU Pitressin diluted in 10 to

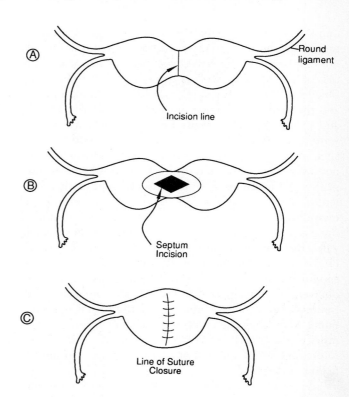

Figure 30–14. Technique for the performance of the Tompkins metroplasty.

50 ml normal saline) is an effective means of inducing vasoconstriction of the microvessels, thus reducing intraoperative blood loss. Of course, neither technique replaces good surgical hemostasis. Finally, following completion of the uterine closure, application of a sheet of Interceed, a finely woven mesh of reconstituted cellulose that precludes fibroblast growth, to the incision site appears to reduce significantly the adherence of bowel and omentum to the healing uterine scar.[24]

The development of improved hysteroscopic equipment, modification of the resectoscope, and the appearance of laser equipment of wavelengths that allow for operation in a liquid environment are advances that have led to the recent interest in incision of the uterine septum by a hysteroscopic approach, now the preferred surgical technique. Clearly, the hysteroscopic approach, as a technique of minimally invasive surgery, has the advantages of avoidance of a large abdominal incision, reduction in the resultant hospital and postoperative recovery periods, and reduction in the potential for the formation of intra-abdominal adhesions that may result in subsequent infertility or chronic pelvic pain.

The hysteroscopic approach should be undertaken in conjunction with laparoscopy to reduce the risk of perforation of the uterine wall and injury to adjacent structures. Operative hysteroscopy is most often performed

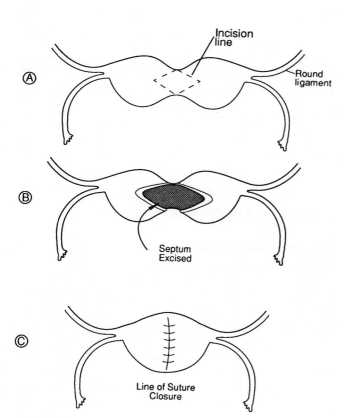

Figure 30–13. Technique for the performance of the Jones metroplasty.

employing Hyskon, saline, or 3 percent glycine for distention of the uterine cavity. Carbon dioxide is usually not employed for operative hysteroscopy because of the risk of embolism as well as the reduced visibility from bleeding. The septum is visualized hysteroscopically and the septum is incised midway between the anterior and posterior uterine walls from the lower aspect upward. (Fig 30–15). In general, there is no need for excision of the septal tissue since spontaneous retraction normally occurs. Incision of the septum may be accomplished with scissors,[25–28] the resectoscope with a wire loop,[29,30] or various laser modalities.[31,32] Hysteroscopic incision of a uterine septum is best undertaken during the early proliferative phase of the endometrial cycle when the endometrium is thin, the risk of bleeding is reduced, and visibility is best. Postoperative management should include therapy with exogenous estrogen to induce endometrial growth and reduce the formation of intrauterine adhesions at the site of the septal incisions. Some surgeons have advocated the short-term use of an intrauterine contraceptive device or an inflatable balloon to prevent approximation of uterine surfaces during the healing process.

Surgical therapy for developmental conditions other than duplication of the uterus and septation of the congenitally small uterine cavity such as a DES uterine defect appear to be of limited value. Attempts at enlarging the uterine cavity by "shaving" of the myometrium under hysteroscopic visualization have not met with success. Additionally, while pregnancy in a rudimentary horn is likely to result in rupture during pregnancy, diagnosis of this condition prior to conception is extremely unlikely. If such a diagnosis were made, surgical extirpation of the rudimentary horn may be indicated. At the present time, surgical therapy to improve reproductive outcome or potential appears not to be effective for women with conditions that result from Müllerian agenesis.

Results of Treatment. The results of various therapeutic approaches to uterine malformation can be expected to differ somewhat based upon the degree of malformation as well as the presence or absence of additional factors that may affect fertility or subsequent maintenance of pregnancy. In one study of 49 patients with various uterine anomalies, successful pregnancy without surgical correction was noted in only 28 percent of those patients with uterus didelphys.[6] At the same time, metroplasty performed in women with bicornuate or septate uteri resulted in an increase in the rate of successful pregnancy from 7 to 75 percent.[6] Rock and Jones reported the results of their extensive experience with surgical correction in women with uterine malformation.[13] They indicated that successful pregnancy occurred in 59 percent of women with a duplicated uterus with conservative management alone. On the other hand,

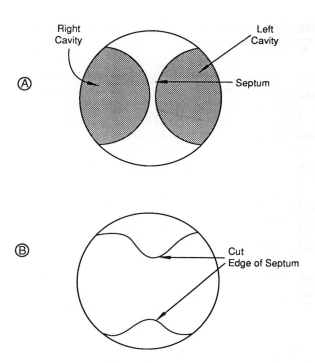

Figure 30–15. Artist's rendition of the hysteroscopic view before and after incision of a uterine septum.

surgical therapy improved pregnancy success rates to 71 and 81 percent, respectively, depending upon whether there was or was not an associated extrauterine abnormality. In addition, hysteroscopically directed techniques are associated with much less perioperative morbidity, and appear to provide successful pregnancy rates that are similar to those obtained following conventional surgical methods, 73 to 82 percent.[25,30] Furthermore, the results with various hysteroscopic methods, (laser, resectoscope versus sharp incision) are similar (Table 30–2).

ACQUIRED ABNORMALITIES

Uterine Leiomyomas

Uterine leiomyomas (also known as uterine fibroids) occur in 1 of every 4 to 5 women during reproductive life. As such, they represent the most common solid tumor of the pelvis in women. They are believed to originate most commonly directly from the myometrium, but may also derive from mesenchymal cells of coelomic lining origin. Townsend demonstrated that each of the cells that comprise a given leiomyoma is of an identical glucose-6-phosphate dehydrogenase subtype, while the cells of two different leiomyomas in the same woman may be of different enzyme subtypes.[33] These data are strongly suggestive of the possibility that each leiomyoma arises from a single aberrant cell.

TABLE 30–2. RESULTS OF SURGICAL CORRECTION OF PARTIAL OR COMPLETE UTERINE DUPLICATION

Author (yr)	Metroplasty Technique	No. Patients	Type of Uterine Defect	Successful Pregnancy Rate	
				Preop (%)	*Postop (%)*
Musich (1978)	Tompkins	11	Didelphys,	57	
	Jones	28	septate/bicornuate	7	75
	Strassman				
Mercer (1981)	Jones	15	Septate,	73	—
	Strassman	2	bicornuate		
Jones (1977)	Jones	76	Double uterus (didelphys, bicornuate, septate)	0–59	1–81
Strassman (1966)	Strassman	128	Double uterus	19	86
Daly (1983)	Hysteroscopy, sharp incision	25	Septate uterus	10	73
Peruro (1987)	Hysteroscopy, sharp incision	24	Septate	11	78.6
DeCherney (1986)	Hysteroscopy	72	Septate	—	80.5
DeCherney (1983)	Hysteroscopy	11	Septate	—	81

It has been suggested that estrogen plays a signal role in the pathogenesis of uterine leiomyomas. First, leiomyomas tend to arise only during the reproductive years (rarely do they develop before puberty or after menopause). Second, leiomyomas tend to grow dramatically during pregnancy when the estrogen concentrations in plasma are high. Third, leiomyomas tend to regress spontaneously and progressively following menopause and the cessation of ovarian estrogen production. Furthermore, the results of recent biochemical investigations are suggestive also of a role of estrogen in the initial development of uterine leiomyomas. While the concentrations of estradiol in plasma of women with leiomyomas are no higher than those of women without leiomyomas,[34] the content of estrogen receptors is higher in the cells of leiomyomas than normal myometrium,[35–37] and the metabolism of estradiol to estrone[38] is greater in leiomyoma cells than in normal myometrium. While there also is evidence that human growth hormone and human chorionic somatotropin act synergistically with estrogen to stimulate the growth of uterine leiomyomas in laboratory animals,[39] there are no data to support such actions of these hormones in women. Finally, it has been proposed that growth factors may explain the development or the various rates of growth of different leiomyomas within the uterus of a given woman.

It is estimated that between 20 and 50 percent of women will experience symptoms directly attributable to leiomyomas. The severity of the symptoms that are experienced appears to be related primarily to the size and location of the leiomyomas. Among the various symptoms that have been reported are menorrhagia, pelvic pain, pelvic pressure, reduced urinary bladder capacity, constipation, infertility, and recurrent pregnancy wastage.

Interestingly, a small percentage of women with leiomyomas of significant size have been found to develop polycythemia or ascites. The mechanism(s) involved remain to be elucidated. It is reasonable to surmise that uterine leiomyomas may occasionally produce erythropoietin-like substance(s) or growth factors that stimulate bone marrow activity. It has been suggested that alterations in the uterine microvasculture result in fluid loss into the abdominal cavity, which leads to ascites.

Infertility. Opinions differ widely regarding the role of uterine leiomyomas in the etiology of infertility. In 1913, Hofmeier suggested that uterine leiomyomas played no role in the etiology of infertility but merely were observed concomitantly with complaints of infertility as a part of some constitutional disease.[40] About that same time, Olshausen reported an incidence of infertility that approached 30 percent among some 1730 married women with uterine leiomyomas.[41] More recently, a number of investigators have sought to determine the role of uterine leiomyomas in infertility. In an accumulated series of 1698 patients treated by myomectomy, the incidence of infertility prior to surgery was 27 percent.[41] Among 677 women with infertility, Buttram reported leiomyomas to be the sole cause of infertility in only 9 percent.[42]

The mechanisms by which uterine leiomyomas might cause infertility are largely hypothetical. In general, it appears that leiomyomas affect fertility by mechanical means. Very large leiomyomas may actually occlude the fallopian tubes or distort tubal architecture in such a manner as to have an adverse effect on tubal function and motility. It has been suggested that leiomyomata in the posterior aspect of the lower uterine segment may alter the normal relationship between the cervical os and the vaginal pool of semen by elevating the cervix into an anterior position behind the symphysis pubis. Coutinho and Maia hypothesized that the action of prostaglandins, derived from seminal plasma, which induce rhythmic uterine contractions thus facilitating transuterine sperm transport is hampered by the presence of large uterine leiomyomas.[43]

Pregnancy Wastage. Leiomyomas may complicate pregnancy and are believed to often result in spontaneous abortion, premature uterine contractions, and uterine irritability. Much like their hypothesized role as causative agents in association with infertility, the exact mechanism(s) by which uterine leiomyomas cause spontaneous abortion remain to be defined. A number of investigators have evaluated the possibility that uterine leiomyomas adversely affect endometrial physiology. Deligdish and Loewenthal studied histologically the endometrium at four sites in uteri that contained submucous leiomyomas: directly over, adjacent, opposite, and at a site distant from the leiomyoma.[44] They found that the endometrium varied significantly within these uteri, depending upon location of the leiomyoma. Atrophy of endometrial glands and stroma, presumably the result of pressure and/or diminished blood flow, was observed in the endometrium overlying or opposite the leiomyoma. At the margin of the leiomyoma, on the other hand, hyperplastic glands were observed, possibly secondary to increased vascularity and thus increased hormone delivery. In leiomyomas located at distant sites, the endometrium appeared to function normally. Farrer-Brown et al confirmed that myomas were associated with ectasia of the venules within the endometrium, the result of vascular obstruction produced by the leiomyomas.[45] This finding of venous dilatation was observed in endometrium overlying as well as adjacent to leiomyoma.

The logical conclusion to draw from these data is that in the presence of a leiomyoma especially in a submucous location, an altered vascularity and disruption of the normal flow of blood to the endometrium may occur. One might envision a situation whereby increased blood flow, and thus hormone delivery, might lead to endometrial hyperplasia as observed in areas adjacent to leiomyomas. At the same time, reduced blood flow, congestion, and the resultant reduction in hormone delivery may well result in atrophy of the endometrium directly over a submucous leiomyoma. While these changes may result in disordered placentation and thus early pregnancy wastage, it is unreasonable to conclude that similar mechanisms may lead to preterm labor or uterine irritability.

Several mechanisms have been invoked to explain the apparent increase in incidence of spontaneous pregnancy loss and uterine irritability associated with uterine leiomyomas. Multiple submucous leiomyomas may well

interfere with expansion of the fetus, or limit the compliance of the uterus as it must expand to accommodate the enlarging fetus. It also has been suggested, but without scientific documentation, that inadequate blood flow to rapidly enlarging leiomyomas within the pregnant uterus results in spontaneous degeneration. The inflammatory response to degeneration is likely associated with increased eicosanoid production that results in decidual activation, myometrial contractibility, and even preterm labor as well as abdominal pain. Whether a similar but less dramatic occurrence results in increased uterine irritability remains to be determined. Finally, there has also been a suggestion that uterine leiomyomas lead to fetal malpresentation because of mechanical limitation to intrauterine change in fetal position.

A final word is in order concerning abnormal bleeding in women with uterine leiomyomas. While it is accepted frequently that leiomyomas are the cause of abnormal uterine bleeding, there are data in the medical literature supportive of a different view. It is true that menorrhagia may be linked frequently with the presence of leiomyomas, but in up to 48 percent of women no such bleeding is observed. One should not expect a pedunculated fundal or subserous leiomyoma to be associated with abnormal bleeding, whereas a submucous location more likely would lead to such signs. Jacobson and Enzer[46] reported no abnormal bleeding in 41 percent of women with submucous leiomyomas. Suffice it to say that the presence of leiomyomas alone is not predictive of the incidence of abnormal uterine bleeding. Furthermore, even if leiomyomas are present, a search for other causes of abnormal bleeding is prudent.

Diagnosis. The ideal technique for evaluation of patients believed to have uterine leiomyomas remains to be defined. Of course, bimanual pelvic examination will always be a gold standard, and yet uterine enlargement may at times be difficult to appreciate. Serial sonographic examination has become a standard method for evaluation and observation of the patient in whom one suspects uterine leiomyomas. This technique clearly offers an objective method for determination of the size, number, and location of uterine leiomyomas. In addition, sonography offers the opportunity for creation of a permanent photographic record against which future assessments can be compared to detect changes in size or number of leiomyomas (Fig 30–16).

While sonographic techniques are inexpensive, readily available, and generally easy to perform, there are limitations. Any solid mass may appear to have the appearance of a leiomyoma on sonographic scanning. Furthermore, determination of exact location of a leiomyoma within the uterus may be difficult even with today's high resolution technology. For these reasons, many clinicians have advocated the use of computed to-

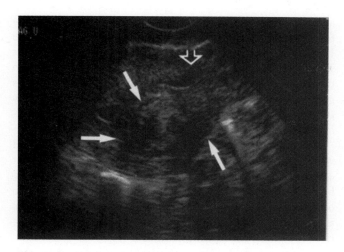

Figure 30–16. Sonogram of the uterus of a woman with a large posterior intramural leiomyoma. The solid arrows point to the margins of the leiomyoma. The open arrow points to the endometrial cavity as a sonolucent area.

mography or magnetic resonance imaging as techniques with greater accuracy and value in the evaluation of women suspected of having leiomyomas.

Hysterosalpingography. The value of hysterosalpingography in the evaluation of women with uterine myomas is questionable. If leiomyomas are large or if multiple leiomyomas are present, one would expect to observe some distortion of the uterine cavity. While there is no argument that hysterosalpingography may allow for easy elucidation of a submucous or pedunculated intracavitary leiomyoma, a striking relationship between preoperative distortion of the uterine cavity and subsequent postoperative outcome has not been observed.[47]

Other Sonographic Techniques. The possibility of endometrial polyps, submucous or intracavitary myomas, or intrauterine adhesions as possible etiologic factors in infertility and pregnancy wastage has prompted investigators to seek ever more accurate and cost-effective techniques to identify potential abnormalities. Sono-hysterography is one of the new tools that allows for highly accurate detection and evaluation of uterine leiomyomas that encroach upon the uterine (endometrial) cavity.[48,49]

Three-dimensional sonography techniques also have been utilized recently for evaluation of uterine anatomy and detection of the presence and location of myomas.[50] A real-time technique, 3D sonography enables the radiologist to evaluate the relationships between myomas, myometrium, and endometrial cavity. This technique may be particularly useful in preoperative evaluation, thereby facilitating the surgeon's selection of the most appropriate approach to surgical treatment.

Treatment

Indications. The indications for myomectomy must be valid or many women will be exposed to needless surgical procedures. The clinician must stand by the admonition that the presence of leiomyomas alone, without symptoms or complaints, is rarely an acceptable indication for surgical intervention. Conception occurs without difficulty in many, if not most, women with uterine leiomyomas and continues without symptomatology or complication in a significant percentage. On the other hand, leiomyomas may be associated with a variety of symptoms of such degree that surgical therapy may be an appropriate option. When leiomyomas result in severe pain, abdominal pressure due to excessive size, bowel or bladder dysfunction, or persistent and uncontrolled hemorrhage, surgical intervention is indicated. When these types of symptoms appear in a woman with uterine leiomyomas during her childbearing years, they are often associated with some disruption of normal reproductive function, frequently recurrent pregnancy wastage and occasionally apparent infertility. Under these circumstances, retention of childbearing potential often is of major import to the woman involved, and conservative surgical therapy is appropriate. Indeed, in several large series, the presence of uterine leiomyomas in women with symptoms of bleeding, infertility, or recurrent spontaneous abortion and a strong desire to retain fertility potential was the most common reason for myomectomy.[42,47–63]

The rapid growth of leiomyomas also may be an acceptable indication for surgical intervention since the possibility of malignant degeneration of uterine leiomyomas, although probably rare, must always be considered. While some authors feel that malignant degeneration occurs within otherwise benign tumors, some pathologists feel that leiomyosarcomas arise primarily and not secondarily from previously benign lesions. Importantly, uterine leiomyosarcomas are not always obvious on gross examination. Hannigan and Gomez reported that 40 percent of patients proven histologically to have a sarcoma appeared to have a simple leiomyoma on gross inspection.[64] For this reason, if the primary indication for surgery is rapid enlargement, myomectomy may be inappropriate.

Size alone may be an indication for surgical intervention, especially if the size itself is considered to be the major etiologic factor in the patient's symptoms. It is not uncommon for a myomatous uterus of greater than 12 to 14 wk gestational size to be associated with symptoms of pelvic pressure, dyspareunia, constipation, or decreased bladder volume and subsequent increase in urinary frequency. Some clinicians hold the view that uterine size greater than that of 12 wk of gestation is an indication for hysterectomy even if symptoms do not exist. This latter view is less widely held today, and probably has no role in the modern management of women with uterine leiomyomas.

Infertility as a primary indication for surgical therapy is probably appropriate only on rare occasions. While several authors have suggested that fertility improves following myomectomy in up to 30 percent of patients,[42,48,49] it is this author's opinion that myomectomy should be considered a reasonable therapeutic modality for fertility only in the woman in whom tubal occlusion is believed to be secondary to the location of the leiomyoma or as a final possibility in the woman with large leiomyomas and no other explanation for failure to conceive. Most importantly, such a patient should be counseled extensively regarding the relatively low rate of improvement in fertility associated with myomectomy, the risks of surgery, and the other options available in her pursuit of fertility (eg, assisted reproduction techniques).

Perhaps the most important indication for conservative surgery in the woman with uterine leiomyomas is recurrent pregnancy loss (see also Chap 34). There is little dispute that large uterine leiomoymas are associated with an increased incidence of preterm labor as well as early pregnancy wastage. Furthermore, a review of the literature is suggestive of an improvement in the rate of fetal salvage following myomectomy (Table 30–3) that varies between 4 and 47 percent. In addition, it appears that the improvement in the rate of fetal salvage that follows myomectomy is greatest when previous history of recurrent loss can be attributed primarily to the presence of uterine leiomyomas.

Medical Therapy. Because of the difficulties inherent in surgical extirpation of uterine leiomyomas, as well as the costs of surgical therapy, whether hysterectomy or myomectomy, in terms of financial and social issues, a search for alternative methods of treatment is ongoing. Because uterine leiomyomas increase in size during pregnancy, a state of relative hyperestrogenism, and decrease in size following the cessation of ovarian estrogen biosynthesis that occurs with menopause, most forms of medical ther-

apy have been directed at either counteraction of the effects of estrogen or reduction in estrogen production. Early studies of the effect of progestational agents were suggestive that such treatment leads to degeneration of the uterine leiomyomas.[65] However, the effect of progestins was found to be unpredictable at low doses, and the side effects associated with therapy with large doses of progestins are intolerable.

A recent advance in the medical treatment of women with uterine leiomyomas derived from the clinical introduction of the long-acting gonadotropin-releasing hormone (GnRH) analogues. Based upon the early works of Knobil,[66] it is apparent that the pituitary responds to the pulsatile presentation of GnRH with pulsatile secretion of follicle-stimulating hormone (FSH) and luteinizing hormone (LH). When GnRH is presented to the pituitary gland, it rapidly becomes refractory to further stimulation by GnRH, and secretion of FSH and LH practically ceases. The mechanism(s) involved are discussed elsewhere in this text. Under these circumstances, stimulation of ovarian folliculogenesis and subsequent ovarian biosynthesis of estrogen and androgens essentially ceases, thereby creating a pseudomenopausal state. With the withdrawal of estrogen, estrogen-dependent diseases can be expected to regress.

GnRH is a decapeptide that is cleared rapidly from the circulation by the action of endopeptidases. The action of these endopeptidases is to cleave circulating peptides, including GnRH, into smaller fragments that lack bioactivity. The primary site of cleavage is the bond between the sixth and the seventh amino acids (L-glycine and L-leucine, respectively) and indeed this appears to be an important recognition point for enzymatic interaction. Consequently, a substitution for either of these amino acids may result in the formation of a GnRH-like peptide that is not recognized by plasma endopeptidases and that remains in the circulation as a long-acting GnRH analogue. To date, there are some 2000 long-acting GnRH analogues that have been synthesized. Relatively few have been tested, however, in the clinical situation.

The first report of the ability of therapy with GnRH analogues to reduce the size of uterine leiomyomas was authored by Filicori et al.[67] Subsequently, a number of reports have appeared in the literature suggesting that therapy with GnRH analogues will reduce predictably the size of uterine leiomyomas.[68–70] Most investigators,[68–70] including this author,[71] have found that treatment with GnRH analogues of women of reproductive age who have uterine leiomyomas is associated with a 40 to 50 percent reduction in size. It has been shown that the reduction in uterine size during such therapy is the result of reduction of both leiomyomatous mass as well as that of the normal myometrium. Therapy results in reduction in cell size, both of the leiomyomas and the my-

**TABLE 30–3. RATES OF FETAL SALVAGE
AMONG WOMEN WITH UTERINE LEIOMYOMATA
BEFORE AND AFTER MYOMECTOMY**

	N	Preop	Postop
Davids	1335	61	88
Ingersoll	139	59	81
Stevenson	107	56	85
Malone	75	50	77
Loeffler	180	55	59
Babaknia	46	24	91
Buttram	59	48	69
TOTAL	1941	59	81

(Modified, with permission, from Buttram & Reiter. Uterine leiomyomata: Etiology, symptomatology, and management. Fertil Steril. 36:433, 1981.)

ometrium, rather than an actual reduction in cell number. Importantly, however, it has been demonstrated also that the uterine leiomyomas begin to increase in size within 2 to 3 mo following the cessation of therapy with a GnRH analog. Indeed, within 12 mo of the cessation of therapy, the leiomyomas attain a size similar to that observed prior to the commencement of therapy.[72] For these reasons, it is recommended that the role of therapy with the GnRH analogues in the treatment of patients with uterine leiomyomas must be primarily as an adjunct to surgical therapy (therapy or hysterectomy).

Theoretically, GnRH analogue therapy may have a role in delaying the need for surgery in a perimenopausal female with uterine leiomyomata in anticipation of the menopausal, hypoestrogenic state expected at the time of menopause. It should also be mentioned that therapy with GnRH analogues might also be of potential benefit in creating a state of amenorrhea in the woman who develops anemia secondary to heavy and persistent uterine bleeding associated with leiomyomas. This might allow natural erythropoeisis sufficient time to restore a normal circulating hemoglobin concentration prior to surgical therapy, thereby avoiding blood transfusion. Finally, therapy with GnRH analogues might prove to be useful even in the patient about to undergo hysterectomy in the sense that such therapy may allow reduction of uterine volume sufficient to allow for a vaginal as opposed to an abdominal approach to hysterectomy.

Surgical Therapy. In general, most clinicians have found that surgical therapy of women with uterine leiomyomas who desire to retain reproductive function is best accomplished following pretreatment with a GnRH analogue only if the uterine size is consistent with that of a 14 to 16 wk gestation or greater. Myomectomy, when the uterine size is less than 14 wk, is not significantly easier or associated with less blood loss following medical pretreatment than without pretreatment. The most important fact to remember, however, is that myomectomy is a more difficult procedure than hysterectomy, and is associated with greater risks of complication.

The surgical approaches to the treatment of women with leiomyomas may be divided into procedures performed at laparotomy, and those performed under laparoscopic or hysteroscopic direction. In general, the latter two approaches tend to be somewhat limited and appropriate under only very specific conditions. Most clinicians feel today that leiomyomas that can be removed satisfactorily using a laparoscopic approach probably are of such size and location as to have little clinical significance. The ability to handle appropriately the uterine dissection involved and subsequent uterine closure required in the removal of large intramural or submucosal leiomyomas is limited presently by the current stage of technical advance in instrumentation. Perhaps in the fu-

ture, laparoscopic myomectomy will become more generally feasible.

At laparotomy, the most important principles of multiple or single myomectomy include gentle handling of tissues, appropriate selection of incision site, and atraumatic repair to limit subsequent adhesion formation. Excessive intraoperative blood loss and postoperative adhesion formation are the principal difficulties to be avoided. A number of authors have described various techniques for myomectomy. It is this author's opinion that the following technique allows the best chance of success with a minimum of complications. Initially, it is necessary to select an appropriate site to incise the uterine serosa. In general, an anterior incision is less likely to adhere to bowel, omentum, tubes, or ovaries, than a posterior one. It is best to place the incision in a location to afford removal of the maximal numbers of leiomyomas through a single incision, to avoid making multiple wounds that increase the chances of postoperative adhesion formation. Once an incision site is selected, the serosa and underlying leiomyomas are injected with a solution of Pitressin (20 IU Pitressin in 10 to 50 ml normal saline) to reduce bleeding at the incision site. An incision is made through the myometrium down to the pseudocapsule of the leiomyoma. Since the majority of blood vessels tend to be compressed to the sides of the leiomyoma, avoidance of blunt dissection reduces the amount of bleeding associated with extirpation of the leiomyoma. For these reasons, the leiomyoma is grasped with a tenaculum or Lahey thyroid clamp and elevated.

The capsular tissue is thus placed under tension. Using either a contact neodymium YAG laser, a KTP laser, an electrocautery needle, or a scalpel, gentle, shallow incision is made across the adventitial tissue, allowing the vessels to retract under tension or with gentle pressure without cutting across the vessels themselves. A similar technique has been recommended for separating pubovesical fascia from vaginal mucosa in the performance of an anterior colporrhaphy. Once the leiomyoma is removed, any large vessels in the resultant cavity are ligated individually. The cavity is closed in layers using an absorbable suture material, making sure not to leave potential spaces for subsequent fluid or blood collection. The serosa is closed employing a running baseball-stitch technique to invert the edges and to expose minimal suture material to the peritoneal cavity. After meticulous hemostasis is obtained, the author routinely places a sheet of Interceed, an absorbable antiadhesion formation barrier, over the incision site.

The technique for performing myomectomy under laparoscopic visualization follows the general principles just described. The serosa overlying the leiomyoma is injected with a dilute solution of Pitressin. An incision is made in the serosa with an electrocautery needle, a laser, or with scissors following blanching and coagulation of the surface with an endocoagulator or some other coagulation device. The leiomyoma is dissected free of the surrounding myometrium and removed. The remaining cavity should be irrigated and any bleeding sites cauterized. If possible, the serosa should then be sutured closed. It is this latter technique that limits the practicality of laparoscopic myomectomy because of the lack of availability of curved needles.

Asherman Syndrome

Amenorrhea traumatica (atretica) has been described in the medical literature by a number of authors. The first report appeared in 1894, and between then and 1933 some 20 case reports were published. In 1948, Asherman published his classic article in which he described 8 cases of intrauterine stenosis.[73] Intrauterine stenosis is most frequently the result of development of adhesions, or synechiae, between the anterior and posterior walls of the uterus that follows partial or total removal of endometrium, thereby exposing the myometrium during vigorous curettage of the uterine cavity. Recall that the uterine cavity is in essence a potential space with the opposing walls of endometrium in approximation. This is visible on ultrasonographic examination as an "endometrial stripe." Intrauterine adhesions may develop following a dilatation and curettage for an incomplete abortion or more often after a curettage following a term delivery. If a significant amount of endometrium is removed and myometrium is exposed, opposing myometrial surfaces are likely to heal together. The result may be the formation of adhesive bands of various size, and may lead to partial or total obliteration of the endometrial cavity. As a result, there is amenorrhea or reduction in quantity of menstrual flow.

Diagnosis. The diagnosis of intrauterine adhesions is suggested by a noticeable decrease in menstrual flow that follows a dilatation and curettage. The subsequent menstrual pattern may be characterized by hypomenorrhea or amenorrhea. Since the etiology of this abnormality is mechanical, hormonal parameters are normal and ovulation occurs. Because of this, patients frequently continue to experience the cyclic, somatic symptoms and premenstrual molimina associated with normal ovarian function. Such a history is important to recognize, since intrauterine adhesions are the most likely cause of amenorrhea following curettage.

When the possibility of intrauterine adhesions is considered, diagnosis can be confirmed by hysterosalpingography or hysteroscopy. Sonography, and even hysterosonography, do not appear to be reliable techniques for evaluation of the uterus for intrauterine adhesions.[48] Hysterosalpingography can be accomplished usually even if the adhesions extend to the internal cervical os. Once the uterus is sounded, instillation of contrast material outlines filling defects within the uterine cavity. The defects may be minimal or extensive and result in failure to demonstrate tubal patency. An example of a hysterosalpingography demonstrative of uterine synechia is shown in Fig 30–17. Hysteroscopic evaluation of the uterine cavity has gained favor rapidly, especially with the development of carbon dioxide insufflation equipment, flexible hysteroscopes, and the ability to perform diagnostic procedures in an office setting. Hysteroscopic evaluation is frequently more accurate than radiographic studies, especially when the degree of intrauterine adhesion formation is minimal and involves only the lateral aspects of the uterine cavity or the lower uterine segment.

Treatment. Management of the woman with intrauterine adhesions has changed greatly over the past 2 to 3 decades. Blind, undirected endometrial curettage followed by insertion of an intrauterine device to keep the opposing intrauterine surfaces opposed was the recommended method of therapy in the 1960s.[74] Hysteroscopy has now become the method of choice for the treatment of intrauterine adhesions. Under direction visualization, uterine adhesions can be lysed and the uterine cavity restored to a normal or near normal configuration. Lysis can be accomplished sharply employing a variety of flexible or rigid scissors, by cautery employing a resectoscope, or by using any of a variety of laser energy wavelengths delivered through quartz fibers. Once hysteroscopic adhesi-

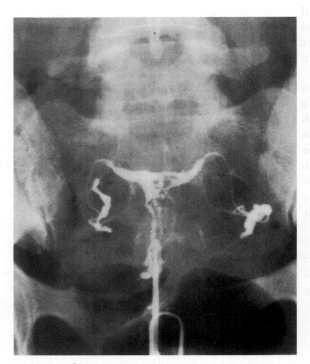

Figure 30–17. Hysterosalpingogram of a woman with Asherman syndrome. Notice the multiple filling defects in the middle and right portions of the uterus. *(Photograph courtesy of S. Karasick, MD.)*

olysis has been accomplished, insertion of an intrauterine device or a small balloon catheter ensures separation of the uterine walls. In addition, treatment with exogenous estrogen to stimulate the growth of endometrial tissue is often recommended. Several authors have reported variations of this method of hysteroscopic treatment.[75,76]

Results of Treatment.   Standard uterine curettage with a hope of lysis of synechia was somewhat effective. Most patients experienced resumption of menses, and over 90 percent demonstrated restoration of the uterine cavity on the basis of subsequent hysterosalpingography. However, in most series of patients with significant degrees of endometrial ablation, the subsequent pregnancy rates were 20 to 25 percent. Using a hysteroscopic approach, on the other hand, pregnancy rates of 40 to 70 percent have been achieved.[75–77]

Uterine Infection

Under ordinary circumstances, the endometrium and the uterine cavity are sterile.[78] Following childbirth or surgical invasion of the endometrial cavity, endometritis may occur as the result of inoculation of bacteria into the cavity. Furthermore, ascending infection from the cervix with organisms such as *Neisseria gonorrhoeae* or *Actinomyces israelii* can result in endometritis.[79] More indolent infections such as *Chlamydia trachomatis* also has been recognized as a potential cause of infertility, since this pathogen may alter endometrial function and result in tubal occlusion or peritubal adhesion formation.[80] If an acute endometrial infection is suspected, appropriate cultures should be taken and therapy with appropriate broad-spectrum antibiotics commenced.

Chronic endometritis is a subject of very limited discussion in the medical literature but one of potential significance in the woman who presents with a complaint of infertility. The most common cause of chronic endometrial infection is tuberculosis, which is rare in developed countries. In underdeveloped countries, the incidence of pelvic tuberculosis is much higher. Indeed, in India, tuberculosis is involved in nearly 15 percent of women with a complaint of primary amenorrhea.[81]

If nontuberculous, chronic endometritis is suspected, cultures should be obtained and broad-spectrum antibiotics should be administered. After antibiotic therapy has been instituted, a gentle uterine curettage may be effective in eliminating the bulk of the infected endometrium. Care should be taken not to curette the endometrial cavity too vigorously, to prevent the development of intrauterine adhesions. Thereafter, it is recommended that administration of estrogen (conjugated estrogen, 2.5 to 10 mg orally, daily, or the equivalent) for 1 to 2 mo be instituted to induce the regeneration of healthy endometrium.

Adenomyosis

Adenomyosis, the finding of endometrial glands and stroma insinuated into the myometrium, is a condition that results in symptoms that may be suggestive of endometriosis—lower abdominal pain, dysmenorrhea, and dyspareunia. While adenomyosis has been referred to in the past as "endometriosis interna," it is clear that adenomyosis and endometriosis are two very different conditions that are found in the same patient only 20 percent or less of the time.[81] Indeed, endometriosis and adenomyosis are similar only in the sense that endometrial glands and stroma are found at ectopic sites. Adenomyosis is derived from aberrant endometrial glands that arise in the basalis layer of the endometrium. As a consequence of the abnormal nature of these glands, the normal proliferative and secretory changes associated with the cyclic ovarian hormone production are not observed in adenomyosis.

The pathogenesis of adenomyosis remains unknown. Since this condition is observed most frequently in the older and multiparous woman, it has been suggested that adenomyosis results from the expansion of spaces between myometrial fibers and resultant insinuation or trapping of endometrial elements during parturition. Serial histologic specimens confirm that the glandular elements of adenomyosis are continuous with the basal layer of the endometrium. Thus, adenomyosis is the result of direct extension of the endometrium. For an unknown reason, the normal barrier between the endometrium and the myometrium is broken. At first, the stromal elements and then the glandular gradually grow into the myometrium. Furthermore, it is generally held that high concentrations of estrogen stimulate the growth of the basal layer of endometrium along the planes of least resistance, which commonly follow alongside lymphatic and vascular channels.[82]

Adenomyosis is diagnosed most commonly as an incidental finding by the pathologist during histologic examination of the hysterectomy specimen. The most common histologic pattern is a diffuse one that involves both the anterior and the posterior walls of the uterus in which one can observe erratically located areas of endometrium. Occasionally, it is possible also to observe a more localized form of the disease, an adenomyoma, in which the areas of ectopic endometrium may be encapsulated.[83] From a clinical point of view, the latter can be mistaken easily for a leiomyoma during physical examination, during sonography, as well as during surgical exploration.

Some imaging techniques are occasionally useful in the detection of adenomyosis. Hysterosalpingography may detect a pattern of "spiculation" of the interface of dye and endometrium suggestive of adenomyosis.[84,85] In addition, "lollipop" diverticuli (collections of dye separated by radiolucency from the endometrial cavity) have also been described.[86] Transvaginal sonography also has proven to be a useful tool providing that the adenomyosis is significant enough to result in the development of anechoic areas in the myometrium.[87] At present, however, magnetic resonance imaging (MRI) is the diagnostic modality of choice when adenomyosis is suspected.[88]

As mentioned previously, it is unusual for the endometrial glands and stroma of adenomyosis to undergo the cyclic changes of the normal endometrium. Indeed, it has even been suggested that there is a relative deficiency of progesterone and estrogen receptors in the adenomyomatous cells compared to endometrial cells. This deficiency may explain the apparent diminished response of this tissue to ovarian hormones as well as to exogenous hormonal therapy.

The standard criterion for the diagnosis of adenomyosis on the basis of histologic examination is the demonstration of endometrial glands and stroma more than one low-powered field (2.5 mm) from the basalis layer of the endometrium. The glands usually exhibit an inactive or proliferative pattern, although cystic hyperplasia or a secretory pattern have been described. Interestingly, the presence of endometrial tissue appears to have a mitogenic action on the surrounding myometrium, since there is often associated hyperplasia and hypertrophy of individual muscle fibers adjacent to the adenomyosis implants.

The majority of women with adenomyosis are asymptomatic or experience only minor symptoms that usually are not bothersome enough to lead them to seek evaluation. Indeed, most patients attribute the increase in dysmenorrhea or menstrual bleeding to the aging process. On the other hand, occasionally adenomyosis can result in a series of complaints that can be frustrating for both patient and physician. Symptomatic adenomyosis usually is observed in the woman between 35 and 50 yr old. The classic symptoms are secondary dysmenorrhea and menorrhagia. Usually, the acquired dysmenorrhea becomes increasingly more severe with the passage of time and the advance of the disease. The uterus tends to enlarge symmetrically and may be found to be globular and tender, especially immediately prior to the onset of menses. But the diagnosis is confirmed only on histologic examination.

No wholly satisfactory treatment exists for adenomyosis. Occasionally, a woman with adenomyosis will respond to therapy with a prostaglandin synthetase inhibitor and may experience diminution in symptoms of pain and bleeding. The nonsteroidal anti-inflammatory agents tend to be most efficacious if therapy is commenced 1 to 2 days before the expected onset of menses. Attempts at hormonal manipulation have not met with much success, although the use of progestin dominant oral contraceptives or cyclic administration of strong progestins with the intent of suppressing pituitary function and thus limiting ovarian estrogen production has

met with limited success. Several investigators have suggested the potential use of gonadotropin-releasing hormone agonists as a means of reducing estrogenic stimulation of the endometrium as well as the adenomyosis.[89] On the other hand, this author's experience with this form of therapy has not been overly positive. It may be that the relative lack of ability of the adenomyosis cells to respond to hormones limits the usefulness of these forms of therapy. For these reasons, hysterectomy is the most commonly successful form of definitive therapy for the patients with adenomyosis. It should be emphasized, however, that the accuracy of making the diagnosis of adenomyosis prior to hysterectomy depends in large part upon the index of suspicion of the clinician. Other potential causes of the symptoms should be eliminated preoperatively.

Abnormal Uterine Bleeding

Abnormal bleeding can be divided into two causes, anovulatory or ovulatory. In anovulatory bleeding, the causes are hormonal, and in ovulatory bleeding, organic. The approach and treatment of these disorders differ significantly.

Abnormal Bleeding in the Anovulatory Woman.

When ovulation fails to occur, for whatever reason, it is expected that the normal pattern of uterine bleeding might be disrupted. If estrogen action is unopposed or fails to be interrupted by the action of progesterone, endometrial growth continues unabated. The result is endometrial hyperplasia,[90] irregular shedding, and abnormal uterine bleeding. In addition to diagnostic testing to determine the cause of anovulation, endometrial sampling may be appropriate to eliminate the possibility of an endometrial malignancy. However, endometrial curettage is, under these circumstances, a diagnostic rather than a therapeutic procedure. If malignancy is not involved, intermittent treatment with progesterone (medroxyprogesterone acetate, 5 to 10 mg orally, daily for 5 to 10 days/mo or norethindrone acetate, 5 mg orally, daily for 5 to 10 days/mo) or cyclic combined oral contraceptives will result in orderly endometrial sloughing and the restoration of regular menstrual bleeding, thus eliminating or reducing the frequency of occurrences of abnormal uterine bleeding.

Occasionally, the anovulatory woman fails to produce adequate quantities of estrogen to maintain endometrial integrity. While the etiology may vary, in general such women experience endometrial atrophy because of hypoestrogenemia. Occasionally, such women may present with a complaint of abnormal uterine bleeding. Again, a search for an endocrine etiology to the patient's anovulation should be conducted. Endometrial sampling to rule out an endometrial malignancy is likely to be suggestive of endometrial atrophy. In such women, intermittent treatment with progestin usually fails to cure the problem and is associated frequently with exacerbation of the atrophic changes within the endometrium that likely will result in increased rather than decreased uterine bleeding. Instead, if the diagnosis of anestrogenic abnormal uterine bleeding is made, the woman should be treated with estrogen (conjugated estrogen, 0.625 to 1.25 mg or the equivalent orally, daily) and progestin (medroxyprogesterone acetate, 5 to 10 mg or the equivalent, orally, daily), in a sequential manner, or cyclic oral contraceptives. These regimens will result in replication of the regular endometrial sloughing, thus eliminating the episodes of abnormal uterine bleeding.

Abnormal Uterine Bleeding in the Ovulatory Woman.

As noted, abnormal uterine bleeding in the ovulatory female is likely the result of an organic lesion within the uterus or endometrial cavity. While hormonal therapy occasionally may cure abnormal uterine bleeding, this can be expected to be temporary, since the organic lesion is still present. When abnormal bleeding reoccurs in spite of hormonal therapy, a search for an organic lesion should be undertaken but not to the exclusion of a thorough evaluation of the patient's endocrine status; it is possible for more than one abnormality to coexist.

When abnormal uterine bleeding occurs in the woman who is ovulatory, the methods available currently for diagnosis include an appropriate physical examination and various imaging techniques including sonography, hysterosalpingography, and hysteroscopy. Traditional dilatation and curettage has been the diagnostic and therapeutic technique of choice for such women, but the limitations of the procedure in patients with abnormal uterine bleeding have been elucidated by a number of authors.[86–95] However, the evolution of endoscopic technologies as well as improved sonographic equipment now allow for highly accurate evaluation of women experiencing abnormal bleeding due to organic causes.

While sonographic techniques are accurate for the demonstration of uterine leiomyomata, as well as other uterine masses, the accuracy of this technique for the visualization of endometrial polyps is less accurate. Hysterosalpingography evaluates the contour of the endometrial cavity, but the exact definition of an intrauterine lesion remains speculative. For instance, a "filling defect" identified by HSG may be a polyp, carcinoma, or leiomyoma. For these reasons, hysteroscopy, which allows for direct visualization, appears to be superior to hysterosalpingography for diagnosis of intrauterine pathology. Furthermore, when combined with the operative instrumentation now available for use with the hysteroscope, hysteroscopy takes on the role of both a diagnostic and a therapeutic procedure.

In this context, hysteroscopy may be performed in an outpatient setting under suitable analgesia with or without light anesthesia. The results of several studies of findings of organic causes of abnormal bleeding are compared in Table 30–4. The difficulty in interpretation of these data lies in the fact that most authors do not segregate their results on the basis of whether or not their patients were ovulatory or anovulatory. Nonetheless, in up to 95 percent of cases, an organic lesion was identified, thus attesting to the value of this diagnostic technique.

If these data are re-evaluated and exclude those women found with anovulatory bleeding, the percentage of patients found to have organic lesions within the uterus is even greater. On this basis, diagnostic hysteroscopy in the woman with abnormal uterine bleeding who experiences normal ovarian function appears to be an accurate and appropriate procedure.

Although outpatient hysteroscopy may occasionally be useful, there is a certain advantage to performing hysteroscopy in a surgical unit employing a liquid medium for distention of the endometrial cavity. The use of carbon dioxide allows for very little in the way of therapeusis, since even a small amount of intrauterine bleeding very quickly obscures the operative field. Operative hysteroscopy is performed, generally employing a liquid distention medium, which allows for continuous inflow and outflow of irrigant, thereby offering unobstructed visualization. Various distention media have been recommended and include Hyskon, 3 percent glycine, lactated

TABLE 30–4. HYSTEROSCOPIC FINDING IN WOMEN WITH ABNORMAL UTERINE BLEEDING

Finding Author	Hamou[96]	Wamsteker[97]	Valle[98]	Barbot[99]	Motashaw[100]
Normal cavity	9 (5%)	85 (43%)	30 (29%)	30 (14%)	124 (34%)
Endometrial polyp(s)	15 (9%)	39 (20%)	42 (40%)	34 (16%)	76 (21%)
Submucous leiomyoma	49 (30%)	16 (8%)	18 (17%)	44 (21%)	42 (11%)
Endometrial carcinoma	1 (.006%)	12 (6%)	—	—	5 (1%)
Hormonally related endometrial abnormality (hyperplasia/atrophy)	63 (38%)	45 (23%)	4 (4%)	45 (21%)	91 (25%)
Other	32 (20%)	3 (2%)	6 (6%)	2 (.009%)	11 (3%)
Total no. cases	164	199	104	213	370

Ringer's solution, or normal saline. Recently, several instrument companies have produced insufflators that deliver the distention medium at a selectable pressure directly at the focus point of the hysteroscopic lens. This serves the function of continuous irrigation of the operative field. At the same time, an outlet port, which is at a site removed from the field of view, allows constant circulation of the distention medium. Accurate volume determinations can be made, thus reducing the likelihood of inadvertent fluid overload during lengthy procedures.

The technique for operative hysteroscopy varies, depending on the operator's experience. Briefly, under general anesthesia or with the combined use of intravenous analgesia and local anesthesia, the cervix is dilated in the routine fashion to a diameter sufficient to accommodate a 5-mm operating sheath through which may be passed a 4-mm diagnostic hysteroscope. The uterine cavity is distended and visualization of the entire endometrial cavity is carried out. If a lesion is identified that is amenable to treatment hysteroscopically, then appropriate instruments may be employed.

The incidence of endometrial polyps varies from 9 to 40 percent. Polyps may be single or multiple and may appear at virtually any age after puberty. The tissue type identified in endometrial polyps may vary from adenomatous to adenomyomatous, fibrous, or telangectasic. Generally benign, the incidence of endometrial carcinoma associated with endometrial polyps in a woman in the postmenopause has been reported to be 15 percent.[101] Telangectasia in an endometrial polyp is a rare occurrence.

Endometrial polyps may be removed by grasping the individual polyp at the base with a rigid or flexible scissors or biopsy forcep, thereafter excising the polyp by pulling it loose from its attachment. Intrauterine pressure should be maintained between 15 and 75 mm Hg. The pressure should be above capillary pressure to ensure a minimum of oozing. On the other hand, excessive intrauterine pressure may lead to vascular intravasation and the potential for fluid overload.

The treatment of uterine leiomyomas has been discussed previously. Uterine leiomyomas, especially if submucous, may be associated with abnormal uterine bleeding. While multiple large leiomyomas may distend the uterine cavity, thereby increasing the endometrial surface and proportionally increasing the volume of menstrual flow, it is the submucous variety that is responsible primarily for intermenstrual spotting or bleeding, as a result of ulceration or poor vascularization of the overlying endometrial layer. Several authors have reported various techniques and series of hysteroscopic myomectomy.[102,103] In general, for leiomyomas less than 3 cm in size, sharp dissection with scissors, a wire loop of a resectoscope, or

with laser energy delivered through a fiber delivery system have met with equal success. If depth of penetration of the leiomyoma into the myometrium is questionable, it may be appropriate to perform hysteroscopic resection under laparoscopic control to avoid inadvertent myometrial perforation and injury to intra-abdominal structures. When a larger leiomyoma is visualized, it is preferable to employ a urologic resectoscope with its heavier wire loop. This technique involves the curettage of fragments from the central portion of the leiomyoma. As this is accomplished, the natural tendency of normal myometrium to contract will cause the remaining myomatous tissue to bulge into the uterine cavity. In this way, the leiomyoma can be shaved down to the pseudo-capsule. As can be imagined, large tumors can take a considerable amount of time to remove in this manner, since instruments must be withdrawn frequently and fragments must be washed away. For these procedures, a liquid distention medium is required and concomitant laparoscopy is recommended.

Endometrial Ablation

With some frequency, the clinician is presented with women who complain of abnormal uterine bleeding but in whom no endometrial or uterine pathology can be identified. Most often these women are anovulatory, and hormonal manipulation is the first choice of therapy. However, hormonal therapy may be unsuccessful in reducing the frequency of episodes of bleeding because of lack of compliance, inability to tolerate medication, contraindication to therapy, or presumably some intrinsic defect in the endometrium. At the same time, some ovulatory women also have no apparent organic abnormality of the uterus to account for the abnormal uterine bleeding. For these patients, hysteroscopically directed endometrial ablation has been suggested as a therapeutic option as opposed to hysterectomy.

While it has been suggested that Fritsch first described post-traumatic intrauterine synechiae in 1894, it was not until 1948 that Asherman published the findings of his series of patients with the syndrome of partial or complete ablation of endometrial cavity that come to bear his name.[73] The symptoms associated with Asherman syndrome include amenorrhea, and it was not long before a number of clinicians began to seek iatrogenic means to create endometrial ablation as a means of treating the woman with menorrhagia or as a means of limiting fertility. Various chemical substances were applied to the uterine cavity in attempts to recapitulate endometrial destruction—paraformaldehyde, methylcyanoacrylate, oxalic acid, and quinacrine.[104–107] Physical agents such as intracavitary radium insertion, direct application of superheated stram, and cryocoagulation also were employed with some limited success.[108] It was not until 1981, when

Goldrath et al published their first series of results of photovaporization of the endometrium by the application of laser energy, that endometrial ablation became a therapeutic modality with reasonable success.[109] Since then, a number of publications have reported success with this form of therapy.[110–112]

The procedure for endometrial ablation varies depending upon the technique utilized—laser, resectoscope with wire loop, or resectoscope with a rollerball. Pretreatment for 1 to 2 mo with danazol (800 mg daily) or a gonadotropin-releasing hormone agonist is effective in reducing estrogenic stimulation of the endometrium. Thereafter, endometrial ablation is performed more efficiently and perhaps more effectively under a condition of endometrial atrophy.

In general, hysteroscopy is performed as described previously. If the laser is employed, ablation should commence in the cornual portion of the uterus, with care to avoid uterine perforation since the myometrium is thinnest in the cornual region. A contact or noncontact technique appears to be equally effective. The surgeon should attempt to vaporize the endometrium to a depth of 0.2 to 0.4 cm, a depth sufficient to eliminate the regenerative layer of basal endometrium. If the resectoscope is utilized, care must be taken to coagulate the endometrium sufficiently to necrose this regenerative layer.

Success rates following endometrial ablation vary depending upon the definition of success. The results in several series are presented in Table 30–5.

It appears that about 50 percent of women will experience amenorrhea following any of the thermal ablation techniques. Of the 50 percent who continue to have menses, about one half experience hypomenorrhea and only half continue to have regular menses.

The major complications associated with endometrial ablation may be classified as immediate versus long term. Fluid overload has been reported to be the most common intraoperative complication. Fortunately, meticulous attention to input and output of distention medium allows for avoidance of this complication.

Hemorrhage, either immediate or delayed, also has been reported.[113] Immediate postoperative bleeding is the result of unroofing of venous sinuses during destruction of the endometrium. This may be managed by placement of a Foley catheter with a 30-cc balloon within the uterine cavity. The balloon should be inflated just until bleeding stops, and may be left in place for 6 to 24 hr.[113]

Delayed bleeding may be the result of necrosis into the primary uterine vessels. For this reason, it is recommended that endometrial ablation be carried down the lower uterine segment no closer to the external cervical os than 4 cm. This is the point at which the cervical branch of the uterine artery enters the myometrium. If thermal injury is sufficiently close to these vessels, delayed necrosis may result in profound bleeding that requires hysterectomy.

The long-term consequences of endometrial ablation remain to be elucidated. The possibility of isolated pockets of active endometrium remaining must be considered and hematometrium may result. In addition, the formation of adenocarcinoma of any remaining endometrium remains a theoretical risk. Of concern is the possibility that malignancy might go undetected because of lack of subsequent uterine bleeding.

The issue of the appropriate indications for endometrial ablation, by whatever technique, remains controversial. For the woman with abnormal uterine bleeding who fails to respond to hormonal manipulation, and for whom no organic cause can be identified, it seems that endometrial ablation is an appropriate option. For the woman with uterine leiomyomata, the appropriateness of this therapeutic modality is less obvious and myomectomy or hysterectomy is recommended. Obviously, before such therapy is offered, a thorough evaluation should be completed, thus ruling out any other explanation for the abnormal uterine bleeding.

SUMMARY

The principal role of the uterus appears to be its capacity to serve as the residence for the developing fetus. Uterine abnormalities whether developmental, acquired, or functional are frequently a reason that women seek gynecological care. This chapter provides a review of developmental processes that give rise to the normal and abnormal uterus. Techniques for evaluation and treatment are provided. Acquired diseases, such as uterine leiomyomata and Asherman syndrome also are discussed. Finally, a review of potential modalities of therapy, short of hysterectomy, is offered. It is hoped that this information will prove to be of significant value to the clinician in caring for women.

TABLE 30–5. LASER ENDOMETRIAL ABLATION: SUMMARY OF REPORTED DATA

Author	No. Patients	Successful Procedures (%)	Amenorrhea No. (%)
Loffer[114]	33	(94)	11 (33)
Davis[104]	25	(52)	3 (12)
Goldrath[109]	335	(87.2)	163 (50)
Gimpelson[93]	23	(96)	10 (43.5)
Lomano[110]	10	(100)	2 (20)
Total	426	86	44

REFERENCES

1. Jarcho J. Malformations of the uterus: Review of the subject, including embryology, comparative anatomy, diagnosis and report of cases. *Am J Surg.* 106, 1946

2. Tarry WF, Duckett JW, Stephens FD. The Mayer-Rokitansky syndrome: Pathogenesis, classification and management. *J Urol.* 136:648, 1986

3. Candiani M, Busacca M, Natale A, Sambruni I. Case report. Bicervical uterus and septate vagina: Report of a previously undescribed Müllerian anomaly. *Hum Reprod.* 11:218, 1996

4. Gruenwald P. The relation of the growing Müllerian duct to the Wolffian duct and its importance for the genesis of malformations. *Anat Rec.* 81:1, 1941

5. McBean JH, Brumsted JR. Septate uterus with cervical duplication: A rare malformation. *Fertil Steril.* 62:415, 1994

6. Acien P, Ruiz JA, et al. Renal agenesis in association with malformation of the female genital tract. *Am J Obstet Gynecol.* 165:1368, 1991

7. Acien P. Embryological observations on the female genital tract. *Hum Reprod.* 7:437, 1992

8. Jones HW. Reproductive impairment and the malformed uterus. *Fertil Steril.* 36:137, 1981

9. Heinonen PK, Pystynen PP. Primary infertility and uterine anomalies. *Fertil Steril.* 40:311, 1983

10. Buttram VC, Gibbons WE. Müllerian anomalies: A proposed classification (an analysis of 144 cases). *Fertil Steril.* 32:40, 1979

11. Mercer CA, Long WN, Thompson JD. Uterine unification: Indications and technique. *Clin Obstet Gynecol.* 24:1199, 1981

12. White MM. Uteroplasty in infertility. *Proc R Soc Med.* 53:1006, 1960

13. Rock JA, Jones HW. The clinical management of the double uterus. *Fertil Steril.* 28:798, 1977

14. Hein P, Stolte T, Esker T, et al. The motility of the non-pregnant congenitally malformed uterus. *Eur J Obstet Gynecol Reprod Biol.* 4:51, 1974

15. Kaufman RH, Adam E, Burder GL, Gerthoffer. Upper genital tract changes and pregnancy outcome in offspring exposed in utero to diethylstilbesterol. *Am J Obstet Gynecol.* 137:299, 1980

16. Barnes AB, Colton T, Gundersen J, et al. Fertility and outcome of pregnancy in women exposed in utero to diethylstilbesterol. *N Engl J Med.* 302:609, 1980

17. Cousins L, Karp W, Lacey C, Lucas WE. Reproductive outcome of women exposed to diethylstilbesterol in utero. *Obstet Gynecol.* 56:70, 1980

18. Schmidt G, Fowler WC Jr, Talbert LM, Edelman DA. Reproductive history of women exposed to diethylstilbesterol in utero. *Fertil Steril.* 33:21, 1980

19. Herbst AL, Hubby MM, Blough RR, Azizi F. A comparison of pregnancy experience in DES-exposed and DES-unexposed daughters. *J Reprod Med.* 24:62, 1980

20. Pennes DR, Bowerman RA, Silver TM. Congenital uterine anomalies and associated pregnancies: findings and pitfalls of sonographic diagnosis. *J Ultrasound Med.* 4:531, 1985

21. Strassmann EO. Fertility and unification of double uterus. *Fertil Steril.* 2:165, 1966

22. Jones HW, Jones GES. Double uterus as an etiological factor in repeated abortion: Indications for surgical repair. *Am J Obstet Gynecol.* 65:325, 1953

23. Tompkins P. Comments on the bicornuate uterus and training. *Surg Clin North Am.* 42:1049, 1962

24. Cohen SM, Franklin RR, Haney AF, et al. Prevention of postsurgical adhesions by Interceed (TC7), an absorbable adhesion barrier: A prospective randomized multicenter clinical study. *Fertil Steril.* 51:6, 1989

25. Daly DC, Walters CA, Sot-Albors CE, Riddick DH. Hysteroscopic metroplasty: Surgical technique and obstetric outcome. *Fertil Steril.* 39:623, 1983

26. Perino A, Mencaglia L, Hamou J, Cittadini E. Hysteroscopy for metroplasty of uterine septa: Report of 24 cases. *Fertil Steril.* 48:321, 1987

27. Chervenak FA, Neuwirth RS. Hysteroscopic resection of the uterine septum. *Am J Obstet Gynecol.* 141:351,1981

28. DeCherney AH, Russell JB, Graebe RA. Resectoscopic management of Müllerian fusion defects. *Fertil Steril.* 46:726, 1986

29. DeCherney A, Polan ML. Hysteroscopic management of intrauterine lesions and intractable uterine bleeding. *Obstet Gynecol.* 61:392, 1983

30. Tadir Y, Fisch B, Ovadia J. Gynecologic laser endoscopy. *Colposc Gynecol Laser Surg.* 4:51, 1988

31. Daniell JF, Osher S, Miller W. Hysteroscopic resection of uterine septi with visible light laser energy. *Colposc Gynecol Laser Surg.* 3:217, 1987

32. Tulandi T, Arronet GH, McInnes RA. Arcuate and biocornuate uterine anomalies and infertility. *Fertil Steril.* 34:362, 1980

33. Townsend DE, Sparkes RS, Baludo MC, McClelland G. Unicellular histogenesis of uterine leiomyomas as determined by electrophoresis of glucose-6-phosphate dehydrogenase. *Am J Obstet Gynecol.* 107:1168, 1970

34. Spellacy WN, LeMaire WJ, Buhi WC, et al. Plasma growth hormone and estradiol levels in women with uterine myomas. *Obstet Gynecol.* 40:829, 1979

35. Pauka MJ, Kontula KK, Kauppila AJI, et al. Estrogen receptors in human myoma tissue. *Mol Cell Endocrinol.* 6:35, 1976

36. Tamaya T, Motoyama T, Ohono Y, et al. Estradiol-17β progesterone and 5α diethylstilbesterol receptors of uterine myometrium and myoma in the human subject. *J Steroid Biochem.* 10:615, 1979

37. Pollow K, Geilfuss J, Boquoi E, Pollow B. Estrogen and progesterone binding proteins in normal human myometrium and leiomyoma tissue. *J Clin Chem Clin Biochem.* 16:503, 1978

38. Pollow K, Sinnecker G, Boquoi E, Pollow B. In vitro conversion of estradiol-17β into estrone in normal human myometrium and leiomyoma. *J Clin Chem Clin Biochem.* 16:493, 1978

39. Grattarola R, Li CH. Effect of growth hormone and its combination with estradiol 17β on the uterus of hypophysectomized and hypophysectomized ovariectomized rats. *Clin Endocrinol.* 65:802, 1959

40. Hofmeier MF. *Handbuch der Frauenkrankheiten.* 15th ed. Leipzig, 1913: 579

41. Olshausen R. *Handbuch der Gynakologie.* 2:791, 1898

42. Buttram VC, Reiter RC. Uterine leiomyomata: Etiology, symptomatology, and management. *Fertil Steril.* 36:433, 1981

43. Coutinho EM, Maia HS. The contractile response of the human uterus, fallopian tubes, and ovary to prostaglandins in vivo. *Fertil Steril.* 22:539, 1971

44. Deligdish L, Loewenthal M. Endometrial changes associated with myomata of the uterus. *J Clin Pathol.* 23:676, 1970

45. Farrer-Brown G, Beilby JO, Tarbit MH. Venous changes in the endometrium of myomatous uteri. *Obstet Gynecol.* 38:743, 1971

46. Jacobson FJ, Enzer N. Uterine myomas and the endometrium: Study of the mechanism of bleeding. *Obstet Gynecol.* 7:206, 1956

47. Babaknia A, Rock JA, Jones HW. Pregnancy success following abdominal myomectomy for infertility. *Fertil Steril.* 30:644, 1978

48. Romano F, Cicinelli E, Anastasio PS, et al. Sonohysterography versus hysteroscopy for diagnosing endouterine abnormalities in fertile women. *Int J Gynecol Obstet.* 45:253, 1994

49. Gaucherand P, Piacenza JM, Salle B, Rudigoz RC. Sonohysterography of the uterine cavity: Preliminary investigations. *J Clin Ultrasound.* 23:339, 1995

50. Jurkovic D, Geipel A, Gruboeck K, et al. Three-dimensional ultrasound for the assessment of uterine anatomy and detection of congenital anomalies: A comparison with hysterosalpingography and two-dimensional sonography. *Ultrasound Obstet Gynecol.* 5:233, 1995

51. Ingersoll FM, Malone LJ. Myomectomy: An alternative hysterectomy. *Arch Surg.* 100:557, 1970

52. Lock FR. Multiple myomectomy. *Am J Obstet Gynecol.* 104:642, 1969

53. Mussey RD, Randall LM, Doyle LW. Pregnancy following myomectomy. *Am J Obstet Gynecol.* 49:508, 1945

54. McCormick TA. Myomectomy with subsequent pregnancy. *Am J Obstet Gynecol.* 75:1128, 1958

55. Berkeley AS, DeCherney AH, Polan ML. Abdominal myomectomy and subsequent fertility. *Surg Obstet Gynecol.* 156:319, 1983

56. Davids AM. Myomectomy in the relief of infertility and sterility and in pregnancy—Technique and results. *Surg Clin North Am.* 37:563, 1957

57. Stevenson CS. Myomectomy for improvement of fertility. *Fertil Steril.* 15:367, 1964

58. Rubin IC. Progress in myomectomy—Surgical measures and diagnostic aids favoring lower morbidity and mortality. *Am J Obstet Gynecol.* 44:196, 1942

59. Ranney B, Frederick I. The occasional need for myomectomy. *Obstet Gynecol.* 53:437,1979

60. Bonney V. Myomectomy as the treatment of election for uterine fibroids. *Lancet.* 2:1060, 1925

61. Finn WF, Muller PF. Abdominal myomectomy: Special reference to subsequent pregnancy and to the reappearance of fibromyomas of the uterus. *Am J Obstet Gynecol.* 60:109, 1950

62. Brown JM, Malkasian GD, Symmonds RE. Abdominal myomectomy. *Am J Obstet Gynecol.* 99:126, 1967

63. Dearnley G. The place of myomectomy in the treatment of primary infertility. President's address. *Proc R Soc Med.* 49:252, 1956

64. Hannigan EV, Gomez LG. A review of prognostic clinical and pathologic features. *Am J Obstet Gynecol.* 134:557, 1979

65. Goldzieher JW, Maqueo M, Ricaud L, et al. Induction of degenerative changes in uterine myomas by high dosage progestin therapy. *Am J Obstet Gynecol.* 96:1078, 1966

66. Knobil E. The neuroendocrine control of the menstrual cycle. *Recent Prog Horm Res.* 36:53, 1980

67. Filicori M, Hall DA, Loughlin JS, et al. A conservative approach to the management of uterine leiomyoma: Pituitary desensitization by luteinizing hormone-releasing hormone analogue. *Am J Obstet Gynecol.* 147:726, 1983

68. Maheux R, Guilloteau C, Lemay A, et al. Regression of leiomyomata uteri following hypoestrogenism induced by repetitive luteinizing hormone-releasing hormone agonist treatment: Preliminary report. *Fertil Steril.* 42:644, 1984

69. Friedman AJ, Barbieri RL, Doubilet PM, et al. A randomized, double-blind trial of gonadotropin-releasing hormone agonist (leuprolide) with or without medroxyprogesterone acetate in the treatment of leiomyomata uteri. *Fertil Steril.* 49:404, 1988

70. Healy DL, Fraser HM, Lawson SL. Shrinkage of uterine fibroid after subcutaneous infusion of a LHRH agonist. *Br Med J.* 289:1267, 1984

71. Coddington CC, Collins RL, Shawker TH, et al. Long-acting gonadotropin hormone-releasing hormone analog used to treat uteri. *Fertil Steril.* 45:624, 1986

72. Letterie GS, Coddington CC, Winkel CA, et al. Efficacy of gonadotropin-releasing hormone agonist in the treatment of uterine leiomyomata: Long-term follow-up. *Fertil Steril.* 51:951, 1989

73. Asherman JG. Amenorrhea traumatica (atretica) *J Obstet Gynaecol Br Emp.* 55:23, 1948

74. Loures NC, Danezis JM, Potifix G. Use of intrauterine devices in treatment of intrauterine adhesions. *Fertil Steril.* 19:509, 1968

75. Sugimoto O. Diagnostic and therapeutic hysteroscopy for traumatic intrauterine adhesions. *Am J Obstet Gynecol.* 131:539, 1978

76. March CM, Israel R, March AD. Hysteroscopic management of intrauterine adhesions. *Am J Obstet Gynecol.* 130:653, 1978

77. Tadir Y, Raif J, Dagan J. Hysteroscope for CO_2 laser application. *Lasers Surg Med.* 4:153, 1984

78. Mishell DR, Moyer DL. Association of pelvic inflammatory disease with the intrauterine device. *Clin Obstet Gynecol.* 12:179, 1969

79. Schiffer MA, Elguezabal A, Sultana M, Allen AC. Actinomycosis infections associated with intrauterine contraceptive devices. *Obstet Gynecol.* 45:67, 1975

80. Mordh PA, Ripe T, Svensson L, Westrom L. *Chlamydia trachomatis* in patients with acute salpingitis. *N Engl J Med.* 296:1377, 1977

81. Emge LA. The elusive adenomyosis of the uterus. *Am J Obstet Gynecol.* 83:1541, 1962

82. Janovski NA, Dubrauszky V. *Atlas of Gynecologic and Obstetric Diagnostic Histopathology.* New York, McGraw-Hill, 1967

83. Bird CC, McElin TW, Manalo-Estrella P. The elusive adenomyosis of the uterus—revisited. *Am J Obstet Gynecol.* 112:583, 1972

84. Marshak RH, Eliasoph J. The roentgen findings in adenomyosis. *Am J Obstet Gynecol.* 64:846, 1955

85. Slezak P, Tillinger KG. The incidence and clinical importance of hysterographic evidence of cavities in the uterine wall. *Radiology.* 118:581, 1976

86. Wolf DM, Spataro RF. The current state of hysterosalpingography. *Radiographics.* 8:1041, 1988

87. Fedele L. Transvaginal ultrasonography in the diagnosis of diffuse adenomyosis. *Fertil Steril.* 58:94, 1992

88. Arnold LL, Ascher SM, Schruefer JJ, Simon JA. Reviews: The nonsurgical diagnosis of adenomyosis. *Obstet Gynecol.* 86:461, 1995

89. Yen SSC. Clinical applications of gonadotropin-releasing hormone and gonadotropin-releasing hormone analogs. *Fertil Steril.* 39:257, 1983

90. Smith DC, Pretice RL, Bauermeister DE. Endometrial carcinoma: Histopathology, survival and exogenous estrogens. *Gynecol Obstet Invest.* 12:169, 1981

91. Gribb J. Hysteroscopy: An aid to gynecologic diagnosis. *Obstet Gynecol.* 15:593, 1960

92. Valle R. Hysteroscopic evaluation of patients with abnormal uterine bleeding. *Surg Gynecol Obstet.* 153:521, 1981

93. Gimpelson R. Panoramic hysteroscopy with directed biopsies vs dilatation and curettage for accurate diagnosis. *J Reprod Med.* 29:575, 1984

94. Stock R, Kanbour A. Prehysterectomy curettage. *Obstet Gynecol.* 45:537, 1975

95. Englund F, Ingleman-Sundberg A, Westin B. Hysteroscopy in diagnosis and treatment of uterine bleeding. *Gynaecologia.* 143:217, 1957

96. Hamou JE. Microhysteroscopy: A new procedure and its original applications in gynecology. *J Reprod Med.* 26:375, 1981

97. Wamsteker K. Hysteroscopy in the management of abnormal uterine bleeding in 199 patients. In: Siegler AM, Lindemann JH, eds. *Hysteroscopy: Principles and Practice.* Philadelphia, J. B. Lippincott, 1984: 128

98. Valle RF, Sciarra JJ. Current status of hysteroscopy in gynecologic practice. *Fertil Steril.* 32:619, 1979

99. Barbot J. L'hystéroscopie de contact. Thesis. Paris, 1975

100. Motashaw ND, Dave S. Therapeutic hysteroscopy in management of abnormal uterine bleeding. *J Reprod Med.* 35:612, 1990

101. Peterson W, Novak E. Endometrial polyps. *Obstet Gynecol.* 8:40, 1956

102. DeCherney AH, Polan ML. Hysteroscopic management of intrauterine lesions. *Obstet Gynecol.* 61:392, 1983

103. Neuwirth RS. Hysteroscopic management of symptomatic submucous fibroids. *Obstet Gynecol.* 62:509, 1983

104. Davis R, Erb R, Kyriazis G, Balin H. Fallopian tube occlusion in rabbits with silicone rubber. *J Reprod Med.* 14:56, 1975

105. Zipper J, Stachetti E, Medel M. Human fertility control by transvaginal application of quinacrine on the fallopian tube. *Fertil Steril.* 12:581, 1970

106. Stevenson T, Talor D. The effect of methyl cyanoacrylate tissue adhesive on the human fallopian tube and endometrium. *J Obstet Gynecol Br.* 79:1028, 1972

107. Shenker JG, Polishuk WZ. Regeneration of rabbit endometrium following intrauterine instillation of chemical agents. *Gynecol Invest.* 4:1, 1973

108. Deoegemueller W, Greer B, Davis J, et al. Cryocoagulation of the endometrium at the uterine cornua. *Am J Obstet Gynecol.* 131:1, 1978

109. Goldrath MH, Fuller TA, Segal S. Laser photovaporization of endometrium for the treatment of menorrhagia. *Am J Obstet Gynecol.* 104:14, 1981

110. Lomano JM. Photocoagulation of the endometrium with the Nd:YAG Laser for the treatment of menorrhagia. A report of 10 cases. *J Reprod Med.* 51:148, 1986

111. Lomano JM, Feste J, Loffer F, Goldrath MH. Ablation of the endometrium with the neodymium:Yag laser: A multicentered study. *Colposc Gynecol Laser Surg.* 2:203, 1986

112. Zumwalt T, Wesseler T, Joffe S. A comparison of artificial sapphire tip with the quartz tips in *in vitro* endometrial ablation. *Colposc Gynecol Laser Surg.* 2:47, 1986

113. Goldrath M. Uterine tamponade for the control of acute uterine bleeding. *Am J Obstet Gynecol.* 147:869, 1983

114. Loffer ED. Hysteroscopic endometrial ablation with the nd:YAG laser during a nontouch technique. *Obstet Gynecol.* 69:679, 1987

Chapter 31

DIAGNOSIS AND MANAGEMENT OF TUBAL DISEASE

Levent M. Senturk and Aydin Arici

FALLOPIAN TUBE PATHOPHYSIOLOGY

Anatomy

The normal fallopian tube extends from the area of ipsilateral ovary anteriorly and medially to its terminus in the posterosuperior aspect of the uterine fundus. During the reproductive years, its length varies usually between 9 and 11 cm.[1] It is the site for ovum retrieval, ovum and sperm transport, sperm capacitation, fertilization, and embryo transport. The Müllerian (paramesonephric) ducts appear between the fifth and sixth embryonic weeks. Each grows caudally, lateral to its ipsilateral Wolffian duct, turning inwards and crossing anterior to the Wolffian duct, and then joining at the back of the urogenital sinus between 7 and 12 wk of gestation. The lower ends form the uterus and the upper portion of the vagina; the upper ends form the fallopian tubes.[2]

The oviduct is made up of five anatomic segments; the fimbria, infundibulum, ampulla, isthmus, and intramural (interstitial) segments (Fig 31–1).

The fimbria, the most distal portion of the oviduct, is 1 to 1.5 cm in diameter and 1 cm long, and is surrounded by approximately 25 irregular finger-like extensions called *fimbriae*. The longest and most prominent of these extensions is called *fimbria ovarica*, which comes into contact with the ipsilateral ovary and plays an important role in ovum pickup. The fimbriae attach to the infundibulum, a 1-cm long trumpet-shaped portion of the fallopian tube. Both the fimbriae and infundibulum are rich in mucosal folds, but poor in muscle fibers with thin outer longitudinal and inner circular layers. The epithelium is densely ciliated (60 to 80 percent), beating uniformly towards the uterus.[3] The ampulla, the longest segment, is two thirds of the total tubal length. The lumen diameter decreases from 1 cm at the ampullary–infundibular junction to 1 to 2 mm at the ampullary–isthmic junction. The mucosa contains 3 to 5 longitudinal major folds. In between the major folds there are numerous minor folds, which are rich in blood vessels and lymphatics. The mucosa has 40 to 60 percent ciliated cells, and their proportion increases towards the apex of the mucosal folds.[3] The muscle fibers are arranged in three layers: an outer longitudinal layer, a middle circular layer, and an incomplete longitudinal spiral layer that diminishes at the ampullary–isthmic junction. The isthmus is approximately one third of the oviduct (3 to 3.5 cm), with a luminal diameter 0.1 to 0.5 mm. The muscle layer is well developed into outer and inner longitudinal layers with a circular layer in between. There are 4 to 5 small mucosal folds in the isthmus, which are slightly rounded. Ciliated cells account for 20 to 25 percent of the epithelial cells. The intramural segment of the tube is short (1 cm) and may have a straight, curved, or convoluted course ending in a rounded or fish-mouthed opening at the cornua of the uterus. The muscular layer is composed of an inner and outer longitudinal layer with an intermediate circular-spiral layer. The 2 or 3 mucosal folds may extend into the uterine cavity. The transition from intramural endosalpinx to cornual endometrium is marked by a transitional area that has, characteristically, a decreased number of ciliated cells and polygonal, elongated (rather than their usual rounded-dome appearance) secretory cells. It is postulated that this region acts as an adrenergic sphincter because of its rich vascular supply and innervation.

The arterial blood supply has a dual origin. A tubal branch of the uterine artery passes in the mesosalpinx laterally from the cornu of the uterus to anastomose with tubal branches of ovarian artery to form an arcade parallel to the fallopian tube. The parietal arteries originate

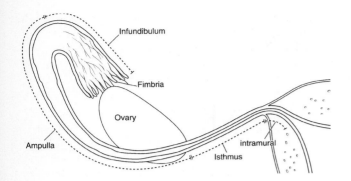

Figure 31–1. Anatomy of the fallopian tube.

individually from this arcade and penetrate the muscularis layer to the mucosa through the antimesenteric side. This vascular bed responds to vasoconstrictor solutions, facilitating hemostasis at the time of the removal of an ectopic pregnancy. The veins, draining the submucosal and muscular venous plexus, follow the arterial pathways. The lymphatic system consists of mucosal, intramuscular, and subserous systems. The mucosal system is highly developed in the fimbriae and ampulla, where they probably play a role in functions such as ovum pickup, transport, and fertilization. The lymph capillaries drain into the intramuscular lymphatic system, forming lymphatic vessels that pass laterally, accompanying the ovarian vessels. On the right side, lymph drains into nodes in the area of the right renal vein and in the inferior vena cava, whereas on the left side, lymph drains into nodes lying between the left ovarian and left renal vein. Lymph also drains into the presacral and common iliac nodes.

The nerve supply of the tube is both sympathetic and parasympathetic. Sympathetic fibers from T10 through L2 synapse in the celiac, aortic, renal, inferior mesenteric, cervicovaginal, and presacral plexuses. The distribution of sympathetic fibers is most dense in the isthmus and ampullary–isthmic junction, particularly in the circular muscle layer, but is scanty and located around blood vessels in the ampulla. Adrenergic neural mechanisms seem to have a role in the mediation of the periovulatory changes in tubal contractility that occur in response to steroid hormone changes. Owing to the rich innervation and vascularization of the intramural segment of the fallopian tube, it is highly responsive to hormonal, pharmacologic, and neurologic stimuli. Estrogens increase ciliation, epithelial height, and mitotic activity. Estrogens also increase the number of alpha receptors, which will increase activity and contraction of the fallopian tubes. Conversely, progesterone decreases ciliation, epithelial folds, and mitotic activity, while increasing the number of beta receptors, resulting in decreased activity and relaxation. Prostaglandin F_2 (PGF_2) stimulates con-

tractions, while PGE_1-E_2 causes relaxation. Alpha adrenoreceptor agonists such as epinephrine and norepinephrine also cause contractions, whereas β_2 agonists such as isoproterenol, isoxsuprine, and terbutaline cause relaxation.[4] Sensory pain fibers pass along with the sympathetic nerves to the spinal cord at the level of T10 to T12. Parasympathetic innervation is supplied in the proximal region by the pelvic nerve formed by fibers derived from the second to fourth sacral segment and in the distal region by the vagal nerve via the ovarian plexus.

A mucosal membrane, a wall of smooth muscle, and a serosal coat make up the three histologic layers of the tube. The serosa is lined by flattened mesothelial cells. Beneath the mesothelium lies a small amount of connective tissue containing a few collagen fibers and blood vessels. The tubal muscularis is composed of two layers that differ in architecture, depending on the tubal segment, as mentioned. The mucosal layer lies directly on the muscularis. It consists of a luminal epithelial lining and a scanty underlying lamina propria containing vessels and angular cells. Angular cells decidualize in 5 to 12 percent of pregnancies and up to 80 percent of ectopic pregnancies.[5]

The epithelial layer of the mucosa is composed of four different cell types. The *ciliated cells* are cuboidal with finely granular cytoplasms and large central round or oval nuclei. The *secretory cells* have a finely granular cytoplasm, narrower than the ciliated cells and oval or wedge-shaped nuclei depending on the phase of the menstrual cycle. During the follicular phase, the epithelium attains its greatest height and secretory and ciliated cells are equally prominent. Late in the luteal phase, the apical parts of the secretory cells rupture, extruding cytoplasmic and nuclear material into the tubal lumen. Subsequently, there is a marked irregularity of the border due to the decrease in the height of the non-ciliated cells. Secretory cells are more plentiful at the base of the mucosal folds whereas ciliated cells are at the apex of them. The *intercalary* or *peg cells* are most numerous in the premenstrual and menstrual phases; frequently, they cannot be distinguished from secretory cells, and these two types of cells are thought to represent different phases of the same cell. *Indifferent cells*, the fourth group, form a small population of the cells that lie along the base of the normal epithelium.[6]

Physiology

The epithelial cells attain maximum height and degree of ciliation during the late follicular and early luteal phases in both the fimbriae and the ampulla, with secretory cells undergoing more height variation than ciliated cells. At the end of the luteal phase, some atrophy and deciliation occur, especially in the fimbriae. Hypertrophy and reciliation occur during the early follicular phase.

Approximately 10 to 12 percent of the cells form new cilia in both the fimbriae and the ampulla during each menstrual cycle. It is postulated that estrogen stimulates and progesterone antagonizes cell hypertrophy, secretion, ciliogenesis, and cell height.[7] It is also suggested that oviductal stromal cells, smooth-muscle cells, and secretory cells all have estrogen and progesterone receptors whereas ciliated cells do not have either receptors.[8] Both steroids are thought to act on ciliated cells via some probable mediators: cytokines or growth factors that are secreted from stromal cells. The morphologic and biochemical changes in the tubal epithelial lining are essential for the transport of the sperm and the egg, and coincide with the period of final oocyte maturation, sperm capacitation, fertilization, and early embryonic development.[7]

The tubal epithelium seems to be a major site for the synthesis of epidermal growth factor (EGF) and its receptor protein and transforming growth factor-α (TGF-α). These factors vary with the phase of the menstrual cycle, cell type, and segment of the tube (ampulla or fimbriae).[9] Growth factors may have a role in the contractile activity of tubal muscle cells, facilitating sperm, oocyte, and embryo transportation in the oviduct. Insulin-like growth factors (IGFs) exhibit insulin-like growth-promoting activities, and their actions are modulated by six different binding proteins (IGFBP-1 to IGFBP-6).[10] IGF-I, IGF-II, and IGFBP-1 to -4 are synthesized by both secretory and ciliated cells of the oviduct, regardless of the site but much more during the early and midluteal phases.[11] TGF-β (isomers 1 to 3 and type I, II, and III receptors),[12] platelet-derived growth factor (PDGF)-AA and its α and β receptors,[13] granulocyte macrophage colony-stimulating factor (GM-CSF) and its α and β receptors,[14] and leukemia inhibitory factor (LIF)[15] are all reported to be synthesized to some extent, depending on the phase of the cycle. Under the influence of ovarian steroids, a variety of growth factors, cytokines, and polypeptide hormones are expressed and synthesized by the oviductal epithelial lining. Due to the presence of the receptors in embryos during development in the tubes, all those factors are postulated to influence sperm, oocyte, sperm–oocyte interaction, and embryo transportation.[16] Moreover, LIF is also believed to have an association with early embryonic development, tubal implantation, and especially ectopic pregnancy pathogenesis.[15] Prostaglandins are products of the oviductal cells and are believed to be the end products of tubal motility and, consequently, it would be safe to use nonsteroidal anti-inflammatory drugs during the menstrual cycle without increasing the risk of tubal pregnancy.[17]

The fallopian tube has the complex task of ensuring the transport of spermatozoa towards the ovary, ova towards the uterus, and subsequently the transport of the zygote towards the normal site of implantation in the uterine endometrium. The fimbriae are directed to the ovulation site by the muscular contractions of the mesosalpinx and tubo-ovarian ligaments. The newly released oocyte, with its sticky cumulus, is swept from the surface of the ovary by the help of fimbriae and propelled towards the tubal peritoneal ostium by the beating of the cilia.[18] During its voyage in the oviduct, the ovum is retained in the ampulla longer than the rest of the tube and in this segment, ovum maturation, fertilization, and early embryo cleavage occur. Both fertilized and unfertilized ova remain in the ampulla for approximately 72 hr.[19] The cilia beat while in contact with the ovum; the peristaltic and segmentary contraction of the tube are all involved in the transportation of the ovum. The secretory activity of the isthmus is maximal at ovulation, and viscous mucus fills the lumen and blocks ovum passage.[20]

Spermatozoa may be found in the oviduct a few minutes after their deposition in the vagina.[21] Only a small portion of the ejaculated spermatozoa, probably 200, enter the oviduct and reach the ampulla, which is the site of fertilization[22] (see Chap 1). The uterotubal junction relaxes as a result of the response of musculature to progesterone, prostaglandins, oxytocin, adrenaline, and other probable mediators and accepts the spermatozoa into the oviduct. The isthmic secretory plug protects the spermatozoa from the beating effect of cilia towards the uterus. After capacitation of spermatozoa during the travel through the female reproductive tract, fertilization and cleavage of the embryo occurs in the ampulla. Cleavage continues on the way to the uterus and occasionally a human embryo enters the uterus as early as the 8- to 12-cell stage.

TUBAL DISEASES IN INFERTILITY

Congenital Tubal Abnormalities
Congenital tubal abnormalities range from 1 in 500 to 700 deliveries.[23] *Complete absence* of the oviduct may occur with or without concomitant absence of the ipsilateral ovary.[24] Bilateral absence of the ampullary muscularis layer results in convoluted or tortuous tubes.[25] Distal *segmental absence* of the oviduct with absence of the ipsilateral ovary or proximal segmental absence has also been reported.[26]

Accessory tubes are small blind-ending cylindrical structures attached to the ampulla of a normal-sized fallopian tube. At their distal end there is a small fimbria-like structure. As the ova may be captured by the fimbriae of the accessory tube, an ectopic pregnancy may result if fertilization occurs. Thus, it is advisable that these structures be removed during infertility surgery. *Accessory ostia* are always located on the mesenteric side

TABLE 31–1. ETIOLOGIES OF PROXIMAL AND DISTAL TUBAL DISEASE

Distal Tubal Obstruction
Hydrosalpinx (thin/thick-walled; hydrosalpinx simplex/follicularis)
Pelvic inflammatory disease

Proximal Tubal Obstruction
Congenital atresia
Debris, viscous secretions
Muscular spasm, stromal edema
Obliterative fibrosis
Salpingitis isthmica nodosa
Chronic tubal inflammation
Intrinsic (intramural) endometriosis
Endosalpingiosis
Tubocornual polyps
Granulomatous salpingitis (genital tuberculosis, actinomycosis,
    schistosomiasis, sarcoidosis, foreign bodies)
Remnants of ectopic pregnancy
Tubal sterilization

of the ampulla. The *immotile cilia syndrome* is characterized by congenitally nonfunctioning cilia.[27] Women with this disorder are thought to have reduced fertility due to lack of cilial activity in the tubal mucosa.[28] It is inherited in an autosomal dominant manner, and women with this syndrome may exhibit the *Kartagener triad* with situs inversus, bronchiectasis, and chronic sinusitis. Among the various *anatomic displacements* of the tube, *torsion* is the most common.

Tubal lesions can be grouped in two major groups: *distal* and *proximal tubal diseases*. Proximal tubal obstruction occurs less frequently than distal obstruction and its etiology and treatment are more controversial (Table 31–1).

Distal Tubal Obstruction

Hydrosalpinx. The most common lesion of distal tubal occlusion, hydrosalpinx is a major cause of infertility. Because of distal blockage, dilatation of the fallopian tube results filled with clear, sterile, and serous fluid. Several authors believe that the obstruction is the end result of pyosalpinx that has become inactive for an extended time, whereas others accept it as a primary lesion that may secondarily result in pyosalpinx.[29] An abnormality in the muscular wall of the tube has also been suggested as a cause. The reason why dilatation can occur when only the distal end of the tube is blocked is not fully understood; but once the tube becomes distended by fluid, its muscular contractions may not be strong enough to empty the lumen.

There are two forms of hydrosalpinx. In *hydrosalpinx simplex*, the tube is dilated but there is a single lumen and no adhesions between the mucosal folds. In *hydrosalpinx follicularis*, the tubal lumen is divided into locules by adhered mucosal folds. Macroscopically, a hydrosalpinx is classified as either thin- or thick-walled. In thin-walled hydrosalpinx, the fallopian tube is grossly distended by copious straw-colored fluid and is translucent, whereas in thick-walled, the wall is fibrous and the smaller lumen contains little fluid. In both entities the tube is totally blocked at the distal end. In general, thin-walled cases have fewer intratubal adhesions, fewer flattened areas in mucosal folds, less desquamation in epithelial cells, and less deciliation in ciliated cells in comparison to the thick-walled cases. In thick-walled cases, numerous agglutinations of the folds cause a characteristic honeycomb appearance. Identification of swollen cilia (megacilia) at the tip is also among the common features of thick-walled hydrosalpinx.

Classification of the extent of the distal tubal obstruction can be made into various stages (Table 31–2).[30] Surgery is capable of restoring patency in more than 75 percent of hydrosalpinges, but the intrauterine pregnancy rate is only 10 to 35 percent.[31] Restoration of tubal patency may partly improve the quality of the mucosa with the loss of pressure on the mucosa, but despite the recovery of the ciliated cells after surgery, it is likely that mucosal damage such as agglutination, adhesion formation, and loss of folds is irreversible. In addition, an important issue is that pregnancy rates are lower for thick-walled cases in comparison to the thin-walled cases after microsurgery.

Pelvic Inflammatory Disease. Damage resulting from infection is the most common cause of tubal infertility. Traditionally, gonorrhea had been considered the major causative agent in pelvic inflammatory disease (PID). Recent studies have demonstrated that PID is polymicrobial in nature, the most common causes being sexually transmitted nonspecific infection and postabortus and postpartum salpingitis.[32] Evidence suggests that *Chlamydia trachomatis*, currently one of the most common sexually transmitted pathogens, plays an increasing role in impaired fertility due to tubal obstruction and salpingitis. Other organisms such as *Mycoplasma hominis*, *Ureaplasma urealyticum*, and group A streptococci may also be implicated in the etiology of salpingitis. Although anaerobes are the most commonly recovered organisms from the upper genital tract of women with PID, they are generally thought to invade secondarily and damage a fallopian tube that is primarily infected by gonococci or chlamydiae.[33] Salpingitis may present in acute or chronic form, or as an acute exacerbation of a chronic infection. Both gonococci and chlamydiae ascend from the lower genital tract via the mucosal surfaces of the endocervix and endometrium to the endosalpinx, causing epithelial damage with loss of ciliation and adhesions between mucosal folds. Streptococci, staphylococci, gram-negative bacteria, and probably mycoplasma reach the tubes via the lymphatic and vascular channels, affecting pri-

TABLE 31–2. CLASSIFICATION OF SEVERITY OF DISEASE IN DISTAL TUBAL OBSTRUCTION

Extent of Disease	Findings
Mild	Absent or small hydrosalpinx <15 mm in diameter Inverted fimbria easily recognized when patency achieved No significant peritubal or periovarian adhesions Preoperative hysterosalpingogram reveals a rugal pattern
Moderate	Hydrosalpinx 15 to 30 mm in diameter Fragments of fimbria not readily identified Periovarian and/or peritubular adhesions without fixation, minimal cul-de-sac adhesions Absence of a rugal pattern on preoperative hysterosalpingogram
Severe	Large hydrosalpinx >30 mm in diameter No fimbria identified Dense pelvic or adnexal adhesions with fixation of the ovary and tube to the broad ligament, pelvic side-wall, omentum, and/or bowel Obliteration of the cul-de-sac Frozen pelvis

(Reproduced, with permission, from Rock JA, Katayama P, Martin EJ, et al. Factors influencing the success of salpingostomy techniques for distal fimbrial obstruction. Obstet Gynecol. *52:591, 1978.)*

marily the tubal wall and parametrium rather than the endosalpinx. Salpingitis can also occur as a result of adjacent organ inflammation such as appendicitis or diverticulitis.

Studies on laparoscopically confirmed salpingitis have shown that with prompt diagnosis and treatment before the development of adnexal swelling and in the absence of recurrent infections, tubal patency and morphology are unlikely to be impaired. Infertility occurs in 13 percent of patients who have had a single infection, 35 percent after two episodes and up to 75 percent after three or more infections.[34] In addition, PID is one of the most common causes of the tubal lesions responsible for ectopic pregnancy. Patients who have had conservative treatment for acute salpingitis have 5- to 6-fold increased risk of ectopic pregnancy. Whatever the etiology, salpingitis may damage the distal portions of the fallopian tubes resulting in hydrosalpinx, pyosalpinx, fimbrial obstruction, or interstitial salpingitis. It may involve the proximal segment, resulting in isthmic and cornual stenosis, or blockage.

Proximal Tubal Obstruction

Proximal lesions of the fallopian tube occur less often than lesions of the distal end. The most common of these are obliterative fibrosis (38 percent), salpingitis isthmica nodosa (24 percent), chronic tubal inflammation (21 percent), intrinsic (intramural) endometriosis (14 percent), and endosalpingiosis.[35,36] The less frequent causes are tubocornual polyps, tuberculosis, and remnants of chronic ectopic pregnancy.

Obliterative Fibrosis. In obliterative fibrosis, collagen fibers are deposited medial to the inner longitudinal layer of the myosalpinx, resulting in the complete occlusion of the lumen and complete destruction of the epithelium. There is minimal involvement of the musculature. Obliterative fibrosis is the most common cause of proximal tubal obstruction and has been postulated to be a nonspecific response of the tubal isthmic or interstitial epithelium to an inflammation or infection.[35]

Salpingitis Isthmica Nodosa. The exact etiology of salpingitis isthmica nodosa (SIN), the second most common lesion of the proximal fallopian tube, is controversial. It is most frequently found in women who have previously had an ectopic pregnancy, and in up to 70 percent of those undergoing tubal surgery for proximal obstruction, and has an age range of 26 to 30 yr.[37,38] A higher incidence has been noted in the black population, especially among Jamaicans.[37,39] Salpingitis isthmica nodosa is identified as the causative histologic abnormality in 23 to 60 percent of cases with occlusive tubal disease.[40,41] In 46 to 57 percent of patients with ectopic pregnancies, the involved tube has been found to carry histopathologic changes of SIN.[37,42] The documentation of SIN in fallopian tubes has implications for future management and follow-up for both fertility and ectopic pregnancy.[43,44]

Lesions of SIN are bilateral in most of the cases (36 to 85 percent). In 50 to 69 percent of SIN, the proximal tube (isthmus) is involved, whereas in 28 percent only the midtubal region and in 7 percent the entire tube is involved.[38,45] The pathologic hallmark of the lesion is the presence of isthmic diverticula or outpouchings of tubal epithelium. These projections, which often communicate with the central tubal lumen, invade the surrounding muscularis and stimulate secondary smooth muscle hypertrophy that results in nodularity. Diverticula typically do not connect with the serosal surface but may be found

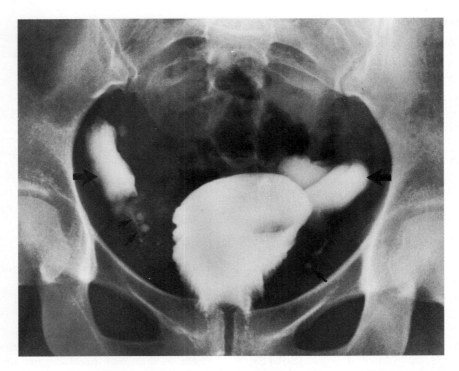

Figure 31–2. Hysterosalpingogram of salpingitis isthmica nodosum. Bilateral small accumulations of contrast medium (small arrows) near the isthmic portion of fallopian tubes and associated bilateral hydrosalpinx (large arrows) are observed.

in close proximity to it.[1] SIN seems to be an acquired disorder, but a variety of etiologies have been proposed: congenital, hormonal, infectious, and adenomyosis-like. So far, current literature has failed to support the congenital theory, and although no cause-and-effect relationship could be shown yet, the infectious theory is the most popular. Salpingitis isthmica nodosa demonstrates invasion of the tubal musculature by tubal epithelium (adenomyosis-like process) with subsequent muscular hypertrophy. Interestingly, unilateral SIN is often accompanied by ipsilateral uterine adenomyosis.[1]

The diagnosis of SIN can be confirmed only by inspection of tubal histology. In recent years, HSG based diagnosis of SIN has been the basis for many studies that explore the incidence and clinical significance of the disease. Typically 2-mm accumulations of contrast medium are observed bilaterally near the isthmic portion of the oviducts (Fig 31–2).[46] Tubal obstruction and hydrosalpinx are commonly associated findings and the incidence of SIN by hysterosalpingography (HSG) varies from 3.8 to 8.7 percent.[47] At laparoscopy, nodular, fusiform enlargement with thickening and induration of the isthmus are characteristic findings. Salpingoscopy via the laparoscopic or hysteroscopic route is another method to confirm diagnosis.[48,49]

Salpingitis isthmica nodosa appears to be a progressive disease, with an initial increase in the size of lesions, eventually leading to complete obliteration

of the tubal lumen despite lack of evidence of a continuous stimulus.[50] Presently, besides assisted reproductive technologies, segmental resection and tubal reanastomosis is the best alternative for patients with obstructed or patent but dysfunctional oviducts.

Chronic Tubal Inflammation. Chronic tubal inflammation is the third most common proximal pathology. The inflammatory process may involve all three layers, causing the epithelium to become atrophic, the submucosal layer to become dense, and the myosalpinx to be thickened. Lesions confined to the proximal tube may extend to the whole fallopian tube in severe cases.

Intrinsic (Intramural) Endometriosis. Intrinsic endometriosis of the fallopian tube has an incidence of 7 to 14 percent.[35,40,41,45] Fertility outcome after tubocornual anastomosis for proximal tubal endometriosis has been reported to be poor, with a high reocclusion rate of 63 percent at the end of the first year.[40,45] Successful use of GnRH analogs in nodular proximal tubal occlusions such as SIN and fallopian tube endometriosis has been recently reported.[51] Recanalization rate with a 6-month GnRH-analog treatment is found to be 87 percent. However, authors have reported that the spontaneous pregnancy rate is dramatically lower (1.8 percent/cycle) with only GnRH-a treatment, and the chance of pregnancy can be enhanced significantly (up to 50 percent/cycle) using assisted reproduction techniques (GIFT) following tubal recatheterization and GnRH-analog administration.

Endosalpingiosis. Endosalpingiosis is characterized by the ectopic location of tubal epithelium with ciliated, nonciliated, and intercalary cells, involving peritoneal surfaces. This disorder was first reported by Sampson in 1928 to describe ectopic tubal mucosa found on the tubal or uterine serosa and thought to have spread locally from the traumatized endosalpinx of patients with a history of partial or total salpingectomy.[52,53] Endosalpingiosis is associated with entities such as chronic pelvic pain, salpingitis, serous tumors, ectopic pregnancy, and endometriosis.[54–56] The incidence of this disorder was reported to be 11.8 percent among women with chronic pelvic pain.[36]

Histologic lesions usually appear as small clear cysts, microscopically lined by fallopian-type epithelium. The endosalpingeal outpouchings can be distinguished from SIN by the absence of characteristic myosalpingeal hypertrophy. The histogenesis is unknown and commonly offered theories include transplantation, coelomic metaplasia, and induction.[52,53,55] It is thought that the development of endosalpingiosis may be mediated hormonally and the related chronic pelvic pain could be managed by removing the foci and administering additional GnRH analogs postoperatively.[36]

Tubocornual Polyps. Tubocornual polyps are detected in 2 to 10 percent of hysterosalpingograms of infertile patients,[57] and in 11 percent in hysterectomy and autopsy studies.[58] Polyps usually occur in the intramural portion and less often in the isthmus. They may arise from the endometrium or tubal mucosa or they may have a fibrous origin. Tubocornual polyps may be attached with a broad base ranging from 2 to 3 mm to 10 mm. They have been reported to be associated with endometriosis in 41 percent of patients,[58] but their association with infertility is controversial.

Tuberculosis. Genital tuberculosis is estimated to have an incidence of 1 percent among infertile women in the United States; it is much more common (20 percent) in developing countries.[59] Genital tuberculosis always occurs secondary to a focus in another organ, usually in the lungs, spreading to the fallopian tubes hematogenously. Spread may also be via lymphatics or directly from the peritoneal cavity. The fallopian tubes are the most common site of the initial infection in genital tuberculosis and the ampulla is the most involved segment of the tube.

Genital tuberculosis rarely produces significant symptoms in early stages and is usually detected by HSG. This disorder presents as primary (94 percent) or secondary (6 percent) infertility.[60] Although the initial oviductal assault is mucosal, later the muscularis and the serosa are involved. At surgery, the tube is rigid

and the ampulla may be dilated, but fimbriae often appear to be normal and the ostium to be open. If adhesions develop between the tube and ovary they either close the fimbrial end or constrict the proximal end of the dilated ampulla, resulting in a characteristic "tobacco pouch" or "pipe-stem" appearance on HSG. The healing process results either in a totally obliterated tubal lumen with infertility or in massive adhesion of mucosal folds and scarring of the endosalpinx with markedly decreased fertility. The resultant extensive tubal damage is such that tubal repair cannot yield functional fallopian tubes. Such an attempt can also reactivate the infection, and if pregnancy does occur there is a high risk of ectopic implantation.[61]

Tuberculosis salpingitis is the predominant manifestation of granulomatous salpingitis. Other causative agents or entities for granulomatous salpingitis are actinomycosis, parasites such as pinworm, and schistosomiasis, sarcoidosis, Crohn's disease, and foreign bodies such as mineral oil, lubricant jelly, starch, and talc powder.[1]

Poststerilization Sequelae. There are various methods for tubal sterilization but those commonly utilized in the last decade include tubal ligation, laparoscopic electrocoagulation, and application of silicone rings or tubal clips. Poststerilization studies have demonstrated abnormalities in 28 percent of tubes after 3 yr, rising to 72 percent after 10 yr.[62] Histologic changes found in the tubal segment remaining after sterilization were flattening and fibrosis of the mucosal folds, deciliation, polyp formation, tuboperitoneal fistulae, and tubal endometriosis.

There is no correlation between the success of microsurgical reversal and the time elapsed since sterilization. However, there is a correlation between tubal lesions and subsequent fertility. Women without tubal lesions in the remaining re-anastomosed tubes, reportedly had up to a 50 to 64 percent chance of pregnancy.[62,63]

DIAGNOSTIC TOOLS IN TUBAL DISEASES

Hysterosalpingography

Hysterosalpingography is probably the most common technique that is undertaken during an infertility investigation. It is best performed towards the end of the first week of the cycle, just after the cessation of menstrual bleeding, when the isthmus is most distensible and the fallopian tubes are most readily filled by contrast medium. Hysterosalpingography is generally the first tubal investigation to be performed as it is considered to be less invasive than endoscopy. Some authors have suggested that it also has a therapeutic effect on infertility, especially when an oil-soluble contrast medium has been used.[64,65] Hysterosalpingography is a test of uterine–tubal anatomy but does not provide information regarding function.

Normally, after the uterus is filled with the contrast medium, the spindle-shaped cornua, then a pretubal bulge, caused by an anatomic fold separating the endometrium from endosalpinx, is seen. The apex of the cornua is seen to be continuous with the lumen of the intramural segment of the tube. The luminal wall of the intramural and isthmic segment should be smooth and uniform in diameter. The mucosal folds of ampulla and spilling of contrast medium from the fimbrial end should be detected on a normal HSG. Occasionally, there may be a genuine tubal spasm in the uterocornual junction. This spasm is more likely caused by a complex response of this area to hormonal, pharmacologic, and neurologic stimuli that may be relieved by administering drugs such as diazepam, amyl nitrite, or glucagon.

In distal tubal obstruction there is a varying degree of ampullary dilatation and no spillage of contrast medium. Sometimes the obstruction is incomplete. There may not be any dilatation of ampulla, and there may be peritubal adhesions causing the medium to have a loculated appearance. Hysterosalpingographic findings of SIN are, characteristically, diverticula of varying size, usually 1 to 2 cm long on one or both tubes. In tubal endometriosis, the isthmus may have a honeycomb appearance with the presence of tubal patency. Genital tuberculosis may mimic the radiologic appearance of SIN, but the nodules are less uniform and the tube is more rigid, with small terminal sacculations. There may be calcifications in the tube, ovaries, or local pelvic lymph nodes. The tubes are frequently blocked on both sides and are usually moderately dilated, with a club-shaped appearance of the ampulla. The tube, typically, may have a rigid "pipe-stem" appearance or be fixed in an abnormal position by adhesions. Rarely, tubointestinal fistulae may be seen. Tubal polyps are seen as oval shadows or filling defects in the intramural segment with contrast medium flowing in a thin line above or below them. In case of a large ovarian cyst, the tube may seem to be stretched over the cyst, distorted and partially obstructed.

Nevertheless, recent studies and meta-analysis have shown that HSG has limited use in demonstrating the absence of distal and proximal tubal obstruction and minimal use in the documentation of peritubal adhesions.[66] However, it is able to detect the presence of proximal, distal obstruction, and hydrosalpinx.

Radionuclide Hysterosalpingography

Brundin et al have described a method to show the function and capacity of the tubal epithelium to transport particles using radionuclide hysterosalpingography (RN-HSG).[67] HSG was carried out using sufficient contrast medium to fill both tubes when they were intact. Approximately 1 to 4 mo later, RN-HSG was performed 1 to 2 days before the ovulation estimated by basal body temperature charts during the 2 preceding mo. Brundin et al have reported that 53 percent of patients with patent tubes on HSG had nonfunctional (functionally obstructed) tubes on RN-HSG and none of the patients were able to achieve pregnancy after a follow-up of 18 mo.[67]

Hysterosalpingo-Contrast Sonography (HyCoSy)

In 1981, Nannini et al were the first to report that saline injected into the uterine cavity allowed intrauterine structures such as endometrium to be observed with ultrasound.[68] The fluid, observed in the pouch of Douglas, indicated that the tubes were patent. Normal fallopian tubes are not visible by ultrasound unless tubal damage such as hydrosalpinx exists. The observations that fluid in the uterus and tubes could enhance the diagnostic power of ultrasonography led to the realization that injecting fluid into the uterus could allow both intrauterine structures and tubal patency to be investigated during an ultrasonographic examination, especially with the use of transvaginal color Doppler.[69–72] Saline or Ringer's solutions that were used initially gave unpredictable, nonreproducible results and could only visualize the proximal part of the tubes. Thereafter, a new saccharide-based echo enhancing agent (Echovist), was determined to be suitable for assessing tubal patency during a transvaginal ultrasonography. Degenhardt et al have recently reported that during evaluation of tubal patency, HyCoSy results were in confirmation with HSG and laparoscopy in 91 and 92 percent of cases, respectively.[73] Although this procedure may be performed on an outpatient basis without anesthesia, lack of information regarding anatomy of tubal and pelvic structures is its major drawback.

Laparoscopy

Laparoscopy is a well-established technique in routine investigation and treatment of infertility. Following inspection of the uterus, the fallopian tubes should be examined in detail, from the cornua to the fimbriae. Proximal obstruction will be evident if dye fails to fill the tubal lumen, and with increasing pressure a blue coloration of the uterine fundus will occur due to extravasation of the dye. Irregularities on the isthmic segment may indicate endometriosis or SIN. The diverticula of SIN can be identified when they fill with dye and small blue spots are seen beneath the tubal serosa during chromopertubation. During examination of the ampulla, its diameter, adhesions that limit its mobility, and surface lesions such as endometriotic spots should be noted carefully. The fimbrial adhesions that might indicate mucosal damage and the fimbria ovarica should be checked before completion of the procedure. In cases of distal obstruction, the dilated ampulla must be examined carefully to determine the type of hydrosalpinx; thin-walled (transparent) or thick-walled (opaque appearance) hydrosalpinx. Large fimbrial cysts interfering with tubal motility should be removed.

Studies comparing findings at laparoscopy with HSG have been reviewed by Maguiness et al.[74] The superior performance of laparoscopy in identifying tubal adhesions is clearly demonstrated by the number of cases of tubal pathology diagnosed in women with an apparently normal HSG (17.4 percent). Overall, there is total agreement on tubal status between the two methods in 73.9 percent and disagreement in 26.1 percent of cases. The disadvantages of laparoscopy are that it is usually performed under general anesthesia and does not give information about the uterine cavity. However, because of the additional information obtained about the pelvic organs, this procedure is now complementary to HSG in assessing the fallopian tubes.

Salpingoscopy

Salpingoscopy is the procedure for performing tubal endoscopy via laparoscopy or laparotomy, and the fimbria is the site of entry. The first successful salpingoscopy was reported in the early 1980s.[75] There are rigid or flexible salpingoscopes that may be used in laparotomy[76] or in laparoscopy.[77] The optical systems currently used in rigid laparoscopes provide sharper images with a panoramic field, but with this instrumentation it is not possible to view the endosalpinx beyond the ampullary–isthmic junction. However, access to the isthmic portion of the tube using a flexible, fiberoptic salpingoscope has been accomplished.[78]

After entering the peritoneal cavity by use of laparotomy or laparoscopy, the endoscope, called a salpingscope, is introduced via the distal tubal opening. Afterwards, a balanced salt solution is given to distend the tubal lumen for visualization. During a normal salpingoscopy, the infundibulum is characterized by several large, radially arranged folds.[79] The ampulla has 3 to 6 major and several minor folds in between, 4 and 1 mm in height, respectively. The ampullary–isthmic junction has several folds that diverge from isthmus toward the ampulla. Fimbrial agglutination, intraluminal synechiae, stenoses, flattening or loss of mucosal folds, and atrophy of the mucosa are the major pathologic findings during salpingoscopy. Unfortunately, no systematic salpingoscopic classification of pathologic findings has been developed.

In the past, the endotubal mucosa of a hydrosalpinx has been assessed by a preoperative HSG before microsurgery but later salpingoscopy has replaced HSG with comparable results. Several studies reported a false negative (normal mucosa with HSG, abnormal with salpingoscopy) rate of 45 percent and a false positive rate (abnormal mucosa with HSG, normal with salpingoscopy) of 30 percent for HSG.[80,81] Salpingoscopy has also been proven to be a good prognostic indicator for tuboplasty in regard to pregnancy outcome. Henry-Suchet et al found a total pregnancy rate of 50 percent, an intrauterine pregnancy rate of 46 percent, and an ectopic pregnancy rate of 8 percent in a group of patients who had normal endotubal mucosa as assessed by salpingoscopy before tuboplasty. These rates were 19, 9, and 55 percent in the salpingoscopically abnormal group, respectively.[82]

In unexplained infertile patients with normal pelvic findings at laparoscopy, salpingoscopic abnormalities may be encountered in 27 to 37 percent of the tubes.[83] Salpingoscopy is also well correlated with histopathologic findings in normal, mild, and severe cases but occasionally underdiagnosing moderate cases.[78]

Falloposcopy

Falloposcopy is the transvaginal technique for tubal microendoscopy of the oviduct that enters the fallopian tube through uterotubal ostium. Kerin et al were the first to report successful falloposcopy.[84] It was first described as a coaxial delivery system using a hysteroscope for visualization of the uterotubal ostium and thus requiring general anesthesia. The coaxial technique involves the passage of small, steerable, tapered guide wires made of stainless steel or Teflon into the fallopian tube. The flexible guide wires, ranging 0.3 to 0.8 mm in outer diameter, can advance in the tube in harmony with its curvatures, minimizing the risk of tubal trauma. After the wire has passed 1.5 cm beyond the uterotubal ostium, flexible Teflon cannulas with an outer diameter of 1.2 to 1.3 mm are introduced over this guide wire. The guide wire is then withdrawn, keeping the Teflon cannula in place, and the falloposcope is introduced into it. Recently, an alternative approach, the *linear everting catheter (LEC)* system, has been developed.[85] This catheter, with an outer diameter of 1.2 mm, consists of inner and outer catheter bodies joined circumferentially at their distal tips by a flexible and distensible membrane. When the membrane is pressurized, the inner membrane inflates and begins to unroll outwards and advance through the tube. This catheter does not require the hysteroscopic guidance, thus eliminating anesthesia. The unrolling action eliminates any sheer forces between the balloon element and the inner walls of the tube. Also, the forward progression concentrates energy at the tip, making it self-guiding. In both methods, the catheter tip is advanced until the fimbrial end of the fallopian tube and then withdrawn slowly while investigating the endotubal mucosa.

During falloposcopy, normal uterotubal ostium is seen with a sharp outline, circular or ovoid in shape, with a 1.3-mm diameter in the relaxed state. As the tube contracts, typical four-segment puckering occurs.[84] The normal intramural segment is 1.5 to 2.5 cm long and 0.8 to 1.4 mm wide, with the narrowest point at the uterotubal junction. It is pale pink and contains 4 to 6 folds. The isthmic lumen is the narrowest extrauterine tubal segment and extends from the uterotubal junction to the ampullary–isthmic junction; it is 1 to 2 mm in diameter and 2 to 3 cm long. Again, it is pink and has 4 to 6 mucosal folds. Beyond the ampullary–isthmic junction, the diameter of the ampulla increases quite rapidly from 1.5 to 10 mm. The color of the epithelium is red because of the well-vascularized secondary epithelial folds.

A falloposcopic classification and scoring system has been developed to standardize the pathologic falloposcopic findings.[86] Parameters such as degree of patency, epithelial and vascular changes, adhesion formation, and amount of dilatation are scored between 1 and 3. A total minimum score of 20 for each tube reflects normality, 20 to 30 reflects mild to moderate endotubal disease, and a score greater than 30 reflects severe endotubal disease. The most common lesions have been reported to be intraluminal nonobstructive adhesions (39 percent), stenoses (19 percent), obstruction (16 percent), and polyps (10 percent), with isthmus as the most common (45 percent) localization for these lesions.[86]

THERAPEUTIC APPROACHES IN TUBAL DISEASES

Tubal Surgery

Reproductive surgery plays an important role in the management of tubal infertility, which is the cause of female infertility in 15 to 25 percent of cases. Selection of the most appropriate approach is a critical part of the surgical management of tubal factor infertility. The results of surgery depend on various factors such as the nature and extent of the tubal damage and periadnexal and pelvic adhesions, the final length of the reconstructed oviduct, and the presence of additional pelvic disease. With the evolution of microsurgery in gynecology in 1970s, a variety of microsurgical procedures were developed. The term "microsurgery" refers not simply to magnification but to meticulous hemostasis, minimized tissue handling, prevention of tissue desiccation, avoidance of contamination with foreign bodies such as talc, and use of fine suture material with minimal reactivity. Surgical techniques were found to give better results when compared with macrosurgical techniques.[87] Relative and absolute contraindications to tubal microsurgery still exist. Some of them are tuberculosis of the oviduct, a frozen pelvis with massive pelvic adhesions, a high-risk patient for surgery, and a patient with a recent attack of salpingitis. A bipolar disease (proximal and distal obstruction, simultaneously) is also a contraindication for reconstructive surgery because surgery in women with bipolar blockage is associated with a poor pregnancy rate of only 12 percent.[88] Since the mid-1980s, laparoscopic surgery has developed extensively for gynecologic and as well as reproductive surgery, allowing good magnification, rapid recovery time, and smaller scars. One major issue is that a history of tubal surgery places the patient in a higher risk group for ectopic pregnancy; 3 to 20 percent of those patients encounter an ectopic pregnancy after the corrective surgery.[89] Also, patients with previous ectopic pregnancy should not be considered for microsurgery owing to the high risk of recurrence and to the reduced chance of intrauterine pregnancy.[90] When the risk of ectopic pregnancy is unacceptably high or when the patient is reluctant to be exposed to a high-risk of ectopic pregnancy, IVF-ET could be offered as an alternative, informing the patient that this procedure can also result in a high 17 percent ectopic pregnancy risk. Considering that tubal patency rates after tubal surgery are higher than pregnancy rates, it has been suggested that postoperative fallopian tubes most likely experience some loss in ciliary function despite the achievement of anatomic patency.[89]

Second Look Laparoscopy. Liberation of adhesions during a second look laparoscopy (SLL) after a previous laparotomy has been suggested to increase the overall pregnancy rate and decrease the ectopic pregnancy rates. Currently, optimal time for such an SLL and salpingo-ovariolysis is accepted to be 4 to 8 wk after a laparotomy. Second look laparoscopy is not performed after 6 or 12 mo, when it is ineffective.[91,92]

Distal Disease

Surgical management of distal tubal occlusion may be performed laparoscopically or by microsurgery via laparotomy. Laparoscopic technique is becoming the procedure of choice, since the pregnancy rates after laparoscopic surgery approach those yielded by microsurgery.[31,93] After microsurgical salpingostomy, live birth rates vary between 20 and 30 percent and ectopic pregnancy rates up to 18 percent.[94,95]

Salpingo-Ovariolysis. In contemporary practice, salpingo-ovariolysis is usually performed laparoscopically. Periadnexal adhesions can be divided with laparoscopic scissors, electrocautery, or a laser beam. The intrauterine pregnancy rate after laparoscopic salpingo-ovariolysis is 62 percent and the ectopic pregnancy rate is 5.4 percent,[96] which compares favorably with the results of laparotomy.[96,97] However, severe and dense adhesions cannot be completely removed by the laparoscopic approach. In vitro fertilization is recommended for those patients due to poor pregnancy rates following salpingo-ovariolysis.[97]

Tulandi et al evaluated pregnancy rates among women with periadnexal adhesions with or without salpingo-ovariolysis and found the cumulative pregnancy rate to be 45 percent in the treated group and 16 percent in the untreated group after a follow-up of 24 mo.[98] The fact that the pregnancy rate in the treated group was higher but ectopic pregnancy rates did not differ between the two groups suggests that the intrinsic damage of the fallopian tube plays a more important role in the development of ectopic pregnancy than do periadnexal adhesions but the presence of adhesions decreases the chance of overall pregnancy.

Fimbriolysis. Fimbriolysis is performed when the fimbrial surface is generally healthy but some fimbriae have become attached and phimotic as a result of inflammatory process, generally as a result of extragenital disease such as appendicitis. A relatively high pregnancy rate of 52 percent and a low ectopic rate of 3.5 percent were reported following microsurgical fimbriolysis.[89]

Fimbrioplasty. In cases of more severe tubal disease, such as tubal phimosis or a mild hydrosalpinx, fimbrioplasty is the surgical procedure performed for repair of the partial obstruction at the fimbriated end. It can be done under magnification at laparotomy or laparoscopically by dividing the adhesions sharply with cautery or laser. Once the serosa is opened, it can be sutured back to the fallopian tube serosa by everting the opening and thus maintaining the tubal patency. Good prognostic factors include a thin tubal wall and a small ampullary dilatation. The intrauterine and extrauterine pregnancy rates were reported to be 68 and 5 percent in laparotomic microsurgery, versus 25 to 50 percent and 5 to 10 percent in laparoscopy.[45,99] Fayez recommends not to use alligator forceps because of the high ectopic pregnancy rates due to probable tubal damage.[100]

Neosalpingostomy. Neosalpingostomy is used to reopen the distal end of a completely occluded fallopian tube by creating a new stoma as a tubal ostium using scissors, electrosurgery, or laser. The occlusion or hydrosalpinx is usually a sequela of PID. The tubal patency rate after neosalpingostomy is approximately 90 to 95 percent, but the overall term pregnancy rate is as low as 20 to 25 percent and the ectopic pregnancy rate is 3 to 11 percent, indicating the important role of intraluminal pathology.[99,101] The intrauterine pregnancy rate yielded by laparoscopic salpingostomy appears slightly lower than those reported after microsurgical salpingostomy. However, the benefits of a laparoscopic salpingostomy are those of a minimally invasive procedure coupled with reduced hospital costs. It is arguable that IVF-ET, rather than tubal surgery, should be offered to those patients with a poor prognosis and at high risk for ectopic pregnancy. Factors affecting surgical outcome include distal ampullary diameter, tubal wall thickness, nature of the tubal epithelium at the neostomy site, and extent and type of adhesions. Poor prognostic factors include thickened tubal walls, an ampullary diameter exceeding 3 cm, and intratubal severe and periadnexal adhesions.[99] Using the Rock classification system for distal tubal obstruction

(Table 31–2), the pregnancy rates were reported to be 80 percent with mild, 31 percent with moderate, and 16 percent with severe disease.[102] Various surgical repair techniques and success rates for tubal disease are summarized in Table 31–3.

Proximal Disease

A tube may be patent despite failure of dye to pass during a HSG due to cornual spasm, a mucous plug, or synechiae obstructing the intramural or isthmic portion of the tube. Selective salpingography or tubal cannulation under hysteroscopic, ultrasonographic, or radiographic guidance will provide a differential diagnosis of such conditions from pathologic obstructions. Several authors have noted a lack of histologic confirmation of luminal occlusion in about 10 to 20 percent of patients despite an apparent cornual block on repeated HSGs or even laparoscopy.[108] Debris, viscous mucous, endometrial polyps, and parasitic infections are the intraluminal reasons for proximal tubal obstruction, whereas muscular spasm, inflammatory fibrosis, tuberculosis, SIN, neoplasia, endometriosis, and congenital atresia are the examples for intramural reasons. Among those, muscular spasm, stromal edema, mucosal agglutination, amorphous debris, and viscous secretions will benefit from various tubal cannulation procedures. Cornual polyps, endometriosis, chronic salpingitis, SIN, and some parasitic infections may also respond to these techniques. Congenital atresia, luminal fibrosis, and tuberculosis are the conditions in which cannulation will be unsuccessful.[109] Generally, microsurgical correction of proximal tubal obstruction resulting from SIN, endometriosis, or postinflammatory fibrosis can yield live birth rates between 37 and 58 percent and ectopic pregnancy rates of 5 to 7 percent. Microsurgical tubotubal anastomosis for reversal of sterilization yields live birth rates of 60 to 80 percent.[99]

TABLE 31–3. VARIOUS SURGICAL TECHNIQUES AND SUCCESS RATES FOR TUBAL DISEASE

	IUP (%)	EP (%)
Distal Disease		
Salpingo-ovariolysis[96]	62	5.4
Fimbriolysis[89]	52	3.5
Fimbrioplasty		
Laparotomy[45]	60–68	2–5
Laparoscopy[99]	25–50	5–10
Neosalpingostomy[30,99,101]	20–25	3–11
Proximal Disease		
Uterotubal implantation[103]	29	N/A
Tubocornual anastomosis[45,104–106]	58–69	6–8
Tubal anastomosis (sterilization reversal)[99,107]	68–80	4.4

IUP, Intrauterine pregnancy; EP, ectopic pregnancy; N/A, not assessed.

Uterotubal Implantation. The traditional treatment of cornual occlusion is uterotubal implantation. The intramural portion of the tube is resected, an opening is created in the uterine cornu, and the remaining distal part of the tube is reimplanted into the uterus. However, this procedure is associated with bleeding and the new uterotubal junction is unphysiologic, yielding a low pregnancy rate of 29 percent.[103]

Tubocornual Anastomosis. In tubocornual anastomosis, the occluded portion of the tube is circumferentially incised from the surrounding myometrium and the tube is then transected with microscissors at 2-mm intervals until the patent portion is found with the help of chromopertubation. The distal segment of the tube is treated in the same way, and the two cut ends of the tube are approximated with several interrupted 8-0 sutures. The pregnancy rate after tubocornual anastomosis is superior (58 percent) to uterotubal implantation.[105] Fayez et al have also confirmed those results, with patency and pregnancy rates for uterotubal anastomosis of 70 and 39 percent and for tubocornual anastomosis of 94 and 69 percent.[106]

Tubal Anastomosis. Microsurgery finds its best application in tubal anastomosis.[63,110] The most frequent cause of midtubal occlusion is a prior tubal sterilization, and tubal anastomosis is performed to reverse tubal sterilization or to remove and reconstruct lesions that are occlusive and affect the tube at sites other than the fimbriated end.

Approximately 1 to 2 percent of women seek a reversal of a previous sterilization. Previously, reversal surgery was performed by macrosurgical techniques with a pregnancy rate of 68 percent and a 4.4 percent tubal pregnancy rate.[107] Hulka and Halme have utilized a microsurgical technique and reported a tubal patency rate of 91 percent.[111] The best results have been obtained following sterilization with Hulka clips or Fallope rings, while the worst outcome results after unipolar cautery. Several studies have concluded that the most important factors affecting the outcome after a sterilization reversal are the length of the remaining tube (at least 4 cm) and the type of sterilization performed. Age, parity, and interval from sterilization to reversal surgery did not affect the overall pregnancy rates.[110,112] Although sterilization by Kroener fimbriectomy was once thought to be irreversible, a technique utilizing cuff eversion and transverse salpingostomy has later been described with a success rate of 40 percent.[113]

Transcervical Tubal Cannulation. Access to the fallopian tubes via the cervix has become easier in the last 10 yr with the advent of specially designed catheter systems. Tubal cannulation is performed now under fluoroscopic, hysteroscopic, and ultrasonographic guidance with ureteral catheters, balloon angiographic catheters, guide wires, and coaxial systems.[114] In one of the largest series utilizing fluoroscopy, 124 of 154 fallopian tubes in 77 patients were reported to be successfully cannulated using a balloon angiocatheter through a coaxial system.[115] The success rate of fluoroscopic transcervical tubal cannulation has been reported at 79 percent with a 5 percent perforation rate.[114] After an average follow-up of 6 mo, the pregnancy rate was 34 percent, comparable with microsurgical anastomosis after cornual resection (40 percent after 12 mo).[116] The drawback of fluoroscopically guided transcervical tubal cannulation is that additional anatomic abnormalities such as adhesions and endometriosis cannot be diagnosed and treated at that time. The procedure can be performed on an outpatient basis without general anesthesia.

Tubal cannulation using hysteroscopy can be performed under laparoscopic guidance. At that time procedures such as adhesiolysis or vaporization of endometriosis foci can also be accomplished. Several studies have demonstrated excellent results with up to 92 percent successful cannulation rate and 81 percent tubal patency on following hysterosalpingograms.[114] The perforation rate was 11 percent and the pregnancy rate 39 percent after 3 to 7 mo follow-up. Term pregnancy rate after microsurgical repair of pathologic uterotubal junction obstructions was 28 percent.[116]

With ultrasonographic guidance, the successful cannulation rate was 87 percent. Sixty-seven percent of fallopian tubes cannulated remained patent, and 29 percent of those patients achieved pregnancy in less than 6 mo.[117,118]

Transcervical tubal cannulation and tuboplasty procedures may also be helpful in the management of SIN. Although a successful guidewire cannulation and balloon tuboplasty has been reported in a case of isthmic stricture secondary to SIN,[84] the most widely accepted recommendation for SIN is the resection of the affected segment and anastomosis of the remaining parts of the fallopian tube in order to yield a better pregnancy rate without ectopic pregnancy occurrence.[42,105,119]

Tubal cannulation techniques are under investigation for use during insemination, gamete and embryo transfers, and evaluation of intratubal milieu.[120–123]

General Considerations

Laparoscopy Versus Laparotomy. Microsurgery was introduced into gynecology primarily to improve the outcome of infertility surgery.[104,124,125] When compared with conventional surgery, the use of microsurgery resulted in the doubling of the success rates associated with salpingostomy, correction of pathologic cornual occlusion, and tubotubal anastomosis.

Laparoscopic access yields several important advantages when a laparotomy is avoided, provided the specific procedure undertaken is completed successfully. Elimination of a laparotomy incision results in less postoperative discomfort, reduced requirements for postoperative analgesia, a shorter convalescence, and quicker return to normal activity.[126] However, the perception that the laparoscopic approach results in less postoperative adhesion formation[127,128] is debatable, because a given peritoneal trauma should produce the same degree of inflammatory response irrespective of the mode of access, as demonstrated in an experimental animal model.[129]

The limitations of operative laparoscopy in performing certain precise procedures have forced surgeons to incorporate microsurgical principles in laparoscopic interventions so that the advantages of minimal access are not negated by the occurrence of greater tissue trauma. The length of the instruments and the cannula in the abdominal wall, acting as a fulcrum, may cause an increase in the force applied to tissue by the working end of the instruments, and this may generate undue trauma.[125] Nevertheless, operating within a closed peritoneal cavity as in laparoscopy largely prevents desiccation of the peritoneal surfaces, eliminating the need to use packs, and prevents the introduction of foreign materials such as talcum powder. The laparoscope provides a degree of magnification and an excellent visibility by bringing the distal end of the laparoscope close to the area of interest. It is possible to carry out intraoperative irrigation of tissues to keep them moistened and expose any bleeding vessels. Furthermore, the pressure effect of the pneumoperitoneum diminishes venous oozing and permits spontaneous coagulation of minor bleeders. However, there are some limitations to the laparoscopic approach. Laparoscopic suturing is awkward and more time consuming. The use of fine sutures is difficult, which frequently leads to the use of larger material and the application of fewer sutures. Hand–eye coordination is somewhat limited by the lack of stereoscopic vision. Many of these limitations are simply technical problems that undoubtedly will be overcome.[125]

The efficacy and safety of the laparoscopic approach was first shown with procedures designed to correct distal tubal occlusion. The results obtained by laparoscopic salpingo-ovariolysis and fimbrioplasty were similar to those by microsurgical techniques, with intrauterine pregnancy rates nearly 60 and 50 percent, respectively.[104–126] However, laparoscopy was assessed to be not appropriate for tubal anastomosis.[130] The laparoscopic approach has also been proven to be effective and safe in the surgical treatment of tubal ectopic pregnancy. In a study of 216 consecutive tubal pregnancies, the operating time and the amount of postoperative analgesia were found to be significantly less with patients treated by laparoscopy compared with those treated by laparotomy.

There was no difference in the rate of postoperative morbidity and the subsequent fertility outcomes between the two routes.[131,132] Other studies have confirmed these findings and also demonstrated a savings of health care costs of approximately $1,500 per patient.[133] However, retained trophoblastic tissue incidence was higher during laparoscopic procedures.[134–136] In addition, the patients usually returned to full activity within 1 wk of the surgery.

In conclusion, the approach that will yield the best outcome for the patient should be sought and selected. Peritoneal trauma will produce the same degree of inflammatory response irrespective of the mode of access; thus, it is essential to incorporate microsurgical principles to the performance of reproductive procedures to reduce postoperative complications and adhesions and preserve the woman's reproductive potential.

Tubal Surgery Versus Assisted Reproduction. The development of operative laparoscopy, microsurgery, and IVF in the last 20 years improved the outlook for couples suffering from tubal infertility. The goal for any infertile couple should be either a live birth or the ability to feel that they have exhausted all reasonable attempts to achieve a pregnancy.[137] Compared with tubal surgery, which has postoperative monthly conception rates of 2 to 4 percent, IVF offers a conception rate close to that seen in the general fertile population (see Chap 33).[138] The most recent data on the outcome of 31,900 IVF cycles have revealed a monthly conception rate of 19.8 percent and an ectopic pregnancy rate of 4.6 percent (see Chap 33).[139]

The relative risk of having an ectopic pregnancy dramatically increases with tubal surgery or with the disorders that lead to tubal surgery. In one study, the relative risk for ectopic pregnancy after tubal surgery was 4.5 and in the presence of pelvic adhesions, 5.6.[140] Moreover, in order to decrease the risk for ectopic pregnancy during an IVF procedure, surgical occlusion of the tube proximally or salpingectomy have been suggested prior to IVF cycles.[141] One group of investigators computed that the cost per live birth was $17,000 after tubal surgery compared with $12,000 after IVF.[142] However, a drawback of IVF is the 20 percent multiple gestation rate with its medical, emotional, and economic consequences.[143]

Another important issue is that the implantation, pregnancy, and live-birth rates are approximately halved in cases with hydrosalpinx, most likely due to hydrosalpinx fluid yielding poor endometrial receptivity.[144,145] For those cases, salpingectomy is recommended prior to IVF procedure. In a recent review on the subject, it is proposed that if there is a small or moderate-sized hydrosalpinx without a history of hydrorrhea or fluid distention of the uterine cavity, a single IVF cycle should be performed as a primary therapy.[146] If the hydrosalpinx is large and if there are subjective or objective signs of fluid leakage to the uterine cavity, the patient should have laparoscopy. Thereafter, reconstructive surgery may be attempted during the surgical procedure. However, in the majority of patients, salpingectomy is indicated and should be performed.[146]

Based on what has been published to date, it appears that, in a young patient, surgery is the first choice for proximal tubal occlusion without severe adhesions or for a distal tubal damage provided that mucosal folds can be detected easily by HSG. For patients with severe disease accompanied by extensive pelvic adhesions, IVF should be the primary approach.[137,147,148] In vitro fertilization clearly represents the only therapeutic option for those with inoperable tubes, with tuberculous salpingitis or bipolar disease (proximal and distal disease simultaneously); in the case of absence of the fallopian tubes; and in the presence of additional factors such as severe male infertility. In older patients, because of the rapid decline of fertility potential with advancing age, therapeutic choice shifts towards the IVF side of the spectrum rather than surgical techniques that would probably cause a delay in achieving pregnancy.

Adhesion Prevention. Postoperative adhesions develop after the majority of gynecologic surgical procedures, with incidences after laparotomy of 55 to 100 percent and after laparoscopy of 97 percent.[149] For many years, the hypothesis has been formulated that normal peritoneal fibrinolytic activity prevents the formation of adhesions by lysis of any fibrin deposits within the first days. Following trauma or insult to the peritoneal surface (surgical, infectious, inflammatory), increased vessel permeability and histamine release from disrupted stromal mast cells produce a transudative cell layer (Fig 31–3).[150] Within hours, this layer is infiltrated with a variety of inflammatory mediators including histiocytes, monocytes, plasma cells, neutrophils, and platelets. A fibrin matrix is formed that covers the area of insult until the plasma mediated fibrinolytic pathway acts to degrade it. In the absence of fibrinolysis, the fibrin matrix persists and accumulates, and as it is invaded by proliferating fibroblasts, vascularization and cellular growth result in the formation of adhesive bridges between peritoneal surfaces. Recent studies have shown that human peritoneum possesses plasminogen activator activity that acts to prevent deposition of intra-abdominal fibrin and its subsequent organizations into fibrous adhesions. In inflammatory conditions, the production of plasminogen activator inhibitors by mesothelial cells, macrophages, and endothelial cells is stimulated by different cytokines (TNF, IL-2, IL-6), leading to a depression of the plasminogen activator activity. The prolonged depression of peritoneal fibrinolysis allows deposition and organization of fibrin deposits and formation of permanent fibrous adhesions.

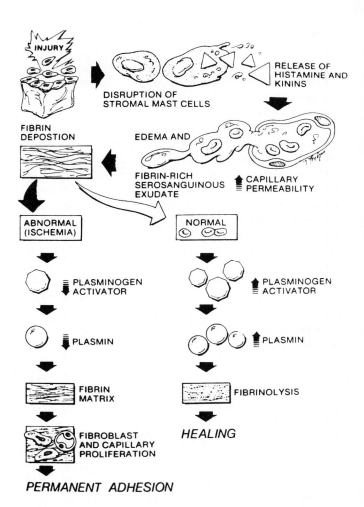

Figure 31–3. Pathophysiology of adhesion formation. *(Reproduced, with permission, from Buttram VC, Reiter RC.* Surgical Treatment of the Infertile Female. *Baltimore, Md., Williams and Wilkins, 1985)*

Adhesions may cause infertility, pelvic pain, ectopic pregnancy, and sometimes bowel obstruction. The most frequent causes of pelvic adhesions are infection, endometriosis, surgery, foreign body, and sometimes neoplasia and radiation. Postoperative adhesions occur primarily at the site of the operative procedure. Tuboperitoneal adhesions caused by PID result in tubal immobilization, obstructive (phimosis), occlusive (hydrosalpinx) lesions, and consequently infertility. Tubal mucosal adhesions are caused by PID, tuberculosis, ectopic pregnancy, and tubal surgery. Postinflammatory periadnexal adhesions and hydrosalpinges are associated with tubal mucosal adhesions in 25 to 65 percent of cases. The risk of ectopic pregnancy in PID is significantly related to the presence of tubal mucosal adhesions. Tubal mucosal adhesions in the absence of periadnexal adhesions are rare (except for genital tuberculosis). The pregnancy outcome in PID and after ectopic pregnancy is more dependent on tubal mucosal than periadnexal adhesions.

Techniques of preventing or reducing adhesions include prevention or decrease of the initial peritoneal injury, prevention of the coagulation of serous exudate, removal of fibrin, keeping apart the fibrin-coated peritoneal surfaces until peritonealization has occurred, and inhibition of the fibroblastic proliferation, once established. Traditionally, various combinations of anti-inflammatory and antifibrinoblastic agents have been used perioperatively. Nonsteroidal anti-inflammatory agents such as ibuprofen, glucocorticoids, and antihistamines were all used to retard the formation and propagation of the initial inflammatory exudate. However, the efficacy of any of those agents has not been proven.[151]

Surface separation (barriers) is the method of choice for the majority of products available today. They reduce adhesion by preventing the formation of fibrin bridges between healing tissues[152] and can be classified as liquid and solid forms.

Liquid Barriers

CRYSTALLOID SOLUTIONS. The most commonly used agent for adhesion prevention is a crystalloid solution such as Ringer's lactate, or phosphate-buffered or normal saline. Absorption of water and electrolytes from the peritoneal cavity is rapid, with up to 500 ml of normal saline being absorbed in less than 18 hr (30 to 37 ml/hr).[153] Because it takes 5 to 8 days for peritoneal surface to reperitonealize after surgery,[154] crystalloids would be absorbed well before the process of fibrin deposition and adhesion formation is completed. Thus, intraperitoneal crystalloids would not be expected to prevent adhesion formation. Clinical studies with crystalloids have revealed 80 to 85 percent failure rates in adhesion prevention.[155,156]

DEXTRAN. Dextran is a water-soluble glucose polymer. In adhesion prevention studies, a 32 percent dextran 70 (Hyskon) solution has been tried, yielding very controversial results. Its beneficial effect was limited and gravity dependent.[157–159] It also has a lot of side effects such as ascites, weight gain, vulvar edema, pleural effusion, and sometimes coagulopathy.

Solid Barriers

INTERCEED (TC7). Interceed is composed of an oxidized regenerated cellulose that has been woven in a special pattern. Once applied to peritoneal surfaces, it adheres without suturing and forms a gel within 2 to 8 hr. Within 20 hr of application, it forms a barrier potentially separating two opposing surfaces. After re-epithelization it undergoes absorption. In various studies including tubal surgery, more than 50 to 60 percent of cases were found to be adhesion free at second look laparoscopy.[160,161] During salpingostomy for ectopic pregnancy, fimbriolysis or adhesiolysis, following hemostasis using pitressin, Interceed is wrapped over the tube. For successful results, it should be applied at the end of the surgical procedure following a complete hemostasis. All irrigation fluid and instillates from the peritoneal cavity should be removed when the patient is put in the reverse Trendelenburg position. It should be applied as large as possible, enough to cover the area and even overlap the margins by 3 to 5 mm. No sutures are needed, and it should be moistened with 2 ml saline per 3 × 4 inches.

PRECLUDE. Preclude (Gore-Tex Surgical Membrane) is a thin, fabric-like polytetrafluoroethylene sheet. It is non-inflammatory, nonabsorbable, and has to be sutured or stapled in place. Although it is recommended to remove the membrane in a second surgical procedure, many surgeons prefer to leave it in its place forever. Second look laparoscopies revealed marked reduction in adhesion formation with both barriers in randomized studies.[162] *Seprafilm Bioresorbable Membrane*, also an adhesion prevention barrier composed of chemically derivatized sodium hyaluronate and carboxymethylcellulose, is now available commercially.

Although those surface barriers were shown to be safe and effective in human clinical studies, their usage did not eliminate adhesions in all patients. It is important to emphasize that the use of those agents is not a substitute for the surgeon's strict attention to the surgical techniques employed.

ECTOPIC PREGNANCY

A pregnancy in which a fertilized ovum implants outside the endometrial lining of the uterus is defined as ectopic pregnancy. Almost all ectopic pregnancies are located in the fallopian tube: 80 percent in the ampullary segment, 12 percent in the isthmic segment, 5 percent around the fimbrial end, and 2 percent on cornual and interstitial sites.[163] Although relatively uncommon, ectopic pregnancies in nontubal sites such as abdominal (1.4 percent), ovarian (0.2 percent), and cervical (0.2 percent) pregnancies are susceptible to major complications such as hemorrhage and have greater mortality rates.[164] There are two forms of abdominal pregnancy; in *primary abdominal pregnancy* the first and only implantation site should be the peritoneal surface with no evidence of recent or remote injury to tubes and ovaries and absence of uteroplacental fistula. In *secondary abdominal pregnancy*, the conceptus implants originally near the tubal ostia, aborting subsequently, and reimplants onto a peritoneal surface. A cervical pregnancy occurs when the developing conceptus implants in the cervical canal, at or below the internal os. *Ligamentous pregnancy* is a secondary form of ectopic pregnancy in which a primary tubal pregnancy, abrading the tube, finds its way into the mesosalpinx between the leaves of the broad ligament. *Heterotopic pregnancy* exists when both intrauterine and extrauterine implantation occur simultaneously. There are also reported cases in which both fallopian tubes carry extrauterine gestations at the same time.[165]

Incidence

There was nearly a fourfold increase in the number of ectopic pregnancies in the United States between 1970 and 1989, from 17,800 to 88,400 ectopic pregnancies with rates from 4.5 to 16.8 per 1000 reported pregnancies. However, at the same time the mortality rate decreased from 35.5 to 3.8 per 10,000 ectopic pregnancies, a decrease of 90 percent, but still remaining as the second leading cause of maternal mortality (12 percent of all maternal deaths).[166–168] The highest rate occurs in women aged 35 to 44 yr, and the risk of ectopic pregnancy among African-Americans and other minorities is 1.6 times greater than the risk among Caucasians. It is also recently suggested that the rates of ectopic pregnancy are lower in the spring and summer than in autumn and winter.[169] One of the major variations in the demographic data of ectopic pregnancy lies in *heterotopic pregnancy*. Natural heterotopic pregnancy, a relatively rare condition with an incidence of 1/30,000 pregnancies, has nowadays dramatically increased with treatments for ovulation induction or superovulation for assisted reproductive technologies (ART), reaching an incidence of 1/100 pregnancies among ART-treated women.[170]

Etiology and Risk Factors

A recent meta-analysis has revealed that risk of ectopic pregnancy is strongly correlated with previous ectopic pregnancy, tubal surgery, documented tubal pathology, and in utero diethylstilbestrol (DES) exposure.[171] Previous genital infections (PID, chlamydia, gonorrhea), infertility, and a lifetime number of sexual partners exceeding 1, are associated with a mildly increased risk. Previous pelvic and/or abdominal surgery, smoking, vaginal douching, and an early age for first sexual intercourse are associated with a slightly increased risk.

Pelvic Infection. The incidence of tubal obstruction increases with successive episodes of PID: 13 percent after the first, 35 percent after the second, and 75 percent after the third episode.[172,173] After the first episode of PID, a woman has a four- to sixfold increase in ectopic pregnancy incidence. Salpingitis damages the endosalpinx, resulting in agglutination of the mucosal folds and subsequent adhesion formation. Circulating chlamydial antibodies, especially with titers greater than 1/64, were reported to be responsible for a greater than twofold increased risk of ectopic pregnancy.[174] A slighter increased risk was found in association with vaginal douching.

Prior Tubal/Abdominal Surgery. A greater than fourfold increased risk of ectopic pregnancy is associated with tubal surgery such as salpingostomy, neosalpingostomy, fimbrioplasty, and anastomosis, leading to an overall ectopic pregnancy rate of 2 to 7 percent and an intrauterine pregnancy rate of 50 percent.[89] An abdominal surgery, irrelevant to the tubes or without a rupture of the appendix, does not increase the ectopic pregnancy rate.[175] Radical or conservative surgery after tubal ectopic pregnancy does not significantly change intrauterine (40 percent) and extrauterine pregnancy rates (12 percent). Preservation of the tubes improves overall total pregnancy rates while not altering the incidence of repeat ectopic pregnancy.[176] The status of the contralateral tube affects the incidence of ectopic pregnancy which is 7 percent with a normal, 18 percent with a damaged, and 25 percent with an absent contralateral tube.[177]

The greatest risk for poststerilization ectopic pregnancy exists during the first 2 yr rather than immediately after the procedure, varying between 5 and 16 percent depending on the technique.[178,179] The overall ectopic risk in women with sterilization is 80 percent less than that in nonsterilized women; however, the relative risk is 3.7 times that of women using oral contraception and 2.8 times that of women utilizing barrier methods.[179] Sterilization reversal after electrocauterization carries a 15 percent risk of ectopic pregnancy, which is much more than the 3 percent risk after Pomeroy or Fallope ring procedures.[111,180]

Method of Contraception. Women who conceive with an intrauterine device (IUD) have a chance of ectopic pregnancy 0.4 to 0.8 times than that of women not using contraception. However, because IUDs prevent implantation more effectively in the uterus than in the tube, a woman conceiving with an IUD in place has a six- to tenfold greater chance of having a tubal pregnancy in comparison to one using no contraception.[181,182] With progesterone IUDs, 17 percent, and with copper IUDs, 4 percent of contraceptive failures end in tubal pregnancy.[183] According to a WHO study, the ectopic pregnancy risk of progesterone IUD is nearly 30 times greater in comparison to the copper-T IUD or Norplant system.[181] Progesterone-only contraceptives such as the mini-pill and Norplant system protect against both intrauterine and extrauterine pregnancy when compared with no contraception, but if a pregnancy occurs, the chance of its being ectopic is 4 to 10 percent for the mini-pill[184] and 30 percent for Norplant system.[185]

Infertility and Assisted Reproductive Technology.

Although the incidence of ectopic pregnancy increases with increasing age and parity, there is also a 2.6-fold increased risk for a nulliparous woman with unexplained infertility.[140] A case control study has concluded that the risk of ectopic pregnancy was increased fourfold with ovulation induction but not further increased when ovulation induction was used for IVF, indicating that the multiple eggs and high hormone levels are the responsible factors.[186,187] The first pregnancy obtained with IVF was a tubal pregnancy.[188] About 2 to 8 percent of IVF conceptions are ectopic pregnancies and tubal factor infertility is associated with a further increased risk of 17 percent.[189,190]

Diethylstilbestrol.

Women exposed to diethylstilbestrol (DES) in utero are more than twice as likely to have a tubal pregnancy; 50 percent of these women have uterine cavity abnormalities.[191,192]

Salpingitis Isthmica Nodosa.

Salpingitis isthmica nodosa (SIN), a noninfectious pathologic condition of the fallopian tubes in which the tubal epithelium extends into the myosalpinx and forms a true diverticulum, was found to be more common among women with tubal pregnancies.[42,193]

Smoking.

Current cigarette smokers have an increased risk of ectopic pregnancy (2.5-fold for 20 cigarettes a day, 1.3-fold for less) compared to nonsmokers. Nicotine is thought to have direct adverse effects on ciliar activity, tubal motility, and blastocyst implantation.[194,195]

Diagnosis

Signs and Symptoms.

Only 14 percent of women who present with the classical clinical triad of abdominal pain, irregular uterine bleeding, and an adnexal mass on physical examination are found to have an ectopic pregnancy. Only half of the women with an ectopic pregnancy have pain, amenorrhea, and irregular vaginal bleeding.[196] The menstrual shedding may be followed by a period of amenorrhea lasting 3 to 10 wk, after which the clinical symptoms of ectopic pregnancy typically become manifest. Abdominal pain, the most common symptom (91 percent), can develop before tubal rupture with varying characteristics. It may be focal or diffuse, unilateral or bilateral, and dull, sharp, or crampy. An adnexal mass may be palpable in up to 38 to 50 percent of cases, and cervi-

cal tenderness may or may not be present. With tubal rupture there may be a transient relief of the pain. Hemoperitoneum will cause shoulder, back pain, and abdominal rebound tenderness due to peritoneal irritation, and at this stage cervical tenderness is usually present. Orthostatic hypotension, tachycardia, and the development of syncope reflect the degree of cardiovascular compromise caused by the hemoperitoneum.

Laboratory Evaluation

Serum Quantitative Human Chorionic Gonadotropin.

HCG is secreted by the syncytiotrophoblasts and reaches a maximal level of 50,000 to 100,000 mIU/ml at 8 to 12 wk of gestation. It can be detected in maternal serum as early as the day after blastocyst implantation. There are three hCG reference standards defined up to now. At the moment, the standard that is used most commonly is the IRP (International Reference Preparation), and it is equal to 0.58 mIU of hCG of the Second International Standard (2nd IS).[197]

Serum hCG concentrations increase exponentially for the first 38 days after ovulation. During the first postovulatory 14 to 17 days, the time required for the doubling of hCG remains constant, with a mean of 1.9 days.[198] It is reported that 85 percent of women with ectopic pregnancies and 15 percent of women with intrauterine pregnancies could expect to have hCG doubling times of greater than 2.7 days when hCG concentrations are below the levels of 6,000 mIU/ml (IRP).[199] Thus, a 66 percent increase in hCG levels over 48 hr represents the lower limit of normal values for viable intrauterine pregnancies, with a 85 percent confidence limit.[200] This means that approximately 15 percent of patients with viable intrauterine pregnancies will have an increase of less than 66 percent, whereas 15 percent of patients with extrauterine pregnancies will have an increase of more than 66 percent in hCG levels over 48 hr. Kadar and Romero have further studied falling hCG values and have concluded that a slow fall with a half-life greater than 7 days is likely to represent an ectopic pregnancy, whereas a rapid fall with a half-life of less than 1.4 days is rarely associated with an ectopic pregnancy.[201] As a general rule, a completed abortion will have a rapidly falling hCG level (50 percent over 48 hr) whereas levels of an ectopic pregnancy will rise or plateau. A *single* hCG measurement has limited use because of considerable overlap between values from normal and abnormal pregnancies. It may be useful only when it is negative and thus excludes the diagnosis of ectopic pregnancy. It is also reported that hCG levels do not correlate with the ectopic site.[202] Recently, β-hCG core fragment concentrations in the urine of patients with ectopic pregnancies were found to be significantly reduced in comparison to normal intrauterine pregnancies.[203]

Serum Progesterone. Serum progesterone levels in patients with ectopic pregnancies are lower than those with normal intrauterine pregnancies. Over 70 percent of patients with a viable intrauterine pregnancy have serum progesterone levels >25 ng/ml (79.5 nmol/L), whereas only 4 percent of patients having abnormal intrauterine pregnancies and 1.5 percent of patients with ectopic pregnancies have serum progesterone levels higher than this level.[196,204,205] A serum progesterone level <5.0 ng/ml is highly suggestive of an abnormal pregnancy. The risk of terminating a viable intrauterine pregnancy with a serum progesterone level <5.0 ng/ml is 1/1500.[206] It has been recently recommended that patients with serum progesterone values >17.5 ng/ml (55.7 nmol/L) could be followed without further diagnostic study because only 8.3 percent of ectopic pregnancies will be above this value.[207] No viable pregnancies occur with a progesterone level less than 2.5 ng/ml, and only 0.16 percent viable pregnancies occur with a level <5.0 ng/ml (15.9 nmol/L), making a diagnostic curettage safer below this level. With the help of these cut-off values it is possible to differentiate between viable and nonviable pregnancies, but it is hard to differentiate between nonviable intrauterine and extrauterine pregnancies.[207] However, it should be remembered that these limits are for spontaneous ovulations with a single corpus luteum, and will be useless in ovulation induction cases with multiple corpora lutea. In conclusion, the value of a single serum progesterone value is to help in making a decision regarding the viability of a possible intrauterine pregnancy prior to curettage. The vast majority of progesterone values are inconclusive, because they fall in the indeterminate region between 5 and 25 ng/ml.

Serum Estradiol. Measurement of serum estradiol may help in the differentiation of ectopic pregnancy from threatened abortion and normal intrauterine pregnancy. Patients with ectopic pregnancies were found to have a significantly lower estradiol level in comparison to normal pregnancies and threatened abortions.[208] Only 1 of 100 patients with ectopic pregnancies had a serum estradiol level above 650 pg/ml, whereas only 1 of 105 patients with intrauterine pregnancies had a level less than that.

Other Endocrinologic and Protein Markers. Maternal serum *creatine kinase* levels were found to be significantly higher in all patients with tubal pregnancy in comparison to patients who had missed abortions or normal intrauterine pregnancies.[209] But recent studies have concluded that concentrations of creatine kinase are not sufficiently discriminative to be of clinical value in the diagnosis of ectopic pregnancy.[210–213] *Relaxin*, a protein hormone produced by the corpus luteum of pregnancy, peaking at 10 wk of gestation, is reported to have decreased levels in ectopic pregnancies and spontaneous abortions in comparison to intrauterine pregnancies.[214]

Recently, serum levels of *placental protein 14* have been reported to be lower than the fifth percentile and to be useful in distinguishing spontaneous abortions from ectopic pregnancies.[215] However, the clinical utility of those markers in diagnosing ectopic pregnancy has not yet been determined.

Ultrasonography. Transvaginal ultrasonography is superior to transabdominal ultrasonography in evaluating pelvic structures. The diagnosis of an intrauterine pregnancy can be made 1 wk earlier with transvaginal than with transabdominal ultrasonography. The various signs of ectopic pregnancy—such as detection of adnexal mass, an empty uterine cavity, and free peritoneal fluid in cul-de-sac—are more reliably and efficiently established with the transvaginal route.[216–218] Vaginal sonography allows excellent visualization of the uterine cavity with two separate endometrial layers. A gestational sac at 33 days after the last menstrual period can be demonstrated as a fluid collection of 1 to 3 mm in diameter located on either side of the endometrium, eccentrically, with respect to the cavity. The sac has an echogenic contour caused by trophoblast invasion into the decidualized endometrium.[219] Some features of a true intrauterine sac are important for the differential diagnosis; a *pseudogestational sac* can be observed in 10 to 20 percent of ectopic pregnancies. Due to intracavitary fluid collection, the pseudosac is usually located centrally, between the two endometrial layers, in contrast to the eccentrically located real gestational sac. The pseudogestational sac is composed of a single decidual layer surrounded by a fluid collection whereas the early gestational sac is encircled by a double layer consisting of the chorionic membrane and decidua parietalis (double ring sign).[219,220]

If no uterine sac is seen or the detected sac is considered to be a pseudogestational sac, thereafter adnexal structures should be carefully examined.[217] A tubal ring is defined as a 1- to 3-cm rounded extraovarian structure consisting of a 2- to 4-mm concentric ring of echogenic tissue surrounding a hypoechogenic center. This is detected in 46 to 71 percent of tubal pregnancy cases if the tube is unruptured, because in case of rupture, bleeding around the sac results in the appearance of nonspecific adnexal mass.[221] The demonstration of adnexal gestational sac with a fetal pole and cardiac activity is the most specific but least sensitive sign of ectopic pregnancy, occurring in only 10 to 17 percent of cases.[221,222] The corpus luteum, which is more eccentrically located within the ovary, should be considered in the differential diagnosis. A thin-walled ovarian follicle, small intestine, and fluid containing structures such as hydrosalpinx should be remembered during differential diagnosis.[217] A hemorrhagic corpus luteum cyst could be differentiated with its hypoechogenic central region.[218] The presence of moderate to large amounts of intraperitoneal fluid is known to correlate with ectopic pregnancy; an echogenic fluid in particular will indicate hemoperitoneum, which may be the only sonographic finding in 15 percent of patients with early unruptured ectopic pregnancies. Free fluid the in cul-de-sac can be detected in both intrauterine (up to 20 percent) and ectopic pregnancies (40 to 83 percent of all cases.).[221]

Human chorionic gonadotropin titer above which a gestational sac can be demonstrated with ultrasonography is defined as *the discriminatory zone*. Previously, with abdominal sonography this was 6,000 to 6,500 mIU/ml (IRP).[199] The absence of an intrauterine sac above this level was associated with ectopic gestations in 87 percent of cases. Normal intrauterine pregnancies exceeding this level could be visualized by the help of transabdominal sonography with a 94 percent sensitivity. However, fewer than 40 percent of suspected ectopic pregnancies present with an hCG concentration above 6,500 mIU/ml.[199] Fortunately, with the advent of vaginal sonography, an intrauterine gestational sac can be visualized as early as 33 to 35 days from the last menstrual period, at which time the hCG level is approximately 1,400 mIU/ml (Table 31–4).[223] Others have reported this discriminatory zone for the vaginal sonography to vary between 1,000 and 2,004 mIU/ml.[224–228] It should be kept in mind that the discriminatory zone in a multiple pregnancy will be a little higher, requiring an extra 2 to 3 days for a gestational sac to become visible. Also, it should be remembered that demonstration of a viable intrauterine pregnancy does not absolutely exclude the possibility of a heterotopic ectopic pregnancy.

Color and pulsed Doppler increases the sensitivity of vaginal ultrasonography. A Doppler analysis in the first trimester shows a high-resistance, low-velocity pattern in the uterine arteries and a high-velocity, low-resistance signal at placental site.[229–231] The pattern, seen near the endometrium, is associated with normal and abnormal intrauterine pregnancies and is designated the peritrophoblastic flow. The use of Doppler techniques allows detection of intrauterine pregnancies at an earlier stage when compared to plain vaginal sonography, which requires detection of a well-developed gestational sac and sometimes cardiac activity for the diagnosis of intrauterine pregnancies. Doppler technique is also helpful in dif-

ferentiating pseudogestational and double decidual sacs.[232] A high-velocity, low-resistance flow around the adnexal region characterizes ectopic pregnancies. The addition of Doppler techniques to vaginal sonography improves the diagnostic sensitivity for ectopic pregnancies from 71 to 87 percent, for nonviable intrauterine pregnancies from 24 to 59 percent, and for normal intrauterine pregnancies from 90 to 99 percent.[224,232,233]

Dilatation and Curettage. Uterine curettage should be performed after assuring of a nonviable pregnancy on the basis of plateauing hCG and a serum progesterone value below 5 ng/ml.[234] Once the tissue is obtained, it can be added to saline, in which it will float. Floating tissue corresponds to chorionic villi, indicating a spontaneous abortion. Because the floating technique is not 100 percent accurate, a rapid frozen section will be valuable in differentiating the tissue.[235] If a frozen section is not available, serum hCG levels should be obtained. The absence of floating tissue that corresponds only to decidua but not villi, and a decrease greater than 15 percent in the levels of hCG 8 to 12 hr after curettage, will imply the diagnosis of complete abortion. Otherwise, with rising or plateauing hCG levels, the diagnosis will be ectopic pregnancy.[234]

Culdocentesis. Culdocentesis has traditionally been used as an important tool in the evaluation of ectopic pregnancy. If nonclotting blood is obtained via aspiration, the test is considered to be positive if the hematocrit of the obtained fluid is greater than 15 percent. If the hematocrit is less than 15 percent or the aspirate is clotted, the test is negative. The procedure is nondiagnostic if no fluid is obtained. The results of culdocentesis do not always correlate with the status of conception. Although 70 to 90 percent of patients with an ectopic pregnancy have a hemoperitoneum demonstrated with culdocentesis, only 50 percent have a ruptured tube.[236] Moreover, approximately 6 percent of patients with positive culdocentesis do not have an ectopic gestation but a hemorrhagic corpus luteum at the time of laparotomy. Therefore, a positive culdocentesis is of little value in deciding whether to treat medically or surgically. At the moment, with the use of quantitative hCG testing and transvaginal ultrasonography, culdocentesis is rarely indicated.

Laparoscopy. Laparoscopy is considered to be the gold standard for the diagnosis of ectopic pregnancy. It allows not only a thorough and direct visualization of the entire pelvis but also helps in carrying out definitive surgical procedures for the treatment of ectopic pregnancy. Even if an ectopic pregnancy is not found at laparoscopy, other pathologic conditions such as adnexal torsion, a corpus luteum cyst, or a pedunculated myoma may be diagnosed and treated. A 3 to 4 percent misdiagnosis rate is mostly due to very early ectopic pregnancies.

TABLE 31–4. TRANSVAGINAL ULTRASONOGRAPHIC FINDINGS IN RELATION TO hCG VALUES

TV-USG Findings	Days From LMP	hCG (mIU/ml) (IRP)
Sac	34.8 ± 2.2	1,398 ± 155
Fetal pole	40.3 ± 3.4	5,113 ± 298
Fetal heart motion	46.9 ± 6.0	17,208 ± 3,772

TV-USG, transvaginal ultrasonography; LMP, last menstrual period; hCG, human chorionic gonadotropin; IRP, International Reference Preparation. *(Reproduced, with permission, from Fossum GT, Davajan V, Kletsky OA. Early detection of pregnancy with transvaginal ultrasound. Fertil Steril. 49:788, 1988.)*

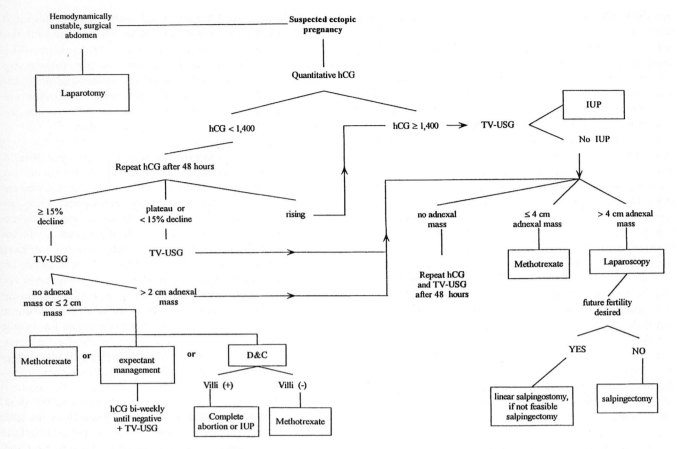

Figure 31–4. Management of ectopic pregnancy. (TV-USG, transvaginal ultrasonography; hCG, human chorionic gonadotropin, mIU/ml in IRP.)

Selective Salpingography. Another new diagnostic approach could be selective salpingography. In patients with equivocal clinical, laboratory, and ultrasonographic findings, selective salpingography may be used in the diagnosis and even in the treatment of an early ectopic pregnancy with methotrexate. Seven ectopic pregnancies were recently detected and successfully treated with local methotrexate injection in 10 patients.[237]

An algorithm useful in the diagnosis and management of ectopic pregnancy is summarized in Figure 31–4.

Treatment

Expectant Management. Approximately one fourth of patients presenting with ectopic pregnancy can be managed expectantly. Garcia et al expectantly followed 13 patients with tubal pregnancies less than 4 cm diameter diagnosed by laparoscopy and reported no ruptures.[238] Human chorionic gonadotropin titers of all patients returned to normal levels within 5 wk of laparoscopy. Seven of ten patients had bilateral tubal patency, verified by a hysterosalpingography 3 mo later.

For the expectant management of a definite tubal pregnancy, an ectopic mass less than 2 cm, a falling hCG with an initial titer less than 1000 mIU/ml, no evidence of rupture or bleeding, and a cul-de-sac fluid less than 100 ml are important criteria established by various studies.[239–243] The summary of these studies resulted in an overall 73 percent success and 82 percent tubal patency rate. An initial hCG titer less than 1,000 mIU/ml is the best independent predictor of spontaneous resolution of an ectopic pregnancy.[241,243] A low and rapidly decreasing hCG level with repeated vaginal sonographies is the accepted hallmark in the expected management of ectopic pregnancy.[239,240] Korhonen et al found the success rate for a spontaneous resolution to be 88 percent when the initial hCG level was less than 200 mIU/ml, but only 25 percent at levels higher than 2,000 mIU/ml.[240] Transvaginal sonography appears useful in recognizing the ectopic pregnancies most likely to resolve spontaneously without complication. A decrease in adnexal mass size on the seventh day has a sensitivity of 84 percent and specificity of 100 percent.[244]

Medical Treatment. Medical treatment for unruptured tubal pregnancies has several advantages such as lower cost, less tubal damage, less adhesion, and increased future fertility. Although methotrexate is the most frequently used agent in the medical management of ectopic pregnancy, other agents such as potassium chloride (KCl), hyperosmolar glucose, prostaglandins, and RU-486 have also been studied.

Methotrexate, a folic acid antagonist, inhibits de novo synthesis of purines and pyrimidines (by inhibiting dihydrofolate reductase, an enzyme that converts dihydrofolic acid to tetrahydrofolic acid), thus interfering with DNA synthesis and cell proliferation. Actively proliferating trophoblasts are vulnerable to methotrexate, and it has been used extensively for the treatment of gestational trophoblastic disease. Uncommonly reported side effects are leukopenia, thrombocytopenia, bone marrow aplasia, ulcerative stomatitis, enteritis, alopecia, dermatitis, pneumonitis, and elevated liver enzymes.[245] Methotrexate, when used with *citrovorum factor* (folinic acid), has been reported to cause no increase in congenital malformations, spontaneous abortions, or secondary tumors after administration.[246,247] Methotrexate was first used to treat an isthmic ectopic pregnancy in Japan.[248] In 1986, Ory et al treated successfully 6 patients with laparoscopically proven unruptured ampullary ectopic pregnancies less than 4 cm in diameter, with four intravenous doses of methotrexate (1 mg/kg) alternating with 4 doses of citrovorum factor (0.1 mg/kg) every other day.[249]

Stovall et al were the first to establish an outpatient methotrexate treatment protocol for laparoscopically confirmed ectopic pregnancies.[250] This protocol, now known as the *multiple-dose systemic methotrexate protocol*, has been shown to be 95 to 96 percent successful.[251,252] The inclusion criteria are (1) a hemodynamically stable, compliant, and healthy patient; (2) no intrauterine pregnancy detected by transvaginal ultrasonography; (3) absence of villi during uterine curettage (if a nonviable intrauterine pregnancy is suspected, ie, hCG <2,000 mIU/ml and progesterone <5 ng/ml); (4) unruptured ectopic pregnancy mass less than 3 or 4 cm in diameter; and (5) hCG titers preferably below 5,000 mIU/ml. Failures have been more common with levels greater than 5,000 mIU/ml. Thus the detection of fetal cardiac activity is generally a contraindication; however, even ectopic pregnancies with fetal cardiac activity have been successfully treated. On the first day of treatment, baseline studies such as ultrasonography, hCG, normal CBC (WBC <2,000/ml and platelet count >100,000/ml), liver enzymes (SGOT), and renal function (BUN, creatinine) should be checked thoroughly. On days 1, 3, 5, and 7, 1 mg/kg methotrexate is given intramuscularly. On days 2, 4, 6 and 8, 0.1 mg/kg citrovorum factor is administered intramuscularly. Beginning on day 4, hCG titers should be checked every day. Treatment is discontinued whenever a decline >15 percent in hCG titers is seen; otherwise, all four doses of the two agents should be accomplished (in case of discontinuation before all four doses are given, corespondent citrovorum factor should be given). On the last (8th) day of the treatment, hCG titers and the other important blood markers listed should be rechecked. Weekly hCG titers should be followed until negative. Approximately 20 percent of patients will require only one dose of methotrexate whereas 20 percent will require all four doses.

The methotrexate regimen defined so far required laparoscopic diagnosis. Although laparoscopy has been the "gold standard" for the diagnosis of ectopic pregnancy, for methotrexate therapy to be acceptable to patients, a non-laparoscopic diagnosis should have been established. Stovall et al designed a non-laparoscopic diagnostic algorithm and applied it successfully with 100 percent accuracy.[251] They also found that a significant number of patients did not require several doses when on the multiple-dose treatment. For the sake of fewer side effects and cost-effectiveness, they established a *single-dose methotrexate protocol*, abandoned the citrovorum factor, and combined the nonsurgical diagnostic algorithm with this single-dose regimen. They obtained encouraging results even with very high hCG levels and the presence of fetal cardiac activity.[253] According to this protocol, methotrexate 50 mg/m^2 is given intramuscularly following baseline laboratory studies and hCG level. After obtaining an hCG level on day 4, a third hCG titer, CBC, and liver and renal function tests are checked on day 7. The hCG titers usually keep rising for the first 3 to 4 days but by day 7 would start to decline. If the hCG titer is lower on day 7 than on day 4, hCG level is observed weekly thereafter until negative. If the hCG titer is higher on day 7 than on day 4, a second methotrexate dose (50 mg/m^2) is given, and the titers are measured again on days 4 and 7. This second dose of methotrexate is needed in 4 percent of cases.

Three to four days after initiation of methotrexate treatments, a symptomatic exacerbation of lower abdominal pain is noted in approximately 60 percent of the patients.[252,254] The pain may represent trophoblastic degeneration with bleeding from the tubal ostia leading to peritoneal irritation, or it may be a symptom caused by methotrexate itself. A nonsteroidal anti-inflammatory agent can be given, but if the pain is not relieved by the medication, a repeat ultrasonography and hemoglobin level should be obtained. The ultrasonographic picture of a mass can persist after hCG titers become negative. The time for the resolution of the mass is variable and often can take several months.[255] Because of the possible pain, patients on methotrexate treatment should avoid gas-producing food such as cabbage, beans, and leeks. They should also avoid alcohol intake, multivitamins containing folic acid, sexual intercourse, and exposure to the sun because of photosensitivity.[256] Patients should use oral contraceptive or barrier methods to prevent pregnancy for at least 2 mo after treatment. Hysterosalpingography can be performed 5 to 6 mo later. Clinicians should always be alert for the possibility of rupture (3 to 4 percent) during medical treatment because a satisfying decline in hCG titers does not guarantee against rupture.[257] The risk of tubal rupture is about 10 percent when the hCG titer is less than 1000 mIU/ml, but rupture is still possible in case of an isthmic pregnancy with hCG levels below 100 mIU/ml.

According to Stovall's experience, using the multiple dose protocol, 95 to 96 percent of patients would be treated successfully with 4 percent mild side effects and 85 percent tubal patency. Among women actively pursuing pregnancy, 62.5 percent would achieve pregnancy and 7 percent of these would be recurrent ectopic pregnancy.[252] After single-dose methotrexate therapy, tubal patency on the ipsilateral side was 82.3 percent, intrauterine pregnancy rate was 60 percent, and the recurrent ectopic pregnancy rate was 8.8 percent.[254] These results match well with the 67 percent intrauterine and 12 percent recurrent ectopic pregnancy rates observed after laparoscopic surgery.[258] Review of the literature suggests that 4 to 8 percent of patients treated with methotrexate will require surgical intervention, a rate similar to the 5 to 15 percent failure rate of laparoscopic salpingostomy.[252,254]

Methotrexate can also be administered orally in a dose of 0.3 mg/kg daily for 4 days. The hCG titers should be followed weekly and in case of raising or plateau, a second course of drug should be administered or the ectopic pregnancy should be treated surgically. Methotrexate has also been used in the treatment of persistent ectopic pregnancy after conservative surgery and cornual pregnancy.[259,260]

There are several other local ways for administering methotrexate in ectopic pregnancy (Table 31–5). *Salpingocentesis* is a technique in which agents such as methotrexate,[261–264] KCl,[265] prostaglandins,[266,267] or hyperosmolar glucose[268,269] are injected into the ectopic pregnancy sac transvaginally using ultrasonographic guidance, by transcervical tubal cannulation (selective salpingography),[237,270] or under laparoscopic guidance. During salpingocentesis various doses of methotrexate (5 to 50 mg) have been used with a successful treatment rate of 78 to 100 percent with 86 to 100 percent tubal patency. Stomatitis and other side effects were only experienced if the chemotherapy was also administered systemically.[271] Although KCl lacks the side effects of methotrexate, its main disadvantage is that it causes fetal death by yielding asystolia of the fetal heart but has no direct inhibitory effect on the growth of trophoblastic tissue. KCl was also used in the treatment of heterotopic pregnancy.[272] Currently, systemic use of methotrexate is the preferred and better-known way in the medical therapy of ectopic pregnancy. Using other routes for administration of methotrexate or other agents is still under investigation and requires expertise.

Surgical Treatment. Gross intra-abdominal hemorrhage in ectopic pregnancy necessitates prompt surgical intervention and in some of those cases laparotomy may

TABLE 31–5. VARIOUS ROUTES OF METHOTREXATE ADMINISTRATION IN ECTOPIC PREGNANCY

	Number of Patients	Successful Treatment (%)	Tubal Patency (%)	Number of Patients Desiring Pregnancy	IUP (%)	EP (%)
Multiple Dose, Systemic						
Stovall, 1991[252]	100	96	49/58 (85)	56	55	7
Single Dose, Systemic						
Stovall, 1993[254]	120	94	51/62 (82)	49	69	10
Glock, 1994[273]	35	86	10/13 (77)	15	20	0
Henry, 1994[274]	61	85	N/A	N/A	N/A	N/A
Local by Laparoscopy						
Pansky, 1989[275]	27	89	18/21 (86)	N/A	N/A	N/A
Zakut, 1989[276]	10	80	7/7 (100)	N/A	N/A	N/A
Kojima, 1990[277]	9	100	9/9 (100)	N/A	N/A	N/A
Kooi, 1990[278]	25	96	N/A	N/A	N/A	N/A
Local by Transvaginal Ultrasonography						
Menard, 1990[261]	17	77	N/A	N/A	N/A	N/A
Tulandi, 1992[279]	40	70	9/11 (82)	N/A	N/A	N/A
Fernandez, 1993[263]	100	83	72/80 (90)	58	54	5

IUP, intrauterine pregnancy; EP, ectopic pregnancy; N/A, not assessed.

be indicated to achieve hemostasis as quickly as possible. Surgical intervention permits confirmation of the diagnosis of tubal pregnancy; assessment of the status of the affected and contralateral tubes and of the other pelvic organs; and effective and instant treatment irrespective of the size of the gestation, tubal rupture, and presence of hemoperitoneum. Surgical treatment of tubal pregnancy can be divided in two main groups, Radical and Conservative, each performed via laparotomy or laparoscopy.

Radical Surgery. The historic approach to management of ectopic pregnancy was removal of the involved tube and ipsilateral ovary in the 1960s.[280] Ipsilateral oophorectomy was usually performed to make sure that ovulation would subsequently occur on the same side as the remaining tube.[281] However, assessing the 15 percent possible migration of the oocyte to the contralateral tube, clinicians later abandoned this practice. Nowadays, a salpingectomy is advisable in cases of extensive distortion of anatomy, uncontrolled bleeding, recurrent ectopic pregnancy in the same tube, and absence of desire for future pregnancies. Cornual resection and uterine preservation is possible in greater than 50 percent of interstitial pregnancies, although the risk of uterine rupture in future pregnancies must be considered when extensive myometrial resection is required. The intrauterine pregnancy rate after unilateral salpingectomy is nearly 40 percent, and the recurrent ectopic pregnancy rate in the contralateral tube varies between 10 and 15 percent.[282] This procedure can be accomplished by both laparotomy and laparoscopy. Hemodynamic instability and cornual ectopic pregnancies are contraindications for laparoscopy; whereas extensive pelvic adhesions, hemoperitoneum, and an ectopic pregnancy greater than 6 cm constitute relative contraindications.[134,282]

Conservative Surgery. Since Stromme's initial report of conservative surgery for ectopic pregnancy in 1953, salpingostomy has replaced salpingectomy.[283] Linear salpingostomy is currently the procedure of choice when the patient has an unruptured ectopic pregnancy and wishes to retain her potential for future fertility. Numerous studies, whether performed by laparoscopy or laparotomy, have demonstrated subsequent intrauterine pregnancy rates of 40 to 70 percent and recurrent ectopic pregnancy rates of 10 to 15 percent with salpingostomy. These reproductive outcome rates are slightly higher in comparison to salpingectomy[284] (Table 31–6). Timonen and Nieminen reported a 49 percent intrauterine pregnancy rate and a 12 percent repeat ectopic rate following salpingectomy compared with a 53 percent intrauterine pregnancy and 16 percent repeat ectopic pregnancy rate after salpingostomy.[280] DeCherney and Kase gave similar rates with 42 percent and 12 percent with salpingectomy

and 40 percent and 12 percent with salpingostomy, respectively.[285] Several investigators have reviewed pregnancy rates in patients who had salpingostomies performed on a sole remaining fallopian tube and found the reproductive parameters to be similar to the early reports.[134,286,287] This implies that normal tubal function can be restored following conservative treatment of ectopic pregnancy. Salpingostomy (without closure) has become the preferred method over *salpingotomy* (one- or two-layer suture closure of the tubal incision) because a similar pregnancy rate but less adhesion has been shown with salpingostomy.[288]

Linear salpingostomy is the preferred technique for unruptured ampullary ectopic pregnancies where the gestation grows in extratubal space, between the serosa and the lumen (inside the wall) of the fallopian tube. In isthmic pregnancies in which the ectopic material is in the lumen of the tube, damaging the endosalpinx, segmental resection may be applied to the affected portion. Following segmental resection, *immediate* and *delayed* anastomosis can be performed, but the latter is preferred because existing tubal edema decreases the success of surgical and reproductive outcome.[296] Although segmental resection with delayed anastomosis previously was the advised surgical method for isthmic pregnancies,[42,297] laparoscopic salpingostomy is now the method of choice, with a 61 percent intrauterine and 19 percent ectopic pregnancy rate.[258,294,298–302] Evacuation of a distal ampullary or a fimbrial gestation by suction or digital expression (*milking*) is not recommended because of the reports of high rates of retained trophoblastic activity and postoperative bleeding,[303] but the spontaneous aborting tissue extruding through the infundibulum may be carefully removed in an atraumatic manner.[304]

Shapiro et al were first to remove successfully a small, unruptured ampullary ectopic pregnancy via the laparoscopic route in 1973.[305] Several investigators later compared salpingostomy by laparotomy versus laparoscopy and found out that the laparoscopic approach provided not only a shorter operating time (average 45 min), shorter hospital stay (average 1.5 days), and lesser peritoneal adhesion, but also better pregnancy and tubal patency rates (Table 31–6).[136,289,306,307] Vermesh et al have compared salpingostomy via laparoscopy versus laparotomy in 60 ampullary ectopic pregnancy patients, divided into two randomized groups prospectively.[282] They found 89 percent ipsilateral tubal patency, 58 percent subsequent pregnancy, and 37 percent recurrent ectopic pregnancy rates with laparotomy. Corresponding figures for laparoscopy were 80, 56, and 10 percent. Persistent trophoblastic disease was seen in 1 patient of each group (3.3 percent). Having found the reproductive parameters to be similar with both techniques, the authors concluded that laparoscopic salpingostomy is

TABLE 31–6. SUCCESS RATES AND REPRODUCTIVE OUTCOME FOLLOWING LAPAROSCOPIC SALPINGOSTOMY FOR UNRUPTURED ECTOPIC PREGNANCY

	Number of Patients	Successful Treatments (%)	Tubal Patency (%)	Number of Patients Desiring Pregnancy	IUP (%)	EP (%)
Bruhat, 1980[289]	60	95	13/18 (72)	25	72	12
Cartwright, 1986[290]	27	96	6/8 (75)	8	50	13
Pouly, 1986[134]	321	95	N/A	118	64	22
Bornstein, 1987[291]	22	100	17/21 (81)	21	24	5
DeCherney, 1987[292]	79	98	N/A	69	52	10
Vermesh, 1989[282]	30	87	16/20 (80)	18	50	6
Mecke, 1991[293]	95	94	N/A	143	58	16
Chapron, 1992[294]	26	96	N/A	11	64	9
Langebrekke, 1993[295]	74	96	N/A	58	66	7
Fernandez, 1995[264]	20	95	16/18 (89)	10	30	0
TOTAL	864	95	68/85/(80)	481	58	14

IUP, intrauterine pregnancy; EP, ectopic pregnancy; N/A, not assessed.

associated with significant reduction in patient morbidity, hospitalization, and length of stay. Reproductive outcome of laparoscopic surgery for ectopic pregnancy can be summarized as follows: subsequent tubal patency rate 80 percent, subsequent intrauterine pregnancy rate 58 percent, subsequent ectopic pregnancy rate 14 percent, and persistent ectopic pregnancy rate 14 percent (Table 31–6).

Persistent Ectopic Pregnancy. Persistent ectopic pregnancy occurs when functional trophoblastic tissue remains in the fallopian tube following (usually), a conservative surgical procedure. Trophoblastic tissue may also disseminate throughout the peritoneal cavity and peritoneal implantation may cause persistent trophoblastic disease.[308–310] It has been reported following 3 to 5 percent of salpingostomies performed by laparotomy and following 5 to 20 percent (~15) of laparoscopic procedures.[135] Pouly reported it to be 4.8 percent (15 patients) among 321 patients who underwent conservative laparoscopy.[134] This complication is more common following linear salpingostomy for very early ectopic pregnancies of 2 cm or less in diameter or less than 42 days of amenorrhea, during which it is difficult to find the plane between the tube and small gestational products.[136] To diagnose this situation early, various studies reported that patients with preoperative hCG levels greater than 3,000 mIU/ml or with postoperative levels greater than 1,000 mIU/ml on the second or seventh postoperative days are prone to have persistent trophoblastic tissue.[311] With appropriate removal of the trophoblastic tissue, serum hCG levels usually decline within 72 hr of surgery to a concentration of 15 to 20 percent of the preoperative value. Vermesh et al suggested

that persistent ectopic pregnancy should be suspected if hCG levels did not fall below 10 percent of the initial value on the 12th postoperative day.[135,282] The average time for hCG to become undetectable varies from 4 to 6 wk; therefore, hCG levels should be followed at least weekly following surgery, especially conservative surgical procedures.

For the treatment of persistent ectopic pregnancy, reoperation, sometimes salpingectomy, is a treatment option; however, systemic (50 mg/m²) or local methotrexate regimens with doses of 12.5 to 50 mg can be used.[312–316]

Rh Immunoglobulin Prophylaxis. Between 8 and 12 wk, 50 μg, and after 12th wk of gestation, 300 μg Rho immune globulin should be administered to the Rh-negative patient with ectopic pregnancy unless the partner is proven to be Rh negative.[317]

Infertility After Ectopic Pregnancy. It has been estimated that approximately 20 percent of women who suffer a tubal pregnancy will subsequently be infertile because of tubal abnormality.[318] The major etiologic factors are tubal dysfunction and tuboperitoneal adhesions. Adhesion formation may occur not only in patients treated at laparotomy for ectopic gestation but also in those treated by laparoscopy.[319] Nevertheless, pregnancy results and reproductive outcome after ectopic pregnancy seem not to differ so much in terms of surgical approach (salpingostomy versus salpingectomy or laparoscopy versus laparotomy). In terms of infertility, it is recommended that patients should be assessed with an HSG after 4 to 6 mo and laparoscopy at 1 yr if pregnancy has not yet occurred.

Another important issue is recurrent ectopic pregnancies and the status of the contralateral tube. It appears that the operative method has no influence on subsequent fertility in women with an intact contralateral tube. Women with an unaffected contralateral tube have a significantly higher live birth rate (76 percent) and lower recurrent ectopic pregnancy rate (7.7 percent) than women with an affected contralateral tube (52 and 56 percent, respectively). The risk of a subsequent ectopic pregnancy for nulliparous women (22 percent) is higher than for parous women (9 percent).[320,321]

Following a second ectopic pregnancy, the intrauterine pregnancy rate is 31 percent. Following the third ectopic pregnancy, the rate is 8 percent.[322] Although these rates favor a conservative intervention in case of recurrent ectopic pregnancy, nowadays, with the fast advent in ART, laparoscopic salpingectomy may even be preferable to conservative approaches such as salpingostomy for the sake of reducing the risk for a subsequent ectopic pregnancy during an IVF cycle.

SUMMARY

The fallopian tube has the complex task of ensuring the transport of spermatozoa towards the ovary, ova towards the uterus, and subsequently the transport of the zygote towards the normal site of implantation in the uterine endometrium. The approach to diagnose and treat various conditions such as tubal infertility and ectopic pregnancy has changed and improved over the past 20 years. Despite the recent advances in assisted reproductive technologies, reconstructive tubal surgery still remains important in the treatment of tubal disease. As the role of various growth factors and cytokines in the tubal environment is understood, we will better overcome reproductive problems.

REFERENCES

1. Wheeler JE. Disease of the fallopian tube. In: Kurman RJ, ed. *Blaustein's Pathology of the Female Genital Tract*, 4th ed. New York, Springer-Verlag, 1994: 529
2. Williams PL. *Gray's Anatomy*, 37th ed. London, Churchill Livingstone, 1989
3. Donnez J, Casanas-Roux F, Caprasse J, et al. Cyclic changes in ciliation, cell height, and mitotic activity in human tubal epithelium during reproductive life. *Fertil Steril.* 43:554, 1985
4. Valle RF. Tubal cannulation. *Obstet Gynecol Clin North Am.* 22:519, 1995
5. Green LK, Kott ML. Histopathologic findings in ectopic tubal pregnancy. *Int J Gynecol Pathol.* 8:255, 1989
6. Pauerstein CJ, Woodruff JD. The role of the "indifferent" cell of the tubal epithelium. *Am J Obstet Gynecol.* 98:121, 1967
7. Verhage HG, Bareither ML, Jaffe RC, Akbar M. Cyclic changes in ciliation, secretion and cell height of the oviductal epithelium in women. *Am J Anat.* 156:505, 1979
8. Gasc JM, Baulieu EE. Steroid hormone receptors: Intracellular distribution. *Biol Cell.* 56:1, 1986
9. Lei ZM, Rao CV. Expression of epidermal growth factor (EGF) receptor and its ligands, EGF and transforming growth factor-alpha, in human fallopian tubes. *Endocrinology.* 131:947, 1992
10. Jones JI, Clemmons DR. Insulin-like growth factors and their binding proteins: Biological actions. *Endocr Rev.* 16:3, 1995
11. Giudice LC, Dsupin BA, Irwin JC, Eckert RL. Identification of insulin-like growth factor binding proteins in human oviduct. *Fertil Steril.* 57:294, 1992
12. Zhao Y, Chegini N, Flanders KC. Human fallopian tube expresses transforming growth factor (TGF beta) isoforms, TGF beta type I-III receptor messenger ribonucleic acid and protein, and contains [125I]TGF beta-binding sites. *J Clin Endocrinol Metab.* 79:1177, 1994
13. Westermark B. The molecular and cellular biology of platelet-derived growth factor. *Acta Endocrinol.* 123:131, 1990
14. Zhao Y, Chegini N. Human fallopian tube expresses granulocyte-macrophage colony stimulating factor (GM-CSF) and GM-CSF alpha and beta receptors and contain immunoreactive GM-CSF protein. *J Clin Endocrinol Metab.* 79:662, 1994
15. Keltz MD, Attar E, Buradagunta S, et al. Modulation of leukemia inhibitory factor gene expression and protein biosynthesis in the human fallopian tube. *Am J Obstet Gynecol.* 175:1611, 1996
16. Adamson ED. Activities of growth factors in preimplantation embryos. *J Cell Biochem.* 53:280, 1993
17. Elder MG, Myatt L, Chaudhuri G. The role of prostaglandins in the spontaneous motility of the fallopian tube. *Fertil Steril.* 28:86, 1977
18. Odor DL, Blandau RJ. EGG transport over the fimbrial surface of the rabbit oviduct under experimental conditions. *Fertil Steril.* 24:292, 1973
19. Croxatto HB. The duration of egg transport and its regulation in mammals. *Basic Life Sci.* 4:159, 1974
20. Jansen RP. Fallopian tube isthmic mucus and ovum transport. *Science.* 201:349, 1978
21. Settlage DS, Motoshima M, Tredway DR. Sperm transport from the external cervical os to the fallopian tubes in women: A time and quantitation study. *Fertil Steril.* 24:655, 1973
22. Ahlgren M. Sperm transport to and survival in the human fallopian tube. *Gynecol Invest.* 6:206, 1975
23. Paterson PJ, Chan CL. Congenital absence of fallopian tube segments. *Aust NZ J Obstet Gynaecol.* 25:130, 1985
24. Bates GW, Abide JK. Bilateral autoamputation of the fallopian tubes. *Fertil Steril.* 38:253, 1982
25. Tulusan AH. Complete absence of the muscular layer of the ampullary part of the Fallopian tubes. *Arch Gynecol.* 234:279, 1984
26. Wanerman J, Wulwick R, Brenner S. Segmental absence of the fallopian tube. *Fertil Steril.* 46:525, 1986

27. Afzelius BA, Camner P, Mossberg B. On the function of cilia in the female reproductive tract. *Fertil Steril.* 29:72, 1978

28. Rott HD. Kartagener's syndrome and the syndrome of immotile cilia. *Hum Genet.* 46:249, 1979

29. Brosens IA, Gordon AG. *Tubal Infertility,* London, Gower Medical Publishing, 1990

30. Rock JA, Katayama KP, Martin EJ, et al. Factors influencing the success of salpingostomy techniques for distal fimbrial obstruction. *Obstet Gynecol.* 52:591, 1978

31. McComb PF, Paleologou A. The intussusception salpingostomy technique for the therapy of distal oviductal occlusion at laparoscopy. *Obstet Gynecol.* 78:443, 1991

32. Westrom L. Incidence, prevalence, and trends of acute pelvic inflammatory disease and its consequences in industrialized countries. *Am J Obstet Gynecol.* 138: 880, 1980

33. Sweet RL, Mills J, Hadley KW, et al. Use of laparoscopy to determine the microbiologic etiology of acute salpingitis. *Am J Obstet Gynecol.* 134:68, 1979

34. Westrom L, Bengtsson LP, Mardh PA. Incidence, trends, and risks of ectopic pregnancy in a population of women. *Br Med J.* 282:15, 1981

35. Fortier KJ, Haney AF. The pathologic spectrum of uterotubal junction obstruction. *Obstet Gynecol.* 65:93, 1985

36. Keltz MD, Kliman HJ, Arici AM, Olive DL. Endosalpingiosis found at laparoscopy for chronic pelvic pain. *Fertil Steril.* 64:482, 1995

37. Majmudar B, Henderson PHD, Semple E. Salpingitis isthmica nodosa: A high-risk factor for tubal pregnancy. *Obstet Gynecol.* 62:73, 1983

38. Creasy JL, Clark RL, Cuttino JT, Groff TR. Salpingitis isthmica nodosa: Radiologic and clinical correlates. *Radiology.* 154:597, 1985

39. Persaud V. Etiology of tubal ectopic pregnancy. Radiologic and pathologic studies. *Obstet Gynecol.* 36:257, 1970

40. Donnez J, Casanas-Roux F. Histology: A prognostic factor in proximal tubal occlusion. *Eur J Obstet Gynecol Reprod Biol.* 29:33, 1988

41. Punnonen R, Soderstrom KO, Alanen A. Isthmic tubal occlusion: Etiology and histology. *Acta Eur Fertil.* 15:39, 1984

42. Homm RJ, Holtz G, Garvin AJ. Isthmic ectopic pregnancy and salpingitis isthmica nodosa. *Fertil Steril.* 48:756, 1987

43. Saracoglu FO, Mungan T, Tanzer F. Salpingitis isthmica nodosa in infertility and ectopic pregnancy. *Gynecol Obstet Invest.* 34:202, 1992

44. Kutluay L, Vicdan K, Turan C, et al. Tubal histopathology in ectopic pregnancies. *Eur J Obstet Gynecol Reprod Biol.* 57:91, 1994

45. Donnez J, Casanas-Roux F. Prognostic factors influencing the pregnancy rate after microsurgical cornual anastomosis. *Fertil Steril.* 46:1089, 1986

46. Thomas ML, Rose DH. Salpingitis isthmica nodosa demonstrated by hysterosalpingography. *Acta Radiol Diagn.* 14:295, 1973

47. Karasick S, Karasick D, Schilling J. Salpingitis isthmica nodosa in female infertility. *J Can Assoc Radiol.* 36:118, 1985

48. Vancaillie T, Schmidt EH. The uterotubal junction. A proposal for classifying its morphology as assessed with hysteroscopy. *J Reprod Med.* 33:624, 1988

49. Gurgan T, Urman B, Yarali H, et al. Salpingoscopic findings in women with occlusive and nonocclusive salpingitis isthmica nodosa. *Fertil Steril.* 61:461, 1994

50. McComb PF, Rowe TC. Salpingitis isthmica nodosa: Evidence it is a progressive disease. *Fertil Steril.* 51:542, 1989

51. Wiedemann R, Sterzik K, Gombisch V, et al. Beyond recanalizing proximal tube occlusion: The argument for further diagnosis and classification. *Hum Reprod.* 11:986, 1996

52. Sampson JA. Endometriosis following salpingectomy. *Am J Obstet Gynecol.* 16:461, 1928

53. Sampson JA. Postsalpingectomy endometriosis (endosalpingiosis). *Am J Obstet Gynecol.* 20:443, 1930

54. Davies SA, Maclin VM. Endosalpingosis as a cause of chronic pelvic pain. *Am J Obstet Gynecol.* 164:495, 1991

55. Zinsser KR, Wheeler JE. Endosalpingiosis in the omentum: A study of autopsy and surgical material. *Am J Surg Pathol.* 6:109, 1982

56. Ryuko K, Miura H, Abu-Musa A, et al. Endosalpingiosis in association with ovarian surface papillary tumor of borderline malignancy. *Gynecol Oncol.* 46:107, 1992

57. Reasbeck J, Wynn-Williams G, Gillett W. Tubal intramural polyps: Incidence and radiographic demonstration. *Australas Radiol.* 32:117, 1988

58. Lisa JR, Gioia J, Rubin IC. Observations of the interstitial portion of the fallopian tube. *Surg, Gynecol Obstet.* 99:159, 1954

59. Schaefer G. Tuberculosis of the female genital tract. *Clin Obstet Gynecol.* 13:965, 1970

60. Nogales-Ortiz F, Tarancon I, Nogales FF, Jr. The pathology of female genital tuberculosis. A 31-year study of 1436 cases. *Obstet Gynecol.* 53:422, 1979

61. Ballon SC, Clewell WH, Lamb EJ. Reactivation of silent pelvic tuberculosis by reconstructive tubal surgery. *Am J Obstet Gynecol.* 122:991, 1975

62. Vasquez G, Winston RM, Boeckx W, Brosens I. Tubal lesions subsequent to sterilization and their relation to fertility after attempts at reversal. *Am J Obstet Gynecol.* 138:86, 1980

63. Gomel V. Microsurgical reversal of female sterilization: A reappraisal. *Fertil Steril.* 33:587, 1980

64. DeCherney AH, Kort H, Barney JB, DeVore GR. Increased pregnancy rate with oil-soluble hysterosalpingography dye. *Fertil Steril.* 33:407, 1980

65. Watson A, Vandekerckhove P, Lilford R, et al. A meta-analysis of the therapeutic role of oil soluble contrast media at hysterosalpingography: A surprising result? *Fertil Steril.* 61:470, 1994

66. Swart P, Mol BW, van der Veen F, et al. The accuracy of hysterosalpingography in the diagnosis of tubal pathology: A meta-analysis. *Fertil Steril.* 64:486, 1995

67. Brundin J, Dahlborn M, Ahlberg-Ahre E, Lundberg HJ. Radionuclide hysterosalpingography for measurement of human oviductal function. *Int J Gynaecol Obstet.* 28:53, 1989

68. Nannini R, Chelo E, Branconi F, et al. Dynamic echohysteroscopy: A new diagnostic technique in the study of female infertility. *Acta Eur Fertil.* 12:165, 1981

69. Mitri FF, Andronikou AD, Perpinyal S, et al. A clinical comparison of sonographic hydrotubation and hysterosalpingography. *Br J Obstet Gynaecol.* 98:1031, 1991

70. Stern J, Peters AJ, Coulam CB. Color Doppler ultrasonography assessment of tubal patency: A comparison study with traditional techniques. *Fertil Steril.* 58:897, 1992

71. Yarali H, Gurgan T, Erden A, Kisnisci HA. Colour Doppler hysterosalpingosonography: A simple and potentially useful method to evaluate fallopian tubal patency. *Hum Reprod.* 9:64, 1994

72. Battaglia C, Artini PG, D'Amibrogio, et al. Color Doppler hysterosalpingography in the diagnosis of tubal patency. *Fertil Steril.* 65:317, 1996

73. Degenhardt E, Jibril S, Gohde M, et al. Die ambulante Hystero-Kontrast-Sonographie (HKSG) als Moglichkeit zur Kontrolle der Tubendurchgangigkeit. *Geburtshilfe Frauenheilkd.* 55:143, 1995

74. Maguiness SD, Djahanbakhch O, Grudzinskas JG. Assessment of the fallopian tube. *Obstet Gynecol Surv.* 47:587, 1992

75. Hamou J. Microhysteroscopy. A new procedure and its original applications in gynecology. *J Reprod Med.* 26:375, 1981

76. Shapiro BS, Diamond MP, DeCherney AH. Salpingoscopy: An adjunctive technique for evaluation of the fallopian tube. *Fertil Steril.* 49:1076, 1988

77. De Bruyne F, Puttemans P, Boeckx W, Brosens I. The clinical value of salpingoscopy in tubal infertility. *Fertil Steril.* 51:339, 1989

78. Hershlag A, Seifer DB, Carcangiu ML, et al. Salpingoscopy: Light microscopic and electron microscopic correlations. *Obstet Gynecol.* 77:399, 1991

79. Brosens I, Boeckx W, Delattin P, et al. Salpingoscopy: A new pre-operative diagnostic tool in tubal infertility. *Br J Obstet Gynaecol.* 94:768, 1987

80. Henry-Suchet J, Tesquiter L, Pez JP, Loffredo V. Prognostic value of tuboscopy vs. hysterosalpingography before tuboplasty. *J Reprod Med.* 29:609, 1984

81. Puttemans P, Brosens I, Delattin P, et al. Salpingoscopy versus hysterosalpingography in hydrosalpinges. *Hum Reprod.* 2:535, 1987

82. Henry-Suchet J, Loffredo V, Tesquier L, Pez JP. Endoscopy of the tube (= tuboscopy): Its prognostic value for tuboplasties. *Acta Eur Fertil.* 16:139, 1985

83. Marana R, Muscatello P, Muzii L, et al. Perlaparoscopic salpingoscopy in the evaluation of the tubal factor in infertile women. *Int J Fertil.* 35:211, 1990

84. Kerin J, Daykhovsky L, Segalowitz J, et al. Falloposcopy: A microendoscopic technique for visual exploration of the human fallopian tube from the uterotubal ostium to the fimbria using a transvaginal approach. *Fertil Steril.* 54:390, 1990

85. Pearlstone AC, Surrey ES, Kerin JF. The linear everting catheter: A nonhysteroscopic, transvaginal technique for access and microendoscopy of the fallopian tube. *Fertil Steril.* 58:854, 1992

86. Kerin JF, Williams DB, San Roman GA, et al. Falloposcopic classification and treatment of fallopian tube lumen disease. *Fertil Steril.* 57:731, 1992

87. Fayez JA, Suliman SO. Infertility surgery of the oviduct: Comparison between macrosurgery and microsurgery. *Fertil Steril.* 37:73, 1982

88. Patton PE, Williams TJ, Coulam CB. Results of microsurgical reconstruction in patients with combined proximal and distal tubal occlusion: Double obstruction. *Fertil Steril.* 48:670, 1987

89. Lavy G, Diamond MP, DeCherney AH. Ectopic pregnancy: Its relationship to tubal reconstructive surgery. *Fertil Steril.* 47:543, 1987

90. Strandell A, Thorburn J. Previous ectopic pregnancy should be considered a contraindication for microsurgery. *Acta Obstet Gynecol Scand.* 75:394, 1996

91. Tulandi T, Falcone T, Kafka I. Second-look operative laparoscopy 1 year following reproductive surgery. *Fertil Steril.* 52:421, 1989

92. Raj SG, Hulka JF. Second-look laparoscopy in infertility surgery: Therapeutic and prognostic value. *Fertil Steril.* 38:325, 1982

93. Dubuisson JB, Bouquet de Joliniere J, Aubriot FX, et al. Terminal tuboplasties by laparoscopy: 65 consecutive cases. *Fertil Steril.* 54:401, 1990

94. Gomel V. Salpingostomy by microsurgery. *Fertil Steril.* 29:380, 1978

95. Boer-Meisel ME, te Velde ER, Habbema JD, Kardaun JW. Predicting the pregnancy outcome in patients treated for hydrosalpinx: A prospective study. *Fertil Steril.* 45:23, 1986

96. Gomel V. Salpingo-ovariolysis by laparoscopy in infertility. *Fertil Steril.* 40:607, 1983

97. Tulandi T. Salpingo-ovariolysis: A comparison between laser surgery and electrosurgery. *Fertil Steril.* 45:489, 1986

98. Tulandi T, Collins JA, Burrows E, et al. Treatment-dependent and treatment-independent pregnancy among women with periadnexal adhesions. *Am J Obstet Gynecol.* 162:354, 1990

99. Gomel V, Wang I. Laparoscopic surgery for infertility therapy. *Curr Opin Obstet Gynecol.* 6:141, 1994

100. Fayez JA. An assessment of the role of operative laparoscopy in tuboplasty. *Fertil Steril.* 39:476, 1983

101. Daniell JF, Diamond MP, McLaughlin DS, et al. Clinical results of terminal salpingostomy with the use of the CO_2 laser: Report of the Intraabdominal Laser Study Group. *Fertil Steril.* 45:175, 1986

102. Schlaff WD, Hassiakos DK, Damewood MD, Rock JA. Neosalpingostomy for distal tubal obstruction: Prognostic factors and impact of surgical technique. *Fertil Steril.* 54:984, 1990

103. Rock JA, Katayama KP, Martin EJ, et al. Pregnancy outcome following uterotubal implantation: A comparison of the reamer and sharp cornual wedge excision techniques. *Fertil Steril.* 31:634, 1979

104. Gomel V. An odyssey through the oviduct. *Fertil Steril.* 39:144, 1983

105. McComb P. Microsurgical tubocornual anastomosis for occlusive cornual disease: Reproducible results without the need for tubouterine implantation. *Fertil Steril.* 46:571, 1986

106. Fayez JA. Comparison between tubouterine implantation and tubouterine anastomosis for repair of cornual occlusion. *Microsurgery.* 8:78, 1987

107. Siegler AM, Hulka J, Peretz A. Reversibility of female sterilization. *Fertil Steril.* 43:499, 1985

108. Sulak PJ, Letterie GS, Coddington CC, et al. Histology of proximal tubal occlusion. *Fertil Steril.* 48:437, 1987

109. Woolcott R. Proximal tubal occlusion: A practical approach. *Hum Reprod.* 11:1831, 1996

110. Rock JA, Guzick DS, Katz E, et al. Tubal anastomosis: Pregnancy success following reversal of Falope ring or monopolar cautery sterilization. *Fertil Steril.* 48:13, 1987

111. Hulka JF, Halme J. Sterilization reversal: Results of 101 attempts. *Am J Obstet Gynecol.* 159:767, 1988

112. Spivak MM, Librach CL, Rosenthal DM. Microsurgical reversal of sterilization: A six-year study. *Am J Obstet Gynecol.* 154:355, 1986

113. Novy MJ. Reversal of Kroener fimbriectomy sterilization. *Am J Obstet Gynecol.* 137:198, 1980

114. Flood JT, Grow DR. Transcervical tubal cannulation: A review. *Obstet Gynecol Surv.* 48:768, 1993

115. Confino E, Tur-Kaspa I, DeCherney A, et al. Transcervical balloon tuboplasty. A multicenter study. *JAMA.* 264:2079, 1990

116. Musich JR, Behrman SJ. Surgical management of tubal obstruction at the uterotubal junction. *Fertil Steril.* 40:423, 1983

117. Deaton JL, Gibson M, Riddick DH, Brumsted JR. Diagnosis and treatment of cornual obstruction using a flexible tip guidewire. *Fertil Steril.* 53:232, 1990

118. Lisse K, Sydow P. Fallopian tube catheterization and recanalization under ultrasonic observation: A simplified technique to evaluate tubal patency and open proximally obstructed tubes. *Fertil Steril.* 56:198, 1991

119. McComb P. The determinants of successful surgery for proximal tubal disease. *Fertil Steril.* 46:1002, 1986. Editorial

120. Balmaceda JP, Gastaldi C, Remohi J, et al. Tubal embryo transfer as a treatment for infertility due to male factor. *Fertil Steril.* 50:476, 1988

121. Seracchioli R, Possati G, Bafaro G, et al. Hysteroscopic gamete intra-fallopian transfer: A good alternative, in selected cases, to laparoscopic intra-fallopian transfer. *Hum Reprod.* 6:1388, 1991

122. Scholtes MC, Roozenburg BJ, Verhoeff A, Zeilmaker GH. A randomized study of transcervical intrafallopian transfer of pronucleate embryos controlled by ultrasound versus intrauterine transfer of four- to eight-cell embryos. *Fertil Steril.* 61:102, 1994

123. Scholtes MC, Roozenburg BJ, Alberda AT, Zeilmaker GH. Transcervical intrafallopian transfer of zygotes. *Fertil Steril.* 54:283, 1990

124. Swolin K. Electromicrosurgery and salpingostomy: Long-term results. *Am J Obstet Gynecol.* 121:418, 1975

125. Gomel V. From microsurgery to laparoscopic surgery: A progress. *Fertil Steril.* 63:464, 1995. Editorial

126. Gomel V. Operative laparoscopy: Time for acceptance. *Fertil Steril.* 52:1, 1989

127. Luciano AA, Maier DB, Koch EI, et al. A comparative study of postoperative adhesions following laser surgery by laparoscopy versus laparotomy in the rabbit model. *Obstet Gynecol.* 74:220, 1989

128. Lundorff P, Hahlin M, Kallfelt B, et al. Adhesion formation after laparoscopic surgery in tubal pregnancy: A randomized trial versus laparotomy. *Fertil Steril.* 55:911, 1991

129. Filmar S, Gomel V, McComb PF. Operative laparoscopy versus open abdominal surgery: A comparative study on postoperative adhesion formation in the rat model. *Fertil Steril.* 48:486, 1987

130. Reich H, McGlynn F, Parente C, et al. Laparoscopic tubal anastomosis. *J Am Assoc Gynecol Laparoscop.* 1:16, 1993

131. Zouves C, Urman B, Gomel V. Laparoscopic surgical treatment of tubal pregnancy. A safe, effective alternative to laparotomy. *J Reprod Med.* 37:205, 1992

132. Urman B, Zouves C, Gomel V. Fertility outcome following tubal pregnancy. *Acta Eur Fertil.* 22:205, 1991

133. Murphy AA, Nager CW, Wujek JJ, et al. Operative laparoscopy versus laparotomy for the management of ectopic pregnancy: A prospective trial. *Fertil Steril.* 57:1180, 1992

134. Pouly JL, Mahnes H, Mage G, et al. Conservative laparoscopic treatment of 321 ectopic pregnancies. *Fertil Steril.* 46:1093, 1986

135. Vermesh M, Silva PD, Sauer MV, et al. Persistent tubal ectopic gestation: Patterns of circulating beta-human chorionic gonadotropin and progesterone, and management options. *Fertil Steril.* 50:584, 1988

136. Seifer DB, Gutmann JN, Doyle MB, et al. Persistent ectopic pregnancy following laparoscopic linear salpingostomy. *Obstet Gynecol.* 76:1121, 1990

137. Benadiva CA, Kligman I, Davis O, Rosenwaks Z. In vitro fertilization versus tubal surgery: Is pelvic reconstructive surgery obsolete? *Fertil Steril.* 64:1051, 1995

138. Penzias AS, DeCherney AH. Is there ever a role for tubal surgery? *Am J Obstet Gynecol.* 174:1218, 1996

139. Assisted reproductive technology in the United States and Canada: 1993 results generated from the American Society for Reproductive Medicine/Society for Assisted Reproductive Technology Registry. *Fertil Steril.* 64:13, 1995

140. Marchbanks PA, Annegers JF, Coulam CB, et al. Risk factors for ectopic pregnancy. A population-based study. *JAMA.* 259:1823, 1988

141. Zouves C, Erenus M, Gomel V. Tubal ectopic pregnancy after in vitro fertilization and embryo transfer: A role for proximal occlusion or salpingectomy after failed distal tubal surgery? *Fertil Steril.* 56:691, 1991

142. Holst N, Maltau JM, Forsdahl F, Hansen LJ. Handling of tubal infertility after introduction of in vitro fertilization: Changes and consequences. *Fertil Steril.* 55:140, 1991

143. Callahan TL, Hall JE, Ettner SL, et al. The economic impact of multiple-gestation pregnancies and the contribution of assisted-reproduction techniques to their incidence. *N Engl J Med.* 331:244, 1994

144. Andersen AN, Yue Z, Meng FJ, Petersen K. Low implantation rate after in-vitro fertilization in patients with hydrosalpinges diagnosed by ultrasonography. *Hum Reprod.* 9:1935, 1994

145. Strandell A, Waldenstrom U, Nilsson L, Hamberger L. Hydrosalpinx reduces in-vitro fertilization/embryo transfer pregnancy rates. *Hum Reprod.* 9:861, 1994

146. Andersen AN, Lindhard A, Loft A, et al. The infertile patient with hydrosalpinges-IVF with or without salpingectomy. *Hum Reprod.* 11:2081, 1996

147. Hull MG, Fleming CF. Tubal surgery versus assisted reproduction: Assessing their role in infertility therapy. *Curr Opin Obstet Gynecol.* 7:160, 1995

148. Mosgaard B, Hertz J, Steenstrup BR, et al. Surgical management of tubal infertility. A regional study. *Acta Obstet Gynecol Scand.* 75:469, 1996

149. Diamond MP, DeCherney AH. Pathogenesis of adhesion formation/reformation: application to reproductive pelvic surgery. *Microsurgery.* 8:103, 1987

150. Buttram VC, Reiter RC. *Surgical Treatment of the Infertile Female.* Baltimore, Md., Williams and Wilkins, 1985

151. diZerega GS, Hodger GD. Prevention of postoperative tubal adhesions. Comparative study of commonly used agents. *Am J Obstet Gynecol.* 136:173, 1980

152. diZerega GS. Contemporary adhesion prevention. *Fertil Steril.* 61:219, 1994

153. Shear L, Swartz C, Shinaberger JA, Barry KG. Kinetics of peritoneal fluid absorption in adult man. *N Engl J Med.* 272:123, 1964

154. diZerega GS, Rodgers KE. *The Peritoneum.* New York, Springer-Verlag, 1992

155. Fayez JA, Schneider PJ. Prevention of pelvic adhesion formation by different modalities of treatment. *Am J Obstet Gynecol.* 157:1184, 1987

156. Gurgan T, Kisnisci H, Yarali H, et al. Evaluation of adhesion formation after laparoscopic treatment of polycystic ovarian disease. *Fertil Steril.* 56:1176, 1991

157. Rosenberg SM, Board JA. High-molecular weight dextran in human infertility surgery. *Am J Obstet Gynecol.* 148:380, 1984

158. Larsson B, Lalos O, Marsk L, et al. Effect of intraperitoneal instillation of 32% dextran 70 on postoperative adhesion formation after tubal surgery. *Acta Obstet Gynecol Scand.* 64:437, 1985

159. Jansen RP. Failure of intraperitoneal adjuncts to improve the outcome of pelvic operations in young women. *Am J Obstet Gynecol.* 153:363, 1985

160. Sekiba K. Use of Interceed(TC7) absorbable adhesion barrier to reduce postoperative adhesion reformation in infertility and endometriosis surgery. The Obstetrics and Gynecology Adhesion Prevention Committee. *Obstet Gynecol.* 79:518, 1992

161. Nordic Adhesion Prevention Study Group. The efficacy of Interceed(TC7) for prevention of reformation of postoperative adhesions on ovaries, fallopian tubes, and fimbriae in microsurgical operations for fertility: A multicenter study. *Fertil Steril.* 63:709, 1995

162. Haney AF, Hesla J, Hurst BS, et al. Expanded polytetrafluoroethylene (Gore-Tex Surgical Membrane) is superior to oxidized regenerated cellulose (Interceed TC7+) in preventing adhesions. *Fertil Steril.* 63: 1021, 1995

163. Breen JL. A 21 year survey of 654 ectopic pregnancies. *Am J Obstet Gynecol.* 106:1004, 1970

164. Atrash HK, Friede A, Hogue CJ. Abdominal pregnancy in the United States: Frequency and maternal mortality. *Obstet Gynecol.* 69:333, 1987

165. Guvener S, Kopera H, Atasu T, Hulagu C. Bilaterale Tubargraviditaten. *Zentralbl Gynakol.* 95:657, 1973

166. Ectopic pregnancy—United States, 1988–1989. *MMWR.* 41:591, 1992

167. Goldner TE, Lawson HW, Xia Z, Atrash HK. Surveillance for ectopic pregnancy—United States, 1970–1989. *MMWR.* 42:73, 1993

168. Atrash HK, Friede A, Hogue CJ. Ectopic pregnancy mortality in the United States, 1970–1983. *Obstet Gynecol.* 70:817, 1987

169. Coste J, Job-Spira N, Aublet-Cuvelier B, et al. Incidence of ectopic pregnancy. First results of a population-based register in France. *Hum Reprod.* 9:742, 1994

170. Tal J, Haddad S, Gordon N, Timor-Tritsch I. Heterotopic pregnancy after ovulation induction and assisted reproductive technologies: A literature review from 1971 to 1993. *Fertil Steril.* 66:1, 1996

171. Ankum WM, Mol BW, van der Veen F, Bossuyt PM. Risk factors for ectopic pregnancy: A meta-analysis. *Fertil Steril.* 65:1093, 1996

172. Westrom L. Influence of sexually transmitted diseases on sterility and ectopic pregnancy. *Acta Eur Fertil.* 16:21, 1985

173. Westrom L, Joesoef R, Reynolds G, et al. Pelvic inflammatory disease and fertility. A cohort study of 1,844 women with laparoscopically verified disease and 657 control women with normal laparoscopic results. *Sex Transm Dis.* 19:185, 1992

174. Chow JM, Yonekura ML, Richwald GA, et al. The association between Chlamydia trachomatis and ectopic pregnancy. A matched-pair, case-control study. *JAMA.* 263: 3164, 1990

175. Ni HY, Daling JR, Chu J, et al. Previous abdominal surgery and tubal pregnancy. *Obstet Gynecol.* 75:919, 1990

176. Hallatt JG. Tubal conservation in ectopic pregnancy: A study of 200 cases. *Am J Obstet Gynecol.* 154:1216, 1986

177. Langer R, Bukovsky I, Herman A, et al. Conservative surgery for tubal pregnancy. *Fertil Steril.* 38:427, 1982

178. McCausland AM. Recanalization and fistulization of the fallopian tubes are thought to be the causes of pregnancies following female sterilization. *Am J Obstet Gynecol.* 139:114, 1981

179. Holt VL, Chu J, Daling JR, et al. Tubal sterilization and subsequent ectopic pregnancy. A case-control study. *JAMA.* 266:242, 1991

180. Lennox CE, Mills JA, James GB. Reversal of female sterilisation: A comparative study. *Contraception.* 35:19, 1987

181. A multinational case-control study of ectopic pregnancy. The World Health Organization's Special Programme of Research, Development and Research Training in Human Reproduction: Task Force on Intrauterine Devices for Fertility Regulation. *Clin Reprod Fertil.* 3:131, 1985

182. Ory HW. Ectopic pregnancy and intrauterine contraceptive devices: New perspectives. The Women's Health Study. *Obstet Gynecol.* 57:137, 1981

183. Sivin I. Dose- and age-dependent ectopic pregnancy risks with intrauterine contraception. *Obstet Gynecol.* 78:291, 1991

184. Liukko P, Erkkola R, Laakso L. Ectopic pregnancies during use of low-dose progestogens for oral contraception. *Contraception.* 16:575, 1977

185. Shoupe D, Mishell DR, Jr., Bopp BL, Fielding M. The significance of bleeding patterns in Norplant implant users. *Obstet Gynecol.* 77:256, 1991

186. Gemzell C, Guillome J, Wang CF. Ectopic pregnancy following treatment with human gonadotropins. *Am J Obstet Gynecol.* 143:761, 1982

187. Fernandez H, Coste J, Job-Spira N. Controlled ovarian hyperstimulation as a risk factor for ectopic pregnancy. Obstet Gynecol. 78:656, 1991

188. Steptoe PC, Edwards RG. Reimplantation of a human embryo with subsequent tubal pregnancy. *Lancet.* 1:880, 1976

189. Herman A, Ron-El R, Golan A, et al. The role of tubal pathology and other parameters in ectopic pregnancies occurring in in vitro fertilization and embryo transfer. *Fertil Steril.* 54:864, 1990

190. Dor J, Seidman DS, Levran D, et al. The incidence of combined intrauterine and extrauterine pregnancy after in vitro fertilization and embryo transfer. *Fertil Steril.* 55:833, 1991

191. Herbst AL, Hubby MM, Blough RR, Azizi F. A comparison of pregnancy experience in DES-exposed and DES-unexposed daughters. *J Reprod Med.* 24:62, 1980

192. Barnes AB, Colton T, Gundersen J, et al. Fertility and outcome of pregnancy in women exposed in utero to diethylstilbestrol. *N Engl J Med.* 302:609, 1980

193. Dubuisson JB, Aubriot FX, Cardone V, Vacher-Lavenu MC. Tubal causes of ectopic pregnancy. *Fertil Steril.* 46:970, 1986

194. Handler A, Davis F, Ferre C, Yeko T. The relationship of smoking and ectopic pregnancy. *Am J Public Health.* 79:1239, 1989

195. Coste J, Job-Spira N, Fernandez H. Increased risk of ectopic pregnancy with maternal cigarette smoking. *Am J Public Health.* 81:199, 1991

196. Stovall TG, Kellerman AL, Ling FW, Buster JE. Emergency department diagnosis of ectopic pregnancy. *Ann Emerg Med.* 19:1098, 1990

197. Storring PL, Gaines-Das RE, Bangham DR. International Reference Preparation of Human Chorionic Gonadotrophin for Immunoassay: Potency estimates in various bioassay and protein binding assay systems; and International Reference Preparations of the alpha and beta subunits of human chorionic gonadotrophin for immunoassay. *J Endocrinol.* 84:295, 1980

198. Kadar N, Freedman M, Zacher M. Further observations on the doubling time of human chorionic gonadotropin in early asymptomatic pregnancies. *Fertil Steril.* 54:783, 1990

199. Kadar N, DeVore G, Romero R. Discriminatory hCG zone: Its use in the sonographic evaluation for ectopic pregnancy. *Obstet Gynecol.* 58:156, 1981

200. Kadar N, Caldwell BV, Romero R. A method of screening for ectopic pregnancy and its indications. *Obstet Gynecol.* 58:162, 1981

201. Kadar N, Romero R. Further observations on serial human chorionic gonadotropin patterns in ectopic pregnancies and spontaneous abortions. *Fertil Steril.* 50:367, 1988

202. Cartwright PS, Moore RA, Dao AH, et al. Serum beta-human chorionic gonadotropin levels relate poorly with the size of a tubal pregnancy. *Fertil Steril.* 48:679, 1987

203. Cole LA, Kardana A, Seifer DB, Bohler HC, Jr. Urine hCG beta-subunit core fragment, a sensitive test for ectopic pregnancy. *J Clin Endocrinol Metab.* 78:497, 1994

204. Stovall TG, Ling FW, Cope BJ, Buster JE. Preventing ruptured ectopic pregnancy with a single serum progesterone. *Am J Obstet Gynecol.* 160:1425, 1989

205. Stovall TG, Ling FW, Andersen RN, Buster JE. Improved sensitivity and specificity of a single measurement of serum progesterone over serial quantitative beta-human chorionic gonadotrophin in screening for ectopic pregnancy. *Hum Reprod.* 7:723, 1992

206. Cowan BD, Vandermolen DT, Long CA, Whitworth NS. Receiver-operator characteristic, efficiency analysis, and predictive value of serum progesterone concentration as a test for abnormal gestations. *Am J Obstet Gynecol.* 166:1729, 1992

207. McCord ML, Muram D, Buster JE, et al. Single serum progesterone as a screen for ectopic pregnancy: Exchanging specificity and sensitivity to obtain optimal test performance. *Fertil Steril.* 66:513, 1996

208. Guillaume J, Benjamin F, Sicuranza BJ, et al. Serum estradiol as an aid in the diagnosis of ectopic pregnancy. *Obstet Gynecol.* 76:1126, 1990

209. Lavie O, Beller U, Neuman M, et al. Maternal serum creatine kinase: A possible predictor of tubal pregnancy. *Am J Obstet Gynecol.* 169:1149, 1993

210. Duncan WC, Sweeting VM, Cawood P, Illingworth PJ. Measurement of creatine kinase activity and diagnosis of ectopic pregnancy. *Br J Obstet Gynaecol.* 102:233, 1995

211. Korhonen J, Alfthan H, Stenman UH, Ylostalo P. Failure of creatine kinase to predict ectopic pregnancy. *Fertil Steril.* 65:922, 1996

212. Vandermolen DT, Borzelleca JF. Serum creatine kinase does not predict ectopic pregnancy. *Fertil Steril.* 65:916, 1996

213. Qasim SM, Trias A, Sachdev R, Kemmann E. Evaluation of serum creatine kinase levels in ectopic pregnancy. *Fertil Steril.* 65:443, 1996

214. Bell RJ, Eddie LW, Lester AR, et al. Relaxin in human pregnancy serum measured with an homologous radioimmunoassay. *Obstet Gynecol.* 69:585, 1987

215. Stabile I, Olajide F, Chard T, Grudzinskas JG. Circulating levels of placental protein 14 in ectopic pregnancy. *Br J Obstet Gynaecol.* 101:762, 1994

216. Cacciatore B, Stenman UH, Ylostalo P. Comparison of abdominal and vaginal sonography in suspected ectopic pregnancy. *Obstet Gynecol.* 73:770, 1989

217. Timor-Tritsch IE, Yeh MN, Peisner DB, et al. The use of transvaginal ultrasonography in the diagnosis of ectopic pregnancy. *Am J Obstet Gynecol.* 161:157, 1989

218. Fleischer AC, Pennell RG, McKee MS, et al. Ectopic pregnancy: Features at transvaginal sonography. *Radiology.* 174:375, 1990

219. Cacciatore B, Tiitinen A, Stenman UH, Ylostalo P. Normal early pregnancy: Serum hCG levels and vaginal ultrasonography findings. *Br J Obstet Gynaecol.* 97:899, 1990

220. Nyberg DA, Laing FC, Filly RA, et al. Ultrasonographic differentiation of the gestational sac of early intrauterine

pregnancy from the pseudogestational sac of ectopic pregnancy. *Radiology.* 146:755, 1983

221. Nyberg DA, Hughes MP, Mack LA, Wang KY. Extra-uterine findings of ectopic pregnancy of transvaginal US: Importance of echogenic fluid. *Radiology.* 178:823, 1991

222. Rottem S, Thaler I, Levron J, et al. Criteria for transvaginal sonographic diagnosis of ectopic pregnancy. *J Clin Ultrasound.* 18:274, 1990

223. Fossum GT, Davajan V, Kletsky OA. Early detection of pregnancy with transvaginal ultrasound. *Fertil Steril.* 49:788, 1988

224. Nyberg DA, Mack LA, Laing FC, Jeffrey RB. Early pregnancy complications: Endovaginal sonographic findings correlated with human chorionic gonadotropin levels. *Radiology.* 167:619, 1988

225. Bernaschek G, Rudelstorfer R, Csaicsich P. Vaginal sonography versus serum human chorionic gonadotropin in early detection of pregnancy. *Am J Obstet Gynecol.* 158:608, 1988

226. Hay DL, de Crespigny LC, McKenna M. Monitoring early pregnancy with transvaginal ultrasound and choriogonadotrophin levels. *Aust NZ J Obstet Gynaecol.* 29:165, 1989

227. Bateman BG, Nunley WC, Jr., Kolp LA, et al. Vaginal sonography findings and hCG dynamics of early intrauterine and tubal pregnancies. *Obstet Gynecol.* 75:421, 1990

228. Cacciatore B, Stenman UH, Ylostalo P. Diagnosis of ectopic pregnancy by vaginal ultrasonography in combination with a discriminatory serum hCG level of 1000 IU/l (IRP). *Br J Obstet Gynaecol.* 97:904, 1990

229. Campbell S, Pearce JM, Hackett G, et al. Qualitative assessment of uteroplacental blood flow: Early screening test for high-risk pregnancies. *Obstet Gynecol.* 68:649, 1986

230. McCowan LM, Ritchie K, Mo LY, et al. Uterine artery flow velocity waveforms in normal and growth-retarded pregnancies. *Am J Obstet Gynecol.* 158:499, 1988

231. Taylor KJ, Ramos IM, Feyock AL, et al. Ectopic pregnancy: Duplex Doppler evaluation. *Radiology.* 173:93, 1989

232. Dillon EH, Feyock AL, Taylor KJ. Pseudogestational sacs: Doppler US differentiation from normal or abnormal intrauterine pregnancies. *Radiology.* 176:359, 1990

233. Emerson DS, Cartier MS, Altieri LA, et al. Diagnostic efficacy of endovaginal color Doppler flow imaging in an ectopic pregnancy screening program. *Radiology.* 183:413, 1992

234. Stovall TG, Ling FW, Carson SA, Buster JE. Serum progesterone and uterine curettage in differential diagnosis of ectopic pregnancy. *Fertil Steril.* 57:456, 1992

235. Kurman RJ, Main CS, Chen HC. Intermediate trophoblast: A distinctive form of trophoblast with specific morphological, biochemical and functional features. *Placenta.* 5:349, 1984

236. Vermesh M, Graczykowski JW, Sauer MV. Reevaluation of the role of culdocentesis in the management of ectopic pregnancy. *Am J Obstet Gynecol.* 162:411, 1990

237. Confino E, Binor Z, Molo MW, Radwanska E. Selective salpingography for the diagnosis and treatment of early tubal pregnancy. *Fertil Steril.* 62:286, 1994

238. Garcia AJ, Aubert JM, Sama J, Josimovich JB. Expectant management of presumed ectopic pregnancies. *Fertil Steril.* 48:395, 1987

239. Ylostalo P, Cacciatore B, Sjoberg J, et al. Expectant management of ectopic pregnancy. *Obstet Gynecol.* 80:345, 1992

240. Korhonen J, Stenman UH, Ylostalo P. Serum human chorionic gonadotropin dynamics during spontaneous resolution of ectopic pregnancy. *Fertil Steril.* 61:632, 1994

241. Fernandez H, Frydman R. Abstention therapeutique dans la grossesse extra-uterine. *Contracept Fertil Sex.* 22:410, 1994

242. Shalev E, Peleg D, Tsabari A, et al. Spontaneous resolution of ectopic tubal pregnancy: Natural history. *Fertil Steril.* 63:15, 1995

243. Trio D, Strobelt N, Picciolo C, et al. Prognostic factors for successful expectant management of ectopic pregnancy. *Fertil Steril.* 63:469, 1995

244. Cacciatore B, Korhonen J, Stenman UH, Ylostalo P. Transvaginal sonography and serum hCG in monitoring of presumed ectopic pregnancies selected for expectant management. *Ultrasound Obstet Gynecol.* 5:297, 1995

245. Berkowitz RS, Goldstein DP, Jones MA, et al. Methotrexate with citrovorum factor rescue: Reduced chemotherapy toxicity in the management of gestational trophoblastic neoplasms. *Cancer.* 45:423, 1980

246. Berkowitz RS, Goldstein DP, Bernstein MR. Ten year's experience with methotrexate and folinic acid as primary therapy for gestational trophoblastic disease. *Gynecol Oncol.* 23:111, 1986

247. Rustin GJ, Rustin F, Dent J, et al. No increase in second tumors after cytotoxic chemotherapy for gestational trophoblastic tumors. *N Engl J Med.* 308:473, 1983

248. Tanaka T, Hayashi H, Kutsuzawa T, et al. Treatment of interstitial ectopic pregnancy with methotrexate: Report of a successful case. *Fertil Steril.* 37:851, 1982

249. Ory SJ, Villanueva AL, Sand PK, Tamura RK. Conservative treatment of ectopic pregnancy with methotrexate. *Am J Obstet Gynecol.* 154:1299, 1986

250. Stovall TG, Ling FW, Buster JE. Outpatient chemotherapy of unruptured ectopic pregnancy. *Fertil Steril.* 51:435, 1989

251. Stovall TG, Ling FW, Carson SA, Buster JE. Nonsurgical diagnosis and treatment of tubal pregnancy. *Fertil Steril.* 54:537, 1990

252. Stovall TG, Ling FW, Gray LA, et al. Methotrexate treatment of unruptured ectopic pregnancy: A report of 100 cases. *Obstet Gynecol.* 77:749, 1991

253. Stovall TG, Ling FW, Gray LA. Single-dose methotrexate for treatment of ectopic pregnancy. *Obstet Gynecol.* 77:754, 1991

254. Stovall TG, Ling FW. Single-dose methotrexate: An expanded clinical trial. *Am J Obstet Gynecol.* 168:1759, 1993

255. Brown DL, Felker RE, Stovall TG, et al. Serial endovaginal sonography of ectopic pregnancies treated with methotrexate. *Obstet Gynecol.* 77:406, 1991

256. Neiman RA, Fye KH. Methotrexate induced false photosensitivity reaction. *J Rheumatol.* 12:354, 1985

257. Tulandi T, Hemmings R, Khalifa F. Rupture of ectopic pregnancy in women with low and declining serum beta-human chorionic gonadotropin concentrations. *Fertil Steril.* 56:786, 1991

258. Pouly JL, Chapron C, Manhes H, et al. Multifactorial analysis of fertility after conservative laparoscopic treatment of ectopic pregnancy in a series of 223 patients. *Fertil Steril.* 56:453, 1991

259. Patsner B, Kenigsberg D. Successful treatment of persistent ectopic pregnancy with oral methotrexate therapy. *Fertil Steril.* 50:982, 1988

260. Henderson P, Lim BH. Management of cornual pregnancy with oral methotrexate. *N Z Med J.* 107:227, 1994

261. Menard A, Crequat J, Mandelbrot L, et al. Treatment of unruptured tubal pregnancy by local injection of methotrexate under transvaginal sonographic control. *Fertil Steril.* 54:47, 1990

262. Shalev E, Peleg D, Bustan M, et al. Limited role for intratubal methotrexate treatment of ectopic pregnancy. *Fertil Steril.* 63:20, 1995

263. Fernandez H, Benifla JL, Lelaidier C, et al. Methotrexate treatment of ectopic pregnancy: 100 cases treated by primary transvaginal injection under sonographic control. *Fertil Steril.* 59:773, 1993

264. Fernandez H, Pauthier S, Doumerc S, et al. Ultrasound-guided injection of methotrexate versus laparoscopic salpingotomy in ectopic pregnancy. *Fertil Steril.* 63:25, 1995

265. Oelsner G, Admon D, Shalev E, et al. A new approach for the treatment of interstitial pregnancy. *Fertil Steril.* 59:924, 1993

266. Feichtinger W, Kemeter P. Treatment of unruptured ectopic pregnancy by needling of sac and injection of methotrexate or PG E2 under transvaginal sonography control. Report of 10 cases. *Arch Gynecol Obstet.* 246:85, 1989

267. Hagstrom HG, Hahlin M, Sjoblom P, Lindblom B. Prediction of persistent trophoblastic activity after local prostaglandin F2 alpha injection for ectopic pregnancy. *Hum Reprod.* 9:1170, 1994

268. Laatikainen T, Tuomivaara L, Kaar K. Comparison of a local injection of hyperosmolar glucose solution with salpingostomy for the conservative treatment of tubal pregnancy. *Fertil Steril.* 60:80, 1993

269. Lang P, Weiss PA, Mayer HO. Local application of hyperosmolar glucose solution in tubal pregnancy. *Lancet.* 2:922, 1989

270. Risquez F, Forman R, Maleika F, et al. Transcervical cannulation of the fallopian tube for the management of ectopic pregnancy: Prospective multicenter study. *Fertil Steril.* 58:1131, 1992

271. Ylostalo P, Cacciatore B, Koskimies A, et al. Conservative treatment of ectopic pregnancy. *Ann N Y Acad Sci.* 626:516, 1991

272. Fernandez H, Lelaidier C, Doumerc S, et al. Nonsurgical treatment of heterotopic pregnancy: A report of six cases. *Fertil Steril.* 60:428, 1993

273. Glock JL, Johnson JV, Brumsted JR. Efficacy and safety of single-dose systemic methotrexate in the treatment of ectopic pregnancy. *Fertil Steril.* 62:716, 1994

274. Henry MA, Gentry WL. Single injection of methotrexate for treatment of ectopic pregnancies. *Am J Obstet Gynecol.* 171:1584, 1994

275. Pansky M, Bukovsky I, Golan A, et al. Tubal patency after local methotrexate injection for tubal pregnancy. *Lancet.* 2:967, 1989

276. Zakut H, Sadan O, Katz A, et al. Management of tubal pregnancy with methotrexate. *Br J Obstet Gynaecol.* 96:725, 1989

277. Kojima E, Abe Y, Morita M, et al. The treatment of unruptured tubal pregnancy with intratubal methotrexate injection under laparoscopic control. *Obstet Gynecol.* 75:723, 1990

278. Kooi S, Kock HC. Treatment of tubal pregnancy by local injection of methotrexate after adrenaline injection into the mesosalpinx: A report of 25 patients. *Fertil Steril.* 54:580, 1990

279. Tulandi T, Atri M, Bret P, et al. Transvaginal intratubal methotrexate treatment of ectopic pregnancy. *Fertil Steril.* 58:98, 1992

280. Timonen S, Nieminen U. Tubal pregnancy, choice of operative method of treatment. *Acta Obstet Gynecol Scand.* 46:327, 1967

281. Jeffcoate TNA. Salpingectomy or salpingo-oophorectomy. *Br J Obstet Gynaecol.* 135:74, 1955

282. Vermesh M, Silva PD, Rosen GF, et al. Management of unruptured ectopic gestation by linear salpingostomy: A prospective, randomized clinical trial of laparoscopy versus laparotomy. *Obstet Gynecol.* 73:400, 1989

283. Stromme WB. Salpingotomy for tubal pregnancy. *Obstet Gynecol.* 1:472, 1953

284. Vermesh M. Conservative management of ectopic gestation. *Fertil Steril.* 51:559, 1989

285. DeCherney A, Kase N. The conservative surgical management of unruptured ectopic pregnancy. *Obstet Gynecol.* 54:451, 1979

286. DeCherney AH, Maheaux R, Naftolin F. Salpingostomy for ectopic pregnancy in the sole patent oviduct: Reproductive outcome. *Fertil Steril.* 37:619, 1982

287. Valle JA, Lifchez AS. Reproductive outcome following conservative surgery for tubal pregnancy in women with a single fallopian tube. *Fertil Steril.* 39:316, 1983

288. Tulandi T, Guralnick M. Treatment of tubal ectopic pregnancy by salpingotomy with or without tubal suturing and salpingectomy. *Fertil Steril.* 55:53, 1991

289. Bruhat MA, Manhes H, Mage G, Pouly JL. Treatment of ectopic pregnancy by means of laparoscopy. *Fertil Steril.* 33:411, 1980

290. Cartwright PS, Herbert CMD, Maxson WS. Operative laparoscopy for the management of tubal pregnancy. *J Reprod Med.* 31:589, 1986

291. Bornstein S, Kahn J, Fausone V. Treatment of ectopic pregnancy with laparoscopic resection in a community hospital. *J Reprod Med.* 32:590, 1987

292. DeCherney AH, Diamond MP. Laparoscopic salpingostomy for ectopic pregnancy. *Obstet Gynecol.* 70:948, 1987

293. Mecke H, Argiriou CSK. Die Behandlung der Tubargravidität per pelviskopiam—Komplikationen, Schwangerschafts- und Rezidivraten. *Geburtshilfe Frauenheilkd.* 51:549, 1991

294. Chapron C, Pouly JL, Wattiez A, et al. Results of conservative laparoscopic treatment of isthmic ectopic pregnancies: A 26 case study. *Hum Reprod.* 7:422, 1992

295. Langebrekke A, Sornes T, Urnes A. Fertility outcome after treatment of tubal pregnancy by laparoscopic laser surgery. *Acta Obstet Gynecol Scand.* 72:547, 1993

296. DeCherney AH, Boyers SP. Isthmic ectopic pregnancy: Segmental resection as the treatment of choice. *Fertil Steril.* 44:307, 1985

297. Senterman M, Jibodh R, Tulandi T. Histopathologic study of ampullary and isthmic tubal ectopic pregnancy. *Am J Obstet Gynecol.* 159:939, 1988

298. Confino E, Gleicher N. Conservative surgical management of interstitial pregnancy. *Fertil Steril.* 52:600, 1989

299. Tulandi T, Monton L. Conservative surgical management of interstitial pregnancy. *Fertil Steril.* 53:581, 1990

300. Nezhat C, Nezhat F. Conservative management of ectopic gestation. *Fertil Steril.* 53:382, 1990

301. Wood C, Hurley V. Ultrasound diagnosis and laparoscopic excision of an interstitial ectopic pregnancy. *Aust NZ J Obstet Gynaecol.* 32:371, 1992

302. Tulandi T, Vilos G, Gomel V. Laparoscopic treatment of interstitial pregnancy. *Obstet Gynecol.* 85:465, 1995

303. Biljan MM, Edwards GJ, Kingsland CR. Delayed haemorrhage of a persistent ectopic pregnancy following expression of ampullar ectopic pregnancy. *Br J Obstet Gynaecol.* 100:1053, 1993

304. Sherman D, Langer R, Herman A, et al. Reproductive outcome after fimbrial evacuation of tubal pregnancy. *Fertil Steril.* 47:420, 1987

305. Shapiro HI, Adler DH. Excision of an ectopic pregnancy through the laparoscope. *Am J Obstet Gynecol.* 117:290, 1973

306. DeCherney AH, Romero R, Naftolin F. Surgical management of unruptured ectopic pregnancy. *Fertil Steril.* 35:21, 1981

307. Brumsted J, Kessler C, Gibson C, et al. A comparison of laparoscopy and laparotomy for the treatment of ectopic pregnancy. *Obstet Gynecol.* 71:889, 1988

308. Thatcher SS, Grainger DA, True LD, DeCherney AH. Pelvic trophoblastic implants after laparoscopic removal of a tubal pregnancy. *Obstet Gynecol.* 74:514, 1989

309. Beck E, Siebzehnrubl E, Jager W, et al. Disseminierte intraperitoneale Trophoblast-Aussaat nach Laparoskopisch behandelter Extrauteringraviditat. *Geburtshilfe Frauenheilkd.* 51:939, 1991

310. Sjogren P, Hansen F. Disseminated implantation of peritoneal trophoblastic tissue secondary to laparoscopic removal of a tubal pregnancy. *Acta Obstet Gynecol Scand.* 75:408, 1996

311. Lundorff P, Hahlin M, Sjoblom P, Lindblom B. Persistent trophoblast after conservative treatment of tubal pregnancy: Prediction and detection. *Obstet Gynecol.* 77:129, 1991

312. Hoppe DE, Bekkar BE, Nager CW. Single-dose systemic methotrexate for the treatment of persistent ectopic pregnancy after conservative surgery. *Obstet Gynecol.* 83:51, 1994

313. Parker J, Thompson D. Persistent ectopic pregnancy after conservative management successful treatment with single-dose intramuscular methotrexate. *Aust NZ J Obstet Gynaecol.* 34:99, 1994

314. Rose PG, Cohen SM. Methotrexate therapy for persistent ectopic pregnancy after conservative laparoscopic management. *Obstet Gynecol.* 76:947, 1990

315. DiMarchi JM, Cyka RE. Oral methotrexate for persistent ectopic pregnancy. A case report. *J Reprod Med.* 37:659, 1992

316. Bengtsson G, Bryman I, Thorburn J, Lindblom B. Low-dose oral methotrexate as second-line therapy for persistent trophoblast after conservative treatment of ectopic pregnancy. *Obstet Gynecol.* 79:589, 1992

317. Grimes DA, Geary FH, Jr., Hatcher RA. Rh immunoglobulin utilization after ectopic pregnancy. *Am J Obstet Gynecol.* 140:246, 1981

318. Mueller BA, Daling JR, Weiss NS, et al. Tubal pregnancy and the risk of subsequent infertility. *Obstet Gynecol.* 69:722, 1987

319. Mecke H, Semm K, Freys I, et al. Incidence of adhesions in the true pelvis after pelviscopic operative treatment of tubal pregnancy. *Gynecol Obstet Invest.* 28:202, 1989

320. Tuomivaara L, Kauppila A. Radical or conservative surgery for ectopic pregnancy? A follow-up study of fertility of 323 patients. *Fertil Steril.* 50:580, 1988

321. Langer R, Raziel A, Ron-El R, et al. Reproductive outcome after conservative surgery for unruptured tubal pregnancy—A 15-year experience. *Fertil Steril.* 53:227, 1990

322. DeCherney AH, Silidker JS, Mezer HC, Tarlatzis BC. Reproductive outcome following two ectopic pregnancies. *Fertil Steril.* 43:82, 1985

Chapter 32

DIAGNOSIS AND MANAGEMENT OF ENDOMETRIOSIS

Michael M. Guarnaccia and David L. Olive

Endometriosis is a disease commonly identified in the reproductive-age woman. Despite its wide prevalence, it remains one of the most enigmatic disorders in gynecology. The literature on endometriosis is extensive, but often contradictory or inadequate. This has led to a number of traditional concepts regarding aspects of the disease that may or may not be based upon facts.

This chapter provides a thorough review of the current state of knowledge we possess for endometriosis. The clinical aspects of the disease will be summarized, as will the theories regarding pathogenesis of both pain and infertility. Finally, treatment options will be evaluated and reasonable conclusions drawn from the available data.

Definition

Endometriosis is defined as the presence of endometrial tissue in an ectopic location. By "ectopic," the implication is that the endometrium is not located within the uterine cavity (normal location) or within the myometrium (adenomyosis). Histologically, authors have required a number of different criteria to make the diagnosis of endometriosis. Most commonly, the presence of both glands and stromal tissue is cited as necessary to identify the disorder, although it is unclear to what degree a single tissue component (when found alone) can act pathologically.

PATHOGENESIS

Pathogenesis of endometriosis consists of several components: histogenesis, etiology, and factors critical for growth and maintenance. Early studies were directed at an understanding of the histogenic origin of the tissue, whereas recent investigation has centered upon etiologic

and growth factors responsible for the development of the ectopic tissue.

Histogenesis

Numerous theories of histogenesis have been proposed by many of the leading investigators in the field.[1] However, three main theories dominate current thinking.

The original theory proposed for the origin of ectopic endometriosis was coelomic metaplasia. This theory states that endometriosis develops from metaplasia of cells lining the pelvic peritoneum. The basis of this concept derives from the observation that Müllerian ducts, germinal epithelium, and pelvic peritoneum all derive from the same source—epithelium of the coelomic wall. The theory was initially advanced by the eminent pathologist Robert Meyer, who provided evidence that tissue differentiation can proceed in selected tissue in the adult.[2,3] However, neither he nor subsequent investigators have been able to demonstrate that differentiated peritoneal cells maintain a capacity for further differentiation.

In addition to our lacking substantive evidence for coelomic metaplasia as the source of endometriotic tissue, there are several issues that create serious doubt as to the validity of the concept. If there were significant potential for metaplastic transformation of peritoneum, the phenomenon should also be seen in males. However, only a handful of such cases have been reported, and each involved prostatic carcinoma treated with high-dose estrogen therapy.[4–7] Such rarities may well represent hyperplasia and spread from endometrial cell rests of the prostatic utricle, a remnant of the Müllerian duct in males. A second issue involves distribution of the disease: If metaplasia of coelomic tissue is the source, then all such tissue should contain the same developmental potential. Although the coelomic membrane covers both the abdominal and thoracic cavities,[8,9] endometriosis is seen primarily in the pelvis. Finally, if the disease tissue derives from a metaplastic process, the incidence should increase with advancing age. In reality, the disease is virtually limited to reproductive-age women. To explain the observed age distribution, a theory of estrogen-induced metaplasia must be involved. However, this is inconsistent with a low incidence in anovulatory women with chronically elevated estrogen levels.

The theory of coelomic metaplasia is a theory that has persisted for many years. However, to date there is no scientific evidence to help validate the theory. It remains for proponents of this idea to demonstrate that coelomic metaplasia can indeed result in endometriosis.

A second theory of histogenesis is transplantation of shed uterine endometrium to ectopic locations.[10] A number of routes of dissemination of the tissue have been proposed, including lymphatic dissemination, vascular spread, iatrogenic transplantation, and retrograde menstruation.

A critical aspect of this theory is that cast-off endometrium cells remain viable and capable of implanting. Furthermore, it proposes that the tissue distribution has the capacity to sustain implantation. Considerable research has established that shed endometrial cells are viable in vitro.[11,12] In fact, such cells have been maintained in culture for up to 2 mo.[13] Early studies designed to determine the implantation capacity of such cells in vivo were disappointing.[14,15] However, subsequent experiments involving both the monkey[16] and human[17,18] have shown that placement of endometrial tissue into ectopic locations will indeed result in endometriosis.

It thus appears that endometrial tissue, when shed, is indeed viable and capable of resulting in endometriosis. However, direct evidence that this process is via implantation of the shed cells is lacking. Further investigation into this aspect of the theory is required to demonstrate its validity definitively.

The induction theory of endometriosis is a combination of the other two proposals. It states that substances from shed endometrium induce undifferentiated mesenchyme to form endometriosis. Several lines of investigation in the rabbit support this theory. First, deposition of both fresh and denatured endometrium into subcutaneous tissue resulted in endometrial cyst formation.[19] Subsequently, endometrium-containing millipore chambers were placed in rabbit peritoneal cavities for up to 39 weeks.[20,21] Upon excision, endometrial-like glands were observed in the tissue adjacent to the chambers. Interestingly, no endometrial stroma was induced in either of these experiments. Whether this induction is merely the well-recognized process of stromal induction of adjacent epithelium,[22] or the induction of complete endometrium capable of growth and development, is unclear and a subject for future investigation.

Etiology

The origin of endometriosis (histogenesis) should not be confused with factors causing the disease (etiology). Regardless of which theory of histogenesis is invoked, additional etiologic factors must be responsible for expression of the disease. Although numerous causative factors have been postulated to play a role in the development of endometriosis, two theories predominate.

Retrograde menstruation is a well-established phenomenon. Data available from women undergoing peritoneal dialysis[23] and laparoscopy[24,25] at the time of menses suggest that 76 to 90 percent of women have retrograde flow. If this occurrence is important to the development of endometriosis, it would follow that women with an increase in such flow should have a greater incidence of endometriosis. This appears to be the case in that women with Müllerian anomalies and outflow tract obstruction have an increased incidence of disease.[26]

Circumstantial evidence supporting the role of retrograde menstruation as an etiologic factor is found in data reporting relative hypotonia of the uterotubal junction in women with endometriosis.[27] Furthermore, endometrial tissue is refluxed into the peritoneal cavity in women with endometriosis more frequently than in controls with patent tubes but no endometriosis.[28] Finally, the anatomic distribution of endometriotic implants clearly supports this hypothesis, as implants are found much more commonly in dependent areas of the pelvis.[29] Taken together, these pieces of evidence strongly implicate retrograde menstruation as an etiologic factor in the development of endometriosis.

Given the near universality of retrograde menstruation, it is likely that additional etiologic factors are responsible for initiation of the disease. Recently, studies have suggested altered immune function to be a contributory factor in the development of endometriosis. Abnormalities in T-cell mediated cytotoxicity,[30,31] B-cell function with autoantibody production,[32,33] and complement deposition[28,34] have been reported. Clearly, there is an association between endometriosis and altered immunity. However, the mechanism(s) by which these immunologic aberrations result in endometriosis awaits further study.

Olive and Hammond suggested that retrograde menstruation and deficient cellular immunity are both important etiologic factors.[35] They proposed that development of endometriosis occurs when the amount of retrograde seeding of endometrial tissue exceeds the capacity of the immune system to eliminate menstrual debris (Fig 32–1). However, this theory has yet to be substantiated; furthermore, it remains a mystery as to why in the nondiseased subject the body would routinely remove autologous tissue despite its ectopic locale.

Several lines of investigation have centered on interleukin-8 (IL-8) and monocyte chemotactic protein-1

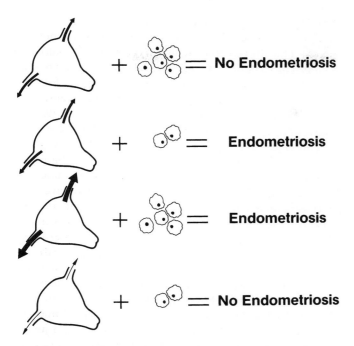

Figure 32–1. Theory for the etiology of endometriosis based upon degree of retrograde menstruation and immunologic response. Women who have either an inadequate response to normal amounts of retrograde flow or those who have a large degree of retrograde flow exceeding their immunologic response capacity would be susceptible to endometriosis. *(Reproduced, with permission, from Olive DL, Henderson DY. Obstet Gynecol. 81:414, 1993.)*

(MCP-1), highly cell-specific chemoattractants in the pathogenesis of endometriosis. IL-8 is a potent angiogenic agent, chemoattractant, and activating cytokine for granulocytes, while MCP-1 is a chemoattractant and activating cytokine for monocytes and macrophages. Sources of these cytokines include endometrium (with retrograde menstrual debris possibly providing sufficient amounts) and peritoneal mesothelium. The concentrations of MCP-1 and IL-8 are elevated in the peritoneal fluids of women with endometriosis compared to disease-free women, and the levels correlate with the severity of the disease.[36,37] These preliminary data serve to explain the process of endometriosis generation. Retrograde menstruation is a mandatory component, with implantation and growth requiring estrogen in conjunction with growth factors from peritoneal macrophages. In turn, these macrophages are recruited via chemoattractants such as IL-8 and MCP-1, which are produced by endometrium and/or peritoneum. Added to this may be a deficiency in the response by cytotoxic T-cells and NK-cells, leading to the passive promotion of endometriosis.

Growth and Maintenance

It is well known that endometrium responds to ovarian steroids in a predictable, cyclic manner in the normal ovulatory female. Estrogen stimulates endometrial prolifera-

tion, whereas progesterone inhibits the proliferative action and creates tissue stability. Recent studies suggest, however, that this mitogenic effect is not merely a direct effect of estrogen but rather a complex interaction involving growth factors.[38] Although our current understanding is far from complete, it appears that endometrium functions similarly to other mesothelial tissues by requiring an initiating stimulus (complement factor) to allow response to mitogenic action (progression factor).[39]

Endometriosis appears in general to behave similarly to endometrium in its response to estrogen. The disease is rarely seen in the hypoestrogenic female, and is frequently treated by creating a functional hypoestrogenic state. More detailed information has been obtained from animal models, however. In the monkey, initiation of growth of transplanted endometrium was not dependent upon ovarian steroids, but either estrogen or progesterone was necessary to sustain the implants.[40] Similar results have been reported in the rat model.[41] Such findings would predict progression of disease with pregnancy. However, there appears instead to be a marked variability in response to pregnancy in both the monkey[42] and human,[43] with the majority of women believed to respond with inhibition of growth or regression of endometrial tissue.

The aberrant, unpredictable response to steroid hormones is seen in the histology of implants. Normal endometrium undergoes cyclic histologic changes in response to ovarian hormonal cyclicity. The majority of endometriotic implants do not demonstrate this typical cyclic histology, and those that do are often asynchronous with active tissue.[44] It is unclear whether this is due to abnormal hormonal responsiveness because of altered steroid receptor populations, an altered epithelial-stromal relationship, aberrant blood supply, or the presence of an associated inflammatory reaction.

An additional variable in the growth of ectopic endometrium is the presence of growth factors. An association between endometriosis and peritoneal macrophages has long been recognized.[45] Macrophages are known producers of growth factors that bestow competence upon mesothelial tissue, allowing response to specific mitogens.[46,47] In endometrium, these macrophage-derived growth factors (MDGFs) allow estrogen to induce cell proliferation (Fig 32–2).[38] It may well be that in women with enhanced MDGF secretion, as well as relative hyperestrogenism, conditions may be optimal for ectopic endometrial implantation and growth. Clearly, given the nature of the hormonal response of endometrial implants, further investigation is needed to clarify this picture.

PREVALENCE AND EPIDEMIOLOGY

Endometriosis appears as a disease nearly exclusively of reproductive-age women. The mean age of diagnosis has

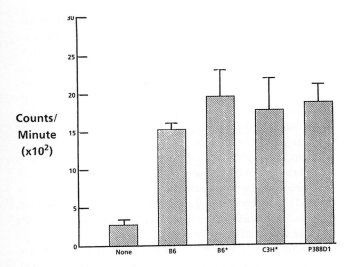

Figure 32–2. Effect of addition of 10 percent macrophage-conditioned media (MCM) on endometrial stromal cell proliferation as measured by [³H] thymidine incorporation. Cells were harvested 48 hr after planting. None = no MCM supplementation; B6* = MCM from peptone-stimulated macrophages of C3H/Hej mice; P388D₁ = MCM from the P388D₁ = murine macrophage-like cell line.) *(Reproduced, with permission, from Olive DL, Montoya I, Riehl RM, Schenken RS. Macrophage-conditioned media enhance endometrial stromal cell proliferation in vitro. Am J Obstet Gynecol. 164: 953–958, 1991.)*

been reported to be from 25 to 29 yr,[48,49] although this figure is largely dependent upon the mechanism by which diagnosis is made. Because accurate diagnosis currently requires laparoscopy, it is likely that the disease is present to a significant extent prior to this age. Indeed, one report places mean onset of endometriosis-related symptoms to age 20.

Endometriosis is rarely found in the pre-menarchal female, and has been reported to be symptomatic in such women. The rate of occurrence in adolescents is unknown but evidently is not rare. In two studies of women under age 20 with chronic pelvic pain or dysmenorrhea unresponsive to medical therapy, endometriosis was found at surgery in 47 to 65 percent of cases.[50,51] Simply considering the teenage years to be a single entity, however, may be misleading, as most documented cases of endometriosis in girls under age 17 are associated with Müllerian anomalies and outflow tract obstruction.[52] Conversely, when the disease is noted in older teens they invariably have normal genital tract development.

Endometriosis is most common during the reproductive years, but it can occur frequently in menopausal women and represents 2 to 4 percent of all women requiring laparoscopy for endometriosis.[53,54] The majority of these cases are a sequela of hormone replacement therapy, but this is not true in all cases.[55]

The "true" prevalence of endometriosis in the general population is difficult to determine. As surgery is required to make the diagnosis definitively, the observed prevalence will vary significantly based upon the indication, type of procedure performed, and skill and experience. The Baylor Gynecologic Collaborative Group found a prevalence of endometriosis of 0.7 percent in women undergoing tubal anastomosis, 1.6 percent at laparoscopic tubal ligation, 11.3 percent at abdominal hysterectomy, and 31 percent at operative laparoscopy.[56] From these data, a 10 percent prevalence in the reproductive-age population can be estimated.

The choice of the population studied has been responsible for the large variations in observed frequency of disease. The prevalence has ranged from 2 to 48 percent in those populations studied, but these figures have been based on the populations studied. The highest rates of endometriosis are found in women undergoing laparoscopy for infertility and pelvic pain, whereas the lowest rates are in those undergoing laparoscopic tubal sterilization.[57]

Endometriosis has long been believed to have a strong racial preponderance. Early studies that purported to show a higher incidence in white women failed to control for potentially confounding variables such as availability of health care, access to contraception, cultural difference in childbearing patterns, attitudes toward menses and pain, and incidence of sexually transmitted diseases. When these factors are controlled, incidence rates appear similar among the races.[58,59] One notable exception to this is Japanese women, in whom there appears to be twice the incidence found in whites, despite similar socioeconomic backgrounds.[60] Investigations undertaken recently have noted an increased rate of endometriosis among Asian women in comparison to other ethnic groups.[57] They noted a higher probability of disease among Asian women (odds ratio, 8.6) compared with Caucasian women after controlling for the effect of age, the number of live births, and income. When other socioeconomic factors were controlled for (marital status, income level, and education), no association with endometriosis was noted.

A familial tendency for endometriosis has been uncovered in a number of reports. Ranney, in 1971, first demonstrated hereditary tendencies for the disease among 53 families retrospectively reviewed.[61] Recent investigations have suggested that genetic transmission is highly likely, with the most probable mode of inheritance being polygenic and multifactorial.[62,63] A current search is ongoing for the endometriosis gene. The OXEGENE project has targeted sister–sister pairs with advanced, documented endometriosis as a source to identify a gene variant unique to this population. Results will be forthcoming.

CLINICAL PRESENTATION AND DIAGNOSIS

Symptoms

Endometriosis is associated with a wide variety of symptoms, although many with the disease are entirely asymptomatic. While some symptoms may strongly suggest the diagnosis, none is indicative of the disease.

A common symptom associated with endometriosis is infertility. Endometriosis has been linked to aberrations in every step of the reproductive process. Moderate to severe disease can lead to marked anatomic alterations and subsequent changes in the tubo-ovarian relationship. Disturbances in ovulation due to intermittent anovulation, abnormal follicular development, and/or luteal phase defects have been suggested as possible mechanisms. The rate of endometriosis in the infertile population undergoing surgical evaluation has ranged from 4.5 to 33 percent, with a mean of 14 percent.[64] One comparative trial found a 21 percent incidence of endometriosis in infertile women undergoing laparoscopic evaluation, whereas only 2 percent of women experiencing laparoscopic tubal sterilization were found to have the disease.[65] Endometriosis thus appears to be well associated with infertility. Unfortunately, the incidence of infertility in women with endometriosis cannot be adequately assessed.

Pelvic pain is also a common complaint in the woman with endometriosis. Secondary dysmenorrhea or worsening primary dysmenorrhea is commonly seen among these patients. Dyspareunia is also a frequent complaint, and is most often reported with uterosacral ligament involvement. Other types of "pelvic" pain include noncyclic lower abdominal pain and backaches. In addition, pain symptoms may be site specific when endometriosis is found in unusual locations outside the pelvis. The heterogeneity of the disease process, however, suggests that a range of pathophysiologic processes are involved. Different types of lesions cause pain via different routes.

Dysfunctional uterine bleeding is often linked to endometriosis. Various studies have reported high rates of abdominal bleeding in these patients, although in most cases associated pelvic pathology was present to explain the bleeding pattern.[55,66] Anovulation rates in women with endometriosis are reported to be 9 to 17 percent.[67,68] However, such studies lack control groups, utilize inconsistent criteria for the diagnosis of anovulation, and have not evaluated the frequency of repetitive anovulatory cycles. Thus, there is no evidence at present that endometriosis is a cause of dysfunctional uterine bleeding.

Physical Findings

Physical findings associated with endometriosis are variable and dependent on the severity and location of disease as well as the character of the population under study. Physical examination may be of limited value in women with endometriosis, as patients with extensive disease often have minimal findings. As disease manifestations often become more pronounced and areas of ec-

topic endometrial implantation more tender during the menses, it is often useful to examine the patient during the perimenstrual period. Common signs include nodularity or tenderness of the cul-de-sac, parametrial thickening, and adnexal masses. A fixed, retrodisplaced uterus may also be seen with extensive disease. Rarely, cutaneous lesions may be present in such locations as the vagina, perineum, and umbilicus, and within surgical scars. Ascites has also been reported.[69]

Diagnostic Methods

Three classes of technology have been used to diagnose and follow patients with endometriosis: serum markers, imaging techniques, and laparoscopic examination of the peritoneal cavity.

The monoclonal antibody OC-125 identifies the antigenic determinant CA-125, originally a product of an ovarian epithelial tumor. The antigen has subsequently been found in most Müllerian derivatives and tissue derived from the coelomic membrane. An elevated concentration of CA-125 has been found in the peripheral blood of some women with endometriosis.[70] Unfortunately, extensive evaluation has revealed that testing for CA-125 levels is insufficiently sensitive or specific to be useful in diagnostic screening for the disease.[71–73] Furthermore, a placebo-controlled trial has questioned the value of following serum CA-125 levels to monitor treatment effectiveness.[74]

Recent development of a second-generation CA-125 assay has increased interest in its use. Hornstein and colleagues recently have compared the serum CA-125 concentrations in women with and without endometriosis using both the older assay and the new CA-125 assay in an effort to determine if the newer assay has improved clinical utility. They found that the sensitivity and specificity of the newer assay was slightly improved; however, they found no significant increase in the rate of detection of endometriosis over the old assay.[75]

Another serum protein, PP14, originates nearly exclusively in human secretory endometrium. The protein is known to vary in concentration throughout the menstrual cycle, and research has demonstrated a significant contribution to serum PP14 levels by active endometriotic tissue.[76] More recently, it has been shown that superficial endometriosis secreted both PP14 and CA-125 into the peritoneal cavity, and that more deeply infiltrating lesions secreted these substances into the blood.[77] Further work is clearly needed to investigate the utility of the protein in the diagnosis of endometriosis.

A third approach to serum screening for endometriosis is the use of endometrial antibody determination.[78,79] To date, this test has failed to provide sufficient sensitivity to allow its use as a diagnostic tool. Current work to improve detection methods may yet prove this assay to be of value in screening for endometriosis.

Imaging techniques have been utilized on occasion in attempts to diagnose endometriosis. Ultrasound has proven to be of value in the diagnosis of endometriomas, although specificity is quite low. Also, this technique cannot reliably identify focal implants.

Magnetic resonance imaging (MRI) has demonstrated its value in the diagnosis of endometriosis,[80,81] based on the difference in signal intensity of endometrium compared to other pelvic tissues. Recently, MRI detection of diffuse endometriosis has undergone refinement with the inclusion of both fat-suppression and fat-saturation techniques. Overall diagnostic sensitivities range from 77 to 89 percent versus conventional MRI.[82,83] Two potential roles for MRI remain to be evaluated. One is the identification of endometriosis obscured by pelvic adhesions, which may prove an important screening tool prior to surgery. Second, MRI has potential utility in the evaluation of the response to medical treatment of endometriosis.

Recently, an attempt at diagnosis of endometriosis using immunoscintigraphy with radiolabeled OC-125 fragments has been made; the method proved highly sensitive but fairly nonspecific.[84]

Today, laparoscopy remains the optimal method for diagnosing endometriosis. However, endometriosis is protean in appearance and often may have been missed by the inexperienced surgeon.[85,86] Interestingly, difficulty in identifying the more subtle manifestations of endometriosis may have resulted in an underestimation of endometriosis in young adults. Recently, a pattern of evolution of the lesions has been identified, with subtle appearance in the teenage years and more traditional red or black foci a decade later (Table 32–1).[87] D'Hooghe and colleagues have demonstrated that endometriosis in captive baboons undergoing repeated laparoscopies is a dynamic and moderately progressive disease with periods of development and regression and active remodeling.[88]

Given this wide variation in the appearance of endometriotic lesions (Fig 32–3), simple visualization cannot be relied upon to rule out the disease. To this end, excision of suspect areas of peritoneum is essential to assess the lesions histologically.[89] Nevertheless, some colorless manifestations are extremely subtle. One technique useful to assist the surgeon in identifying these lesions is the "painting" of peritoneal surfaces with bloody peritoneal fluid (Fig 32–4). By allowing the fluid to flow across the peritoneal surface, colorless endometriotic lesions will be highlighted as the red blood cells stream around them.[90] The suspect area can then be excised and histologically examined. A good rule of thumb is that if the peritoneal surface looks unusual, it is endometriosis until proven otherwise.

PATHOLOGY

Peritoneal implants of endometriosis have most commonly been described as bluish-gray "powder burns." This color appears to represent a late manifestation of the evolution of the lesion, and is attributed to some degree of menstrual cyclicity. This bleeding results in eventual encapsulation by fibrotic tissue, as well as hemolysis of the debris.

Additional presentations of ectopic endometrium include non-pigmented, clear vesicles; white plaques; and reddish petechiae or flame-like areas. These implants range from several mm to 2 cm in diameter and may be superficial or invasive.

Endometriotic cysts occur frequently in the ovary. In many, cyclic hemorrhage results in a dark, tarry, "chocolate brown" fluid within the cyst. This fluid appears to be retained by the cyst due to slow absorption by the surrounding cyst wall.

With metabolically active endometriotic lesions, a chronic irritation can develop in the surrounding tissue. This may result in a fibrous reaction, with formation of local scarring and adhesion formation. Foci of endometriosis are frequently found at the base of such adhesions.

TABLE 32–1. EVOLUTION OF COLOR APPEARANCE OF ENDOMETRIOSIS WITH AGE

Color Appearance	No. of Patients	Mean Age (yr) ± SD	Age Range (yr)
Clear papules only	6	21.5 ± 3.5	17–26
Clear papules plus other clear lesions	8	23.0 ± 4.0	17–28
Clear plus any others	14	23.4 ± 4.7	17–31
Red only	16	26.3 ± 5.4	16–38
Red plus any others	22	26.9 ± 5.7	17–43
All nonblack	55	27.9 ± 7.2	17–42
White plus any others	24	28.3 ± 6.9	17–43
Black plus any others	34	28.4 ± 5.8	17–43
White only	8	29.5 ± 5.9	20–39
Black only	48	31.9 ± 7.5	20–52

(Reproduced, with permission, from Redwine DB, Age-related evolution in color appearance of endometriosis. Fertil Steril. 48:1062, 1987)

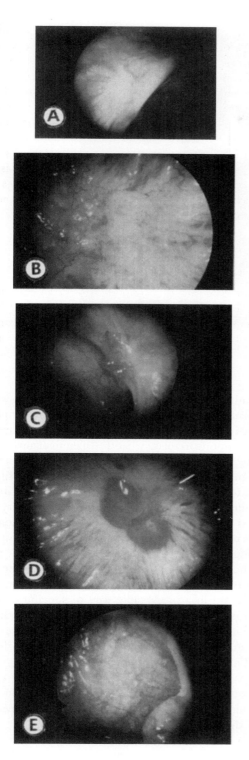

Figure 32–3. Wide variation in appearance of endometriotic lesions. **A.** Circumscribed and thickened patches of specified white peritoneum. **B.** Thickened white peritoneum in the right ovarian fossa with nodular, glistening lesions medially. **C.** Raised, glassy, transluscent, gland-like lesions. **D.** Raised, red, flamelike lesions of the cul-de-sac. **E.** Vesicular superficial excrescences in the right ovarian fossa. *(Reproduced, with permission, from Jansen RPS, Russell P. Nonpigmented endometriosis: clinical, laparoscopic, and pathologic definition. Am J Obstet Gynecol. 155:1154, 1986)*

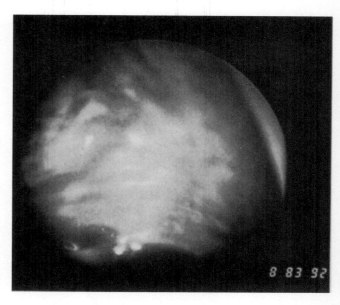

Figure 32–4. Peritoneal blood painting to diagnose endometriosis. Bloody peritoneal fluid has been "painted" onto walls of the right cul-de-sac. Two areas of abnormal peritoneum are highlighted by erythrocytes that stream around them. Both areas were confirmed as endometriosis following excision. *(Reproduced, with permission, from Redwine DB. Peritoneal blood painting: An aid in the diagnosis of endometriosis. Am J Obstet Gynecol. 161:865, 1989)*

Peritoneal pockets have been described as associated with endometriosis for over 60 yr.[91] These pockets are found in roughly 18 percent of women with endometriosis, and two thirds of the structures have endometriotic implants either around the rim or at the base of the defect.[92] Such pockets are thought to represent a primary developmental formation defect of the pelvic peritoneum; the ontologic relationship between these pockets and endometriosis, if any, has yet to be delineated.

Despite the recognition that endometriosis is frequently difficult to identify, recent data suggest the disease may be missed completely due to its presence only as microscopic lesions in visually normal peritoneum.[93] In the otherwise normal pelvis, such lesions were found in 6 percent of women.[94] This finding, however, has been disputed by others who claim "microscopic" disease merely represents "unrecognized" lesions.[95] Clearly, more investigation is needed to determine the validity and significance of this finding.

Microscopically, endometriotic implants should contain endometrial glandular tissue and endometrial stroma and may be accompanied by adjacent fibrosis and hemorrhage (Fig 32–5). Endometromas are quite nondescript, with simple cuboidal epithelium and fibrous tissue surrounding the cyst wall. There may be little evidence of cyclicity aside from the hemorrhagic debris filling the cyst.

Ultrastructurally, endometriotic lesions may or may not demonstrate cycle-dependent changes seen in normal endometrium.[96,97] These include giant mitochondria

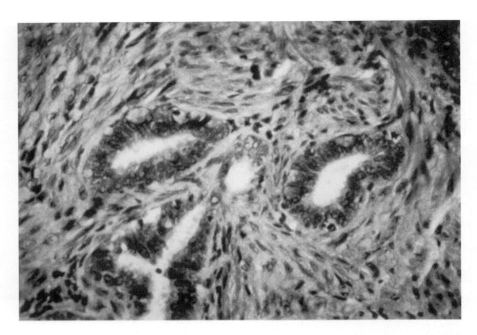

Figure 32–5. Histologic components of peritoneal endometriosis. Endometrial glands and stroma are present, surrounded by fibrovascular tissue. (H&E, original magnification × 275.)

and the appearance of nuclear channel systems coinciding with ovulation. Frequently, collagen fibrils surround the implant with obliteration of standard histologic features. Recently, though estrogen and progesterone receptor content was evaluated in both normal endometrium and peritoneal endometriotic implants. The estrogen receptor content was found to be lower in the endometriotic tissue when compared with endometrium, but the cyclic pattern was similar in both tissues. Progesterone receptor content was similar in both tissues, except during the late secretory phase in ectopic glandular epithelium in which high, persistent progesterone receptor content was observed.[98] It is unclear whether this is due to abnormal hormonal responsiveness because of altered steroid receptor populations, an altered epithelial–stromal relationship, an aberrant blood supply, or the presence of an associated inflammatory reaction.

CLASSIFICATION

Over the years, many classification schemes have been proposed for endometriosis. Early attempts centered around descriptions derived from surgical or histopathologic findings. Riva and colleagues[99] were the first to attempt to quantify the severity of disease by applying scalar criteria to their classification method. This attempt was the forerunner of current classification schemes.

Modern attempts at staging endometriosis have focused less upon the physical manifestations of the disease and more upon the prognosis of affected women. Acosta and associates[100] were the first to correlate the extent of dis-

ease with subsequent pregnancy rates following surgical treatment. Over the next 5 yr, a number of similar approaches to classifying endometriosis were undertaken, each attempting to relate what was seen to chances of conception.[101–103] In 1978, the American Fertility Society convened an expert panel to develop a consensus classification system for the disease. The result was an innovative approach utilizing a scalar scoring system with arbitrary values assigned to each disease locus.[104] In 1985, this scheme was revised to reflect more importance for adnexal adhesions and deep endometriotic invasion (Fig 32–6).[105]

The basic reason for formulating classification systems is to identify similar manifestations of a disease that will respond in a predictable way to specific treatment plans, resulting in reproducible outcome. Unfortunately, all schemes developed to date (including those of the American Fertility Society) have failed to fulfill this purpose. The reasons for this are multiple:

All classification schemes thus far are based upon clinical opinion rather than sophisticated statistical evaluation of the data.

In scalar systems each site endometriosis/adhesions has been arbitrarily assigned points that may or may not reflect true relative risk.

Cutoff thresholds for severity categories are arbitrarily chosen.

The accuracy or precision of these staging systems has never been assessed.

All staging schemes deal exclusively with fertility prognosis, while ignoring other symptoms of the disease.

Patient's Name _____   Date _____

Stage I   (Minimal)   · 1-5
Stage II (Mild)   · 6-15
Stage III (Moderate) · 16-40
Stage IV (Severe)   · >40
Total _____

Laparoscopy _____ Laparotomy _____ Photography _____
Recommended Treatment _____

Prognosis _____

PERITONEUM	ENDOMETRIOSIS	<1cm	1-3cm	>3cm
	Superficial	1	2	4
	Deep	2	4	6
OVARY	R Superficial	1	2	4
	Deep	4	16	20
	L Superficial	1	2	4
	Deep	4	16	20

	POSTERIOR CULDESAC OBLITERATION	Partial	Complete
		4	40

	ADHESIONS	<1/3 Enclosure	1/3-2/3 Enclosure	>2/3 Enclosure
OVARY	R Filmy	1	2	4
	Dense	4	8	16
	L Filmy	1	2	4
	Dense	4	8	16
TUBE	R Filmy	1	2	4
	Dense	4*	8*	16
	L Filmy	1	2	4
	Dense	4*	8*	16

*If the fimbriated end of the fallopian tube is completely enclosed, change the point assignment to 16

Additional Endometriosis _____   Associated Pathology _____

To Be Used with Normal Tubes and Ovaries

To Be Used with Abnormal Tubes and/or Ovaries

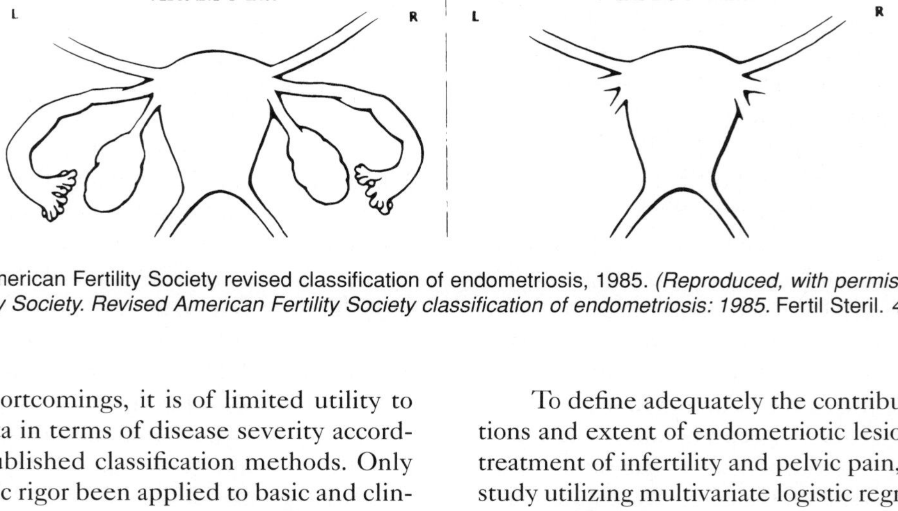

Figure 32–6. American Fertility Society revised classification of endometriosis, 1985. *(Reproduced, with permission, from American Fertility Society. Revised American Fertility Society classification of endometriosis: 1985.* Fertil Steril. *43:351, 1985)*

Given these shortcomings, it is of limited utility to report treatment data in terms of disease severity according to any of the published classification methods. Only recently has scientific rigor been applied to basic and clinical investigation into endometriosis, as anecdotal reports and retrospective surveys appeared in an attempt to pass for treatment trials. The reproducibility of the revised AFS classification scheme for endometriosis has been called into question. Hornstein and colleagues found that the comparison of intraobserver and interobserver scores resulted in a change in endometriosis staging in 38 and 52 percent of patients, respectively. The variability was found to be high for ovarian endometriosis and cul-de-sac subscores when the revised classification was utilized.[106]

To define adequately the contribution of various locations and extent of endometriotic lesions to the successful treatment of infertility and pelvic pain, a large, prospective study utilizing multivariate logistic regression analysis is required. Palmisano and Adamson evaluated the use of endometriosis staging systems to predict pregnancy rates in a cohort of infertile women. Their results showed that no anatomic site or type significantly affected prognosis, and staging systems based solely on anatomic site and the type of lesion are insufficient for predicting fertility.[107]

The relationship of pelvic pain to the stage and type of endometriotic lesions requires a different scheme, with this best illustrated by the surgical trial undertaken by Sutton and colleagues. In their study assessing the efficacy of laser laparoscopic surgery in the treatment of pain associated with minimal, mild, and moderate endometriosis, they observed the poorest results in those patients with stage 1 disease. Conversely, patients with stage II and III disease experienced marked and prolonged relief of symptoms.[108] Clearly, the standard classification of endometriosis as it relates to pelvic pain had no bearing on the severity of symptoms or surgical outcome.

PATHOPHYSIOLOGY

Pain

Noncyclic pelvic pain, dyspareunia, and dysmenorrhea are common complaints of women with endometriosis. Unfortunately, little investigation has been performed to determine the origin or mechanism of such pain symptoms. Endometriotic lesions may cause noncyclic pain by a number of potential mechanisms.[109]

Vulvar or lower vaginal endometriosis may elicit pain when touched.
Ruptured or leaking endometriomas may cause peritoneal irritation and acute pain.
Peritoneal endometriotic implants may secrete factors (histamines) that irritate the peritoneal surface.
Pelvic adhesions with scarring or retractions may cause pain transmitted by somatic fibers of the peritoneum.
Retroverted uteri or ovaries adherent in the cul-de-sac may cause dypareunia due to compression of these structures or tension on surrounding peritoneum.
Uterosacral nodules may cause pain when touched due to compression or stretching of surrounding peritoneum.
Invasion of the urinary or gastrointestinal tract with or without obstruction may elicit visceral pain.

Each of the mechanisms, while imminently logical, based upon our knowledge of pain transmission, has yet to be looked at in a scientifically rigorous manner. Thus, these pathophysiologic mechanisms remain speculative.

Recently, investigation into endometriotic implant depth revealed that increased penetration by such lesions often results in pain.[110] Deep implants were found more often in the posterior cul-de-sac and along uterosacral ligaments, and were more often hormonally responsive than their superficial counterparts.

Very deep implants appear to be more active and may be found exclusively in patients with pain. Cornillie and co-workers found that nearly all women with lesions deeper than 1 cm suffer from severe pain.[111] In this study, women with superficial (<1 mm), intermediate (2 to 4 mm), or deep (5 to 10 mm) infiltration had pain in 17, 53, and 37 percent of cases, respectively. Total lesion volume, however, has not been found to be directly related to patient symptoms. Most recently, Vercellini and

co-workers found that the frequency and severity of deep dyspareunia and the frequency of dysmenorrhea were less in the patients with only ovarian endometriosis than in those with lesions at other sites. The presence of vaginal endometriosis was associated with more frequent and severe deep dyspareunia.[112] Further studies of these areas may prove fruitful in understanding the relationship between endometriosis and pain.

The cause of dysmenorrhea in women with endometriosis has remained speculative. Retrograde menstruation, once thought to be an etiologic factor in the pain, did not appear to cause dysmenorrhea in a controlled trial.[25] Prostaglandins, a prime candidate for factors involved in dysmenorrhea, have been linked to endometriotic implants. It is well established in humans and experimental animals that endometriotic tissue contains and produces prostaglandins.[113–115] However, it has yet to be firmly established that such prostaglandin production results in dysmenorrhea or other symptoms of endometriosis.

One argument solidifying the relationship between endometriosis and pelvic pain is the apparent effectiveness of medical treatment. Virtually all hormonal therapies directed at resolution of implants have been proven effective in relieving endometriosis-associated pain. In addition, a placebo-controlled trial of prostaglandin synthetase inhibitors in the treatment of pain demonstrated that such medications substantially reduce symptoms.[116] Thus, it is likely that endometriotic lesions do, in fact, cause pain. Future investigations will be needed to further delineate the importance of location, depth of penetration, and secretory activity in the generation of this disorder.

Infertility

The association of infertility with endometriosis has long been noted (see Chap 27). As many as 20 to 50 percent of infertile women have been noted to have endometriosis, and infertility is a common finding among women with endometriosis.[109] However, despite the apparent association, the question remains as to whether endometriosis can actually *cause* infertility.

Certainly, when endometriosis produces anatomic distortion of the pelvic viscera or fallopian tube obstruction, the result is often infertility. Existing studies in animal models support this notion.[117,118] In addition, the efficacy of surgical therapy for treatment of endometriosis-associated infertility with severe disease (extensive pelvic adhesions) lends credence to this concept.

A more intriguing question is whether or not endometriotic implants alone, in the absence of adhesions, can cause infertility. Experimental animal models of endometriosis have been used by several investigators to address this question. In both the rabbit[119] and monkey[117] models, transplanted endometrium has been shown to decrease fertility. However, in both experiments this was apparently due to pelvic adhesion formation; in the absence of such anatomic distortion, there was no change in fertility.

Clinical investigators also recently addressed this issue. Jansen prospectively analyzed 91 women undergoing artificial insemination with donor sperm who had no other apparent infertility factor.[120] All had husbands with azoospermia or severe oligospermia. Of the 91, 7 had endometriosis upon screening laparoscopy. Subsequent fertility was significantly lower in the women with infertility. However, several problems exist with the study. First, the number of endometriosis patients was small, enabling small errors in diagnostic accuracy to have a potentially substantial effect. Along these lines, multiple referring physicians performed the laparoscopies; thus, it is unlikely that uniform criteria for the diagnosis of endometriosis were applied. Second, the monthly rate of conception among women with endometriosis in this donor program was less than 4 percent, a figure far lower than that seen in most endometriosis-associated infertility.[121] Thus, this study must be considered suggestive at best.

Conflicting evidence is presented by Rodriguez-Escudero and colleagues.[122] In a population of 21 donor sperm recipients with endometriosis, they were able to demonstrate a monthly probability of pregnancy in excess of 20 percent. A recent study by Chauhan and associates[123] also investigated women undergoing donor insemination. Presentation of their data required grouping those women with oligospermic and azoospermic husbands; in doing so, recalculation of their monthly probability of pregnancy revealed a 9.3 percent rate among women with treated endometriosis versus a 9.9 percent monthly rate among those without identifiable infertility factors. Finally, a comprehensive multivariate investigation into potential pathogenic factors affecting fertility in 731 infertile women determined that endometriosis without adhesions did not alter the cumulative conception rate.[124] Furthermore, data demonstrate a lack of efficacy of medical treatment in enhancing conception among women with endometriosis-associated infertility. These studies, taken together, seriously question the concept that implants alone can be a primary cause of infertility.

Despite the absence of evidence that endometriosis can result in infertility, numerous mechanisms for such a cause–effect relationship have been proposed.[109] Aside from the aforementioned anatomic distortion, such hypothesized mechanisms include:

Anovulation, luteal phase defects, and hormonal abnormalities
Galactorrhea/hyperprolactinemia
Luteinized unruptured follicles

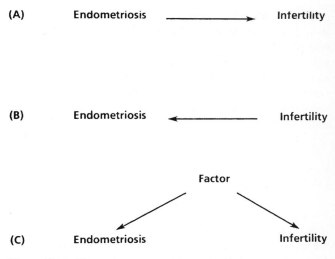

Figure 32–7. Theoretical relationships to explain the association between endometriosis and infertility. **A.** Endometriosis causes infertility. **B.** Infertility causes endometriosis. **C.** An unidentified factor leads to both endometriosis and infertility.

Autoimmunity
Peritoneal macrophages and the peritoneal inflammatory response
Peritoneal fluid prostaglandins
Spontaneous abortion

One or more studies exist to demonstrate associations between each of these factors and endometriosis in infertile women. However, in each case there is little or no evidence to demonstrate that endometriosis is the reason for the apparent relationship. Thus, in no case has the cause–effect relationship been proven.

Given the absence of data implicating endometriotic implants as a cause of infertility, it may well be that the association of the two is a result of the reverse: Infertility may well lead to endometriosis. Such a relationship would be consistent with existing data, and would explain the failure of treatment directed at endometriosis to enhance fertility. Another potential model would be one in which some pathologic process produces both endometriosis and infertility (Fig 32–7). Further investigation into these pathophysiologic options is clearly needed to clarify the relationship between infertility and endometriosis.

TREATMENT

Study Design and Analysis

Assessing the value of a given treatment modality for endometriosis is a complex process as there are multiple measurable outcomes. One commonly utilized outcome to assess treatment is anatomic extent of disease, with published studies often citing a lessening of visible endometriosis following treatment. Using such an outcome in an uncontrolled fashion assumes that endometriosis is a relentlessly progressive disease. However, longitudinal data in untreated women tend to dispute this concept. In 17 such patients followed for 6 mo, 29 percent showed a decrease in the extent of the endometriosis, 24 demonstrated no change, and 47 percent proved to have worsening of disease.[125]

A second commonly used outcome parameter is relief of pelvic pain. Two points are critical in using this outcome: Pain relief is time dependent (ie, there is a recurrence rate that increases with time following discontinuation of therapy), and there is a notable placebo effect.[126]

A third possible outcome is fertility rate following treatment intervention. Although infertility has been associated with endometriosis, the infertility is not absolute, except in extreme cases of extensive pelvic adhesions with tubal obstruction. In most such women, there is a relative decrease in fertility reflected in a lower (but finite) rate of conception than that seen in the general population. Such conceptions are also a time-dependent phenomenon: The longer the time of follow-up, the greater the chance of conceiving.

Given the nature of these outcome measures, it is readily apparent that uncontrolled or poorly controlled trials are of limited value. To generate meaningful information, randomized prospective trials are optimal, with a controlled comparative design a minimum requirement. Thus, only these types of studies will be considered in evaluating therapies.

Therapy Directed Against Endometriosis

Medical strategies for combating endometriosis have centered upon altering cyclic ovulation in the female. Thus, medications currently available have been designed to create a pseudopregnancy, postmenopausal state, or chronic anovulatory pattern.

Danazol is an isoxazol derivative of 17-alpha-ethinyl testosterone. It was originally thought to produce a pseudomenopause, but subsequent studies have revealed the drug to act primarily by diminishing the midcycle luteinizing hormone (LH) surge, creating a chronic anovulatory state.[127,128] Additional actions include inhibition of multiple enzymes in the steroidogenic pathology[129] and increase in free serum testosterone.[130] Side effects of danazol are numerous and frequent.[131] Most result from androgenic effects of the drug, and some may be irreversible.

An effect of danazol upon endometriotic implants has been consistently observed. Uncontrolled trials have demonstrated implant resolution in the vast majority of treated patients.[132,133] Questionable studies have shown a mean decrease of 61 to 89 percent of implant volume[134,135] and a 43 percent decrease in classification score.[136] A placebo-controlled prospective trial examined the effect upon implants 6 mo following completion of

drug therapy,[137] with resolution of implants in 18 percent of the placebo group and 60 percent of the danazol treatment group.

Pain relief has also been well demonstrated with danazol, with 84 to 92 percent of women responding.[138] A recent trial proved danazol reduced pain significantly better than placebo for up to 6 mo following discontinuation of the drug (Fig 32–8).[137] No good data exist for longer follow-up periods.

Given the side-effect profile of danazol, investigators treated endometriosis patients with moderate to severe pelvic pain with very low-dose danazol, 50 mg/day for 9 mo, or depot leuprolide acetate for 3 mo followed by very low-dose danazol at 50 mg/day for 6 mo. They noted a significant improvement in dysmenorrhea, deep dyspareunia, and nonmenstrual pain in both treatment groups.[139]

Two randomized, prospective trials have evaluated the effects of danazol upon fertility. In women with minimal endometriosis, 37.2 percent of the danazol-treated women conceived within 1 yr, whereas 57.4 percent of the untreated group became pregnant (Fig 32–9).[140] A second study included women with all stages of disease, finding a 33 percent 30-mo pregnancy rate in those taking danazol versus 46 percent in those taking placebo.[141] Thus, there is no evidence that danazol will enhance rates of conception in women with endometriosis-associated infertility.

Progestational drugs have also been used extensively to treat endometriosis. Their mechanism of action is believed to be via initial decidualization of endometrial tissue with eventual atrophy. Side effects are highly variable and depend upon the specific progestogen, dosage, treatment duration, and route of administration. Common side effects include abnormal bleeding, nausea, breast tenderness, and fluid retention.[142] All of these side effects resolve with discontinuation of the medication.

Medroxyprogesterone has been clearly shown to reduce the extent of disease. Six mo following discontinuation of the drug, resolution of implants is comparable to the results of danazol therapy and better than placebo treatment.[137] Pain relief also appears to be good with this class of drugs. Uncontrolled trials suggest relief in roughly 90 percent regardless of the progestogen used.[143–146] In a prospective, randomized trial, high-dose medroxyprogesterone relieved pain symptoms to a degree comparable to danazol and significantly better than placebo.[137]

Conversely, the efficacy of progestogens in treating infertility is as yet unproven. In a concurrent, nonrandomized, comparative trial of women with early-stage endometriosis, medroxyprogesterone produced a pregnancy rate similar to danazol therapy and expectant management over a 30-mo period.[147] A second study, involving women with all stages of disease, also failed to show a difference in conception rates among medroxyprogesterone, danazol, and placebo.[141]

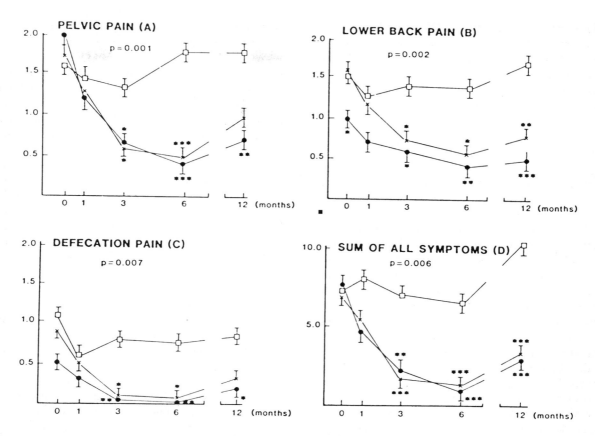

Figure 32–8. Comparison of the effects of medroxyprogesterone acetate (MPA) (X), danazol (•), and placebo (▫) on **(A)** pelvic pain alone (*P* = .001 in analysis of variance), **(B)** lower back pain alone (*P* = .002), **(C)** defecation pain alone (*P* = .007), and **(D)** on the six endometriosis-associated symptoms altogether (pelvic pain, lower back pain, defecation pain, dysuria, dyspareunia, diarrhea) (*P* = .006) before, during, and after treatments. Values are given as mean ± SEM of the scores. Asterisks indicate statistical significances of differences between MPA and placebo and danazol and placebo at different time points (Bonferroni test). (**P* <.05, ***P* <.01, ****P* <.001.) *(Reproduced, with permission, from Telimaa S, et al, Placebo-controlled comparison of danazol and high-dose medroxyprogesterone acetate in the treatment of endometriosis. Gynecol Endocrinol. 1:13, 1987)*

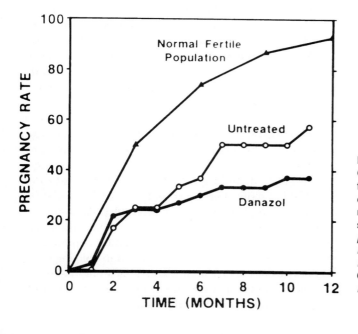

Figure 32–9.
Cumulative pregnancy rates in danazol-treated and untreated patients with minimal endometriosis. The cumulative pregnancy rate in an ideal fertile population is also shown for comparison. *(Reproduced, with permission, from Bayer SR, Seibel MM, Medical treatment: Danazol. In: Schenkel RS, ed.* Endometriosis: Contemporary Concepts in Clinical Management. *Philadelphia, J. B. Lippincott, 1989: 169–187)*

TABLE 32–2. THE STRUCTURES OF COMMONLY USED GnRH AGONISTS

GnRH	pGlu-His-Trp-Ser-Tyr-Gly-Leu-Arg-Pro-Gly-NH₂	
Leuprolide	D-leu	NHEt
Buserelin	D-Ser(tBu)	aza-Gly
Nafarelin	D-Nal(2)	
Histrelin	D-His(Bzl)	NHEY
Goserelin	D-Ser(tBu)	aza-Gly

A more recent development in the medical treatment of endometriosis is the use of gonadotropin-releasing hormone (GnRH) analogs. These medications are modifications of GnRH (Table 32–2) and function to downregulate the pituitary gland. The net effect is a decline in gonadotropins and resultant "medical oophorectomy." A decline in serum estradiol is seen in roughly 3 to 6 wk. Side effects are numerous and are similar to those experienced in the menopausal years.[142]

The effect of GnRH analogs on endometriotic implants is impressive in both animals[148] and humans. In two comparative trials, GnRH analogs have been shown to produce a degree of regression of implants similar to that produced by danazol.[136,149] However, although the implants appear inactive during treatment, they are capable of later growth.[150]

Pain relief in uncontrolled studies appears to be seen in roughly 80 percent of those treated with GnRH analogs. In a randomized trial comparing a GnRH analog to danazol, the two drugs produced an equivalent amount of pain relief.[136] Recurrence rates have been noted to be as low as 20 percent at 6 mo posttherapy[150] but nearly 50 percent by 1 yr.[149]

Pregnancy rates following GnRH agonist therapy have been reported by numerous investigators. However, most studies suffer from small sample size, inconsistent staging, and variable length of follow-up. In comparative trials with danazol, no difference in pregnancy rates has been detected at 1 yr[136] or at 18 mo follow-up.[149]

The combination of estrogen and a progestogen for treatment of endometriosis, the so-called "pseudopregnancy regimen," has been utilized for 30 yr and today remains the most popular medical treatment for endometriosis. Like progestational therapy, combination treatment acts via initial decidualization, followed by atrophy. Side effects are numerous, and include androgenic, estrogenic, and progestogenic effects. These have lessened, however, with the advent of the low-dose oral contraceptive pill (OCP). Unfortunately, the efficacy of this popular treatment remains a mystery, as no properly controlled studies assessing extent of disease, pain relief, or fertility enhancement exist. Adamson and associates, using life-table analysis, were able to show that treatment with OCPs had a less favorable effect on the pregnancy rate than surgical treatment or no treatment for the groups analyzed (ie,

presence or absence of adnexal lesions, anatomic structures involved, and specific types of lesions.)[151]

Apart from its controversial role in pregnancy termination, mifepristone (RU 486) may well prove to be of value in a wide variety of gynecologic disorders, including endometriosis. The drug is an anti-progestational and anti-glucocorticoid that can inhibit ovulation and disrupt endometrial integrity. Daily doses of the medication range from 50 to 100 mg, with side effects ranging from hot flashes to fatigue, nausea, and transient elevation in liver transaminases. No effect on lipid profiles or bone mineral density has been reported. The ability of mifepristone to produce a regression of endometriotic lesions has been variable and apparently dependent upon duration of treatment, with 6 mo being the minimal amount of time required to produce results.[152]

Additional medications exist for the treatment of endometriosis. Gestrinone is currently a popular treatment in Europe. Methyltestosterone and diethylstilbestrol have been used in the past, although neither is utilized with any frequency today. New drugs currently under development or testing include antiestrogens such as tamoxifen and GnRH antagonists.

Medical therapy directed at endometriosis appears to be of some value, depending upon the goal of treatment. If the objective is to diminish the anatomic extent of disease (exclusive of pelvic adhesions) or reduce pain symptoms, all the drugs thus far evaluated appear efficacious. However, few data are available regarding the long-term effectiveness of such therapies, and there is some suggestion that, in some instances, recurrence may be substantial.

The role of medical therapy in the promotion of fertility, however, appears to be less clear-cut. To date, there is no evidence that any medical therapy alone can increase the rate of conception among women with endometriosis-associated infertility.

Surgery is the most commonly used treatment for endometriosis. The goals of this type of intervention are to restore pelvic anatomy and remove visible endometriotic lesions. Such surgery is termed "conservative" when the ability to conceive is retained, and may be performed either laparoscopically or via laparotomy.

The techniques of conservative surgery have been well described,[153] and space does not permit a thorough description of them here. A variety of surgical instruments have also been utilized. Sharp dissection, cauterization, endocoagulation, and vaporization have been used to remove endometriotic implants and lyse adhesions.[154] No clear advantage has been demonstrated by any one approach, and it is recommended that the surgeon utilize the instruments with which he or she feels most comfortable.

The success of surgical intervention in ablating endometriotic lesions and restoring normal anatomy is initially quite high. However, a recurrence risk exists for both implants and adhesions. Wheeler and Malinak[155] noted a

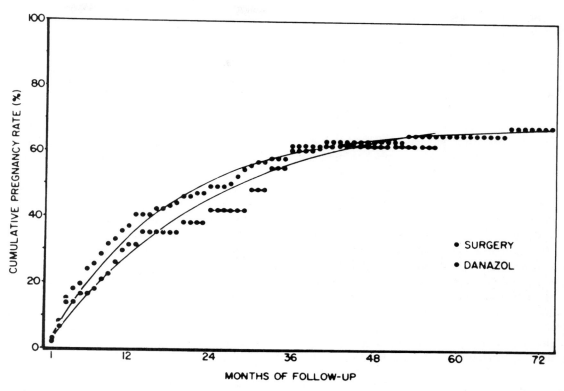

Figure 32–10. Cumulative pregnancy rates for patients with mild or moderate endometriosis treated with conservative surgery or danazol. *(Reproduced, with permission, from Guzick DS, Rock JA, A comparison of danazol and conservative surgery for the treatment of infertility due to mild or moderate endometriosis. Fertil Steril. 40:580, 1983)*

40 percent recurrence of symptomatic disease at 9-yr follow-up.[153] A second study found recurrent disease in 28 percent at 18 mo or longer postoperatively.[156] Lysis of adhesions is also only marginally successful, with 40 to 50 percent of women demonstrating significant reformation.[154,157,158]

The efficacy of conservative surgery for the treatment of pelvic pain is unclear. Uncontrolled trials generally report immediate relief in 70 to 100 percent.[153,154] One report also notes 82 percent of women had complete relief 1 yr postsurgery.[159] However, whether this is due to removal of implants and adhesions or other adjunctive procedures directed at pain relief is unclear. Sutton and colleagues assessed the efficacy of laser laparoscopic surgery in the treatment of pain associated with minimal, mild, and moderate endometriosis. They found that laser laparoscopic removal of endometriosis in conjunction with uterosacral nerve ablation resulted in statistically significant pain relief compared with those patients undergoing sham laparoscopy up to 6 mo after surgery.[108]

Conservative surgery has been used extensively in an attempt to enhance fertility. Most studies, however, are uncontrolled. Two comparative (albeit retrospective) trials have been reported. Guzick and Rock[160] compared pregnancy rates in 224 women with early-stage endometriosis treated with either danazol or conservative surgery; no difference between therapies was noted in terms of subsequent conception rates (Fig 32–10). Olive and Lee[161]

compared conservative surgery to expectant management and found them to be equally efficacious for mild or moderate disease. However, for severe endometriosis surgery produced significantly better results than did no treatment.

One prospective study of laparoscopic cauterization of implants has been published.[162] Women with otherwise unexplained infertility and 8 mo of failed expectant management underwent laparoscopy and, if found to have early-stage disease, were randomized to cautery versus no cautery of implants. The treated group proved to have a significantly higher rate of conception (Table 32–3). These results suggest that specific subgroups of early-stage endometriosis patients may exist that will benefit from conservative surgery, although they may require careful selection.

TABLE 32–3. PREGNANCY AND LIVE BIRTH RATES IN WOMEN WITH STAGE 1 OR 2 ENDOMETRIOSIS AND INFERTILITY AT 8-MO FOLLOW-UP

	n	Pregnant	Live Birth
No treatment	69	42 (61%)[a]	37 (54%)[b]
Fulguration	54	10 (18%)	10 (18%)

[a]$P < .00001$.
[b]$P < .00001$.
(Reproduced, with permission, from Nowroozi K, et al, The importance of laparoscopic coagulation of mild endometriosis in infertile women. Int J Fertil. 32:442, 1987)

Clearly, conservative surgery can be efficacious in the reduction of disease and relief of pain. However, it is not a panacea for enhancing fertility. The procedure seems to be optimal for advanced disease as a means of correcting anatomic relationships. However, in the absence of such anatomic distortion the value of surgical intervention to treat infertility is debatable.

Meta-analysis encompassing studies from 1982 to 1994 carried out by Adamson and Pasta showed that either no treatment or surgery alone is superior to medical treatment for minimal and mild endometriosis associated with infertility.[163] They found that medical treatment merely delays the possibility of pregnancy by the duration of therapy, typically 3 to 6 mo. Similarly, meta-analysis was also carried out by Hughes and associates on 25 randomized controlled trials and cohort studies. They found possible treatment benefit from laparoscopic conservative surgery, but overall they concluded that medical treatment via ovulation suppression was ineffective in the treatment of endometriosis-associated infertility.[164] Although these medications may be considered to be an empiric intervention following the exhaustion of other treatments, the numerous side effects and the creation of the mandatory period of amenorrhea during medical treatment make the wisdom of this approach questionable.

When hysterectomy with salpingo-oophorectomy is performed for endometriosis, the procedure is referred to as definitive surgery. Such surgery, in conjunction with excision of existing endometriotic lesions, is believed to eliminate endometriosis-associated pain in a high proportion of cases, although limited data are available to substantiate this.

Often, there is the desire with definite procedures to preserve one or both ovaries. Recurrence of disease in such cases has ranged from 0 to 85 percent, with a mean of 7 percent among published reports.[165] More recently, patients undergoing definitive surgery with ovarian preservation were found to have a 6.1 times greater risk of developing recurrent pain and an 8.1 times greater risk of reoperation.[166] However, with advanced disease as many as one third of women will suffer recurrence if oophorectomy is not performed. Based upon extensive clinical experience, Ranney has suggested four criteria that should mandate removal of both ovaries:

1. Hilar areas are involved bilaterally.
2. Extensive endometriosis is present that cannot be resected.
3. A hemoperitoneum is present, necessitating emergency surgery.
4. Associated pelvic pathology is present, necessitating removal of the ovaries.[167]

Given the potential advantages of medical and surgical therapy, many clinicians favor combining the two to combat the disease. Although such practice is relatively common, there are few data to assess the value of this approach. Two randomized, comparative trials addressing this issue have been published. In early-stage disease, Chong and associates found no differences in fertility rates after treatment with danazol, laparoscopic laser vaporization, or laser surgery followed by danazol.[168] For patients with advanced disease, conservative surgery has been combined with danazol, medroxyprogesterone, and placebo and the results compared.[169] Although pregnancy rates were similar in the three groups, pain relief proved significantly better in the women undergoing combination medical–surgical therapy (Fig 32–11). Thus, it appears that the primary role of the combined medical–surgical approach lies in the treatment of pain symptoms in women with extensive disease.

Therapy Directed Against Symptoms

Although the majority of treatments for endometriosis are directed at eliminating the lesions themselves, some treatment regimens are designed to bypass the implants and attack the symptoms directly. Pain resulting from endometriosis can be treated in this manner in a variety of ways.

A medical approach to pain relief is the use of nonsteroidal anti-inflammatory drugs (NSAIDs). These medications act by inhibiting prostaglandin synthetase, thereby reducing prostaglandin production. In addition, some of these drugs antagonize prostaglandins at their receptors. The effect of such drugs on endometriosis-associated pain has been variable. In a randomized, placebo-controlled study, neither aspirin, indomethacin, nor tolfenamic acid (a fenamate) decreased the premenstrual pain experienced by women with endometriosis.[170] Tolfenamic acid resulted in a significant decrease in dysmenorrhea, whereas the other medications failed to outperform placebo.[170,171] In a second trial, naproxen sodium proved significantly better at providing relief of dysmenorrhea compared to placebo.[172] These data suggest that some NSAIDs may play a role in the treatment of selected aspects of endometriosis-associated pain.

Pelvic pain may be approached surgically by performing a presacral neurectomy (PSN) or uterosacral nerve ablation. Each of these procedures may be carried out either laparoscopically or via laparotomy. Although the PSN has been implemented for many years, only recently has its value been critically assessed. In a randomized, prospective study, PSN by laparotomy proved highly effective at relieving dysmenorrhea; by contrast, patients not having the procedure experienced no relief of dysmenorrhea pain (Table 32–4).[173] Interestingly, the effect of PSN on lateral pain, back pain, and dyspareunia proved inconsistent. Conversely, in a randomized controlled study by Candiani et al, the addition of presacral neurectomy to conservative surgery for moderate or se-

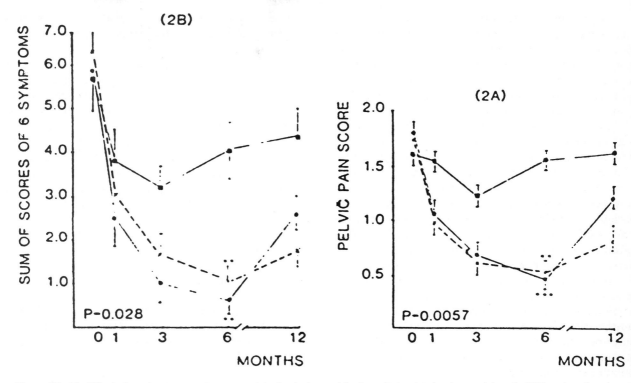

Figure 32–11. Effect of medroxyprogresterone acetate (x-x), danazol (•-•), and placebo (■-■) on pelvic pain (2A) and on the six endometriosis-associated symptoms (pelvic pain, lower back pain, defecation pain, dysuria, diarrhea, and dyspareunia) (2B) evaluated by symptom scores before, during, and after treatments. Results are given as mean ± SEM of the scores. The P value indicates the statistical significance of difference between the treatment and placebo groups during the whole trial in analysis of variance. Asterisks indicate statistical significances of differences between the treatment and placebo groups at different time points in the modified Bonferroni test: $^{*}P < .05$, $^{**}P < .001$. *(Reproduced, with permission, from Telimaa S, et al, Placebo-controlled comparison of danazol and high-dose medroxyprogesterone acetate in the treatment of endometriosis after conservative surgery. Gynecol Endocrinol. 1:363, 1987)*

vere endometriosis did not result in a greater reduction of pelvic pain than did conservative surgery alone.[174] Thus, the role of PSN in relief of endometriosis-associated pain remains controversial.

Uterosacral nerve ablation has recently been popularized due to its simplicity as performed through the laparoscope. Studies evaluating the success rates of LUNA in the treatment of endometriosis-associated dysmenorrhea have shown marked improvement of dysmenorrhea ranging from 70 to 90 percent. When the effect of LUNA was evaluated in patients with severe incapacitating dys-

menorrhea who had no pelvic pathology at laparoscopy, significant pain relief was noted in the treated group.[175] Of note, though, only 44 percent of women had continued relief from dysmenorrhea 12 mo after surgery. In another study, by Sutton and colleagues, women with minimal endometriosis were evaluated after either diagnostic laparoscopy followed by expectant management or LUNA with ablation of endometriosis. At 6 mo after surgery, a significantly greater proportion of patients in the latter group (62 percent) had improvement or resolution of pain compared with the former group (23 percent).[108]

TABLE 32–4. INCIDENCE AND LOCATION OF PAIN

	Midline No. (%)	Back No. (%)	Lateral No. (%)	Dyspareunia No. (%)
Protocol				
PSN (n = 4)	4 (100)	1 (25)	2 (50)	1 (25)
Non-PSN (n = 4)	4 (100)	3 (75)	2 (50)	1 (25)
Nonprotocol				
PSN (n = 13)	13 (100)	13 (100)	9 (70)	10 (78)
Non-PSN (n = 5)	5 (100)	5 (100)	4 (80)	4 (80)

PSN-presacral neurectomy group; non-PSN-nonpresacral neurectomy group.
(Reproduced, with permission, from Tjaden B, et al, The efficacy of presacral neurectomy for the relief of midline dysmenorrhea. Obstet Gynecol. 76:89, 1990)

An option for the treatment of endometriosis-associated infertility is the use of advanced reproductive technologies. Patients with relatively mild disease may be approached similarly to couples with unexplained infertility, with the empiric use of controlled ovarian hyperstimulation combined with intrauterine insemination. Such an approach results in a monthly rate of conception of 17 percent.[176] The use of in vitro fertilization (IVF) and gamete intrafallopian transfer (GIFT) in these women has proven highly efficacious, with conception rates comparable to those seen in women with unexplained infertility or tubal obstruction.

In women with more advanced stages of disease, pelvic adhesions generally preclude the use of controlled ovarian hyperstimulation and intrauterine insemination or GIFT. Experience with IVF for patients with endometriosis has been evaluated, and no difference was found with regards to stimulation between patients with male factor only, tubal factor only, or unexplained infertility versus patients with endometriosis. Investigators found that there was no difference in mean number of ampules of HMG administered, estradiol concentration on the day of HCG administration, number of days of HMG administration, mean number of oocytes retrieved and retrieval rate, fertilization rate, number of normally fertilized embryos, number of transferred embryos per cycle, or implantation rate. More importantly, the pregnancy rates were similar, as were the miscarriage rates. Additionally, they separated the endometriosis patients based on staging, according to the revised AFS classification, and found no difference in results between stage I–II and III–IV disease.[177] Thus, the previously held belief that endometriosis adversely affected the success rates of IVF appears to be in doubt. Additionally, the original data suggesting a difference was based on laparoscopic oocyte retrieval; therefore, a lower number of oocytes were retrieved in those patients with advanced endometriosis. The advent of transvaginal oocyte retrieval has eliminated any difference with regard to stage of disease and lower pregnancy rates.

CONCLUSIONS

Endometriosis is a common disorder of substantial interest to gynecologists. Numerous investigators are rapidly advancing our knowledge of the disease, yet as we learn more about endometriosis it becomes increasing apparent how little we truly understand about this disorder. The pathogenesis of the disease, its prevalence in the population, and risk factors for endometriosis are all far from determined. Classification methods, although improved over several decades ago, still have severe shortcomings. Pathophysiologic mechanisms for the production of endometriosis-associated pain and infertility are undefined. Finally, optimal treatment for the disorder is often unclear, with conflicting data and a plethora of poorly constructed studies.

Given this situation, what should be the future course of endometriosis research? Clearly, the answer lies in basic investigation designed to elucidate the precise mechanisms by which endometriosis is created and maintained, and by which it alters normal physiologic processes. This must be supplemented by well-constructed, prospective clinical trials to carefully test specific hypotheses, enabling the formation of sensible conclusions. Only then, by carefully pairing both basic and clinical investigative efforts, are we likely to uncover the secrets of this enigmatic disease.

REFERENCES

1. Schenken RS, ed. Pathogenesis. In: *Endometriosis: Contemporary Concepts in Clinical Management*. Philadelphia, J. B. Lippincott, 1989: 1–48
2. Meyer R. Uber den stand der frage der adenomyositis und adenomome im allegemeinen und ins besondere uber adenomyositis seroephithelialis und adenomyometritis sarcomatosa. *Zentralbl Gynakol*. 36:745, 1919
3. Meyer R. Uber endometrium in der tube, sowie uber die hierausentstenhenden wirklichen und vermantlichen folgen. *Zentralbl Gynakol*. 51:1482, 1927
4. Melicow MM, Pachter MR. Endometrial carcinoma of the prostatic utricle (uterus masculinus). *Cancer*. 20:1715, 1967
5. Oliker AJ, Harns AE. Endometriosis of the bladder in a male patient. *J Urol*. 106:858, 1971
6. Pinkert TC, Catlow CE, Strauss R. Endometriosis of the urinary bladder in a man with prostatic carcinoma. *Cancer*. 43:1562, 1979
7. Schrodt GR, Alcorn MD, Ibanez J. Endometriosis of the male urinary system: A case report. *J Urol*. 124:722, 1980
8. Maximow A. Uber die mesothel (deckzellen der serosen haut) und die zellen der serosen exsudate: Untersuchungen an entzudetem gewebe und an gewebskulturen. *Arch Exp Zellforsch*. 4:1, 1927
9. Filatow D. Uber die bildung des anfangsstadiums bei der extremitatenntwicklung. *Roux Arch Entw Mech Organ*. 127:776, 1933
10. Sampson JA. Perforating hemorrhagic (chocolate) cysts of the ovary. *Arch Surg*. 3:245, 1921
11. Geist SH. The viability of fragments of menstrual endometrium. *Am J Obstet Gynecol*. 25:751, 1933
12. Keettell WC, Stein RJ. The viability of the cast-off menstrual endometrium. *Am J Obstet Gynecol*. 61:440, 1951
13. Mungyer G, Willemsen WNP, Rolland R, et al. Cells of the mucous membrane of the female genital tract in culture: A comparative study with regard to the histogenesis of endometriosis. *In Vitro Cell Dev Biol*. 23:111, 1987
14. Heim H. Ueber die entwicklung der endometriose am ort und stelle. *Arch Gynakol*. 125:269, 1933
15. Markee JE. Menstruation in intraocular endometrial transplants in the rhesus monkey. *Contrib Embryol*. 28:23, 1940

16. TeLinde RW, Scott RB. Experimental endometrium. *Am J Obstet Gynecol.* 60:1147, 1950

17. Ridley JH. The validity of Sampson's theory of endometriosis. *Am J Obstet Gynecol.* 82:777, 1961

18. Ridley JH, Edwards IK. Experimental endometriosis in the human. *Am J Obstet Gynecol.* 76:783, 1958

19. Lavender G, Normal P. The pathogenesis of endometriosis. An experimental study. *Acta Obstet Gynecol Scand.* 34:366, 1955

20. Merrill JA. Experimental induction of endometriosis across millipore filters. *Surg Forum.* 14:397, 1963

21. Merrill JA. Experimental induction of endometriosis across millipore filters. *Am J Obstet Gynecol.* 94:780, 1966

22. Cunha GR, Chung LWK, Shannon JM, Reese BA. Stroma-epithelial interactions in sex differentiations. *Biol Reprod.* 22:19, 1980

23. Blumenkrantz MU, Gallagher N, Bashore RA, Tenckhoff H. Retrograde menstruation in women undergoing chronic peritoneal dialysis. *Obstet Gynecol.* 94:780, 1966

24. Halme J, Hammond MG, Hulka JF, et al. Retrograde menstruation in healthy women and in patients with endometriosis. *Obstet Gynecol.* 64:151, 1984

25. Liu DTY, Hitchcock A. Endometriosis: Its association with retrograde menstruation, dysmenorrhea and tubal pathology. *Br J Obstet Gynaecol.* 93:859, 1986

26. Olive DL, Henderson DY. Endometriosis and müllerian anomalies. *Obstet Gynecol.* 69:412, 1987

27. Ayers JWT, Friedenstab AP. Utero-tubal hypotonia associated with pelvic endometriosis (abstr). *41st Annual Meeting of American Fertility Society. Abstracts of the Scientific and Poster Sessions.* Birmingham, Ala., American Fertility Society, 1985: 131

28. Bartosik D, Jacobs S, Kelly IJ. Endometrial tissue in peritoneal fluid. *Fertil Steril.* 46:796, 1986

29. Jenkins S, Olive DL, Haney AF. Endometriosis: Pathogenetic implications of the anatomic distribution. *Obstet Gynecol.* 67:335, 1986

30. Dmowski WP, Steele RW, Baker GF. Deficient cellular immunity in endometriosis. *Am J Obstet Gynecol.* 141:377, 1981

31. Steele RW, Dmowski WP, Marmer DJ. Immunologic aspects of human endometriosis. *Am J Reprod Immunol.* 6:33, 1984

32. Badawy SZA, Cuenca V, Stitzel A, et al. Autoimmune phenomena in infertile patients with endometriosis. *Obstet Gynecol.* 63:271, 1984

33. Mathur S, Peress MR, Williamson HO, et al. Autoimmunity to endometrium and ovary in endometriosis. *Clin Exp Immunol.* 50:259, 1982

34. Weed JC, Arguembourg PC. Endometriosis: Can it produce an autoimmune response resulting in infertility? *Clin Obstet Gynecol.* 23:885, 1980

35. Olive DL, Hammond CB. Endometriosis: Pathogenesis and mechanisms of infertility. *Postgrad Obstet Gynecol.* 5:1, 1985

36. Arici A, Attar E, Tazuke S, et al. Monocyte chemotactic protein-1 (MCP-1) in human peritoneal fluid and modulation of MCP-1 expression in human mesothelial cells. 51st Annual Meeting of the American Society of Reproductive Medicine. Seattle, October 7–12, 1995: S80

37. Arici A, Tazuke SI, Attar E, et al. Interleukin-8 concentration in peritoneal fluid of patients with endometriosis and modulation of interleukin-8 expression in human mesothelial cells. *Mol Hum Reprod.* 2:404, 1996

38. Olive DL, Montoya I, Riehl RM, Schenken RS. Macrophage-conditioned media enhance endometrial stromal cell proliferation in vitro. *Am J Obstet Gynecol.* 1991; 164:953

39. Wharton W, Gillespie GY, Russell SW, Pledger WJ. Mitogenic activity elaborated by macrophage-like cell lines act as competence factor(s) for BALB/c3T3 cells. *J Cell Physiol.* 110:93, 1982

40. DiZerega GS, Barber DL, Hodgen GD. Endometriosis: Role of ovarian steroids in initiation, maintenance, and suppression. *Fertil Steril.* 33:649, 1980

41. Sharpe KL, Bertero MC, Homm RJ, Vernon MW. Effects of exogenous steroid administration or GnRH antagonist-suppressed endometriosis in the rat. *Fertil Steril.* 54:544, 1990

42. Schenken RS. Effect of pregnancy on surgically induced endometriosis in cynomolgus monkeys. *Am J Obstet Gynecol.* 157:1392, 1987

43. McArthur JW, Ufelder H. The effect of pregnancy upon endometriosis. *Obstet Gynecol Surv.* 20:709, 1965

44. Metzger DA, Olive DL, Haney AF. Limited hormonal responsiveness of ectopic endometrium: Histologic correlation with intrauterine endometrium. *Hum Pathol.* 19:1417, 1988

45. Haney AF, Muscato JJ, Weinberg JB. Peritoneal fluid cell populations in infertility patients. *Fertil Steril.* 35:696, 1981

46. Bitterman PB, Rennard SI, Hunningnhake GW. Human alveolar macrophage growth factor for fibroblasts. *J Clin Invest.* 70:806, 1982

47. Leslie CC, Mussen RA, Hanson PM. Production of growth factor activity for fibroblasts by human monocyte-derived macrophages. *J Leukocyte Biol.* 36:143, 1984

48. Norwood GE. Sterility and fertility in women with pelvic endometriosis. *Clin Obstet Gynecol.* 3:456, 1960

49. Olive DL, Haney AF. Endometriosis. In DeCherney AH, ed. *Reproductive Failure.* New York, Churchill Livingstone, 1986: 153–201

50. Goldstein DP, deCholnoky C, Emans SJ, Leventhal JM. Laparoscopy in the diagnosis and management of pelvic pain in adolescents. *J Reprod Med.* 24:251, 1980

51. Chatman DL, Ward AB. Endometriosis in adolescents. *J Reprod Med.* 27:156, 1982

52. Huffman JW. Endometriosis in young teen-age girls. *Pediatr Ann.* 10:44, 1981

53. Kempers RD, Dockerty MB, Hunt AB. Significant postmenopausal endometriosis. *Surg Gynecol Obstet.* 111:348, 1960

54. Punnonen R, Klemi P, Nikkanen V. Postmenopausal endometriosis. *Eur J Obstet Gynaecol Reprod Biol.* 11:195, 1980

55. Djursing H, Peterson K, Weberg E. Symptomatic postmenopausal endometriosis. *Acta Obstet Gynecol Scand.* 60:529, 1981

56. Wheeler JM. Epidemiology of endometriosis-associated infertility. *J Reprod Med.* 34:41, 1989

57. Sangi-Haghpeykar H, Poindexter A. Epidemiology of endometriosis among parous women. *Obstet Gynecol.* 85:983, 1995

58. Scott RB, TeLinde RW. External endometriosis—The scourge of the private patient. *Ann Surg.* 131:697, 1950

59. Lloyd FP. Endometriosis in the Negro woman. *Am J Obstet Gynecol.* 89:468, 1954

60. Metzger DA, Haney AF. Endometriosis: Etiology and pathophysiology of infertility. *Clin Obstet Gynecol.* 31:801, 1988

61. Ranney B. Endometriosis IV. Hereditary tendencies. *Obstet Gynecol.* 37:734, 1971

62. Simpson JL, Elias S, Malinak LR, Buttram VC Jr. Heritable aspects of endometriosis. I. Genetic studies. *Am J Obstet Gynecol.* 137:327, 1980

63. Malinak LR, Buttram VC Jr, Elias S. Heritable aspects of endometriosis. II. Clinical characteristics of familial endometriosis. *Am J Obstet Gynecol.* 137:332, 1980

64. Pauerstein CJ. Clinical presentation and diagnosis. In: Schenken RS, ed. *Endometriosis: Contemporary concepts in Clinical Management.* Philadelphia, J. B. Lippincott, 1989: 127–144

65. Strathy JH, Molgaard CA, Coulam CB, Melton LJ III. Endometriosis and infertility: A laparoscopic study of endometriosis among fertile and infertile women. *Fertil Steril.* 38:667, 1982

66. Ranney B. Endometriosis. III. Complete operations. Reasons, sequelae, treatment. *Am J Obstet Gynecol.* 109:1137, 1971

67. Soules MR, Malinak LR, Bury R, Poindexter A. Endometriosis and anovulation: A coexisting problem in the infertile female. *Am J Obstet Gynecol.* 125:412, 1976

68. Radwansak E, Rane D, Dmowski WP. Management of infertility in women with endometriosis and ovulatory dysfunction. *Fertil Steril.* 41:775, 1984

69. Jenks JE, Artisan LE, Haoskins WJ, Miremadi AK. Endometriosis with ascites. *Obstet Gynecol.* 63:755, 1984

70. Pittaway DE, Fayez JA. The use of CA-125 in the diagnosis and management of endometriosis. *Fertil Steril.* 46:790, 1986

71. Malkasian GD Jr, Podratz KC, Stanhope CR, et al. CA-125 in gynecologic practice. *Am J Obstet Gynecol.* 155:515, 1986

72. Patton EP, Field CS, Harms RW, Coulam CB. Ca-125 levels in endometriosis. *Fertil Steril.* 45–770, 1986

73. Gurgan T, Kisnisci H, Yarali H, et al. Serum and peritoneal fluid CA-125 levels in early stage endometriosis. *Gynecol Obstet Invest.* 30:105, 1990

74. Kauppila A, Telimaa S, Ronnberg L, Vucri J. Placebo-controlled study on serum concentrations of CA-125 before and after treatment of endometriosis with danazol or high-dose medroxyprogesterone acetate alone or after surgery. *Fertil Steril.* 49:37, 1988

75. Hornstein MD, Harlow BL, Thomas PP, Check JH. Use of a new CA-125 assay in the diagnosis of endometriosis. *Hum Reprod.* 10:932, 1995

76. Telimaa S, Kauppila A, Ronnberg L, et al. Elevated serum levels of endometrial secretory protein PP14 in patients with advanced endometriosis. *Am Obstet Gynecol.* 161:866, 1989

77. Koninckx PR, Riittinen L, Seppala M, Cornillie FJ. CA-125 and placental protein 14 concentrations in plasma and peritoneal fluid of women with deeply infiltrating pelvic endometriosis. *Fertil Steril.* 57:523, 1992

78. Wild RA, Shiver CA. Antiendometrial antibodies in patients with endometriosis. *Am J Reprod Immunol Microbiol.* 8:84, 1985

79. Chihal HJ, Mathur S, Hatty GL, Williamson HO. An endometrial antibody assay in the clinical diagnosis and management of endometriosis. *Fertil Steril.* 46:408, 1986

80. Zawin M, McCarthy S, Scoutt L, Comite F. Endometriosis: Appearance and detection at MR imaging. *Radiology.* 171:693, 1989

81. Togashi K, Nishimura K, Kimura I, et al. Endometrial cysts: Diagnosis with MR imaging. *Radiology.* 180:73, 1991

82. Takahashi K, Okada S, Ozaki T, et al. Diagnosis of pelvic endometriosis by magnetic resonance imaging using "fat-saturation" technique. *Fertil Steril.* 62:973, 1994

83. Ha HK, Lim YT, Kim HS, et al. Diagnosis of pelvic endometriosis: Fat-suppressed T1-weighted vs conventional MR images. *Am J Roentgenology.* 163(1):127–31, 1994

84. Kennedy SH, Mojiminiyi OA, Soper NDW, et al. Immunoscintigraphy of endometriosis. *Br J Obstet Gynaecol.* 97:667, 1990

85. Jansen RPS, Russell P. Nonpigmented endometriosis: Clinical, laparoscopic, and pathologic definition. *Am J Obstet Gynecol.* 155:1154, 1986

86. Stripling MC, Martin DC, Chatman DL, et al. Subtle appearance of pelvic endometriosis. *Fertil Steril.* 49:427, 1988

87. Redwine DB. Age-related evolution in color appearance of endometriosis. *Fertil Steril.* 48:1062, 1987

88. D'Hooghe TM, Bambra CS, Raeymaekers BM, Koninckx PR. Serial laparoscopies over 30 months show that endometriosis in captive baboons (*Papio anubis, Papio cynocephalus*) is a progressive disease. *Fertil Steril.* 65:645, 1996

89. Martin DC, Zwagg RV. Excision techniques for endometriosis with the CO_2 laser laparoscope. *J Reprod Med.* 32:753, 1987

90. Redwine DB. Peritoneal blood painting: An aid in the diagnosis of endometriosis. *Am J Obstet Gynecol.* 161: 865, 1989

91. Sampson JA. Peritoneal endometriosis due to the menstrual dissemination of endometrial tissue into the peritoneal cavity. *Am J Obstet Gynecol.* 14:422, 1927

92. Redwine DB. Peritoneal pockets and endometriosis: Confirmation of an important relationship, with further observations. *J Reprod Med.* 34:270, 1989

93. Murphy AA, Green WR, Bobbie D, et al. Unsuspected endometriosis documented by scanning electron microscopy in visually normal peritoneum. *Fertil Steril.* 46:522, 1986

94. Nisolle M, Paindaveine B, Bourdon A, et al. Histologic study of peritoneal endometriosis in infertile women. *Fertil Steril.* 53:984, 1990

95. Redwine DB. Is "microscopic" peritoneal endometriosis invisible? *Fertil Steril.* 50:665, 1988

96. Ferenczy A. Studies on the cystodynamics of human endometrial regeneration. I. Scanning electron microscopy. *Am J Obstet Gynecol.* 124:64, 1976

97. Ferenczy A. Studies on the cytodynamics of human endometrial regeneration. II. Transmission electron microscopy and histochemistry. *Am J Obstet Gynecol.* 124:582, 1976

98. Nisolle M, Casanas-roux F, Wyns C, et al. Immuno-histochemical analysis of estrogen and progesterone receptors in endometrium and peritoneal endometriosis: A new quantitative method. *Fertil Steril.* 62:751, 1994

99. Riva HL, Kawasaki DM, Messenger AJ. Further experience with norethynodrel in the treatment of endometriosis. *Obstet Gynecol.* 19:111, 1962

100. Acosta AA, Buttram VC Jr, Besch PK, et al. A proposed classification of pelvic endometriosis. *Obstet Gynecol.* 42:19, 1973

101. Ingersoll FM. Selection of medical and surgical treatment of endometriosis of endometriosis. *Clin Obstet Gynecol.* 20:849, 1977

102. Kistner RW, Siegler AM, Behrman SJ. Suggested classification for endometriosis: Relationship to infertility. *Fertil Steril.* 28:1008, 1987

103. Buttram CV Jr. An expanded classification of endometriosis. *Fertil Steril.* 28:1008, 1987

104. American Fertility Society. Classification of endometriosis. *Fertil Steril.* 32:633, 1979

105. American Fertility Society. Revised American Fertility Society classification of endometriosis: 1985. *Fertil Steril.* 43:351, 1985

106. Hornstein MD, Gleason RE, Orav J, et al. The reproducibility of the revised American Fertility Society classification of endometriosis. *Fertil Steril.* 59:1015, 1993

107. Palmisano GP, Adamson GD, Lamb EJ. Can staging systems for endometriosis based on anatomic location and lesion type predict pregnancy rates? *Int J Fertil Menopausal Stud.* 38:241, 1993

108. Sutton CJG, Ewen SP, Whitelaw N, et al. Prospective, randomized, double-blind, controlled trial of laser laparoscopy in the treatment of pelvic pain associated with minimal, mild, and moderate endometriosis. *Fertil Steril.* 62:696, 1994

109. Burns WN, Scheneken RS. Pathophysiology. In: Schenken RS, ed. *Endometriosis: Contemporary Concepts in Clinical Management.* Philadelphia, J. B. Lippincott, 1989: 83–126

110. Cornillie FJ, Oosterlynck D, Lauweryns JM, Koninckx PR. Deeply infiltrating pelvic endometriosis: Histology and clinical significance. *Fertil Steril.* 53:978, 1990

111. Cornillie FJ, Oosterlynck D, Lauweryns J, et al. Deeply infiltrating pelvic endometriosis: Histology and clinical significance. *Fertil Steril.* 53:978, 1990

112. Vercellini P, Trespidi L, DeGiorgi O, et al. Endometriosis and pelvic pain: Relation to disease stage and localization. *Fertil Steril.* 65:299, 1996

113. Moon YS, Leung PCS, Yuen BH, Gomel V. Prostaglandin F in human endometriotic tissue. *Am J Obstet Gynecol.* 141:344, 1981

114. Schenken RS, Asch RH, Williams RF, Hodgen GD. Etiology of infertility in monkeys with endometriosis. Measurement of peritoneal fluid prostaglandins. *Am J Obstet Gynecol.* 150:349, 1984

115. Vernon MS, Beard JS, Graves K, Wilson EA. Classification of endometriotic implants by morphologic appearance and capacity to synthesize prostaglandin F. *Fertil Steril.* 46:801, 1986

116. Kauppila A, Puolakka J, Ylikorkala O. Prostaglandin biosynthesis inhibitors and endometriosis. *Prostaglandins.* 18:655, 1979

117. Schenken RS, Asch RH, Williams RF, Hodgen GD. Etiology of infertility in monkeys with endometriosis. *Fertil Steril.* 41:122, 1984

118. Werlin LB, DiZerega GS, Hodgen GD. Endometriosis: Effect of ovulation, ovum pickup, and transport in monkeys: An interim report. *Fertil Steril.* 35:263, 1981. Abstract

119. Kaplan CR, Eddy CA, Olive DL, Schenken RS. Effect of ovarian endometriosis on ovulation in rabbits. *Am J Obstet Gynecol.* 160:40, 1989

120. Jansen RPS. Minimal endometriosis and reduced fecundability: Prospective evidence from an artificial insemination by donor program. *Fertil Steril.* 46:141, 1986

121. Olive DL, Haney AF. Endometriosis-associated infertility: A critical review of therapeutic approaches. *Obstet Gynecol Surv.* 41:538, 1986

122. Rodriguez-Escudero FJ, Neyro JL, Corcosteugui B, Benito JA. Does minimal endometriosis reduce fecundity? *Fertil Steril.* 50:522, 1988

123. Chauhan M, Barratt CLR, Cooke SMS, Cook ID. Differences in the fertility of donor insemination recipients—A study to provide prognostic guidelines as to its success and outcome. *Fertil Steril.* 51:815, 1989

124. Dunphy BC, Key R, Barratt CLR, Cooke ID. Female age: The length of involuntary infertility prior to investigation and fertility outcome. *Hum Reprod.* 4:527, 1989

125. Cooke ID, Thomas EJ. The medical treatment of mild endometriosis. *Acta Obstet Gynecol Scand.* 150(suppl.):27, 1989

126. Kauppila A, Puolakka J, Ylikorkala O. Prostaglandin biosynthesis inhibitors and endometriosis. *Prostaglandins.* 18:655, 1979

127. Floyd WS. Danazol: Endocrine and endometrial effects. *Int J Fertil.* 25:75, 1980

128. Goebel R, Rjosk HK. Laboratory and clinical studies with the new antigonadotropin, danazol. *Acta Endocrinol.* 85:134, 1977

129. Barbieri RL, Canich JA, Makris A, Todd RB. Danazol inhibits steroidogenesis. *Fertil Steril.* 28:809, 1977

130. McGinley R, Casey JH. Analysis of progesterone in un-extracted serum: A method using danazol-A blocker of steroid binding to proteins. *Steroids.* 33:127, 1979

131. Buttram VC Jr, Belue JB, Reiter R. Interim report of a study of danazol for the treatment of endometriosis. *Fertil Steril.* 37:478, 1982

132. Dmowski WP, Cohen MR. Treatment of endometriosis with an antigonadotropin, danazol: A laparoscopic and histologic evaluation. *Obstet Gynecol.* 46:147, 1975

133. Barbieri RL, Evans S, Kistner RW. Danazol in the treatment of endometriosis: Analysis of 100 cases with a 4 year follow-up. *Fertil Steril.* 37:737, 1982

134. Doberl A, Jeppsson S, Rannevik G. Effect of danazol on serum concentrations of pituitary gonadotropins in postmenopausal women. *Acta Obstet Gynecol Scand.* 123(suppl.): 95, 1984

135. Buttram VC Jr, Reiter RC, Ward S. Treatment of endometriosis with danazol: Report of a six-year prospective study. *Fertil Steril.* 43:353, 1985

136. Henzl MR, Corson SL, Moghissi K, et al. Administration of nasal nafarelin as compared with oral danazol for endometriosis. *N Engl J Med.* 318:485, 1988

137. Telimaa S, Puolakka J, Ronnberg L, Kaupilla A. Placebo-controlled comparison of danazol and high-dose medroxyprogesterone acetate in the treatment of endometriosis. *Gynecol Endocrinol.* 1:13, 1987

138. Bayer SR, Seibel MM. Medical treatment: Danazol. In: Schenkel RS, ed. *Endometriosis: Contemporary Concepts in Clinical Management.* Philadelphia, J. B. Lippincott, 1989: 169–187

139. Vercellini P, Trespidi L, Panazza S, et al. Very low dose danazol for relief of endometriosis-associated pelvic pain: A pilot study. *Fertil Steril.* 62:1136, 1994

140. Bayer SR, Seibel MM, Saffan DS, Berger MJ. The efficacy of danazol treatment for minimal endometriosis in an infertil population: A prospective, randomized study. *J Reprod Med.* 33:179, 1988

141. Telimaa S. Danazol and medroxyprogesterone acetate inefficacious in the treatment of endometriosis associated with infertility. *Fertil Steril.* 50:872, 1988

142. Olive DL. Medical treatment: Alternatives to danazol. In: Schenken RS, ed. *Endometriosis: Contemporary Concepts in Clinical Management.* Philadelphia, J. B. Lippincott, 1989:189–211

143. Timonen S, Johansson CJ. Endometriosis treated with lynestrenol. *Ann Chir Gynaecol Fenn.* 57:144, 1968

144. Johnston WI. Dihydrogesterone and endometriosis. *Br J Obstet Gynaecol.* 83:77, 1976

145. Moghissi KS, Boyce CRK. Management of endometriosis with oral medroxyprogesterone acetate. *Obstet Gynecol.* 47:265, 1976

146. Schlaff WD, Dugoff L, Damewood MD, Rock JA. Megestrol acetate for treatment of endometriosis. *Obstet Gynecol.* 75:646, 1990

147. Hull ME, Moghissi KS, Magyar DF, Hayes MF. Comparison for different treatment modalities of endometriosis in infertile women. *Fertil Steril.* 47:40, 1987

148. Werlin LB, Hodgen GD. Gonadotropin-releasing hormone agonist suppresses ovulation, menses, and endometriosis in monkeys: An individualized, intermittent regimen. *J Clin Endocrinol Metab.* 56:844, 1983

149. Fedele L, Bianchi S, Arcaini L, et al. Buserelin versus danazol in the treatment of endometriosis-associated infertility. *Am J Obstet Gynecol.* 161:871, 1989

150. Lemay A, Maheux R, Faure N, Jean C. Reversible pseudomenopause induced by repetitive luteinizing-hormone-releasing hormone agonist administration (Buserelin): A new approach to the treatment of endometriosis. In: Raynaud JP, Ojasoo T, Martini L, eds. *Medical Management of Endometriosis.* New York, Raven Press, 1984: 263

151. Adamson GD, Frison L, Lamb EJ. Endometriosis: Studies of a method for the design of a surgical staging system. *Fertil Steril.* 38:659, 1982

152. Kettel LM, Murphy AA, Morales AJ, et al. Treatment of endometriosis with the antiprogesterone mifepristone (RU 486). *Fertil Steril.* 65:23, 1996

153. Olive DL. Conservative surgery. In: Schenken RS, ed. *Endometriosis: Contemporary Concepts in Clinical Management.* Philadelphia, J. B. Lippincott, 1989: 213–247

154. Vancaillie T, Schenken RS. Endoscopic surgery. In: Schenken RS, ed. *Endometriosis: Contemporary Concepts in Clinical Management.* Philadelphia, J. B. Lippincott, 1989: 249–266

155. Wheeler JM, Malinak LR. Recurrent endometriosis: Incidence, management, and prognosis. *Am J Obstet Gynecol.* 146:247, 1983

156. Gordts S, Boeckx W, Brasens I. Microsurgery of endometriosis in infertile patients. *Fertil Steril.* 42:520, 1984

157. Adhesion Study Group. Reduction in postoperative pelvic adhesions with intraperitoneal 32% dextran 70: A prospective, randomized clinical trial. *Fertil Steril.* 40:612, 1983

158. Diamond MP, Daniell JF, Martin DC, Feste J. Tubal patency and pelvic adhesions at early second-look laparoscopy following intra-abdominal use of the carbon dioxide laser: Initial report of the intra-abdominal laser study group. *Fertil Steril.* 42:717, 1984

159. Nezhat C, Hood J, Winer JW, et al. Videolaseroscopy and laser laparoscopy in gynaecology. *Br J Hosp Med.* 38:219, 1987

160. Guzick DS, Rock JA. A comparison of danazol and conservative surgery for the treatment of infertility due to mild or moderate endometriosis. *Fertil Steril.* 40:580, 1983

161. Olive DL, Lee KL. Analysis of sequential treatment protocols for endometriosis-associated infertility. *Am J Obstet Gynecol.* 154:613, 1986

162. Nowroozi K, Chase JS, Check JH, Wu CH. The importance of laparoscopic coagulation of mild endometriosis in infertile women. *Int J Fertil.* 32:442, 1987

163. Adamson GD, Pasta DJ. Surgical treatment of endometriosis-associated infertility: Meta-analysis compared with survival analysis. *Am J Obstet Gynecol.* 171:1488, 1994

164. Hughes EG, Fedorkow DM, Collins JA. A quantitative overview of controlled trials in endometriosis-associated infertility. *Fertil Steril.* 59:963, 1993

165. Walters MD. Definitive surgery. In: Schenken RS, ed. *Endometriosis: Contemporary Concepts in Clinical Management.* Philadelphia, J. B. Lippincott, 1989: 267–278

166. Namnoum AB, Hickman TN, Goodman SB, et al. Incidence of symptom recurrence after hysterectomy for endometriosis. *Fertil Steril.* 64:898, 1995

167. Ranney B. Endometriosis. III. Complete operations. Reasons, sequelae, treatment. *Am J Obstet Gynecol.* 109:1137, 1971

168. Chong AP, Keene ME, Thornton NL. Comparison of three modes of treatment for infertility patients with minimal pelvic endometriosis. *Fertil Steril.* 53:407, 1990

169. Telimaa S, Ronnberg L, Kaupila A. Placebo-controlled comparison of danazol and high-dose medroxyprogesterone acetate in the treatment of endometriosis after conservative surgery. *Gynecol Endocrinol.* 1:363, 1987

170. Ylikorkala O, Viinikka L. Prostaglandins and endometriosis. *Acta Obstet Gynecol Scand.* 113(suppl.):105, 1983

171. Kauppila A, Puolakka J, Ylikorkala O. Prostglandin biosynthesis inhibitors and endometriosis. *Prostaglandins.* 18:655, 1979

172. Kaupilla A, Ronnberg L. Naproxen sodium in dysmenorrhea secondary to endometriosis. *Obstet Gynecol.* 65:379, 1985

173. Tjaden B, Schlaff WD, Kimball A, Rock JA. The efficacy of presacral neurectomy for the relief of midline dysmenorrhea. *Obstet Gynecol.* 76:89, 1990

174. Candiani GB, Fedele L, Vercellini P, et al. Presacral neurectomy for the treatment of pelvic pain associated with endometriosis: A controlled study. *Am J Obstet Gynecol.* 167:100, 1992

175. Lichten EM, Bombard J. Surgical treatment of primary dysmenorrhea with laparoscopic uterine nerve ablation. *J Reprod Med.* 32:37, 1987

176. Dodson WC, Whitesides DB, Hughes CL Jr, et al. Superovulation with intrauterine insemination in the treatment of infertility: A possible alternative to gamete intrafallopian transfer and in vitro fertilization. *Fertil Steril.* 48:441, 1987

177. Geber S, Paraschos T, Atkinson G, et al. Results of IVF in patients with endometriosis: The severity of the disease does not affect outcome, or the incidence of miscarriage. *Hum Reprod.* 10:1507, 1995

Chapter 33

ASSISTED REPRODUCTIVE TECHNOLOGY

Michael P. Steinkampf, Owen K. Davis, and Zev Rosenwaks

Until recently, the success of virtually all infertility treatments was limited by the ability of the oviduct to transport egg and sperm to the distal ampulla, with conveyance of the resulting preimplantation embryo to the uterus. Assisted reproductive technology (ART) collectively refers to infertility treatments that involve the retrieval of oocytes, bypassing part or all of the natural pickup and transport of gametes/embryos. Although originally designed to treat women with absent or irreparably damaged fallopian tubes, ART procedures have since been developed to deal with a wide variety of infertility problems. The rapid development and sophistication of ART procedures has been a milestone in the treatment of the infertile couple, but the ethical dilemmas resulting from these new treatment options have called into question whether society should somehow limit how humans reproduce.

IN VITRO FERTILIZATION AND EMBRYO TRANSFER: THE PROTOTYPE ART PROCEDURE

The concept of achieving fertilization by placing egg and sperm in a culture dish ("in vitro" is Latin for "under glass") is not a new concept. In vitro fertilization was first attempted as early as 1878 (see reference 1 for review), but success eluded investigators until it was realized that IVF required processing of sperm to achieve capacitation, enabling the subsequent acrosome reaction and penetration of the egg. By 1959, the first births (in rabbits) from IVF had been reported.[2] In humans, successful in vitro fertilization with subsequent embryo cleavage was first reported in 1944,[3] but a successful human IVF pregnancy was not achieved until 1978.[4] Since then, hundreds of IVF programs have sprung up across the world, and more than 9000 deliveries occur annually in North America from this procedure (Fig 33–1).

Indications and Patient Selection

As noted, IVF was designed to treat women with damaged fallopian tubes who had not conceived after reconstructive surgery. Pregnancy rarely occurs after the repair of occluded tubes with extensive pelvic adhesions or severe tubal damage,[5] and proceeding directly to IVF in these patients has been recommended by some. However, there is a growing consensus that the presence of hydrosalpinges has a deleterious effect on implantation following IVF and embryo transfer (ET).[6–9] This finding has prompted some clinicians to offer pretreatment salpingostomies or salpingectomies to such patients, or to consider salpingectomy in the event that one or more prior IVF cycles have failed. Thus, even the patient with severely damaged tubes may ultimately require some surgical treatment. Infertility due to pelvic adhesions or endometriosis in which pregnancy has not resulted after surgical treatment is also amenable to IVF, as is infertility due to immunologic or unexplained causes.

The initial use of IVF for male factor infertility was disappointing. Fertilization with conventional IVF is unlikely to occur when there are fewer than 3 million motile sperm in the ejaculate,[10] or when motility or the percentage of normal forms is severely decreased. However, the recent development of microsurgical fertilization techniques has dramatically improved the success of IVF for male infertility (discussed later).

Although the age of the male does not appear to be associated with the chance of pregnancy after IVF, the age of the female partner is a critical determinant of outcome (Fig 33–2). This age-related decline in fertility is most apparent beginning at about age 38.[11] The decreased chance for viable pregnancy following IVF-ET in older women is primarily due to ovarian senescence rather than the aging uterine milieu, as suggested by work utilizing donor eggs.[12] Study of biopsied embryos analyzed with techniques such as fluorescence in situ hybridization has

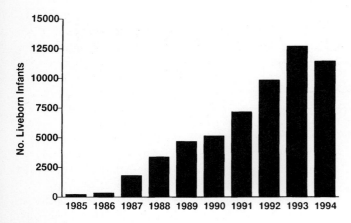

Figure 33–1. Number of liveborn infants in US and Canada resulting from assisted reproductions procedures. *(Reproduced, with permission, from* Fertil Steril. *66:697, 1996.)*

demonstrated sharply increased rates of numeric chromosomal abnormalities with advancing age,[13] suggesting that embryonic aneuploidy is responsible for the maternal age-related decline in IVF success rates in particular, and fecundity in general. In addition, the inexorable depletion of oocytes with increasing age results in fewer embryos available for transfer.

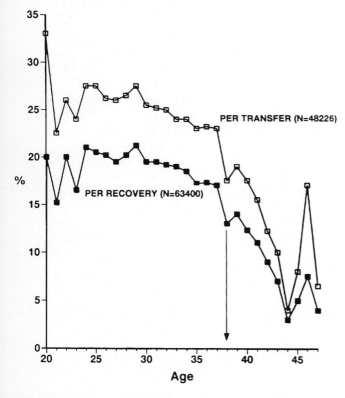

Figure 33–2. Maternal age versus chance of pregnancy via IVF. *(Reproduced, with permission, from* Fertil Steril. *59:587, 1993.)*

These effects translate into higher rates of cancellation, lower rates of pregnancy, and a higher risk of spontaneous abortion in older IVF patients. In the 1994 Society for Assisted Reproductive Technology Registry, women 40 years of age and older (with no male factor) experienced a 6.9 percent delivery rate per cycle start, compared to a 21.5 percent delivery rate for women younger than 40.[14] Very few births from conventional IVF occur after the age of 42.

Ovarian reserve may be assessed by measuring basal follicle-stimulating hormone (FSH) and estradiol levels early in the follicular phase (eg, day 3). An elevated FSH and/or estradiol level may indicate incipient ovarian failure and a reduced chance for success following IVF.[15] Some investigators have suggested that an exaggerated rise in FSH levels following the administration of a standard dose of clomiphene citrate also denotes a guarded prognosis.[16,17]

IVF candidates should undergo a thorough review of their prior fertility evaluation and any therapy, including prior IVF. This evaluation may uncover deficiencies in the fertility workup or suggest alternative therapy. Examination of the female includes assessment of uterine size and position, often including a uterine sounding with a transfer catheter, to determine uterine depth and to anticipate any potential technical difficulty prior to actual embryo transfer. Papanicolaou smears and cervical cultures (eg, chlamydia) may be obtained at this time, but routine culture of the semen does not appear to be of value.[18] Hysterosalpingogram films should be reviewed to evaluate for intrauterine pathology, including submucous myomata, polyps, synechiae, or a septum, which might impede blastocyst implantation or increase the risk of spontaneous abortion.[19] Significant filling defects should be further assessed by hysteroscopy and surgically corrected.

A complete semen analysis should be performed in the IVF program's andrology laboratory to evaluate for a possible male factor. Abnormalities may prompt additional testing such as semen culture or assay for antisperm antibodies or plans for assisted fertilization at the time of IVF.

Ovarian Stimulation

The first human IVF pregnancy resulted from retrieval of a single oocyte in a spontaneous menstrual cycle.[4] This approach ultimately proved laborious because of the need for round-the-clock blood and urine sampling to identify the spontaneous luteinizing hormone (LH) surge and the possibility of an oocyte retrieval occurring at any time of the day or night, 25 to 29 hr following onset of the surge. Pregnancy rates were limited due to the replacement of single embryos. In general, IVF success rates improve as the number of transferred embryos is increased, and virtually all programs now routinely utilize ovarian hyperstimulation protocols to effect multiple follicular recruitment.

Drugs that have been used for ovarian stimulation in IVF include clomiphene, human menopausal gonadotropins (hMGs), purified follicle-stimulating hormone, and analogs of gonadotropin-releasing hormone (GnRH). Gonadotropin use affords the maturation of more eggs than clomiphene, but at considerably higher cost (the details of clomiphene and gonadotropin treatment can be found in Chap 29). The standard protocol at most IVF centers has come to be a combination of a GnRH analog and gonadotropins. Parenteral administration of a long-acting GnRH agonist results in an initial surge of gonadotropin release from the anterior pituitary followed by downregulation of gonadotropin secretion. GnRH antagonists have also been developed, and have the advantage of inducing immediate suppression of FSH and LH secretion without an initial agonistic effect. The clinical applicability of GnRH antagonists has been hampered by histaminic side effects, and these agents are not commercially available as of this writing.

Initially, GnRH analogs were used only with patients who manifested premature LH surges during previous ovarian stimulation, leading either to cycle cancellation or the retrieval of poor quality oocytes due to premature follicular luteinization. GnRH analog use also allows more convenient scheduling of egg retrievals, thus reducing costs and limiting the need for weekend egg retrievals. More recently, the routine use of GnRH analog-gonadotropin protocols has been shown to improve pregnancy rates,[20,21] predominantly by reducing the cancellation rate from premature ovulation but also by increasing the number of oocytes obtained.[22]

In the United States, the GnRH agonist most widely used in IVF is leuprolide acetate (Lupron). This agonist is administered as a daily subcutaneous dose of 0.5 to 1 mg. If leuprolide is started in the midluteal phase of the preceding cycle ("long protocol"), ovarian suppression is usually complete by the onset of menses, approximately 1 wk later. Alternatively, the GnRH analog may be begun with the onset of menses and an estradiol level checked about 10 days later to assess response. Once pituitary suppression has been achieved, gonadotropins are then administered concomitantly and the leuprolide is discontinued on the day of the human chorionic gonadotropin (hCG) injection. Leuprolide and gonadotropins may, alternatively, be initiated in the early follicular phase (short or "flare" protocol); here, the agonist phase of the GnRHa stimulates the ovaries in an additive manner with the gonadotropins, prior to pituitary downregulation, which occurs in time to obviate a premature LH surge.[23] Although success has been reported with both protocols, midluteal GnRHa initiation is probably the more commonly used approach.[24]

The principal disadvantages of adjunctive GnRH analog use for IVF are (1) an increased total dosage requirement for hMG and/or FSH (although this is not a problem with the "flare" protocol); (2) the potential for oversuppression of the ovaries with a subsequent failure of response (more likely to be seen in women approaching menopause); and (3) a possibly increased risk of ovarian hyperstimulation syndrome in high responders.

Some clinicians have evinced a renewed enthusiasm for IVF in spontaneous or clomiphene-stimulated cycles,[25,26] prompted by cost factors and concerns regarding the risks of gonadotropin use. However, the low per-cycle pregnancy rates with this approach has led to its use predominantly in the "low responder" who repeatedly recruits a single dominant follicle despite high-dose gonadotropin treatment.

Egg maturation in vitro may be another alternative to gonadotropin stimulation for IVF. Several births have been reported with IVF using immature eggs obtained by excision from ovarian tissue or by follicle aspiration,[27–29] but low pregnancy rates and the need for intensive laboratory manipulation have limited enthusiasm for this approach.

Oocyte Retrieval

Recovery of the oocytes is generally performed 34 to 36 hours following hCG administration. This interval allows the resumption of meiosis I, with extrusion of the first polar body occurring near the time of the egg retrieval. Initially, laparoscopic follicular aspiration was the standard method for oocyte retrieval. Ultrasound-directed techniques were first developed for use in cases where ovaries were inaccessible to the laparoscope, as in patients with severe pelvic adhesions.[30,31] As equipment was refined and operators developed greater expertise, ultrasound-directed techniques have virtually replaced the endoscopic approach except in cases in which cannulation of the fallopian tubes is required (reviewed later), when a diagnostic examination of the pelvis is indicated, or when the ovaries are located above the pelvic brim.

Several sonographic techniques have been reported, including percutaneous transvesical, transurethral-transvesical, and transvaginal aspiration, with either transabdominal or transvaginal scanning. Transvaginal follicle aspiration with a vaginal ultrasound transducer has become the prevalent technique at most centers. For this procedure, the patient is placed in the dorsal lithotomy position, and the vagina is prepped with an antiseptic cleanser followed by copious saline irrigation, although one study suggests that better results are obtained if the vaginal antiseptic is omitted.[32] Intravenous sedation and analgesia are adequate for most transvaginal oocyte retrievals. Although the benefit of prophylactic antibiotics is not clearly proven, some authors have recommended

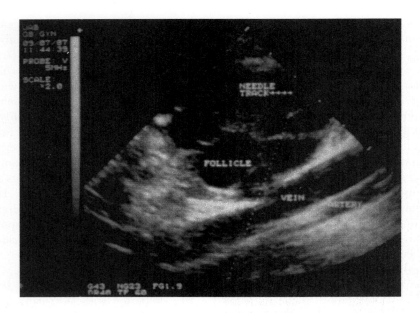

Figure 33–3. Ultrasound view of transvaginal follicle aspiration for egg retrieval.

their routine use,[33] because postretrieval pelvic infections can be severe.[34] A transvaginal ultrasound probe housing a high-frequency transducer (typically 5 to 7 MHz) is introduced with a fixed needle guide. The maximum diameter of each follicle is aligned with the puncture line on the screen, and the needle is advanced into the follicle along the shortest path. A negative pressure of 100 to 120 mm Hg is applied to the needle just prior to follicle puncture (higher negative pressures increase the risk of oocyte disruption). Collapse of the follicle is visualized on the ultrasound screen (Fig 33–3), and the machine-scored needle tip may be used to curette the follicle. Following aspiration of each follicle, the needle may either be advanced to the next follicle or kept in place until the oocyte is identified by the embryologist so as to facilitate further flushing and reaspiration. A typical oocyte retrieval will be completed within 15 to 45 min, depending on the number of follicles to be aspirated and the speed with which oocytes can be identified.

Classification of Oocyte Maturity

Oocyte classification is based on characteristics of the oocyte–corona–cumulus complex, including the extent of mucification and dispersal of the corona radiata and cumulus, and the presence or absence of a nuclear membrane (germinal vesicle) or polar body. An estimate of oocyte maturity based solely on an assessment of cumulus and corona dispersal is generally sufficient when performing conventional IVF.

A mature preovulatory oocyte displays extensive dispersal of the surrounding granulosa cells, with an expanded cumulus and corona radiata. Presence of the first polar body indicates that an oocyte is in metaphase II. An oocyte of intermediate maturity is marked by a slightly dense corona with a dispersed cumulus. Neither a germinal vesicle nor a polar body can be identified. An immature oocyte has a compact corona, with a cumulus composed of only a few cell layers. The germinal vesicle may be easily visualized in a grossly immature oocyte. An atretic oocyte characteristically displays a sparse, unexpended cumulus with a dark and irregularly shaped ooplasm.

In Vitro Insemination and Culture

The operation of a successful in vitro fertilization laboratory requires meticulous attention to detail. Quality control includes testing of instruments, media, and plasticware for potential embryo toxicity. The following is a general overview of insemination and culture procedures; the specific details vary from program to program, and a given laboratory will adopt those procedures with which it has enjoyed the greatest success.

The sperm sample is obtained just before or shortly after oocyte recovery. Semen is obtained in a sterile plastic jar or occasionally with the use of a Silastic condom. The seminal fluid is allowed to liquefy at room temperature and the sperm is then prepared for insemination. Although a variety of techniques are in use, the most common is the "swim-up," in which an aliquot of semen is diluted with culture medium and centrifuged. The supernatant is discarded, and the sperm pellet is resuspended in fresh medium. After a second centrifugation, sperm from the pellet is allowed to migrate into a small aliquot of overlain culture

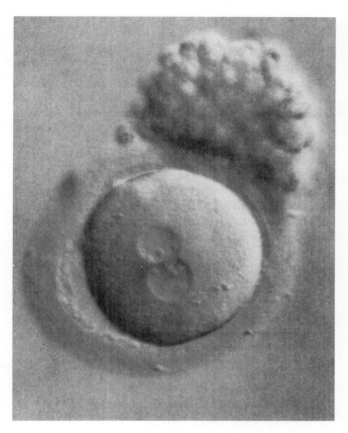

Figure 33–4. A normal zygote displaying paternal and maternal pronuclei. *(Courtesy of J. Cohen.)*

medium for 30 to 60 min. This highly motile fraction is then pipetted off and used for insemination of the oocytes. Mature preovulatory oocytes are usually preincubated for 2 to 8 hr prior to insemination, as this is thought to improve fertilization rates versus immediate insemination. In some programs, immature oocytes are incubated for up to 36 hr before insemination in order to allow further maturation.

Typically, each oocyte is inseminated with roughly 100,000 to 200,000 motile sperm, although the sperm density is sometimes increased to as many as 500,000 per oocyte in an effort to enhance fertilization. The sperm and oocytes are coincubated for 12 to 18 hr in 5 percent CO_2 with 98 percent relative humidity, at a temperature of 37 °C. The oocytes are then examined for evidence of fertilization, which is confirmed by the presence of two pronuclei (male and female) or by extrusion of the second polar body (Fig 33–4). It is important to look for possible polyspermic fertilization, signaled by the presence of more than two pronuclei per oocyte (Fig 33–5). A polyploid embryo may subsequently cleave normally and could be missed unless identified at the pronuclear stage.

The incidence of polyspermia after conventional IVF is approximately 10 percent; contributing factors may include high concentrations of sperm and postmaturity or immaturity of the oocytes.[35–37]

Assisted Fertilization

Fertilization rates with IVF using mature oocytes generally exceed 80 percent. Of the oocytes that fertilize, over 85 percent will subsequently cleave. However, in men with severe sperm abnormalities, fertilization rarely occurs with conventional IVF. In recent years, microsurgical techniques have been developed to achieve fertilization in these difficult cases. A brief history of the evolution of microsurgically assisted fertilization technology underscores the rapid pace of innovation in this field. The first technique, developed to overcome the barrier to fertilization posed by the zona pellucida, involved the creation of a physical gap in the zona pellucida, thus facilitating the entrance of motile sperm into the perivitelline space. Variations of this procedure have been described, ranging from chemical "drilling" with acidic Tyrodes solution[38] to mechanical incision of the zona. The most successful variation of this initial approach was partial zona dissection (PZD).[39] Using a micromanipulator, the oocyte was stabilized with a suction micropipette, and a surgical incision was introduced into the zona with a glass microneedle. PZD resulted in the first human pregnancies from micro-surgical fertilization.[40] A subsequent and more effective method of microsurgical fertilization involved the direct insertion of sperm under the zona (subzonal insertion).[41] As only a few motile spermatozoa were needed for each oocyte, this technique was applied to men with more marked degrees of oligospermia.

The major disadvantages of these earlier techniques were an increased risk of polyspermic fertilization (as increased numbers of sperm had unimpeded access to the oolemma), and relatively low fertilization rates. A more effective procedure is direct injection of a single sperm into the ooplasm.[42] This procedure, known as intracytoplasmic sperm injection (ICSI), involves denuding the oocytes of their surrounding cumulus cells with hyaluronidase, followed by injection of the metaphase II oocytes with a single, motile (ie, viable) sperm (Fig 33–6). This technique has been successfully extended to the treatment of men with unreconstructable obstructive azoospermia using sperm aspirated from the epididymis or the testis.[43,44]

There are several potential risks inherent in microsurgical fertilization. Theoretically, perforation of the zona could increase the risk of invasion of the transferred embryos by bacteria and/or inflammatory cells. Indeed, one study indicated that the administration of a short course of oral antibiotics and glucocorticoids in

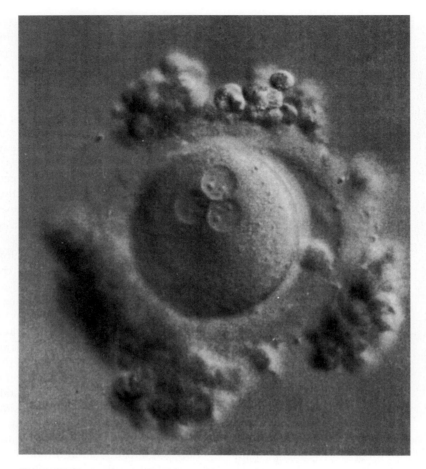

Figure 33–5. A polyspermic embryo with three pronuclei. *(Courtesy of J. Cohen.)*

the peritransfer period improved the implantation rates of zonamanipulated embryos.[45] ICSI can mechanically damage oocytes, but this is infrequent in experienced hands. Finally, concerns have been raised as to whether ICSI might increase the incidence of congenital malformations in offspring, given the somewhat arbitrary selection of a single sperm by the operator and the intrinsic invasiveness of the technique. However, a recent review of 987 ICSI cycles at Cornell indicated a frequency of malformations lower than that observed in offspring born after standard IVF.[46] Nonetheless, certain types of male factor infertility are associated with transmissible genetic abnormalities. Men with congenital bilateral absence of the vas deferens have a high incidence of cystic fibrosis gene mutations, thus mandating screening of such couples with genetic counseling prior to sperm aspiration and ICSI. Men with nonobstructive azoospermia may have karyotypic abnormalities (eg, Klinefelter syndrome) or microdeletions of the Y chromosome, which might be transmitted to male offspring. Genetic testing and counseling

about these risks is appropriate for couples contemplating ICSI.

EMBRYO CULTURE

The optimal culture conditions for human preimplantation eggs and embryos have not been established, and most techniques for human IVF have been developed using embryos from other species, which may have different nutritional requirements.[47] In most U.S. programs, a complex media such as Ham's F-10 or HTF (a media designed to mimic human tubal fluid) is used for both sperm processing and embryo culture. These media contain bicarbonate and require equilibration with an atmosphere containing 5 percent CO_2 to achieve a physiologic pH (7.4). Protein derived from human or animal serum is generally used to supplement the media. Although human fetal serum obtained from the placenta at delivery was once considered a superior supplement,[48] it has been supplanted by autologous serum or commercially

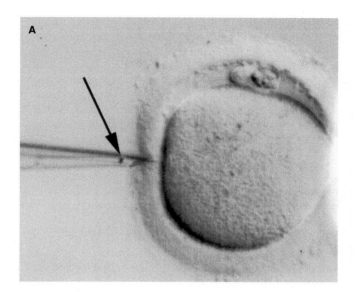
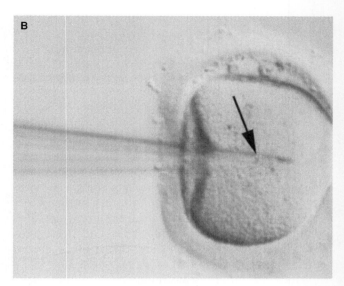
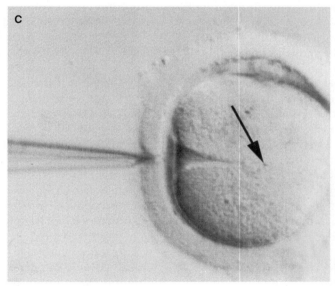

Figure 33–6. Techniques of intracytoplasmic sperm injection (ICSI). Black arrow indicates location of sperm. A: Sperm loaded in injection pipette. B: Insertion of pipette into ooplasm. C: Pipette withdrawn after sperm injected (*Courtesy of Michael Tucker.*)

available products based on human albumin.[49] The concentration of protein in the culture medium is sometimes varied based on the developmental stage of the embryo, although there are few data to indicate whether this is beneficial.

Embryo Transfer

Pregnancies have been reported after the transfer of embryos ranging from the pronuclear to blastocyst stage. At most IVF programs, transfer is performed 48 to 72 hr after oocyte retrieval. Prior to transfer, embryo quality is assessed on the basis of morphologic criteria (cell number, symmetry and shape of the blastomeres,

and the presence and extent of cytoplasmic fragmentation). Healthy embryos will reach the 4- to 8-cell stage within 36 to 48 hr following insemination; rapidly dividing embryos with symmetrical blastomeres and little fragmentation are most likely to implant. Despite refinements in the approach to embryonic grading, estimation of embryo viability remains an inexact science, as even "low-quality" embryos may implant and culminate in live births.

Pregnancy rates improve as the number of embryos replaced is increased,[50] but the rate of multiple pregnancy increases as well. In Great Britain, the maximum number of embryos allowed for transfer (three) is specified by law, while in the United States, most centers base the number of embryos to be transferred on embryo quality and the age of the patient in order to optimize the chance of pregnancy while limiting the risk of multiple gestation. Typically, three or four embryos are transferred in women under 40 yr of age.

A variety of transfer catheters are available. All are composed of nontoxic plastic, but they differ in length, caliber (most are 18- to 20-gauge), stiffness, and location of the distal opening (end versus side loading). Some catheters are inserted through a rigid introducer while others are threaded directly into the uterus without an outer sheath. Embryo transfers are typically done with the patient in the dorsal lithotomy position, although some programs employ the knee–chest position for an anteverted uterus and dorsal lithotomy for retroversion.

Once the patient is positioned on the table, a sterile speculum is inserted and the cervix is cleansed with culture medium to remove excess cervical mucus. Although rarely necessary, using a tenaculum or allowing the bladder to fill[51] may straighten the uterine axis if difficulty is encountered in negotiating the cervical canal. The embryos are loaded into a sterile catheter in a small volume (20 to 50 µl) of transfer medium, and the catheter is inserted through the cervical os toward the uterine fundus. The embryos are slowly injected using a small syringe attached to the catheter. The catheter is then microscopically examined and flushed with medium in an effort to identify any retained embryos for retransfer. The patient is transferred to a holding area where she remains supine for an interval of 30 min or more prior to discharge, although the length of this post-transfer rest period has not been shown to affect the cycle outcome.

Luteal Phase Management

Surveillance of the luteal phase may be limited to a serum β-hCG measurement two weeks after transfer. Some programs favor a more extensive protocol for luteal monitoring, with serial determinations of estradiol, progesterone, and β-hCG levels, but this has not been shown to improve cycle outcome.

Although most clinicians agree that luteal phase hormonal support is beneficial following adjunctive GnRH agonist therapy, it is less clear whether routine, empiric luteal supplementation is needed when GnRH agonists are not used.

Follicular aspiration for oocyte recovery disrupts and evacuates a small percentage of the granulosa cells lining the follicles. Theoretically, this "debulking" of the total mass of granulosa cells could lead to diminished hormonal secretion in the luteal phase. It is probable, however, that the multiple corpora lutea resulting from

ovarian hyperstimulation more than compensate in terms of net steroid secretion; peak luteal estradiol and progesterone levels following IVF cycles often far exceed those in the natural cycle.

Guided by these concerns, and supported by some clinical evidence that the incidence of histologic luteal phase defect is increased in canceled IVF cycles,[52] most programs routinely implement exogenous luteal support. Progesterone or hCG is most commonly used, although hCG increases the risk of ovarian hyperstimulation syndrome (OHSS) in some patients.[53] A recently published meta-analysis indicates that luteal support in IVF cycles does appear to improve pregnancy rates overall.[54]

Pregnancy Outcome—Results of IVF-ET

Pregnancy following IVF-ET is documented by an elevated serum hCG level 12 to 14 days following retrieval. Serial titers may be obtained to demonstrate a normal rise. Ultrasound examination is performed 3 to 6 wk after transfer in order to document viability and to assess for multiple gestation. With transvaginal ultrasound, fetal heart activity can often be seen as early as 4 wk after embryo transfer; exogenous luteal support is generally discontinued at that time.

Because the term "pregnancy" can connote anything from a transient rise in serum hCG levels to a live, term delivery, it is important to strictly define terms in any discussion of IVF outcomes. A "biochemical" pregnancy refers to a preclinical pregnancy identified by the secretion of hCG, with resorption or early spontaneous abortion prior to sonographic documentation. A "clinical" pregnancy is viable at least to the point where a gestational sac can be identified by sonography, or products of conception are obtained with uterine curettage. Spontaneous abortion rates occur in about 25 percent of clinical pregnancies after IVF, but can exceed 50 percent in women over 40 yr old.[55] "Ongoing" pregnancies typically include all undelivered pregnancies that have progressed beyond the first trimester. Finally, success rates may be reported exclusively in terms of "deliveries," which generally include all live births (regardless of whether the infants survive the neonatal period).

Most centers express pregnancy rates as clinical pregnancies or deliveries as a percentage of cycle starts, oocyte retrievals, or embryo transfers. The 1994 Society of Assisted Reproductive Technology (SART) IVF-ET Registry (249 clinics) recorded an overall delivery rate of 20.7 percent per retrieval.[14] Cumulative IVF pregnancy rates rise with repeated cycles; it is unclear whether the per-cycle pregnancy rate declines in patients who fail to conceive with the initial attempt.[56]

The incidence of ectopic gestation in the United States is approximately 1 percent of clinical pregnancies, while about 4 percent of IVF pregnancies are ectopic.[14] Heterotopic, cervical, and abdominal pregnancies have been reported following IVF-ET.[57–59] The rate of heterotopic gestation after assisted reproduction far exceeds the 1 in 30,000 risk for spontaneous pregnancies. A high index of suspicion and early sonographic evaluation of all IVF pregnancies is in the patient's best interest.[60]

Probably the most common significant complication of assisted reproductive technology is the increased incidence of multiple gestations. Multiple gestations can comprise more than 30 percent of the clinical pregnancies in an IVF program, and about 7 percent of IVF deliveries are triplets or higher.[14] The recent development of ultrasound-guided multifetal pregnancy reduction offers an alternative to couples with high-order multiple gestations.[61] Infants born after IVF-ET do not appear to be at an increased risk for congenital malformation or other morbidity when compared with spontaneously conceived infants when controlling for maternal age and multiple pregnancy.[62–64]

ART VARIATIONS AND REFINEMENTS

Assisted Hatching

Another application of zona micromanipulation technology has been the development of assisted hatching, a technique applied to embryos prior to transfer. Based on the observation that cleaved embryos with thinned areas on their zonae have higher implantation rates, it was hypothesized that one factor limiting success rates in IVF may be a failure of blastocyst hatching from the zona, a prerequisite for implantation. One randomized clinical trial showed that the per embryo implantation rate for assisted hatching embryos was 22 percent, versus 13 percent for the control group ($P < 0.05$).[65] Other studies have yielded conflicting results,[65–68] but there is a growing consensus that assisted hatching, now generally performed by zona drilling, may enhance implantation in selected patients, especially older women (>38 yr).

Embryo Co-culture

Because the optimal conditions for in vitro growth of human preimplantation embryos remain obscure, some have proposed that the culture of embryos with somatic "feeder" cells may be beneficial. The rationale for this approach is to mimic the environment of the fallopian tube. This embryo co-culture technique has been shown to improve the embryo growth in a variety of mammalian species.[69] Interestingly, cells from nonreproductive tissues also seem to promote preimplantation embryo growth.[70] It has been proposed that the beneficial effects of embryo co-culture occur via secretion of embryotrophic growth factors, or by elimination of embryotoxins present in the culture media or produced by the embryo itself. Technical challenges in culturing somatic cells in IVF programs and the lack of large-scale clinical trials demonstrating efficacy of embryo co-culture have limited the popularity of this technique.[71]

Embryo Biopsy

Zona drilling is also performed in embryo biopsy procedures, permitting removal of one or more blastomeres for preimplantation genetic diagnosis.[72] Adjunctive techniques such as fluorescence in situ hybridization (FISH) and polymerase chain reaction (PCR) permit the diagnosis of aneuploidy, gender in cases of X-linked disorders, and specific genetic disorders (eg, cystic fibrosis, Tay–Sach's disease), thus allowing transfer of normal embryos in couples at risk.[73] However, the expense of repeated IVF cycles and the technical challenges involved with reliably analyzing a single cell have limited the popularity of this approach to prenatal diagnosis.

Embryo and Oocyte Cryopreservation

Trounsen reported the first human pregnancy resulting from transfer of a cryopreserved and thawed embryo in 1983.[74] Prior to the availability of embryo cryopreservation, IVF programs had to deal with a quandary of "excess" oocytes and embryos that resulted from multifollicular stimulation. If selective insemination of oocytes was performed, normal eggs might be wasted, while if all oocytes were inseminated, embryos in excess of the usual number transferred might be obtained, leading to the dilemma of whether to discard potentially viable embryos or transfer them all, with the attendant risk of high-order multiple gestation. Embryo cryopreservation allows insemination of all recovered oocytes, thus maximizing the chance of transferring an optimal number of viable embryos, with the ability to freeze extra embryos for future transfer. Embryo cryopreservation increases the cumulative pregnancy rate per oocyte retrieval,[75] although some pregnancies from embryo cryopreservation occur in women who had already conceived in the original IVF cycle.

Human embryos may be cryopreserved at virtually any developmental stage from pronuclear (zygote) to blastocyst.[76] Freezing and thawing protocols vary with embryonic stage. In addition to a liquid nitrogen supply and storage facility, a controlled biologic freezer capable of cooling in increments of 0.10 to 0.5 °C per min is required.

Cryoprotectants, chemical agents used to replace cellular water, are required in order to minimize embryo damage caused by intracellular ice crystal formation during freezing and thawing. The choice of cryoprotectant is determined by the embryonic stage due to differences in cell permeability. Propanediol is generally used for pronuclear and 2-cell embryos, dimethyl sulfoxide (DMSO) for 4- to 12-cell embryos, and glycerol for blastocysts.

The cryoprotectant is added by pipetting the embryos through increasing concentrations of the agent. The embryos are then sealed in plastic straws or glass ampules and cooled to a temperature just below freezing to initiate the crystallization of freezing (seeding). The temperature is then reduced at a closely regulated rate to between −30 and −110 °C before they are plunged into liquid nitrogen (−196 °C). Embryo thawing is achieved by reversing the freezing process. The cryoprotectant is gradually removed by sequentially decreasing its concentration, and the embryos are then cultured for an interval prior to transfer.

Transfer of frozen embryos is usually performed in a natural menstrual cycle, with monitoring of serum and/or urine LH levels in order to detect the onset of the surge. Alternatively, the patient's ovarian function can be suppressed with a GnRH agonist and endometrial maturation controlled with an estrogen and progesterone replacement regimen.[76] The goal is to transfer the embryos into endometrium synchronized with their postinsemination age.

Overall, approximately 60 to 70 percent of cryopreserved embryos survive thawing. Of the 6,901 frozen ET procedures reported in the 1994 SART Registry, the clinical pregnancy and delivery rates were 19.2 and 15.6 percent overall.[14] As with fresh embryos, pregnancy after transfer of cryopreserved per transfer of cryopreserved embryos associated with increasing numbers of embryos frozen and with decreasing degree of embryo fragmentation. In addition, implantation is more likely to occur if a pregnancy resulted from the transfer of fresh embryos (from the same cohort) in the original IVF treatment cycle.

Oocyte Cryopreservation

Experience with cryopreservation of unfertilized human eggs has been limited. Only a few human pregnancies have resulted from cryopreserved oocytes.[77,78] Oocyte freezing protocols are analogous to those applied to embryos; a cryoprotectant (eg, DMSO) and controlled cooling are usually employed. A major concern regarding oocyte cryopreservation is the possibility of microtubule depolymerization with mitotic spindle damage. This could lead to chromatid nondisjunction at fertilization and result in aneuploidy. One approach to circumvent this problem is to freeze immature ooctyes, which are less susceptible to spindle disruption,[79,80] but the technique of in vitro maturation of cryopreserved oocytes has not yet been perfected.

Oocyte Donation

Artificial insemination with donor sperm has been a valuable option for couples with refractory male factor infertility. Before the advent of IVF and related techniques, no similar option existed for women with premature ovarian failure. Although donor oocyte IVF was initially primarily used to treat functionally agonadal women, other indications include hereditable genetic disorders, prior failed IVF due to poor oocyte quality, and, increasingly, advanced maternal age and incipient ovarian failure (reflected by persistently elevated basal FSH levels). Therefore, donor oocyte candidates can be divided into two general categories: those with and without endogenous ovarian function.

Oocyte donors may be anonymous or not (eg, sisters). Anonymous donors principally include other IVF patients willing to donate excess oocytes and women who volunteer to undergo stimulation and oocyte retrieval expressly for the purpose of oocyte donation. Potential donors must be thoroughly screened with a history and physical examination, including a genetic history and communicable disease evaluation comparable to that used for sperm donors. It is preferred that oocyte donors be younger than 35 yr of age.

Oocyte recipients are treated with sequential estrogen and progestin in order to achieve a fully developed secretory endometrium. In women with residual ovarian function, a GnRH analog is generally given to facilitate coordinating the donor and recipient cycles. A number of steroid replacement protocols have been described, most of which employ estradiol and progesterone given orally, vaginally, intramuscularly, or (in the case of estradiol) transdermally.[81,82] The recipient's "follicular phase" may be shortened or extended in order to facilitate synchronization with the egg donor's cycle. The first day of progesterone administration is defined as day 15. Serial measurement of serum estradiol and progesterone levels and a midluteal (days 20 to 21) endometrial biopsy and/or midcycle sonographic measurement of endometrial thickness may be performed in a preparatory cycle in order to document the adequacy of the regimen,[81] although the value of this is uncertain. If pregnancy occurs, estradiol and progesterone support are maintained through the first trimester.

The success of oocyte donation depends on synchronization of the recipient's endometrium with embryonic development. Immature or overly advanced endometrium is unlikely to support implantation. Pregnancy rates are highest when the 4- to 6-cell embryo is transferred on days 17, 18, or 19 of the recipient's simulated cycle.[81]

Success rates following donor oocyte ET have been very favorable. The 1994 SART Registry reported an overall 41.8 percent clinical pregnancy rate and 34.4 percent live delivery rate, following 2758 donor transfers. Although frozen donor embryos allow the advantage of quarantining the samples to allow more rigorous HIV screening, the decreased success associated with cryopreservation has limited the popularity of this approach.

As noted, failure to achieve pregnancy in young women with poor embryo quality in repeated IVF attempts has been proposed as an indication for oocyte donation. The etiology for impaired embryo development in such patients is unknown but may be due to deficient function of cytoplasmic organelles. Recently, the successful transfer of microscopic aliquots of cytoplasm from fertile egg donors to infertile recipients with poor embryo quality in previous IVF attempts has been reported.[83] After cytoplasmic transfer, ICSI was performed, with culture and subsequent transfer of the resulting embryos. Such a technique may provide the high success rate of egg donor IVF while maintaining the genetic composition of the recipient.

Gamete Intrafallopian Transfer

One factor thought to limit the success of IVF is the requirement for fertilization and early embryo development to occur in an artificial environment—-the culture dish. One approach to overcome this is gamete intrafallopian transfer (GIFT),[84] in which oocytes and sperm are immediately transferred to the fallopian tubes after egg retrieval. Ovarian stimulation protocols are identical to those used for IVF, and egg retrieval can be accomplished laparoscopically, using sonographic guidance, or rarely by minilaparotomy. Although ultrasound-guided transcervical techniques for fallopian tube cannulation have been developed,[85] pregnancy rates appear to be lower than when gamete transfer is accomplished laparoscopically.[86]

Because of the requirement for at least one patent fallopian tube, GIFT is performed most frequently in women with infertility due to endometriosis or unexplained causes. Although the success of GIFT appears to be higher than that of IVF (Fig 33–7), some clinicians argue that this may be due to patient selection or the inadequacies of certain embryo laboratories. A large-scale randomized trial of GIFT versus IVF has yet to be performed.

Tubal Embryo Transfer

Tubal embryo transfer (TET) combines IVF with the intrafallopian replacement of fertilized oocytes.[87] This procedure is sometimes referred to as PROST (pronuclear stage tubal transfer) or ZIFT (zygote intrafallopian transfer) if embryo transfer is performed before embryo cleavage begins. TET combines the techniques of IVF and GIFT, allowing confirmation of fertilization before transfer while providing at least some of the benefit of the fallopian tube environment. Patient selection criteria are similar to those for GIFT, although TET may be preferable to GIFT for women with circulating antisperm antibodies, because fertilization occurs in vitro in an "antibody-free" environment. Pregnancy rates with TET are comparable to GIFT,[14] but because the procedure requires two operative procedures (egg retrieval followed by laparoscopy 1 to 3 days later), its popularity in North America is declining.[14]

CONCLUSIONS

The development of assisted reproductive techniques represents the most important advance in the management of the infertile couple in this century. It has allowed the routine establishment of pregnancy with couples in whom success would be otherwise considered impossible, while offering an unparalleled opportunity to observe the

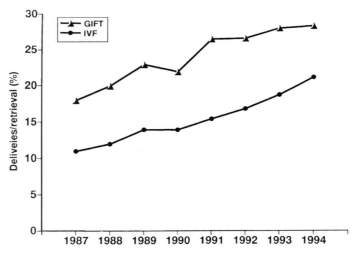

Figure 33–7. GIFT versus IVF delivery rates in US and Canada 1988–1994. *(Reproduced, with permission, from Fertil Steril. 66:697, 1996.)*

early reproductive events in humans. At the same time, the bewildering array of new infertility treatment options has challenged society's notions of what parenthood really means. It is likely that the rapid development of reproductive technology will continue, as will controversy about its appropriate use.

REFERENCE

1. Perone N. In vitro fertilization and embryo transfer—a historical perspective. *J Reprod Med.* 39:695, 1994
2. Chang MC. Fertilization of rabbit ova in vitro. *Nature.* 184:446, 1959
3. Rock J, Menkin MF. In vitro fertilization and cleavage of human ovarian eggs. *Science.* 100:105, 1944
4. Steptoe PC, Edwards RG. Birth after reimplantation of a human embryo. *Lancet.* 2:366, 1978
5. Boer-Meisel ME, Te Velde ER, Habbema JD. Predicting the pregnancy outcome in patients treated for hydrosalpinx: A prospective study. *Fertil Steril.* 45:23, 1986
6. Anderson AN, Yue Z, Meng FJ, Peterson K. Low implantation rate after in-vitro fertilization in patients with hydrosalpinges diagnosed by ultrasonography. *Hum Reprod.* 9:1935, 1994
7. Vandromme J, Chasse E, Lejeune B, et al. Hydrosalpinges in in-vitro fertilization: An unfavourable prognostic feature. *Hum Reprod.* 10:576, 1995
8. Katz E, Akman MA, Damewood MD, Garcia JE. Deleterious effect of the presence of hydrosalpinx on implantation and pregnancy rates with in vitro fertilization. *Fertil Steril.* 66:122, 1996
9. Fleming C, Hull MG. Impaired implantation after in vitro fertilization treatment associated with hydrosalpinx. *Br J Obstet Gynecol.* 103:268, 1996
10. Van Uem JFHM, Acosta AA, Swanson RG, et al. Male factor evaluation in in vitro fertilization: Norfolk experience. *Fertil Steril.* 44:375, 1985
11. French National IVF Registry. Analysis of 1986 to 1990 data. *Fertil Steril.* 59:587, 1993
12. Sauer MV, Paulson RJ, Lobo RA. A preliminary report on oocyte donation extending reproductive potential to women over 40. *N Engl J Med.* 51:651, 1990
13. Munne S, Alikani M, Tomkin G, et al. Embryo morphology, developmental rates, and maternal age are correlated with chromosome abnormalities. *Fertil Steril.* 64:382, 1995
14. Society for Assisted Reproductive Technology and the American Society for Reproductive Medicine. Assisted reproductive technology in the United States and Canada: 1994 results generated from the American Society for Reproductive Medicine/Society for Assisted Reproductive Technology Registry. *Fertil Steril.* 66:697, 1996
15. Scott RT, Oehninger S, Toner JP, et al. Follicle-stimulating hormone levels on cycle day 3 are predictive of in vitro fertilization outcome. *Fertil Steril.* 51:651, 1989
16. Navot D, Rosenwaks Z, Margolioth ES. Prognostic assessment of female fecundity. *Lancet.* 2:645, 1987
17. Laumaye E, Billion JM, Mine JM, et al. Prediction of individual response to controlled ovarian hyperstimulation by means of clomiphene citrate challenge test. *Fertil Steril.* 53:295, 1990
18. Liversedge NH, Jenkins JM, Keay SD, et al. Antibiotic treatment based on seminal cultures from asymptomatic male partners in in-vitro fertilization is unnecessary and may be detrimental. *Hum Reprod.* 11:1227, 1996
19. Lavergne N, Aristizabal J, Zarka V, et al. Uterine anomalies and in vitro fertilization: What are the results? *Eur J Obstet Gynecol Reprod Biol.* 68:29, 1996
20. Meldrum DR, Wisot A, Hamilton F, et al. Routine pituitary suppression with leuprolide before ovarian stimulation for oocyte retrieval. *Fertil Steril.* 5:455, 1989
21. Hughes EG, Fedorkow DM, Daya S, et al. The routine use of gonadatropin-releasing hormone agonist prior to in vitro fertilization and gamete intrafallopian transfer: A meta-analysis of randomized controlled trials. *Fertil Steril.* 58:888, 1992
22. Liu HC, Lai YM, Davis O, et al. Improved pregnancy outcome with gonadotropin-releasing hormone agonist (GnRHa) stimulation is due to the improvement of oocyte quantity rather than quality. *J Assist Reprod Genet.* 9:338, 1992
23. Garcia JE, Padilla SL, Bayati J, et al. Follicular phase gonadotropin releasing hormone agonist and human gonadotropins: A better alternative for ovulation induction in in vitro fertilization. *Fertil Steril.* 53:302, 1990
24. San Roman GA, Surrey ES, Judd HL, Kerin JF. A prospective randomized comparison of luteal phase versus concurrent follicular phase initiation of gonadotropin-releasing hormone agonist for in vitro fertilization. *Fertil Steril.* 58:744, 1992
25. Foulot H, Ranoux C, Dubuission JB, et al. In vitro fertilization ovarian stimulation: A simplified protocol applied in 80 cycles. *Fertil Steril.* 52:617, 1989
26. Steinkampf MP, Kretzer PA, McElroy E, Conway-Myers BA. A simplified approach to in vitro fertilization. *J Reprod Med.* 37:199, 1992
27. Cha KY, Koo JJ, Ko JJ, et al. Pregnancy after in vitro fertilization of human follicular oocytes collected from non-stimulated cycles, their culture in vitro and their transfer in a donor oocyte program. *Fertil Steril.* 55:109, 1991
28. Trounson A, Wood C, Kauscher A. In vitro maturation and the fertilization and developmental competence of oocytes recovered from untreated polycystic ovarian patients. *Fertil Steril.* 62:353, 1994
29. Russell JB, Knezevich KM, Fabian KF, Dickson JA. Unstimulated immature oocyte retrieval: Early versus midfollicular endometrial priming. *Fertil Steril.* 67:616, 1997
30. Lenz S, Lauritsen JG, Kjellow M. Collection of human oocytes for IVF by ultrasonically guided follicular puncture. *Lancet.* 1:1163, 1981
31. Gleicher N, Friberg S, Fullan N, et al. Egg retrieval for in-vitro fertilization by sonographically controlled vaginal culdocentesis. *Lancet.* 2:508, 1993
32. Van Os HC, Roozenburg BJ, Janssen-Caspers HA, et al. Vaginal disinfection with povidon iodine and the outcome of in-vitro fertilization. *Hum Reprod.* 7:349, 1992

33. Meldrum DR. Antibiotics for vaginal oocyte aspiration. *J In Vitro Fert Embryo Transf.* 6:1, 1989. Editorial

34. Howe RS, Wheller C, Mastroianni LJ, et al. Pelvic infection after transvaginal ultrasound-guided ovum retrieval. *Fertil Steril.* 49:726, 1988

35. Diamond MP, Rogers BJ, Webster BW, et al. Polyspermy: Effect of varying stimulation protocols and inseminating sperm concentrations. *Fertil Steril.* 43:777, 1985

36. Van der Ven HH, Al-Hasani S, Hamerich U, et al. Polyspermy in in vitro fertilization of human oocytes: frequency and possible causes. *Ann NY Acad Sci.* 442:88, 1985

37. Ho PC, Yeung WS, Chan YF, et al. Factors affecting the incidence of polyploidy in a human in vitro fertilization program. *Int J Fertil Menopausal Stud.* 39:14, 1994

38. Gordon JW, Talansky BE. Assisted fertilization by zona drilling: A mouse model for correction of oligospermia. *J Exp Zool. 239:347, 1986*

39. Malter HE, Cohen J. Partial zona dissection of the human oocyte: A nontraumatic method using micromanipulation to assist zona pellucida penetration. *Fertil Steril.* 51:139, 1989

40. Cohen J, Malter H, Fehilly C, et al. Implantation of embryos after partial opening of oocyte zona pellucida to facilitate sperm penetration. *Lancet.* 2:162, 1988

41. Ng SC, Bongso TA, Ratman SS, et al. Pregnancy after transfer of multiple sperm under the zona. *Lancet.* 2:790, 1988

42. Palermo G, Joris H, Devroey P, van Steirteghem AC. Pregnancies after intracytoplasmic injection of single spermatozoon into an oocyte. *Lancet.* 340:17, 1992

43. Silber SJ, Nagy ZP, Liu J, et al. conventional in-vitro fertilization versus intracytoplasmic sperm injection for patients requiring microsurgical sperm aspiration. *Hum Reprod.* 9:1705, 1994

44. Silber SJ, Van Steirteghem AC, Liu J, et al. High fertilization and pregnancy rate after intracytoplasmic sperm injection with spermatozoa obtained from testicle biopsy. *Hum Reprod.* 10:148, 1995

45. Cohen J, Malter H, Elsner C, et al. Immunosuppression supports implantation of zona pellucida-dissected human embryos. *Fertil Steril.* 53:662, 1990

46. Palermo GD, Colombero LT, Schattman GL, et al. Evolution of pregnancies and initial follow-up of newborns delivered after intracytoplasmic sperm injection. *JAMA.* 276:1893, 1996

47. Menezo YJR, Khatchadourian CJ. The laboratory culture media. *Assist Reprod Rev.* 1:136, 1991

48. Leung PCS, Gronow MJ, Kellow GN, et al. Serum supplement in human in vitro fertilization and embryo development. *Fertil Steril.* 41:36, 1984

49. Dugan KJ, Shalika S, Smith RD, Padilla SL. Comparison of synthetic serum substitute and fetal cord serum as media supplements for in vitro fertilization: A prospective, randomized study. *Fertil Steril.* 67:166, 1997

50. Muasher S, Wilkes C, Garcia JE, et al. Benefits and risks of multiple transfer with in vitro fertilization. *Lancet.* 1:570, 1954

51. Lewin A, Schenker JG, Avrech O, et al. The role of uterine straightening by passive bladder distension before embryo transfer in IVF cycles. *J Assist Reprod Genet.* 14:32, 1997

52. Graf MJ, Reyniak JV, Baffle-Mutter P, et al. Histologic evaluation of the luteal phase in women following follicle aspiration for oocyte retrieval. *Fertil Steril.* 49:616, 1988

53. Herman A, Ron-El R, Golan A, et al. Pregnancy rate and ovarian hyperstimulation after luteal human chorionic gonadotropin in in vitro fertilization stimulated with gonadotropin-releasing hormone analog and menotropins. *Fertil Steril.* 53:92, 1990

54. Soliman S, Daya S, Collins J, Hughes EG. The role of luteal phase support in infertility treatment: a meta-analysis of randomized trials. *Fertil Steril.* 61:1068, 1994

55. Romeu A, Muasher SJ, Acosta A, et al. Results of in vitro fertilization attempts in women 40 years of age and older: The Norfolk experience. *Fertil Steril.* 47:130, 1987

56. Padilla SL, Garcia JE. Effect of maternal age and number of in vitro fertilization procedures on pregnancy outcome. *Fertil Steril.* 52:270, 1989

57. Dimitry ES, Subak-Sharpe R, Mills M, et al. Nine cases of heterotopic pregnancies in four years of in vitro fertilization. *Fertil Steril.* 53:107, 1990

58. Bayati J, Garcia JE, Dorsey JH, et al. Combined intrauterine and cervical pregnancy from in vitro fertilization and embryo transfer. *Fertil Steril. 51:725, 1989*

59. Oehninger S, Kreiner D, Bass MJ, et al. Abdominal pregnancy after in vitro fertilization and embryo transfer. *Obstet Gynecol.* 72:499, 1988

60. Rein MS, Disalvo DN, Friedman AJ. Heterotopic pregnancy associated with in vitro fertilization and embryo transfer: A possible role for routine vaginal ultrasound. *Fertil Steril.* 51:1057, 1989

61. Lynch L, Berkowitz RL, Chitkara U, et al. First-trimester transabdominal multifetal pregnancy reduction: A report of 85 cases. *Obstet Gynecol.* 75:735, 1990

62. Saunders K, Spensley J, Munro J, Halasz G. Growth and physical outcome of children conceived by in vitro fertilization. *Pediatrics.* 97:688, 1996

63. Olivennes F, Kerbrat V, Rufat P, et al. Follow-up of a cohort of 422 children aged 6 to 13 years conceived by in vitro fertilization. *Fertil Steril.* 67:284, 1997

64. D'Souza SW, Rivlin E, Cadman J, et al. Children conceived by in vitro fertilization after fresh embryo transfer. *Arch Dis Child Fetal Neonatal Ed.* 76:F70, 1997

65. Cohen J, Elsner C, Kort H, et al. Impairment of the hatching process following IVF in the human and improvement by assisted hatching using micromanipulation. *Hum Reprod.* 5:7, 1990

66. Bider D, Livshits A, Yonish M, et al. Assisted hatching by zona drilling of human embryos in women of advanced age. *Hum Reprod.* 12:317, 1997

67. Chao KH, Chen SU, Chen HF, et al. Assisted hatching increases the implantation and pregnancy rate of in vitro fertilization (IVF)-embryo transfer (ET), but not that of IVF-tubal ET in patients with repeated IVF failures. *Fertil Steril.* 67:904, 1997

68. Tucker MJ, Morton PC, Wright G, et al. Enhancement of outcome from intracytoplasmic sperm injection: Does co-culture or assisted hatching improve implantation rates? *Hum Reprod.* 11:2434, 1996

69. Wiemer KE, Cohen J. Co-culture of mammalian embryos. In: Evers JHL, Heineman MJ, eds. *From Ovulation to Implantation.* New York, Elsevier, 1990: 297

70. Thibodeaux JK, Godke RA. In vitro enhancement of early-stage embryos with co-culture. *Arch Pathol Lab Med.* 116:364, 1992

71. Bavister BD. Co-culture for embryo development: Is it really necessary? *Hum Reprod.* 7:1339, 1992

72. Handyside AH, Kontogianni EH, Hardy K, Winston RML. Pregnancies from biopsied human preimplantation embryos sexed by Y-specific DNA amplification. *Nature.* 344 :768, 1990

73. Verlinsky Y, Munne S, Simpson JL, et al. Current status of preimplantation diagnosis. *J Assist Reprod Genet.* 14:72, 1997

74. Trounsen AO, Mohr L. Human pregnancy following cryopreservation, thawing and transfer of an eight-cell embryo. *Nature.* 305:707, 1983

75. Cohen J, De Vane GH, Elsner CW, et al. Cryopreservation of zygotes and early cleaved human embryos. *Fertil Steril.* 49:283, 1988

76. Queenan JT, Veeck LL, Muasher SJ. Clinical and laboratory aspects of cryopreservation. *Semin Reprod Endocrinol.* 13:64, 1995

77. Chen C. Pregnancy after human oocyte cryopreservation. *Lancet.* 1:884, 1986

78. Van Uem JF, Seibzehurubl ER, Schuh B, et al. Birth after cryopreservation of unfertilized oocytes. *Lancet.* 1:752, 1986

79. Baka SG, Toth TL, Veeck LL, et al. Evaluation of the spindle apparatus of in-vitro matured human oocytes following cryopreservation. *Hum Reprod.* 10:1816, 1995

80. Contvrindt R, Smitz J, Van Steirteghem AC. A morphological and functional study of the effect of slow freezing followed by complete in-vitro maturation of primary mouse ovarian follicles. *Hum Reprod.* 11:2648, 1996

81. Rosenwaks ZR. Donor eggs: Their application in modern reproductive technologies. *Fertil Steril.* 47:895, 1987

82. Droesch K, Navot D, Scott R, et al. Transdermal estrogen replacement in ovarian failure for ovum donation. *Fertil Steril.* 50:931, 1988

83. Cohen J, Scott RT Jr, Levron J, Willadsen S. Birth of infant after transfer of anucleate donor oocyte cytoplasm into recipient eggs. *Lancet.* 350:186, 1997

84. Asch RH, Balmaceda JP, Ellsworth LR, et al. Preliminary experiences with gamete intrafallopian transfer (GIFT). *Fertil Steril.* 45:366, 1986

85. Jansen RPS, Anderson JC, Sutherland PD. Nonoperative embryo transfer to the fallopian tube. *N Engl J Med.* 319:288, 1988

86. Jansen RPS, Anderson JC. Nonsurgical gamete intrafallopian transfer. *Semin Reprod Endocrinol.* 13:72, 1995

87. Yovich JL, Blackledge DG, Richardson PA, et al. Pregnancies following pronuclear stage tubal transfer. *Fertil Steril.* 48:851, 1987

1.8 to 4.6 percent of couples, or as a fetal chromosomal anomaly in 20 to 50 percent of products of conception from women with RPL. Endocrinologic abnormalities have been reported in 5 to 29 percent of women with pregnancy loss. Immunologic factors have been associated with RPL in 15 to 50 percent of couples. Anatomic abnormalities, of both the congenital and acquired nature, have been reported in 5 to 28 percent of women with RPL. While microbiologic factors have not been shown to be a cause of multiple pregnancy loss, infectious agents are a factor in some cases of sporadic pregnancy loss. Psychologic factors, which undoubtedly play a role in couples who have experienced the grief and suffering of even a single pregnancy loss, are more difficulty to quantitate but often lend themselves to individual or group support sessions.

The etiology attributed to the various causes of recurrent pregnancy loss is difficult to ascertain from published reports. Differences in definition make direct comparisons between various studies impossible. For example, some authors define recurrent pregnancy loss as the consecutive loss of two (as opposed to three) pregnancies. Other investigators do not completely evaluate what might be considered a basic workup of pregnancy loss before assigning "unknown" as the etiology. After basic evaluation for recurrent pregnancy loss is completed, as described later in this chapter, an etiology can be determined in about 60 percent of all couples.[12]

Genetic Factors

Losses attributed to genetic reasons can be divided into two large categories: fetal and parental. The causes of single spontaneous abortion have been investigated by many groups, and several large studies concur that fetal chromosomal abnormalities account for the majority of all cases. The frequency of karyotypically abnormal fetal tissue is about 60 percent at 12 gestational wk, 45 percent by 16 wk, 12 percent at 20 wk, and 6 percent by 24 wk. At term, the incidence of chromosomal anomalies in a live-born is only 0.5 percent.

The chromosomal defects that occur as a percent of all genetic causes of single pregnancy loss have been thoroughly investigated. As a group, the autosomal trisomies comprise the most frequent chromosomal complement in first-trimester spontaneous abortions. Of these, trisomy 16 occurs most frequently and is uniformly lethal. Trisomy 21 (Down syndrome) is usually the result of meiotic nondisjunction: The extra chromosome is maternal 80 percent of the time, which suggests a greater frequency of nondisjunction in oocytes than in spermatocytes. Monosomy X (45,X or Turner syndrome) is the most frequent individual karyotype found in the abortus of women with a single pregnancy loss. Triploidy (3n = 69) is the next most frequent group of chromosomal anomalies. The supernumerary haploid chromosome set

originates from a paternal source in 80 percent of cases, suggesting polyspermia is a possible mechanism. Tetraploidy (4n = 92), translocations, and mosaicisms occur less frequently. In addition, it has been shown that a correlation exists between the chromosomal complement of different spontaneous miscarriages in the same couple.[17-19] A pregnancy loss with a normal karyotype is most likely to result in a normal karyotype in the next pregnancy, whether it is a loss or a delivery. Furthermore, there is no increased risk of trisomy from a previous trisomic fetus. Finally, a nontrisomic but aneuploid loss results in an increased risk of nontrisomic aneuploid in the next pregnancy.

Parental genetic structural anomalies can also be the cause of pregnancy loss. In recurrent pregnancy loss, a parental chromosomal anomaly (usually a balanced translocation) can be identified approximately 2 to 4 percent of the time.[20] The distribution of chromosomal abnormalities according to the sex of the carrier has been analyzed (Table 34–5).[21] Overall abnormalities were identified twice as frequently in the female partner out of 16,661 couples studied. Certainly, a karyotype on both partners should be included in the workup for RPL.

Endocrinologic Factors

Defective function of the corpus luteum with resultant reproductive failure was first postulated by Jones.[22] Widely divergent estimates of the significance of this "luteal phase deficiency" syndrome in RPL have been described. Initial estimates ranged from 20 to 60 percent,[23] but two recent studies of RPL have noted a 15 to 20 percent incidence of a lag in endometrial maturation of 2 or more days in two consecutive cycles.[24,25] It is also of interest that evaluation of late luteal phase endometrial biopsies performed on regularly menstruating, fertile

TABLE 34–5. DISTRIBUTION OF CHROMOSOME ABNORMALITIES ACCORDING TO THE SEX OF THE CARRIER

Abnormality	Males (n = 16,661) No. (%)	Females (n = 16,661) No. (%)	Both (n = 33,322) No.
Reciprocal translocations	150 (36.1)	265 (63.9)	415
Robertsonian translocations	58 (30.4)	133 (69.6)	191
Inversions	25 (41.7)	35 (58.3)	60
Sex chromosome aneuploidy	7 (26.9)	19 (73.1)	26
Supernumerary chromosome	2 (18.2)	9 (81.8)	11
TOTAL ABNORMALITIES	242 (34.4)	461 (65.6)	703

(Reproduced, with permission, from DeBraekeleer M, Dao TN. Cytogenetic studies in couples experiencing repeated pregnancy losses. Hum Reprod. 5:519, 1990.)

women with no history of pregnancy loss reveals a 26.7 percent incidence of at least a 2-day lag in sequential cycles.[26] These results bring into question the association of a luteal phase defect with RPL as postulated by several authors.

The optimal means of diagnosing a luteal phase defect is also uncertain. Basal body temperature measurements may aid in identifying a short luteal phase, but controversy exists regarding the appropriate criterion to be used.[27] The use of serum progesterone levels and of timed endometrial biopsies have both been championed, and some authors require both.[28,29] In general, if a mid-luteal serum progesterone level is in excess of 10 ng/ml, an endometrial biopsy performed near the end of this cycle is unlikely to demonstrate a time lag greater than 2 days.[30] Biopsy studies appear to be more sensitive, but they are less specific. A diagnosis of luteal phase defect is generally reserved for those cases in which at least two consecutive biopsies have shown results consistent with a 2-day or greater lag in endometrial maturation.[31] Establishing ovulation more objectively via sonography or luteinizing hormone (LH) monitoring has been urged as a means to improve diagnostic testing and validity.[32]

Various treatments have been prescribed for luteal phase deficiency,[23] including ovulation induction with either clomiphene citrate or human menopausal gonadotropins, hCG injection at the time of expected ovulation, and progesterone supplementation both during the luteal phase and up to 8 wk of gestation. Bromocriptine therapy is recommended if the luteal phase dysfunction is thought to be secondary to elevated prolactin levels.[33]

Despite the numerous publications discussing clinical experience of luteal phase defects treated with these and other agents, the actual scientific evidence of these data may be inadequate to support any valid conclusion. Only limited conclusions can be drawn from the majority of these studies because study group sizes were smaller than required to achieve significant statistical power.[34]

There is less information regarding other endocrinopathies and early pregnancy loss. Diabetes is more often associated with late pregnancy loss or stillbirth. Significant thyroid and adrenal disorders usually result in infertility. However, both hypo- and hyperthyroidism are associated with both early and late pregnancy loss, but data are insufficient to correlate thyroid disorders and recurrent early pregnancy loss.

Anatomic Factors

Women with a history of RPL have been determined to have a significantly greater incidence of abnormalities in uterine anatomy. This diagnostic group encompasses not only congenital uterine anomalies[35] but also acquired abnormalities such as intrauterine synechiae, leiomyomatas, and the functional abnormality termed cervical incompetence. Müllerian anomalies have been diagnosed in 2 to 6

percent of women in populations with normal reproductive histories.[36–38] An even greater percentage of women evaluated for RPL have been found to have abnormalities of the upper genital tract.[37,39] A modified classification system of these upper genital tract anomalies has been presented by the American Fertility Society.[40] The majority of Müllerian anomalies most likely originate from polygenetic or multifactorial causes, but some types of Müllerian malformations have been associated with in utero diethylstilbestrol (DES) exposure.[41] All of these DES-exposed patients suffer increased rates of spontaneous abortion, preterm delivery, and ectopic pregnancy.[42,43] Unfortunately, data on the benefit of surgical therapy in patients with Müllerian anomalies are inconclusive because the majority of studies present the outcomes for groups of nonrandomized patients.[44–46] Patients with a history of DES exposure or the diagnosis of a unicornuate uterus are generally thought to be unimproved by metroplasty. Some investigators have advocated the liberal use of cerclage in patients with RPL, particularly for individuals with a history of second-trimester losses.[47,48] Women with RPL and a uterus didelphys or a bicornuate uterus can be considered for a cerclage or a Strassman unification procedure. Following confirmation of two separate horns by either sonography, magnetic resonance imaging (MRI), or laparoscopy, a cerclage (for late losses) or Strassman procedure has been performed with apparent improvement in subsequent outcome. Operatively, hysteroscopy is the most popular therapy for a septate uterus when this anomaly is identified in a patient with RPL.[49,50] It is important to remember that these recommendations are based on favorable outcomes for patients carefully selected before surgery. Without data from a randomized, prospective trial, the true benefit of these procedures for fertility and pregnancy maintenance remain uncertain. One recent retrospective analysis of pregnancy outcomes has even found no difference between those treated expectantly or surgically.[51] A complete evaluation for other causes of RPL should be performed before recommending metroplasty.

Intrauterine synechiae are found in approximately 5 percent of women with RPL.[52] Whether these adhesions and/or the accompanying uterine curettage are causative of, or secondary to, pregnancy loss is unknown. The majority of cases of Asherman syndrome appear to result from uterine instrumentation. Good success rates have been reported following hysteroscopic removal of intrauterine adhesions,[53] and one earlier study of pregnancy outcome would seem to confirm a much greater rate of abortion and early delivery in untreated cases.[52]

The importance of leiomyomas as a cause of RPL is not well documented. The diagnosis and best treatment for cervical incompetence also remain areas of controversy rather than subjects of appropriately randomized clinical trials, although women with histories most clearly suggestive of cervical incompetence demonstrate excellent rates of term pregnancy achievement following an early-gestation cervical cerclage procedure.[54,55]

Immunologic Factors

Much speculation has centered on the potential importance of the immune system as a piece of the RPL puzzle. Two primary pathophysiologic models have evolved. The first is that some women's immune systems may produce phospholipid or other autoantibodies, which are thought to have a variety of deleterious effects on pregnancy. This is the "autoimmune" theory of RPL. The classical "alloimmune" theory is the model in which normal pregnancy maintenance requires that the immune system recognize an implanting embryo as "foreign" in order to protect the embryo from attack by the maternal system.[56] More recently various alloimmune theories have been invoked to explain fetal loss including T-helper embryo-toxic cytokine factors, CD56 positive natural killer cells, and antipaternal cytotoxic antibodies.[57–59]

Autoimmune Association. An association between certain autoimmune conditions and RPL is now well established. Since the mechanism(s) responsible for pregnancy loss in these disorders is unknown, management remains controversial. During the past decade, the antiphospholipid syndrome (APS) has emerged as a heterogeneous autoimmune disorder associated with substantial risk for fetal loss.[60] The diagnosis of APS requires both clinical and serologic features as outlined in Table 34–6. The syndrome is designated as primary in patients with no apparent underlying disease and secondary when systemic lupus erythematosus (SLE) or a lupus-like disorder is also present. Women with antiphospholipid antibodies (APA) but no clinical features and those with fetal deaths and thromboembolic events but no laboratory abnormalities are not currently classified. The most significant APA have specificity against negatively charged phospholipids and are most commonly detected by determining lupus anticoagulant (LA) and anticardiolipin antibody (ACA) activity. Women with both previous early fetal loss and high levels of ACA may suffer a recurrent loss rate of 70 percent.[61] In referral populations of women with recurrent pregnancy loss, an approximate incidence of 15 percent positive APA has been reported.[11] However, only 2 percent of low-risk obstetrical patients with no history of recurrent loss will have LA or ACA.[62,63] The presence of LA must be confirmed by two additional tests when one identifies a prolonged phospholipid-dependent clotting assay.[64] Failure to correct the prolonged test with appropriate mixing studies and confirmation of phospholipid dependence are essential steps necessary to conclude that LA is present.

Lupus anticoagulant produces a paradoxic prolongation of phospholipid-dependent clotting assays, which is not corrected on mixing with normal plasma. Tests commonly used to screen for LA are the activated partial thromboplastin time (aPTT), dilute Russell viper venom time (dRVVT), and the kaolin clotting time (KCT).[65] The LA inhibitor is present when clotting is prolonged beyond two standard deviations above the control mean. In contrast, anticardiolipin antibody (aCL) is detected in an enzyme-linked immunosorbent assay (ELISA) using cardiolipin as antigen. For the results from a laboratory to be reliable, the aCL assay must be properly standardized.[66,67]

LA and aCL have closely related specificities and are the same family of autoantibodies detected by two different types of assays. Many APS patients have both LA and aCL, but they are not always concordant in a given patient. Therefore, both a coagulation assay for LA and an immunoassay for aCL should be performed if the presence of antiphospholipid antibodies is suspected. Low levels of IgG aCL or IgM aCL may represent nonspecific binding and are of questionable clinical significance.[68]

Some authors have suggested that autoantibodies other than LA or aCL, contribute to the diagnosis or management of patients with recurrent autoimmune pregnancy loss.[69] Beta-2 glycoprotein is a co-factor for phospholipid binding, but its relevance to recurrent pregnancy loss is uncertain.[7] Women with recurrent pregnancy loss have a higher frequency of positive antinuclear antibody (ANA) titers, but their next pregnancy outcomes do not differ from women with negative ANAs.[70,71] The value of routine "profiles" for other phospholipids, nucleotides, histones, and their isotypes is still under investigation.[72–75] As many as 10 to 15 percent of

TABLE 34–6. SUGGESTED CLINICAL AND LABORATORY CRITERIA FOR THE ANTIPHOSPHOLIPID SYNDROME[a]

Clinical Features	Laboratory Features

Pregnancy loss
  Fetal death
  Recurrent pregnancy loss
	Lupus anticoagulant

Thrombosis
  Venous
  Arterial, including stroke
	IgG anticardiolipin antibodies (≤20 GPL)

Autoimmune thrombocytopenia	

Other
  Coombs' positive
    hemolytic anemia
  Livedo reticularis
	IgM anticardiolipin antibodies (≤ 20 MPL)

[a]Patients with antiphospholipid syndrome should have at least one clinical and one laboratory feature at some time in the course of their disease. Laboratory tests should be positive on at least two occasions more than 8 wk apart.

normal pregnant women have low ANA titers,[71] and 2 to 4 percent of healthy individuals have detectable antiphospholipid antibodies.[61–63] The statistical chance of obtaining false positive results in normal patients increases with the number of antigens and their isotypes tested. An independent association between each antibody and pregnancy loss must be proven in properly designed studies before it can be used as a screening test.

Autoantibodies to thyroglobulin and thyroid peroxidase or microsomal antigen are found in patients with Hashimoto's thyroiditis, Graves' disease, postpartum thyroiditis, and in some normal individuals. A correlation between the presence of thyroid antibodies and first-trimester pregnancy loss has been reported, but other causes of miscarriages were not ruled out.[76–78] The incidence of antithyroid antibodies was reported as 17 percent in normal pregnant women compared to 30 percent in women with a history of recurrent miscarriages.[76,79] Recurrent miscarriage patients with antithyroid antibodies had a higher rate of fetal loss with their next pregnancy than those without the antibodies.[80] Antithyroid antibodies may be a marker for other autoimmune diseases, or may identify a subgroup of women who may not meet the increased demand for thyroid hormones in early pregnancy, but the etiology of thyroid antibody-related pregnancy loss remains largely theoretical. More studies are needed to determine if effective treatment can be identified, and to resolve whether these screening tests have any utility in the routine evaluation of patients with RPL.

Preconceptional counseling of the APS patient regarding the risk for serious medical problems is essential. In populations of women referred to perinatologists, 30 to 50 percent have histories of thromboembolic events including stroke, and over 85 percent occur during pregnancy, the postpartum period, or while taking oral contraceptives.[81] However, in women referred to reproductive endocrinologists with APS and histories of early pregnancy loss, the prevalence of prior thromboembolic events is much less frequent.[82] Other pregnancy complications include pre-eclampsia, fetal growth restriction, fetal distress, and a rare but serious postpartum cardiopulmonary syndrome.[64]

Approximately 15 percent of women with RPL have APA.[11,64] Death of an embryo or fetus earlier determined to have cardiac activity is characteristic for APS, and about 15 to 40 percent of these occur after 13 wk of gestation.[82,83] Pregnancy loss in untreated patients with LA is as high as 90 percent, and it is about 40 to 50 percent in women with more than 20 GPL units of IgG aCL. The previous obstetric history is also important from a prognostic standpoint. A firm relationship between fetal loss and antiphospholipid antibodies has been demonstrated in patients with a prior history of thrombosis, fetal death, or other autoimmune manifestations.

Deciding on the optimum treatment for an individual patient is not always easy. Some patients have achieved live births without specific medical therapy. However, the prognosis is less favorable when previous pregnancies have been unsuccessful in the presence of LA or high levels of aCL. Comparison of studies is limited because of differences in study design, patient selection, and regimens utilized; however, relevant studies are summarized in Table 34–7.[81,82,84-89] Inclusion criteria used to select studies for this analysis were (1) a study design that included a treated and control group, (2) patients with at least two prior fetal losses, and (3) patients with serologic proof of LA or IgG aCL above 20 GPL.[21–30] All treatments appeared to improve the live birth rate, but heparin and low-dose aspirin were superior to prednisone and low-dose aspirin when considering maternal and fetal complications.[89] Heparin has been shown to bind aCL in vitro, and this may partially explain the decreased levels of aCL reported in women treated with heparin during a successful pregnancy.[90]

It should be noted that low-dose aspirin was used in patients with fewer previous pregnancy losses in some studies, which may bias the results. Heparin was associated with fewer side effects than prednisone in some but not all studies. The evidence indicates that 10,000 to 20,000 units of heparin daily in two divided doses is effective. Supplemental calcium of 1.5 g/day may reduce the increased risk of osteopenia associated with higher doses. Concomitant use of prednisone and heparin is not recommended because this combination has not been shown to be better than either alone in achieving a live birth, and fracture risk may increase in women treated with the combination regimen.

Some pregnant women with APS have now been treated with intravenous immune globulin (IVIG). This therapy is based on anecdotal reports of successful pregnancy outcomes, lowered APL levels, and fewer adverse effects than either prednisone or heparin.[91,92] However, IVIG for APS remains experimental at this time and larger randomized clinical trials are necessary to prove its efficacy.

Alloimmune Association. Alloimmunity refers to immunologic differences between individuals of the same species. One example is the major histocompatibility antigen system. As an embryo is the product of both maternal and paternal genomes, it is antigenically different from the mother. One rationale for an alloimmune cause for RPL is the assumption that unless the maternal immune system is suppressed, it would normally reject an implanting embryo. The process of blocking embryo rejection is believed to be maternally mediated. Alloimmune mediated pregnancy rejection has been hypothesized to be due to the absence of dissimilarities between paternal and maternal antigens (ie, HLA sharing). In this

TABLE 34–7. COMPARISON OF TREATMENTS AND PREGNANCY OUTCOME IN APS PATIENTS

Author (yr)	Inclusion Criteria	Treatments Compared[a]	Live Birth Rate	Number (%)	P Value
Laskin (1996)	≤2 Fetal losses LA or aCL >20 GPL	Pred 0.5-0.8 mg/kg and ASA 100 mg	25/42	(47.8)	0.57
		Placebo	24/46	(52.4)	
Hasegawa (1992)	≥2 Fetal losses LA or aCL >33 GPL	Pred 40 mg and ASA 81 mg	13/17	(76.5)	0.01
		No treatment	1/12	(8.3)	
Passaleva (1992)	≥2 Fetal losses/SAB LA or aCL	Pred 20 mg and ASA 100 mg	5/5	(100.0)	
		No treatment	1/6	(17.0)	
		ASA 100 mg	9/11	(81.8)	
Kutteh (1996)	≥3 Pregnancy losses aCL >20 GPL	Heparin 10,000-30,000 U and ASA 81 mg	20/25	(80.0)	0.02
		ASA 81 mg	11/25	(44.0)	
Cowchock (1992)	≥2 Fetal losses LA or aCL	Heparin 20,000 U and ASA 81 mg	9/12	(75.0)	1.00
		Pred 40 mg and ASA 81 mg	6/8	(75.0)	
Branch (1992)	≥2 Fetal losses LA or aCL >20 GPL[b]	Heparin 15,000-20,000 U and ASA 81 mg	14/19	(73.7)	0.17
		Pred 40 mg and ASA 81 mg	21/39	(53.8)	
Kutteh (1996)	≥3 Pregnancy losses aCL >20 GPL	Low-dose heparin and ASA 81 mg	19/25	(76.0)	0.50
		High-dose heparin and ASA 81 mg	20/25	(80.0)	
Rai (1997)	≥3 Pregnancy losses LA or aCL	Heparin 10,000 U and ASA 81 mg	32/45	(71.0)	0.01
		ASA 81 mg	19/45	(42.0)	

[a] Converted to equivalent prednisone dose.
[b] Some patients had previous thromboembolic events but no prior pregnancy loss.

case, the maternal immune system would not identify the embryo as foreign, and the resulting unregulated immune system would destroy the embryo. One might hypothesize that the presence of a significant amount of HLA sharing between partners would increase the chances for an alloimmune-mediated mechanism for recurrent abortion. However, laboratory tests such as HLA-typing or blocking antibodies are of no value in identifying patients with alloimmune-mediated pregnancy losses.[93,94] More recently, several tests have been reported to be useful in identifying women with autoimmune abnormalities associated with RPL.[57–59] Tests that identify T-helper embryotoxic cytokine factors, such as interferon-gamma and tumor necrosis factor-alpha, are being investigated. These cytokines have been reported in supernatants from peripheral blood leukocytes of some women with RPL stimulated with trophoblast antigens.[57] Immunophenotypes of endometrial cells from women with RPL compared to normal fertile controls demonstrate alterations in large granular lymphocytes identified as natural killer cells.[95,96] One recent analysis suggesting an association between elevated levels of peripheral blood natural killer cells (CD 56+) and RPL needs

to be expanded and confirmed.[58] Antipaternal cytotoxic antibody assays (leukocyte antibody detection) are also being evaluated as a possible marker for autoimmune-associated RPL.[59]

If one can assume that alloimmune problems are a common cause of otherwise unexplained RPL, then therapies that appropriately modify the immune system might prove to be efficacious in the treatment of unexplained RPL. Animal models of partner-specific RPL demonstrate that protective immunity may be induced by presentation of paternal antigens or by stimulation of the maternal immune system with a nonspecific adjuvant.[97,98] To this end, even though definitive tests to diagnose patients with alloimmune-mediated RPL are lacking, two modes of alloimmunotherapy have been studied. These therapies are immunization with allogeneic blood mononuclear cells, an active immunization; and administration of IVIG, a passive immunization.

With leukocyte immunization, the patient with RPL is given either paternal or donor leukocytes before conception. Leukocytes have been administered intravenously, subcutaneously, intradermally, and in combination. The majority of studies are descriptive case-series reports, but a few reports of randomized, controlled trials have been published (Table 34–8).[99–102] These controlled studies and 19 case-series reports were analyzed by meta-analysis in a review.[103] Two of the controlled studies compared outcome with the administration of paternal leukocytes or maternal leukocytes, and a third study compared the administration of paternal leukocytes with administration of normal saline infusion. A fourth study compared trophoblast membrane infusion treatment with a control group receiving Intralipid intravenously. Only one of the first two studies observed a significantly greater incidence of live births in the treatment group.[99] Because three trials used paternal leukocytes as therapy but the major differences in outcome were in the control groups (control group success rates varied from 37 to 76 percent), the authors of the meta-analysis concluded that immunotherapy does not significantly improve pregnancy outcome.[103]

The results of a retrospective worldwide observational study and meta-analysis on allogenic leukocyte immunization therapy for RPL coordinated by the Ethics Committee for Immunotherapy of the American Society of Reproductive Immunology have been published.[104] The compilation of over 400 cases has demonstrated a marginal improvement for immunized women. Perhaps all that can be concluded at this time is that roughly 60 percent of patients with RPL who have received paternal leukocyte immunization therapy have had successful pregnancies. From two independent analyses, the conclusion was reached that 11 patients have to be immunized to achieve one additional live birth.[104] The considerable expense and potential morbidity associated with immunization therapy make full disclosure of relevant information and informed consent all the more important.[105,106]

The administration of IVIG has been evaluated as an alternative to allogeneic blood leukocyte therapy for the treatment of RPL. The mechanism by which IVIG modulates immune function is not known. The results from the three randomized clinical trials evaluating the efficacy of IVIG for RPL are shown in Table 34–9.[107–109] The first is a multicenter trial from the German Recurrent Spontaneous Abortion IVIG Group (GRSA/IVIGG). Both the GRSA/IVIGG trial and the study by Christiansen began therapy after conception and continued for up to 34 wk of gestation. The study by Coulam began therapy during the month of anticipated conception and continued until 32 wk of gestation. The study results differed and only the study by Coulam demonstrated a significant benefit.[47] Moreover, the live birth rate in the control groups in the studies by Coulam and Christiansen were less than 40 percent, while one might expect higher spontaneous success rates. Enthusiasm over this possibly safer treatment scheme should await the outcome of an appropriately designed, randomized, controlled trial for the use of IVIG for RPL.

Microbiologic Factors

Maternal infections by a variety of organisms have been linked to pregnancy loss, including *Mycoplasma* (*M hominis*),[110] *Ureaplasma* (*U urealyticum*), group B β-hemolytic streptococci, *Chlamydia*,[111] *Treponema pallidum, Toxoplasma*, and viruses such as rubella, cytomegalovirus, herpes, and coxsackievirus. Most investigators interested in RPL have focused on *M hominis* and *U urealyticum* as possible causative agents. Two studies have reported a higher incidence of infection by these organisms in women with a history of multiple losses as compared with control

TABLE 34–8. PUBLISHED AND UPDATED TRIALS OF LEUKOCYTE THERAPY FOR RECURRENT SPONTANEOUS ABORTION

Author (yr)	Treatments (no. of subjects)	Route	Dose(s)	Live Birth Rate (%)	*P* Value	Power to Detect 50% Increase Over Baseline	Updated RR (95% CI)
Mowbray (1985)	Pat WBC (22) vs Mat WBC(27)	3/5 IV 1/5 SC 1/5 ID	1	77 37	0.01	0.26	1.45 (0.95–2.21)
Ho (1991)	Pat/Donor WBC (50) vs Mat WBC (49)	ID	>1	78 65	0.16	0.48	1.20 (0.93–1.56)
Cauchi (1991)	Pat WBC (21) vs Saline (25)	1/2 IV 1/4 SC 1/4 ID	1	62 76	0.31	0.23	0.89 (0.59–1.35)
Gatenby (1993)	Pat WBC (19) vs Mat WBC	3/5 IV 1/5 SC 1/5 ID	1	68 47	0.14	0.19	1.14 (0.71–1.82)

Pat = paternal; Mat = maternal; WBC = leukocytes; IV = intravenous; SC = subcutaneous; ID = intradermal; RR = relative risk; CI = confidence interval.

TABLE 34–9. IMMUNOGLOBULIN THERAPY FOR RECURRENT SPONTANEOUS ABORTION

Study (yr)	Treatments Compared (no. of subjects)	Dose Frequency	Therapy Interval (wk gestation)	Live Birth Rate (%)	P Value
GRSA/IVIGG (1994)	Immunoglobulin (33) vs Albumin (31)	q 21 days	8–25	60.6 67.7	0.173
Coulam (1995)	Immunoglobulin (29) vs Albumin(32)	q 28 days	0–32	62 38	0.04
Christiansen (1995)	Immunoglobulin (17) vs Albumin (17)	q 7–14 days	5–34	52.9 29.4	0.16

women,[112,113] and two other nonrandomized studies have reported a higher proportion of good pregnancy outcomes following antibiotic therapy for infections of these organisms in women with RPL.[114,115] However, conclusive cause-and-effect relationships between *M hominis* and *U urealyticum* infection, antibiotic therapy, and RPL cannot be assumed.[116]

Other Factors

It has been postulated that RPL is caused by maternal exposure to a variety of environmental factors.[117,118] Few of the suggested agents have been conclusively demonstrated to be causative of abortion, however, except for ionizing radiation and several drugs such as antimetabolites (eg, methotrexate), isotretinoin, and mifepristone.[117] Alcohol consumption and cigarette smoking have both been observed to increase the occurrence of pregnancy loss.[119–121] Controversy continues over the association of caffeine use with spontaneous pregnancy loss.[122–125]

Recently, retrospective studies have focused on video display terminals and their possible link to miscarriage. Two reports indicate that the use of video terminals and exposure to the accompanying electromagnetic fields do not put a woman at risk for spontaneous abortion.[126,127]

Several investigators have presented results suggesting that psychological stress may be directly involved with RPL.[14,128] A selected subset of a group of patients with RPL who received supportive counseling demonstrated a better pregnancy outcome than those patients not receiving this support. Interesting theoretical models linking stress to biologic changes detrimental to fetal development have been described.[129]

SUMMARY

Evaluation of a couple with RPL includes a directed history, physical examination, and laboratory evaluation.

RPL by definition involves women who have had three or more losses, but factors such as advanced age or patient desire may sometimes prompt evaluation of women with two losses. Both the evaluation and treatment must involve a sensitivity to psychological stresses that invariably accompany this problem. Appropriate counseling may lessen patient distress and marital dysfunction and may even improve the prognosis.[14,128]

When the decision to begin an evaluation is made, the complete evaluation should be recommended to all women (Table 34–10). Many have multiple factors contributing to RPL that can be identified only after a complete evaluation. Laboratory evaluations almost universally accepted include a karyotype of the woman and her partner, some assessment of luteal phase adequacy and, when indicated, serum thyrotropin and prolactin levels. An assessment of uterine structure is important by hysterosalpingogram, hysteroscopy, or sonohysterogram.[130] Immunologic screening is complete only with appropriately performed assays for LA and aCL, such as the dRVVT and the ELISA. Cervical cultures for *Chlamydia* and *Mycoplasma* are often included and may be an occasional cause of miscarriage, but rarely would be associated with multiple losses.[116] Data from several well-designed studies argue against the use of expensive tests such as HLA typing (including HLA-DQα),[131] antipaternal antibody titers, or mixed lymphocyte "blocking factor" testing.[93,94] The role of tests for antithyroid antibodies, embryotoxic factors, and peripheral blood immunophenotypes remains unclear.

The use of alloimmunotherapy for unexplained RPL remains controversial.[59] At present, neither therapy can be recommended for routine clinical use for the treatment of recurrent spontaneous abortion. Thus, only patients who have had a complete evaluation that was negative and who have given informed consent should be considered for either leukocyte or IVIG therapy. A randomized, multicenter trial sponsored by the National Institutes of Health to evaluate the efficacy of leukocyte therapy for RPL is currently ongoing.

TABLE 34–10. DIAGNOSIS AND MANAGEMENT OF RECURRENT PREGNANCY LOSS

Etiology	Diagnostic Evaluation	Therapy
Genetic	Karyotype partners	Genetic counseling
		Donor gametes
Anatomic	Hysterosalpingography	Septum transection
	Hysteroscopy	Remove polyp
	Sonohysterography	Resect synechiae
Endocrinologic	Endometrial biopsy	Progesterone
	Midluteal progesterone	Clomiphene citrate
	Thyrotropin	Thyroxine
	Prolactin	Bromocriptine
Immunologic	Lupus anticoagulant	Prednisone
	Antiphospholipid	Heparin
	antibodies	Aspirin
	(? Antithyroid antibodies)	(? IV immunoglobulin)
	(? Embryotoxic factors)	
Microbiologic	Cervical cultures	Antibiotics
Psychologic	Interview	Support group, counseling
Environmental	Exposure to tobacco, ethanol, toxins	Eliminate consumption, eliminate exposure

Clearly, a large number of couples with RPL experience profound grief, anger, and depression as a result of their reproductive failure. The ensuing sense of desperation may lessen their ability to cogently weigh pros and cons of various therapies. Couples with RPL who are having great difficulty dealing with their losses should be encouraged to undergo psychologic counseling and join specific support groups such as SHARE.[132] Physicians are responsible for helping them resist the temptation of treatments that have not been scientifically validated. Finally, on an optimistic note, the couple should be reminded that 60 to 70 percent of women with a completely negative evaluation for RPL will ultimately deliver healthy offspring.[133]

REFERENCES

1. Plouffe L, Tho SPT, Hansen K. Basic workup of the couple with recurrent pregnancy loss. *Infert Reprod Med Clin North Am.* 7:825, 1996
2. Cunningham FG, MacDonald PC, Gant NF, et al. Abortion. In: Cunningham FG, McDonald PC, Gant NF, et al, eds. *Williams Obstetrics*, 19th ed. Norwalk, Conn, Appleton & Lange, 1993: 661–689
3. Doubilet PM, Benson CB. Embryonic heart rate in the first trimester: What rate is normal? *J Ultrasound Med.* 14:431, 1995
4. Gilmore DH, McNay MB. Spontaneous fetal loss rate in early pregnancy. *Lancet.* 1:107, 1985
5. Warburton D, Fraser FC. Spontaneous abortion risks in man: Data from reproductive histories collected in a medical genetics unit. *Am J Hum Genet.* 16:1, 1964
6. Wilcox AJ, Weinberg CR, O'Connor JF, et al. Incidence of early pregnancy loss. *N Engl J Med.* 319:189, 1988
7. Mills JL, Simpson JL, Driscoll SG, et al. Incidence of spontaneous abortion among normal women and insulin-dependent diabetic women whose pregnancies were identified within 21 days of conception. *N Engl J Med.* 319:1617, 1988
8. Miller JF, Williamson E, Glue J, et al. Fetal loss after implantation: A prospective study. *Lancet.* 2:554, 1980
9. Poland BJ, Miller JR, Jones DC, Trimble BK. Reproductive counseling in patients who have had a spontaneous abortion. *Am J Obstet Gynecol.* 127:685, 1977
10. Stirrat GM. Recurrent miscarriage. I. Definition and epidemiology. *Lancet.* 336:673, 1990
11. Kutteh WH, Pasquarette MM. Recurrent pregnancy loss. *Adv Obstet Gynecol.* 2:147, 1995
12. Harger JH, Archer DF, Marchese SG, et al. Etiology of recurrent pregnancy losses and outcome of subsequent pregnancies. *Obstet Gynecol.* 62:574, 1983
13. Stirrat GM. Recurrent miscarriage. II. Clinical associations, causes, and management. *Lancet.* 336:728, 1990
14. Stray-Pederson B, Stray-Pederson S. Etiologic factors and subsequent reproductive performance in 195 couples with a prior history of habitual abortion. *Am J Obstet Gynecol.* 148:140, 1984
15. Tho PT, Byrd JR, McDonough PG. Etiologies and subsequent reproductive performance of 100 couples with recurrent abortion. *Fertil Steril.* 32:389, 1979
16. Stephenson M. Frequency of factors associated with habitual abortion in 197 couples. *Fertil Steril.* 66:24, 1996
17. Hassold TJ. A cytogenetic study of repeated spontaneous abortions. *Am J Hum Genet.* 32:723, 1980
18. Warburton D, Kline J, Stein Z, et al. Does the karyotype of a spontaneous abortion predict the karyotype of a subsequent abortion? Evidence from 273 women with two karyotyped spontaneous abortions. *Am J Hum Genet.* 41:465, 1987
19. Geraedts JPM. Chromosomal anomalies and recurrent miscarriage. *Infertil Reprod Med Clin North Am.* 7:677, 1996

20. Castle D, Berstein R. Cytogenetic analysis of 688 couples experiencing multiple spontaneous abortions. *Am J Med Genet.* 39:549, 1988

21. DeBraekeleer M, Dao TN. Cytogenetic studies in couples experiencing repeated pregnancy losses. *Hum Reprod.* 5:519, 1990

22. Jones GS. The luteal phase defect. *Fertil Steril.* 27:351, 1976

23. Doody KJ, Carr BR. Diagnosis and treatment of luteal dysfunction. In: Hillier SG, ed. *Ovarian Endocrinology.* Oxford, U.K., Blackwell Scientific, 1991:260

24. Tulppala M, Björses UM, Stenman UH, et al. Luteal phase defect in habitual abortion: Progesterone in saliva. *Fertil Steril.* 56:41, 1991

25. Baird DD, Weinberg CR, Wilcox AJ, et al. Hormonal profiles in natural conception cycles ending in early, unrecognized pregnancy loss. *J Clin Endocrinol Metab.* 72:793, 1991

26. Davis OK, Berkeley AS, Naus GJ, et al. The incidence of luteal phase defect in normal, fertile women, determined by serial endometrial biopsies. *Fertil Steril.* 51:582, 1989

27. McNeely MS, Soules MR. The diagnosis of luteal phase deficiency: A critical review. *Fertil Steril.* 50:1, 1988

28. Rosenfeld DL, Garcia CR. A comparison of endometrial histology with simultaneous plasma progesterone determinations in infertile women. *Fertil Steril.* 27:1256, 1976

29. Koninckx PR, Goddeeris PG, Lauweryns JM, et al. Accuracy of endometrial biopsy dating in relation to the midcycle luteinizing hormone peak. *Fertil Steril.* 28:443, 1977

30. Heinsleigh PA, Fainstat T. Corpus luteum dysfunction: Serum progesterone levels in diagnosis and assessment of therapy for recurrent and threatened abortion. *Fertil Steril.* 32:396, 1979.

31. Noyes RW. Uniformity of secretory endometriosis. *Obstet Gynecol.* 7:221, 1956

32. Peters AJ, Lloyd RP, Coulam CB. Prevalence of out-of-phase endometrial biopsy specimens. *Am J Obstet Gynecol.* 166:1738, 1992

33. Pozo ED, Wyss H, Tolis G, et al. Prolactin and deficient luteal function. *Obstet Gynecol.* 53:282, 1979

34. Karamardian LM, Grimes DA. Luteal phase deficiency: Effect of treatment on pregnancy rates. *Am J Obstet Gynecol.* 167:1391, 1992

35. Rock JA. Diagnosing and repairing uterine anomalies. *Contemp Obstet Gynecol.* 1:17, 1981

36. Cooper JM, Houck RM, Rigberg HS. The incidence of intrauterine abnormalities found at hysteroscopy in patients undergoing elective hysteroscopic sterilization. *J Reprod Med.* 28:659, 1983

37. Portuondo JA, Clmara MM, Echanojauregui AD, et al. Müllerian abnormalities in fertile women and recurrent aborters. *J Reprod Med.* 31:616, 1986

38. Greiss FC, Mauzy CH. Genital anomalies in women: An evaluation of diagnosis, incidence and obstetrical performance. *Am J Obstet Gynecol.* 82:330, 1961

39. Buttram VC, Gibbons WE. Müllerian anomalies: A proposed classification (an analysis of 144 cases). *Fertil Steril.* 32:40, 1979

40. American Fertility Society. The American Fertility Society classifications of adnexal adhesions, distal tubal occlusion, tubal occlusion secondary to tubal ligation, tubal pregnancies, Müllerian anomalies and intrauterine adhesions. *Fertil Steril.* 49:944, 1988

41. Kaufman RH, Adam E, Binder GL, et al. Upper genital tract changes and pregnancy outcome in offspring exposed in utero to diethylstilbestrol. *Am J Obstet Gynecol.* 137:299, 1980

42. Senekjean EK, Potkul RK, Frey K, et al. Infertility among daughters either exposed or not exposed to diethylstilbestrol. *Am J Obstet Gynecol.* 158:493, 1988

43. Stillman RJ. In utero exposure to diethylstilbestrol: Adverse effects on the reproductive tract and reproductive performance in male and female offspring. *Am J Obstet Gynecol.* 142:905, 1982

44. Heinoven PK, Saarikoski S, Pystynen P. Reproductive performance of women with uterine anomalies. *Acta Obstet Gynecol Scand.* 61:157, 1982

45. Thompson JP, Smith RA, Welsch JS. Reproductive ability after metroplasty. *Obstet Gynecol.* 28:363, 1966

46. Rock JA, Jones HW Jr. The clinical management of the double uterus. *Fertil Steril.* 28:798, 1977

47. Ludmir J, Landon B, Gabbe SG, et al: Management of the diethylstilbestrol exposed pregnant patient: A prospective study. *Am J Obstet Gynecol.* 157:655, 1987

48. Abromovici H, Faktor JH, Pascal B. Congenital uterine malformations as indications for cervical suture (cerclage) in habitual abortion and premature delivery. *Int J Fertil.* 28:161, 1983

49. March CM, Israel R. Hysteroscopic management of recurrent abortion caused by septate uterus. *Am J Obstet Gynecol.* 156:834, 1987

50. Perino A, Mencaglia C, Hamou J, et al. Hysteroscopy for metroplasty of uterine septa: Report of 24 cases. *Fertil Steril.* 48:321, 1987

51. Kirk EP, Chuong CJ, Coulam CB, et al. Pregnancy after metroplasty for uterine anomalies. *Fertil Steril.* 59:1164, 1993

52. Schenker JG, Margalioth EJ. Intrauterine adhesions: An updated appraisal. *Fertil Steril.* 37:593, 1982

53. Lancet M, Kessler I. A review of Asherman's syndrome, and results of modern treatment. *Int Fertil.* 33:14, 1988

54. Golan A, Barnan R, Wexier S, et al. Incompetence of the uterine cervix. *Obstet Gynecol Surv.* 44:96, 1989

55. Harger JH. Comparison of success and morbidity in cervical cerclage procedures. *Obstet Gynecol.* 56:543, 1980

56. Coulam CB, Moore SB, O'Fallon WM. Association between major histocompatibility antigen and reproductive performance. *Am J Reprod Immunol Microbiol.* 14:54, 1987

57. Hill JA, Polgar K, Anderson DJ. T-helper 1-type immunity to trophoblast antigens in women with recurrent spontaneous abortion. *JAMA.* 273:1933, 1995

58. Beer AE, Kwak JYM, Ruiz JE. Immunophenotype prophiles of peripheral blood lymphocytes in women with recurrent pregnancy loss and in infertile women with multiple failed in vitro fertilization cycles. *Am J Reprod Med.* 35:376, 1996

59. Coulam CB. Immunotherapy for recurrent spontaneous abortion. Early pregnancy. *Biol Med.* 1:13, 1995

60. Lockshin MD. Antiphospholipid antibody syndrome. *Rheum Dis Clin North Am.* 20:45, 1994

61. Dudley DJ, Branch W. Antiphospholipid syndrome: A model for autoimmune pregnancy loss. *Infertil Reprod Med Clin North Am*. 2:249, 1991

62. Lockwood CJ, Romero R, Feinberg RF, et al. The prevalence and biological significance of lupus anticoagulant and cardiolipin antibodies in a general obstetric population. *Am J Obstet Gynecol*. 161:369, 1989

63. Lockshin DW. Answers to the antiphospholipid antibody syndrome? *N Engl J Med*. 332:1025, 1995

64. Brandt JT, Triplett DA, Alving B, Scharrer I. Criteria for the diagnosis of lupus anticoagulants: an update. *Thromb Haemost*. 74:1185, 1995

65. Martin BA, Branch DW, Rodgers GM. Sensitivity of the activated partial thromboplastin time, the dilute Russell's viper venom time and the kaolin clotting time for the detection of the lupus anticoagulant. A direct comparison using plasma dilutions. *Blood Coag Fibrinolysis*. 7:31, 1996

66. Peaceman AM, Silver RK, MacGregor SN, et al. Interlaboratory variation in antiphospholipid antibody testing. *Am J Obstet Gynecol*. 166:1780, 1992

67. Kutteh WH, Wester R, Kutteh CC. Multiples of the median: An alternative method for reporting antiphospholipid antibodies in women with recurrent pregnancy loss. *Obstet Gynecol*. 84:811, 1994

68. Silver RM, Porter TF, Greenhill AE, et al. Anticardiolipin antibodies: Clinical consequences of "low titers." *Obstet Gynecol*. 87:494, 1996

69. Gleicher N, Pratt D, Dudkiewicz A. What do we really know about autoantibody abnormalities and reproductive failure? A critical review. *Autoimmunity*. 16:115, 1993

70. Osasawaram MM, Aoki K, Yagami Y. Are antinuclear antibodies predictive of recurrent miscarriage? *Lancet*. 347:1183, 1996

71. Harger JH, Rabin BS, Marchese SG. The prognostic value of antinuclear antibodies in women with recurrent pregnancy losses: A prospective controlled study. *Obstet Gynecol*. 73:419, 1989

72. Ober C, Karrison T, Harlow L, et al. Autoantibodies and pregnancy history in a healthy population. *Am J Obstet Gynecol*. 169:143, 1993

73. Cowchock FS, Fort UG. Can tests for IgA, IgG or IgM antibodies to cardiolipin or phosphatidylserine substitute for lupus anticoagulant assays in screening for antiphospholipid antibodies? *Autoimmunity*. 17:119, 1994

74. Yetman DL, Kutteh WH. Antiphospholipid antibody panels and recurrent pregnancy loss: Prevalence of anticardiolipin antibodies compared to other phospholipid antibodies. *Fertil Steril*. 66:540, 1996

75. Branch DW, Silver R, Pierangeli S, et al. Antiphospholipid antibodies other than lupus anticoagulant and anticardiolipin antibodies in women with recurrent pregnancy loss, fertile controls, and antiphospholipid syndrome. *Obstet Gynecol*. 89:549, 1997

76. Stagnaro-Green A, Roman SH, Cobin RH, et al. Detection of at-risk pregnancy by means of a highly sensitive assay for thyroid autoantibodies. *JAMA*. 264:1422, 1990

77. Gilnoer D, Soto MF, Bourdoux P, et al. Pregnancy in patients with mild thyroid abnormalities: Maternal and neonatal repercussions. *J Clin Endocrinol Metab*. 73:421, 1991

78. Singh A, Dantas ZN, Stone SC, et al. Presence of thyroid antibodies in early reproductive failure: Biochemical versus clinical pregnancies. *Fertil Steril*. 63:277, 1995

79. Pratt D, Novotny M, Kaberlein G, et al. Antithyroid antibodies and the association with non-organ-specific antibodies in recurrent pregnancy loss. *Am J Obstet Gynecol*. 168:837, 1993

80. Pratt DE, Kaberlein G, Dudkiewicz A, et al. The association of antithyroid antibodies in euthyroid nonpregnant women with recurrent first trimester abortions in the next pregnancy. *Fertil Steril*. 60:1001, 1993

81. Branch DW, Silver RM, Blackwell JL, et al. Outcome of treated pregnancies in women with antiphospholipid syndrome: An update of the Utah experience. *Obstet Gynecol*. 80:614, 1992

82. Kutteh WH. Antiphospholipid antibody-associated recurrent pregnancy loss: Treatment with heparin and low-dose aspirin is superior to low-dose aspirin alone. *Am J Obstet Gynecol*. 174:1584, 1996

83. Branch DW. Thoughts on the mechanism of pregnancy loss associated with the antiphospholipid syndrome. *Lupus*. 3:275, 1994

84. Laskin C, Bombardier C, Mandel F, et al. A randomized controlled trial of prednisone and ASA in women with autoantibodies and unexplained recurrent fetal loss. Presented at Society of Perinatal Obstetricians Meeting, Kamuela, Hawaii, February 5–10, 1996

85. Hasegawa I, Takakuwa R, Goto S, et al. Effectiveness of prednisolone/aspirin therapy for recurrent aborters with antiphospholipid antibody. *Hum Reprod*. 7:203, 1992

86. Kutteh WH, Ermel LD. A clinical trial for the treatment of antiphospholipid antibody associated recurrent pregnancy loss with lower dose heparin and aspirin. *Am J Reprod Immunol*. 35:402, 1996

87. Passaleva A, Massai G, D'Elios MM, et al. Prevention of miscarriage in antiphospholipid syndrome. *Autoimmunity*. 14:121, 1992

88. Rai R, Cohen H, Dave M, Regan L. Randomized, controlled trial of aspirin and aspirin plus heparin in pregnant women with recurrent miscarriage associated with phospholipid antibodies (or antiphospholipid antibodies). *Br Med J*. 314:253, 1997

89. Cowchock FS, Reece EA, Balaban D, et al. Repeated fetal losses associated with antiphospholipid antibodies: A collaborative randomized trial comparing prednisone with low-dose heparin treatment. *Am J Obstet Gynecol*. 166:1318, 1992

90. Ermel LD, Marshburn PB, Kutteh WH. Interaction of heparin with antiphospholipid antibodies (APA) from the sera of women with recurrent pregnancy loss (RPL). *Am J Reprod Immunol*. 33:14, 1995

91. Spinnato JA, Clark AL, Pierangeli S, et al. Intravenous immunoglobulin for the antiphospholipid syndrome in pregnancy. *Am J Obstet Gynecol*. 172:690, 1995

92. Valensise H, Vaquero E, de Carolis C, et al. Normal fetal growth in women with antiphospholipid syndrome treated with high-dose intravenous immunoglobulin (IVIG). *Prenat Diagn*. 15:509, 1995

93. Coulam CB. Immunologic tests in the evaluation of reproductive disorders: A critical review. *Am J Obstet Gynecol.* 167:1844, 1992

94. Cowchock FS, Smith JB. Predictors for live births after unexplained spontaneous abortions: Correlations between immunologic test results, obstetric histories, and outcomes of next pregnancy without treatment. *Am J Obstet Gynecol.* 167:1208, 1992

95. Clark DA, Vince G, Flanders KC, et al. CD56+ lymphoid cells in first trimester pregnancy decidua as a source of novel transforming growth factor-β2-related immunosuppressive factors. *Hum Reprod.* 9:2270, 1994

96. Lachapell MH, Miron P, Hemmings R, Roy DC. Endometrial T, B, and NK cells in patients with recurrent spontaneous abortion. *J Immunol.* 156:4027, 1996

97. Toder V, Strassgurger D, Irlin Y, et al. Immunopotentiation and pregnancy loss: Complete Freund's adjuvant reverses high fetal resorption rates in CBA x DBA/2J mouse combination. *Am J Reprod Immunol.* 24:63, 1990

98. Chaouat G, Clark DA, Wegmann TG. Genetic aspects of the CBA × DBA/2 and B10 × B10.A models of murine pregnancy failure and its prevention by leukocyte immunization. In: Beard RW, Sharp F, eds. *Early Pregnancy Failure: Mechanisms and Treatment.* Ashton-under-Lyme, U.K. Peacock Press, 1988: 89–102

99. Mowbray JF, Liddel H, Underwood JL, et al. Controlled trial of treatment of recurrent spontaneous abortion by immunization with paternal cells. *Lancet.* 1:941, 1985

100. Ho H-N, Gill TJ, Hsieh HE, et al. Immunotherapy for recurrent spontaneous abortions in a Chinese population. *Am J Reprod Immunol.* 25:10, 1991

101. Cauchi MN, Lim D, Young DE, et al. Treatment of recurrent aborters by immunization with paternal cells controlled trial. *Am J Reprod Immunol.* 25:16, 1991

102. Gatenby PA, Cameron K, Simes RJ, et al. Treatment of recurrent spontaneous abortion by immunization with paternal lymphocytes: Results of a controlled trial. *Am J Reprod Immunol.* 29:88, 1993

103. Fraser EJ, Grimes DA, Schulz KF. Immunization as therapy for recurrent spontaneous abortion: A review and metaanalysis. *Obstet Gynecol.* 82:854, 1993

104. The Recurrent Miscarriage Immunotherapy Trialists Group. Worldwide Collaborative Observational Study and Meta-Analysis on Allogenic Leukocyte Immunotherapy for Recurrent Spontaneous Abortion. *Am J Reprod Immunol.* 32:55, 1994

105. Bux J, Westphal E, de Sousa F, et al. Alloimmune neonatal neutropenia is a potential side effect of immunization with leukocytes in women with recurrent spontaneous abortions. *J Reprod Immunol.* 22:299, 1992

106. Katz I, Ovadia J, Fisch B, et al. Cutaneous graft-versus-host–like reaction after paternal lymphocyte immunization for prevention of recurrent abortion. *Fertil Steril.* 57:927, 1992

107. The German RSA/IVIG Group. Intravenous immunoglobulin in the prevention of recurrent miscarriage. *Br J Obstet Gynecol.* 101:1072, 1994

108. Coulam CB, Krysa L, Stern JJ, Bustillo M. Intravenous immunoglobulin for treatment of recurrent pregnancy loss. *Am J Reprod Immunol.* 34:333, 1995

109. Christiansen OB, Mathiesen O, Husth M, et al. Placebo-controlled trial of treatment of unexplained secondary recurrent spontaneous abortions and recurrent late spontaneous abortions with I.V. immunoglobulin. *Hum Reprod.* 10:2690, 1995

110. Riley LR, Tuomala RE. Infectious disease and recurrent pregnancy loss. *Infertil Reprod Med Clin North Am.* 2:165, 1991

111. Witkin SS, Ledger WJ. Antibodies to chlamydia trachomatis in sera of women with recurrent spontaneous abortion. *Am J Obstet Gynecol.* 167:135, 1992

112. Stray-Pederson B, Eng J, Reikvam T. Uterine T-mycoplasma colonization in reproductive failure. *Am J Obstet Gynecol.* 130:307, 1978

113. Quinn PA, Shewchuk AB, Shuber J, et al. Serologic evidence of Ureaplasma urealyticum infection in women with spontaneous pregnancy loss. *Am J Obstet Gynecol.* 145:245, 1983

114. Quinn PA, Shewchuk AB, Shubr J, et al. Efficacy of antibiotic therapy in preventing spontaneous pregnancy loss among couples colonized with genital mycoplasmosis. *Am J Obstet Gynecol.* 145:239, 1983

115. Toth A, Lessen ML, Brooks-Toth CW, et al. Outcome of subsequent pregnancies following antibiotic therapy after primary or multiple spontaneous abortions. *Surg Gynecol Obstet.* 163:243, 1986

116. Summers PR. Microbiology relevant to recurrent miscarriage. *Clin Obset Gynecol.* 37:722, 1994

117. Polifka JE, Friedman JM. Environmental toxins and recurrent pregnancy loss. *Infertil Reprod Med Clin North Am.* 2:195, 1991

118. Verp MS. Environmental causes of repetitive spontaneous abortion. *Semin Reprod Endocrinol.* 7:188, 1989

119. Harlap S, Shiono PH. Alcohol, smoking, and incidence of spontaneous abortions in the first and second trimester. *Lancet.* 2:173, 1980

120. Kline J, Shrout P, Stein Z, et al. Drinking during pregnancy and spontaneous abortion. *Lancet.* 2:176, 1980

121. Kline J, Stein ZA, Susser M, et al. Smoking and the occurrence of congenital malformations and spontaneous abortions: Multivariate analysis. *Am J Obstet Gynecol.* 145:61, 1983

122. Mills JL, Holmes LB, Aarons JH, et al. Moderate caffeine use and the risk of spontaneous abortion and intrauterine growth retardation. *JAMA.* 269:593, 1993

123. Kline J, Levin B, Silverman J, et al. Caffeine and spontaneous abortion of known karyotype. *Epidemiology.* 2:409, 1991.

124. Fenster L, Eskenazi B, Windham GC, et al. Caffeine consumption during pregnancy and spontaneous abortion. *Epidemiology.* 2:168, 1991

125. Infante-Rivard C, Fernandex A, Gauthier R, et al. Fetal loss associated with caffeine intake before and during pregnancy. *JAMA.* 270:2940, 1993

126. Roman E, Beral V, Pelerin M, et al. Spontaneous abortion and work with visual display units. *Br J Indust Med.* 49:507, 1992

127. Schnorr TM, Grajewski BA, Hornung RW, et al. Video display terminals and the risk of spontaneous abortion. *N Engl J Med.* 324:727, 1991

128. Vlanderen W, Treffers PE. Prognosis of subsequent pregnancies after recurrent spontaneous abortion in first trimester. *Br Med J.* 295:92, 1987

129. Lapple M. Stress as an explanatory model for spontaneous abortions and recurrent spontaneous abortions. *Zentralbl Gynakol.* 110:325, 1988

130. Keltz MD, Olive DL, Kim AH, Arici A. Sonohysterography for screening in recurrent pregnancy loss. *Fertil Steril.* 67:670, 1997

131. Townson DD, Nelson L, Scott JR, et al. Human leukocyte antigen DQ sharing is not increased in couples with recurrent miscarriage. *Am J Reprod Immunol.* 34:209, 1995

132. SHARE, Pregnancy and Infant Loss Support, Inc., St. Joseph Health Center, 300 First Capitol Drive, St. Charles, MO 63301

133. Hargar JH, Archer DF, Marchese SG, et al. Etiology of recurrent pregnancy losses and outcome of subsequent pregnancies. *Obstet Gynecol.* 62:574, 1983

Chapter 35

INFERTILITY AND PREGNANCY LOSS

Psychological Aspects of Treatment

Patricia Honea-Fleming and Richard E. Blackwell

Couples seeking treatment for infertility and pregnancy loss have matured in a society that requires achievement and perfection from its successful members. Nurtured on such expectations, these couples not only intend to be able to have a child, they intend to be able to have it when they wish. They also expect that the child will be perfectly formed with a perfect delivery, which will also be timed appropriately to their needs. They expect their physicians, as bearers of all the truth and power of science, to be able to quickly correct any variation from these expectations.

Coming to terms with the limits of their bodies, their ability to control their own lives, and the abilities of the medical profession is only *one* aspect of the emotional challenge facing these couples. While the medical treatment of infertility and recurring pregnancy loss is exquisitely complex, the emotional experience of the couple coping with these medical conditions is equally complicated.

Many couples report that infertility is the most significant stress in their lives.[1,2] While this may reflect the relative ease of these couples' lives, more likely it is an accurate reflection of the emotional valence attached to the desire to bear children. As Glazer and Cooper[3] note, most couples "approach conception with delight and with optimism." The inability to conceive sends a shock throughout their entire world view, as well as challenging their self-concept and marriage.

This chapter reviews the emotional experiences of infertility and pregnancy loss from the perspective of a couple pursuing treatment. The role of the physician and medical team in helping the couple address these aspects of infertility and pregnancy loss is crucial to the couple's ability to cope effectively. The last section of this chapter addresses specific ways in which the medical team can support and guide couples.

UNDERSTANDING THE INFERTILE COUPLE'S EXPERIENCE

Identification of Infertility and Early Evaluation/Treatment

The necessity to employ medical assistance to conceive causes significant stress for both the husband and wife, as well as placing strain on their marriage.[4,5] This couple, generally beginning with a visit by the wife to her gynecologist, must make the transition in their own minds from being a healthy, normal husband and wife to being patients who must seek help to complete the most basic human act of procreation. They must choose to view themselves as patients. These newly self-ordained patients seek help in knowing *why* they have not conceived.

Often, early in the evaluation process couples are experiencing both shock and denial. As the awareness that something may be wrong with one or both of them creeps into recognition, couples vacillate between surprise that this is happening to them and a refusal to acknowledge that it *may* be happening to them. Although not always present, denial can function effectively as a protective mechanism in early diagnosis. It allows the couple to gradually adjust to the pain of the losses associated with being infertile. Long-term denial, however, may produce problems for the marriage, as well as interfere with seeking treatment.

In a world of science, we are taught to believe everything has a cause. When bodies do not function perfectly, reasons are sought. Blame and guilt may be close behind. When the body's malfunction pertains to sexuality, the blame/guilt tendency is especially likely. As a diagnosis begins to emerge, it is not uncommon for the member of the couple who carries the causal "factor" (ie, *male* factor) to also carry feelings of guilt and inadequacy. These feelings may be compounded with presumed blame from the spouse and consequent fears of rejection. Even though assigning blame is impossible usually and is damaging to the couple's relationship, most members of an infertile couple do consider it, if only within the privacy of their own thoughts. Whether rational or not, the possibility of assigning blame is an effort to restore the belief that there are specific causes and that someone is responsible. This line of thinking can be viewed as an attempt to renew a sense of order and control to the world. The loss of control over one's body is one of the most deeply felt identity issues of the infertility experience.

This loss of control is particularly salient regarding issues of sexuality. Women, even though adjusted to the annual gynecologic exam, generally experience the intense physical examination of their bodies and the careful review of their sexual experience as an emotional and physical invasion. While most women come to view this frequent probing as an acceptable means to a desired end, some experience prolonged reactions to this process. Glazer and Cooper[3] speak for women on the examining table: "Some of the embarrassment at being naked with one's feet in stirrups diminishes with time, but the sense of helplessness and vulnerability persists as the work up (and later treatment) progresses."

These feelings can be minimized by appropriate application of examinations when necessary; establishment of a sound, logical plan of diagnosis and treatment; continuous patient education; and involvement of the couple in participating in the testing process, such as discussing sonar findings while the procedure is being carried out.

Especially in the early stages of infertility assessment, it is common for the wife to feel uncomfortable involving her husband in the physical and emotional examinations necessary to appropriately evaluate infertility. The need to produce a semen sample by masturbation may arouse feelings of guilt, inadequacy, and anxiety in the husband.[6] Feelings of self-worth and virility are frequently attached to the outcome of testing for the husband. As Menning noted, negative outcome can threaten even the most secure ego.[1]

While production of the semen analysis may produce anxiety on the part of the male, to forego this test is a breach of the standard of care. For those who object to masturbation, silicon condoms are available for collection, which can be used at home during intercourse. If continued resistance is met, the physician must consider that the husband may not be committed to achieving a pregnancy, that he has a previous history of infertility unknown to his wife, or in the most unfortunate circumstances, that he may have undergone a vasectomy. Likewise, extreme reluctance to undergo fallopian tube evaluation by the female may suggest previous tubal sterilization.

Standard diagnostic procedure requires at least six cycles of unprotected intercourse at the time of ovulation. The necessity for daily assessment of basal body temperature carries with it daily hope and fear. The necessity for sexual intercourse, as dictated by the basal body temperature (BBT) chart, often begins with humor and good-natured hope. But, after several unsuccessful cycles hope and good humor can be replaced by despair and frustration. Sexuality becomes a job, a duty, rather than an expression of desire and love. Planned intercourse was reported by all couples in one study to have had a negative effect on sexual life.[6] Postcoital tests and the requirement for sexual intercourse during ovulation can also create performance expectations that can lead to temporary impotence[7] and may produce a midcycle pattern of sexual dysfunction.[8]

As the early evaluation of infertility continues, responsibility and causality become entangled with fears and doubts about sexuality and performance. Even deeper emotional responses begin to emerge. As shock and denial begin to fade, feelings of anger, isolation, and depression begin to affect the wife and husband and, consequently, their marriage. Once the loss of the choice to become parents is accepted, it often enrages many couples.[3] Unexpressed anger may develop into overt hostility toward care providers, produce a feeling of isolation from "the fertile world,"[1] and may lead to more pervasive feelings of depression.

The physician should remember that the anger felt by an infertile couple will rarely be directed at him or her, but at other members of the infertility team and business group. Health care providers may also receive misdirected anger for the cost of infertility therapy.

Exclusion from the fertile world is one of the most common scenarios to infertility. Women feel surrounded by others who are pregnant, not because the event is more common, but because they are more attuned to it. Couples tend to avoid social engagements with others who have children, as discussions invariably involve child-rearing dilemmas. Further, many infertile women are extremely reluctant to attend such events as baby showers, and in fact may become isolated from the probing questions of well-meaning family members.

The pattern of emotional expression in response to the infertility workup is determined largely by the outcome and diagnosis. Should the initial workup indicate a cause of infertility that is not treatable, the couple should be expected to mourn the losses of procreation.[9] They have lost the potential for a child of their own. They have lost their own reproductive health either as an individual or as a couple. They may feel betrayed by their bodies and may be unprepared to grieve the depth of their losses. They have lost the potential to share pregnancy and birth. They have lost the easiest, most assured route to the assigned status of adult in our culture. Some of these couples may pursue other avenues of parenthood but their losses deserve and require both the acknowledgment of their health care team and the time to heal. Further discussion of these losses and the grieving process follow.

Should the initial workup yield a diagnosis of treatable infertility, the couple may experience a wide range of emotions: hope, apprehension, frustration, and conflict. As more treatment options are developed and as patients become ever more educated regarding these new possibilities to conceive, the journey of infertility can extend over many years. Should the initial workup conclude with a diagnosis of unexplained infertility, the couple faces all the emotional challenges of treatable infertility *and* all the uncertainty of the potential loss of never conceiving. When secondary infertility faces a couple, they will experience many of the same emotional reactions as those couples who have no children. They, too, will face a recognition of the loss of reproductive health and the choice to conceive. They, too, will face the limits of their ability to control life events and the limits of medicine to produce a perfect outcome.

It is important to be aware that the range of emotional responses to infertility may be taking place inside a couple who present themselves to health care providers as model patients: composed, cooperative, articulate, and compliant. The medical team needs to be aware that these feelings may be operating at a subtle level in their patients and may not be verbalized. These couples are learning, many for the first time, how to negotiate the medical system. As Salzer notes, this may be the first crisis of a couple's life and most likely is their first intensive contact with the medical profession.[10] Couples frequently refrain from expressing their emotional concerns and responses for fear that it might influence the care they receive. Please refer to the last section of this chapter for suggestions in helping couples cope with these feelings.

Long-term Treatment and Emotional Losses

The early losses that accompany a diagnosis of infertility are an overture for the losses that occur throughout the treatment of long-term infertility. Many couples pursue treatment for years, suffering many surgeries, repeated evaluations, and eagerly accepting any new diagnostic or treatment modality. Over the years of extended treatment, infertility has an impact on both members of the couple. Infertility and its treatment:

Are a source of stress.
Have a profound impact on identify and self-esteem.
Produce widespread losses.

Stress. As discussed in Mahlstedt,[4] long-term infertility meets *both* of the common definitions of stress: (1) a major life experience that creates the need for change in a per-

son's life, and (2) a prolonged series of everyday irritations. Threatened with the losses detailed below, couples readily acknowledge infertility as a critical focal point in their lives. Regardless of the outcome, each of them and their relationship are changed forever. The daily irritations of infertility include temperature taking, sex scheduling, leave taking from work, explaining one's own sexual and reproductive reality to healthcare providers, as well as family and friends, and waiting—waiting for test results, for ultrasound results, for nurses, for physicians, for an appointment day, for more test results, and for a baby.

Balancing these stresses with the emotional turmoil they engender adds to the tension. Preparing for and enduring surgery and other painful procedures is a source of anxiety and fear—even though these interventions are eagerly sought as a means to the desired pregnancy. Over the years of treatment, these stresses accumulate and compound. Although most couples develop an ability to tolerate the stress of infertility, some couples respond to these difficulties by simply not returning for a scheduled appointment. They drop out of treatment without resolving their infertility. The need to restore control and normalcy to their lives takes precedence over the desire to have a child.

Identity and Self-Esteem. In addition to causing stress, infertility creates a challenge to identity for both the wife and husband. Identity is an internal definition of oneself. It is the answer to the question "Who am I?" Commonly thought to be completed in adolescence, current research[11,12] supports the experience of most adults: Identity is an ongoing creation, the result of an internal dialogue that responds to the changing external realities of life. Most women have developed their identity with consideration of motherhood.[13] Most women still respond to their own internal desires and societal expectations to be mothers. Most men who choose to marry still harbor the belief that having children is a choice they may make. Rarely have either husband or wife considered that the option to procreate may not be theirs. As treatment extends, this possibility grows more real. The inner dialogue about the self is forced to attend to this external potential reality.[13]

This is often an extremely difficult task for the career woman or upwardly mobile couple, as they have invariably been able to overcome life's adversities and succeed by hard work and determination. They will usually attempt to apply the same solution to the infertility problem, and care must be exercised on the professional's part to keep this from becoming an all-consuming obsession.

A woman begins to ask herself: Who am I as a woman if my body will not respond?; who am I as a wife if I cannot give my husband a child?; who are we as a couple if we cannot reproduce?; are we truly adult members of our society? A man begins to ask himself these questions also, whether male factor is present or not. Regardless of the source of infertility, both members of the couple must reconsider their own identity. Over time, over tests, and over many treatment procedures, self-definition begins to focus on this one, critical task. This funneling effect is a consequence of the widespread effect of infertility on the lives of those pursuing treatment (Fig 35–1).

Prior to treatment, most individuals identify themselves in relation to many other people (daughter or son, husband or wife, sister or brother) and many other goals or abilities. If infertility continues without success, each of these aspects of identity is re-examined and reformulated. For some couples, or sometimes one member of a couple, withdrawal from other important aspects of themselves and from relationships that have become painful is a coping choice. This withdrawal becomes a way of avoiding feelings of failure and of being unacceptable. As the funnel effect takes hold, identity issues will likely focus on the critical goal of achieving pregnancy. The longer this intense focus is sustained, the higher the likelihood of serious disturbance if pregnancy does not occur. The isolated couple begins to retreat further and further from life. Couples struggling with infertility must address the difficult challenge of redefining the purpose of life it they cannot achieve this critical goal of having their own child.

Closely linked to identity and self-concept is the evaluative component of self-regard or self-esteem. A man with a low sperm count may feel that his masculinity is faltering along with his sperm count. He may feel that he is worth less to his wife as a man because he cannot provide sperm to create a child. He may feel that he is worth less to society at large because he cannot father a child. The vulnerability of both husband and wife, regardless of etiology, is perhaps greatest regarding self-esteem as a sexually effective adult. Under normal conditions, we are given little guidance in the development of a positive sense of sexual self-esteem. When fertility is at question, the cultural link between sexual efficacy and fertility emerges with full force. Friends may insensitively imply that couples simply do not know what to do; that they should relax; even suggesting their willingness to assist. Although usually intended to help ease the difficulty of coping with infertility, these comments substantiate the link between fertility and sexual worthiness. Even with the recognition that such thoughts are not rational, couples sometimes feel that if they cannot create a child they must be worth less as sexual persons and sexual partners.

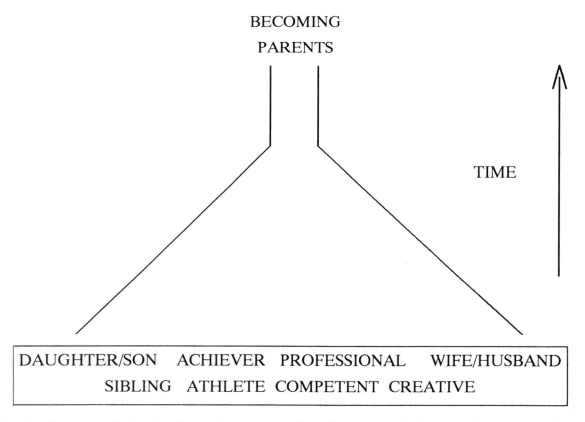

Figure 35–1. Infertility's funnel effect on identity. Long-term treatment of infertility diminishes identity complexity as all effort is focused on achieving pregnancy.

Because sexuality, fertility, self-esteem, and identity are so closely and intensely related, the actual experience of sex itself is greatly changed by infertility. Each expression of sexuality can carry the reminder of the inability to conceive whether it occurs at midcycle or not. Making love can begin to seem like work. No longer is it an expression of the desire to give and receive pleasure and to create love between husband and wife. It becomes the job of procreating. Like any job, it requires scheduling and like most jobs the schedule is not determined by choice. Much effort must be expended to determine when ovulation is occurring and to arrange "coverage." Not only must the couple know *when*, they must be ready and able to alter their priorities, choosing not to attend a professional meeting, for example, so that they can "be home." All this effort must be expended even in the face of so much previous ineffectiveness. It is common for resentment to build as the costs for pursuing this goal rise. Performance in the bedroom becomes more critical with so much invested.

This performance aversion can be minimized by patient education. The recent observation by Wilcox et al, evaluating 625 menstrual cycles for which the dates of ovulation could be estimated in evaluating 192 pregnancies that were initiated, suggests that nearly all pregnancies could be attributed to intercourse during a 6-day period, ending on the day of ovulation. Therefore, the couple should be encouraged to "cover" a fertile zone and should be discouraged from the frequently advised pattern of daily or every other day intercourse unless it suits their sexual needs.[14]

And, sometimes the bedroom seems more crowded. Couples have reported that so much attention to when and how they make love can lead to the feeling that physicians and nurses are almost present during their most intimate moments. A not uncommon outcome is a protective reduction in the intimacy expressed with sex. When the other emotional reactions to infertility are active (anger, depression, isolation), they can reduce the desire for sexual expression. With recognition, support, and guidance, most couples are able to face the sexual difficulties of infertility. For some, however, the costs are high and long lasting. For those unable to overcome the change in their sexual relationship, the attempt to have a child may cost them an intimate and nurturing sexual relationship.

Loss. The necessity to reconstruct an identity and the challenge of sustaining a satisfying sexual relationship are the result of the loss of fertility. While fertility *may* be restored with the appropriate medical intervention, the experience of its loss is not removed. Losses are widespread and broadly effect the various components of couples' lives. Losses are experienced across the entire time span of infertility treatment and remain active even after treatment is concluded.

The monthly grieving that begins before any treatment is sought continues throughout the years of extended treatment. Each menstrual period, normally a reminder of health and womanhood, now serves as a reminder of disease and the doubt of fertility.

When the couple must use services such as artificial insemination or other assisted reproductive technologies, they experience a loss that is rarely acknowledged by well-motivated physicians and nurses. Frequently, this loss is obscured by the couple's own hope and expectation of success. Assistance in conception means that the traditionally intimate and sacred act of creating new life, normally private and special, is joined by strangers, takes place in a strange setting, and is more clinical than sacred. Even though couples may willingly sacrifice "conception in the marriage bed, the way it's supposed to be," the loss is still felt.

In many ways, couples *actually* lose control over their bodies, sexuality, marriage goals, and life choices. This loss of control is especially disturbing to individuals who are expected to set goals, manage both themselves and others toward fulfilling those goals, and succeed. These individuals, who have identified themselves as achievers, are likely to be deeply threatened by this loss.[15,16] Once this challenge to control is acknowledged, the effect of that challenge may spread through the entire belief system. Their confidence in the future ability to control life events may erode. Their naive belief that their bodies are healthy is lost and with it the belief that they have control over their bodies. Even the control over the nature of their lives has been lost. For many couples, this loss of control is very disturbing and requires a complete reformulation of their belief system.[17]

Throughout long-term infertility, the necessity to reformulate identity, tolerate the everyday stress of treatment, emotionally respond to loss, cope with repeated challenges to self-esteem, and adjust sexual expression take their toll on the couple. These tasks are present as a background against which the hopes and victories of treatment take place.

Concluding Treatment

Treatment may end in many ways. Most couples expect to be among the successful, and for many treatment ends with a pregnancy. It is important to remember that even these couples will continue to carry the losses associated with impaired infertility. Complemented with the joys of parenthood, the experience of infertility can be viewed as an opportunity for emotional and marital growth.

But, for some couples the tension of treatment is simply too great and resolution too complicated to achieve. These couples simply drop out of treatment.

Some may seek support from Resolve or from individual counselors, while others attempt to regain a normal life alone. Some of these couples may return for treatment after reorganizing their lives and relationship.

For some couples, the decision to end treatment without having an ongoing pregnancy is critical to their efforts to restructure their lives. Unlike those who simply drop out, these couples may discuss their decision to stop with their physician in great detail. The decision to stop may even be made in the face of new treatments that may offer potential success. Most of these couples have carefully evaluated their life goals and immediate needs. For them it is best to put down this dream and return to more available choices. Many couples who continue long-term infertility treatment might make this decision with the guidance and support of their physicians. When the medical options are limited or extreme, physicians must provide not only information for the couple's decision process but *permission* to stop as well. Couples know that the final losses of infertility can be avoided by continuing treatment.

The physician can help the couple resolve the infertility problem by stating at the outset of the evaluation that the goals of therapy are to find out the cause of infertility if possible, help the couple achieve a pregnancy, help the couple achieve adoption, or help them resolve or reconcile their therapy and loss. It can't be emphasized too strongly that a logical, efficient game plan that seeks the most common cause of infertility in the most cost-effective manner by the safest route is perhaps the greatest thing a physician can offer to help a couple achieve a pregnancy and resolve their infertility problem.

The final, long-dreaded losses of infertility are profound. At the most immediate level, the couple loses their now comfortable status as a patient. For some, this relationship with physicians and nurses has become an important source of support and direction. These are the people who have been helping them, directing their efforts to fulfill their goal, supporting them in times of loss, and providing a safe harbor from the fertile world.

At the same time, most must squarely face the loss of their own biologic child. The depth of this loss is reflected by the effort they have expended in avoiding it. For those who "try everything," the loss of their own biologic heir is deeply painful. Being denied the physical experience of pregnancy and birth is a loss that is difficult to even describe. The loss of the possibility of creating another human life from the loving union of husband and wife is still powerful even after living with so much doubt. The couple is also losing a relationship with their long-sought child. For those acknowledging this loss, the experience is one of losing a precious fantasy, the belief that a child will be there to structure time, give meaning to life, and make one feel worthwhile. When couples end their treatment, whether by choice or necessity, they must face the deep experience of grief. Please refer to the discussion of the grief process that follows for a detailed review of this experience.

Adoption offers some couples the great joys and satisfactions of parenting. For others, the carefully considered choice of using donor gametes may provide pregnancy and birth experiences as well as parenting. But, even with these excellent options these couples must grieve their losses also. It is important to remember that losses are experienced regardless of the outcome of treatment. Even during the most satisfying times the old loss may flicker deep within. Resolving infertility, regardless of the outcome, is a psychological task[10] that requires emotional attention. The couple must renew their relationship and create a new view of their future. They must acknowledge the stigma of infertility[13] and work through the process of separating it from themselves. They must create a new identity of themselves that incorporates the losses they have experienced. They must make some sort of peace with themselves. For most couples, this process or recreation is slow and occurs at a subtle level of awareness. For some, resolution requires a more public recognition of the experience of infertility.

ADOPTION

Adoption is often suggested to infertile couples as a means of resolving their infertility. Folk literature suggests that couples who adopt are more likely to achieve a biologic pregnancy; however, prospective studies have shown this to be false on several occasions. Adoption satisfies a couple's need for parenting, but not for being pregnant, undergoing delivery, and participating in its ancillary activities. The adopting couple may receive a newborn, a multiple gestation, or a sibling combination. While the adoptive couple may wait many years to receive their child, the arrival is usually on short notice, and one does not have a traditional 9-mo period to prepare for parenthood. Adoption agencies, either private or state, use the "home study" to help prepare couples for parenting. While adoptions may be handled privately or through an agency, all of them will ultimately be handled by similar legal mechanisms. Therefore, it is suggested that the prospective adoptive couple attempt to work with an adoption agency to benefit from their experience, even if they ultimately receive a child through private adoption.

Adoption, like infertility and pregnancy loss, can evoke tremendous stress in a couple. If the adoption is a private one, extreme care must be taken in choosing legal counsel, as this law is a highly specialized art. Private adoptions are fraught with hazards, particularly when dealing with a minor female, an unknown or absent father, intrusive relatives, or an interstate or international arrangement. If the legal process is not handled appropriately, the couple risks losing the child, either before birth or sometimes many years after adoption. In case of agency adoptions, minors are virtually always declared adults by the court, partners relinquish rights to the child, the courts sever maternal ties, and after an appropriate waiting period the issuance of an interlocutory decree will usually ensure the success of the adoption. The final adoption usually occurs a yr and a day after placement, and one should consider that adoption laws are not uniform among states.

Couples will frequently be discouraged from adoption when they call an agency seeking a newborn child of a particular sex and eye color. These types of demands suggest to the caseworker that the couple has not seriously considered this situation and they will usually be told that a wait of 5 yr or more is the rule. However, a couple should realize that the adoption rolls will shrink rapidly as many people conceive, adopt through other agencies, receive children through private adoptions, or move to other locations. Further, most couples will register with multiple adoption agencies and they are under no obligation to commit to a particular agency until a home study is carried out.

The home study is an interesting experience in which usually 10 or more couples will meet with a caseworker or two to discuss a variety of adoption issues including various parenting scenarios dealing with difficult children. The couple will take an opportunity to explore their own feelings and those of their partners regarding the adoptive process. Often, they will be asked to write essays about each other, their likes and dislikes, and will be asked to disclose an extremely detailed financial statement. The home visit usually takes place at the agency and virtually never at home, although a one-time visit may be in order. These home study sessions may range from 8 to 12 in number and usually occur each wk. The home study is a useful time for exploring one's feelings about adoption; it is not uncommon for up to half of the participants to withdraw once they recognize that they are more concerned with pregnancy than with being parents.

A special note should be made regarding the couple who receives a child through private adoption. The family court will order a home study by the Department of Pensions and Securities prior to placement of a child. This often puts pressure on caseworkers and agencies as well as extra stress on the potential adoptive parents. Further, it should be realized that the findings of the agency and the opinion of the court will determine whether a private adoption occurs or not; therefore, it is again recommended that couples contemplate private adoption, work through an agency, and receive their home study and approval for adoption before such activities have to be court directed.

UNDERSTANDING THE EXPERIENCE OF PREGNANCY LOSS

For physicians treating infertility, pregnancy loss is a significant and common event. Because rates for miscarriage in a "natural" milieu are between 15 to 20 percent,[18] early loss of pregnancy occurs frequently and remains within the domain of infertility care. Loss at later stages of pregnancy is also part of infertility treatment because those couples who were in treatment for infertility prior to the pregnancy often elect to return to try again. Indeed, it is important to recognize that the pain of pregnancy loss covers a wide spectrum of experience. At the early end of the spectrum is the couple who has had a successful transfer of viable embryos in an in vitro fertilization (IVF) cycle. Should the IVF "pregnancy" not continue, they may feel many of the same losses as those suffering a later miscarriage. An ectopic pregnancy, most frequently diagnosed as both a pregnancy and a loss simultaneously, presents a painful juxtaposition of hope and despair. At the most complex end of the spectrum is repeated later pregnancy loss. This couple experiences these losses as both unique and cumulative ends. *All* of these couples are feeling grief at the loss of their potential child.

At all points on this spectrum, the loss is of a *specific* potential child, one the potential parents have begun to relate to as an individual, a dream made real, *their* child. Bonding, particularly for the mother, begins early in childhood when fantasies of motherhood initiate the internalization of her identity as a mother. The bonding becomes increasingly immediate and intense as planning, conception, and acceptance of pregnancy occur.[19] Clinical experience suggests that the identification with a *specific* potential child is developed earlier with the diagnostic methods used with infertile couples.[20] Yet, data comparing the grief response of women who suffered miscarriage, stillbirth, and neonatal death suggest that the reaction to loss is as great in early miscarriage as it is in neonatal loss.[21] Physicians can significantly aid in the healing of these couples by openly acknowledging that they have suffered a real loss and by acknowledging that the couple may consider themselves to actually *be* parents to their lost child.

The Grief Process

A thorough understanding of the grief process and its special manifestations for pregnancy loss is essential for physicians dealing with infertility. Much has been made of the stage theory of grief, which suggests that the suffering person progresses neatly through denial, isolation, anger, grief, and resolution.[22,23] Yet, it is clear to those who have experienced loss that these feelings and many more complex emotional clusters present themselves in a less ordered way. For the couple who is experiencing the loss of a pregnancy, an immediate emotional need is to create some sense out of the loss, to understand what has happened, to have a reason. Especially in very early pregnancy, the likelihood of having any explanation is very low. Even with later losses, the medical team is frequently unable to provide an explanation. So, the couple may search for any activity that may have initiated the loss.[24] Sometimes sexual intercourse is targeted by the couple as a cause with mutual guilt and blame resulting.[25]

For some women, the frustration of this loss may be manifested in anger. The anger may be directed toward herself if she feels that her body has failed or it may be directed toward her physician and other caregivers. Feelings of guilt, inadequacy, and failure are common. For infertile couples especially, the loss of a pregnancy will reinstate the fears and panic of being out of control of their own life. For these couples, who were expecting joy and the beginning of life, the loss of a pregnancy is a cruel jolt.

Accompanying these intense feelings are a range of physical responses. Normal somatic responses include loss of appetite, malaise, and sleeplessness, as well as bouts of weeping and shortness of breath. Cognitive alterations are also part of the grief reaction and include such difficulties as sustaining attention or remembering, a sense of unreality, and a dislocation in time. It is not only a baby or hoped-for baby that has been lost. At this time, when loss is all there is, the couple feels that they have lost a life as parents to *this* child, they have lost their dream of everything that *might* have been real.

Impact on Marriage and Sexuality

While the marriage may be expected to be a source of support and strength during most crises, the pain of losing a pregnancy may not be eased by a loving partner. Husband and wife grieve differently and they may not have the energy to care for each other. They do not experience the same feelings, and many use different coping skills to ease their pain. While a wife may wish to talk and review her feelings, a husband may seek comfort in the distraction of more work. Studies suggest that men tend to have fewer symptoms of grief and experience their symptoms for a shorter time than women do when a baby has died.[26]

Because it is the wife who carries the child and experiences the physical distress of miscarriage or stillbirth and because women in our culture are permitted the luxury of openly expressing emotion, it is the wife who most frequently assumes the role of the "designated griever." It is important to remember that although he is expected to be the strong one,[27] the husband also experiences deep

loss and is grieving in his own way. Indeed, resolving his loss may be impeded by his position of strength. Especially when the husband is expected to be the problem solver of the couple, the experience of pregnancy loss can be complicated. He may also experience the nagging frustration of needing to be both strong *and* expressive of his grief. He, like others, is actually helpless to change the painful reality of their loss.

Grief of any sort has the effect of decreasing sexual interest. For the couple who has lost a pregnancy, sexual expression is usually saturated with loss. The association of sexuality, conception, and loss is a poignant deterrent to sexual desire. Each time they make love, they may recall the loss of their child. Yet, over time, in a nurturing and intimate marriage, sexual expression may offer much-needed support and comfort.

Unfortunately, couples dealing with infertility must realize that this state has a profound negative impact on marriage, and divorces among infertile couples are more common than in the population at large. Members of the infertile couple may consciously or unconsciously feel that changing partners may enhance their likelihood of reproduction, particularly if the cause of infertility appears unclear.

Conceiving Again

When the loss has occurred late in the pregnancy, some couples are reluctant to complete their grief because they feel they are abandoning the lost child.[28] Sometimes, even early in the experience, well-meaning comments by medical personnel or friends seek to minimize their loss ("You can always try again"). After a short period, most of their support begins to suggest that the grief should be ending. When couples do choose to begin treatment again, most are simultaneously experiencing both loss and hope. They may relive the events of the first pregnancy with all its old pain made fresh. Yet, the hope and uniqueness of *this* pregnancy brings them forward. The fear of a reoccurrence of their loss, however, is ever present.

Special mention should be made of the concerns of the male regarding pregnancy loss. Often, the husband will tend to minimize the importance of pregnancy to his wife and the physician after a loss or series of recurrent losses. As it has been pointed out, men probably do not network as well as women and our society tends to thwart the exploration of inner feelings by the male. However, many men use this defense mechanism not so much to protect themselves, but to protect their wives. After all, they may have witnessed their spouse going through painful labor, bleeding excessively, and being treated with emergent health care.

Factors affecting the rate of recovery for a couple suffering a pregnancy loss are many. Clearly, even though the initial loss may be comparable, recovery from an early miscarriage would be expected to proceed more quickly than a loss in delivery of a full-term child. Repeated miscarriages or ectopic pregnancies, which damage the reproductive capability as well as producing a specific loss, might be expected to take a more significant recovery toll. Support from spouse, friends, and relatives can greatly decrease the isolation and speed recovery. Personal qualities of the individual such as effective coping skills, positive self-esteem, and a diversity of interests and commitments are deciding factors influencing the grief process. As we have seen, couples who have experienced long-term infertility may have little in reserve to cope with the demands of effectively grieving pregnancy loss. Sensitive physicians who provide guidance, permission, and information play a central role in preparing the grieving couple for their next step.

PHYSICIAN'S ROLE IN ADDRESSING EMOTIONAL CONCERNS

As primary care provider, the physician must accept responsibility to provide for both the physical as well as emotional health of the couple. This may seem to require shifting from a results/success perspective to a more integrated "softer" approach to care. Yet, even with high-stress treatment such as IVF clinical experience suggest that the effect of recognizing and addressing emotional needs is improved tolerance of treatment and consequently improved success. Particularly with end-phase, assisted reproductive technologies where success rates are low, it is crucial to recognize the objective of treatment is not only the pregnancy/baby/success rate but also an effective negotiation of the experience of infertility for the couple. The medical professionals who direct this experience are critical to couples' healthy resolution of infertility. The physician treating a couple for infertility has significant power to shape what may be a long and powerful episode of their lives. By truly understanding the basic emotional issues that affect these couples, empowering them to regain control of their lives, and securing support for their emotional needs, the medical team can facilitate a couple's resolution.

Physicians can best serve their patients' emotional needs by being honest with themselves and their patients about their level of interest in dealing with this difficult problem, their competence, and referring patients to infertility subspecialists in a timely manner. They need to have a command of the literature, understand the success and failures of various therapies, and be prepared to advise couples frankly and honestly about the chance of conception. When these forms of therapies do not result in pregnancy, couples should be moved on to more advanced treatment rather than undergoing redundant

therapy with multiple ovulation induction cycles and surgeries that are unlikely to produce conception.

A recent survey by Louis Harris and Associates (111 Fifth Avenue, New York, NY 10003; study number 954011) evaluated the quality of care in fertility treatment. Couples, physicians, and other health care providers were surveyed including 165 patients, 279 medical professionals including 100 doctors, 103 nurses, and 76 pharmacists. Fifty-nine percent of patients and their partners felt that their doctor spent too little time counseling them about emotional issues. Sixty-nine percent of physicians admitted that they spent only some or a small amount of time counseling patient fears, and they relied on nursing personnel 43 percent of the time to deal with these issues. Forty-nine percent of the nurses indicated that they spent a huge amount of time counseling patients on emotional issues. This survey would seem to confirm that physicians would be wise to invest a greater amount of their time addressing emotional concerns.

Recognizing Central Emotional Issues

Earlier in this chapter, the emotional experiences of infertility and pregnancy loss were reviewed. All members of the medical team *and* the support staff who interact with patients should be aware of the emotional milieu of those to whom they are offering services. They should understand that the couple in their care is experiencing both emotional pain and medical need.[4] And, they should remember that both husband and wife are their patients. Infertility is a *couple's* medical problem and both need to be respected. Both should be aware of the plan of treatment. Should other physicians be involved in treatment of a spouse, regular communication between treating physicians ensures that couples are not following different treatment protocols.[10] In addition to understanding the emotional concomitant of infertility, it is important for those providing care to be clear about two other fundamental aspects of the experience:

For most couples pursuing treatment, stress is the result of infertility, not the cause.

The desire for privacy is not relinquished when the couple agrees to undertake treatment.

Cause. Generations of physicians have believed that (what we now call) stress can cause infertility. In the past it was believed that 62 percent of infertility was caused by stress; a more contemporary figure would suggest less than 2 percent of infertility is secondary to this cause. At its most damaging, this belief resulted in countless referrals to psychiatrists who provided in-depth analysis for such stress as a woman's conflict over giving up her career or her deep hostility toward her own mother. While a reasonable effort to address what was believed to be a genuine deterrent to conception, these referrals, for conditions such as tubal occlusion or sperm antibodies, now medically diagnosed, caused much stress themselves. Often, leading a woman to what might have been real psychological issues, this approach did not identify the real reasons for failing to conceive. Yet, the approach did leave the patient unfairly accountable for her infertility.

The inference then, *and* for some less aware physicians *now*, is that the woman herself is exercising some intrapsychic control to prevent pregnancy. While conflict over having children may well manifest itself at the level of sexual exposure when either partner abstains from sexual relations, an in-depth literature review has concluded that no evidence convincingly demonstrates a specific psychological factor affecting fertility.[29] Contemporary researchers, with the advantage of sophisticated diagnostic techniques, are able to ascribe medical causes to 90 percent of infertility cases. Yet, the tendency to attribute infertility to psychological factors remains a convenient answer for both layperson and professional.

Despite these feelings, it is extremely difficult to separate the psychological from the physiologic. As discussed in the chapters dealing with ovulation induction and ovulatory dysfunction, a decrease in body weight can be associated with subtle disorders of ovulation to the extreme of amenorrhea. Conditions such as anorexia nervosa would represent the extreme case; however, many women in American society function at the bottom of their height/weight range. One frequently encounters the patient who is underweight for her height, carries little body fat, and has ovulatory dysfunction. In addition, one may encounter the patient who participates in extreme forms of physical activity. It should be noted that long-distance running appears to have the greatest effect on menstrual function. Finally, stress results in the release of many neuroactive compounds that can disrupt menstrual function. Stress is particularly damaging in the patient with a low body weight and a small amount of body fat, who exercises greater than average.

Perhaps the close association of infertility and stress leads those without medical evidence to conclude a causal direction in which stress produced infertility. Most contemporary studies, however, suggest that the association between stress and infertility is correct but the causal direction is reversed.[30,31] Indeed, as now understood, is it the condition of being infertile and the experience of pursuing treatment that causes the stress. It is precisely in those instances where infertility is without a medical diagnosis that highest levels of emotional disturbance are found.[32] The lack of explanation, the inexplicable loss of control over their lives and choices, is the source of increased stress.

It is important for providers to understand this causal direction because the cost of confusion is high.

Patients who are told that their own inner thoughts are to blame for their infertility suffer deeply. Even the suggestion that "you just relax, let nature take her course" infers a control and willfulness residing with the patients that is maddening to people so thoroughly *out of control*. As we have seen, blame and guilt are common responses as couples seek to restore control and order to their lives. The slightest implication of "emotional resistance" as a cause of organic infertility is fuel for that fire. At the same time, physicians should be sensitive to indecision or confusion regarding the desire for pregnancy whether it originates from husband or wife. Should hesitancy be observed, frank and careful counseling is appropriate. If the couple needs help resolving this issue, appropriate referral to a counseling professional is suggested.

Privacy. When a couple initiates treatment for infertility, they have little idea how much it will penetrate their lives. They quickly become aware that the intimate details of their sexual lives, both past and present, are the data with which their medical team works. They soon understand that their bodies and their sexual relationship are now a group project. They struggle to sustain some sense of dignity and self-regard even "with six strangers standing between my open legs."[33] Insemination has little to do with the emotional and sacred act of intimacy between husband and wife.

Yet, it is the physician whose work necessitates this data and these procedures who can restore to the couple the sense of privacy. By simply acknowledging the discomfort of collecting a semen specimen and providing a private and appropriate setting, the physician treats the husband with respect.[34] By simply acknowledging the difference between insemination and "conception in the marriage bed" and treating both the woman *and* the event with respect and dignity, the physician helps her cope with her own loss of privacy. It is worth noting, however, that some women prefer to keep their treatment procedures and the intimate sexual relationship separate as much as possible. For these women, the presence of their husbands at an insemination or an IVF transfer presents more conflict than comfort. As with all patient care, the individual's needs and preferences are the ultimate criteria for action. It is necessary for the physician and the medical team to *know* their patients to treat them with respect and to be able to respond to their individual needs.

It is difficult for a physician treating hundreds of active patients to sustain a sensitivity to privacy issues and regard each of these patients as individuals. It is easier and emotionally safer for the physician to relate to his or her patients as *results, success rates, types of surgeries,* and *types of treatment.* Many physicians are not prepared for the extent of loss they must confront in the practice of infertility care. It is imperative for physicians to carefully review their own attitudes toward sexuality and grief. It is unlikely that a physician who experiences his or her own discomfort when discussing sexuality will be able to convincingly honor and respect the sexual relationship of the couple across the desk. Physicians who are intimidated by loss and grief will be hard pressed to lead their patients to an effective resolution of infertility.

The delicate balance between sensitivity and respect is difficult to sustain. Physicians must be knowledgeable about the emotional aspects of infertility and aware of their own issues regarding sexuality and loss. They must be attuned to patients' emotional needs and ready to respond to any emotional conflict that may arise. Yet, they must also respect that many couples reserve the right to handle their emotional issues themselves and do *not* wish to review them with their physician. They must also learn to set limits for patients and return responsibility for some aspects of treatment to the patients. And this is the *background* against which they must practice the technical and procedural aspects of medicine.

Empowering the Couple

By guarding against the tendency to ascribe the cause of infertility to psychological conflict and remaining sensitive to the couple's need for privacy, the physician and medical team are able to view their patients as fellow human beings. But, as we have seen, the patients, themselves, may not consider themselves to be worthy adults. The condition and treatment of infertility has made them feel powerless and ineffectual. The loss of control or helplessness has been associated with depression, as well as reduced immune function.[35] Even the perception of control, whether it is true or not, has been shown to have a positive effect.[36] The physician and medical team are in a decisive position to restore a sense of control to the couple.

Communicate With Care. By discussing the treatment and outcome with a patient in the office rather than at the examining table, where she is unclothed and lying down, the physician conveys respect. Be refraining from insensitive use of humor with those who take their infertility as a loss, the physician conveys caring. By communicating knowledge of the discomfort and pain associated with some infertility procedures, the physician prepares the patient to face the reality of what she may experience. By having an accessible staff who can communicate promptly and courteously with patients, the physician enables the patient to retain a sense of control. By being honest and realistic with patients, the physician enables them to make appropriate choices for themselves.

The way we discuss a patient's condition carries subtle but potent meaning. While we may refer to those we treat as "couples," there are times when it is appro-

priate at refer to them as a family. Doing so empowers them to view themselves as a legitimate family unit rather than as two people waiting to be made a family. The value of recognizing the couple as a family is perhaps most critical in the case of pregnancy loss, particularly loss late in pregnancy. By acknowledging this couple as parents, even if their child lived only briefly, they are empowered to claim their experience. Talking about the lost child and expressing sorrow can facilitate recovery. In one recent discussion, a patient shared that her infertility specialist was the first medical care provider to ask the name of her son who had died late in pregnancy.[33] She noted that this open acknowledgment of her as a parent gave her a sense of worth she greatly needed.

In an effort to ease the pain of loss, whether of a canceled IVF cycle, an ectopic, or simply a "not missed" menstrual period, we sometimes use expressions that minimize the couple's experience. "It was only a zygote." "Perhaps it was all for the best." "You'll have fun trying again." While perhaps crass to the sensitive ear, these comments are common and usually well intended. Care must be taken to educate oneself and one's staff regarding the power of such comments.

Finally, we must recognize the tendency within the practice of reproductive endocrinology to use an evaluative language that aggravates the fault/blame tendency among patients and consequently feeds their fears of inadequacy. The mixture of medical terminology and evaluative assessment in such phrases as *incompetent* cervix, a *failed* cycle, and *achieving* a pregnancy can have a significant though subtle impact on the individuals to whom they refer. While some expressions of this type are technical and are not likely to be altered, care to avoid the implication of failure or fault must be taken when discussing such medical conditions with those who have them. Some expressions, however, are simply conventions that develop in a specific practice and can be altered.

Enable Decision Making. The opportunity to make decisions regarding their own care is an important way of empowering infertile patients. While it may seem obvious that the patients are the final arbitrators of their medical choices, many physicians do not treat their patients as such. With the increased consumer awareness surrounding infertility treatment, it is important to realize that many patients *expect* to be given these choices. The physician can help the couple regain a sense of control by looking for opportunities for decision making. They should expect and encourage questions. They must also be prepared to repeat answers or explain them in a different way. Couples are often overwhelmed with information and may need extra help with technical information.

Counseling regarding both the medical and emotional aspects of infertility should be provided *early* in the treatment process.[4] Medical counseling should provide an overview of the entire diagnostic procedure and possible treatment options. Prior to any delivery of a chosen treatment, couples should be counseled regarding the specific medical procedures to be used *and* about the usual emotional or physical experience of the procedure. As an example, couples should clearly understand exactly what will happen during a hysterosalpingogram, what will be learned from the procedure, *and* that most women undergoing this procedure experience mild to extreme discomfort. Countless women have shared with the author that they were told that this procedure would be painless. They were not only shocked at their own experience but sometimes deeply concerned that they might be more "diseased" than expected.

When advising couples about various treatment options, outcome data should be presented in a format they can understand. This is particularly important for assisted reproductive technologies such as IVF. Information should be provided in discussion and these meetings should be supplemented with written material the couple can read at home. Many physicians address the need for preparation and information by assigning this responsibility to specially trained members of their nursing staff. While helpful and efficient, basic medical counseling and review of the emotional features of infertility should be conducted by the physician when decisions must be made.

Most physicians find that recommending reading helps couples understand their experience better. The American Society for Reproductive Medicine (1209 Montgomery Highway, Birmingham, Alabama 35216-2809, phone 205-978-5000) produces a series of booklets that are especially helpful and can be ordered directly from the Society. These booklets address medical conditions (male infertility, endometriosis), treatment options (ovulation drugs, IVF, and gamete intrafallopian transfer [GIFT]), and emotional and decision making aspects of infertility (if you are having trouble conceiving, adoption). Most couples are particularly eager to find support in the experience of others. Many "self-help" books, some written by authors who have experienced infertility, are available and helpful to patients (see Table 35–1). Any of these books would also be helpful to providers in further understanding both the patients' experience and their developing expectations of the healthcare professional.

Physicians who provide opportunity and guidance for decision making can help the couple regain a sense of control over their lives. It is important to include both the husband and wife in decision making as often as possible. By including the husband early in the diagnostic and treatment process, improved communication between partners and increased compliance with treatment result.

TABLE 35–1. SUGGESTED READING FOR PATIENTS

Becker G. *Healing the Infertile Family: Strengthening Your Relationship in the Search for Parenthood.* New York, N.Y., Bantam Books, 1990

Carter JW, Carter M. *Sweet Grapes: How to Stop Being Infertile and Start Living Again.* Indianapolis, Ind., Perspective Press, 1989

Glazer ES. *The Long Awaited Stork: A Guide to Parenting After Infertility.* Lexington, Mass., Lexington Books, 1990

Glazer ES, Cooper SL. *Without Child: Experiencing and Resolving Infertility.* Lexington, Mass., Lexington Books, 1988

Lasker JN, Borg S. *In Search of Parenthood: Coping with Infertility and High-Tech Conception.* Boston, Mass., Beacon Press, 1987

Noble E. *Having Your Baby by Donor Insemination.* Boston, Mass., Houghton-Mifflin, 1987

Salzer LP. *Infertility: How Couples Can Cope.* Boston, Mass., G.K. Hall & Co., 1986

Smith JL. *In Pursuit of Pregnancy.* New York, N.Y., Newmarket Press, 1987

The physician is also able to identify any potential conflict between the couple early in treatment. Finally, the physician must assume responsibility for reading the patient's tolerance for information and accept that some decisions will require lengthy discussion and deliberation between the husband and wife.

Appropriate Support and Referral

The physician should inquire on a regular basis regarding the impact of treatment on the couple's marital and sexual relationship[4,6] and be tolerant of repeated discussion of these issues. But, it is also necessary to recognize the couple's need for privacy and possible need to separate these issues from their medical treatment. Referral to a counseling professional with whom the physician has an established relationship is recommended in these cases. A recent study showed that the majority of infertility patients surveyed endorsed the need for psychological services.[37] Counseling opportunities may be provided to the couple in a number of settings.[38] These include supportive counseling provided by a clinic's staff, services provided by a professional counselor either on staff or as a consultant, and community settings such as support groups and private counselors. Care should be taken in referring a couple to outside counselors. It is imperative that these professionals have a working knowledge of infertility that includes both the emotional *and* medical aspects of treatment. A couple seeking therapy does not need to educate their therapist. Developing an open and mutually supportive relationship between a physician and a consulting counseling professional is in the best interest of all—and especially in the interest of the patient.

Couples are most likely to need referral for counseling services for help in coping with specific issues. Physicians should be alert to this need when loss issues are intense or repeated, when signs of depression are present, when either of the couple express concerns regarding their sexual relationship, or when the couple must make significant decisions in their treatment—such as ending treatment or using assisted reproductive technologies. Whenever a patient manifests signs of withdrawal or major changes in affect, such as increased crying or anger, the opportunity to address emotional concerns should be taken. These changes are most likely to be noted by the nursing staff, who generally have more contact with the patient and with whom the patient is most likely to express these emotions.

Whenever a patient explicitly requests a referral for supportive counseling, it should be honored. Whenever a patient's emotional needs are beyond their own ability to resolve and especially when these needs are manifested as inappropriate reliance on the medical staff, the physician needs to offer the more effective services of a counseling professional. Referral to a professional counselor should be offered with respect and the clear acknowledgment that coping with infertility is difficult and exhausting emotionally.

Perhaps the most profound statement of the complex decisions involved in infertility and the emotional turmoil for patients pursuing treatment is the organization Resolve (1310 Broadway, Somerville, MA 02144-1731). Founded by Barbara Eck Menning, a former infertility patient, this self-help patient group has had a significant effect in shaping not only the experience of the patients whom they advise but the actual delivery of medical services as well. The national Resolve office coordinates the services of local chapters. These local chapters provide an opportunity for couples to share their experiences and learn from those of others. All couples should be offered information about Resolve whether a local chapter is available or not.

Financial Stress of Infertility Therapy

Infertility unfortunately is often treated by the insurance industry and employers not as a series of disease processes that affect reproduction, but as a condition that should be ignored. Treatment for infertility is often considered elective and is omitted from many benefit plans, or severely restricted. Only a handful of states including Massachusetts, Illinois, and Maryland have mandated coverage for infertility, and these statutes are under attack for repeal in various legislatures. The Harris survey showed that 49 percent of patients and their partners felt that doctors spent too little time discussing reimbursement issues, and 54 percent of pharmacists said they spent a great deal of time with patients discussing costs and reimbursement issues. Therefore, healthcare providers should take the time to discuss these sensitive issues with patients and their family members. Further,

the cost of adoption should be discussed as an alternative and patients should be encouraged to consider the impact of finances on their overall life goals in making decisions whether to utilize certain forms of advanced infertility therapy or, in fact, continue therapy. This issue is particularly pertinent for the couple with secondary infertility, where expenditure of large amounts of family resources may have a deleterious effect on the upbringing and education of other siblings.

SUMMARY

Coping with the emotional aspects of infertility is a complex and difficult challenge. Couples seeking medical treatment rely upon their medical professionals for acknowledgment, guidance, and support in dealing with these issues. An informed physician and medical team who strive to sustain a compassionate and respectful attitude toward those in their care can greatly aid these couples to resolve their infertility experience. Relating to these couples as individuals whose feelings are part of their health enables them to take responsibility for themselves. Remembering and conveying the belief that most of these couples are healthy people coping with a powerful life challenge can give much-needed perspective to physician and patient alike.

Unfortunately, despite the best efforts of the health care provider and couple, infertility can extract a terrible toll. Some couples become so obsessed with achieving pregnancy that it becomes an end in itself. Once a child is conceived, the cost of this endeavor may be viewed by one or both partners as too extreme, and the child may be resented. Unfortunately, the long quest may end in divorce, perpetual bitterness, or, in the worst case, suicide. The couple who does not conceive at times emerges with a stronger relationship and sense of self; unfortunately, many others harbor an obsession that seems to have no resolution. These couples will try any therapy and go to any means to attempt conception, even beyond the age of advanced menopause.

REFERENCES

1. Menning B. *Infertility*. Englewood Cliffs, N.J., Prentice Hall, 1997
2. Kraft AD, Palombo J, Mitchell D, et al. The psychological dimensions of infertility. *Am J Orthopsychiatry*. 50:618, 1980
3. Glazer E, Cooper S. *Without Child: Experiencing and Resolving Infertility*. Lexington, Mass., Lexington Books, 1988
4. Mahlstedt P. The psychological component of infertility. *Fertil Steril*. 43:335, 1985
5. Shapiro CH. *Infertility and Pregnancy Loss*. San Francisco, Calif., Jossey-Bass, 1988

6. Lalos A, Lalos O, Jacobsson L, von Schoultz B. Psychological reactions to the medical investigation and surgical treatment of infertility. *Gynecol Obstet Invest.* 20:209, 1985

7. Rosenfeld DL, Mitchell E. Treating the emotional aspects of infertility: Counseling services in an infertility clinic. *Am J Obstet Gynecol.* 135:177, 1979

8. Drake TS, Grunert GM. A cyclic pattern of sexual dysfunction in the infertility investigation. *Fertil Steril.* 32:542, 1979

9. Shapiro CH. The impact of infertility on the marital relationship. *Social Casework.* 63:387, 1982

10. Salzer LP. *Infertility: How Couples Can Cope.* Boston, Mass., G.K. Hall, 1986

11. Fiske M. Changing hierarchies of commitment in adulthood. In: Smelser NJ, Erikson E, eds. *Themes of Work and Love in Adulthood.* Cambridge, Mass., Harvard University Press, 1988

12. Peck T. Women's self-definition in adulthood: From a different model? *Psy Women Q.* 10:274, 1986

13. Josselson R. *Finding Herself: Pathways to Identity Development in Women.* San Francisco, Calif., Jossey-Bass, 1987

14. Wilcox A, Weinberg C, Baird D. Timing of sexual intercourse in relation to ovulation. *N Engl J Med.* 333:1517, 1995

15. Becker G. *Healing the Infertile Family: Strengthening Your Relationship in the Search for Parenthood.* New York, N.Y., Bantam Books, 1990

16. McCormick RM. Out of control: One aspect of infertility. *J Obstet Gynecol Neonat Nurs.* 2:205, 1980

17. Platt JJ, Ficher I, Silver MJ. Infertile couples: Personality traits and self-ideal concept discrepancies. *Fertil Steril.* 24:972, 1973

18. Jones HW, Jones GS. *Novaks' Textbook of Gynecology.* Baltimore, Md., Williams and Wilkins, 1981

19. Peppers L. Grief and elective abortion: Implications for the counselor. In: Doka K, ed. *Disenfranchised Grief: Recognizing Hidden Sorrow.* Lexington, Mass., Lexington Books, 1989

20. Stephany TM. Early miscarriage: Are we too quick to dismiss the pain? *RN.* 45:89, 1982

21. Peppers L, Knapp R. Maternal reaction to involuntary fetal/infant death. *Psychiatry.* 43:155, 1980

22. Kubler-Ross E. *On Death and Dying.* New York, N.Y., MacMillan, 1969

23. Clapp D. Emotional responses to infertility: Nursing interventions. *J Obstet Gynecol Neonat Nurs.* 14:6, 1985

24. Bowers N. Early pregnancy loss in the infertile couple. *J Obstet Gynecol Neonat Nurs.* 14:6, 1985

25. Borg S, Lasker J. *When Pregnancy Fails: Families Coping With Miscarriage, Stillbirth, and Infant Death.* Boston, Mass., Beacon Press, 1981

26. Nichols JA. Perinatal death: Bereavement issues. *Arch Found Thanatol.* 6, 1987

27. Ryan DR, Raymond D: Underestimated grief. In: Doka K, ed. *Disenfranchised Grief: Recognizing Hidden Sorrow.* Lexington, Mass., Lexington Books, 1989

28. Nichols JA. Perinatal death. In: Doka K, ed. *Disenfranchised Grief: Recognizing Hidden Sorrow.* Lexington, Mass., Lexington Books, 1989

29. Noyes RW, Chapnick E. Literature on psychology and infertility: A critical analysis. *Fertil Steril.* 15:543, 1964

30. Pantesco V. Nonorganic infertility: Some research and treatment problems. *Psych Rep.* 58:731, 1986

31. Seibel MM, Taymor ML. Emotional aspects of infertility. *Fertil Steril.* 37:137, 1982

32. McEwan KL, Costello CG, Taylor PJ. Adjustment to infertility. *J Abnorm Psych.* 96:108, 1987

33. Honea-Fleming P. Personal communication from counseling client, 1991

34. Honea-Fleming P. The psychologist role in delivery of in vitro fertilization services. *Symposium Presentation, Experiencing Infertility: Psychological Concomitants, Coping Processes, and Adaptational Outcomes.* American Psychological Association, Annual Meeting, New York, 1987

35. Kiecolt-Glaser JK, Glaser R. Psychological moderators of immune function. *Ann Behav Med.* 9:2, 1987

36. Brier A, Albus M, Pickar D, et al. Controllable and uncontrollable stress in humans: Alterations in mood and neuroendocrine and psychophysiological function. *Am J Psychiatry.* 144:11, 1987

37. Daniluk JC. Infertility: Intrapersonal and interpersonal impact. *Fertil Steril.* 49:6, 1988

38. US Congress, Office of Technology Assessment. Infertility: Medical and Social. OTA-BA-358. Washington D.C., U.S. Government Printing Office, 1988

Chapter 36

CONTRACEPTION

Michael P. Steinkampf, Bruce R. Carr, and Richard E. Blackwell

It has been estimated that 95 percent of the 54 million American women between the ages of 15 and 44 who have intercourse use some form of contraception.[1] The choice of contraceptive method is affected not only by the perceived efficacy and convenience of the technique but whether additional risks or benefits are associated with its use. While the combined estrogen/progestin oral contraceptive pill remains the single most popular method of reversible pregnancy prevention in the United States, permanent sterilization, barrier contraception, vaginal spermicides, intrauterine devices, and periodic abstinence are viable alternatives for women whose social circumstances or medical condition contraindicate hormonal methods of birth control (Fig 36–1).[2]

HISTORIC METHODS

Many picturesque methods of contraception have been used to achieve family planning.[3] The earliest methods involve physical contraception and written records show that such techniques were practiced some 3,000 yr ago. One early method was the use of a pessary made out of a mixture of honey and crocodile dung. Apparently, the honey mechanically inhibits sperm motility and has some bacteriostatic and bactericidal properties. However, these properties were not assigned to concentrated sugars until the mid-1600s. Some of the early forerunners of vaginal contraception are rock salt, alum, and quinacrine, which possess strong spermicidal properties. In addition, the Chinese employed systemic contraception consisting of fried quicksilver in oil or swallowed 14 live tadpoles 3 days after menstruation. Other systemic approaches consisted of eating the uterus of mules. In addition, various charms and potions were used to prevent conception. For instance, Byzantine women attached tubes of cat liver to the left foot; potions were prepared from willow leaves, slag, iron rust, clay, and the kidneys of mules; and in the 16th century European brides were taught to sit on their fingers while riding in their coach or place walnuts in the bosom, one for every barren year desired. Some forerun-

ners of current contraceptive agents include sea sponges, which were used for centuries to soak up semen, medicated steams in various douches, which were used to instill "antihuman seed medicants," the precursor to the cervical caps and diaphragms produced in China and Japan, and the disk of oil silk paper placed against the cervix. Subsequently, in Europe molded wax wafers and finally linen cloths were used as a diaphragm on occasions.

BARRIER CONTRACEPTION

Condoms

The forerunner of the condom was the primitive male counterpart to the female chastity belt. A metal ring was passed through the prepuce, which served as an impediment to intercourse. In ancient Rome, bladders of animals were fashioned into primitive condoms. It is of interest that the early Egyptians dyed these sheaths various colors, which is reminiscent of today's condoms. In 1838, the vulcanization of rubber was discovered. Subsequently, modern-day condoms could be constructed from latex or silicone. However, the prototype of the modern condom was introduced in the 16th century by the Italian Fallopius, who devised a linen sheath for the penis and advised its use for the prevention of syphilis. It was described as the armor against enjoyment and a spider web against danger. Casanova, although employing the condom in his exploits, said "I do not care to shut myself up in a piece of dead skin in order to prove I am perfectly alive."

The current condom enjoys a 17 percent use among those that employ contraception. It has an accidental pregnancy rate of 12 percent in the first yr of use (Table 36–1).[4] Condoms may be transparent or opaque, colored, lubricated or dry, with plain or reservoir tip. It may be ribbed, have a contoured or rough surface, and is available in a variety of sizes including the magnum model. Its advantages include easy use and expense, it does not require a prescription, and it is protective against a variety

Percentage of Women Ages 15-50

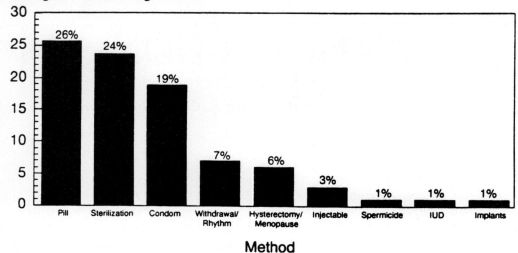

Figure 36–1. Contraceptive use in the United States, 1995. *(Reproduced, with permisson, from Ortho Pharmaceuticals, 1995, Annual Birth Control Study.)*

TABLE 36–1. CONTRACEPTIVE FAILURE AND CONTINUING USE, UNITED STATES

Method	Women Experiencing an Accidental Pregnancy Within First Year of Use		Women Continuing Use at 1 Yr (%)
	Typical Use (%)	*Perfect Use* (%)	
Chance	85	85	
Spermicides	21	6	43
Periodic abstinence	20		67
Calendar		9	9
Ovulation method		3	
Sympto-thermal		2	
Post-ovulation		1	
Withdrawal	19	4	
Cap			
Parous women	36	26	45
Nulliparous women	18	9	58
Sponge			
Parous women	36	20	45
Nulliparous women	18	9	58
Diaphragm	18	6	58
Condom			
Female (Reality)	21	5	56
Male	12	3	63
Pill	3		72
Progestin only		0.5	
Combined		0.1	
IUD			
Progesterone T	2.0	1.5	81
Copper T 380A	0.8	0.6	78
LNg 20	0.1	0.1	81
Depo-Provera	0.3	0.3	70
Norplant (6 capsules)	0.09	0.09	85
Female sterilization	0.4	0.4	100
Male sterilization	0.15	0.10	100

(Reproduced, with permission, from Hatcher RA, Trussell J, Stewart F, et al. Contraceptive Technology, 16th ed. New York, N.Y., Irvington, 1994: 113; and Trussell J, Hatcher RA, Cates W, et al. Contraceptive failure in the United States: An update. Stud Fam Plann. 21:51, 1995.)

of sexually transmitted diseases including acquired immunodeficiency syndrome (AIDS).[5] The disadvantages appear to be deterioration of the rubber, particularly when stored in hot areas or areas with high humidity, and the possibility of breakage during use. If used properly and consistently, the efficacy of a condom is 97 percent, and if used in conjunction with contraceptive jelly or cream, a 99 percent success rate can be obtained. The condom is the most widely used form of contraception throughout the world with in excess of 900 million units being sold annually in the United States alone. Many objections have been raised to the condom including the necessity for applying the sheath during sexual foreplay, decreased sensation to both partners during intercourse, inability of women to sense the ejaculatory process, and its tendency to rupture during intercourse. The condom remains the only reversible means of male contraception with the exception of coitus saxonicus, which consists of compression of the male urethra at the base of the penis at the time of ejaculation, causing retrograde ejaculation into the bladder; coitus reservatus, where control is exercised over the act of coitus so that even after prolonged intercourse ejaculation does not take place; and coitus interruptus, the oldest method of contraception, in which the male withdraws his penis prior to ejaculation. Unfortunately, the average pregnancy rate with this technique is 19 per 100 woman yr.

Latex condoms are generally 0.3 to 0.8 mm thick. Sperm are 0.003 mm in diameter, and therefore cannot penetrate the condom. Likewise, organisms that cause sexually transmitted disease and AIDS are excluded by the latex matrix. Latex is highly distensible and strong, and commercial tests involve inflating condoms with either water or air to gigantic proportions prior to rupture. Nevertheless, sensitivity is a function of membrane thickness as well as lubrication and the ability of the film to slide across the organ. Polyurethanes are a family of inherently strong polymers that are being evaluated for use in condoms by various manufacturers. Thus far the development of these products has been restricted by the lack of elasticity of the condoms. Therefore, it is hoped that a new generation of condoms will be available which could be used by those individuals who have an allergy to latex-absorbed antigens.

Intermediate between the diaphragm and condom is a new generation of products called the female condom. These are polyurethane (nonlatex) devices that are composed of an outer and inner ring surrounding an inverted condom. The inner ring is inserted much like a diaphragm trapping the cervix while the outer ring surrounds the vulva. The product is intended for use in the prevention of pregnancy and sexually transmitted diseases including HIV transmission. The Reality female condom is made by Chartrex International, in

London, and distributed by Wisconsin Pharmaceuticals, Jackson, Wisconsin. The female condom has a failure rate of 13 percent during the first six mo and 26 percent per yr.[6]

Diaphragms

Dr. Frederick Wilde is credited with inventing the diaphragm in 1858. The diaphragm is used by 4 to 6 percent of contraceptive users and has an accidental pregnancy rate in the first yr of 2 to 23 percent (Table 36–1).[4] It is composed of a soft rubber cup, usually surrounding a wound metal spring, and is used in combination with contraceptive jelly or cream that is placed in the diaphragm. It is protective against certain sexually transmitted diseases; however, women who use the diaphragm are more prone to bladder infections and allergic reactions to the rubber or cream.[7] Diaphragms generally do not rupture but may be dislodged during intercourse. Commercial diaphragms range between 50 and 105 mm in size and must be properly fitted by a health care professional. They should be carefully inspected for wear and punctures and must be replaced periodically.

Recent studies by Bounds et al evaluated 216 women for efficacy of diaphragms with and without spermicide. Eighty-four women were randomized to a diaphragm-only group, and 80 to a diaphragm and spermicide group. Typical user 12-mo failure rates for the diaphragm-only group were 28.6 per hundred women, and for diaphragm with spermicide group, 21.2. The 12-mo consistent user failure rates were 19.3 per hundred women for the diaphragm-only group as compared with 12.3 per hundred women for users of a diaphragm with spermicide.[8]

As with condoms, efforts are being made to develop polyurethane diaphragms. These products may be used a single time or repetitively. The matrix may be infused with a detergent such as nonoxynol-9, and used as a disposable contraceptive device. Such a device might be fitted or used in a one-size-fits-all mode, which would allow it to be distributed through the over-the-counter market.

Cervical Cap

Although introduced in the United States in the early part of the century, cervical caps fell from acceptance because of their difficulty of insertion and extraction. The cervical cap is a variation of the diaphragm and is placed over the cervix and remains in place by suction. Cervical caps must be tailor fitted to each cervix to allow the devices to remain in place. Many women have difficulty feeling their cervix and therefore have trouble fitting the cap. The caps can be left in place for up to 48 hr, allowing for spontaneous intercourse, whereas diaphragms are generally removed after 6 to 8 hr.[7]

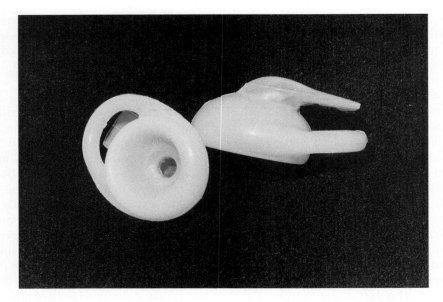

Figure 36–2. Lea shield. *(Photograph courtesy of David Archer, M.D., Eastern Virginia Medical School, Norfolk, VA.)*

Although there are several types of cervical caps, the cavity rim cap (Prentif) is approved in the United States. The Femcap, which is made of silicone rubber, is said to allow a better fit over the cervix and vaginal fornices. It is shaped like a sailor's hat and may ultimately prove to be more user friendly.[9]

The Lea shield is a barrier contraceptive agent that fits over the cervix (Fig 36–2). It is held in place by vaginal wall pressure, composed of silicone, and one size fits all. A flexible valve communicates with a 9-mm opening, which allows equalization of air pressure during insertion and drainage of cervical discharge. The posterior part of the device fits into the fornix which stabilizes the spermicide. The device is generally used in conjunction with a spermicide and may be left in place up to 48 hr after intercourse.[10]

VAGINAL CONTRACEPTIVES

Sponges

Until recently, natural sponges were used for contraception. These have been replaced by latex rubber and polyethylene foams. These devices are used by 3 percent of contraceptive users and have an accidental pregnancy rate in the first year of 18 percent. Sponges are inserted into the vagina prior to intercourse and release spermicides such as nonoxynol-9. The sponge is a one-time use device over 24 hr, does not require a prescription, and may be protective against sexually transmitted diseases such as herpes. The disadvantage of sponge use appears to be allergic reaction and difficulty of removal. There is a slight risk of toxic shock syndrome occurring with sponge use.[11]

Unfortunately, the Today's sponge has been removed from the U.S. market. It can be speculated that the demise of this product was due to improper use rather than lack of efficacy or safety. It was necessary to expose this product to water and to induce a foam prior to insertion. It appears that this was not being done. It is hoped that the demise of this product will not deter development of medicated vaginal rings or other implants to replace this product.

Spermicides

Vaginal spermicides are used by approximately 2 percent of the contraceptive-using population and have an accidental pregnancy rate the first year of 21 percent (Table 36–1.)[4] These preparations are sold in the form of foams, creams, jellies, tablets, and suppositories that are inserted into the vagina prior to intercourse. They inactivate the sperm by detergent activity and mechanically prevent sperm from entering the cervical mucus. Most of these items are nonprescription and may have a protective effect against sexually transmitted disease; however, contact dermatitis has been shown to occur with their use. Nonoyxnol-9 has been reported to be associated with a twofold increased risk in selected congenital birth defects. However, these studies have not been confirmed.[12]

There is considerable interest in the development of new vaginal contraceptive agents. Concern still exists that nonoxynol-9 may have undesirable long-term side effects. However, no product has appeared to replace it. D-propanolol has antispermicidal properties, but its development has been terminated.

INTRAUTERINE DEVICES

Approximately 85 million women worldwide use the intrauterine device (IUD), including more than 59 million women in China. The IUD was first used in antiquity, but modern use was initiated with the development of intrauterine rings. Two types of IUD are now used worldwide: (1) unmedicated (Lippes loop, single-coil stainless steel ring); and (2) medicated, containing copper (Copper-7, TCu-200B, TCu-380A) or hormone (Progestasert). In the United States, IUDs are used only by 3 percent of women using contraceptives (Fig 36–1). Recently, there has been an increased interest in IUDs in this country, but the only two devices currently marketed are Progestasert and a copper-containing IUD (TCu-380A). The TCu-380A contains 380 mm^2 of exposed copper wrapped around the vertical stem and arms of the plastic device to enhance contraceptive effectiveness, and is currently approved for 10 yr of continuous use. Progestasert, also a T-shaped plastic device, contains 38 mg of progesterone, which is released at a daily rate of 65 μg. IUDs may be inserted at any time of the menstrual cycle but are usually inserted at the time of menstrual bleeding to enhance the ease of insertion and to diminish the chance of pregnancy.

New devices containing longer-acting progestogens are available in Europe and may be available in the future in the United States.[13] All devices used worldwide are roughly equal in contraceptive effectiveness, with failure rates ranging from 1.4 to 4 per 100 women at 1 yr after insertion. The major advantages of the copper-containing IUDs are (1) a smaller increase in menstrual blood flow than with the unmedicated IUDs, (2) a lower expulsion rate, and (3) less pain after insertion. The progesterone-containing IUD is associated with a decrease in both menstrual bleeding and dysmenorrhea. The drawback of the progesterone-containing IUDs compared with the TCu-380A IUD is the necessity for yearly replacement.[14]

The precise mechanism by which the IUD acts as a contraceptive is unclear. The devices may prevent fertilization by impairing sperm transport and by damaging sperm directly. Another action is thought to result from an induction of an endometrial inflammatory response, so that the endometrium is unfavorable for implantation. Copper appears to increase the inflammatory action, and the progesterone-containing IUD interferes with the hormonal response of the endometrium. Complications of IUD use include excessive bleeding, infection, and expulsion. Approximately 5 to 15 percent of women discontinue its use within the first yr because of bleeding and pain.[13]

A potentially serious complication of IUD use is the development of pelvic inflammatory disease, which usually occurs soon after insertion. To minimize the risk of infection most physicians administer prophylactic antibiotics (500 mg tetracycline by mouth) prior to insertion of the IUD. This issue is important both because of the acute morbidity and because of an increased risk of infertility related to tubal obstruction. Current IUD users are 1.6 times more likely to be hospitalized with pelvic inflammatory disease than women utilizing no forms of contraception, and 4.5 times more likely than oral contraceptive users. Indeed, the incidence of pelvic inflammatory disease may actually be reduced in women using barrier contraceptives or oral contraceptives. Potential mechanisms for the increased incidence of pelvic inflammatory disease include the entry of bacteria into the endometrium at the time of or shortly after insertion, and promotion of bacterial growth by the increased volume and duration of menstrual bleeding. The highest rates of pelvic inflammatory disease occurred with the Dalkon Shield device. Retrospective and prospective studies suggest a lower but still significant risk of pelvic inflammatory disease in women using currently available IUDs compared with nonusers, but it should be emphasized that the risk of infection in IUD users is related to the number of sexual partners. There does not appear to be an increased risk of infection in IUD users who are monogamous.[15]

If pregnancy occurs, the IUD should be removed (if the string is visible) to reduce the incidence of spontaneous abortion, severe infection, and occasional maternal death in IUD users. If the IUD string is not visible, the choice of abortion is offered, and if abortion is not acceptable, the patient should be observed for signs of infection. Such pregnancy is more likely to be extrauterine than intrauterine, because the IUD reduces the incidence of intrauterine pregnancies more efficiently than that of ectopic pregnancies.[13]

Women who are nulligravid should use other forms of contraception. In addition, women with a history of pelvic inflammatory disease or who have multiple sex partners run an increased risk of developing pelvic inflammatory disease and also should use an alternative form of contraception. A rare complication is perforation at the time of insertion, which is an indication for surgical removal. Absolute contraindications for IUD use include active or previous pelvic infection, abnormalities or distortion of the uterine cavity, undiagnosed genital bleeding, uterine or cervical malignancy, history of ectopic pregnancy, increased susceptibility to infection (leukemias, diabetes, valvular heart disease, acquired immunodeficiency syndrome, and long-term glucocorticoid therapy), genital actinomycosis, allergies to copper or Wilson disease (for copper-containing IUDs), and known or suspected pregnancy.[13]

SURGICAL STERILIZATION

Vasectomy

Vasectomy is used among 14 percent of individuals seeking contraception. It has a failure rate of 0.15 percent. This is a permanent method of contraception that prevents sperm from traveling from the testicles to the penis. It is carried out as an outpatient surgical procedure and minor complications include pain and swelling around the incision sites; epididymitis occurs in 1 to 2 percent of patients. The process can be reversed in about 50 percent of cases. The highest success rate occurs if the procedure is done within 2 yr of the original operation. Approximately half the individuals who undergo a vasectomy develop an antibody to some sperm antigens; however, this is not thought to be associated with the development of autoimmune diseases.[16]

The no-scalpel technique has been perfected in China. It is faster, less invasive, and requires simple instruments. In Bangkok, for instance, 680 vasectomies were performed in one day with 3 complications, versus 523 vasectomies performed with standard technique which resulted in 16 complications. Reversal is no easier than with other techniques of vasectomy.[17]

Tubal Ligation

Female sterilization is carried out in approximately 19 percent of those individuals seeking contraception and has a failure rate of approximately 0.4 percent during the first year following surgery.[4] This is designed as a permanent mode of contraception and involves interruption of the fallopian tubes with either plastic bands, clips, electrocautery, or ligation. The procedure can be carried out laparoscopically, by laparotomy, or transvaginally. It produces an extremely low failure rate if properly done; however, it can be associated with anesthetic or surgical complications that may be as severe as vascular injury and death or bowel perforation.[18] Although it is a permanent means of contraception, tubal ligations can be successfully reversed.[19] Factors affecting the reversibility of a tubal ligation include the age of the patient, overall fertility status of the couple, length of fallopian tubes to be reanastomosed, and site of anastomosis. While tubal ligation is relatively simple to perform, reanastomosis is a major operative procedure usually lasting between $1^1/_2$ and 4 hr.

Other Surgical Procedures

Various other forms of surgery may be used to induce female sterilization including vaginal or abdominal hysterectomy, laser or roller ball ablation of the uterine lining, ablation of the tubal ostium, and the introduction of various plastics, caustic chemicals, or silicans into the fallopian tube via hysteroscopy. These surgical procedures are generally carried out for other indications and are not approved for fertility control. The hysteroscopic procedures at this juncture are experimental and have a high failure rate incompatible with use in the United States.

RHYTHM METHOD

Natural family planning or rhythm method is a form of controlled periodic abstinence. It is used by approximately 4 percent of couples seeking contraception and has a 20 percent failure rate in the first yr.[4] This method involves avoidance of intercourse at the time of ovulation and during the fertile period. Because ovulation frequently occurs between days 12 to 16 and sperm may live in the cervical mucus for at least up to 2 days, this requires a relatively long period of either abstinence or the use of another form of contraception. One could combine the use of the rhythm method with the use of basal body temperature charting or an ovulation predictor kit to enhance its efficacy.

HORMONAL CONTRACEPTION

Oral Contraceptives

The development of hormonal forms of contraception represents one of the greatest advances of modern gynecology. The concept of pregnancy prevention from administration of hormones originated with the realization that ovulation was inhibited by the presence of the corpus luteum. Ludwig Haberlandt, a professor of physiology in Innsbruck, Austria, demonstrated in 1919 that fertile adult rabbits became sterile after receiving subcutaneous transplants of ovaries from pregnant does. A number of investigators showed that extracts of ovaries, and later progesterone or estrogen, inhibited ovarian function.[20] Progestins were shown to inhibit ovulation; the addition of estrogen was found both to regulate menstrual bleeding and increase contraceptive effectiveness. The first clinical trials of oral contraceptives were described in 1958 by Pincus, Rock, and Garcia,[21] with approval for marketing in the United States obtained in 1960. Within 5 yr of its introduction, more than 30 million prescriptions for oral contraceptives were being prescribed annually, making it one of the most common medications in use.

Physiology of Hormonal Contraceptives. Current formulations of hormonal contraceptives rely upon the effects of estrogen and/or progestin. These hormones have both direct and indirect actions on the reproductive tract (Table 36–2). Both estrogen and progestin prevent ovulation by suppression of follicle-stimulating hormone (FSH) and luteinizing hormone (LH) secretion. This occurs by inhibition of hypothalamic gonadotropin-

**TABLE 36–2. MECHANISM OF ACTION
OF ESTROGEN/PROGESTIN CONTRACEPTIVES**

Inhibition of ovulation by suppression of FSH and LH

Alteration of cervical mucus to inhibit sperm transport

Interference with ovum transport

Inhibition of implantation by suppression of normal endometrial development

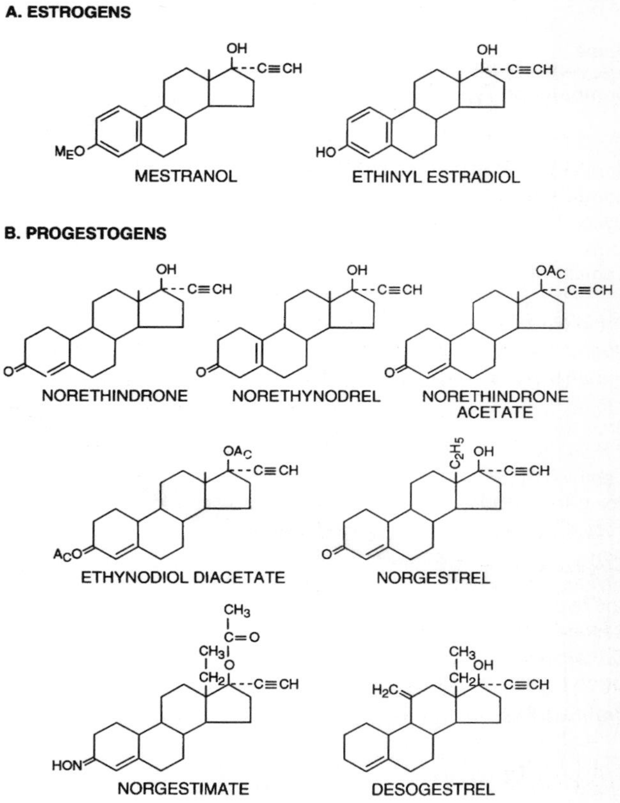

Figure 36–3. Structural formulas of contraceptive hormones approved for use in the United States.

releasing hormone (GnRH) release and possibly by a direct effect on the pituitary.[22] In users of combination estrogen/progestin contraceptives, levels of LH, FSH, progesterone, and estradiol are suppressed.[23] Progestins induce the formation of thick, viscid cervical mucus, which limits the penetrability of sperm. Both estrogen and progestin alter motility of the fallopian tube,[24] but the importance of this effect in women is not known. Normal endometrial development is interrupted by estrogen and progestin; this effect may be important in progestin-only contraceptives or when estrogen/progestin combinations are used for postcoital contraception.[25]

Current Formulations of Hormonal Contraceptives.
While both estrogens and progestins affect many different organs, producing a broad range of clinical effects, comparisons of these compounds have frequently been based upon isolated hormonal or biochemical effects. In addition, the clinical effects of these compounds given in combination are markedly different than when administered alone. The high steroid doses in early oral contraceptives were chosen because of the effects of the isolated components to prevent pregnancy in laboratory animals, with the synergistic effects of combined estrogen/progestin formulations recognized only some years later.[26] Thus, the rational approach to the evaluation of contraceptive steroids relies more upon the results of comparative clinical trials than studies of isolated effects in animals or humans.

COMBINED ORAL CONTRACEPTIVES. Orally active contraceptives contain either a combination of estrogen and progestin or a progestin alone. Only two types of estrogen are currently used: ethinyl estradiol and its 3-methyl ether, mestranol (Fig 36–3). These compounds share an ethinyl group in the 17-α position that inhibits hepatic metabolism of the molecule, thus enhancing oral potency. Mestranol does not bind to estrogen receptors and must undergo conversion to ethinyl estradiol to become biologically active. Oral contraceptives containing 50 μg mestranol produce plasma ethinyl estradiol concentrations approximately equivalent to those containing 35 μg ethinyl estradiol.[27] No oral contraceptive containing less than 50 μg mestranol has been marketed in the United States, while the dose of ethinyl estradiol in currently available pills ranges from 20 to 50 μg.

Removal of the 19-carbon from testosterone converts the major hormonal effect from androgenic to progestational, with addition of a 17-α ethinyl group giving an orally active compound. The seven progestins currently marketed for contraceptive use in the United States are all 17-α ethinyl analogs of 19-nortestosterone (Fig 36–3). Concomitant with the hormonal effects associated with progesterone, synthetic progestins exhibit varying degrees of estrogenic and androgenic side effects. Levonorgestrel, the most potent contraceptive progestin currently available, is the biologically active stereoisomer of norgestrel and is thus about twice as potent as the racemic mixture. Norgestrel is generally considered the most androgenic progestin, while norgestimate has been shown to have less androgenic side effects than other derivatives of 19-nortestosterone.[28] This effect may be of considerable importance because many of the adverse effects of steroid contraceptives are thought to be mediated by the androgenic actions of progestins. Desogestrel has clinical profiles similar to norgestimate.[29]

TABLE 36–3. COMPOSITION OF ORAL CONTRACEPTIVES

Name	Estrogen	μg	Progestogen	mg
Combination Type				
		Estrogen Content = 50 μg		
Ortho-Novum 1/50	Mestranol	50	Norethindrone	1.0
Norinyl 1 + 50	Mestranol	50	Norethindrone	1.0
Norethin 1/50M	Mestranol	50	Norethindrone	1.0
Ovcon-50	Ethinyl estradiol	50	Norethindrone	1.0
Ovral	Ethinyl estradiol	50	Norgestrel	0.5
Demulen 1/50	Ethinyl estradiol	50	Ethynodiol diacetate	1.0
		Estrogen Content <50 μg		
Ortho-Novum 1/35	Ethinyl estradiol	35	Norethindrone	1.0
Norinyl 1 + 35	Ethinyl estradiol	35	Norethindrone	1.0
Norethin 1/3SE	Ethinyl estradiol	35	Norethindrone	1.0
Modicon	Ethinyl estradiol	35	Norethindrone	0.5
Brevicon	Ethinyl estradiol	35	Norethindrone	0.5
Ovcon-35	Ethinyl estradiol	35	Norethindrone	0.4
Demulen 1/35	Ethinyl estradiol	35	Ethynodiol diacetate	1.0
Loestrln 1 .5/30[a]	Ethinyl estradiol	30	Norethindrone acetate	1.5
Loestrin 1/20[a]	Ethinyl estradiol	20	Norethindrone acetate	1.0
Nordette	Ethinyl estradiol	30	Levonorgestrel	0.15
Levlen	Ethinyl estradiot	30	Levonorgestrel	0.15
Lo/Ovral	Ethinyl estradiol	30	Norgestrel	0.3
Desogen	Ethinyl estradiol	30	Desogestrel	0.15
Ortho-Cept	Ethinyl estradiol	30	Desogestrel	0.15
Ortho-Cyclen	Ethinyl estradiol	35	Norgestimate	0.25
Biphasic Type				
Ortho-Novum 10/11				
First 10 d	Ethinyl estradiol	35	Norethindrone	0.5
Next 11 d	Ethinyl estradiol	35	Norethindrone	1.0
Jenest-28				
First 7 d	Ethinyl estradiol	35	Norethindrone	0.5
Next 14 d	Ethinyl estradiol	35	Norethindrone	1.0
Triphasic Type				
Ortho-Novum 7/7/7				
First 7 d	Ethinyl estradiol	35	Norethindrone	0.5
Second 7 d	Ethinyl estradiol	35	Norethindrone	0.75
Third 7 d	Ethinyl estradiol	35	Norethindrone	1.0
Tri-Norinyl				
First 7 d	Ethinyl estradiol	35	Norethindrone	0.5
Next 9 d	Ethinyl estradiol	35	Norethindrone	1.0
Next 5 d	Ethinyl estradiol	35	Norethindrone	0.5
Ortho Tri-Cyclen				
First 7 d	Ethinyl estradiol	35	Norgestimate	0.18
Next 7 d	Ethinyl estradiol	35	Norgestimate	0.215
Next 7 d	Ethinyl estradiol	35	Norgestimate	0.25
Tri-Levlen				
First 6 d	Ethinyl estradiol	30	Levonorgestrel	0.05
Next 5 d	Ethinyl estradiol	40	Levonorgestrel	0.075
Next 10 d	Ethinyl estradiol	30	Levonorgestrel	0.125
Triphasil				
First 6 d	Ethinyl estradiol	30	Levonorgestrel	0.05
Next 5 d	Ethinyl estradiol	40	Levonorgestrel	0.075
Next 10 d	Ethinyl estradiol	30	Levonorgestrel	0.125
Progestogen Only				
Micronor	None		Norethindrone	0.35
Nor-Q.D.	None		Norethindrone	0.35
Ovrette	None		Norgestrel	0.075

[a]Also available with iron (Loestrin 1/20 Fe, Loestrin 1.5/20 Fe).

(Reproduced, with permission, from Carr BR, Griffin JA. Fertility control and its complications. In: Wilson JD, Foster DF, eds. Williams Textbook of Endocrinology, 9th ed. Philadelphia, Pa., W. B. Saunders, 1997.)

The specific formulations of hormonal contraceptives are given in Table 36–3. Combination estrogen/progestin oral contraceptives are available with a wide range of hormone types and dosages. Several brands of oral contraceptives contain doses of estrogen and/or progestin that vary throughout the treatment cycle ("multiphasic" formulations). These products provide comparable efficacy and side effect profiles with slightly less progestin than most monophasic preparations.

Progestin-only Contraceptives. Current oral progestin-only formulations available in the United States contain either norethindrone or norgestrel (Table 36–3). These drugs have found limited acceptance due to problems with irregular vaginal bleeding and efficacy slightly less than that of combined oral contraceptives. They may be useful for lactating women or for patients intolerant of estrogen.

Noncontraceptive Benefits of Hormonal Contraceptives

Hormonal contraceptives have other salutary effects on the reproductive system besides prevention of pregnancy. In particular, oral contraceptives have been widely used therapeutically in a variety of gynecologic conditions, even though noncontraceptive uses are not specifically approved by the FDA. It has been estimated that as many as 50,000 hospital admissions are prevented annually because of the noncontraceptive benefits of these drugs.[30] While many of these health benefits were described among users of higher-dose oral contraceptives, it is likely that women taking progestin-containing agents that inhibit ovulation will derive similar advantages.[31]

Regulation of Menstrual Dysfunction. Oral contraceptives are useful for the management of irregular bleeding associated with anovulatory states such as polycystic ovary syndrome, in which unopposed estrogen exposure results in prolonged endometrial proliferation. Patients with menorrhagia not associated with a demonstrable organic cause have been shown to respond to oral contraceptive treatment with 52 percent reduction in menstrual blood loss.[32,33]

Menstrual pain is also significantly decreased in women with primary dysmenorrhea treated with oral contraceptives, and some women also report lessening in premenstrual discomfort. Because ovulation is blocked with combined oral contraceptives, periovulatory discomfort (mittelschmerz) is relieved. The effect is of considerable importance in women with coagulopathies, in which normal ovulation may result in shock from intra-abdominal bleeding.

Endometriosis. Progestins have long been used for the treatment of symptoms associated with endometriosis, either alone or combined with estrogens as part of a "pseudopregnancy" regimen. Although this approach to therapy has been superseded by the development of danazol and GnRH analogs, progestins or estrogen/progestin combinations are still useful for the long-term treatment of patients with symptomatic endometriosis who wish to preserve fertility but are not actively attempting pregnancy.

Functional Ovarian Cysts. In a study of 17,000 women enrolled in a family planning program, Vessey and colleagues[34] noted a 78 percent reduction in corpus luteum cysts and 49 percent reduction in follicular cysts among monophasic combination oral contraceptive users. While it has been suggested that multiphasic pills may not be as effective as higher-dose formulations in the prevention of cyst formation,[35] this has not been established with certainty. Oral contraceptives have been advocated to hasten the resolution of functional ovarian cysts[36]; however, the efficacy of such therapy was not confirmed in a recent randomized clinical trial, and estrogen/progestin treatment appears to have little effect on the course of such cysts once they have developed.[37]

Androgen Excess. Estrogen treatment increases hepatic synthesis of sex hormone-binding globulin (SHGB), and both estrogen and progestin limit ovarian androgen production by suppression of pituitary LH release. These effects result in decreased free (and hence biologically active) testosterone levels, which can limit symptoms such as acne or hirsutism caused by androgen excess. Patients treated with oral contraceptives specifically for this problem benefit most from pills containing at least 35 μg ethinyl estradiol and a progestin with limited androgenic activity such as norethindrone or norgestimate.

Reproductive Tract Tumors. Perhaps the most important noncontraceptive benefit of hormonal birth control is the prevention of genital tract neoplasms. Data from the Oxford Family Planning Clinic Study indicated a 30 percent decrease in the incidence of uterine leiomyomata in oral contraceptive users.[38] The risk for developing endometrial or ovarian cancer is decreased by about one half with oral contraceptive use. This protective effect seems to be more profound in nulliparas, and appears to persist long after pills are discontinued.[39,40] In the United States, about 1700 cases of ovarian cancer are averted every year by the use of oral contraceptives.[32] Current users of oral contraceptives have a 50 percent reduction in the incidence of chronic breast cysts and an 85 percent decrease in the incidence of breast fibroadenomas.[41]

Pelvic Inflammatory Disease. The risk of hospitalization for pelvic inflammatory disease (PID) is reduced by 50 percent in users of oral contraceptives.[42] The mechanism for this effect is not clear but is most likely due to progestin-induced changes in cervical mucus and decreased menstrual blood flow. Whether the effect of oral contraceptives on the incidence of PID involves only gonococcal or chlamydial infections has not been resolved.[43,44]

Other Benefits. The decreased blood flow associated with hormonal contraceptive use diminishes the risk of iron-deficiency anemia. A protective effect on the development of rheumatoid arthritis among current users of oral contraceptives was reported in 1978.[45] This effect has been confirmed in some[46,47] but not other studies.[48–50] It is possible that oral contraceptive use may prevent only the development of severe arthritic disease[51,52]; the progression of the disorder does not appear to be affected in women treated with oral contraceptives who already have developed rheumatoid arthritis.[53]

Adverse Effects of Hormonal Contraceptives

Pregnancy. Hormonal contraceptives are among the most effective methods for preventing pregnancy (Table 36–1). While the theoretical risk of pregnancy is lowest with combined oral contraceptives, long-acting injections and contraceptive implants achieve higher efficacy in actual use because compliance is assured. Progestin-only contraceptives are more effective in preventing intrauterine than ectopic pregnancies; thus, among progestin-only contraceptive failures the ratio of ectopic to intrauterine pregnancies is higher than in women who are not receiving oral contraceptives.

Early retrospective studies suggested that oral contraceptive use during pregnancy was associated with an increased risk of fetal limb reduction defects or cardio-vascular anomalies. Prospective surveys have failed to confirm these initial observations (Table 36–4); warnings about possible birth defects with oral contraceptive use in pregnancy were ordered removed from package inserts by the FDA in 1989.

Norethindrone in high doses (10 to 40 mg/day) in early pregnancy can cause labioscrotal fusion, urethral displacement, and clitoral hypertrophy in female fetuses.[54,55] Less is known about the virilization potential of other 19-nortestosterone derivatives, although similar effects could be expected at high doses. Masculinization of female fetuses has not been reported as a result of modern hormonal contraceptive use, most likely because of the small amounts of progestins in the formulations.[56]

A temporary delay in pregnancy after discontinuation of oral contraceptives has been observed; one recent study found that the chance of conception was significantly decreased for the first six cycles after pill discontinuation and that the delay in conception was longer in users of higher-dose ($\geq$50 µg) estrogen pills.[57]

Circulatory Disorders. Disorders of the cardiovascular system represent the most serious complication of hormonal contraceptive use. Early studies suggested that the incidence of myocardial infarction is increased by two to six times among users of oral contraceptives.[58,59] Concurrent cigarette smoking appears to be responsible for much of the excess risk, especially in patients older than 30 yr of age (Fig 36–4).[60,61] Recent studies in which women with known risk factors for cardiovascular disease were excluded failed to demonstrate an increased incidence of myocardial infarction with low-dose combined

TABLE 36–4. ORAL CONTRACEPTIVE EXPOSURE IN PREGNANCY AND MAJOR CONGENITAL MALFORMATIONS: PUBLISHED PROSPECTIVE STUDIES

Author(s)	Year	Exposed Cases/Total Exposed	Unexposed Cases/Total Unexposed	RR	95% Confidence Interval
Peterson	1969	1/14	15/401	1.91	0.25, 14.46
Robinson	1971	1/46	24/1204	1.09	0.15, 8.06
Haller	1974	2/50	36/1396	1.55	0.37, 6.44
Oechsli	1976	2,77	192/4334	0.59	0.15, 2.36
Royal College of General Practitioners	1976	2/102	95/4420	0.91	0.22, 3.70
Heinonen et al	1977	10/278	1383/50,004	1.30	0.70, 2.42
Rothman and Louik	1978	11/1448	31/4087	1.00	0.50, 1.99
Vessey et al	1979	1/38	19/496	0.69	0.09, 5.13
Kasan and Andrews	1980	81/2859	225/7395	0.93	0.72, 1.20
Harlap and Eldor	1980	10/122	242/2872	0.97	0.52, 1.83
Linn et al	1983	4/223	46/1654	0.64	0.23, 1.79
Harlap et al	1985	19/850	83/4904	1.32	0.80, 2.17
Typical estimated RR				0.99	0.83, 1.19

(Adapted, with permission, from Bracken MB. Oral contraception and congenital malformations in offspring: A review and meta-analysis of the prospective studies. Obstet Gynecol. 76:552, 1990.)

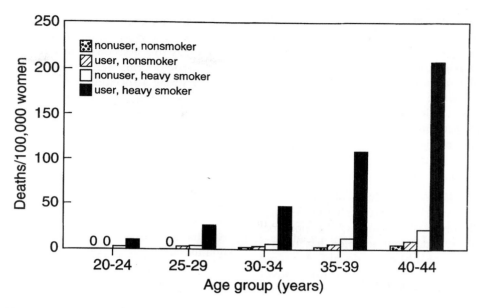

Figure 36–4. Number of deaths from cardiovascular diseases per 100,000 women by smoking status or non-use of oral contraceptives. *(Reproduced, with permission, from Kost K, et al.* Family Plan Perspect. *23:54, 1991.)*

oral contraceptive use.[62,63] Contraceptive progestins decrease in high-density lipoprotein (HDL), probably due to activation of hepatic lipase activity, and limit the estrogen-induced diminution of low-density lipoprotein (LDL). These effects are related to the androgenic activity, dose, and route of administration of progestin, with low-dose progestin-only pills and injectable progestins having little or no effect on lipoprotein levels.[64,65] Combined oral contraceptives containing desogestrel, norgestimate, or low-dose norethindrone are associated with the most favorable lipoprotein profiles[66]; whether these differences are clinically significant has not been established because most women who have sustained a myocardial infarction while on oral contraceptives do not have angiographic or postmortem evidence of coronary atherosclerosis.[67] Thus, it is likely that estrogen-induced coronary artery thrombosis or spasm rather than adverse lipoprotein changes may be responsible. Although one study has indicated a relationship between progestin dose and myocardial infarction risk,[68] it is likely that patients on higher progestin formulations were at increased risk because of more advanced age.[69]

The risk of venous thromboembolism among users of hormonal contraceptives is directly related to the estrogen dose.[69,70] This effect probably occurs by alterations in the coagulation/fibrinolysis system, but changes in venous blood flow or endothelial proliferation may also be responsible.[71] Combined oral contraceptive use in the month before surgery increases the risk of postoperative thromboembolism.[72] If feasible, oral contraceptives should be discontinued at least 4 wk before and for 2 wk after elective surgery of a type associated with an in-creased risk of thromboembolism and during periods of prolonged immobilization.

The risk of cerebrovascular events (thrombotic and hemorrhagic strokes) is increased among oral contraceptive users, although most of the excess risk is among older, hypertensive women who smoke cigarettes.[73] However, there appears to be little risk with pills containing 35 μg of ethinyl estradiol or less. Progestin-only contraceptives do not appear to increase the risk of stroke, but may play a role in its development when combined with estrogen.[72,74]

The incidence of clinically significant hypertension is slightly increased in users of oral contraceptives, with increased progestin dose and patient age being associated risk factors.[39] Interestingly, parenterally administered progestins do not appear to affect blood pressure.[74,75] Activation of the renin–angiotensin system by an increase in renin substrate (angiotensinogen) is thought to be the mechanism of blood pressure elevation seen with oral contraceptive use. This effect is reversed with the discontinuation of oral contraceptives.

Abnormal Uterine Bleeding. Irregular genital bleeding is the side effect most commonly responsible for discontinuation of hormonal contraceptives. Midcycle spotting occurs in users of low-dose oral contraceptives due to inadequate estrogen stimulation of the endometrium. This problem often resolves after the second treatment cycle, but if bleeding is particularly bothersome a pill containing more estrogen can be used or oral estrogens can be temporarily administered. Irregular bleeding is a common and frequently persistent problem among users of progestin-only formulations.

Carbohydrate Intolerance. Impaired glucose tolerance has been observed with use of combined or progestin-only oral contraceptives.[76,77] Progestins induce a decrease in insulin receptors on the cell membrane[78]; orally administered norgestrel seems to have the most pronounced effect,[79] while injectable levonorgestel and MPA induce little or no alteration in carbohydrate metabolism.[80,81] Thus, patients with diabetes who desire hormonal contraception might benefit from a parenteral formulation.

Neoplasms. Given the responsiveness of some malignancies to sex steroids and the association between reproductive status and tumor development, the potential neoplastic effect of steroidal contraception has been a continuing concern to health professionals. As noted above, current formulations of hormonal contraceptives appear to be protective against the development of endometrial and ovarian cancer. The effects on the incidence of other tumors are less certain. There is no current consensus as to whether cancers of the breast, cervix, colon, and skin are influenced by oral contraceptive use. Early studies[82,83] suggesting a protective effect of oral contraceptive use on breast cancer development have not been confirmed, and further analysis indicated that certain subgroups of women might be at increased risk. However, the findings from a number of investigations have been inconsistent and contradictory. Prospective studies, in general, have shown no change in breast cancer in women who have used oral contraceptives.[84–86] In a comprehensive survey of research dealing with breast cancer and oral contraceptives, Harlap[87] concluded that oral contraceptive use does not increase the risk of breast cancer in women over age 45. Controversy still exists as to the risk in younger women, but the lack of consistency among investigations argues against a causal relationship between oral contraceptive use and the development of breast cancer. Little can be said with confidence about the risk of breast cancer with other hormonal contraceptive formulations due to limited patient experience; although depot MPA has been shown to increase the development of breast nodules in beagle dogs, this was not confirmed in case-control studies in humans.[88]

The results of several studies have suggested an increase in the development of cervical cancer in users of oral contraceptives.[89–91] Vessey and colleagues[90] found the risk of cervical neoplasia (including dysplasia and cancer) to be about 70 percent higher among oral contraceptive users as compared to IUD users. However, potential confounding factors such as age at first intercourse, number of sexual partners, and the frequency of Pap smear screening have not been fully controlled for in these investigations. The use of control patients who employ barrier methods that prevent the transmission of papillomavirus, thought to be a precursor of cervical neoplasia, is another potential source of bias in these surveys. It is likely that hormonal contraception does not in itself induce the development of cervical neoplasia.

A strong association exists between oral contraceptive use and the development of benign heptatic adenomas. An increase in incidence of 3.3 cases per 100,000 users has been estimated, with the risk further increasing after 4 or more yr of use, especially with oral contraceptives of higher doses.[92] Data from Great Britain have indicated an increased risk of hepatocellular carcinoma with oral contraceptive use,[93,94] but a large multicenter study was unable to confirm these observations.[95] Due to the rarity of these tumors, the attributable risk (if it exists) has been estimated to be less than one case per million users.[96]

Gallbladder Disease. Early studies of oral contraceptive users reported a twofold increase in gallstones and cholecystitis.[97] More recent data indicate a minimal effect,[98,99] probably due to the low hormone doses in newer formulations. The increased risk of gallbladder disease with progestin-only formulations is not precisely known, but is probably less than that seen with combined oral contraceptive use.

Other Potential Adverse Effects. A number of minor side effects have been ascribed to oral contraceptive use, including nausea, amenorrhea, edema, facial pigmentation (chloasma), breast tenderness and enlargement, lactation, cholestatic jaundice, migraine, mental depression, and change in corneal curvature. The precise mechanism(s) of these changes has not been elucidated. Galactorrhea develops in up to 10 percent of combined oral contraceptive users,[100] and it has been suggested that combination oral contraceptives may promote the growth or development of prolactinomas; however, this was not confirmed in a multicenter case-control study.[101]

Combined oral contraceptive use in the postpartum period can decrease milk production and may affect infant growth if feedings are not supplemented,[102] but progestin-only formulations have no significant effect on lactation.[103,104] The amount transferred to infants of mothers taking currently available formulations is clinically negligible (the equivalent of about one pill for every 4 yr of full lactation).[105]

Accelerated metabolism of steroidal contraceptives has been reported with concurrent use of drugs such as rifampin or anticonvulsants that induce microsomal liver enzymes[106,107] or increase SHBG levels. Breakthrough bleeding and contraceptive failure are more likely to occur in hormonal contraceptive users who take these drugs, and it has been suggested that such patients be placed on oral contraceptives containing at least 50 µg

TABLE 36–5. POTENTIAL EFFECTS OF COMBINED ORAL CONTRACEPTIVES ON LABORATORY TEST RESULTS

Group	Specific Tests and Potential Alteration of Lab Value	
	Increased	*Decreased*
Carbohydrate	FBS and 2 hr pp	Glucose tolerance
Metabolism	Insulin level	
Hematologic/coagulation	Coagulation factor II, VII, XIII, IX, time; plasma volume, plasmin, and plasminogen; platelet count, platelet aggregation, and platelet adhesiveness; prothrombin time	Antithrombin III; erythrocyte count (total); hematocrit; prothrombin time
Lipid metabolism	Cholesterol; lipoproteins (pre-β, β, and α); phospholipids, total; total lipids; triglycerides	
Liver function/gastrointestinal tests	Alkaline phosphatase; bilirubin, SGOT, SGPT; cephalin flocculation; formiminoglutamic acid excretion after histidine (urine); γ-glutamyl *trans*-peptidase; leucine aminopeptidase; proto-porphyrin, coproporphyrin excretion (urine); uroporphyrin excretion (urine); sulfobromoph-thalein retention	Alkaline phosphatase; etiocholanolone excretion (urine); haptoglobin (serum); urobilinogen excretion (urine)
Metals	Copper and ceruloplasmin; iron, iron binding capacity, and transferrin	Magnesium; zinc
Thyroid function	Butanole extractable iodine; protein bound iodine; thyroid-binding globulin; tri-iodothyronine (serum)	Triiodothyronine resin (serum); free thyroxine
Vitamins	Vitamin A (blood and plasma)	Folate (serum); vitamin B_2 (red blood cell and urine excretion); vitamin B_6; vitamin B_{12}; vitamin C
Other hormones/enzyme measurements	Aldosterone (blood and urine); angioten-sinogen; angiotensin I and II; cortisol (blood and urine); growth hormone; prolactin; tes-tosterone (serum); total estrogens	Estradiol and estriol; FSH (urine), LH (blood and urine); gonadotropin excretion (urine); 17-hydroxycorticosteroid excretion (urine); 17-ketosteroid excretion (urine); pregnanediol excretion (urine); renin (serum); tetrahydro-cortisone
Miscellaneous laboratory	α-1 Antitrypsin; antinuclear antibody; bilirubin; complement-reactive protein; globulins a-1, a-2; lactate; lupus erythematosus cell preparation; pyruvate; sodium	Albumin; α-amino nitrogen; calcium (serum) and calcium excretion (urine); complement reactive protein; immunoglobulin A, G, and M

Adapted, with permission, from Hatcher et al, Contraceptive Technology, *16th ed. New York, N.Y., Irvington, 1994*

ethinyl estradiol to ensure contraceptive efficacy.[108–110] Disturbance of enterohepatic circulation of steroids by alteration of gut flora has been suggested as a cause for contraceptive pill failure among users of antibiotics,[111,112] but controlled trials have failed to document a consistent effect on contraceptive steroid serum levels.[113–115]

Physicians who care for patients on hormonal contraceptives should be aware of changes in clinical laboratory values induced by sex steroid use (Table 36–5).

Prescribing Hormonal Contraceptives: A Practical Approach.
The benefits of hormonal contraceptives outweigh the risks for most women. A thorough history and physical examination should be performed, and testing of cholesterol and fasting blood sugar may be appropriate, especially in older women. Contraindications for hormonal contraceptive use should be considered and periodically reviewed (Table 36–6). All patients should be

encouraged to stop smoking and achieve their ideal body weight. Many clinicians feel that the initial choice of an oral contraceptive for most women should be one containing 35 μg ethinyl estradiol or less. Patients should be reassured that mortality among healthy nonsmokers who use oral contraceptives is decreased relative to women who use no contraception (Fig 36–5). Consideration should be given to long-acting parenteral formulations in women who have difficulty complying with daily pill use. Patients with multiple sexual partners should be encouraged to use condoms to minimize the transmission of sexually transmitted diseases.

Other Contraceptive Techniques

Postcoital Contraception (Interception).
The risk of pregnancy from unprotected midcycle intercourse ranges up to 30 percent, and postcoital contraceptive or interception

TABLE 36–6. POSSIBLE CONTRAINDICATIONS TO USE OF COMBINED ORAL CONTRACEPTIVE PILLS

Absolute Contraindications
1. Thrombophlebitis or thromboembolic disorder
2. Past history of deep vein thrombophlebitis or thromboembolic disorders
3. Cerebrovascular or coronary artery disease
4. Known or suspected breast carcinoma
5. Known or suspected estrogen-dependent neoplasia
6. Pregnancy
7. Benign or malignant liver tumor
8. Known impaired liver function
9. Previous cholestasis during pregnancy or with prior pill use

Strong Relative Contraindications
10. Severe headaches, particularly vascular or migraine headaches, that start after initiation of oral contraceptives
11. Hypertension with resting diastolic BP of 140 mm Hg or greater on three or more separate visits or an accurate measurement of 110 mm Hg diastolic or more on a single visit
12. Mononucleosis, acute phase
13. Elective major surgery or major surgery requiring immobilization planned in next 4 wk
14. Long-leg cast or major injury to lower leg
15. Over 40 yr old, accompanied by a second risk factor for the development of cardiovascular disease (such as diabetes or hypertension)
16. Over 35 yr old and currently a heavy smoker (15 or more cigarettes/day)
17. Abnormal genital bleeding

Other Considerations
Diabetes, prediabetes, or a strong family history of diabetes
Sickle cell disease or sickle C disease
Active gallbladder disease
Congenital hyperbilirubinemia (Gilbert's disease)
Undiagnosed, abnormal genital bleeding
Over 50 yr old
Completion of term pregnancy within past 10 to 14 days
Weight gain of 10 lb or more while on the pill
Cardiac renal disease (or history thereof)
Conditions likely to make patient unreliable at following pill instructions (mental retardation, major psychiatric illness, alcoholism or other chemical abuse, history of repeatedly taking oral contraceptives or other medication incorrectly)
Lactation
Family history of death of a parent or sibling due to myocardial infarction before age 50; **myocardial infarction in a mother or sister is especially significant and indicates a need for lipid evaluation**
Family history of hyperlipidemia

(Adapted, with permission, from Hatcher et al, Contraceptive Technology, 16th ed. New York, N.Y., Irvington, 1994.)

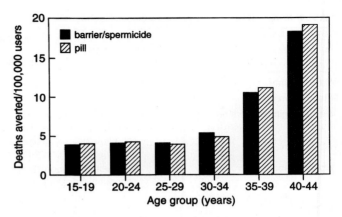

Figure 36–5. Estimated deaths averted annually per 100,000 current users of barrier and spermicide or oral contraceptives. *(Reproduced, with permission, from Kost K, et al. Family Plan Perspect. 23:54, 1991.)*

mended dosage is two tablets within 72 hr of exposure and two more tablets 12 hr later.[118] Mifepristone as a 600-mg oral dose appears to be effective as a postcoital contraceptive, but was not approved for this use in the United States as of 1996.[119]

Long-acting Contraceptive Steroids. A variety of long-acting steroid contraceptives have been developed as alternatives to oral agents. Some of these methods are being utilized extensively in developing countries. Originally, they were developed to eliminate the estrogen component of the oral contraceptives; however, agents containing only progestogen cause significant amenorrhea, breakthrough bleeding, and other deleterious side effects, as discussed earlier.

Injectable Steroids. The principal long-acting injectable contraceptives are medroxyprogesterone acetate (150 mg IM every 3 mo) and norethindrone enanthate (200 mg IM every 8 wk for 6 mo, then every 12 wk).[120] Slightly higher pregnancy rates occur with norethindrone enanthate than with medroxyprogesterone acetate, and the pregnancy rates with both treatment methods are higher shortly after the first injection. The mechanism of action of long-acting progestational agents includes inhibition of ovulation; production of a thick, unfavorable cervical mucus; induction of a decidual reaction, which results in an unfavorable endometrium; and possibly delayed ovum transport. Depot medroxyprogesterone acetate is the only injectable contraceptive approved for use in the United States. Its benefits include better compliance and reduced incidence of endometrial cancer; side effects include irregular uterine bleeding and spotting, weight gain, depression, decrease in HDL cholesterol levels, and possibly breast cancer.[121,122] A number of progestogens are being tested as long-activating injectable agents in the form of

pill is occasionally indicated,[116] for example, after rape. Historically, women have used a variety of agents to avoid pregnancy after unprotected midcycle intercourse. Modern posthormonal interception, often called the morning-after pill, involves administration of high-dose estrogens.[117] Although these agents are effective, their use is associated with nausea, vomiting, and menstrual disturbances. The use of 50 µg of ethinyl estradiol and 0.5 mg of norgesrel is equally effective and results in fewer side effects. The recom-

microspheres or microcapsules that release hormones slowly at a constant rate and are effective for 1 to 6 mo.[120] To reduce vaginal spotting and bleeding problems with pure progestogens, monthly estrogen–progestogen formulations are used in some developing countries.[120]

Implants. Subdermal implantation of polydimethysiloxone (Silastic) capsules or rods containing a variety of progestogens has been used for contraception.[120,123] Such an implant containing levonorgestrel is available in the United States. The capsules are implanted through a small incision on the forearm or inguinal or gluteal surfaces and must be removed after the steroid has been released. The levonorgestrel is released in a constant fashion, and the implant is effective for 5 yr.[120] Thus, a major advantage of this contraceptive is compliance. Although implants are effective, they require removal and are associated with breakthrough bleeding and amenorrhea similar to that seen when agents are injected. Progestogen implants may be less effective in the obese. Biodegradable implants containing progestogens that do not require removal are in the developmental phase, as are biodegradable pellets.[120]

Progesterone Antagonists. The development of a synthetic competitive progesterone antagonist, mifepristone (RU-486), has opened new approaches to fertility control. Mifepristone prevents ovulation in women, induces luteolysis and premature menstruation,[124] and is used as a postcoital contraceptive.[119] This form of medication is not associated with any major side effects and may be used in the future as a contraceptive until women reach menopause. Mifepristone has also been used to induce early abortions when combined with prostaglandins.

Hormonal Contraception in Men
The success of hormonal contraception in women has not been duplicated in men. It is apparently easier to disrupt the maturation, release, or fertilization of a single egg than to completely arrest the development of millions of sperm produced by the fertile male. A recent multicenter study by the World Health Organization found that periodic injections of testosterone enanthate (200 mg intramuscularly per week) induced azoospermia after 6 mo of treatment in only 65 percent of volunteers; however, once sperm production had been blocked the pregnancy rate with continued treatment was only 0.8/100 person-years.[125] Comparable results have been obtained with long-acting GnRH analogs combined with androgen replacement.[126] The use of long-acting androgens for male contraception may be limited by the adverse change in lipoproteins observed with these treatments.[127] Gossypol, a pigment of cottonseed, interferes with spermatogenesis without alteration of sex steroid production, but its acceptance has been limited by occasional symptomatic hypokalemia and a 10 percent chance of irreversible azoospermia.[128] A number of compounds have been identified that in experimental animals interfere with spermatogenesis, sperm maturation or transport, and accessory gland function,[129] but the utility of these agents in humans is unknown.

The Future of Hormonal Contraception
Further improvements in hormonal contraception are expected. The development of alternate delivery systems such as transdermal patches may result in improved compliance, increased contraceptive efficacy, and avoidance of harmful side effects, while circumventing problems with discontinuation of treatment found with currently available implants.[130,131] The steroid RU-486 (mifepristone) was discussed previously, but resentment against its abortifacient properties may restrict its availability in the United States.

Immunologic approaches to contraception involving administration of antibodies to the egg or its attachments,[132] spermatozoa,[133] or reproductive hormones[134,135] have been demonstrated in experimental animals. Clinical trials with a vaccine against the β-subunit of human chorionic gonadotropin have begun,[136] but the abortifacient aspect of this approach to birth control may limit its acceptance.

REFERENCES

1. Forrest JD. Has she or hasn't she? U.S. women's experience with contraception. *Fam Plann Perspect.* 19:133, 1987
2. Forrest JD, Fordyce RR. U.S. women's contraceptive attitudes and practice. How have they have changed in the 1980's? *Fam Plann Perspect.* 20:112, 1988
3. Tatum HJ, Connell-Tatum EB. Barrier contraception: A comprehensive overview. In: Wallach EE, Kempers RD, eds. *Modern Trends in Infertility and Conception Control.* Chicago, Ill., Year Book, 1982; 2: 436–447
4. Trussell J, Hatcher RA, Cates W, et al. Contraceptive failure in the United States: An update. *Stud Fam Plann.* 21:51, 1990
5. Rietmeijer CAM, Krebs JW, Feorino PM, et al. Condoms as physical and chemical barriers against human immunodeficiency virus. *JAMA.* 259:1851, 1988
6. Trussell J, Sturgen K, Strickler J, et al. Comparative efficacy of the female condom and other barrier methods. *Fam Plann Perspect.* 26:66, 1994
7. Connell EB. Barrier methods of contraception: A reappraisal. *Int J Gynaecol Obstet.* 16:479, 1979
8. Bounds W, Guillebaud J, Dominik R, Dalberth B. The diaphragm with and without spermicide: A randomized comparative efficacy trial. *J Reprod Med.* 40:11; 764, 1995
9. Shihata A, Trussell J. New female intervaginal barrier contraceptive device. *Contraception.* 44:11, 1991
10. Archer D, Muck C, Viniegra-Sibal A, Anderson FD. Lea shield: A phase I postcoital study of a new contraceptive study barrier device. *Contraception.* 52:162, 1995

11. National Research Council Institute of Medicine. In: Mastroianni L, Donaldson PJ, Kane TT, eds. *Developing New Contraceptives: Obstacles and Opportunities*. Washington, D.C., National Academy Press, 1990: 18

12. Einarson TR, Koren G, Mattice D, et al. Maternal spermicide use and adverse reproductive outcome: A meta-analysis. *Am J Obstet Gynecol.* 162:655, 1990

13. Population Reports. IUDs: A New Look. Series B, no. 5. *Intrauterine Devices*. Baltimore: The Johns Hopkins University, 1988: 1–31

14. American College of Obstetricians and Gynecologists. The intrauterine devices and pelvic inflammatory disease: An international perspective. *Lancet.* 339:785, 1992

15. Grimes DA. The intrauterine device, pelvic inflammatory disease and infertility: The confusion between hypothesis and knowledge. *Fertil Steril.* 58:670, 1992

16. Alexander NJ, Anderson DJ. Vasectomy: Consequences of autoimmunity to sperm antigens. In: Wallach EE, Kempers RD, eds. *Modern Trends in Infertility and Conception Control.* Chicago, Ill., Year Book, 1982; 2: 448–455

17. Li S, Golten M, Zhu J, Huber D. The no scalpel vasectomy. *Gen Urology.* 145:341, 1991

18. Huggins GR, Sondheimer SJ. Complications of female sterilization: Immediate and delayed. In: Wallach EE, Kempers RD, eds. *Modern Trends in Infertility and Conception Control.* Chicago, Ill., Year Book, 1982; 3: 492–510

19. Stergachis A, Kirkwood K, Shy MD, et al. Tubal sterilization and the long-term risk of hysterectomy. *JAMA.* 264:2893, 1990

20. Goldzieher JW, Rudel HW. How the oral contraceptives came to be developed. *JAMA.* 230:421, 1974

21. Pincus G, Rock J, Garcia CR. Effects of certain 19-nor steroids upon the reproductive process. *Ann NY Acad Sci.* 71:677, 1958

22. Spellacy WN, Kalra PS, Buhi WR, et al. Pituitary and ovarian responsiveness to a graded gonadotropin releasing factor stimulation test in women using a low estrogen on a regular type of oral contraceptive. *Am J Obstet Gynecol.* 137:109, 1980

23. Carr BR, Parker CR Jr, Madden JD, et al. Plasma levels of adrenocorticotropin and cortisol in women receiving oral contraceptive steroid treatment. *J Clin Endocrinol Metab.* 49:346, 1979

24. Greenwald GS. In vivo recording of intraluminal pressure changes in the rabbit oviduct. *Fertil Steril.* 14:666, 1963

25. Rowlands S, Kubba AA, Guillebaud J, Bounds W. A possible mechanism of action of danazol and an ethinyl estradiol/norgestrel combination used as postcoital contraceptive agents. *Contraception.* 33:539, 1986

26. Goldzieher JW, De La Pena A, Chenault CB, Woutersz TB. Comparative studies of the ethynyl estrogens used in oral contraceptives II. Antiovulatory potency. *Am J Obstet Gynecol.* 122:619, 1972

27. Goldzieher JW. Pharmacokinetics and metabolism of ethynyl estrogens. In: Goldzieher JW, Fotherby K, eds. *Pharmacology of the Contraceptive Steroids.* New York, N.Y., Raven Press, 1994: 127–151

28. Hatcher RA, Trussel J, Stewart F, et al. *Contraceptive Technology,* 16th ed. New York, N.Y., Irvington, 1994

29. Fotherby K. Pharmacokinetics and metabolism of progestins in humans. In : Goldzieher JW, Fotherby K, eds. *Pharmacology of the Contraceptive Steroids.* New York, N.Y., Raven Press, 1994: 99–126

30. Ory HW. The noncontraceptive health benefits from oral contraceptive use. *Fam Plann Perspect.* 14:182, 1982

31. Baird DT, Glasier AF. Hormonal contraception. *N Engl J Med.* 328:1543, 1993

32. Speroff L, Darney PD. *A Clinical Guide for Contraception.* Baltimore, Md., Williams and Wilkins, 1992: 1–50

33. Nilsson L, Rybo G. Treatment of menorrhagia. *Am J Obstet Gynecol.* 110:713, 1971

34. Vessey M, Metcalfe A, Wells C, et al. Ovarian neoplasms, functional ovarian cysts, and oral contraceptives. *Br Med J.* 294:1518, 1987

35. Cailloutte JC, Koehler AL. Phasic contraceptive pill and functional ovarian cysts. *Am J Obstet Gynecol.* 156:1538, 1987

36. Spanos WJ. Preoperative hormonal therapy of cystic adnexal masses. *Am J Obstet Gynecol.* 116:551, 1973

37. Stenikampf MP, Hammond KR, Blackwell RE. Hormonal treatment of functional ovarian cysts: A randomized, prospective study. *Fertil Steril.* 54:775, 1990

38. Vessey MP, McPherson K, Johnson B. Mortality among women participating in the Oxford/Family Planning Association Contraceptive Study. *Lancet.* 2:731, 1977

39. Cancer and Steroid Hormone Study of the Centers for Disease Control and the National Institute of Child Health and Human Development. Combined oral contraceptive use and the risk of endometrial cancer. *JAMA.* 257:796, 1987

40. Rossenberg L, Shapiro S, Slone D, et al. Epithelial ovarian cancer and combination oral contraceptives. *JAMA.* 274:3210, 1982

41. Brinton LA, Vessey MP, Flavel R, et al. Risk factors for benign breast disease. *Am J Epidemiol.* 113:203, 1981

42. Grimes DA, Cates W Jr. Family planning and sexually transmitted diseases. In: Holmes KK, Mardh P-A, Sparling PF, et al, eds. *Sexually Transmitted Diseases,* 2nd ed. New York, N.Y., McGraw-Hill, 1990

43. Wolner-Hanssen P, Svensson L, Mardh PA, et al. Laparoscopic findings and contraceptive use in women with signs and symptoms suggestive of acute salpingitis. *Obstet Gynecol.* 66:233, 1985

44. Wolner-Hanssen P, Eschenbach DA, Paavonen J, et al. Decreased risk of symptomatic chlamydial pelvic inflammatory disease associated with oral contraceptive use. *JAMA.* 263:54, 1990

45. Royal College of General Practitioners Oral Contraceptive Study. Reduction of incidence of rheumatoid arthritis associated with oral contraceptives. *Lancet.* 1:569, 1978

46. Hazes JM, Dijkmans BC, Vandenbroucke JP, et al. Reduction of the risk of rheumatoid arthritis among women who take oral contraceptives. *Arthritis Rheum.* 33:173, 1990

47. Spector TD, Roman E, Silman AJ. The pill, parity, and rheumatoid arthritis. *Arthritis Rheum.* 33:782, 1990

48. Del Junco DJ, Annegers JF, Luthra HS, et al. Do oral contraceptives prevent rheumatoid arthritis? *JAMA*. 254:1938, 1985

49. Vessey MP, Villarld-Mackintosh L, Yeates D. Oral contraceptives, cigarette smoking and other factors in relation to arthritis. *Contraception*. 35:457, 1987

50. Moskowitz MA, Jick SS, Burnside S, et al. The relationship of oral contraceptive use to rheumatoid arthritis. *Epidemiology*. 1:153, 1990

51. Van Zeben D, Hazes JM, Vandenbroucke JP, et al. Diminished incidence of severe rheumatoid arthritis associated with oral contraceptive use. *Arthritis Rheum*. 33:1462, 1990

52. Spector TD, Hochberg MC. The protective effect of the oral contraceptive pill on rheumatoid arthritis: An overview of the analytic epidemiological studies using meta-analysis. *J Clin Epidemiol*. 43:1221, 1990

53. Hazes JM, Dijkmans BA, Vandenbroucke JP, Cats A. Oral contraceptive treatment for rheumatoid arthritis: An open study in 10 female patients. *Br J Rheumatol*. 28(suppl. 1):28, 1989

54. Jacobson BD. Hazards of norethindrone therapy during pregnancy. *Am J Obstet Gynecol*. 84:962, 1962

55. Wilkins L. Masculinization of female fetuses due to use of orally given progestins. *JAMA*. 172:1028, 1960

56. Carson SA, Simpson JL. Virilization of female fetuses following maternal ingestion for progestational and androgenic steroids. In: Mahesh VB, Greenblatt RB, eds. *Hirsutism and Virilism*. Boston, Mass., John Wright-PSG, 1983: 177–188

57. Bracken MB, Hellenbrand KG, Holford TR. Conception delay after oral contraceptive use: The effect of estrogen dose. *Fertil Steril*. 53:21, 1990

58. Mann JI, Inman WH. Oral contraceptives and death from myocardial infarction. *Br Med J*. 2:245, 1975

59. Royal College of General Practitioners' Oral Contraception Study. Further analysis of mortality in oral contraceptive users. *Lancet*. 1:541, 1981

60. Goldbaum GM, Kendrick FS, Hogelin GC, Gentry EM. The relative impact of smoking and oral contraceptive use on women in the United States. *JAMA*. 258: 1339, 1987

61. Kost K, Forrest JD, Harlap S. Comparing the health risks and benefits of contraceptive choices. *Fam Plann Perspect*. 23:54, 1991

62. Porter JB, Jick H, Walker AM. Mortality among oral contraceptive users. *Obstet Gynecol*. 70:29, 1987

63. Hirronen E, Heikkila-Idanpen J. Cardiovascular death among women under 40 years of age using low-estrogen oral contraceptives and intrauterine devices in Finland from 1975 to 1984. *Am J Obstet Gynecol*. 163:281, 1990

64. Godsland IF, Crook D, Simpson R, et al. The effects of different formulations of oral contraceptive agents on lipid and carbohydrate metabolism. *N Engl J Med*. 323: 1375, 1990

65. Holma P, Robertson DN. Cholesterol and HDL-cholesterol values in women during use of subdermal implants releasing levonorgestrel. *Contraception*. 32:163, 1985

66. Speroff L, DeCherney A. Evaluation of a new generation of oral contraceptives. The advisory board for the new progestins. *Obstet Gynecol*. 81:1034, 1993

67. Engel HJ, Engel E, Lichtlen PR. Coronary atherosclerosis and myocardial infarction in young women—Role of oral contraceptives. *Eur Heart J*. 4:1, 1983

68. Meade TW, Greenberg G, Thompson SG. Progestogens and cardiovascular reactions associated with oral contraceptives and a comparison of the safety of 50- and 30-μg oestrogen preparations. *Br Med J*. 280:1157, 1980

69. Thorneycroft IH. Oral contraceptives and myocardial infarction. *Am J Obstet Gynecol*. 163:1393, 1990

70. Meade TW, Greenberg G, Thompson SC. Progestogens and cardiovascular reactions associated with oral contraceptives and a comparison of the safety of 50- and 30-mcg oestrogen preparations. *Br Med J*. 280: 1157, 1980

71. Stadel BV. Oral contraceptives and cardiovascular disease (first of two parts). *N Engl J Med*. 305:612, 1981

72. Vessey MP, Doll R, Fairbairn AS, Glober G. Postoperative thromboembolism and the use of oral contraceptives. *Br Med J*. 3:123, 1970

73. Collaborative Group for the Study of Stroke in Young Women. Oral contraceptives and stroke in young women: Associated risk factors. *JAMA*. 231:718, 1975

74. Ginsburg KA, Moghissi KS. Alternate delivery systems for contraceptive progestogens. *Fertil Steril*. 49:16S, 1988

75. Black HR, Leppert P, DeCherney A. The effect of medroxyprogesterone acetate on blood pressure. *Int J Gynaecol Obstet*. 17:83, 1979

76. Spellacy WN, McLeod AGW, Buhi WC, et al. Medroxyprogesterone acetate and carbohydrate metabolism: Measurement of glucose, insulin, and growth hormone during 6 months' time. *Fertil Steril*. 21:457, 1970

77. Spellacy WN, Buhi WC, Birk SA, McCreary SA. Metabolic studies in women taking norethindrone for 6 months' time (measurement of blood glucose, insulin, triglyceride concentrations). *Fertil Steril*. 24:419, 1973

78. Depirro R, Forte F, Bertoli A, et al. Changes in insulin receptors during oral contraception. *J Clin Endcrinol Metab*. 52:29, 1981

79. Spellacy WN, Buhi WC, Birk SA. Prospective studies of carbohydrate metabolism in "normal" women using norgestrel for eighteen months. *Fertil Steril*. 35:167, 1981

80. Singh K, Viegas OA, Ratnam SS. A three-year evaluation of metabolic changes in Singaporean Norplant-2 rod acceptors. *Adv Contracept*. 6:71, 1990

81. Liew DF, Ng CS, Young YM, Ratnam SS. Long-term effects of Depo-Provera on carbohydrate and lipid metabolism. *Contraception*. 31:51, 1985

82. Sartrwell PE, Arthea FG, Tonascia JA. Exogenous hormones, reproductive history and breast cancer. *J. Natl Cancer Inst*. 59:1589, 1979

83. Ravnihar B, Seigel DB, Lindtner J. An epidemiologic study of breast cancer and benign breast neoplasias in relation to the oral contraceptive and estrogen use. *Int J Cancer*. 15:395, 1979

84. Lipnick RJ, Buring JE, Hennekens CH, et al. Oral contraceptives and breast cancer: A prospective cohort study. *JAMA*. 255:58, 1986

85. Kay CR, Hannaford PC. Breast cancer and the pill: A further report from the Royal College of General Practitioners Oral Contraception Study. *Br J Cancer.* 58:675, 1988

86. Vessey MP, McPherson K, Villard-Mackintosh L, et al. Oral contraceptives and breast cancer: Latest findings in a large cohort study. *Br J Cancer.* 59:613, 1989

87. Harlap S. Oral contraceptives and breast cancer—Cause and effect? *J Reprod Med.* 36:374, 1991

88. World Health Organization. Depot-medroxyprogesterone acetate (DMPA) and cancer: Memorandum from a WHO meeting. *Bull WHO.* 64:375, 1986

89. Ory H, Naib Z, Conger SB, et al. Contraceptive choice and prevalence of cervical dysplasia and carcinoma in situ. *Am J Obstet Gynecol.* 124:573, 1976

90. Vessey MP, Lawless M, McPherson K, Yeates D. Neoplasia of the cervix uteri and contraception: A possible adverse effect of the pill. *Lancet.* 2:930, 1983

91. WHO Collaborative Study of Neoplasia and Steroid Contraceptives. Invasive cervical cancer and combined oral contraceptives. *Br Med J.* 290:961, 1985

92. Rooks JB, Ory HW, Ishak KG, et al. Epidemiology of hepatocellular adenoma: The role of oral contraceptive use. *JAMA.* 242:644, 1979

93. Henderson BE, Preston-Martin S, Edmondson HA, et al. Hepatocellular carcinoma and oral contraceptives. *Br J Cancer.* 48:437, 1983

94. Forman D, Vincent TJ, Doll R. Cancer of the liver and oral contraceptives. *Br J Med.* 292:1357, 1986

95. World Health Organization. Combined oral contraceptives and liver cancer. *Int J Cancer.* 43:254, 1989

96. *Physicians' Desk Reference.* Oradell, N.J., Medical Economics Data, 1991: 1601

97. Boston Collaborative Drug Surveillance Program. Oral contraceptives and venous thromboembolic disease, surgically confirmed gall-bladder disease, and breast tumours. *Lancet.* 1:1399, 1973

98. Layde PM, Vessey MP, Yeates D. Risk of gallbladder disease: A cohort study of young women attending family planning clinics. *J Epidemiol Community Health.* 36:274, 1982

99. Storm BL, Tamragouri RT, Morse ML, et al. Oral contraceptives and other risk factors for gallbladder disease. *Clin Pharmacol Ther.* 39:335, 1986

100. Holtz G. Galactorrhea in oral contraceptive users. *J Reprod Med.* 27:210, 1982

101. Pituitary Adenoma Study Group. Pituitary adenomas and oral contraceptives: A multicenter case-control study. *Fertil Steril.* 39:753, 1983

102. Croxatto HLB, Diaz S, Peralta O, et al. Fertility regulation in nursing women: IV long term influence of a low dose combined oral contraceptive initiated at day 30 postpartum upon lactation and infant growth. *Contraception.* 27:13, 1983

103. Tankeyoon M, Dusitsinn N, Chalapatis S, et al. Effects of hormonal contraceptives on milk volume and infant growth. *Contraception.* 30:505, 1984

104. Koetsawang S. The effects of contraceptive methods on the quality and quantity of breast milk. *Int J Gynaecol Obstet.* 258:115, 1987

105. Labbok MH. Consequences of breastfeeding for mother and child. *J Biosoc Sci.* 9(suppl.):43, 1985

106. Conney AH. Pharmacological implications of microsomal enzyme induction. *Pharmacol Rev.* 19:317, 1967

107. Guengerich FP. Oxidation of 27-alpha-ethinyl estradiol by human liver cytochrome P-450. *Mol Pharmacol.* 33:500, 1988

108. Back DJ, Bates M, Bowden A, et al. The interaction of phenobarbital and other anticonvulsants with oral contraceptive steroid therapy. *Contraception.* 22:495, 1980

109. Diamond MP, Green JW, Thompson JM, et al. Interaction of anticonvulsants and oral contraceptives in epileptic adolescents. *Contraception.* 31:623, 1985

110. Haukkamaa M. Contraception by Norplant subdermal capsules is not reliable in epileptic patients on anticonvulsant treatment. *Contraception.* 33:559, 1986

111. Silber TJ. Apparent oral contraceptive failure associated with antibiotic administration. *J Adolesc Health Care.* 4:287, 1983

112. Barnett ML. Inhibition of oral contraceptive effectiveness by concurrent antibiotic administration. *J Periodontol.* 56:18, 1985

113. Back DJ, Breackenridge AM, MacIver M, et al. The effects of ampicillin on oral contraceptive steroids in women. *Br J Clin Pharmacol.* 14:43, 1982

114. Friedman CI, Humeke AL, Kim MH, Powell J. The effect of ampicillin on oral contraceptive effectiveness. *Obstet Gynecol.* 55:33, 1980

115. Neely JL, Abate M, Swinder M, D'Angio R. The effect of doxycycline on serum levels of ethinyl estradiol, norethindrone, and endogenous progesterone. *Obstet Gynecol.* 77:416, 1991

116. Glasier A, Baird DT. Postovulatory contraception. *Baillieres Clin Obstet Gynecol.* 4:283, 1990

117. Silvestre L, Bouali Y, Ulmann A. Postcoital contraception: Myth or reality? *Lancet.* 338:39, 1991

118. Yuzpe AA, Smith RP, Rademaker AW. A multicenter clinical investigation employing ethinyl estradiol combined with DL-norgestrel as a postcoital contraceptive agent. *Fertil Steril.* 37:508, 1982

119. Glasier A, Thong KJ, Dewar M, et al. Mifepristone (RU 486) compared with high-dose estrogen and progestogen for emergency postcoital contraception. *N Eng J Med.* 327:1041, 1992

120. Population Reports. *Hormonal Contraception: New Long-Acting Methods.* Series K, no. 3. *Injectables and Implants.* Baltimore, Md., The Johns Hopkins University, K57-K87, 1987

121. Garza-Flores J, De la Cruz DL, Valles de Bourges V, et al. Long term effects of depot-medroxyprogesterone acetate on lipoprotein metabolism. *Contraception.* 44:61, 1991

122. Skegg DCG, Noonan EA, Paul C. Depot medroxyprogesterone acetate and breast cancer. *JAMA.* 273:799, 1995

123. Segal SJ. Contraceptive implants. In: Mishell DR, ed. *Advances in Infertility Research.* New York, N.Y., Raven, 1982; 2: 117–127

124. Bauleiu EE. RU-486 as an antiprogesterone steroid. *JAMA.* 262:1808, 1989

125. World Health Organization Task Force on Methods for the Regulation of Male Fertility. Contraceptive efficacy of testosterone-induced azoospermia in normal regulation of male fertility. *Lancet*. 336:955, 1990

126. Swerdloff RS, Steiner BS, Bhasin S. Gonadotropin releasing hormone (GnRH) agonists in male contraception. *Med Biol*. 63:218, 1986

127. Wallace EM, Wu FC. Effect of depot medroxyprogesterone acetate and testosterone oenanthate on serum lipoproteins in man. *Contraception*. 41:63, 1990

128. Wooley RJ. Contraception—A look forward, part II: Mifepristone and gossypol. *J Am Board Family Pract*. 4:103, 1991

129. Zaneveld LJ, Waller DP. Nonhormonal mediation of male reproductive tract damage: Data from contraceptive drug research. *Prog Clin Biol Res*. 302:129, 1989

130. Catz P, Friend DR. In vitro evaluations of transdermal levonorgestrel. *Drug Des Deliv*. 6:49, 1990

131. Friend DR. Transdermal delivery of contraceptives. *Crit Rev Ther Drug Carrier Syst*. 7:149, 1990

132. Tesarik J, Testart J, Leca G, Nome F. Reversible inhibition of fertility in mice by passive immunization with anticumulus oophorus antibodies. *Biol Reprod*. 43:385, 1990

133. Primakoff P, Lathrop W, Woolman L, et al. Fully effective contraception in male and female guinea pigs immunized with sperm protein PH-20. *Nature*. 335:543, 1988

134. Roberts AJ, Reeves JJ. Reproductive and endocrine changes in ewes actively immunized against luteinizing hormone. *J Reprod Immunol*. 16:187, 1989

135. Ladd A, Tsong YY, Prabhu G, Thau R. Effects of long-term immunization against LHRH and androgen treatment on gonadal function. *J Reprod lmmunol*. 15:85, 1989

136. Talwar GP, Hingorani V, Kumar S, et al. Phase I clinical trials with three formulations of anti-human chorionic gonadotropin vaccine. *Contraception*. 41:301, 1990

Chapter 37

PHYSIOLOGY OF THE CLIMACTERIC

Brian W. Walsh and Isaac Schiff

Menopause denotes the permanent cessation of menses. This is but one aspect of the climacteric, during which time women undergo endocrine, somatic, and psychological changes. These changes are related both to aging and to estrogen depletion; it is not possible to quantify the respective effects of each. This chapter addresses the consequences of declining estrogen production in postmenopausal women; the development of conditions that are troublesome (hot flashes and urogenital atrophy) and those that have serious morbidity and mortality (atherosclerosis and oesteoporosis).

AGING OF THE OVARY

The mean age of women at menopause is 51 yr,[1] with approximately 4 percent of women undergoing a natural menopause prior to age 40 (Fig 37–1). Menopause is not delayed by prolonged periods of hypothalamic amenorrhea, multiple pregnancies, or oral contraceptive use. Because the average age at menopause has not changed since antiquity,[2] increases in life expectancy mean that American women today will spend one third of their lifetime after ovarian failure.

The aging process of the ovary appears to begin during fetal development. Although 7 million oogonia are present at 20 wk gestation, only 700,000 remain at birth.[3] Following birth, the number of oocytes continues to decline even before the onset of puberty (Fig 37–2). After puberty, many oocytes are lost each month, with typically only one oocyte undergoing ovulation out of an entire cohort recruited.

For several years prior to menopause, estradiol and progesterone production decline despite the occurrence of ovulatory cycles.[4] This waning of ovarian estradiol and inhibin secretion reduces the negative feedback inhibition on the hypothalamic–pituitary system, resulting in a gradual rise in follicle-stimulating hormone (FSH). The remaining ovarian follicles are increasingly less responsive to FSH: Menopause occurs when the residual follicles are refractory to elevated concentrations of FSH. FSH thus reflects the biologic age of the ovary. Indeed, women who have regular menses but also have elevated FSH levels have poor outcome from in vitro fertilization, presumably because their oocytes are senescent.[5]

Postmenopausal women do have some circulating estrogen despite the fact that estrogen production by the postmenopausal ovary is minimal (Fig 37–3). The major source of postmenopausal estrogens is adrenal androgens, particularly androstenedione, which undergoes aromatization by peripheral tissues to estrone. On average, 2.8 percent of androstenedione is converted to estrone, but higher rates are seen in obese women, who have more adipose tissue to aromatize androgens.[6] This explains in part why obese women have fewer menopausal symptoms in comparison to thin women.[7] Because the major source of postmenopausal estrogens is peripheral aromatization of androstenedione, the mean postmenopausal concentration of estrone, 35 pg/ml, exceeds the mean concentration of estradiol, 13 pg/ml.[8] This estradiol is not secreted by the ovary: It is produced by peripheral conversion from estrone.

Although the postmenopausal ovary no longer ovulates, it continues to produce testosterone and androstenedione, primarily from stromal and hilar cells (Fig 37–4). The mean concentration of testosterone in postmenopausal women (approximately 250 pg/ml) is minimally lower than that seen in premenopausal women. In contrast, the mean postmenopausal concentration of androstenedione, 850 pg/ml, is less than that of premenopausal women, 1500 pg/ml.[8] This reflects diminishing adrenal production of androstenedione by the aging adrenal gland. Because these postmenopausal androgens are no longer opposed by estrogens, they may lead to increased hair growth on the upper lip and chin.

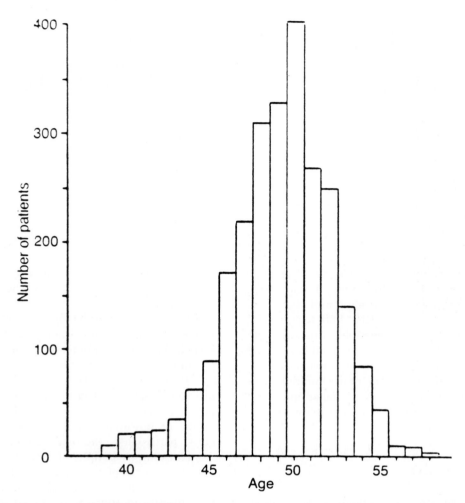

Figure 37–1. Age of menopause in 2000 women during a natural menopause. *(Reproduced, with permission, from Gambrell RD, Jr. The menopause: Benefits and risks of estrogen–progesterone replacement therapy.* Fertil Steril. *37:457, 1982.)*

VASOMOTOR FLUSHES

One of the most frequent and troublesome symptoms for women at the climacteric are vasomotor flushes: More than 80 percent of women will note hot flashes within 3 mo of a natural or surgical menopause. Of those women, 85 percent will have them for more than 1 yr and 25 to 50 percent for up to 5 yr.[9] Hot flashes will lessen in frequency and intensity with advancing age, unlike other sequelae of the menopause, which progress with time.

Definitions and Pathophysiology

A hot flash is the subjective sensation of intense warmth of the upper body, which typically lasts for 4 min but may range in duration from 30 sec to 5 min.[10] This may follow a prodrome of palpitations or headache and is frequently accompanied by weakness, faintness, or vertigo. This episode usually ends in profuse sweating and a cold sensation.

When hot flashes occur at night, they may awaken patients from sleep. This was shown by simultaneously recording finger temperature and skin resistance as objective indices of vasomotor flushes, while monitoring the stages of sleep using a sleep polygraph (electroencephalogram, electromyelogram, and electrooculogram)[11] (Fig 37–5). The waking episodes were indeed highly correlated with the occurrence of hot flashes. The resultant poor quality of sleep results in fatigue, which may then lead to such symptoms as irritability, poor concentration, and impaired memory.

A vasomotor flush is the objective component of this phenomenon, characterized by a visible ascending flush of the thorax, neck, and face. The first event is an increase in peripheral blood flow, particularly to the fingers. This increase in blood flow is limited to the skin and does not involve blood flow to muscle; for this reason, blood pressure does not decline during a flush. However, the cutaneous vasodilatation does cause core temperature to fall.[12] The

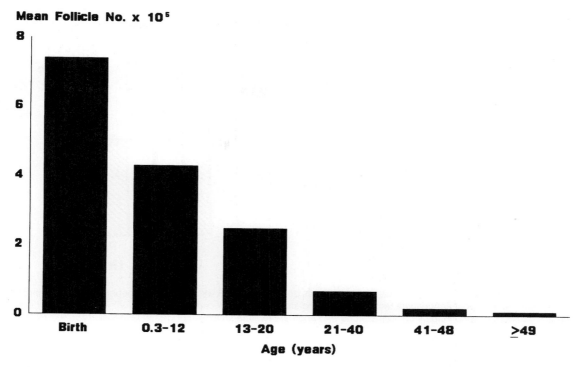

Figure 37–2. Number of primordial oocytes in women throughout the life cycle. *(Reproduced, with permission, from Nicosia SV. Morphological changes of the human ovary throughout life. In: Serra GB, ed.* The Ovary. *New York, N.Y., Raven Press, 1983:*

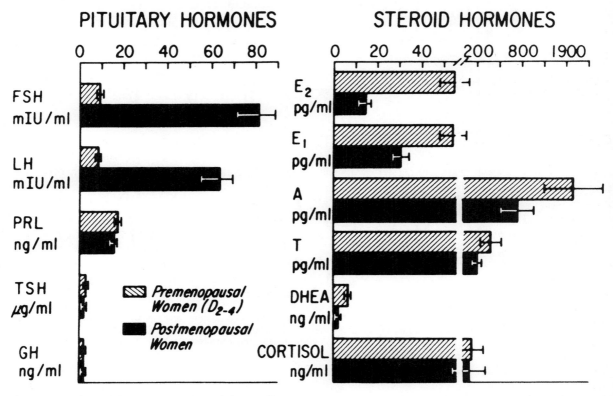

Figure 37–3. Circulating concentrations of pituitary and steroid hormones in premenopausal (menstrual cycle days 2 to 4) and postmenopausal women. *(Reproduced, with permission, from Yen SSC. The biology of menopause.* J Reprod Med. *18:28,*

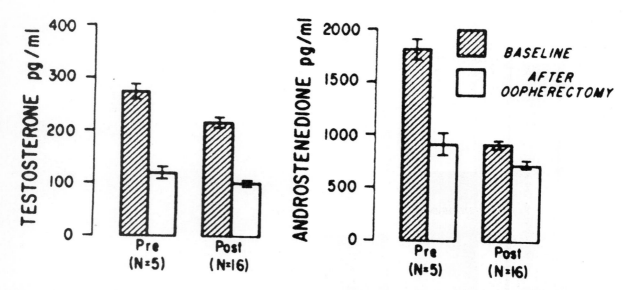

Figure 37–4. Serum testosterone and androstenedione levels before and 6 to 8 wk after bilateral oophorectomy. Five pre-menopausal (pre) and 16 postmenopausal (post) women were studied. *(Reproduced, with permission, from Judd HL, Lucas WE, Yen SSC. Effect of oophorectomy on testosterone and androstenedione levels.* Am J Obstet Gynecol. *118:793, 1974.)*

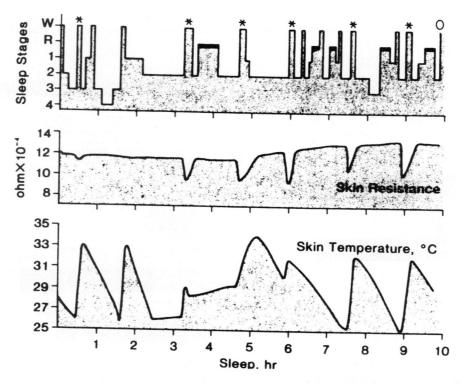

Figure 37–5. Sleepgram and recordings of skin resistance and temperature in a postmenopausal subject with severe hot flashes. Asterisks denote objectively measured hot flashes. *(Reproduced, with permission, from Erlik Y, Tataryn IV, Meldrum DR, et al. Association of waking episodes with menopausal hot flushes.* JAMA. *245:1741, 1981.)*

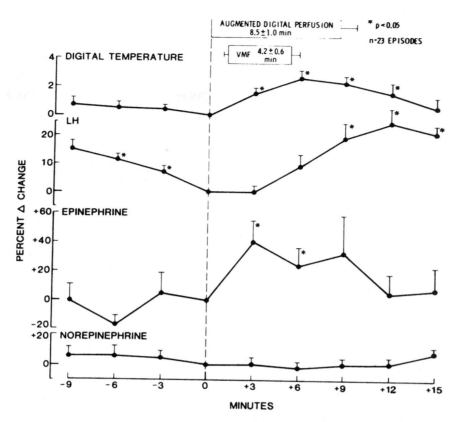

Figure 37–6. Composite graph of objective parameters obtained in five symptomatic postmenopausal women. Data are normalized to the beginning of augmented digital perfusion (0 time). *(Reproduced, with permission, from Mashchak CA, Kletsky OA, Artal R, et al. The relation of physiological changes to subjective symptoms in postmenopausal women with and without hot flushes. Maturitas. 6:301, 1985.)*

subjective sensation of the hot flash follows the increase in blood flow by 1¹/₂ min. Skin temperature reaches its maximum approximately 5 min later (Fig 37–6). A rise in plasma luteinizing hormone (LH) is the final event, reaching its peak 12 min after increased skin perfusion begins. Vasomotor flushes thus appear to result from a sudden lowering of the hypothalamic thermoregulatory set point; core temperature is reduced by activating cutaneous vasodilatation, which causes increased cutaneous blood flow and, consequently, heat loss.

Etiology

Hot flashes result from a sudden reduction of estrogen levels rather than from hypoestrogenism per se. They are therefore associated with menopause, whether it be natural, surgical, or "medical" (ie, hypoestrogenism induced by the use of long-acting gonadotropin-releasing hormone agonists or by danazol). The discontinuation of exogenous estrogens may also precipitate flushes: Women with Turner syndrome, who are hypoestrogenic, do not have hot flashes unless exogenous estrogens have been prescribed and are later withdrawn.[13]

Men also may have hot flashes, but as a consequence of testosterone withdrawal. In fact, 73 percent of men following orchiectomy for prostatic cancer will have flashes.[14] Treatment with estrogens will provide relief, but they may return if estrogen treatment is discontinued.[15] Androgens per se, independent of conversion to estrogen, suppress hot flashes because the use of a nonaromatizable androgen, fluoxymesterone, was as active as methyltestosterone in relieving flashes in a male with testosterone insufficiency.[16]

Obese women tend to be less troubled by hot flashes: Erlik et al found asymptomatic women to weigh considerably more than severely symptomatic ones, even when matched for age, ovarian status, and years since menopause.[7] Obese women are relatively "protected" from hot flashes as they are relatively less hypoestrogenic, for two reasons: (1) Their increased adiposity allows for greater peripheral conversion of adrenal androgens into estrogens[6]; and (2) their sex hormone-binding globulin levels are typically lower[17] and so a greater proportion of their estrogens are unbound and are free to act on target tissues (Fig 37–7).

At one time, LH was thought to play a role in the initiation of vasomotor flushes because LH pulses were coincident with vasomotor flushes. This hypothesis was disproven when the use of exogenous LH (as in human

CONTROL SUBJECTS

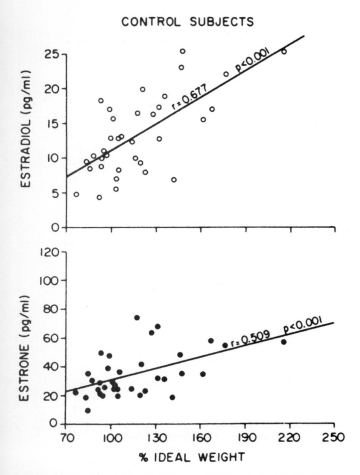

Figure 37–7. Correlation of plasma estradiol and estrone levels with percentage of ideal weight in postmenopausal women. *(Reproduced, with permission, from Judd HL, Davidson BJ, Frumar AM, et al. Serum androgens and estrogens in post-menopausal women. Am J Obstet Gynecol. 136:859, 1980.)*

menopausal gonadotropins) was not found to cause flashes. Careful analysis of the chronology of hot flashes subsequently identified the LH peak to be a late component (see above). Moreover, vasomotor flushes do not require an intact pituitary: A total hypophysectomy will not prevent their occurrence.[18] Vasomotor flushes therefore appear to be caused by an acute lowering of the hypothalamic thermoregulatory set point, precipitated by estrogen withdrawal. The associated LH peaks merely result from stimulation of adjacent hypothalamic centers controlling LH release.

The presence of estrogen may serve to "stabilize" the thermoregulatory center by maintaining hypothalamic opioid activity. The loss of estrogen at menopause may cause a hypothalamic "opioid withdrawal," leading to thermoregulatory instability. This hypothesis is supported by the observation that estrogen prescribed in physiologic quantities induces hypothalamic opioid activity.[19]

Estrogen's effect on the hypothalamic thermoregulatory center may also be mediated by neurotransmitters, such as norepinephrine (NE). As shown in Figure 37–8,[20] the intraneuronal level of NE is regulated by the balance between the enzymes tyrosine hydroxylase (the rate-limiting step of NE synthesis from tyrosine) and monoamine oxidase (which irreversibly degrades NE to inactive metabolites). After synthesis, NE is stored in prejunctional vesicles. When released into the synaptic cleft, NE binds to postjunctional receptors to propagate a response, either excitatory or inhibitory. This action is terminated by the rapid reuptake of NE back into the postjunctional neuron.

In animals, estrogen has been found to have multiple effects on NE neurons. Estrogen stimulates tyrosine hydroxylase activity,[21] thereby increasing NE synthesis. In addition, estrogen reduces monoamine oxidase activity[22] and so retards NE degradation. Both of these actions will increase the intraneuronal level of NE. Estrogen has also been shown to augment NE release[23] and inhibit NE reuptake,[24] thereby potentiating its effect on postjunctional receptors. Last, estrogen also appears to increase the number of hypothalamic α_2-postsynaptic receptors.[25] All of these actions serve to enhance α_2-adrenergic activity. Because this work has been performed in animals, it is not definitively known if estrogen has the same effects in humans. Nevertheless, these findings do suggest that estrogens enhance α_2-adrenergic activity and that estrogen withdrawal may lead to vasomotor flushes due to reduced α_2-adrenergic activity.

This hypothesis is supported by the finding that α_2-agonists, such as clonidine,[26] aldomet (after conversion to its active form, methylnorepinephrine),[27] and lofexidine,[28] have all been shown to reduce hot flashes. This also would explain why estrogen replacement does not produce immediate relief of flashes but requires 2 to 4 wk for its maximal effect[29]; altering central NE metabolism would not be expected to be an instantaneous process. Furthermore, this alteration of NE metabolism would be expected to persist for a short time after estrogen withdrawal, explaining why hot flash relief continues after estrogens are discontinued.

Diagnosis

A careful history and physical examination should be sufficient to make the diagnosis and exclude other conditions such as thyrotoxicosis, carcinoid tumor, pheochromocytoma, anxiety, diabetic insulin reaction, alcohol withdrawal, and diencephalic epilepsy. Menopause may be confirmed, if necessary, by demonstrating an elevated serum FSH. However, the finding of a low serum estradiol level is not diagnostic of menopause because premenopausal women frequently have low levels at the time of their menses.

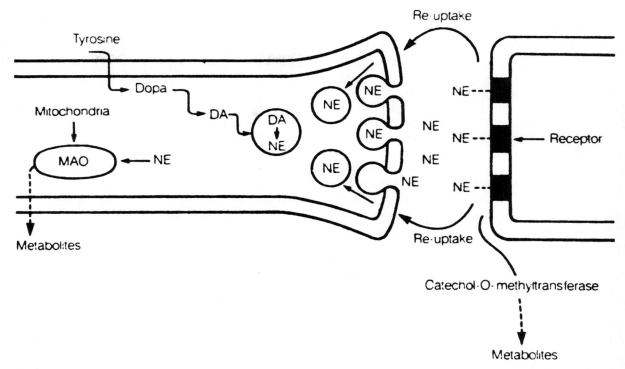

Figure 37–8. Schematic representation of an adrenergic junction. Tyrosine is converted by the enzyme tyrosine hydroxylase to 3,4-dihydroxyphenylalanine (DOPA), decarboxylated to dopamine (DA), hydroxylated to form norepinephrine (NE), and stored in vesicles. Upon release, NE interacts with adrenergic receptors. This action is terminated by reuptake of NE back into the prejunctional neurons. NE is degraded into inactive metabolites by monoamine oxidase (MAO) and catechol-*O*-methyl transferase. (*Reproduced, with permission, from Berkow R, ed.* The Merck Manual of Diagnosis and Therapy. *Rathway, N.J., Merck Sharp & Dohme Research Laboratories, 1987, p. 2472.*)

COGNITIVE FUNCTIONING

Estrogen may favorably affect cognitive functioning in women. First, estrogen promotes the growth of cholinergic neurons, increasing the levels of acetylcholine, a neurotransmitter that may facilitate memory.[30] Second, animal studies indicate that estrogens increase the number of neural synapses in the hippocampus; the hippocampus is believed to play an important role in memory and learning. Gould et al found that the castration of female rats was followed by a decrease in the number of dendritic spines of hippocampal pyramidal cells.[31] This decrease was prevented by administering estradiol.

Whether postmenopausal estrogen use prevents against the development of Alzheimer's disease is presently uncertain. One case-control study found that women with Alzheimer's disease were less likely to have been estrogen users, compared to control women.[32] Two cohort studies prospectively followed healthy postmenopausal women for several years. The Leisure World Study found that the risk of Alzheimer's disease was lower in estrogen users; the relative risk was 0.69 (confidence interval, 0.46 to 1.03), and was proportional to both the dose and duration of estrogen use.[33] A second cohort study found the relative risk of Alzheimer's disease among estrogen users to be 0.40 (CI, 0.22 to 0.85).[34] It is important to note that these were not randomized clinical trials; the possibility exists that women who select estrogen treatment may be less predisposed to develop this condition. To determine if estrogen prevents Alzheimer's disease, randomized, placebo-controlled, double-blind studies are needed.

OSTEOPOROSIS

Definition/Etiology

Osteoporosis is the progressive reduction in bone mass without qualitative abnormalities. It affects trabecular bone earlier than cortical bone, and its major consequence is fracture. The most frequent sites of fracture are the vertebral bodies, distal radius, and femoral neck. It develops when the rate of bone resorption exceeds the rate of bone formation.

Primary osteoporosis results from estrogen deficiency and constitutes 95 percent of all cases. Estrogen receptors are present in bone, and so estrogen may act on bone directly to reduce bone resorption.[35] Estrogen has also been theorized to act by any of the following mechanisms:

(1) by decreasing the sensitivity of bone to parathyroid hormone (PTH) without changing the amount of circulatory PTH; (2) by increasing calcitonin—this is consistent with the facts that (a) high estrogen states such as oral contraceptives and pregnancy are associated with elevated calcitonin,[36] (b) men, who have greater bone mass than women, have higher calcitonin levels as well,[37] and (c) calcitonin levels decline with age[38] and menopause and rise with estrogen replacement[39]; or (3) by directly increasing intestinal calcium absorption.

Secondary osteoporosis, which constitutes a minority of cases, may result from any of the following disorders: glucocorticoid or heparin use, renal failure, hyperthyroidism, primary hyperparathyroidism, hyperadrenalism, dietary calcium deficiency, or upper gastrointestinal (GI) surgery.

Incidence

Peak bone mass is achieved at age 30, with women at all ages having less bone mass than men. After age 40, both sexes progressively lose bone mass with aging, at a rate of approximately 1 to 2 percent per yr.[40] This loss is accelerated at the time of menopause, averaging 3.9 percent per yr for 6 yr[41] (Fig 37–9).

Individuals with a lower peak bone mass are more likely to develop significant osteoporosis. Thus, women are at a higher risk than men, whites and Orientals more than blacks,[42] and thin women more than obese ones.[43] This greater bone mass of obese women may be due to their increased weight, placing additional mechanical stress on their axial skeleton. An alternative explanation is that these women have greater endogenous estrogens due to: (1) increased peripheral aromatization of androstenedione to estrone[6]; and (2) lower sex hormone-binding globulin with greater free estradiol levels.[17]

The rate of bone loss varies greatly among individuals: Women who smoke, drink alcohol, are sedentary, or consume low-calcium, high-protein, or high-phosphate diets lose bone mass more quickly.[44–47] Genetic factors are also at play because family history is a significant risk factor for osteoporosis.

Twenty-five percent of women beyond age 60 will show vertebral fractures on x-ray, as will 50 percent of women beyond age 75.[48,49] Twenty-five percent of women beyond age 80 will have a hip fracture,[50] with the annual incidence of 1.3 percent per yr after age 65 and 3.3 percent per yr after age 85.[51] One of six women with hip fractures will not be alive 3 mo later.[52] The annual healthcare cost in the United States for these fractures is estimated to be 7 billion dollars.

Diagnosis

Once osteoporosis has occurred, it may not be significantly reversed. For that reason, a number of radiologic modalities have been used to detect early losses of bone

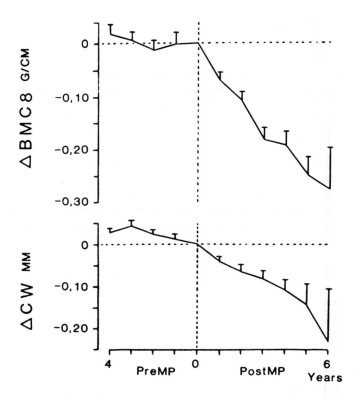

Figure 37–9. Mean (± SEM) changes in bone mass, measured as bone mineral content (g/cm) of the proximal (BMC8) forearm and mean cortical width (CW) (mm) of metacarpals 2,3, and 4 of both hands. (Δ), changes from the last premenopausal (PreMp) year. The **broken horizontal line** gives values for the last premenopausal year (0) and the **broken vertical line** indicates the last premenopausal year. *(Reproduced, with permission, from Falch JA, Oftebro H, Haug E. Early postmenopausal bone loss not associated with decrease in vitamin D. J Clin Endocrinol Metab. 64:836, 1987.)*

mass before significant osteoporosis has developed. The objective is to initiate treatment in women showing early bone loss before fractures occur. A low bone density predicts the likelihood of a future osteoporosis-related fracture. For example, the relative risk for a fracture is 1.4 to 1.6 *for each* standard deviation decrease from peak bone density.[53] Because osteoporosis affects trabecular bone earlier than cortical bone, those modalities that preferentially measure trabecular bone will be the most useful; however, these techniques frequently require greater expense and radiation exposure.

Single-photon absorptiometry of the distal radius is inexpensive, easy to perform, and requires only 5 mrem of radiation. However, it measures 75 percent cortical bone and 25 percent trabecular bone and so may not detect early bone loss. In skilled hands, it has an accuracy within 5 percent and a precision of 2 to 4 percent.[54]

Dual-photon absorptiometry of the second to fourth vertebral body offers an advantage as it measures 60 percent cortical bone and 40 percent trabecular bone. It is more expensive, requires 5 to 15 mrem, and has an accuracy within 5 to 7 percent with a precision of 2 to 5 percent.[54]

Computed tomography of the vertebral body measures 5 percent cortical bone and 95 percent trabecular bone and so may detect changes over an interval as short as 6 mo.[55] It has the greatest radiation exposure (200 mrem) and expense, and has a precision of 1 to 3 percent.

The most recent modality to be developed, quantitative digital radiography (QDR), is the technique of choice. It provides high-resolution images with excellent precision (1 to 2 percent) and much lower radiation exposure (1 to 3 mrem).[56] QDR requires less than 8 min per study, considerably faster than the 20 to 45 min needed for dual-photon absorptiometry.

Patients found to have osteoporosis or osteoporosis related fractures should undergo careful history and physical examination to exclude an underlying etiology. Measurement of serum calcium, phosphate, alkaline phosphatase, sedimentation rate, or serum protein electrophoresis may assist in identifying any of those disorders, but will be normal in patients with primary osteoporosis.

GENITAL ATROPHY

Pathogenesis

The tissues of the lower vagina, labia, urethra, and trigone are of common embryonic origin, derived from the urogenital sinus, and are all estrogen dependent.[57] The loss of estrogen at menopause causes the vaginal walls to become pale, due to diminished vascularity, as well as thin, typically only three or four cells thick. The vaginal epithelial cells contain less glycogen, which prior to menopause had been metabolized by lactobacilli to create an acidic pH, thereby protecting the vagina from bacterial overgrowth. Loss of this protective mechanism leaves the thin, friable tissue vulnerable to infection and ulceration. The vagina also loses its rugae and becomes shorter and inelastic.

Patients may complain of symptoms secondary to vaginal dryness, such as dyspareunia and vaginismus, which may ultimately lead to diminished libido. They may also present with symptoms secondary to vaginal ulceration and infection, such as vaginal discharge, burning, itching, or bleeding.

The urethra and urinary trigone undergo atrophic changes similar to that of the vagina. Dysuria, urgency, frequency, and pubic pain may occur in the absence of infection. Presumably this occurs because the markedly thin urethral mucosa allows urine to come in close contact with sensory nerves. In addition, the menopausal loss of the resistance to urinary flow by a thick, well-vascularized urethral mucosa has been hypothesized to contribute to urinary incontinence.[58]

Diagnosis

Atrophic vaginitis is usually diagnosed by its typical appearance. Atrophy may be confirmed, if necessary, by a vaginal cell maturation index, obtained by scraping the lateral vaginal wall at the level of the cervix. The exfoliated cells can then be classified by degree of maturation, with a small proportion of superficial cells indicating a high degree of vaginal atrophy. If any atypical lesions are present, they should be biopsied for diagnosis. If any discharge is present, it should be evaluated for pathogens such as *Candida*, *Neisseria gonorrhoeae*, *Chlamydia*, *Trichomonas*, and *Gardnerella*. If *Candida* is found, the patient should be screened for diabetes because the low glycogen content of unestrogenized vaginal epithelial cells will not ordinarily support its growth.

Atrophic urethritis/trigonitis is diagnosed by ruling out the presence of infection. Urethroscopy is usually not necessary, but would reveal a pale, atrophic urethra.

ATHEROSCLEROSIS

Estrogens have been hypothesized to protect against atherosclerosis because the incidence of cardiovascular disease (CVD) is lower in women than in men at all age groups. This sex difference is greatest during the premenopausal years, when women have approximately one fifth the CVD mortality of men. However, after menopause female mortality rapidly rises to become half that of men[59] (Fig 37–10). One explanation for this relative increase in mortality is that a premenopausal woman's estrogen confers protection, which is lost at menopause. This is supported by the observation that women who undergo a premature surgical menopause (ie, bilateral oophorectomy) and do not use postmenopausal estrogens have significantly more CVD compared to age-matched premenopausal controls. If they use postmenopausal estrogens, however, their incidence of CVD is the same as premenopausal women of the same age. Premature natural menopause, in contrast, has not been found to increase CVD risk when controlled for age, smoking, and estrogen use.[60]

If estrogens do protect against CVD, one would expect postmenopausal estrogen users to have less CVD compared to nonusers. Many epidemiologic studies have thus compared the incidence of CVD between these two groups. Retrospective case control studies[61–63] provided inconsistent results although most found estrogen use to be associated with less CVD. Prospective cohort studies, which have fewer sources of bias as compared to case control studies, generally showed estrogen use to reduce CVD.[64–67] One notable exception is the Framingham study, which demonstrated an adverse effect[68] or no effect[69] of estrogen treatment depending upon the inclusion criteria for CVD and the multiple regression model

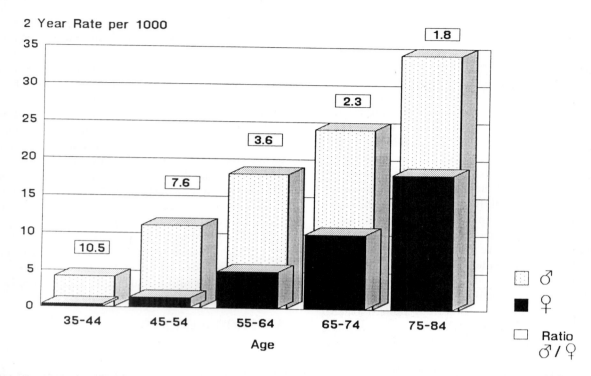

2 Year Rate per 1000

Figure 37–10. Incidence of myocardial infarction by age and sex (female, solid bar; male, stippled bar): 26 years of follow-up, Framingham study. Ratios of male to female myocardial infarctions for each age group are noted at top of graph. (*Adapted, with permission, from Lerner DJ, Kannel WB. Patterns of coronary disease morbidity and mortality: A 26-year follow-up of the Framingham population.* Am Heart J. *111:383, 1986.*)

employed. In contrast, the Nurses Health Study,[70] the largest cohort study, following 59,000 postmenopausal women for up to 16 yr, identified 770 cases of nonfatal myocardial infarction (MI) or fatal coronary heart disease. The relative risk of coronary heart disease with current estrogen use was significantly reduced to 0.6 (95 percent CI: 0.4 to 0.8). The addition of a progestin to estrogen treatment did not alter its apparent cardioprotective effect: The relative risk of heart disease was 0.4 (CI, 0.2 to 0.8). This was most reassuring, since there has been a concern that progestins may detract from the cardioprotective actions of estrogens. Adjustment for a number of cardiovascular risk factors did not alter these findings, arguing against any major physician bias to prescribe estrogens to healthier women. Therefore, the weight of evidence suggests that postmenopausal estrogen replacement protects against CVD.

The only attempts to reduce CVD by estrogen treatment have all been performed in men. Early trials, enrolling men after an MI, showed estrogen treatment to reduce serum cholesterol but not the incidence of a second event.[71,72] The Coronary Drug Project, consisting of 1011 MI survivors, was terminated when excess thrombotic events were seen in the estrogen-treated group; CVD incidence was not reduced.[73] This experience is similar to that seen in men with prostatic cancer treated with an estrogen, diethylstilbestrol, which appears to in-

crease CVD, possibly by causing excessive fluid accumulation, leading to congestive heart failure, or by promoting hypercoagulability, thereby predisposing thromboembolic disease.[74] This adverse action of estrogen in men may have been the consequence of the high estrogenic potency of the doses used and thus would not reflect the physiologic action of estrogens.

Because men and women have an equal incidence of CVD when matched for lipoprotein concentrations,[75] the sex difference in CVD may be a consequence of the characteristic sex differences in serum lipoprotein concentrations. Thus, premenopausal women appear to be protected against CVD by their typically lower low-density lipoprotein (LDL) levels and higher high-density lipoprotein (HDL) levels compared to men of the same age (Fig 37–11). As women pass through menopause, however, their HDL levels fall and LDL levels rise so that their LDL levels exceed those of men.[76] A longitudinal prospective study found a 5 percent net increase in LDL and a 5 percent decrease in HDL in women undergoing menopause compared to age-matched women who remained premenopausal.[77] It has been suggested that the loss of estrogen at menopause causes these increases in LDL and decreases in HDL. This is consistent with the known effects of postmenopausal estrogen replacement to lower LDL by 14 to 19 percent and raise HDL by 15 to 18 percent.[78] However, it should be rec-

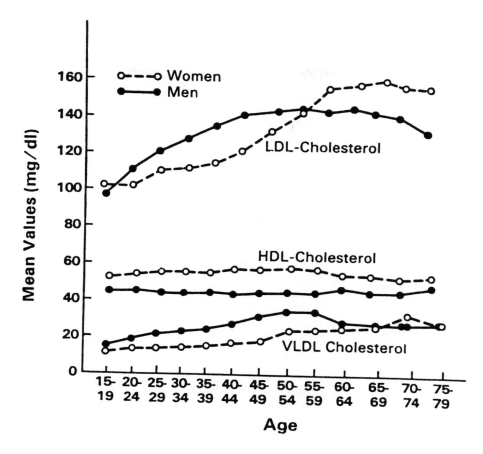

Figure 37–11. Age and sex trends in lipoprotein cholesterol fractions, Framingham study. *(Reproduced, with permission, from Kannel WB. Risk factors for coronary disease in women. Perspective from the Framingham study.* Am Heart J. *114:413, 1987.)*

ognized that oral estrogens may have an additional pharmacologic action on the liver because high portal estrogen concentrations are presented to the liver following intestinal absorption.

An alternative explanation has been proposed for the sex difference in CVD because a semilogarithmic plot of female cardiovascular deaths against age shows that the rate of increase in the rate of CVD is constant throughout a woman's lifetime and is not accelerated after menopause. In contrast, a similar analysis of male CVD shows a decline in the rate of increase after the onset of the "male climacteric," when testosterone levels wane[79] (Fig 37–12). This decline in androgens may therefore be the major factor responsible for the lower female/male CVD ratio seen with increasing age. Androgens are known to adversely affect serum lipoproteins: both exogenous use (eg, testosterone enanthate and methyltestosterone) and endogenous increases in androgens (occurring during puberty) have been found to lower HDL and raise LDL.[80–82]

Approximately half the observed reduction in CVD of estrogen users (compared to nonusers) can be explained by their higher HDL and lower LDL levels.[83] Thus, estrogens have been postulated to reduce CVD by ways other than their beneficial changes in lipoprotein levels. This is also suggested by the observation that primates given an estrogen combined with norgestrel, an androgenic progestin, had substantially less atherosclerosis upon autopsy compared to control animals despite marked reductions in HDL levels induced by the norgestrel.[84] Multiple alternative mechanisms for the protective action of estradiol have been proposed:

1. Estrogens may prevent the oxidation of LDL, which will thus reduce its atherogenicity.
2. Estrogens may alter prostaglandin metabolism, increasing prostacyclin levels and decreasing thromboxane levels[85]; both of these actions will promote vasodilatation.
3. Estrogens may act directly on vessel walls to induce vasodilatation,[86,87] biologically plausible because estrogen receptors have been located at multiple sites throughout the vascular system.

Work is currently underway to provide evidence for these hypotheses.

CONCLUSION

Women today spend one half their adult lifetime after menopause, in an estrogen-deficient state. This menopausal loss of estrogen has multiple sequelae; hot flashes, urogenital atrophy, osteoporosis, and atherosclerosis. The

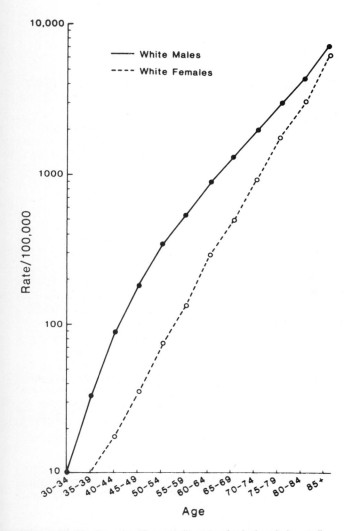

Figure 37–12. Age-specific mortality rates for ischemic heart diseases by sex (whites only, United States, 1977). *(Reproduced, with permission, from Ross RK, Paganini-Hill A. Estrogen replacement therapy and coronary heart disease. Semin Reprod Endocrinol. 1:19, 1983.)*

development of osteoporosis and atherosclerosis causes substantial morbidity and mortality. As detailed in Chapter 38, estrogen replacement can significantly relieve or prevent these conditions, and may allow women to lead long and productive lives.

REFERENCES

1. McKinlay S, Jeffreys M, Thompson B. An investigation of the age of menopause. *J Biosoc Sci.* 4:161, 1972
2. Amundsen DW, Diers CJ. The age of menopause in classical Greece and Rome. *Hum Biol.* 42:79, 1970
3. Schiff I, Wilson E. Clinical aspects of aging of the female reproductive system. In: Schneider EL, ed. *The Aging Reproductive System.* New York, N.Y., Raven Press, 1978: 9–28
4. Sherman BW, West JH, Korenman SG. The menopausal transition: Analysis of LH, FSH, estradiol, and progesterone concentrations during menstrual cycles of older women. *J Clin Endocrinol Metab.* 42:629, 1976
5. Toner JP, Philput CB, Jones GS, Muasher SJ. Basal follicle-stimulating hormone levels is a better predictor of in vitro fertilization performance than age. *Fertil Steril.* 55:784, 1991
6. Grodin JM, Siiteri PK, MacDonald PC. Source of estrogen production in postmenopausal women. *J Clin Endocrinol Metab.* 36:207, 1973
7. Erlik Y, Meldrum DR, Judd HL. Estrogen levels in postmenopausal women with hot flushes. *Obstet Gynecol.* 59:403, 1982
8. Vermeulen A. The hormonal activity of the postmenopausal ovary. *J Clin Endocrinol Metab.* 42:247, 1976
9. Thompson B, Hart SA, Durno D. Menopausal age and symptomatology in general practice. *J Biol Sci.* 5:71, 1973
10. Chang RJ, Judd HL. Elevation of skin temperature of the finger as an objective index of postmenopausal hot flushes: Standardization of the techniques. *Am J Obstet Gynecol.* 135:713, 1979
11. Erlik Y, Tataryn IV, Meldrum DR, et al. Association of waking episodes with menopausal hot flushes. *JAMA.* 245:1741, 1981
12. Mashchak CA, Kletsky OA, Artal R, et al. The relation of physiological changes to subjective symptoms in postmenopausal women with and without hot flushes. *Maturitas.* 6:301, 1985
13. Yen SSC. The biology of menopause. *J Reprod Med.* 18:28, 1977
14. Frodin T, Alund G, Varenhurst E. Measurement of skin blood-flow to assess hot flushes after orchiectomy. *Prostate.* 7:203, 1985
15. Huggins C, Stevens RE, Hodges CU. Studies of prostatic cancer. II. The effects of castration in advanced carcinoma of the prostate. *Arch Surg.* 43:209, 1941
16. DeFazio J, Meldrum DR, Winer JH, et al. Direct action of androgen on hot flushes in the human male. *Maturitas.* 6:8, 1984
17. Davidson BJ, Gambone JC, Lagasse LD. Free estradiol in postmenopausal women with and without endometrial cancer. *J Clin Endocrinal Metab.* 52:404, 1981
18. Larson IF. Hot flushes after hypophysectomy. *Br J Med.* 2:1356, 1977
19. D'Amico JF, Greendale GA, Lu JK, Judd HL. Induction of hypothalamic opiod activity with transdermal estradiol administration in postmenopausal women. *Fertil Steril.* 55:754, 1991
20. Berkow R (ed). *The Merck Manual of Diagnosis and Therapy.* Rahway, N.J., Merck Sharp & Dohme Research Laboratories, 1987, p. 2472
21. Beattie CW, Rodgers CH, Soyka LF. Influence of ovariectomy and ovarian steroids on hypothalamic tyrosine hydroxylase activity in the rat. *Endocrinology.* 91:276, 1972
22. Luine VN, McEwen BS. Effect of estradiol on turnover of type A monomine oxidase in brain. *J Neurochem.* 28:1221, 1977

23. Paul SM, Axelrod J, Saadvedra JM, et al. Estrogen in-duced efflux of endogenous catecholamines from the hy-pothalmus in vitro. *Brain Res.* 178:499, 1979

24. Nixon RL, Jamowsky DS, David JM. Effectsof proges-terone, estradiol, and testosterone on the uptake and metabolism of ^{3}H-norepinephrine, ^{3}H-dopamine, and ^{3}H-serotonin in rat synaptosomes. *Res Comm Chem Pathol Pharmacol.* 7:233, 1974

25. Johnston AE, Nock B, McEwen B, et al. Estradiol modu-lation of noradrenergic receptors in the guinea pig brain assessed by tritium-sensitive film autoradiography. *Brain Res.* 336:153, 1985

26. Clayden JR, Bell JW, Pollard P. Menopausal flushing: Double-blind trial of a nonhormonal medication. *Br Med J.* 1:409, 1974

27. Hammond MG, Hatley L, Talbert LM. A double-blind study to evaluate the effect of methyldopa on menopausal vasomotor flushes. *J Clin Endocrinol Metab.* 58:1158, 1984

28. Jones KP, Ravnikar VA, Schiff I. Effect of lofexidine on vasomotor flushes. *Maturitas.* 7:135, 1985

29. Haas S, Walsh B, Evans S, et al. The effect of transdermal estradiol on hormone and metabolic dynamics over a six-week period. *Obstet Gynecol.* 71:671, 1988

30. Bartus RT, Dean RL 3rd, Beer B, Lippa AS. The cholin-ergic hypothesis of geriatric memory dysfunction. *Science.* 217:408, 1982

31. Gould E, Woolley CS, Frankfurt M, McEwen BS. Gonadal steroids regulate dendritic spine density in hip-pocampal pyramidal cells in adulthood. *J Neurosci.* 10:1286, 1990

32. Henderson VW, Paganini-Hill A, Emanuel CK, et al. Estrogen replacement therapy in older women. Comparisons between Alzheimer's disease cases and nondemented control subjects. *Arch Neurol.* 51:896, 1994

33. Paganini-Hill A, Henderson VW. Estrogen deficiency and risk of Alzheimer's disease in women. *Am J Epidemiol.* 140:256, 1994

34. Tang MX, Jacobs D, Stern Y, et al. Effect of oestrogen during menopause on risk and age at onset of Alzheimer's disease [see comments]. *Lancet.* 348:429, 1996

35. Komm BS, Terpening CM, Benz DJ, et al. Estrogen bind-ing, receptor mRNA, and biologic response in osteoblast-like osteosarcoma cells. *Science.* 241:81, 1988

36. Lindsay R, Sweeney A. Urinary cyclic AMP in osteoporo-sis. *Scott Med J.* 21:231, 1976

37. Hillyard CJ, Stevenson JC, MacIntyre I. Relative defin-ciency of plasma calcitonin in normal women. *Lancet.* 1:961, 1978

38. Deftos LJ, Weisman MH, Williams G, et al. Influence of age and sex on plasma calcitonin in human beings. *N Engl J Med.* 302:1351, 1980

39. Stevenson JC, Abeyasekera G, Hillyard CJ, et al. Calcitonin and the calcium-regulating hormones in postmenopausal women: Effect of estrogens. *Lancet.* 1:693, 1981

40. Heanly RP. Estrogens and postmenopausal osteoporosis. *Clin Obstet Gynecol.* 19:791, 1976

41. Horsman A, Simpson M, Kirby PA. Nonlinear bone loss in oophorectomized women, *Br J Radiol.* 50:504, 1977

42. Smith DM, Nance WE, Kang KW. Genetic factors in determining bone mass. *J Clin Invest.* 52:2800, 1973

43. Dalen J, Hallberg D, Lamke B. Bone mass in obese sub-jects. *Acta Med Scand.* 197:353, 1975

44. Daniell HW. Osteoporosis and the slender smoker. *Arch Intern Med.* 136:298, 1976

45. Aloia JF, Cohn SH, Ostuni JA, et al. Prevention of involu-tional bone loss by exercise. *Ann Intern Med.* 89:356, 1978

46. Matkovic V, Kostial K, Simonovic, I, et al. Bone status and fracture rates in two regions of Yugoslavia. *Am J Clin Nutr.* 32:540, 1979

47. Licata AA, Bou E, Bartter FC, West F. Acute effects of di-etary protein on calcium metabolism in patients with os-teoporosis. *J Geronotol.* 36:14, 1981

48. Alffam PH. An epidemiologic study of cervical and inter-trochanteric fractures of the femur in suburban popula-tion. *Acta Orthop Scand.* 65:1, 1964

49. Iskrant AP. The etiology of fractured hips in females. *Am J Public Health.* 54:485, 1968

50. Gordon G, Vaughan C. *Clinical Managment of the Osteo-poroses.* Acton, Mass., Publishing Sciences Group, 1976

51. Lindsay R, Dempster DW, Clemens T, et al. Incidence, cost and risk factors of fracture of the proximal femur in the USA. In: Christiansen C, et al, eds. *Osteoporosis.* Denmark, Aalborg Stoftsbogturkkeri, 1984: 311–315

52. Gallagher JC, Nordin BEC. Oestrogens and calcium me-tabolism. *Front Horm Res.* 2:98, 1973

53. Melton LJ 3rd, Atkinson EJ, O'Fallon WM, et al. Long-term fracture prediction by bone mineral assessed at dif-ferent skeletal sites. *J Bone Miner Res.* 8:1227, 1993

54. Dequeker JV, Johnston CC. *Noninvasive Bone Measurements.* Oxford, U.K. IRL Press, 1981

55. Cann CE, Genant HK, Ettinger B. Spinal mineral loss in oophorectomized women. Determination by quantitative computer tomography. *JAMA.* 244:2056, 1980

56. Kelly TL, Slovik DM, Schoenfeld DA, et al. Quanti-tative digital radiography vs. dual photon absorptiometry of the lumbar spine. *J Clin Endocrinol Metab.* 67:839, 1988

57. Iosif CS, Batra S, Ek A, Astedt B. Estrogen receptors in the human female lower urinary tract. *Am J Obstet Gynecol.* 141:817, 1981

58. Zinner NN, Sterlin AM, Ritter RC. Role of urethral soft-ness in urinary incontinence. *Urology.* 6:115, 1980

59. Lerner DJ, Kannel WB. Patterns of coronary disease mor-bidity and mortality: A 26-year follow-up of the Framingham population. *Am Heart J.* 111:383, 1986

60. Coldnitz GA, Willett WC, Stampfer MJ, et al. Menopause and the risk of coronary heart disease in women. *N Engl J Med.* 316:1105, 1987

61. Pfeffer RI, Whipple GH, Kurosaki TT, et al. Coronary risk and estrogen use in postmenopausal women. *Epidemiology.* 107:479, 1978

62. Ross RK, Paganini-Hill A, Mack TM, et al. Menopausal estrogen therapy and protection from death from ischemic heart disease. *Lancet.* 1:858, 1981

63. Bain C, Willett WC, Hennekins CH, et al. Use of post-menopausal hormones and risk of myocardial infarction. *Circulation.* 64:42, 1981

64. Hammond CB, Jelousek FR, Leck L, et al. Effects of long term estrogen replacement therapy. *Am J Obstet Gynecol.* 133:525, 1979

65. Bush TL, Cavan LD, Barrett-Connor E. Estrogen use and all-cause mortality. *JAMA.* 249:903, 1983

66. Burch JC, Byrd BF, Vaughn WK. The effects of long-term estrogen on hysterectomized women. *Am J Obstet Gynecol.* 118:778, 1974

67. Petitti DB, Wingerd J, Pellegrin F, et al. Risk of vascular disease in women: Smoking, oral contraceptives, non-contraceptive estrogens and other factors. *JAMA.* 242:1150, 1979

68. Wilson PWF, Garrison RJ, Castelli WP. Postmenopausal estrogen use, cigarette smoking, and cardiovascular morbidity in women over 50. *N Engl J Med.* 313:1038, 1985

69. Eaker ED, Castelli WP. Coronary heart diease and its risk factors among women in the Framingham study. In: Eaker Ed, Packard B, Wenger NK, eds. *Coronary Heart Disease in Women.* New York, N.Y., Haymarket Doyma, 1987: 122–130.

70. Grodstein F, Stampfer MJ, Manson JE, et al. Postmeno-pausal estrogen and progestin use and the risk of cardio-vascular disease (see comments). *N Engl J Med.* 335: 453, 1996

71. Stamler J, Katz LN, Pick R, et al. Effects of long-term es-trogen therapy on serum cholesterol-lipid lipoprotein lev-els and mortality in middle aged men with previous myocardial infarction. *Circulation.* 22:658, 1980

72. Oliver MF, Boyd GS. Endocrine aspects of coronary scler-osis. *Lancet.* 2:1273, 1956

73. DeVogt HJ, Smith PH, Davone-Macaluso M, et al. Cardiovascular side effects of diethylstilbestrol, cypro-terone acetate, and medroxyprogesterone acetate used for treatment of prostatic cancer. *J Urol.* 135:303, 1986

74. The Coronary Drug Project Research Group. Findings leading to discontinuation of the 2.5 mg/day estrogen group. *JAMA.* 226:652, 1973

75. Gordon T, Castelli WP, Hjortland MC, et al. High density lipoprotein as a protective factor against coronary heart disease. *Am J Med.* 62:707, 1977

76. Kannel WB. Risk factors for coronary disease in women. Perspective from the Framingham study. *Am Heart J.* 114:413, 1987

77. Matthews KA, Meilahn E, Kuller LH, et al. Menopause and risk factors for coronary heart disease. *N Engl J Med.* 321:641, 1989

78. Walsh BW, Schiff I, Rosner B, et al. Effects of post-menopausal estrogen replacement on the concentrations and metabolism of plasma lipoproteins. *N Engl J Med.* 325:1196, 1991

79. Heller RF, Jacobs HS. Coronary heart disease in relation to age, sex, and the menopause. *Br Med J.* 1:472, 1978

80. Orchard TJ, Rodgers M. Changes in blood lipids and blood pressure during adolescence. *Br Med J.* 280:1563, 1980

81. Kirkland RT, Keenan BS, Probstfield JL, et al. Decrease in plasma high-density lipoprotein cholesterol levels at puberty in boys with delayed adolescence: Correlation with plasma testosterone levels. *JAMA.* 257:502, 1987

82. Oliver MF, Boyd GS. Influence of reduction of serum lipids on prognosis of coronary heart disease: A five year study using estrogen. *Lancet.* 2:499, 1961

83. Bush TL, Barrett-Connor E, Cowan LD, et al. Cardio-vascular mortality and non-contraceptive estrogen use in women:Results from the Lipid Research Clinics' Program Follow-up Study. *Circulation.* 75:1002, 1987

84. Adams MR, Clarkson TB, Koritnik DR, Nash HA. Contraceptive steroids and coronary artery atherosclerosis in cynomolgus macaques. *Fertil Steril.* 47:1010, 1987

85. Steinleitner A, Stanczyk FZ, Levin JH, et al. Decreased in vitro production of 6-keto-prostaglandin by uterine ar-teries from postmenopausal women. *Am J Obstet Gynecol.* 161:1677, 1989

86. Lieberman EH, Gerhard MD, Uehata A, et al. Estrogen improves endothelium-dependent flow-mediated vasodi-lation in postmenopausal women. *Ann Intern Med.* 121: 936, 1994

87. Rosano GM, Sarrel PM, Poole-Wilson PA, Collins P. Beneficial effect of oestrogen on exercise-induced my-ocardial ischaemia in women with coronary artery disease [see comments]. *Lancet.* 342:133, 1993

Chapter 38

38 *Chapter 38*

HORMONAL TREATMENT OF MENOPAUSAL WOMEN: RISKS AND BENEFITS

Ian H. Thorneycroft

BENEFITS

General Symptoms of Menopause

Figure 38–1 summarizes the major symptoms of menopause and the approximate age at which they appear. The pathophysiology of menopause and these symptoms have been outlined in Chapter 37.

Early Symptoms

Hot flashes are an annoying symptom of menopause. The pathophysiology of these has been outlined in Chapter 37. Women wake up, even from rapid eye movement (REM) sleep, with every hot flash resulting in insomnia, sweating, depression, and irritability. In many randomized prospective double-blinded studies, estrogens have been shown to prevent hot flashes and the resultant insomnia, depression, and irritability. All general symptoms are relieved by estrogens. It is important that any study of hot flashes and any general symptom have a placebo group as there is a high placebo effect.

Virtually any estrogen if given in a sufficient dose will relieve hot flashes. The route of administration is of no importance. Frequently, higher doses of estrogens will initially be required to control hot flashes, particularly in young women. The most common initial dose of estrogen replacement therapy (ERT) includes 0.625 mg qd conjugated equine estrogens (Premarin), 1.25 qd conjugated esterified estrogen (Estratab), estrone sulfate (Ogen), 1 mg qd micronized estradiol (Estrace), and 0.05 mg transdermal estradiol patch (Estraderm). The dose may need to be increased to levels as high as 2.5 mg Premarin or its equivalent to control flashes.[1]

Intermediate Symptoms

Urogenital Atrophy. Reduced estrogen levels for long periods of time result in atrophy of the vaginal, urethral, and bladder trigone epithelium. Estrogen receptors have been demonstrated in the vagina, urethra, trigone of the bladder, and pubococcygeus. Furthermore, estrogens by stimulating α-adrenergic receptors and collagen content of the urethra result in increased urethral tone.[2]

Vagina. Vaginal atrophy results in fewer sloughed vaginal cells and an elevation of vaginal pH between 6 and 8. Infection (atrophic vaginitis) is more common and the vagina becomes friable and easily bleeds. The latter is a cause of postmenopausal bleeding.[3] ERT increases the thickness of the vaginal epithelium and the number of sloughed cells. The normal protective acidic vaginal pH of 4 to 5.5 is restored by the lactobacillus producing more lactic acid from the breakdown of glycogen in the sloughed vaginal cells, and the vagina is less likely to be colonized with anaerobic bacteria.[4]

A sexual history is important in menopausal women as the thin, inflamed, and less distensible menopausal vagina can produce dyspareunia. Vaginal symptoms can be relieved by small doses of estrogen such as 0.3 mg oral or 1 g vaginal conjugated equine estrogen cream. Once changes have been reversed, administration 2 to 3 times per wk is sufficient. Vaginal estrogens may be more

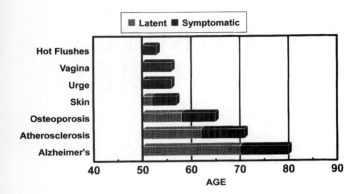

Figure 38–1. Symptoms of menopause and their approximate onset. *(Reproduced, with permission, from Van Keep PA, Kellerhals J. The aging woman. In: Van Keep PA, Lauritzen C, eds. Aging and Estrogens. Basel, Karge, 1973; 2:1600.)*

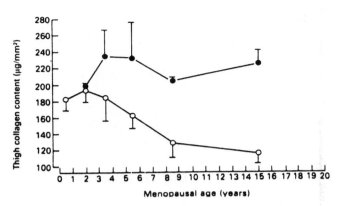

Figure 38–2. Relation between thigh skin collagen content and menopausal age in 51 patients treated with sex hormone implants (●) and in 77 untreated patients (○). *(Reproduced, with permission, from Brincat M, et al. Long-term effects of the menopause and sex hormones on skin thickness. Br J Obstet Gynaecol. 92:256, 1985.)*

effective than oral estrogens in relieving vaginal symptoms.[5]

Stress Incontinence. It has long been thought that stress urinary incontinence (SUI) was aggravated by the lower estrogen levels associated with menopause.[6] The mechanism by which menopause aggravates SUI was thought to be due to decreased urethral pressure from a thinner urethral epithelium and decreased urethral tone by reduced urethral smooth muscle α-adrenergic receptors. ERT was thought to reverse these effects.[7] A recent meta-analysis and a double-blinded prospective study have had difficulties demonstrating an increase in SUI with menopause or improvement with ERT.[8,9] SUI increases primarily with aging and not necessarily with estrogen deficiency. It is worthwhile to attempt ERT in the face of SUI, but due to the most recent data, medical therapy should only be given a short trial before resorting to surgery. Therapy should be given for at least 6 wk using oral doses equivalent to 1.25 mg/day of conjugated equine estrogens. There is evidence that combination of adrenergic agents and estrogens is the most effective regimen.[6]

Urge continence and the urethral syndrome are increased in menopause and are relieved by estrogens.[10] The mechanism is presumably by increasing the thickness and decreasing the inflammation of the urethra and bladder trigone. There is some evidence that there is a lower incidence of urinary tract infections (UTIs) in women on ERT versus placebo.[11] Patients who have been evaluated for urge and UTI-like symptoms with negative workups are good candidates for ERT.

Weight Gain. There is a natural weight gain after menopause, which is confused by many women as being due to ERT/HRT. There is no weight gain from ERT/HRT.[12–14]

Skin Changes. The collagen, proteoglycan, and water content of skin are all decreased in menopausal women and increased by ERT (Fig 38–2). The skin is thicker, less wrinkled, and has more turgor. This is a little publicized benefit of ERT. Interestingly, once collagen is lost from the skin it can indeed be restored by estrogen.[15,16] This is in contradistinction, as we point out later, to bone. Once bone is lost, it cannot be regained.

LONG-TERM BENEFITS

Osteoporosis

Osteoporosis is a reduction in bone density and a normal aging phenomenon in both men and women. Women undergo an additional accelerated rate of bone loss at menopause due to the withdrawal of estrogen. Women lose about 1 to 3 percent of their bone per annum after menopause. When bone mass reaches 2 (NIH) or 2.5 standard deviations (WHO) below those seen in young normals, the patient is considered to have osteoporosis. This is commonly referred to as a t-score. A z-score is when the results are compared to age-matched controls.

The consequences of osteoporosis are fractures,[17] with colles, femoral neck, and vertebral crush fractures the most common sites. The lower the levels of circulating estrogen, the more likely a patient will develop fractures and osteoporosis.[18–20] The hip is the most serious fracture and the incidence goes up logarithmically in the 60s, 70s, and 80s (Fig 38–3). One third of women suffering a hip fracture are dead within 6 mo and half the survivors require nursing home care.[21,22] Osteoporosis is a lethal consequence of the hypoestrogenism of the menopause environment, and ERT prevents osteoporosis and fractures.[23–32]

Osteoporosis unfortunately is difficult to detect. Patients have lost about 25 percent of their bone by the time it can be detected by an ordinary radiograph. By the time a woman has a fracture, even more bone has been

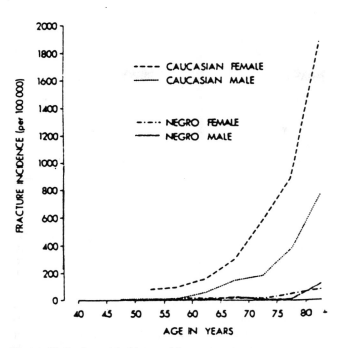

Figure 38–3. Annual incidence of femoral neck fractures in the Johannesburg population over 40 yr old. *(Reproduced, with permission, from Solomon L. Lancet. 2:1327, 1979.)*

lost. To be clinically useful, a technique needs to detect bone loss prior to clinical symptomatology. It is important that the technique also differentiate between cortical and trabecular bone loss as there is more loss of trabecular than cortical bone in the menopause. Two commonly used methods are computed topography (CT) scanning and single- and dual-energy x-ray absorptiometry (DXA or DEXA). CT bone densitometry can accurately differentiate between cortical and trabecular bone. Single-beam absorptiometry is performed in the distal radius, calcaneus, and os calcis. The single beam of γ or x-rays allows one to only quantify the cortical bone and must be performed in an area free of fat that also absorbs gamma rays. DEXA is a technique that uses x-rays of two different energies. Fat tissue, which also absorbs radiation, absorbs the two beams differently than bone. Fat absorption can be subtracted by a series of mathematical equations leaving only bone absorption. Both cortical and trabecular bone density is measured. There has been much discussion as to which technique is best. CT scanning in general requires a more expensive instrument and results in a higher radiation dose than DEXA. The routine use of bone densitometry is controversial not because of accuracy and precision but because of cost.[33–35]

Ovariectomized and menopausal women lose bone rapidly, whereas those replaced with estrogen maintain their bone density. Women in whom there was a delay in starting ERT maintain their bone density but do not re-

gain the lost bone.[36,37] The study by Christiansen et al clearly demonstrated patients not on estrogen lost bone and those on estrogen slightly increased their bone density. Re-randomization after 2 yr showed those on estrogen lost bone when taken off estrogen, and those initially not given estrogen slightly increased their bone density when placed on estrogen. Those never on estrogen continued to lose bone (Fig 38–4).[38] The explanation for the slight increase in bone with ERT is that patients losing bone are both building and breaking down bone at a higher rate. Estrogen only prevents breakdown, while building remains temporarily at a higher level until a new equilibrium is reached. It is therefore important to initiate ERT as early in menopause as possible and preferably within 3 yr.[25] The rate of development of osteoporosis can only be prevented by estrogen. Figure 38–5 illustrates that not only is bone loss prevented by estrogen but also the incidence of fractures is reduced. Almost any form of estrogen (provided the correct dose is given) will prevent osteoporosis. Figure 38–6 illustrates the doses of various estrogens available in the United States that prevent bone loss after natural or surgical menopause. The dose to be used is the one that prevents hip bone loss.

Premarin has a steep dose–response curve, as shown in Figure 38–7. Premarin at 0.15 mg is ineffective for osteoporosis, at 0.3 mg slightly effective (not statistically significant), and at 0.625 mg completely effective. A dose of 1.25 mg was no more effective than 0.625 mg.[39] Estragel at 3 mg/day administered transdermally will also prevent osteoporosis. This preparation produces high estradiol values (190 pg/ml).[40] Estriol is probably not effective in the prescribed doses.[41]

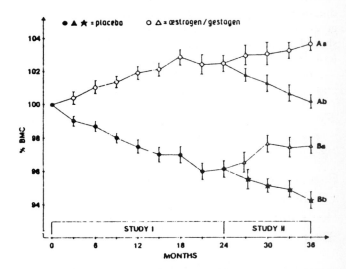

Figure 38–4. Bone mineral content as a function of time and treatment in 94 (study I) and 77 (study II) women soon after menopause. *(Reproduced, with permission, from Christiansen C, et al. Bone mass in postmenopausal women after withdrawal of œstrogen/gestagen replacement therapy. Lancet. 1:459, 1981.)*

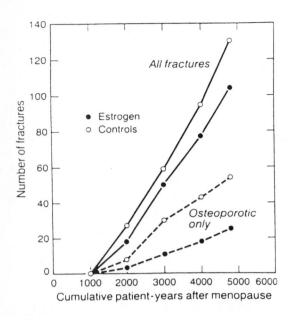

Figure 38–5. Cumulative fractures and osteoporotic fractures by postmenopausal patient-years at risk in 245 women who used estrogen and matched controls. *(Reproduced, with permission, from Ettinger B, et al. Long-term estrogen replacement therapy prevents bone loss and fractures.* Ann Intern Med. *102:319, 1985.)*

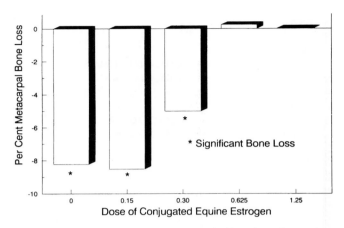

Figure 38–7. Bone loss in patients treated with various doses of conjugated equine estrogen. *(Adapted, with permission, from Lindsay R, et al. The minimum effective dose of estsrogen for prevention of postmenopausal bone loss.* Obstet Gynecol. *63:759, 1984.)*

Menopausal women require 1500 mg of calcium per day, which is 500 mg/day more than premenopausal women; however, many studies have failed to show the utility of calcium in and by itself in preventing osteoporosis. Neither 0.3 mg of Premarin nor 1500 mg calcium will prevent osteoporosis but in combination will prevent osteoporosis. This study needs to be confirmed before prescribing the lower dosage of estrogen for osteoporosis.[42]

It is not known exactly how long one should administer estrogen for the prevention of osteoporosis. Clearly, the goal is to maintain the bone density for long enough such that when discontinued the patient will die of another cause before enough bone is lost to suffer a fracture. It would therefore seem reasonable to continue ERT for osteoporosis for 10 to 15 yr after menopause or until age 70 before stopping therapy. The bone density would have been maintained at such a level that subsequent loss would not result in a fracture before the patient succumbs of other medical complications of aging. Another frequently asked question: How many years postmenopause or in how old a patient should one still consider initiating ERT? Figure 38–8 demonstrates when ERT is started late the bone density is maintained at the level where initiated but bone loss is not regained. Thus, starting ERT several years after menopause at least maintains bone density at the starting level and further loss is prevented. Initiating ERT up to the age of 70 has been demonstrated to be effective. There are other benefits of ERT for which lifelong administration or starting late in life provides, as discussed in the next sections.

Cardiovascular

Myocardial infarctions are about six times less common in premenopausal women than in men of equivalent age. However, as a woman goes through menopause her risk of infarction is almost equal to that of men by age 70 to 80. When menopausal women are compared to pre-menopausal women of the same age, those who are menopausal have a higher cardiovascular disease rate.[43] Low-density lipoprotein (LDL) cholesterol increases in boys after puberty and in women after menopause. During reproductive life, women have lower LDL cholesterol than men. High-density lipoprotein (HDL) cholesterol becomes higher after puberty in girls but does not change greatly at menopause in cross-sectional studies.[44] In a longitudinal study, HDL did decrease slightly as women went through menopause.[45] The increased myocardial infarction rate or the acceleration thereof and

	Spine	**Hip**
Premarin	0.625 mg	0.625 mg
Ogen	.625	1.25
Estrace	0.5-1mg	1 mg*
Estraderm	0.05 mg	0.05 mg*
Climara	**	**
Estratab	0.625 mg	0.625 mg
Estratest	Yes	Yes

* With concurrent progestin
** Probably the same as Estraderm

Figure 38–6. Doses of estrogens that prevent bone loss at the spine and hip.

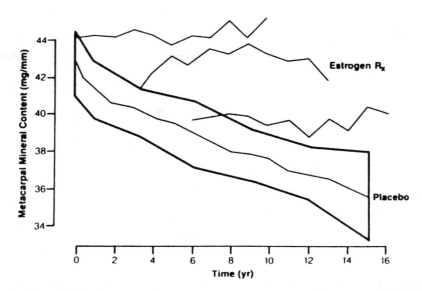

Figure 38–8. Bone loss after initiating estrogen replacement therapy at various times after menopause. *(Reproduced, with permission, from Lindsay R, et al. Interrelationship of bone loss and its prevention and fracture expression. In: Christiansen C, ed. Osteoporosis I—International Symposium on Osteoporosis. Copenhagen, Osteo Press, 1987: 508–512.)*

the rising LDL cholesterol levels after menopause would seem to be related to low estrogen levels.

All estrogens, if given in a high enough dose, will lower LDL cholesterol (Fig 38–9). Oral estrogens appear more potent in this respect, probably due to the first-pass liver effect; however, it is not an exclusive property of oral estrogens.[46] If a sufficiently high dose of a potent estrogen is given non-orally, it can have similar effects on the liver to one given orally, as was well illustrated for the potent estrogen ethinyl estradiol given vaginally by Goebelsmann et al.[46] Oral estrogens are potent in increasing HDL cholesterol, a pharmacologic effect, as HDL cholesterol does not change or only slightly changes with menopause.[47] Oral estrogens are more potent in increasing HDL cholesterol than non-oral estrogens.[48] Oral estrogens also increase triglycerides. If the baseline triglyceride level is greater than 500 mg/dl, then ERT can increase to 1000 mg/dl or greater, which can result in pancreatitis. Such patients should be prescribed transdermal estrogens[49–51]; however, triglyceride levels should be closely monitored. Estratest reduces triglycerides.[52] The changes are probably not sufficient to have any clinical significance. The unfavorable lipid profile of menopause can therefore be reversed and the HDL cholesterol increased with oral estrogens (Fig 38–9).

Cardiac catheterization studies have shown that women taking estrogen have less extensive atherosclerotic heart disease.[53–55] Virtually all studies looking at the effects of ERT on cardiovascular disease have demonstrated about a 50 percent reduction in cardiovascular disease, including stroke.[47,56–83] Importantly, some studies have shown that women with a prior myocardial infarction were less likely to suffer a subsequent myocardial infarction if they were taking estrogens.[63,76] A prior cardiovascular event is not a contraindication to ERT. Fortifying the later statement are some data by Sullivan et al, who followed menopausal women up to 10 yr after the initial catheterization. Those with minimal to no cardiovascular disease accrued virtually no benefit from ERT, but the more severe the cardiovascular disease at the time of original catheterization the more pronounced the benefit of estrogen (Fig 38–10).[81] This would make sense: Women not forming plaques initially are less likely to respond to the antiatherogenic effects of estrogens. Women who had extensive plaque formation would logically be the most benefitted by estrogens.

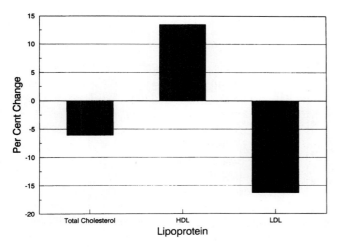

Figure 38–9. Lipid levels after conjugated equine estrogen. *(Adapted, with permission, from Barnes RB, et al. Comparisons of lipid and androgen levels after conjugated estrogen or depo-medroxy progesterone acetate treatment in postmenopausal women. Obstet Gynecol. 66:216, 1985.)*

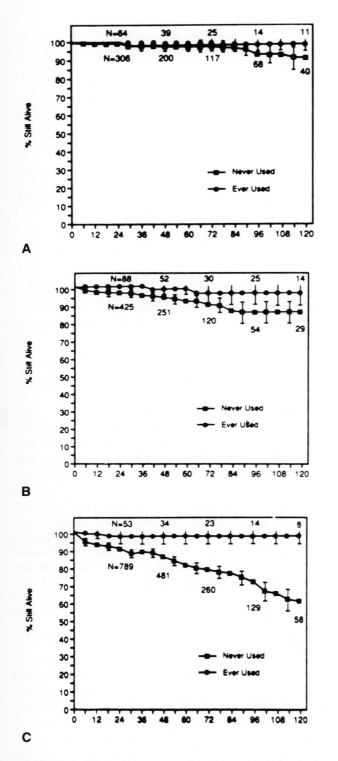

A

B

C

Figure 38–10. Effect of estrogen on the 10-yr survival of patients after cardiac catheterization of patients with **(A)** initially normal coronary arteriograms, **(B)** women whose coronary stenosis varied between detectable and 69 percent, and **(C)** those with left main coronary stenosis that was 50 percent or greater or other stenosis of 70 percent or greater. *(Adapted, with permission, from Sullivan JM, et al. Estrogen replacement and coronary artery disease: Effect on survival in postmenopausal women.* Arch Intern Med. *150:2557, 1990.)*

The longer a patient is treated with estrogen, the more the cardioprotection. It would seem reasonable to treat almost indefinitely with estrogen. Oral estrogens appear to have greater effects on HDL cholesterol and may in the long run provide more cardioprotection. The latter consideration is theoretical; no study has been conducted.

Mechanism of Action. Estrogens decrease LDL cholesterol and raise HDL cholesterol, creating a favorable non-atherogenic profile in women. Bush and Barrett-Connor analyzed lipid data and could not completely explain the benefits of estrogen based upon lipids alone.[63] Their data would indicate only 50 percent of the cardioprotective effect of estrogens is mediated by lipids. Estrogens have a direct effect by inhibiting plaque formation at the level of the coronary artery. Coronary arteries have estrogen receptors, and LDL cholesterol incorporation into the artery wall is inhibited by estrogens.[82] LDL cholesterol must be oxidized before being incorporated into macrophages, which leads to atheroma development.[84] Estrogens are anti-oxidants. The β-ring unsaturated estrogens (equilin, equilenin) are more potent than estradiol or estrone (Fig 38–11).[84] These anti-oxidant properties probably explain the non-lipid-mediated coronary effects of estrogen.[85]

With the utilization of progestogens to prevent endometrial carcinoma, the concern has been raised that the progestogen may interfere with the beneficial effects of estrogens on cardiovascular disease. There are two types of progestogen: Those derived from testosterone, such as norethindrone and norgestrel, and those derived from 17-α-hydroxyprogesterone, such as megestrol acetate and medroxyprogesterone acetate. It would be expected that these two different classes of progestogens would have different effects on lipids. The data of Hirvonen et al in Figure 38–12 illustrate the negative ef-

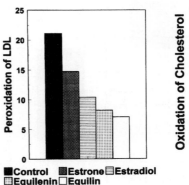

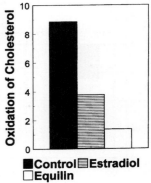

Figure 38–11. Relative anti-oxidant potencies of various estrogens. *(Adapted, with permission, from Subbiah M, Kessel B, Agrawal M, et al. Antioxidant potential of specific estrogens on lipid peroxidation.* J Clin Endocrinol Metab. *77:1095, 1993.)*

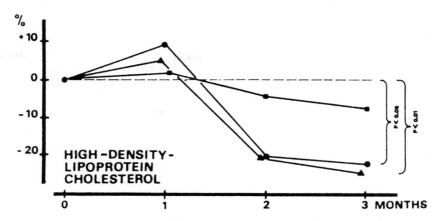

Figure 38–12. Percentage of change in HDL cholesterol during treatment with estradiol valerate 2 mg alone for 1 mo and after the addition of various progestins for 2 mo. Solid circles were given norethindrone acetate 10 mg, solid squares medroxyprogesterone acetate 10 mg, and solid triangles norgestrel 0.5 mg. *(Reproduced, with permission, from Hirvonen E, et al. Effects of different progestogens of lipoproteins during postmenopausal replacement therapy.* N Engl J Med. *304:560, 1981.)*

fect of high doses of norethindrone and norgestrel and virtually no effect of medroxyprogesterone acetate.[86]

Progestins either sequentially or cyclically reduce the increase in HDL and decrease in LDL seen with ERT.[87] Several studies, illustrated in Figure 38–13, have reported no effect on myocardial infarction by the added progestin.[88–91] This apparent paradox is probably largely explained by the anti-oxidant properties of estrogens. Estrogens also increase coronary blood flow. Subjects with angina had less angina and were less likely to have S-T segment depression if they received sublingual estradiol versus placebo prior to a treadmill electrocardiogram.[92] The lack of an effect of an added progestin is probably also explained by this.

Smoking and ERT. Oral contraceptives use in nonsmokers does not increase the rate of myocardial infarction. Women who smoke heavily and use birth control pills are at higher risk for myocardial infarction than women who only smoke.[93] Concern has been raised about menopausal women who smoke and are on ERT.

Women who smoke and take estrogen are more protected than women who smoke and do not take estrogen.[63] Therefore, the magnification effect seen with oral contraceptives is *not* seen with ERT.

Cerebrovascular Accidents. Strokes do not appear to be affected by ERT or HRT. The Nurses' Health Study, which demonstrated no increase or decrease in stroke with ERT or HRT, also showed a significant decrease in MIs with ERT and HRT.[88] A number of studies investigating the role of ERT and HRT on the incidence of stroke confirm these results (Fig 38–14).[94–97]

Summary. Cardiovascular disease increases with menopause and appears to be due to increased LDL cholesterol and the increased incorporation of LDL cholesterol into coronary artery walls secondary to reduced estradiol levels. ERT reduces cardiovascular disease about 50 percent and is the major benefit of ERT.[98]

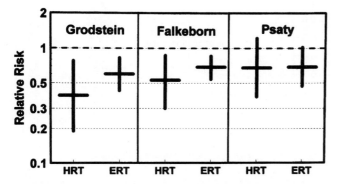

Figure 38–13. Relative risks and 95 percent confidence intervals for myocardial infarction from three separate epidemiologic studies that compared patients given ERT and HRT.

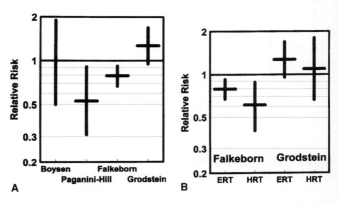

Figure 38–14. Summary of the literature addressing the risk of stroke with ERT and HRT. Figure **(A)** is ERT and **(B)** compares HRT with ERT. Bars are the relative risks and the 95 percent confidence interval of stroke.

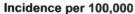

Incidence per 100,000

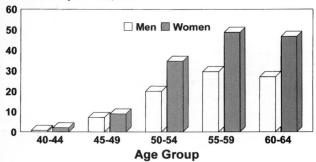

Figure 38–15. Incidence by age and sex for Alzheimer's disease. *(Adapted, with permission, from McGonigal G, Thomas B, McQuade C, et al. Epidemiology of Alzheimer's presenile dementia in Scotland, 1974–88. BMJ. 306:680, 1993.)*

Alzheimer's Disease

Women are more likely than men, and thin women are more likely than obese women, to develop Alzheimer's disease (AD) (Fig 38–15). Androgens are converted to estrogens in the brain. Men experience a gradual drop in their androgen levels with age, unlike the dramatic fall in estrogens in women. Obese women make more estrogen than thin women. For these reasons, it is suspected that estrogen deprivation may play a role in the development of AD and that ERT may reverse or retard its onset. The only currently available therapies for AD disease are cholinesterase inhibitors. AD is characterized by relatively low levels of acetylcholine. Figure 38–16 lists the potential mechanisms by which estrogens could modulate the development and progression of AD. Additionally, there is a specific lesion of the CA nucleus of the hippocampus seen in ovariectomized rats that is also present in AD patients and is a very specific lesion of AD patients. Estrogen reverses the lesion in ovariectomized rats.[99,100]

Figure 38–17 lists the epidemiologic studies that have addressed the effects of estrogen on AD. Some show protection; others show no effect. The problem with AD studies is diagnosis and a sufficient number of very elderly subjects to allow statistically significant results. Two recent studies are of particular note because they studied popula-

► **Regulates amyloid precursor protein processing**
► **Lowers apolipoprotein-E**
► **Increases cerebral blood flow**
► **Enhances cerebral glucose utilization**
► **Cholinesterase inhibitor**
► **Enhances cholinergic activity**
► **Blunts stress induced cortisol elevation**
► **Moderates acute phase inflammation response**
   – Implicated in plaque formation

Figure 38–16. Potential mechanisms by which estrogen can prevent or improve Alzheimer's disease.

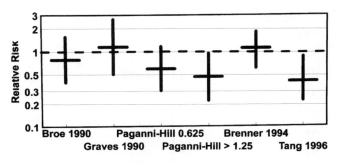

Figure 38–17. Relative risks with 95 percent confidence intervals for Alzheimer's disease in women who ever used ERT.

tions with sufficiently elderly patients and had a large enough number of cases for statistical validity. The USC Leisure World study showed a benefit with estrogens; only the 1.25-mg dose of Premarin was statistically significant. Interestingly, estrogen had to be taken for 7 yr to reach statistical significance although lower doses also reduce the incidence.[101] Tang et al followed a cohort of 1282 women for 1 to 5 yr. None had AD at the beginning of the study. Women who took estrogen for greater than 1 yr (average 13.6 yr) had a significant reduction in the incidence of AD. These results are shown graphically in Figure 38–18. Estrogen appeared to delay the onset of disease.[102] The dose and kind of estrogen was only specified as "the vast majority took conjugated equine estrogens."

Future epidemiology studies should address dose and duration of administration. Criticism of epidemiologic studies is that estrogen tends to be given to highly educated women who are at lower risk of AD, and ERT would probably be withheld from AD patients. Counterbalancing

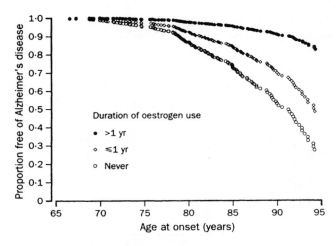

Figure 38–18. Survival analysis plot of the distribution by age of the proportion of individuals remaining unaffected according to duration of estrogen use. *(Reproduced, with permission, from Tang M, Jacobs D, Stern Y, et al. Effect on oestrogen during menopause on risk and age at onset of Alzheimer's disease. Lancet. 348:1, 1996.)*

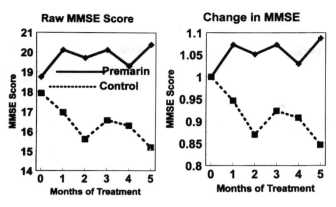

Figure 38–19. Effects on cognitive function in menopausal patients with Alzheimer's disease by Premarin. *(Adapted, with permission, from Ohkura T, Isse K, Akazawa K, et al. Low-dose estrogen replacement therapy for Alzheimer disease in women. Menopause. 1:125, 1994.)*

these confounding factors is the tendency to give estrogen more frequently to thin women.

There have been several small prospective studies that have given estrogens to patients with AD. A placebo-controlled trial is illustrated in Figure 38–19. Those given estrogen maintained their MMSE score whereas those not given estrogen had declines in their score.[103] Larger prospective trials are needed, but the preliminary results are very encouraging. The impact for nursing home costs and quality of life are impressive.

Figure 38–20 illustrates the results of a reanalysis of the Tacrin trials. Women treated with estrogen plus Tacrin did much better than women treated with Tacrin alone. In fact, only the women given estrogen and Tacrin had clinically significant effects.[104]

In summary, preliminary epidemiology indicates a probable benefit of ERT in delaying the onset of the disease. Long-term treatment, possibly with higher doses, may be important. ERT in AD patients appears to im-

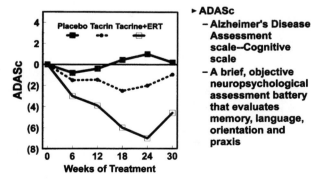

Figure 38–20. Effects of added estrogen to the response of patients with Alzheimer's disease to Tacrin. *(Adapted, with permission, from Schneider L, Farlow M, Henderson V, Pogoda J. Effects of estrogen replacement therapy on response to tacrine in patients with Alzheimer's disease. Neurology. 46:1580, 1996.)*

prove their cognitive functioning or slow further decline. Clearly, prospective treatment studies are needed before estrogen can be strongly advocated as a treatment of AD; however, with all of the other benefits of estrogen, ERT should not be withheld from AD patients. Further epidemiology studies are needed with large numbers of elderly patients and with databases that allow type, dose, and duration of ERT to be analyzed. In addition to ERT being important for cardiovascular and osteoporosis protection, it may be important to slow the development or progression of AD.

Adenocarcinoma of Colon and Rectum

Current studies suggest that ERT and HRT reduce the risk of adenocarcinoma of the colon and rectum.[105,106] Evidence supporting the etiology includes reduction in bile acids, an anti-oxidant effect, and in vitro inhibition of a human cancer cell line.[107,108]

RISKS AND POTENTIAL RISKS

Endometrial Cancer

Beginning in 1976, many articles showed an increased risk of endometrial carcinoma with unopposed estrogens. The risk is related to both duration of use and dose.[109] The relative risks have ranged between 1.8- and 20-fold, with most studies falling between 2 and 4. Whether estrogen is an initiator or promoter of endometrial cancer is still debated. It is probably a promoter. Studies of endometrial cancer and estrogens suffer from a detection bias. Patients on ERT are more likely to have vaginal bleeding and consequently more likely to have an endometrial biopsy performed. Endometrial cancer not related to ERT would therefore be more likely detected. Women not on estrogen and not bleeding may have cancer that remains undetected. In an autopsy series published by Horwitz and Feinstein, 60 percent of all endometrial carcinomas at the time of autopsy were unknown at the time of death, supporting the potential for a detection bias. Correcting for this detection bias, the relative risk decreased from 12 to 1.8.[110,111] The addition of a progestogen significantly decreases the increased risk of endometrial cancer[71,112,113] and hyperplasia.[114,115]

Patients with endometrial cancer and previously using estrogens have a much longer survival than those not using estrogen and not developing endometrial cancer. Either the disease is detected earlier or the biology of the cancer is different in patients using ERT. In fact, the survival of patients with endometrial cancer and taking estrogens is the same as those on estrogen and not developing endometrial cancer (Fig 38–21), again pointing out a different biology of cancer in women on estrogens. The longer survival of patients with endometrial cancer taking estrogens than nonusers without cancer is

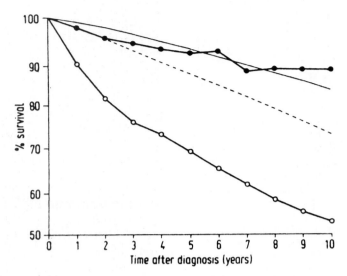

Figure 38–21. Survival of women with endometrial cancer and history of estrogen use. Estrogen users with endometrial cancer ●———●, estrogen user controls (age-adjusted mortality) ———, women with endometrial cancer who were not estrogen users ○———○, and nonestrogen user controls (age-adjusted mortality) – – – – . *(Reproduced, with permission, from Collins J, et al. Oestrogen use and survival in endometrial cancer.* Lancet. *61:964, 1980.)*

probably explained by the cardiovascular and osteoporosis benefits.[116,117]

It would appear, then, that the initial concern about endometrial carcinoma and estrogens is no longer a concern, as concomitant administration of a progestogen will remove the increased risk. Even if an endometrial cancer develops, it is usually well differentiated with an excellent prognosis.

The dose of progestogen to prevent endometrial cancer is not well studied. Ten days of a progestin per month would appear to be the minimum dose.[118] The dose to prevent endometrial hyperplasia is better studied and the data of Whitehead et al would indicate that doses as low as 0.7 to 1 mg norethindrone for 10 days/mo prevents endometrial hyperplasia.[119] Most studies show 10 mg medroxyprogesterone acetate for 10 or more days will prevent endometrial hyperplasia, whereas 5 mg/day for 10 to 14 days does not completely prevent hyperplasia in all studies.[120,121] Duration is as or more important than dose of progestogen in preventing hyperplasia. Lower doses such as 2.5 mg medroxyprogesterone acetate or 0.7 mg norethindrone can be used in continuous combined therapy (estrogen and progestogen every day).[119]

Use of Estrogens in Women With a Previous Diagnosis of Endometrial Cancer.

Two retrospective studies demonstrated women with stage I grade I endometrial carcinoma survived longer and had fewer recurrences than those not treated with estrogens.[122,123] The results from the study by Creasman et al are illustrated in Figure 38–22. Patients with stage I grade I disease can

probably be treated with estrogens immediately, with appropriate informed consent.[124] More advanced disease should probably be allowed 2 to 3 yr of observation for recurrence. If the patient is disease free then, with proper informed consent and for severe symptoms ERT could be initiated. Recently, a small study with stage I and II disease revealed no differences in survival or recurrences in those given ERT/HRT compared to nonusers.[125] The

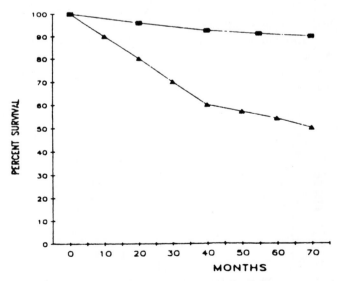

Figure 38–22. Six-year survival rates of patients with endometrial carcinoma, stage I, grade III. (▲) No estrogen replacement; (■), estrogen replacement. *(Reproduced, with permission, from Creasman WT, et al, Estrogen replacement therapy in the patient treated for endometrial cancer.* Obstet Gynecol. *67:326, 1986.)*

benefits of ERT far outweigh the theoretical and un-proven adverse effects on increasing recurrent disease.

Cholelithiasis

Women are more likely to have gallstones than men, with the incidence increasing at puberty. Estrogens are clearly lithogenic.[126–129] Estrogens via any route of administration decrease bile acids and increase the likelihood of a cholesterol stone. Therefore, gallstone formation is not the exclusive domain of oral estrogens, although oral estrogens may be more likely to induce gallstones than non-oral estrogens. There are no studies comparing oral to non-oral estrogens.

Gallstones were initially thought to be 2.5 times as common in women on ERT.[130] This was a similar phenomenon to that noted in oral contraceptive users. More recent studies have shown that the increased risk of gallstones is not as high as originally shown by the Boston Collaborative Study and more data are needed.[131] Cholelithiasis was increased initially in oral contraceptive users but not with longer duration of use. Apparently, the estrogen in oral contraceptives accelerated the time of presentation in women predestined to have a stone.[132] Cholelithiasis is an uncommon complication of ERT, and as can be seen later has little impact on the overall risk–benefit ratio of ERT.

Venous Thrombosis

Until 1996, all of the literature on deep venous thrombosis (DVT) with ERT showed no effect on DVT or pulmonary embolus.[130,133–135] Three articles were published in 1996. Two showed an increase in DVT and one an increase in pulmonary embolus. Figure 38–23 summarizes the literature on DVT and ERT. Taking *all* articles into account, there would not appear to be an increase.[136–138]

Hypertension

Some oral contraceptive users have an increased risk of developing hypertension, and it was assumed that ERT users

would also. A small number of patients will have an idiosyncratic reaction and develop hypertension.[139–142] All patients must be carefully monitored for hypertensive episodes. In a study by Wren and Routledge, there was a small, statistically significant decrease in blood pressure in women on ERT. The change was statistically significant but of no biologic consequence.[142] ERT does not increase hypertension nor is it contraindicated in hypertensive patients. Hypertensive patients treated with ERT have lower rates of myocardial infarction than those not treated.[57]

Breast Cancer

Despite the many benefits of estrogen replacement therapy, there is concern that exogenous estrogen may increase the risk of developing breast cancer. A number of epidemiologic studies have examined the relationship between breast cancer and estrogen replacement therapy with mixed results. A large number of studies have demonstrated no increase in breast cancer risk.[143–154] Of studies including past users, only two have demonstrated an increased risk of developing breast cancer.[155,156] Only one group has demonstrated an increased risk in women with surgical menopause,[157,158] while four studies have demonstrated an increased risk with natural menopause.[156–159] Another area of concern is whether dose and duration of use increase the risk of breast cancer. Five studies have demonstrated an increased risk with increasing dose and duration of use.[156–160] A number of studies demonstrate a duration-related increase in breast cancer, but these were primarily observed in specific subgroups of women and not in all users.[143,147,148,150,155,161–163] Current users have consistently been shown to be at increased risk by the Nurses Health Study but not by others.[153,154]

Other subgroups that demonstrate an increased risk of developing breast cancer include women receiving injectable estrogens (relative risk [RR], 4.0)[155] and those with a history of diethylstilbestrol (DES) use (RR, 1.97) (confidence interval [CI], 1.2 to 3.3).[164] High-risk subgroups include women with a history of benign breast disease and those with a family history of breast cancer. These studies have similar methodologic problems and are limited by their small numbers.

By the nature of their design, epidemiologic studies performing subgroup analysis are subject to several limitations. The small number of cases in the subgroup frequently results in wide confidence intervals, making it impossible to distinguish a true association from a chance finding. Also, by splitting groups into small subgroups statistical significance can frequently be demonstrated. The significance of these findings in a small subgroup of patients requires discretion and can only be applied to the general population if a similar subgroup in multiple studies demonstrate similar findings. Confounding variables and bias due to the patient population can frequently

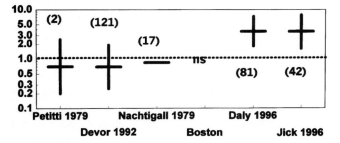

Figure 38–23. Summary of the literature for the development of DVT on ERT. Bars represent the relative risks and 95 percent confidence intervals. Numbers in parentheses are the numbers of cases.

skew the results. This is especially evident in studies that use more than one control group.[146,160,165] Also, retrospective studies can be affected by faulty patient recall. The limitations discussed with subgroup analysis require the reader to review individual studies carefully, and rather than depending upon one study, to determine whether several studies demonstrate similar findings before altering prescribing practices.

Given the variable results demonstrated between studies and the resultant difficulty in interpreting the clinical significance of individual studies, investigators have proposed combining studies and analyzing the pooled data. The statistical tool used to accomplish this utilizes meta-analysis. Meta-analysis allows one to combine results and is especially useful when results from several studies do not agree, when subgroup size is too small to demonstrate significance, or when a large trial is too costly or time consuming to perform.[166,167] Figure 38–24 summarizes all the studies of the relationship between ERT and breast cancer.[168] There is no increase in ever users of ERT. Figure 38–25 is taken from a meta-analysis by Collins that clearly shows that studies with less than 300 cases have too much variability to be able to accurately determine the risk.[169] At most, the risk may be an increase of 10 to 20 percent. Although meta-analysis is reassuring in a low-risk population, there are still a number of issues that remain to be resolved regarding type of estrogen used, combination estrogen and progestin therapy, and effect of estrogen in women with a history of benign breast disease or a family history of breast cancer. Most women in these studies received conjugated estrogen, and it is not known whether other estrogen formulations will yield similar risk estimates. Discussion regarding the effect of estrogen replacement therapy on breast cancer risk must be done in the context of overall mortality in postmenopausal women. The leading cause of death in menopausal women is cardiovascular disease. Fifty-year-old white menopausal women have a 31 percent risk of death from cardiovascular disease and only a 2.8 percent risk of death from breast cancer.[170] In an earlier discussion, it was shown that postmenopausal estrogen use decreases cardiovascular disease risk by approximately 50 percent. It has also been shown that current users have a 40 percent decrease in all cause mortality and women who have used estrogen for at least 30 yr have a 30 percent reduction in all cause mortality.[79] Given Steinberg et al's data suggesting a 30 percent increased risk of developing breast cancer after 15 yr of estrogen use, it is clear that the increased risk of breast cancer is small compared to the potential benefits. Interestingly, there is a 19 percent reduction in breast cancer mortality among estrogen users, again suggesting that the potential benefits outweigh the risks.[79]

It has been suggested that the addition of a progestin may protect the breast in a fashion similar to that

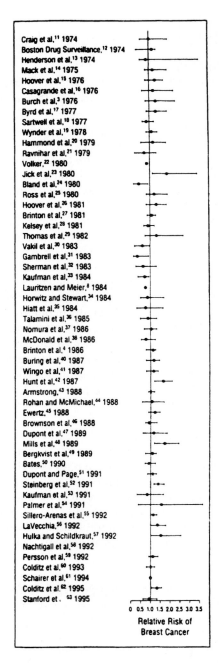

Figure 38–24. Relative risks and 95 percent confidence intervals for ever use of estrogen and developing breast cancer. *(Reproduced, with permission, from Gambrell JR. Hormone replacement therapy and breast cancer risk. Arch Fam Med. 5:341, 1996.)*

which occurs with endometrial cancer. Unfortunately, few data are available to either support or refute a protective role for progestins in breast cancer. Gambrell et al demonstrated a risk of developing breast cancer of 0.3 (CI, 0.1 to 0.8) in women receiving combination estrogen and progestin therapy vs 0.7 (CI, 0.5 to 1.1) in women receiving estrogen alone.[149] A statistically significant differ-

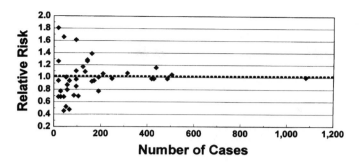

Figure 38–25. Relationship between the relative risk of developing breast cancer from ever use of estrogen as a function of the number of cases in the study. *(Redrawn, with permission, from Collins J. A meta-analysis of breast cancer and estrogen replacement therapy.* J Soc Obstet Gynaecol Can. *17:837, 1995.)*

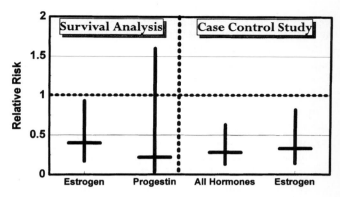

Figure 38–26. Risk of developing a recurrence of breast cancer if given HRT. Bars represent the relative risk and 95 percent confidence intervals. *(Adapted and redrawn, with permission, from Eden J, Bush T, Nand S, Wren B. A case-control study of combined continuous estrogen–progestin replacement therapy among women with a personal history of breast cancer.* Menopause. *2:67, 1995.)*

ence could not be demonstrated between the two groups. Bergkvist et al demonstrated an increased risk of developing breast cancer in menopausal women using combination estrogen and progestin therapy (RR, 4.4) (CI, 0.9 to 22.4).[171] The wide 95 percent CI makes interpretation of this finding difficult. Two studies published in 1995 did not confirm an increase or decrease in breast cancer with the addition of a progestin agent.[153,154] Thus far, the literature does not support the addition of a progestin to protect the breast in women who have undergone hysterectomy.

In summary, in low-risk patients there may be a relationship between estrogen replacement and breast cancer, but the potential benefits far outweigh the risks. Benign breast disease remains a controversial area but estrogen should not be withheld until more definitive data is available. The lowest possible dose of estrogen should always be used. Conjugated estrogens are the most thoroughly studied, and few data are available on other formulations.

Use of Estrogens in Women With a Previous Diagnosis of Breast Cancer

Symptomatic menopausal women with a past history of breast cancer have traditionally been denied the benefit of estrogen replacement therapy. The concern that exogenous estrogen may stimulate a recurrence is appropriate but seems to be unfounded based upon a review of the literature. In fact, it appears that women with breast cancer and on estrogen have a higher survival than those not receiving estrogen.[163] Also, the overall survival in these patients is much better, with a relative risk of 0.55.[172] Because freedom from a recurrence can never be guaranteed, there will be patients who develop recurrent disease while on estrogen. The argument as to whether or not estrogen stimulated the reoccurrence will continue for some time because little information is available on estrogen replacement therapy in this high-risk group. The results of

one observational study with controls demonstrates a good prognosis of patients treated with ERT.[173] A well-conducted epidemiologic study demonstrated that treatment with the equivalent of 0.625 mg of Premarin daily, and the equivalent of 50 mg/day of MPA, reduced the recurrence of breast cancer when compared to controls (Fig 38–26).[174] Given the current literature, it appears that estrogen replacement therapy is not contraindicated in the well-counseled symptomatic menopausal woman with no evidence of active disease. The patient should be thoroughly counseled on the risks versus benefits of estrogen replacement, and should play an active role in the decision.

ESTROGEN REPLACEMENT REGIMENS

Sequential Regimens

Estrogens are given for either the first 21 or 25 days per mo or every day. A progestogen agent is added for 10 to 14 days of the mo. In regimens giving estrogen for 21 or 25 days/mo, the progestogen is given on the terminal 10 to 14 days of that regimen and the patient has a period following the last pill. If the estrogen is given every day, the progestogen agent is usually added on the first 10 to 14 days of the mo and the woman will have a period after the last progestogen pill. This latter regimen is usually easier for women to remember, and the rest period from estrogens in the other regimens has never been shown to have any benefits with either breast or endometrial carcinoma.[175]

Continuous Combined Regimen

In this regimen, the estrogen and progestogen are taken together every day. The vast majority of women will become amenorrheic, and smaller doses of progestogen

(2.5 to 5.0 versus 10 mg medroxyprogesterone acetate) are utilized. Data by Prough et al comparing the bleeding patterns between sequential and continuous combined regimens of Premarin and medroxyprogesterone acetate demonstrated less bleeding with continuous combined regimens. The initial breakthrough bleeding was 40 percent and dropped to 20 percent by 6 mo. The number of bleeding episodes were less on the continuous combined regimen.[176] Those who have breakthrough bleeding find that unacceptable and either prefer to switch to the sequential regimen or discontinue the progestogen or ERT altogether. One small study has shown no increase in hyperplasia when 10 mg of MPA is given for 14 days every 3 mo.[177] This is another acceptable regimen for patients not wishing a monthly bleed or breakthrough bleeding.

Women without a uterus do not need a progestogen. There is no advantage to adding a progestogen to protect breasts, and there are no adequate data to substantiate progestogens added to ERT have any other benefits on osteoporosis. Many patients wish to avoid bleeding and will choose to use unopposed estrogen. Such patients need to have adequate informed consent and an annual biopsy to rule out endometrial hyperplasia and carcinoma. Patients treated with unopposed estrogen have a high rate of breakthrough bleeding.[177]

Endometrial Biopsies. Endometrial biopsies are not generally considered necessary as a pretreatment therapy. The incidence of endometrial hyperplasia or carcinoma is so low that it is not cost effective to perform routine pretreatment biopsies. It may be clinically indicated due to bleeding irregularities, a strong family history, or strong risk factors for endometrial cancer. If bleeding occurs after 7 days of progestogen therapy, the endometrium is usually secretory and biopsy is not necessary.[178] This has been recently challenged.[179] If the patient bleeds while on estrogen alone or in the early part of progestogen therapy, an endometrial biopsy is indicated to rule out endometrial hyperplasia or carcinoma. Patients bleeding heavily for 6 mo have a high probability of submucous fibroids and polyps and should probably have a hysteroscopy or sonohysterography.[180] An endometrial biopsy performed once in patients with persistent breakthrough bleeding is a good idea. It reassures the patient and physician that no pathology exists. Further, biopsies are not indicated unless the clinical presentation changes. A vaginal probe ultrasound can probably be substituted. If the endometrium is less than 5 mm, no further workup is necessary. An endometrial biopsy would be necessary for a thickness greater than 5 mm.

Another reason for not giving progestogens to women without a uterus is that it has a high incidence of negative mood scores.[181] Women also complain of bloating while on progestogens, and a history of premenstrual tension may reoccur in those women who had it prior to menopause.

CONTRAINDICATIONS TO ESTROGEN THERAPY

Estrogens are generally contraindicated in any of the conditions described in the next sections. Interestingly, in no circumstance is an ovariectomy required for any of these circumstances.

Known or Suspected Cancer of the Breast, Except in the Appropriately Selected Patients Treated for Metastatic Disease

The previous section discussed the lack of solid scientific evidence prohibiting the use of estrogens in women with breast cancer.

Women With Known or Suspected Estrogen-Dependent Neoplasia

ERT can be given for both breast and endometrial carcinoma under certain circumstances, as has been outlined in the sections on breast and endometrial cancer.

Known or Suspected Pregnancy

Pregnancy is unlikely in the menopausal patient, and therefore this warning has no relevance. This warning stems from the DES-induced vaginal adenosis and vaginal clear cell carcinoma of the vagina associated with use during pregnancy.

Undiagnosed Abnormal Genital Bleeding

Any abnormal genital bleeding in a menopausal patient is cancer until proven otherwise, and an endometrial biopsy or dilation and curettage (D&C) and hysteroscopy should be performed before initiation of ERT.

Active Thrombophlebitis or Thromboembolic Disorders

Estrogens in high doses do cause thrombosis, but ERT probably does not. Medicolegally, it makes no sense during an active thrombotic episode to give estrogen.

Past History of Thrombophlebitis Thrombosis or Thromboembolic Disorders Associated With Previous Estrogen Use

Again, the doses used in menopause are not associated with thrombosis. Transdermal estrogens are not associated with increased serum clotting parameters and would seem on this basis the preferred estrogen if one absolutely had to give estrogen to these women. Doses as low as 0.625 mg oral conjugated equine estrogens are not thrombotic and could also be given. One publication found no increase in patients with a previous thrombosis.[133] There are no studies demonstrating these patients to be at increased risk due to ERT. It may be medicolegally prudent to use transdermal estrogens in such patients if the decision to use ERT has been made.

The above are considered absolute contraindications, and the practicing physician should not give estrogen to such patients without a careful informed consent and exhaustion of other alternatives. In the next section, non-estrogen alternatives to ERT will be discussed.

MANAGEMENT OF MENOPAUSE WHEN ESTROGEN IS CONTRAINDICATED

In a prior section, contraindications to estrogen therapy were discussed. Management of menopausal symptoms in these patients poses a significant problem. A number of agents are available that can be used for vasomotor symptoms and osteoporosis prevention. Unfortunately, no alternative is available that not only treats vasomotor symptoms but also beneficially affects both cardiovascular and osteoporosis risk.

Treatment of Vasomotor Symptoms

A number of both steroid and nonsteroidal agents are available to treat vasomotor symptoms. Common problems encountered when reviewing the data include a prominent placebo effect and interstudy variability. Of the alternative agents, the most commonly employed and most effective appears to be medroxyprogesterone acetate. Oral and depot formulations appear to be equally effective.

In a double-blind crossover placebo study, 20 mg medroxyprogesterone acetate per day decreased vasomotor flushes by 90 percent, decreased temperature elevations by 67 percent, and decreased mean serum luteinizing hormone (LH) levels by 21 percent.[182] Another randomized double-blind placebo-controlled study examined the effectiveness of three different (50, 100, and 150 mg) depot medroxyprogesterone acetate doses in relieving vasomotor symptoms.[183] All doses used were effective, although the best results were obtained in patients receiving 150 mg. In these patients, hot flushes decreased from an average of 45/wk pretreatment to 5 after 12 wk of therapy. In a randomized study comparing 150 mg depot medroxyprogesterone acetate with 0.625 mg Premarin, both agents were equally as effective in relieving hot flushes.[184] The factors limiting widespread use of these agents are their side effects, which can include irregular uterine bleeding (43 percent), depression (10 percent), headache (7 percent), and vaginal atrophy.[185] Megace 20 mg bid has also been used to prevent hot flushes in 70 to 85 percent of menopausal women and hypogonadal males.[186,187]

Other agents that can be used to treat hot flushes include clonidine, methyldopa, danazol, clomiphene citrate, tamoxifen, naloxone, and bellergal. Success with clonidine has been variable depending upon the investigator. It appears that a minimum daily dose of 0.1 mg is required. Most patients require a higher dose and up to 0.4 mg/day may be necessary.[188] The side effects encountered with higher doses can be significant and can include dry mouth, insomnia, and hypotension. Investigators report up to a 60 percent improvement in vasomotor symptoms.[189] Clonidine relieves hot flushes by diminishing peripheral vascular responsiveness to vasodilator and vasoconstrictor stimuli. Clonidine does not affect LH levels and patients on this treatment will be at risk for vaginal atrophy and osteoporosis.

Methyldopa has been used to treat vasomotor symptoms with good results. In a double-blind placebo-controlled study, women on 250 to 500 mg/day noted a 50 to 60 percent improvement in hot flushes and a 77 percent improvement in well-being.[190] Unfortunately, the large percentage of patients complaining of side effects (fatigue 50, dry mouth 30 percent) limits methyldopa's usefulness. In a small, randomized, double-blinded study of eight patients receiving 100 mg danazol a day, three patients noted 98.5, 80, and 34.7 percent fewer hot flushes, respectively.[191] These results need to be confirmed in a larger group of patients before danazol can be routinely recommended as an alternative to estrogen.

Other drugs that have been advocated in the treatment of hot flushes include naloxone and bellergal. Naloxone is of limited usefulness because it must be given intravenously. Also, naloxone infusion does not appear to effect skin temperature or peripheral vascular resistance, suggesting that it is not effective in relieving hot flushes.[192] In our experience, bellergal, a combination drug consisting of atropine, ergotamine, and phenobarbital, is not useful in treating vasomotor symptoms.

Treatment of Osteoporosis

Maintenance of bone in these patients poses a real problem. A number of agents can be used, including medroxyprogesterone acetate, exercise, calcium supplements, fluoride, vitamin D, calcitonin, and the diphosphinates alendronate and etidronate.

Progestins. A great deal has been written about the beneficial effects of combination estrogen–progestin regimens on bone mineral content, but relatively little is known about progestins when used alone. Lindsay has suggested that progestins may act by increasing new bone formation rather than decreasing bone resorption.[37] Women treated with either 0.625 mg Premarin or 150 mg depot medroxyprogesterone acetate demonstrated a similar decline in urinary calcium/creatinine and hydroxyproline/creatinine ratios. Given the limited information available, it appears that progestins may be helpful in preventing bone loss and should be used if not contraindicated.

Exercise. There is increasing evidence that exercise can be beneficial to bone. Unfortunately, it is difficult to compare studies, because they all employ different exercise regimens. The type of exercise is important, and walking or dynamic bone loading exercises seem to be the best.[193–195] Exercise also gives one a sense of well-being.

Calcium. The average daily calcium intake for adult women is 500 mg. This is well below the minimum daily requirement of 1000 mg for premenopausal women and 1500 mg for postmenopausal women not receiving estrogen. High-dose dietary calcium supplementation does not appear to be as effective an alternative to estrogen or progestin replacement in the prevention of early postmenopausal bone loss.[196] In fact, women receiving high-dose calcium (2000 mg/day) continue to lose bone at a rate similar to controls not receiving treatment.[196] Calcium should be used in conjunction with other therapies to maximize their beneficial effects.

Tamoxifen. Tamoxifen is both an estrogen and an anti-estrogen. It has been demonstrated in many studies to prevent bone loss in menopausal breast cancer patients. It may cause bone loss in premenopausal women.[197,198]

Fluoride. Sodium fluoride (75 mg daily) is a potent stimulator of bone formation and increases in trabecular bone density have been observed with this therapy. Although trabecular bone density increases, cortical bone density decreases. There is also evidence that the new bone formed is structurally abnormal. Clinical evidence that confirms these theories includes the fact that new vertebral fractures are the same in study and control groups and that the number of non-vertebral fractures is higher in the treatment group.[199] Side effects with fluoride therapy are prominent and limit its use. Pak et al suggested that intermittent slow-release fluoride (25 mg bid) and calcium supplementation (1500 mg daily) produces structurally normal bone and decreases vertebral fractures.[200] Also, the slow-release formulation markedly decreases side effects. Before widespread use of this regimen is advocated, these findings must be confirmed by other investigators.

Vitamin D. Although few scientific data are available, a number of therapeutic regimens have included vitamin D. It does not appear that vitamin D is useful in the routine management of osteoporosis.

Calcitonin. Synthetic salmon calcitonin has been approved by the Food and Drug Administration for treat-

ment of postmenopausal osteoporosis. Calcitonin binds to high-affinity receptors on osteoclasts and profoundly inhibits their activity. Long-term studies (2 yr) using 50 to 100 IU three times per wk demonstrated a reduction in bone loss comparable to that seen with estradiol.[201] Side effects are usually mild (dizziness, flushing, gastrointestinal upset, nausea) and can be minimized by starting with a low dose (10 to 25 IU). Unfortunately, it is expensive and is given as a subcutaneous injection or an intranasal spray.

Biphosphonates. Biphosphonates are useful in the treatment of osteoporosis.[202,203] Biphosphonates appear to exert their effects by inhibiting osteoclast-mediated bone resorption. Watts et al in a randomized placebo-controlled multicenter study of 429 osteoporotic patients receiving intermittent cyclic phosphate and etidronate therapy, demonstrated increased bone mass and decreased rates of new vertebral fractures.[202] Each study patient received 1.0 g phosphate twice daily for 3 days, and 400 mg etidronate for the next 14 days, followed by 500 mg calcium daily for the next 74 days. This cycle was repeated every 91 days.

Alendronate (Fosamax) at a dose of 10 mg/day prevents bone loss and prevents fractures at all sites in patients with osteoporosis and at least one vertebral fracture.[204] Recently, a 5-mg dose has been shown to be as effective in preventing bone loss as estrogen.[205] Esophagitis has been reported if alendronate is not taken correctly.[206] Fosamax is the drug of choice when estrogen is contraindicated, refused, or not tolerated.

Cardioprotection

Patients given tamoxifen 20 mg/day had a lower rate of myocardial infarction than those given placebo. Tamoxifen is an anti-oxidant and lowers LDL and lipoprotein (a).[207–210] Raloxifene, currently an experimental drug related to tamoxifen, may have similar properties.[211] Exercise and a low-cholesterol and low saturated-fat diet should also be prescribed for women unable to tolerate estrogen to improve cardiac protection.

Summary of Non-Estrogen Alternatives

The suggestions in this section should not be considered alternatives to estrogen; they are indicated only when estrogen is contraindicated, refused, or not tolerated. No other agent gives all the benefits of estrogen such as cardioprotection, osteoporosis prevention, urogenital atrophy relief, and possibly a delay in the onset of Alzheimer's disease as well as colon and rectal cancer. Most patients with breast cancer are treated with tamoxifen and therefore have osteoporosis protection and cardiac protection. Tamoxifen does increase the rate of endometrial cancer. The endometrium should be monitored by an annual endometrial biopsy. Alendronate protects only bone.

CONCLUSION

Menopause is a state of ovarian failure with reduced estrogen levels. Many adverse consequences of these low estrogen levels have been discussed and how ERT can prevent them. The major problems of menopause are increased cardiovascular disease and osteoporotic fractures, both of which are lethal and both of which can be reduced with a concomitant reduction in mortality by ERT.

Estrogens do have some adverse side effects. Endometrial cancer is the main one, but it can be reduced by concomitant administration of progestogen. The link between breast cancer and estrogens is not definitely established and appears to be limited to patients who used high doses for long periods of time.

What is most important in putting together the role of ERT in the menopausal patient is the overall risk:benefit ratio. Even taking into account a small increase in breast cancer, an increase in endometrial cancer, and cholelithiasis, the cardiovascular and osteoporotic benefits far outweigh any of the adverse consequences.[212] The risk:benefit ratio is very much in favor of the liberal use of estrogen in menopausal women.[79,213]

REFERENCES

1. Lauritzen C. Clinical use of oestrogens and progestogens. *Maturitas.* 12:199, 1990
2. Miodrag A, Castleden CM, Vallance TR. Sex hormones and the female urinary tract. *Drugs.* 36:491, 1988
3. Notelovitz M. Gynecologic problems of menopausal women, part 1. Changes in genital tissues. *Geriatrics.* 33:24, 1978
4. Ginkel P, Soper D, Bump R, Dalton H. Vaginal flora in postmenopausal women: The effect of estrogen replacement. *Infect Dis Obstet Gynecol.* 1:94, 1993
5. Geola FL, Frumar AM, Tataryn IV, et al. Biological effects of various doses of conjugated equine estrogens in postmenopausal women. *J Clin Endocrinol Metab.* 51:620, 1980
6. Biesland HO. Urethral sphincteric insufficiency in postmenopausal females: Treatment with phenylpropanolamine and estriol separately and in combination. A urodynamic and clinical evaluation. *Urol Int.* 39:211, 1984
7. Jolleys JV. Reported prevalence of urinary incontinence in women in a general practice. *Br Med J (Clin Res).* 296:1300, 1988
8. Fantl J, Bump R, Robinson D, et al. Efficacy of estrogen supplementation in the treatment of urinary incontinence. The Continence Program for Women Research Group. *Obstet Gynecol.* 88:745, 1996
9. Fantl J, Cardozo L, McClish D. Estrogen therapy in the management of urinary incontinence in postmenopausal women: A meta-analysis. First Report of the Hormones and Urogenital Therapy Committee. *Obstet Gynecol.* 83:12, 1994
10. Ishigooka M, Hashimoto T, Tomaru M, et al. Effect of hormonal replacement therapy in postmenopausal women with chronic irritative voiding symptoms. *Int Urogynecol J.* 5:208, 1994
11. Raz R, Stamm WE. A controlled trial of intravaginal estriol in postmenopausal women with recurrent urinary tract infections. *N Engl J Med.* 329:753, 1993
12. Hassager C. Soft tissue body composition during prevention and treatment of postmenopausal osteoporosis assessed by photon absorptiometry. *Dan Med Bull.* 38:380, 1991
13. Kritz-Silverstein D, Barrett-Connor E. Long-term postmenopausal hormone use, obesity, and fat distribution in older women. *JAMA.* 275:46, 1996
14. Rubin GL, Peterson HB, Lee MD, et al. Estrogen replacement therapy and the risk of endometrial cancer: Remaining controversies. *Am J Obstet Gynecol.* 162:148, 1990
15. Brincat M, Moniz CJ, Studd JWW, et al. Long-term effects of the menopause and sex hormones on skin thickness. *Br J Obstet Gynaecol.* 92:256, 1985
16. Maheux R, Naud F, Rioux M, et al. A randomized, double-blind, placebo-controlled study on the effect of conjugated estrogens on skin thickness. *Am J Obstet Gynecol.* 170:642, 1994
17. Melton LJ, Wahner HW, Richelson LS, et al. Osteoporosis and the risk of hip fracture. *Am J Epidemiol.* 124:254, 1986
18. Laufer LR, Davidson BJ, Ross RK, et al. Physical characteristics and sex hormone levels in patients with osteoporotic hip fractures or endometrial cancer. *Am J Obstet Gynecol.* 145:585, 1983
19. Cauley JA, Gutai JP, Sandler RB, et al. The relationship of endogenous estrogen to bone density and bone area in normal postmenopausal women. *Am J Epidemiol.* 124:752, 1986
20. Johnston C, Hui SL, Witt RM, et al. Early menopausal changes in bone mass and sex steroids. *J Clin Endocrinol Metab.* 61:905, 1985
21. Jensen JS, Tondevold E. Mortality after hip fractures. *Acta Orthop Scand.* 50:161, 1979
22. Alfram PA. An epidemiologic study of cervical and trochanteric fractures of the femur in an urban population. *Acta Orthop Scand.* 65(suppl): 9, 1964
23. Rodysill KJ. Postmenopausal osteoporosis—Intervention and prophylaxis. A review. *J Chron Dis.* 40:743, 1987
24. Riggs BL, Melton LJ III. Involutional osteoporosis. *N Engl J Med.* 314:1676, 1986
25. Nachtigall LE, Nachtigall RH, Nachtigall RD, Beckman EM. Estrogen replacement therapy I: A 10 year prospective study in the relationship to osteoporosis. *Obstet Gynecol.* 53:277, 1979
26. Hutchinson TA, Polansy SM, Feinstein AF. Postmenopausal oestrogens protect against fractures of hip and distal radius: A case-control study. *Lancet.* 2:705, 1979
27. Ettinger B, Genant HK, Cann CE. Long-term estrogen replacement therapy prevents bone loss and fractures. *Ann Intern Med.* 102:319, 1985

28. Kiel DP, Felson DT, Anderson JJ, et al. Hip fracture and the use of estrogens in postmenopausal women. *N Engl J Med.* 317:1169, 1987

29. Weiss NS, Ure CL, Ballard JH, et al. Decreased risk of fractures of the hip and lower forearm with post-menopausal use of estrogen. *N Engl J Med.* 303:1195, 1980

30. Kreiger N, Kelsey JL, Holford TR, O'Connor T. An epidemiologic study of hip fracture in postmenopausal women. *Am J Epidemiol.* 116:141, 1982

31. Lindsay R, Hart DM, Forrest C, Baird C. Prevention of spinal osteoporosis in oophorectomized women. *Lancet.* 2:1152, 1980

32. Al Azzawi F, Hart DM, Lindsay R. Long-term effects of oestrogen replacement therapy on bone mass as measured by dual photon absorptiometry. *Br Med J.* 294:1261, 1987

33. Cann CE, Genant HK, Ettinger B, Gordan GS. Spinal mineral loss in oophorectomized women. *JAMA.* 244:2056, 1980

34. Roos BO. Dual photon absorptiometry in lumbar vertebrae II. Precision and reproducibility. *Acta Radiol Ther Phys Biol.* 13:291, 1974

35. Roos BO, Skoldborn H. Dual photon absorptiometry in lumbar vertebrae I. Theory and method. *Acta Radiol Ther Phys Biol.* 13:266, 1974

36. Lindsay R, Hart DM, Aitken JM, et al. Long-term prevention of postmenopausal osteoporosis by oestrogen: Evidence for an increased bone mass after delayed onset of oestrogen treatment. *Lancet.* 1:1038, 1976

37. Lindsay R, Hart DM, Abdalla H, Al-Azzawi F. Interrelationship of bone loss and its prevention and fracture expression. In: Christiansen C, ed. *Osteoporosis I—International Symposium on Osteoporosis.* Copenhagen, Osteo Press, 1987: 508–512

38. Christiansen C, Christensen MS, Transbol I. Bone mass in postmenopausal women after withdrawal of œstrogen/gestagen replacement therapy. *Lancet.* 1:459, 1981

39. Lindsay R, Hart DM, Clark DM. The minimum effective dose of estrogen for prevention of postmenopausal bone loss. *Obstet Gynecol.* 63:759, 1984

40. Riis BJ, Thomsen K, Strom V, Christiansen C. The effect of percutaneous estradiol and natural progesterone on post-menopausal bone loss. *Am J Obstet Gynecol.* 156:61, 1987

41. Christiansen C, Redbro P. Does oestriol add to the beneficial effect of combined hormonal prophylaxis against early postmenopausal osteoporosis? *Br J Obstet Gynaecol.* 91:489, 1984

42. Ettinger B, Genant HK, Cann CE. Postmenopausal bone loss is prevented by treatment with low-dosage estrogen with calcium. *Ann Intern Med.* 106:40 1987

43. Gordon T, Kannel WB, Hjortland MC, McNamara PM. Menopause and coronary heart disease: The Framingham study. *Ann Intern Med.* 89:157, 1978

44. Lipid Research Clinics Program. *Lipid Research Clinics Population Studies Data Book*, vol. 1. *The Prevalence Study.* Washington, D.C., U.S. Department of Health and Human Services, Public Health Service, National Institutes of Health. NIH Publications, 1980, no. 80-1527

45. Matthews KA, Meilahn E, Kuller LH, et al. Menopause and Risk Factors for Coronary Heart Disease. *N Engl J Med.* 321:641, 1989

46. Goebelsmann U, Mashchak A, Mishell DR. Comparison of hepatic impact of oral and vaginal administration of ethinyl estradiol. *Am J Obstet Gynecol.* 151:868, 1985

47. Colditz GA, Willett WC, Stampfer MJ, et al. Menopause and the risk of coronary heart disease in women. *N Engl J Med.* 316:1105, 1987

48. Fahraeus L, Wallentin L. High density lipoprotein sub-fractions during oral and cutaneous administration of 17β-estradiol to menopausal women. *J Clin Endocrinol Metab* 56:797, 1983

49. Chetkowski RJ, Meldrum DR, Steingold KA. Biologic effects of transdermal estradiol. *N Engl J Med.* 314:1615, 1986

50. Slowinska-Srzednicka J, Zgliczynski S, Chotkowska E. Effects of transdermal 17β-oestradiol combined with oral progestogen on lipids and lipoproteins in hypercholesterolaemic postmenopausal women. *J Int Med.* 234:447, 1993

51. Glueck CJ, Scheel D, Fishback J. Estrogen-induced pancreatitis in patients with previously covert familial type V hyperlipoproteinemia. *Metabolism.* 21:657, 1972

52. Watts NB, Notelovitz M, Timmons MC, et al. Comparison of oral estrogens and estrogens plus androgen on bone mineral density, menopausal symptoms, and lipid-lipoprotein profiles in surgical menopause. *Obstet Gynecol.* 85:529, 1995

53. McFarland KF, Boniface ME, Hornung CA, et al. Risk factors and noncontraceptive estrogen use in women with and without coronary artery disease. *Am Heart J.* 117:1209, 1989

54. Sullivan JM, Vander Zwagg R, Hughes JP, et al. Postmenopausal estrogen use and coronary atherosclerosis. *Ann Intern Med.* 108:358, 1988

55. Gruchow HW, Anderson AJ, Barboriak JJ, Sobocinski KA. Postmenopausal use of estrogen and occlusion of coronary arteries. *Am Heart J.* 115:954, 1988

56. Criqui MH, Suarez L, Barrett-Connor E, et al. Postmenopausal estrogen use and mortality: Results from a prospective study in a defined, homogeneous community. *Am J Epidemiol.* 128:606, 1988

57. Bush TL, Barrett-Connor E, Cowan LD, et al. Cardiovascular mortality and noncontraceptive use of estrogen in women: Results from the 1987 Lipid Research Clinics Program Followup Study. *Circulation.* 75:1102, 1988

58. Barrett-Connor E, Wingard DL, Criqui MH. Postmenopausal estrogen use and heart disease risk factors in the 1980s. *JAMA.* 261:2095, 1989

59. Bush TL, Cowan LD, Barrett-Connor E, et al. Estrogen use and all-cause mortality: Preliminary results from the Lipid Research Clinics program follow-up study. *JAMA.* 249:903, 1983

60. Bain C, Willett W, Hennekens CH, et al. Use of postmenopausal hormones and risk of myocardial infarction. *Circulation.* 64:42, 1981

61. Adam S, Williams V, Vessey MP. Cardiovascular disease and hormone replacement treatment: A pilot case-control study. *Br Med J.* 282:1277, 1981

62. Burch JC, Byrd BF, Vaughn WK. The effects of long-term estrogens on hysterectomized women. *Am J Obstet Gynecol.* 118:778, 1974

63. Bush TL, Barrett-Connor E. Noncontraceptive estrogen use and cardiovascular disease. *Epidemiol Rev.* 7:80, 1985

64. Henderson BE, Ross RK, Paganini-Hill A, Mack TM. Estrogen use and cardiovascular disease. *Am J Obstet Gynecol*. 154:1181, 1986

65. Hunt K, Vessey M, McPherson K, Coleman M. Long-term surveillance of mortality and cancer incidence in women receiving hormone replacement therapy. *Br J Obstet Gynecol*. 94:620, 1987

66. Henderson BE, Paganini-Hill A, Ross RK. Estrogen replacement therapy and protection from acute myocardial infarction. *Am J Obstet Gynecol*. 159:312, 1988

67. Gordon T, Kannel WB, Hjordand MC, McNamara PM. Menopause and coronary heart disease: The Framingham study. *Ann Intern Med*. 89:157, 1978

68. Jick H, Dinan B, Rothman KJ. Noncontraceptive estrogen and non-fatal myocardial infarction. *JAMA*. 239:1407, 1978

69. Pfeffer RI, Wipple GH, Kurosaki TT, Chapman JM. Coronary risk and estrogen use in postmenopausal women. *Am J Epidemiol*. 107:479, 1978

70. Petitti DB, Wingerd J, Pellegrin F, Ramchuran S. Risk of vascular disease in women: Smoking oral contraceptives, noncontraceptive estrogens, and other factors. *JAMA*. 242:1150, 1979

71. Nachtigall LE, Nachtigall RH, Nachtigall RD, Beckman EM. Estrogen replacement therapy II: A prospective study in the relationship to carcinoma and cardiovascular and metabolic problems. *Obstet Gynecol*. 54:74, 1979

72. Stampfer MJ, Willett WC, Colditz GA, et al. A prospective study of postmenopausal estrogen therapy and coronary heart disease. *N Engl J Med*. 313:1044, 1985

73. Ross RK, Paganini-Hill A, Mack TM, Henderson BE. Cardiovascular benefits of estrogen replacement therapy. *Am J Obstet Gynecol*. 160:1069, 1979

74. Rosenberg L, Armstrong B, Jick H. Myocardial infarction and estrogen therapy in postmenopausal women. *N Engl J Med*. 294:1256, 1976

75. Rosenberg L, Sloane D, Shapiro S, et al. Noncontraceptive estrogens and myocardial infarction in young women. *JAMA*. 224:339, 1980

76. Ross RK, Paganini-Hill A, Mack TM, et al. Menopausal oestrogen therapy and protection from death from ischemic heart disease. *Lancet*. 1:858, 1981

77. Szklo M, Tonascia J, Gordis L, Bloom I. Estrogen use and myocardial infarction risk: A case-control study. *Prev Med*. 13:510, 1984

78. Wilson PWF, Garrison RJ, Castelli WP. Postmenopausal estrogen use, cigarette smoking, and cardiovascular morbidity in women over 50. *N Engl J Med*. 313:1038, 1985

79. Henderson BE, Paganini-Hill A, Ross RK. Decreased mortality in users of estrogen replacement therapy. *Arch Intern Med*. 151:75, 1991

80. Barrett-Connor E, Bush TL. Estrogen and coronary heart disease in women. *JAMA*. 265:1861, 1991

81. Sullivan JM, Vander Zwaag R, Hughes JP, et al. Estrogen replacement and coronary artery disease: Effect on survival in postmenopausal women. *Arch Intern Med*. 150:2557, 1990

82. Adams MR, Clarkson TB, Koritnik DR, Nash HA. Contraceptive steroids and coronary artery atherosclerosis in cynomologous macaques. *Fertil Steril*. 47:1010, 1987

83. Barrett-Connor E, Wingard DL, Criqui MH. Postmenopausal estrogen use and heart disease risk factors in the 1980s. Rancho Bernardo, Calif revisited. *JAMA*. 261:2095, 1989

84. Ravi Subbiah MT, Kessel B, Agrawal M, et al. Antioxidant potential of specific estrogens on lipid peroxidation. *J Clin Endocrinol Metab*. 77:1095, 1993

85. Steinberg D, Parthasarathy S, Carew TE, et al. Modifications of low-density lipoprotein that increases its atherogenicity. *N Engl J Med*. 320:915, 1989

86. Hirvonen E, Malkonen M, Manninen V. Effects of different progestogens of lipoproteins during postmenopausal replacement therapy. *N Engl J Med*. 304:560, 1981

87. The Writing Group for the PEPI Trial. Effects of estrogen or estrogen/progestin regimens on heart disease risk factors in postmenopausal women. The Postmenopausal Estrogen/Progestin Interventions (PEPI) Trial. *JAMA*. 273:199, 1995

88. Grodstein F, Stampfer MJ, Manson JE, et al. Postmenopausal estrogen and progestin use and the risk of cardiovascular disease. *N Engl J Med*. 335:453, 1996

89. Falkeborn M, Persson I, Adami H, et al. The risk of acute myocardial infarction after oestrogen and oestrogen-progestogen replacement. *Gynaecology*. 99:821, 1992

90. Hunt K, Vessey M, McPherson K, Coleman M. Long-term surveillance of mortality and cancer incidence in women receiving hormone replacement therapy. *Br J Obstet Gynaecol*. 94:620, 1987

91. Psaty B, Heckbert S, Atkins D, et al. The risk of myocardial infarction associated with the combined use of estrogens and progestins in postmenopausal women. *Arch Intern Med*. 154:1333, 1994

92. Rosano G, Sarrel P, Poole-Wilson P, Collins P. Beneficial effect of oestrogen on exercise-induced myocardial ischaemia in women with coronary artery disease. *Lancet*. 342:133, 1993

93. Croft P, Hannaford PC. Risk factors for acute myocardial infarction in women: Evidence from the Royal College of General Practitioners' oral contraception study. *Br Med J*. 298:165, 1989

94. Falkeborn M, Ingemar P, Terent A, et al. Hormone replacement therapy and the risk of stroke: Follow up of a population-based cohort in Sweden. *Arch Intern Med*. 153:1201, 1993

95. Boysen G, Jorgen N, Appleyard M, et al. Stroke incidence and risk factors for stroke in Copenhagen, Denmark. *Stroke*. 19:1345, 1988

96. Paganini-Hill A, Ross RK, Henderson BE. Postmenopausal oestrogen treatment and stroke: A prospective study. *BMJ*. 297:20, 1988

97. Petitti DB, Wingerd J, Pellegrin F, Ramcharan S. Risk of vascular disease in women: Smoking, oral contraceptives, noncontraceptive estrogens, and other factors. *JAMA*. 242:1150, 1979

98. Rijpkema AHM, van der Sanden AA, Roijs AHC. Effects of postmenopausal oestrogen–progestogen replacement therapy on serum lipids and lipoproteins: A review. *Maturitas*. 12:259, 1990

99. Sherwin B. Estrogen, the brain, and memory. *Menopause*. 3:97, 1996

100. Gould E, Woolley C, Frankfurt M, McEwen B. Gonadal steroids regulate dendritic spine density in hippocampal pyramidal cells in adulthood. *Neurosci.* 10:1286, 1990

101. Paganini-Hill A, Henderson V. Estrogen deficiency and risk of Alzheimer's disease in women. *Am J Epidemiol.* 140:256, 1994

102. Tang M, Jacobs D, Stern Y, et al. Effect on oestrogen during menopause on risk and age at onset of Alzheimer's disease. *Lancet.* 348:1, 1996

103. Ohkura T, Isse K, Akazawa K, et al. Low-dose estrogen replacement therapy for Alzheimer's disease in women. *Menopause.* 1:125, 1994

104. Schneider L, Farlow M, Henderson V, Pogoda J. Effects of estrogen replacement therapy on response to tacrine in patients with Alzheimer's disease. *Neurology.* 46:1580, 1996

105. Newcomb PA, Storer BE. Postmenopausal hormone use and risk of large-bowel cancer. *J Natl Cancer Inst.* 87:1067, 1995

106. Calle EE, Miracle-McMahill HL, Thun MJ, et al. Estrogen replacement therapy and risk of fatal colon cancer in a prospective cohort of postmenopausal women. *J Natl Cancer Inst.* 87:517, 1995

107. Domenico MD, Castoria G, Bilancio A, et al. Estradiol activation of human colon carcinoma-derived Caco-2 cell growth. *Cancer Res.* 56:4516, 1996

108. McMichael AJ, Potter JD. Reproduction, endogenous and exogenous sex hormones, and colon cancer: A review and hypothesis. *J Natl Cancer Inst.* 65:1201, 1980

109. Hulka BS. Replacement estrogens and risk of gynecologic cancers and breast cancer. *Cancer.* 60:1960, 1987

110. Horwitz RI, Feinstein AR. Alternative analytic methods for case-control studies of estrogens and endometrial cancer. *N Engl J Med.* 299:1089, 1978

111. Horwitz RI, Feinstein AR, Horowitz SM, Robroy SJ. Necropsy diagnosis of endometrial cancer and detection bias in case control studies. *Lancet.* 1:66, 1981

112. Gambrell RD Jr. Prevention of endometrial cancer with progestins. *Maturitas.* 8:159, 1986

113. Persson I, Adami HO, Bergkvist L, et al. Risk of endometrial cancer after treatment with oestrogen alone or in conjunction with progestogens: Results of a prospective study. *Br J Med.* 298:147, 1989

114. The Writing Group for the PEPI Trial. Effects of hormone replacement therapy on endometrial histology in postmenopausal women. The Postmenopausal Estrogen/Progestin Interventions (PEPI) Trial. *JAMA.* 275:370, 1996

115. Woodruff J, Pickar J. Incidence of endometrial hyperplasia in postmenopausal women taking conjugated estrogens (Premarin) with medroxyprogesterone acetate or conjugated estrogens alone. *Am J Obstet Gynecol.* 170:1213, 1994

116. Collins J, Donner A, Allen LH, Adams O. Oestrogen use and survival in endometrial cancer. *Lancet.* 61:964, 1980

117. Chu J, Schweid AI, Weiss NS. Survival among women with endometrial cancer: A comparison of estrogen users and nonusers. *Am J Obstet Gynecol.* 143:569, 1982

118. Perrson I, Adami H, Bergkvist L, et al. Risk of endometrial cancer after treatment with oestrogens alone or in conjunction with progesterones: Results of a prospective study. *BMJ.* 147, 1989

119. Whitehead MI, Townsend PT, Pryse-Davies J, et al. Effects of estrogens and progestins on the biochemistry and morphology of the postmenopausal endometrium. *N Engl J Med.* 305:1599, 1983

120. Weinstein L, Bewtra C, Gallagher JC. Evaluation of a continuous low dose regimen of estrogen–progestin for treatment of the menopausal patient. *Am J Obstet Gynecol.* 162:1534, 1990

121. Whitehead MI, Studd J. Selection of patients for treatment: Which therapy and for how long? In: Studd J. Whitehead MI, eds. *The Menopause.* Blackwell Scientific, Oxford, U.K., 1988: 116–129

122. Creasman WT, Henderson D, Hinshaw W, Clarke-Pearson DL. Estrogen replacement therapy in the patient treated for endometrial cancer. *Obstet Gynecol.* 67:326, 1986

123. Lee RB, Burke TW, Park RC. Estrogen replacement therapy following treatment for stage I endometrial cancer. *Gynecol Oncol.* 36:189, 1989

124. American College of Obstetricians and Gynecologists. Estrogen replacement therapy and endometrial cancer. Committee opinion: Committee on Gynecologic Practice. 126, 1993

125. Chapman JA, DiSaia PJ, Osann K, et al. Estrogen replacement in surgical stage I and II endometrial cancer survivors. *Am J Obstet Gynecol.* 175:1195, 1996

126. Bennion LJ, Knowler WS, Mou DM, et al. Development of lithogenic bile during puberty in Pima indians. *N Engl J Med.* 300:873, 1979

127. Henriksson P, Einarsson K, Eriksson A, et al. Estrogen-induced gallstone formation in males. Relation to changes in serum and biliary lipids during hormonal treatment of prostatic carcinoma. *J Clin Invest.* 84:811, 1989

128. Everson GT, McKinley C, Kern F Jr. Mechanisms of gallstone formation in women. Effects of exogenous estrogen (Premarin) and dietary cholesterol on hepatic lipid metabolism. *J Clin Invest.* 87:237, 1991

129. Honore LH. Increased incidence of symptomatic cholesterol cholelithiasis in perimenopausal women receiving estrogen replacement therapy. A retrospective study. *J Reprod Med.* 25:187, 1980

130. Boston Collaborative Drug Surveillance Program, Boston University Medical Center. Surgically confirmed gallbladder disease, venous thromboembolism, and breast tumors in relation to postmenopausal estrogen use. *N Engl J Med.* 290:15, 1974

131. Kakar F, Weiss NS, Strite SA. Non-contraceptive estrogen use and the risk of gallstone disease in women. *Am J Public Health.* 78:564, 1988

132. Royal College of General Practitioners Oral Contraceptives and Health. An interim report from the oral contraceptive study of the Royal College of General Practitioners. New York, N.Y., Pitman Medical Publishing, 1974

133. Devor M, Barrett-Connor E, Renvall M, et al. Estrogen replacement therapy and the risk of venous thrombosis. *Am J Med.* 92:275, 1992

134. Nachtigall LE, Nachtigall RH, Nachtigall RD, Beckman E. Estrogen replacement therapy II: A prospective study in the relationship to carcinoma and cardiovascular and metabolic problems. *Obstet Gynecol.* 54:74, 1979

135. Pettiti D, Wingerd J, Pellegrin F, Ramcharan S. Risk of vascular disease in women smoking, oral contraceptives, noncontraceptive estrogens, and other factors. *JAMA.* 242:1150, 1979

136. Daly E, Vessey M, Hawkins M, et al. Risk of venous thromboembolism in users of hormone replacement therapy. *Lancet.* 348:977, 1996

137. Grodstein F, Stampfer M, Goldhaber S, et al. Prospective study of exogenous hormones and risk of pulmonary embolism in women. *Lancet.* 348:981, 1996

138. Jick H, Derby L, Myers M, et al. Risk of hospital admission for idiopathic venous thromboembolism among users of postmenopausal oestrogens. *Lancet.* 348:981, 1996

139. Nachtigall LE, Nachtigall RH, Nachtigall RD, Beckman EM. Estrogen replacement therapy II: A prospective study in the relationship to carcinoma and cardiovascular and metabolic problems. *Obstet Gynecol.* 54:74, 1979

140. Hassager C, Riis BJ, Strom V, et al. The long-term effect of oral and percutaneous estradiol on plasma renin substrate and blood pressure. *Circulation.* 76:753, 1987

141. Hassager C, Christiansen C. Blood pressure during oestrogen/progestogen substitution therapy in healthy postmenopausal women. *Maturitas.* 9:315, 1988

142. Wren BG, Routledge AD. The effect of type and dose of oestrogen on the blood pressure of post-menopausal women. *Maturitas.* 5:135, 1983

143. Sartwell PE, Arthes FG, Tonascia JA. Exogenous hormones, reproductive history, and breast cancer. *J Natl Cancer Inst.* 59:1589, 1977

144. Kelsey JL, Fischer DB, Holford TR, et al. Exogenous estrogens and other factors in the epidemiology of breast cancer. *J Natl Cancer Inst.* 67:327, 1981

145. Sherman B, Wallace R, Bean J. Estrogen use and breast cancer. *Cancer.* 51:1527, 1983

146. Horwitz RJ, Stewart KR. Effect of clinical features on the association of estrogens and breast cancer. *Am J Med.* 76:192, 1984

147. Kaufman DW, Miller DR, Rosenberg L, et al. Noncontraceptive estrogen use and the risk of breast cancer. *JAMA.* 252:63, 1984

148. McDonald JA, Weiss NS, Daling JR, et al. Menopausal estrogen use and the risk of breast cancer. *Breast Cancer Res Treat.* 7:193, 1986

149. Gambrell RD Jr, Maier RC, Sanders BI. Decreased incidence of breast cancer in postmenopausal estrogen–progestogen users. *Obstet Gynecol.* 62:435, 1983

150. Buring JE, Hennekens CH, Lipnick RH, et al. A prospective cohort study of postmenopausal hormone use and risk of breast cancer in US women. *Am J Epidemiol.* 125:939, 1987

151. Dupont WD, Page DL. Menopausal estrogen replacement therapy and breast cancer. *Arch Intern Med.* 151:67, 1991

152. Hammond CB, Jelovsek FR, Lee KL, et al. Effects of long-term estrogen replacement therapy. *Am J Obstet Gynecol.* 133:537, 1979

153. Colditz G, Hankinson S, Hunter D, et al. The use of estrogens and progestins and the risk of breast cancer in postmenopausal women. *N Engl J Med.* 332:1589, 1995

154. Stanford J, Weiss N, Voight L, et al. Combined estrogen and progestin hormone replacement therapy in relation to risk of breast cancer in middle-aged women. *JAMA.* 274:137, 1995

155. Hulka BS, Chambless LE, Dembner DC, Wilkinson WE. Breast cancer and estrogen replacement therapy. *Am J Obstet Gynecol.* 143:638, 1982

156. La Vecchia C, Decarli A, Parazzini F, et al. Noncontraceptive estrogens and the risk of breast cancer in women. *Int J Cancer.* 38:853, 1986

157. Hoover R, Gray LA Sr, Cole P, MacMahon B. Menopausal estrogens and breast. *N Engl J Med.* 295:401, 1976

158. Hoover R, Glass A, Finkle WD, et al. Conjugated estrogens and breast cancer risk in women. *J Natl Cancer Inst.* 67:815, 1981

159. Ross RK, Paganini-Hill A, Gerkins VR, et al. Case-control study of menopausal estrogen therapy and breast cancer. *JAMA.* 243:1635, 1980

160. Thomas DB, Persing JP, Hutchinson WB. Exogenous estrogens and other risk factors for breast cancer in women with benign breast diseases. *J Natl Cancer Inst.* 69:1017, 1982

161. Ewertz M. Influence of non-contraceptive exogenous and endogenous sex hormones on breast cancer risk in Denmark. *Int J Cancer.* 42:832, 1988

162. Rohan TE, McMichael AJ. Non-contraceptive exogenous estrogen therapy and breast cancer. *Med J Aust.* 148:217, 1988

163. Bergkvist L, Adami H-O, Persson I, et al. Prognosis after breast cancer diagnosis in women exposed to estrogen and estrogen-progestogen replacement therapy. *Am J Epidemiol.* 130:221, 1989

164. Brinton LA, Hoover R, Fraumeni JF Jr. Menopausal estrogens and breast cancer risk: An expanded case-control study. *Br J Cancer.* 54:825, 1986

165. Nomura AMY, Kolonel LN, Hirohara T, Lee J. The association of replacement estrogens with breast cancer. *Int J Cancer.* 37:49, 1986

166. Armstrong estrogen therapy after the menopause—Boon or bane? *Med J Aust.* 148:213, 1988

167. Steinberg KK, Thacker SB, Smith J, et al. A meta-analysis of the effect of estrogen replacement therapy on the risk of breast cancer. *JAMA.* 265:1985, 1991

168. Gambrell Jr. Hormone replacement therapy and breast cancer risk. *Arch Fam Med.* 5:341, 1996

169. Collins J. Meta-analysis of the relationship of estrogen replacement therapy and breast cancer. *J Soc Obstet Gynaecol Can.* 17:837, 1995

170. Cummings SR, Black DM, Rubin SM. Lifetime-risk of hip, colles', or vertebral fracture and coronary heart disease among white postmenopausal women. *Arch Intern Med.* 149:2445, 1989

171. Bergkvist L, Adami H-O, Persson I, et al. The risk of breast cancer after estrogen and estrogen–progestin replacement. *N Engl J Med.* 321:293, 1989

172. Hunt K, Vessey M, McPherson K, Coleman M. Long-term surveillance of mortality and cancer incidence in women receiving hormone replacement therapy. *Br J Obstet Gynaecol.* 94:620, 1987

173. Wile A, Opfell R, Margileth D. Hormone replacement therapy in previously treated breast cancer patients. *Am J Surg.* 165:372, 1993

174. Eden J, Bush T, Nand S, Wren B. A case-control study of combined continuous estrogen–progestin replacement therapy among women with a personal history of breast cancer. *Menopause.* 2:67, 1995

175. Schiff I, Komarov H, Cramer D, et al. Endometrial hyperplasia in women on cyclic or continuous estrogen regimens. *Fertil Steril.* 37:79, 1982

176. Prough SG, Aksel S, Wiebe RH, Shepherd J. Continuous estrogen/progestin therapy in menopause. *Am J Obstet Gynecol.* 157:1449, 1987

177. Ettinger B, Genant HK, Cann C. Postmenopausal bone loss is prevented by treatment with low-dosage estrogen with calcium. *Ann Intern Med.* 106:40, 1987

178. Padwick ML, Pryse-Davis J, Whitehead MI. A simple method for determining the optimal dosage of progestin in postmenopausal women receiving estrogens. *N Engl J Med.* 315:930, 1986

179. Sturdee D, Barlow D, Ulrich L, et al. Is the timing of withdrawal bleeding a guide to endometrial safety during sequential oestrogen-progestogen replacement therapy? *Lancet.* 343:979, 1994

180. Townsend D, Fields G, McCausland A, Kauffman K. Diagnostic and operative hysteroscopy in the management of persistent postmenopausal bleeding. *Obstet Gynecol.* 82:419, 1993

181. Holst J, Backstrom T, Hammarback S, Schoultz BV. Progestogen addition during oestrogen replacement therapy—Effects on vasomotor symptoms and mood. *Maturitas.* 11:13, 1989

182. Albrecht BH, Schiff I, Tulinchinsky D, Ryan KJ. Objective evidence that placebo and oral medroxyprogesterone acetate therapy diminish menopausal vasomotor flushes. *Am J Obstet Gynecol.* 136:631, 1981

183. Morrison JC, Martin DC, Blair RA, Anderson GD, et al. The use of medroxyprogesterone acetate for relief of climacteric symptoms. *Am J Obstet Gynecol.* 138:99, 1980

184. Lobo RA, McCormic W, Singer F, Roy S. Depomedroxyprogesterone acetate compared with conjugated estrogens for the treatment of postmenopausal women. *Obstet Gynecol.* 63:1, 1984

185. Gambrell RD. Clinical use of progestins in the menopausal patient. *J Reprod Med.* 27:531, 1983

186. Smith JA. A prospective comparison of treatments for symptomatic hot flushes following endocrine therapy for carcinoma of the prostate. *J Urol.* 152:132, 1994

187. Loprinzi CL, Michalak JC, Quella SK, et al. Megestrol acetate for the prevention of hot flashes. *N Engl J Med.* 331:347, 1994

188. Laufer LR, Erlik Y, Meldrum DR, Judd HL. Effect of clonidine on hot flashes in postmenopausal women. *Obstet Gynecol.* 60:583, 1982

189. Nagamani M, Kelver ME, Smith ER. Treatment of menopausal hot flashes with transdermal administration of clonidine. *Am J Obstet Gynecol.* 156:561, 1987

190. Nesheim BI, Saetre T. Reduction of menopausal hot flushes by methyldopa. *Eur J Clin Pharamacol.* 20:413, 1981

191. Foster GV, Zacur HA, Rock JA. Hot flushes in postmenopausal women ameliorated by danazol. *Fertil Steril.* 43:401, 1984

192. DeFazio J, Verhuegen C, Cherkowski R, et al. The effects of naloxone on hot flushes and gonadotropic secretion in postmenopausal women. *J Clin Endocrinol Metab.* 58:578, 1984

193. Ayalon J, Simkin A, Leichner I, Raifmann S. Dynamic bone loading exercises for postmenopausal women: Effect on the density of the distal radius. *Arch Phys Med Rehab.* 68:280, 1987

194. White MK, Martin RB, Yearer RA, et al. The effects of exercise on the bones of postmenopausal women. *Int Orthoped.* 7:209, 1984

195. Krolner B, Toft B, Nielsen SP, Tondevold E. Physical exercise as prophylaxis against involutional vertebral bone loss: A controlled trial. *Clin Sci.* 64:541, 1983

196. Riis B, Thomsen K, Christiansen C. Does calcium supplementation prevent postmenopausal bone loss? *N Engl J Med.* 316:173, 1987

197. Fornander T, Rutqvist LE, Wilking N, et al. Oestrogenic effects of adjuvant tamoxifen in postmenopausal breast cancer. *Eur J Cancer.* 29:497, 1993

198. Powles TJ, Hichish T, Kanis JA, et al. Effect of tamoxifen on bone mineral density measured by duel-energy x-ray absorptiometry in healthy premenopausal and postmenopausal women. *J Clin Oncol.* 14:78, 1996

199. Riggs BL, Hodgson SF, O'Fallon WM, Chao EYS, et al. Effect of fluoride treatment of the fracture rate in postmenopausal women with osteoporosis. *N Engl J Med.* 322:802, 1990

200. Pak CYS, Sakhaee K, Zerwekh JE, Parcel C, et al. Safe and effective treatment of osteoporosis with intermittent slow release sodium fluoride: Augmentation of vertebral bone mass and inhibition of fractures. *J Clin Endocrinol Metab.* 68:150, 1989

201. MacIntyre I, Whitehead MI, Banks LM, Stevenson JC, et al. Calcitonin for prevention of postmenopausal bone loss. *Lancet.* i:900, 1988

202. Watts, NB, Harris ST, Genant HK, Wasnich RD, et al. Intermittent cyclical etidronate treatment of postmenopausal osteoporosis. *N Engl J Med.* 323:7379, 1990

203. Reginster JY, Deroisy R, Denis D, Collette J, et al. Prevention of postmenopausal bone loss by tiludronate. *Lancet.* ii:1469, 1989

204. Black DM, Cummings SR, Karpf DB, et al. Randomised trial of effect of alendronate on risk of fracture in women with existing vertebral fractures. *Lancet.* 348:1535, 1996

205. Hosking D, McConnell M, Ravn P, et al. Alendronate in the prevention of osteoporosis: EPIC study two-year results. American Society for Bone and Mineral Research, 1996 annual meeting

206. Rimmer DE, Rawls DE. Improper alendronate administration and a case of pill esophagitis. *Am J Gastroenterol.* 91:2648, 1996. Letter

207. Wiseman H, Cannon M, Arnstein HR, Barlow DJ. The structural mimicry of membrane sterols by tamoxifen: Evidence from cholesterol coefficients and molecular-modelling for its action as a membrane anti-oxidant and an anti-cancer agent. *Biochimica Biophysica Acta.* 1138:197, 1992

208. McDonald CC, Alexander FE, Whyte BW, et al. Cardiac and vascular morbidity in women receiving adjuvant Tamoxifen for breast cancer in a randomised trial. The Scottish Cancer Trials Breast Group. *BMJ.* 311:977, 1995

209. Elisaf M, Bairaktari E, Nicolaides C, et al. The beneficial effect of tamoxifen on serum lipoprotein-A levels: An additional anti-atherogenic property. *Anticancer Res.* 16:2725, 1996

210. Love RR, Wiebe DA, Newcomb PA, et al. Effects of tamoxifen on cardiovascular risk factors in postmenopausal women. *Ann Intern Med.* 115:860, 1991

211. Kauffman RF, Bensch WR, Rondebush RE, et al. Hypocholesterolemic activity of raloxifene (LY139481): Pharmacological characterization as a selective estrogen receptor modulator. *J Pharmacol Exp Ther.* 280:146, 1997

212. Henderson BE, Paganini-Hill A, Ross RK. Decreased mortality in users of estrogen replacement therapy. *Arch Intern Med.* 151:75, 1991

213. Hillner BE, Hollenberg JP, Pauker SG. Postmenopausal estrogens in prevention of osteoporosis. *Am J Med.* 80: 1115, 1986

INDEX